Spine Care

VOLUME ONE

VOLUME ONE
Diagnosis and Conservative Treatment

VOLUME TWO
Operative Treatment

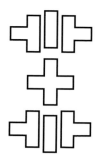

Spine Care
VOLUME ONE

Editor

Arthur H. White, M.D.

Medical Director
San Francisco Spine Institute
SpineCare Medical Group
Daly City, California

Associate Editor

Jerome A. Schofferman, M.D.

Director, Research and Education
San Francisco Spine Institute
SpineCare Medical Group
Daly City, California

with 1918 illustrations including 6 color plates

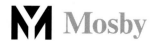 Mosby

St. Louis Baltimore Boston Carlsbad Chicago Naples New York Philadelphia Portland
London Madrid Mexico City Singapore Sydney Tokyo Toronto Wiesbaden

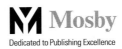

Publisher: Anne Patterson
Editor: Robert Hurley
Developmental Editor: Eugenia A. Klein
Project Manager: Barbara Bowes Merritt
Design, Editorial and Production: York Production Services
Manufacturing Supervisor: Theresa Fuchs

ONE EDITION

Printed in the United States of America
Composition by York Graphic Services, Inc.
Printing/binding by Maple-Vail Book Manufacturing Group

Mosby-Year Book, Inc.
11830 Westline Industrial Drive
St. Louis, Missouri 63146

Library of Congress Cataloging in Publication Data
Spine care: editor, Arthur H. White; associate editor, Jerome A. Schofferman.
    p. cm.
    Includes bibliographical references and index.
    ISBN 0-8016-6328-8
    1. Spine—Diseases. 2. Spine—Wounds and injuries. 3. Backache.
I. White, Arthur H., II. Schofferman, Jerome A.
    [DNLM: 1. Spinal Diseases—therapy. 2. Spinal Diseases—diagnosis.
3. Back Pain—therapy. 4. Back Pain—diagnosis. WE 725 S75915 1995]
RD768; .S673 1995
617.3'75—dc20
DNLM/DLC   94-40833
for Library of Congress   CIP

93 94 95 96 97 / 9 8 7 6 5 4 3 2 1

Contributors

David J. Anderson, M.D.
Department of Psychiatry
SpineCare Medical Group
Daly City, California
Chapt 4: The Psychologic Cascade
Chapt 17: Psychiatric Evaluation of the Chronic
    Pain Patient
Chapt 38: Understanding the Chronic Spine Pain
    Patient: The Attachment Theory

Charles N. Aprill, M.D.
Magnolia Diagnostics
New Orleans, Louisiana
Chapt 14: Discography
Chapt 21: Diagnostic Blocks of Spinal Synovial Joints
Chapt 22: Epidural Steroid Injections

Bruce D. Beynnon, Ph.D.
Research Assistant Professor
Department of Orthopaedics and Rehabilitation
University of Vermont
Burlington, Vermont
Chapt 87: The Vermont Spinal Fixator for
    Posterior Application to Short Segments of the
    Thoracic, Lumbar, or Lumbosacral Spine.

Ronald Blackman, M.D.
Director, Spinal Deformity Clinic
Kaiser Permanente Medical Center
Oakland, California
Chapt 73: Arthroscopic Microdiscectomy:
    Lumbar and Thoracic (section on "Endoscopic
    Thoracic Spine Surgery")

**Nikolai Bogduk, B.Sc. (Med), M.B. B.S., Ph.D.,
M.D., Dip Anat, Hon F.A.C.R.M.**
Professor of Anatomy
Director
Cervical Spine Research Unit
Faculty of Medicine
University of Newcastle
Newcastle, New South Wales, Australia
Chapt 14: Discography
Chapt 21: Diagnostic Blocks of Spinal Synovial Joints
Chapt 22: Epidural Steroid Injections
Chapt 60: Anatomy of the Spine

Richard S. Brower, M.D.
Instructor in Orthopaedic Surgery
Department of Orthopaedics
Northeastern Ohio Universities
College of Medicine
Akron, Ohio
Chapt 99: Cervical Spondylotic Radiculopathy and
    Myelopathy: Posterior Approach

Bobbi Buell
Documedics
San Bruno, California
Appendix: Practical Guide to Billing

Charles V. Burton, M.D.
Medical Director
Department of Neurosurgery
Institute for Low Back Care
Minneapolis, Minnesota
Chapt 79: The Controversy of "Large Vs. Small":
    The Present Role of Minimally Invasive Surgery
    of the Spine

Peter N. Capicotto, M.D.
Orthopaedic Surgeon
St. Vincent Hospital
Indianapolis, Indiana
Chapt 111: Clinical Cervical Deformity and Post
    Laminectomy Kyphosis

Kenichi Chatani, M.D., Ph.D.
Fellow
Department of Orthopaedic Surgery
Kyoto Prefectural University in Medicine
Kyoto City, Kyoto, Japan
Chapt 8: Anatomy, Biochemistry, and Physiology
    of Low-Back Pain

Andrew J. Cole, M.D.
Director
Spine Rehabilitation Services
The Tom Landry Sports Medicine and Research
    Center
Baylor University Medical Center
Dallas, Texas
Chapt 55: Swimming

Patrick J. Connolly, M.D.
Assistant Professor
Department of Orthopaedic Surgery
State University of New York
    Health Science Center at Syracuse
Syracuse, New York
Chapt 101: Anterior Instrumentation of the
    Cervical Spine
Chapt 104: Cervical Spine Fractures

Howard B. Cotler, M.D., F.A.C.S.
Clinical Associate Professor
Department of Orthopaedic Surgery
University of Texas
Houston, Texas
Chapt 100: Cervical Fusions: Arthrodesis and
    Osteosynthesis of the Cervical Spine

Tracy P. Cotter, M.D.
Assistant Professor
Department of Anesthesiology
University of Wisconsin
Madison, Wisconsin
Chapt 68: Anesthesia in Cervical Spine Surgery

Ramon Cuencas-Zamora, Ph.D.
Behavioral Medicine Specialist
Department of Health Psychology and Behavioral
    Medicine
Dallas Spine Rehabilitation Center
Dallas, Texas
Chapt 67: Pyschological Preparation for Surgery

P. Dean Cummings, M.D.
Department of Orthopaedics
Penn State
College of Medicine
The Milton S. Hershey Medical Center
Hershey, Pennsylvania
Chapt 102: Sports Injuries of the Head and
    Cervical Spine

W. Bradford DeLong, M.D., F.A.C.S.
Assistant Clinical Professor
Department of Neurosurgery
University of California, San Francisco;
Neurological Consultant
St. Mary's Spine Center
San Francisco, California;
Neurological Consultant
SpineCare Medical Group
Daly City, California
Chapt 69: Positioning the Patient for Lumbar
    Spine Surgery
Chapt 75: Microsurgical Discectomy and Spinal
    Decompression

Richard Derby, Jr., M.D.
Chief
Department of Anesthesia, Diagnostic Spinal
    Procedures
SpineCare Medical Group
Daly City, California;
Co-Founder
International Spinal Injection Society
Daly City, California
Chapt 14: Discography
Chapt 21: Diagnostic Blocks of Spinal Synovial Joints
Chapt 22: Epidural Steroid Injections

Susan J. Dreyer, M.D.
Diplomate
American Board of Physical Medicine
Clinical Assistant Professor
Department of Medicine and Rehabilitation
Emory University
Atlanta, Georgia
Chapt 56: Weight Lifting

James Dwyer, M.D.
Medical Director
New Jersey Spine Institute
Bedminster, New Jersey;
Clinical Assistant Professor
Orthopaedic Surgery
The New Jersey Medical School
Newark, New Jersey
Chapt 58: History of Spine Surgery

Richard A. Eagleston, M.A., P.T., A.T.C.
Strength Training and Rehabilitation Physical
    Therapy
Redwood City, CA
Chapt 55: Swimming

Sanford E. Emery, M.D.
Assistant Professor, Spine Section
Department of Orthopaedics
Case Western Reserve University
University Hospitals of Cleveland
Cleveland, Ohio
Chapt 98: Cervical Spondylotic Radiculopathy and
    Myelopathy: Anterior Approach and Pathology

William T. Evans, M.D.
Associate Medical Director
Center for Spine Rehabilitation
Colorado Neurological Institute
Englewood, Colorado
Chapt 23: Education: The Primary Treatment of
    Low-Back Pain

Frank J. E. Falco, M.D.
Physiatrist
Georgia Spine and Sports Physicians
Smyrna, Georgia
Chapt 56: Weight Lifting

Joseph P. Farrell, P.T., M.S.
Redwood Orthopaedic Physical Therapy, Inc.
Castro Valley, California;
Senior Clinical Faculty
Kaiser Hayward Physical Therapy Residency
Program in Advanced Manual Therapy
Kaiser Permanente Medical Center
Hayward, California
Chapt 30: The Role of Manual Therapy in Spinal
    Rehabilitation

John G. Finkenberg, M.D., D.C.
Spine Specialist
Department of Orthopedics
Johns Hopkins Hospital
Baltimore, Maryland
Chapt 110: Adult Scoliosis

Kevin S. Finnesey, M.D.
Attending Orthopedic Surgeon
Department of Orthopedics
Mills Peninsula Hospitals
San Mateo County General Hospital
San Mateo, California
Chapt 49: Golf
Chapt 93: The Use of Electrical Stimulation for
    Spinal Fusion

Joseph D. Fortin, D.O.
Clinical Assistant Professor
Department of Rehabilitation
Louisiana State University
New Orleans, Louisiana
Chapt 47: Figure Skating

Robert W. Gaines, Jr., M.D.
Professor
Department of Orthopaedic Surgery
University of Missouri Health Sciences Center
Columbia, Missouri
Chapt 109: Spinal Deformity in Children,
    Adolescents, and Young Adults

Robert J. Gatchel, Ph.D.
Professor of Psychiatry and Rehabilitation Science
Department of Psychiatry
University of Texas Southwestern Medical Center
Dallas, Texas
Chapt 36: Psychosocial Correlates of the
    Deconditioning Syndrome

Stanley D. Gertzbein, M.D.
Director
Department of Research and Education
Texas Back Institute;
Associate Professor
Department of Orthopaedics
University of Texas
Houston, Texas
Chapt 100: Cervical Fusions: Arthrodesis and
    Osteosynthesis of the Cervical Spine

Patricia H. Gibbs, M.D.
Medical Director
San Francisco Free Clinic
San Francisco, California
Chapt 46: Dance

Richard D. Gibbs, M.D.
Supervising Physician
San Francisco Ballet
San Francisco, California
Chapt 46: Dance

Richard G. Gillette, M.S., Ph.D.
Associate Professor
Department of Physiology
Basic Science Division
Western States Chiropractic College
Portland, Oregon
Chapt 9: Neurophysiology of Chronic Idiopathic
    Back Pain

Susan L. Goelzer, M.D.
Associate Professor
Departments of Anesthesiology and Internal
  Medicine
University of Wisconsin
Madison, Wisconsin
Chapt 68: Anesthesia in Cervical Spine Surgery

Erwin G. Gonzalez, M.D.
Director
Department of Physical Medicine and
  Rehabilitation
Professor
Department Rehabilitation Medicine
Mt. Sinai School of Medicine
Beth Israel Medical Center
New York, New York
Chapt 13: Somatosensory and Motor Evoked
  Potential

Matthew F. Gornet, M.D.
Department of Orthopaedic Surgery-Spine
DePaul Health Center
St. Louis, Missouri
Chapt 107: Spinal Infection

Serge Gracovetsky, M.D., Ph.D.
Associate Professor
Department of Electrical Engineering
Concordia University
President
Spinex Medical Technologies
Montreal, Quebec, Canada
Chapt 10: Biomechanics of the Spine

**Alexander G. Hadjipavlou, M.D., M.Sc.,
  F.R.C.S. (C), F.A.C.S.**
Professor
Department of Surgery
Section of Orthopedic Surgery
University of Arizona Health Sciences Center
Tucson, Arizona
Chapt 20: Principles of Assessment of
  Osteometabolic Bone Disease
Chapt 62: Osteoporosis of the Spine and Its
  Management
Chapt 113: Paget's Disease

John A. Handal, M.D.
Assistant Clinical Professor
Department of Orthopedic Surgery
University of Texas Southwestern Medical Center;
Dallas Spine Group
Dallas, Texas
Chapt 2: The Structural Degenerative Cascade
  The Cervical Spine
Chapt 96: Degenerative Disc Disease of the
  Cervical Spine: Degenerative Cascade and the
  Anterior Approach

Gregory A. Hanks, M.D.
Clinical Assistant Professor
Department of Orthopedic Surgery
Temple University
Philadelphia, Pennsylvania;
Pennsylvania Orthopedics, P.C.
Camp Hill, Pennsylvania
Chapt 102: Sports Injuries of the Head and
  Cervical Spine

Robert J. Henderson, M.D.
Spine Surgeon
Medical Arts Hospital
Dallas, Texas
Chapt 42: Use of the Morphine Pump for Pain
  Control
Chapt 82: Anterior Approach for Lumbar Fusions
  and Associated Morbidity

Harry N. Herkowitz, M.D.
Chairman
Department of Orthopaedic Surgery
William Beaumont Hospital
Royal Oak, Michigan
Chapt 99: Cervical Spondylotic Radiculopathy and
  Myelopathy: Posterior Approach

Robert H. Hines, Jr., M.D.
Psychiatrist
Department of Psychiatry
SpineCare Medical Group
Daly City, California
Chapt 38: Understanding the Chronic Spine Pain
  Patient: The Attachment Theory

Betsy A. Holland, M.D.
Co-Medical Director
San Francisco Neuroskeletal Imaging;
Medical Director
Marin Magnetic Imaging;
Assistant Clinical Professor
Department of Radiology
University of California
San Francisco, California
Chapt 11: Imaging of the Spine

Ken Y. Hsu, M.D.
Director of Orthopaedic Services
St. Mary's Spine Center
St. Mary's Hospital and Medical Center
San Francisco, California
Chapt 63: Bone Grafts and Implants

Susan J. Isernhagen, B.S., P.T.
President
Isernhagen and Associates, Inc.;
Isernhagen Clinics, Inc.;
Duluth, Minnesota
Chapt 16: Physical Therapy Approach to
    Diagnosing the Patient with Work Related Injury

Donald R. Johnson, II, M.D.
Medical Director
Carolina Spine Institute
Clinical Assistant Professor
Department of Orthopaedic Surgery
Medical University of South Carolina
Charleston, South Carolina
Chapt 58: History of Spine Surgery

Parviz Kambin, M.D.
Clinical Associate Professor
Department of Orthopaedic Surgery
University of Pennsylvania
School of Medicine;
Chief
Division of Spine Surgery
Director
Disc Treatment and Research Center
The Graduate Hospital
Philadelphia, Pennsylvania
Chapt 71: Selection of Surgical Treatment by
    Analysis of Pain Generators
Chapt 73: Arthroscopic Microdiscectomy
    Lumbar and Thoracic
Chapt 77: Arthroscopic Lumbar Interbody Fusion

Mamoru Kawakami, M.D., Ph.D.
Assistant
Department of Orthopedic Surgery
Wakayama Medical College
Wakayama City, Wakayama, Japan
Chapt 8: Anatomy, Biochemistry, and Physiology
    of Low-Back Pain

Gerald P. Keane, M.D.
Department of Sports Orthopaedics and
    Rehabilitation
Menlo Park, California;
Clinical Instructor
Department of Physical Medicine and
    Rehabilitation
Stanford University
Palo Alto, California
Chapt 18: Multidisciplinary Evaluation

Jeffrey A. Knapp, M.D.
Department of Orthopedics
Naval Hospital, Portsmouth
Portsmouth, Virginia
Chapt 2: The Structural Degenerative Cascade
    The Cervical Spine

Martin H. Krag, M.D.
Associate Professor
Department of Orthopaedics and Rehabilitation
University of Vermont
Burlington, Vermont
Chapt 87: The Vermont Spinal Fixator for
    Posterior Application to Short Segments of the
    Thoracic, Lumbar, or Lumbosacral Spine

Ronald C. Kramis, Ph.D.
Research Scientist
Department of Neurosurgery
Good Samaritan Hospital and Medical Center
Portland, Oregon
Chapt 9: Neurophysiology of Chronic Idiopathic
    Back Pain

Philip H. Lander, M.D.
Associate Professor
Department of Radiology
McGill University
Montreal, Quebec, Canada
Chapt 20: Principles of Assessment of
    Osteometabolic Bone Disease
Chapt 62: Osteoporosis of the Spine and Its
    Management
Chapt 113: Paget's Disease

Casey K. Lee, M.D.
Professor
Department of Orthopaedics
New Jersey Medical School
Newark, New Jersey
Chapt 61: Clinical Biomechanics of the Lumbar
    Spine

Jonathan P. Lester, M.D.
Georgia Spine and Sports Physicians
Atlanta, Georgia
Chapt 56: Weight Lifting

Michael J. Martin, M.D.
Orthopaedic Spine Surgeon
Puget Sound Spine Institute
Tacoma, Washington
Chapt 45: Bicycling

Tom G. Mayer, M.D.
Clinical Professor
Department of Orthopedic Surgery
Southwestern Medical School
University of Texas;
Medical Director
PRIDE
Dallas, Texas
Chapt 35: Physical Correlates of the
    Deconditioning and Dehabilitation Cascade

C. E. McCoy, M.D.
Chairman of the Board
Dallas Spinal Rehabilitation Center
Dallas, Texas
Chapt 67: Psychological Preparation for Surgery

**Marion McGregor, B.Sc., D.C., F.C.C.S.(c),
    M.Sc.**
Associate Professor
Department of Research
National Course of Chiropractic
Lombard, Illinois
Chapt 29: Validity and Basis of Manipulation

Frances A. McManemin, Ph.D.
Psychologist
Department of Behavioral Medicine
Dallas Spinal Rehabilitation Center
Dallas, Texas
Adjunct Professor (Biofeedback)
Department of Psychology
University of North Texas
Denton, Texas
Chapt 67: Psychological Preparation for Surgery

John N. McMillin, M.D.
Battlefield Orthopedics, Inc.
Springfield, Missouri
Chapt 81: Posterior Lumbar Interbody Fusion:
    Biomechanical Selection for Fusions

Henrik Mike-Mayer, M.D.
Orthopaedic Spine Surgeon
Altoona, Pennsylvania
Chapt 100: Cervical Fusions: Arthrodesis and
    Osteosynthesis of the Cervical Spine

Fujio Mita, M.D.
Chairman
Mita Orthopaedic Clinic;
Assistant Professor
Jichi Medical School
Department of Orthopaedic Surgery;
Joysan Orthopaedic Association
Tokyo, Japan
Chapt 78: Myeloscopy and Endoscopic
    Nucleotomy

Vert Mooney, M.D.
Professor
Department of Orthopaedics
University California, San Diego;
Medical Director
USCD OrthoMed Center
LaJolla, California
Chapt 15: Diagnostic Tests for the Patient with
    Work Related Injuries

David B. Morris, Ph.D.
Associate Editor
Literature and Medicine
Kalamazoo, Michigan
Chapt 33: Pain and Its Meaning: A Biocultural
    Model

Marilou Moschetti
Executive Director
AquaTechnics Consulting Group
Aptos, California
Chapt 55: Swimming

Michael H. Moskowitz, M.D., M.P.H.
Psychiatry and Psychosomatics
Department of Psychiatry
SpineCare Medical Group
Daly City, California
Chapt 39: Transcutaneous Electrical Nerve
    Stimulation, Acupuncture, Biofeedback,
    Hypnotherapy, and Spine Pain

Eugene J. Nordby, M.D.
Associate Clinical Professor
Department of Orthopaedics
University of Wisconsin Medical School
Madison, Wisconsin
Chapt 72: Chemonucleolysis

Richard B. North, M.D.
Associate Professor
Department of Neurosurgery
Johns Hopkins Hospital
Baltimore, Maryland
Chapt 41: Neurosurgical Approaches to Chronic
    Pain

Paul J. Nugent, M.D.
Orthopaedic Spine Surgeon
Fresno, California
Chapt 103: Surgical Treatment of Spinal Tumors

Kelly O'Neal, M.D.
Department of Surgery
Kaiser Permanente Medical Center
Oakland, California
Chapt 73: Arthroscopic Microdiscectomy: Lumbar
    and Thoracic (section on "Endoscopic Thoracic
    Spine Surgery")

Gary M. Onik, M.D.
Chairman
Department of Minimally Invasive Therapy
Princeton Hospital
Orlando, Florida
Chapt 74: Automated Percutaneous Lumbar
    Discectomy

Yoshio Ooi, M.D., Ph.D.
Professor and Chairman
Department of Orthopaedic Surgery and
    Rehabilitation Center
Jichi Medical School
Tochigi Pref., Japan
Chapt 78: Myeloscopy and Endoscopic
    Nucleotomy

John H. Peloza, M.D.
Clinical Assistant Professor
Department of Orthopedic Surgery
University of Texas Southwestern Medical Center;
Dallas Spine Group
Dallas, Texas
Chapt 86: Instrumented Posterior Lumbar Surgery

Mark S. Pfeil, B.S., P.T.
Physical Therapist—Trainer
Department of Sports Medicine
Milwaukee Bucks
Milwaukee, Wisconsin
Chapt 44: Basketball

George Picetti, III, M.D.
Clinical Instructor
Department of Orthopaedic Surgery
University of California, Davis
Sacramento, California
Chapt 73: Arthroscopic Microdiscectomy: Lumbar
    and Thoracic (section on "Endoscopic Thoracic
    Spine Surgery")

Peter B. Polatin, M.D.
Associate Clinical Professor
Department of Psychiatry
University of Texas
Southwest Medical Center at Dallas;
Associate Medical Director
PRIDE
Dallas, Texas
Chapt 32: Work Simulation, Work Hardening, and
    Functional Restoration

Steven C. Poletti, M.D.
Assistant Clinical Professor
Department of Orthopaedic Surgery
Medical University of South Carolina;
Carolina Spine Institute
Charleston, South Carolina
Chapt 2: The Structural Degenerative Cascade
    The Cervical Spine
Chapt 96: Degenerative Disc Disease of the
    Cervical Spine: Degenerative Cascade and the
    Anterior Approach

Carol P. Prentice
Alexander Technique Teacher
Alexander Training Institute
San Francisco, California
Chapt 28: Cervicothoracic Muscular
    Stabilization Techniques

Joel M. Press, M.D.
Director
Sports Rehabilitation Program
Rehabilitation Institute of Chicago;
Assistant Professor
Department of Clinical Physical Medicine and
    Rehabilitation
Northwestern University Medical School
Chicago, Illinois
Chapt 12: Electrodiagnostic Evaluation of Spine
    Problems
Chapt 26: The Physiologic Basis of Therapeutic
    Exercise
Chapt 44: Basketball

Charles D. Ray, M.S., M.D., F.A.C.S.
Chief
Department of Neuroaugmentive Surgery
Associate Director
Institute for Low Back Care;
Minneapolis, Minnesota
Past President
North American Spine Society
Chapt 65: Graft Materials to Prevent Lumbar
    Spine Postoperative Adhesions
Chapt 69: Positioning the Patient for Lumbar
    Spine Surgery
Chapt 80: Lumbar Spinal Stenoses: Reliable
    Methods of Decompression
Chapt 88: Posterior Lumbar Interbody Fusions by
    Implanted Threaded Titanium Cages
Chapt 90: Lumbar Pathoanatomy: Soft- and Hard-
    Tissue Decompression

R. Charles Ray, M.D.
Director
Scoliosis Program
Mary Bridge Children's Hospital
Tacoma, Washington
Chapt 85: Anatomic Strategies of Internal Fixation

Thomas S. Renshaw, M.D.
Professor
Department of Orthopaedic Surgery
Yale University
New Haven, Connecticut
Chapt 108: Congenital Spinal Deformity

James B. Reynolds, M.D.
Orthopedic Surgeon
SpineCare Medical Group
Daly City, California
Chapt 91: Degenerative Spondylolisthesis
Chapt 92: Spondylolisthesis: Isthmic, Congenital,
    Traumatic, and Post-Surgical

William J. Richardson, M.D.
Assistant Professor of Surgery
Department of Orthopaedic Surgery
Duke University Medical Center
Durham, North Carolina
Chapt 9: Neurophysiology of Chronic Idiopathic
    Back Pain
Chapt 95: Surgical Approaches to the Cervical
    Spine

**William J. Roberts, Ph.D.,
    M.S.**
Senior Scientist
R.S. Dow Neurological Sciences Institute
Good Samaritan Hospital and Medical Center
Portland, Oregon
Chapt 9: Neurophysiology of Chronic Idiopathic
    Back Pain

**Robin S. Robison, M.S.,
    B.S.**
Spine Coordinator
Department of Physical Therapy
HEALTHSOUTH
Outpatient Services
Stanford University
Menlo Park, California
Chapt 27: Low-Back School and Stabilization:
    Aggressive Conservative Care

Thomas E. Rudy, Ph.D.
Associate Professor
Departments of Anesthesiology and Psychiatry
University of Pittsburgh Medical Center
Pittsburgh, Pennsylvania
Chapt 37: Cognitive-Behavioral Treatment of the
    Chronic Pain Patient

Damon C. Sacco, M.D.
Diagnostic Radiologist
Department of Magnetic Resonance Imaging
California Advanced Imaging
San Francisco, California
Chapt 11: Imaging of the Spine

Richard M. Salib, M.D.
Associate Medical Director
Institute for Low Back Care
Minneapolis, Minnesota
Chapt 83: Anterior Lumbar Interbody Fusion and
    Combined Antero-posterior Fusion

Yukichi Satoh, M.D., Ph.D.
Lecturer
Jichi Medical School
Chief
Tsowa Hospital
Department of Orthopaedic Surgery
Jichi Medical School
Yakushiji, Minamikawachi-Machi,
Kawachi-Gun, Tochigi Prefecture,
Japan
Chapt 78: Myeloscopy and Endoscopic
    Nucleotomy

J.A. Sazy, M.D.
Spine Fellow
Chicago Spine Fellowship
Rush-Presbyterian-St. Luke's Hospital
Rush Medical College of Rush University
Chicago, Illinois
Chapt 76: Laser Surgery

Jonathan L. Schaffer, M.D.
Instructor, Orthopedic Surgery
Orthopedic Surgery
Harvard Medical School and Brigham & Womens
    Hospital
Boston, Massachusetts
Chapt 78: Myeloscopy and Endoscopic
    Nucleotomy

Guido F. Schauer
Founder
LifeWell™
San Francisco, California
Chapt 51: Spine Defense and the Martial Arts

John D. Schlegel, M.D.
Associate Professor
Division of Orthopedic Surgery
University of Utah School of Medicine
Salt Lake City, Utah
Chapt 89: Anterior Lumbar Instrumentation and
    Fusion
Chapt 105: Thoracolumbar Fractures

Rand L. Schleusener, M.D.
Assistant Professor
Division of Orthopedic Surgery
University of Utah Medical Center
Salt Lake City, Utah
Chapt 89: Anterior Lumbar Instrumentation and
    Fusion
Chapt 105: Thoracolumbar Fractures

Carson Schneck, M.D., Ph.D.
Professor of Anatomy and Cell Biology
Professor of Diagnostic Imaging
Department of Anatomy and Cell Biology
Temple University
Philadelphia, Pennsylvania
Chapt 94: Clinical Anatomy of the Cervical Spine

Jerome A. Schofferman, M.D., F.A.C.P.M.
Pain Management and Internal Medicine
SpineCare Medical Group
Director
Research and Education
San Francisco Spine Institute
Daly City, California
Chapt 1: Introduction
Chapt 2: The Structural Degenerative Cascade
    Applied Neurophysiology of Pain
Chapt 5: Diagnostic Decision Making
Chapt 6: Lumbar Spine Disorders: Taking and
    Interpreting the History
Chapt 7: Physical Examination
Chapt 24: Evaluation of Outcome Studies
Chapt 34: Use of Medications for Pain of Spinal
    Origin

David K. Selby, M.D.
Dallas Spine Group
Dallas, Texas
Chapt 2: The Structural Degenerative Cascade
    The Lumbar Spine
Chapt 86: Instrumented Posterior Lumbar Surgery

Henry H. Sherk, M.D.
Professor and Chief
Division of Orthopedic Surgery
Medical College of Pennsylvania
Philadelphia, Pennsylvania
Chapt 76: Laser Surgery

Robert M. Shugart, M.D.
Orthopaedic Surgery and Spine
Fort Wayne Orthopaedics
Fort Wayne, Indiana
Chapt 48: Football

Chris C. Shulenberger, M.S. Engr.
Ergonomist
Occupational Management Systems, Inc.
Pleasant Hill, California
Chapt 31: Ergonomic Intervention for the
    Prevention and Treatment of Spinal Disorders

Edward D. Simmons, M.D., B.Sc., C.M., M.Sc., F.R.C.S.(C)
Clinical Assistant Professor
Department of Orthopaedic Surgery
Buffalo General Hospital
State University of New York at Buffalo
Buffalo, New York
Chapt 111: Clinical Cervical Deformity and Post
Laminectomy Kyphosis

Edward H. Simmons, M.D., B.Sc. (Med), F.R.C.S. (C), M.S. (Tor), F.A.C.S.
Professor of Orthopaedic Surgery
Head, University Orthopaedic Spine Service
State University of New York at Buffalo
Buffalo, New York
Chapt 112: Arthritic Spinal Deformity: Ankylosing
Spondylitis

James W. Simmons, Jr., M.D., F.A.C.S.
Spinal Surgeon
Alamo Bone and Joint Clinic
San Antonio, Texas
Chapt 64: Bone Banking
Chapt 72: Chemonucleolysis
Chapt 81: Posterior Lumbar Interbody Fusion:
Biomechanical Selection for Fusions

Dennis R. Skogsbergh, D.C.
Assistant Professor
Chairman
Department of Diagnostic Imaging and Clinical
Orthopedics
National College of Chiropractic
Lombard, Illinois
Chapt 29: Validity and Basis of Manipulation

Paul J. Slosar, M.D.
Spine Surgeon
Mercy Hospital and Medical Center
Chicago, Illinois
Chapt 50: Ice Hockey
Chapt 53: Snow Skiing
Chapt 91: Degenerative Spondylolisthesis
Chapt 92: Spondylolisthesis: Isthmic, Congenital,
Traumatic, and Post-Surgical

George F. Smith, M.D.
Departments of Pain Management, Spinal
Diagnostics, and Internal Medicine
SpineCare Medical Group
Daly City, California
Chapt 19: Medical Evaluation of the Spine Patient
Chapt 70: Perioperative Care of the Spine Patient

Janet Y. Soto, B.S. P.T.
Private Practitioner
Berkeley Physical Therapy
Berkeley, California
Senior Faculty Member
Physical Therapy Residency
Program in Advanced Orthopedic Manual Therapy
Kaiser Permanente Medical Center
Hayward, California
Chapt 30: The Role of Manual Therapy in Spinal
Rehabilitation

Robert J. Spinner, M.D.
Resident
Division of Orthopaedic Surgery
Duke University Medical Center
Durham, North Carolina
Chapt 95: Surgical Approaches

E. Shannon Stauffer, M.D.
Professor and Chairman
Department of Surgery
Division of Orthopaedics and Rehabilitation
Southern Illinois University
School of Medicine
Springfield, Illinois
Chapt 106: Management of the Spinal Cord-
Injured Patient

Lisa A. Steinkamp, M.S., P.T.
Director and Owner
Functional Rehabilitation and Sports Therapy
Palo Alto, California
Chapt 54: Soccer

Tara B. Sweeney, P.T.
Physical Therapist
Precision Biomechanics
Goleta, California
Chapt 28: Cervicothoracic Muscular
Stabilization Techniques

Charles S. Szabo, M.D., Ph.D.
Associate Director
San Francisco Center for Comprehensive Pain
Management
San Francisco, California
Chapt 40: Pain Management by Electrical Implant

James R. Taylor, M.D., Ph.D.
Professor
Department of Anatomy and Human Biology
University of Western Australia
Nedlands, Australia
Chapt 59: Development and Growth of the
Cervical and Lumbar Spine

Carol Jo Tichenor, M.A., P.T.
Director
Physical Therapy Residency Program in Advanced
    Orthopedic Manual Therapy
Kaiser Permanente Medical Center
Hayward, California
Chapt 30: The Role of Manual Therapy in Spinal
    Rehabilitation

William W. Tomford, M.D.
Associate Professor
Orthopaedic Surgery
Harvard Medical School
Director
Massachusetts General Hospital Bone Bank
Department of Orthopaedic Surgery
Massachusetts General Hospital
Boston, Massachusetts
Chapt 64: Bone Banking

John J. Triano, M.A., D.C., Ph.D.
Staff Physician
Texas Back Institute
Plano, Texas
Chapt 29: Validity and Basis of Manipulation

Dennis C. Turk, Ph.D.
Professor
Department of Psychiatry, Anesthesiology, and
    Behavioral Science
Director
Pain Evaluation and Treatment Institute
University of Pittsburgh
School of Medicine
Pittsburgh, Pennsylvania
Chapt 37: Cognitive-Behavioral Treatment of the
    Chronic Pain Patient

**Lance Twomey, B.A.pp.Sc. (WAIT), B.Sc.
    (Hons), Ph.D. (WAust), T.T.C., M.A.P.A.**
Deputy Vice-Chancellor and Professor
Department of Physiotherapy
Curtin University of Technology
Perth, Western Australia, Australia
Chapt 59: Development and Growth of the
    Cervical and Lumbar Spine

Mark W. Van Dyke, D.O., M.P.H.
Medical Director
Department of Occupational Medicine
Center for Occupational Health
St. Margaret Memorial Hospital
Pittsburgh, Pennsylvania
Chapt 18: Multidisciplinary Evaluation

Paul P. Vessa, M.D.
Somerset Orthopaedic Associates
Bridgewater, New Jersey
Chapt 57: Wrestling

Robert G. Watkins, M.D.
Associate Clinical Professor
Department of Orthopaedics
University of Southern California School of
    Medicine;
Kerlin-Jobe Orthopaedic Clinic
Los Angeles, California
Chapt 43: Baseball
Chapt 84: Results of Anterior Interbody Fusion

James N. Weinstein, D.O.
Professor
Department of Orthopaedic Surgery
Director
Spine Diagnostic and Treatment Center
University of Iowa College of Medicine
Iowa City, Iowa
Chapt 8: Anatomy, Biochemistry, and Physiology
    of Low-Back Pain

F. Todd Wetzel, M.D.
Associate Professor and Director
Department of Orthopaedics and Rehabilitation
University of Chicago Spine Center
University of Chicago
School of Medicine
Chicago, Illinois
Chapt 97: Degenerative Disc Disease of the
    Cervical Spine: Posterior Approach
Chapt 102: Sports Injuries of the Head and
    Cervical Spine

Arthur H. White, M.D.
Medical Director
San Francisco Spine Institute
SpineCare Medical Group
Daly City, California
Chapt 1: Introduction
Chapt 3: The Socioeconomic Cascade
Chapt 18: Multidisciplinary Evaluation
Chapt 25: Conservative Care—Pulling It all
    Together
Chapt 52: Running
Chapt 63: Bone Grafts and Implants
Chapt 66: Surgical Decision Making for
    Degenerative Disease
Appendix: Dynamic Lumbar Stabilization Exercises

Robert E. Windsor, M.D.
President
Georgia Spine and Sports Physicians, P.C.
Smyrna, Georgia
Chapt 56: Weight Lifting

Jeffrey L. Young, M.D., M.A.
Assistant Professor
Department of Physical Medicine and
    Rehabilitation
Northwestern University Medical School;
Attending Physician
Sports Rehabilitation Program
Rehabilitation Institute of Chicago
Chicago, Illinois
Chapt 12: Electrodiagnostic Evaluation of Spine
    Problems
Chapt 26: The Physiologic Basis of Therapeutic
    Exercise
Chapt 44: Basketball

Hansen A. Yuan, M.D.
Professor
Departments of Orthopaedic Surgery and
    Neurological Surgery
Chief
Division of Spinal Surgery
SUNY Health Science Center at Syracuse,
    New York
State University of New York Health Science
    Center at Syracuse
Syracuse, New York
Chapt 89: Anterior Lumbar Instrumentation and
    Fusion
Chapt 101: Anterior Instrumentation of the
    Cervical Spine
Chapt 104: Cervical Spine Fractures
Chapt 105: Thoracolumbar Spine Fractures

James F. Zucherman, M.D.
Director
Department of Orthopaedics
St. Mary's Spine Center
San Francisco, California
Chapt 63: Bone Grafts and Implants

Foreword

Leon L. Wiltse

There are many books on spinal disorders. What to do about any given situation is well documented. I have found none, however, which offers a better framework from which to view the entire patient with all of his complexities than does this one.

The spine specialist needs to be a total doctor, not just a surgical technician or rehabilitationist. Spine medicine is extremely complex. In order to be a good spine specialist, the physician must be well-schooled in many subspecialities, including rehabilitation, surgery, psychiatry, internal medicine, radiology and diagnostics.

Because of the wide range of subjects covered, especially the non-operative, this book will have a strong appeal to all health care professionals who treat the spine. The formation of the International Society for the Study of the Lumbar Spine in 1973 was a landmark in the development of spine medicine and surgery. This organization pioneered the idea of comprehensive care. It selected its members from all health care disciplines which have an interest in the spine. Its membership includes the following: orthopedic surgeons, neurosurgeons, neuroradiologists, neurologists, physiatrists, psychologists, psychiatrists, rheumatologists, epidemiologists, pathologists, engineers, basic scientists, statisticians, chiropractors, and physical therapists.

Other spine organizations which have come along since, in particular, the North American Spine Society, have carried on the same tradition. This book is the embodiment of that concept.

Patient education in the care of the spine is stressed and a neck school is described as well as the more traditional low back school. There is a chapter on the basic theories of spinal manipulation and a chapter on clinical manipulation.

Chapters 43 to 57 are interesting. This section is devoted to sport-specific injuries, including those associated with baseball, basketball, ballet, skating, football, golf, hockey, martial arts, running, skiing, soccer, swimming, lifting, and wrestling. The editors have obviously been very aware of the fact that for conditions in the spine, but especially in the lumbar and cervical spines, pain is the thing that brings the patient to the doctor. But for pain, few would come near us. As a result, a fairly large share of the book is devoted to the treatment of pain, both the basic science of pain, e.g., neurophysiology, and the clinical management of pain.

We are all familiar with Dr. Kirkaldy-Willis' degenerative cascade, but the idea of a socioeconomic cascade (Chapter 3) and a psychological cascade (Chapter 4) would seem unique.

This book gives the reader a framework and a philosophy on which to base his practice. The practice of spine care that this book advocates works. It has been derived from many decades of many spine specialists' lifetime practice experiences.

I have watched this practice style develop out of the teachings of our leading spine luminaries; Philip Newman, Bill Kirkaldy-Willis, Homer Pheasant, Harry Farfan, Harry Crock, Bernie Finneson, and Vert Mooney (to name just a few). These men and many others have progressively added to our current concept of the practice of spinal medicine, which is brought to you in this book.

Foreword

Scott Haldeman

The treatment of patients with spinal symptoms used to be easy, enjoyable, and satisfying. If one was a family physician, most patients seemed to get better with anti-inflammatory medications and bed rest. If one was a chiropractor, one simply looked for subluxations and adjusted them. If one was a surgeon, most patients were diagnosed as having disc herniations and, when unresponsive to other treatments, underwent laminectomy and discectomy. If one was a consultant in neurology, rheumatology, or psychiatry, one simply examined the patient and proclaimed the presence or absence of disease within one's specialty and where appropriate treated (or more likely, declared untreatable) the disease. Unlike this book, textbooks on the topic were small and simplistic, usually concentrating on unproven and often unquestioned theories and then describing the technical method of treatment preferred by the author. Since clinicians from different specialties and professions rarely spoke to each other or attended meetings outside their specialty, everyone was comfortable with the situation and assumed that their method of managing patients was the most effective.

This level of comfort has been gradually eroding over the past two decades. The primary motivation for the change has been the realization that, at least in the Western industrialized nations, back pain disability has reached epidemic proportions. The number of patients claiming disability as a result of spinal problems has increased each year. This has occurred despite a proliferation in the number of clinicians and increased complexity and sophistication of the methods of diagnosing and treating this problem. This text brings these specialties and philosophies together in a usable fashion.

There has also been a rapid, almost exponential, increase in the cost of both treatment and indemnity associated with back pain disability. This, in turn, has been the motivating factor for the growing importance of research into all aspects of spine pathophysiology and management. Whereas there were virtually no scientific peer-reviewed journals devoted to publishing research on spinal disorders in 1976 when "Spine" was first established, it is no longer possible for clinicians, or even scientists, to keep abreast of the twenty or more journals which publish original scientific papers which relate to the spine and its associated structures. The international societies on the lumbar spine, cervical spine and scoliosis used to be the only forums for the presentation of original research for peer review. These organizations must now compete with the North American Spine Society and other national associations with much larger membership, for the best research papers. Furthermore, most of these societies have become interdisciplinary, accepting membership from clinicians and scientists with greatly differing backgrounds and experience.

All this research and debate has resulted in serious questioning of prior theories and models for back pain. Prior simplistic concepts have given way to complex models which combine the increasing number of factors which seem to influence and predict the disability that patients are likely to experience when their back hurts. The new models are attempts to incorporate current knowledge obtained from laboratory experimentation, epidemiology, sociology, psychology and clinical outcome studies. The concept of a structural degenerative cascade, a socioeconomic cascade and a psychological cascade as outlined in the early chapters of this text represent modern efforts at interpreting this data. These modes, in turn, are increasingly being used as a basis for the management of patients with back pain.

Recent emphasis on so-called managed care and costs of health care has forced clinicians to justify the effectiveness of their diagnosis and treatment methods. In the past, the simple observation that a patient or group of patients felt better following a particular treatment approach was sufficient to justify that treatment. In order to be compensated, it has become increasingly important to prove, by means of controlled clinical trials, that a treatment is successful. In the same way a diagnosis test used to be considered important if it revealed information about a patient. It is now necessary to demonstrate that a test will influence the outcome of a patient's treatment for it to be considered reasonable. Professional and governmental expert panels have been convened to provide guidelines on the management of patients with back pain. They have inevitably relied on controlled clinical trials and outcome studies rather than case reports, anecdotal observations, and uncontrolled or retrospective studies when issuing recommendations. This has caused somewhat of a panic among clinicians, but at the same time, has led to the establishment of increasingly sophisticated clinical trials on a wide variety of diagnostic tests and treatment methods. The documentation in this text parallels these scientific directions.

Recent research has also challenged some of the more classic concepts of treatment. There are a large number of studies which have shown a breakdown in the previously perceived relationship between spinal abnormalities on x-rays, MRI and other imaging studies and symptoms. This has changed the emphasis on ordering routine x-rays and early expensive testing unless the study is likely to influence management. The observation that patients with well-defined disc herniations can and do respond to non-surgical approaches not only with reduction of symptoms, but also in the size of the herniation, has led to a de-emphasis of the surgical approach to these patients. At the same time, research on the intervertebral disc as a primary source of pain through the release of inflammatory agents has resulted in an increase in the use of surgery for the treatment of discogenic pain.

More than anything, however, the research has lead to greater understanding of the role of patient social attitudes and habits as a predictor of disability. Increasingly, rehabilitation and preventative interventions are focusing on changing the lifestyle of the patient with back pain. The impact of smoking, exercise and a well-designed work site is being recognized. Patient habits and attitude also appear to

influence the response to treatment. For example, the fusion rates following surgery are diminished if the patient is a smoker, while effects of motivation, psychological depression and litigation on the rehabilitation process is the subject of an increasing number of studies. This knowledge is now being incorporated in work- and sports-related activities in an attempt to reduce the frequency and severity of back injuries. The fact that this text has a whole section of sports-specific injuries reflects the importance of these issues.

It is no longer possible to state that the treatment of back pain is easy. The complexity of the issue has reduced the comfort level and, to some extent, the confidence of many clinicians in dealing with patients with these problems. Furthermore, as this text illustrates, the books on the topic have gotten considerably thicker and more detailed. There is, however, no doubt that spine care has become more interesting and challenging to both the clinician and the scientist. Those of us, including many of the authors in this text, who have had the privilege of watching and participating in the expansion of knowledge on the spine over the past two decades recognize that our understanding of the spine is far from complete. The hope is that by laying out everything we do know in a text such as this, we can begin to see the areas of future research which will clarify and consolidate current knowledge. This is expected to lead to more well-defined and clear-cut models for the understanding and management of patients with spinal problems. At that time, spine care should, once again, become satisfying and enjoyable while, at the same time, more scientifically valid, cost-effective and beneficial to our patients.

Preface

The practice of spinal medicine is in chronic disarray and facing serious jeopardy. This is due to the disorganized and unscientific fashion in which the subspecialties deal with the vague etiologies of back pain and the impatience of the managed care organizations, the government, and the public, with our inefficient, expensive, and disorganized care.

As a result, there may be mandatory restructuring of the spinal medicine delivery system which may set back the quality of spine care twenty years. If we can present a unified approach to a high quality and efficient practice of spine care, we can salvage our subspecialty and have a more rewarding, successful, and enjoyable practice than we now have.

This book presents an answer to our dilemma. It brings together all subspecialty philosophies into a common concept of total spine care. It offers systematic methods of diagnosis and treatment which are efficient and already acceptable to the demands of managed care and government agencies.

We present strong scientific evidence for the source and preferred treatment of back pain. Rather than a compilation of individual opinions, we provide a model which is complete and easy to follow. It takes into consideration not only the physical structural sources of low-back pain, but the psychological, social, and cultural ramifications.

We hope that this book will serve as a catalyst for a unified approach to spine care which will be more beneficial for our individual patients and for society, as a whole.

Arthur H. White, M.D.
Jerome A. Schofferman, M.D.

Acknowledgements

All of the authors of the chapters in this book have devoted considerable time and effort to produce palatable, state of the art spine care information for you, the reader. Several of the authors deserve special thanks because of their voluminous contributions, each of which could have been separate books on their own. These authors are Nicholas Bogduk, M.D., Charlie Ray, M.D., and Jerome Schofferman, M.D. I would like to thank Robert Gaines, for creating at the last minute, a chapter on spinal deformity in children, adolescents, and young adults, which is a distillation of an entire field of spinal medicine. In future revisions of this book he will hopefully expand that chapter to the multiple chapters the subject deserves. Dr. Ken Hsu from San Francisco deserves special thanks for many of the drawings that are found throughout this book.

Most of all I would like to thank Eugenia Klein for the years of effort and consultation that she has provided as well as her valuable editorial support concerning the design and organization of this work.

Arthur H. White, M.D.

I would like to thank Arthur White, MD, who first gave me the opportunity to work with spine patients many years ago and thereby introduced me to an area of medicine that has been so enjoyable and fruitful. I would like to thank the patients with whom I have worked for teaching me the lessons that are not in any book and challenging me to search for better ways to do things. I thank my colleagues and staff at SpineCare whose support allowed me the time and energy to work on this book. Most of all I thank my wife, Sally, for her love and support as well as the encouragement to explore better ways to live. It is perhaps too easy in life to remain static, to accept things as they are, to "gel." Working on this book has kept me fluid professionally. Living with Sally has kept me fluid personally.

Jerome A. Schofferman, M.D.

Contents

VOLUME ONE
Diagnosis and Conservative Treatment

Section 4

Sport-Specific Structural Injuries

VOLUME TWO

Operative Treatment

PART VI

Surgical Treatment

Section 1

General Considerations

Section 2

Minimally Invasive Surgery of the Lumbar Spine

Section 3

Open Surgery of the Lumbar Spine

Section 4

Open Surgery of the Cervical Spine

PART VII

Tumor, Trauma, Infection, Deformity, and Other Conditions

Section 1

Tumors

Section 2

Trauma

Section 3

Infection

Section 4

Deformity

Section 5

Other Conditions

Appendix

Color Plates

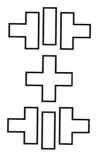

PART I

The Multidisciplinary Approach to Spine Practice

Chapter 1
Introduction

Arthur H. White
Jerome A. Schofferman

The treatment of patients with pain of spinal origin can be extremely interesting and rewarding. However, some patients with low-back or neck pain can be difficult to treat, and care of these patients is often quite challenging. The clinician who is well prepared can offer a patient much more than one who is functioning on an old knowledge base. If the clinician does not have a solid foundation in modern spine medicine, treatment of patients with spinal problems may seem tedious and difficult. It is the purpose of *Spinal Care: Diagnosis and Treatment* to provide a comprehensive framework for the evaluation and treatment of patients with spinal pain at each stage of the problem. This book takes the practitioner through the process alongside the patient in a step-by-step fashion. By providing the in-depth information necessary to increase the chances of a favorable outcome and by anticipating problems that might arise, the authors and editors have attempted to make care of these patients enjoyable.

Low-back pain affects more than 80% of the adult population, and cervical spine pain affects a large number of patients as well. Patients with spinal pain are seen by clinicians of all disciplines, not just orthopedists or neurosurgeons. Therefore, it is important for generalists and specialists alike to have an understanding of this common clinical condition. Many clinicians do not like to see patients with back or neck pain because they feel they have nothing to offer unless surgery is indicated. This book will change that perception.

There are many excellent textbooks available on the spine. Each has a format based on the philosophy of the editors. Most of these books grew from practices that are university-based. Often the editors are academicians first and clinicians second. Many of their patients are seen by residents and fellows, with the attending physician available to provide consultation and advice. Books of this type are rich in literature citations but may lack the clinical substance of the examination room so necessary to teach the art of clinical spine practice. They describe techniques and procedures in detail and offer excellent descriptions of the radiologic findings in different disease states. However in most books, despite the fact that most patients do not require surgery and are treated conservatively, nonoperative treatment is covered only superficially. This type of book is useful if the clinician already knows what is wrong with the patient. It becomes less useful in the actual clinical setting when the clinician has only the patient's symptoms and signs on which to base a diagnostic and therapeutic plan.

Spine Care: Diagnosis and Treatment is different. Each chapter is written by knowledgeable practitioners who are clinicians first and academicians second. First and foremost, the clinical experience and treatment model of each author is reflected in the approach to the patient, which is thoroughly described in this textbook.

The format is patient-oriented. It teaches the reader to formulate a working diagnosis based on the history and physical examination and to use this working diagnosis to initiate treatment. It shows how to revise and update the working diagnosis according to changes in the patient's condition and response to therapy. The book will guide the reader through each stage of the problem from the initial visit through definitive diagnosis, nonoperative and operative treatment, completion of rehabilitation, and eventually discharge. The book is user-friendly for the novice but also sophisticated for the experienced spine clinician.

There are many types of clinicians who treat spine problems just as there are many types of patients with spine problems. Each type of clinician sees a different group of patients. It is not necessary or even desirable for every clinician to have detailed knowledge of every aspect of spinal medicine. However, every clinician who regularly sees spine patients needs to have an overview of current concepts of testing and currently available treatment options. Each clinician must know when a patient requires specialty consultation and the best physician to provide that help. A rehabilitation specialist must know the indications for surgical referral as well as the types of surgical options available for a particular problem. A surgeon should be skilled in multiple surgical techniques in order to fit the operation to the patient, but he/she must also have an adequate understanding of psychology to recognize when not to operate despite structural pathology. In addition, all clinicians must recognize the importance of rehabilitation in the overall treatment plan. This book is designed to provide this comprehensive overview.

In our clinical practices and teaching, we have found it extremely helpful to think of our patients and their problem in terms of cascades. A cascade according to the *American Heritage Dictionary* is "a succession or series of processes, operations, or units. . . the output of each serving as the input for the next." In the area of spinal disorders, there are multiple cascades. We have concentrated on three, the structural degenerative cascade, the psychologic cascade, and the socioeconomic cascade.

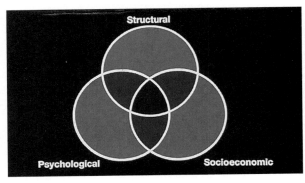

Fig. 1-1

A patient may be symbolized as a series of overlapping circles, each of which represents one cascade.

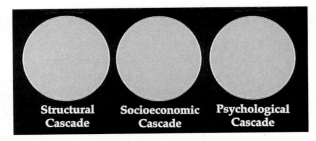

Fig. 1-2

In order to diagnose and treat a patient, the circles or cascades must be separated from each other and analyzed individually.

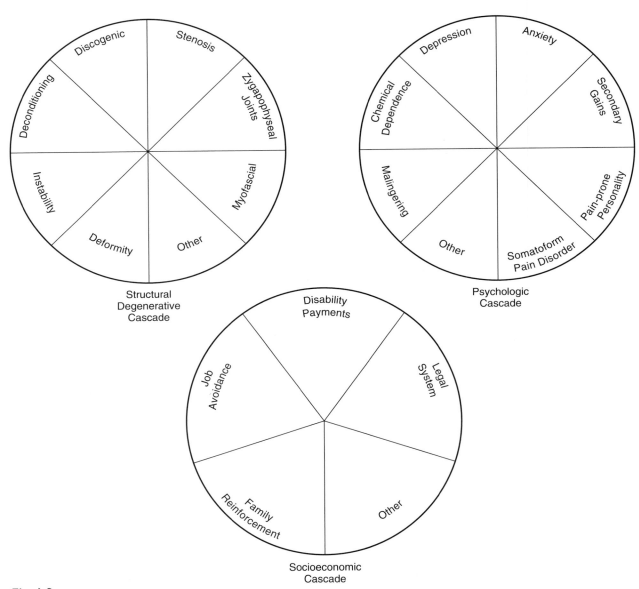

Fig. 1-3

The potential contributing factor(s) to each circle or cascade must be considered.

The patient can be pictured as resembling a set of circles which form a Venn diagram (Fig. 1-1). Each circle represents one cascade. When the patient is first seen the circles are overlapping and the boundaries may be blurred. It is the task of the evaluating clinician to separate the circles (Fig. 1-2). The majority of patients are involved in multiple cascades simultaneously. However, at any time one or more cascades may dominate the clinical picture. In a very straightforward patient, only one cascade may be active. In the complex patient who was injured on the job and has had three prior surgeries, all three cascades may be important.

The next job is to analyze the components of each cascade. Each can be thought of as a pie (Fig. 1-3). The slices of the pie in turn represent the individual components of each cascade. Only when the contribution of each component of each cascade is sorted out and understood can a clinician establish a comprehensive treatment program. This may require consultation with other physicians, physical therapists, and industrial-claims adjusters. Patients with complex problems might best be treated by specialty clinics.

The foundation of working with patients with spinal problems is a thorough history-taking and physical examination. After the initial visit, the clinician will have formulated a working diagnosis. The working diagnosis will include the contributions from the structural degenerative cascade, the psychologic cascade, and the socioeconomic cascade. Having a working diagnosis will permit the clinician to initiate a treatment program that is appropriately matched to the needs of each individual patient.

Patients with simple problems may need only back school and stabilization training. Others may require surgery. Still others will require psychotherapy and a functional restoration program. This process is pictured in algorithm form in Fig. 1-4.

Structural Degenerative Cascade

The structural degenerative cascade is the series of pathoanatomic changes that occur over time. This cascade may manifest clinically by symptoms, signs, or abnormal radiologic studies and surgically by inspection. The process begins with micro or macro trauma, often augmented by biochemical changes, in the disc or facet joints and results in structural alteration of the vertebral motion segment. As the process continues, structural degeneration may eventually manifest as disc degeneration or herniation, spinal instability, malalignment, facet arthrosis, stenosis and/or other structural abnormality, any or all of which may be painful.

Most patients with pain of spinal origin seen in ordinary clinical practice suffer from some form of degenerative disc disease. As described so well by Kirkaldy-Willis, disc degeneration progresses in a longitudinal manner over time. However, patients may or may not be symptomatic at any stage, leading to the variation in clinical presentations. A clinician must be well versed in this "degenerative cascade" to evaluate and treat each patient.

A subcategory of the degenerative cascade is the deconditioning spiral. Many patients with pain become progressively less active. Their musculature becomes weaker through disuse and they become progressively less fit aerobically. The deconditioning may be exacerbated by a clinician who prescribes bed rest. As the patient becomes weaker it becomes more painful to do even ordinary activities, and the patient does even less. The amount of disability becomes greater than expected based on the structural pathol-

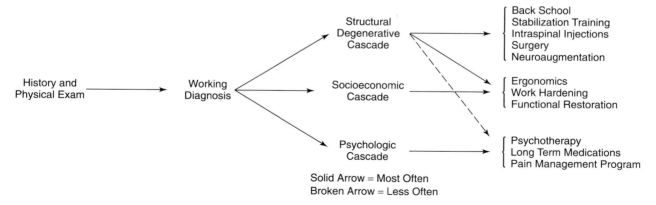

Fig. 1-4
Algorithm for evaluation and treatment of back pain patients.

ogy. Eventually this severe deconditioning becomes a major obstacle to rehabilitation and recovery.

Psychologic Cascade

Psychologic problems may have been present before the spinal disorder or may have arisen as a result of the spinal disorder. Both must be considered.

Psychologic problems that were present before pain or injury may have been active in some individuals and not in others. There are two categories of premorbid psychologic problems—psychologic predisposition toward chronic pain (pain-prone personality) and a psychologic disorder that is a direct cause of the pain.

It is well recognized that there are people with "pain-prone personalities," who appear predisposed to have more pain and disability than others with similar structural pathology. These patients suffer a true mechanical injury but do not recover. It is as if they are predisposed to become patients with chronic pain who have pain and disability far out of proportion to the structural pathology.

There are several psychologic illnesses that present with pain as the predominant symptom. These are somatization disorder, conversion disorder, hypochondriasis, and somatoform pain disorder. In addition, psychoactive substance use disorder may predispose to chronic pain problems.

There are psychologic problems that occur as a direct result of the pain and injury. The longer pain and disability are present, the more likely psychologic problems will appear. The pain of degenerative spinal disease may cause or augment significant psychologic problems that in turn worsen the pain, disability, and dysfunction.

Pain may take a heavy toll on people's lives. It can lead to depression, which in turn makes pain even worse. Patients may become dependent on alcohol, opioid analgesics, or sedative hypnotics, which may worsen the depression. Some patients become hopeless about ever feeling well again.

In addition to depression, there are other forms of psychologic problems that develop as a direct result of the pain and injury. Many of these are lumped under the term *secondary gains*. Patients may unconsciously use pain to avoid unpleasant aspects of their lives or to gain pleasant things that are not otherwise available to them. Pain may allow them to avoid going to a job they hate. Pain may serve to influence a spouse to show affection and lavish increased attention not otherwise attainable.

Learned abnormal pain behavior may develop. Some of these behaviors may be seen during the physical examination. Unconsciously, patients may display awkward and unphysiologic movements when examined. They may grimace or cry out. Range of motion may be ratchety. Muscle weakness may appear that is not physiologic. Patients may limp or display other unusual gait disturbances. Some of these learned behaviors arise out of fear of causing more pain. Others arise out of an unconscious need to prove they are hurting.

Other learned pain behaviors include less and less time up and active. Patients may spend more time in a recliner or bed. They become weaker and deconditioned. They learn to spend more time at home, and they become less interactive.

When the psychologic cascade is a major part of a patient's problem, it must be treated in order for the patient to recover.

Socioeconomic Cascade

The downhill spiral of a patient with a work-related injury who is in the workers' compensation system or of a patient who is in the throes of a personal injury claim are well known. Although the socioeconomic cascade usually begins with a legitimate injury, the structural problems may be superseded by social or economic problems. Some patients who are injured while working are straightforward and their recovery is not delayed by socioeconomic factors. Other patients, however, become entangled in a web of doctors with differing opinions, attorneys, employers, and claims adjusters. As time goes on the web becomes thicker and progressively more difficult to untangle. Just as the patient is caught in this web, so might be the treating physician, especially if he or she is not experienced with the workers' compensation system and work-related spine problems.

Other social problems may follow. Patients who are unable to work often suffer significant financial hardship. Relationships with family, friends, and co-workers often become strained. Patients may spend long hours at home alone and become withdrawn and lonely. Negative social issues have an impact on the psychologic state of the patient and perpetuate the downhill spirals.

It is also important to look at the socioeconomic cascade from a cultural perspective. A hundred years ago a patient with spine pain would be thought of quite differently. There were no effective treatments and no reliable tests available. There were no news reports of miracle surgical cures and no advertisements for pain-relieving drugs. There were no disability or insurance systems. There were only friends or relatives to provide relief or respite. Therefore, a person had little choice but to go out and work or stay at home and not be able to care for or provide for the family.

Summary

Spinal medicine is a young and exciting area of clinical practice. Even clinicians who completed training just a few years ago did not receive comprehensive education in this area. There have been major advances in our understanding of the degenerative process, in our understanding of how psychologic factors affect the perception of pain and disability, and in our knowledge of the social factors that compound the problem, which we must understand.

Economic factors are strongly influencing the way we practice spinal medicine today and will get progressively more important in the near future. If clinicians who treat spine problems do not become part of the solution to the problems of increasing health care and disability costs, we will find our practices controlled by third parties. To avoid this, we must practice spinal medicine that encompasses the structural, psychologic, social, and economic issues described above.

The first section of this book will help the clinician gather information, categorize each patient into one or more cascades, formulate a working diagnosis, and initiate treatment. The remainder of the book will provide the diagnostic and treatment options available for each patient at each stage of the problem. At each stage, structural, psychologic, and socioeconomic issues will be considered.

PATIENT EVALUATION

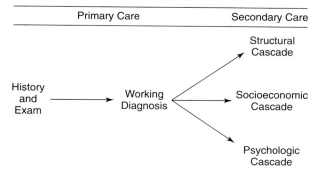

Chapter 2
The Structural Degenerative Cascade

THE LUMBAR SPINE*
David K. Selby

Anatomy of the Motion Segment

In order to understand spine clinical syndromes it is extremely useful to think in terms of the motion segment, which is the basic functional unit of the spine. Each motion segment is composed of two adjacent vertebrae with their intervertebral disc. The disc and the two facet joints at the same level function as a trijoint complex. Over time and with micro or macro trauma there is a natural progression of degeneration of the motion segment with corresponding anatomic, biochemical, and clinical findings.

The bony anatomy is represented by an anterior vertebral body composed of a large volume of trabecular bone (Fig. 2-1). The vertebral body is the major weight-bearing portion of the motion segment. The lumbar vertebrae are more oval than round, with the convexity facing posteriorly. This oval shape lends additional support to the disc in flexion around the center of rotation, which is located at a point at the posterior third of the disc. The oval shape also puts the forces during flexion at the posterior-lateral aspect of the vertebra, which makes the nerve root more susceptible to contact with an abnormal disc.

The posterior elements consist of the lamina, pars interarticularis, and superior and inferior articular processes. The posterior elements bear less weight than the anterior portion. In sitting, the anterior elements bear over 90% of the weight versus 80% in standing. As the degenerative cascade progresses, the relative anterior to posterior weight-bearing changes to 50% each.

The facet or zygapophyseal joints are oriented obliquely to the sagittal plane. Their joint surfaces anteriorly are oriented toward the coronal plane and posteriorly toward the sagittal plane. This orientation offers a greater relative resistance to torsional stress posteriorly and anterior-posterior shear stresses anteriorly. Patients who have more sagittally oriented facet joints may be predisposed to degenerative spondylolisthesis with advanced disc degeneration.

The thecal sac and the beginnings of the exiting nerve roots are contained in the central canal. The central canal protects the spinal cord and the cauda equina (Fig. 2-2). The exiting nerve traverses through the lateral nerve canal, usually referred to as the neural foramen. The neural foramen can be divided into three segments—the entrance zone, the middle zone, and the exit zone. The entrance portion of the canal contains the segment called the "lateral recess" and is bordered by the medial aspect of the superior articular facet. The middle zone is beneath the pars interarticularis and runs along the pedicle and contains the large-diameter dorsal root ganglion. The exit zone is bordered by the superior articular facet on one side and the body of the ver-

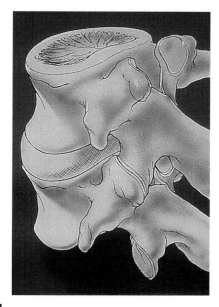

Fig. 2-1

Structural anatomy of motion segment showing two vertebral bodies, intervertebral disc, lamina, pars interarticularis, superior and inferior articular processes, and facet joints. *(From Selby DK, Saal JS: The degenerative cascade: anatomy and pathophysiology of the lumbar spine, Camp International, Inc. Used with permission.)*

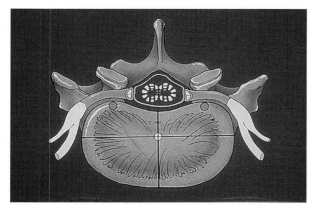

Fig. 2-2

Thecal sac, exiting nerve roots, and dorsal-root ganglia are shown in relationship to bony anatomy. *(From Selby DK, Saal JS: The degenerative cascade: anatomy and pathophysiology of the lumbar spine, Camp International, Inc. Used with permission.)*

---

*Modified from Selby DK, Saal JS: The degenerative cascade: anatomy and pathophysiology of the lumber spine. With permission of Camp International, Inc., Jackson, MI.

tebra on the other. Degenerative hypertrophy of these bony structures can lead to entrapment of the various neural structures.

The spine functions best within a realm of static and dynamic stability. The bony architecture and attendent specialized soft-tissue structures, especially the disc, provide a static stability. Dynamic stability, however, is accomplished via a system of muscular and ligamentous support with distinct postural attendant mechanisms. The overall resolution of forces determines the structural integrity of the trijoint complex. The net shear forces must be maintained below a critical minimum in order to maintain integrity. Persistent or recurrent forces to the motion segment outside this range leads to repetitive microtrauma to the disc and facet joints, which over time trigger and maintain the degenerative process. Repetitive or persistent abnormal forces lead to structural failure, and a painful clinical condition may result. Loss of disc height and structural integrity can create instability.

Intervertebral Disc

In addition to the vertebral body the anterior column also contains the disc (Fig. 2-3). The intervertebral disc is composed of an outer anulus fibrosis, which surrounds the nucleus pulposus. The anulus has two distinct layers. The outer anulus is composed of type I collagen (as is found in tendon) and inserts into the vertebral body via Sharpies fibers. It has both neurogenic and vascular supply. It provides strength to the disc in bending. The inner anulus is composed of Type II collagen (as in hyaline cartilage) and is a cephalocaudal extension of the vertebral end plate. The inner anulus-vertebral end plate combined structure encapsulates the nucleus. It provides the disc with extra strength during compression. The disc nucleus is the remnant of the embryologic notochord. The disc structure is analogous to cartilage. Histologically, the material is described as fibrocartilage, although biochemically there are distinct differences.

Support of the load applied across a disc is a function of the swelling pressure inherent to the water-proteoglycan matrix (Fig. 2-4). Seventy-two percent of the compressive load on a healthy disc is borne by the nucleus. The anulus bears the remainder. In addition to the nucleus, the anulus, particularly the inner layer, is able to imbibe water and thereby add to the support.

The nucleus pulposus makes up two thirds of the surface area of the disc. From youth into the third decade of life, it is composed of 90% water. Over the

next four decades, the water content gradually diminishes to approximately 60 to 65%. The hydration of the nucleus and anulus depends on the amount of proteoglycan present.

The anulus covers approximately a third of the surface area of the disc. It is composed of 65% water. Collagen, Type I primarily but with some Type II, is woven into lamellae, between which there is proteoglycan-rich ground substance. The collagen bundles are oriented approximately 30 degrees to

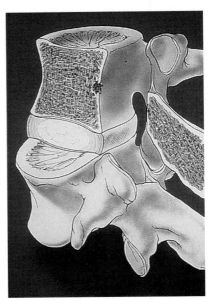

Fig. 2-3
Cutaway view of motion segment with its two vertebrae, intervertebral disc, and posterior elements. *(From Selby DK, Saal JS: The degenerative cascade: anatomy and pathophysiology of the lumbar spine, Camp International, Inc. Used with permission.)*

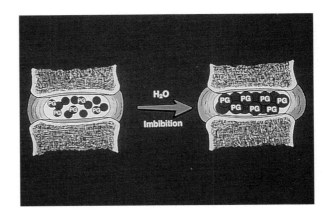

Fig. 2-4
Proteoglycan-rich nucleus imbibes water, which leads to increased swelling pressure, which enables disc to support increased load. *(From Selby DK, Saal JS: The degenerative cascade: anatomy and pathophysiology of the lumbar spine, Camp International, Inc. Used with permission.)*

the horizontal, with a mirror image reversal at each successive layer.

Proteoglycans are megamolecules and are the largest molecules in the human body. They have a large capacity to imbibe water and can thereby increase their weight by approximately 250%. They are synthesized by chondrocytes within the nucleus and are slowly turned over by the low-grade metabolic processes of the disc. The major components are glycosaminoglycans, chondroition-2-sulfate, and keretan-4-sulfate bound to a backbone of hyaluronic acid by a link protein. Proteoglycans are not found free within other spaces of the body but are localized to the matrix of the nucleus. They may be capable of inciting an inflammatory response when exposed to mucosal surfaces such as the epidural space.

Innervation of the Motion Segment

The innervation of the lumbar spine has been beautifully demonstrated by Bogduk and others (Fig. 2-5). The various clinical patterns of pain are due to the richness of innervation. The zygapophyseal or facet joints are innervated by a branching network from the dorsal ramus with overlap to the level above and below via the medial branch of the dorsal ramus. The dorsal root ganglion (DRG) lies in the middle zone of the intervertebral foramen. It is the signal processing center for all afferent input. The DRG plays a critical role in the genesis and modulation of spine pain syndromes. The outer anulus is richly innervated as well.

The outer anulus of the disc has afferent nociceptive and proprioceptive nerve endings. There are also sympathetic efferents that arise from the sinovertebral nerve, a branch of the dorsal ramus (posterior primary ramus). Also, the gray ramus communicans, a connection between the sympathetic trunk and the dorsal ramus, provides innervation directly to the outer anulus. This does not imply direct connection to the sympathetic trunk with the dorsal ramus as the fibers travel down the vertebral ramus as efferent sympathetic nerves to distal structures.

Arterial Supply and Venous Drainage

The arterial supply to the vertebrae is via an arterial grid in the centrum vertically oriented (Fig. 2-6). The branches course past the end plate and anulus. Venous drainage of the disc is provided by a subarticular collecting system that drains to the central

vein of the vertebra and then to Batson's plexus (Fig. 2-7).

The disc is the largest avascular structure in the body. Nutrition to the disc nucleus depends on diffusion of small molecular substances across the end plate (Fig. 2-8). The outer third of the anulus receives blood supply from the epidural space. Disc degeneration is a function of proteoglycan breakdown

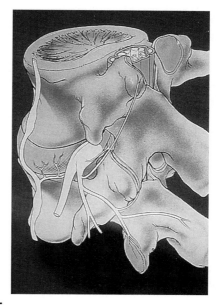

Fig. 2-5
Global innervation of motion segment. Facet joints are innervated by branches of dorsal ramus with overlap to level above and below via medial branches. Dorsal-root ganglion lies in midzone of intervertebral foramen. *(From Selby DK, Saal JS: The degenerative cascade: anatomy and pathophysiology of the lumbar spine, Camp International, Inc. Used with permission.)*

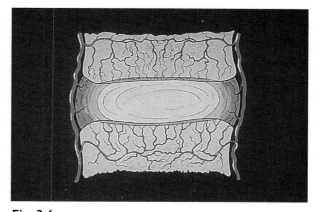

Fig. 2-6
Arterial supply of anterior part of motion segment. *(From Selby DK, Saal JS: The degenerative cascade: anatomy and pathophysiology of the lumbar spine, Camp International, Inc. Used with permission.)*

with associated loss of the cross linkage of collagen proteins. This results in a lowered capacity to imbibe and hold water. The resultant desiccated disc is not as flexible or strong.

Beginnings of the Degenerative Process

Changes in the anterior and posterior columns are intimately related in the degenerative process. The mechanical properties of the disc play an important role in the degenerative cascade. In response to repetitive micro trauma, usually eccentric loading or torsional loading, the disc begins to show signs of mechanical failure that is the start of the degenerative cascade. Repeated micro trauma results in the development of circumferential tears in the outer anular layers (Fig. 2-9). Tears may be followed by or accompanied by end plate separation or failure, with interruption of blood supply, eventually leading to loss of nuclear nutrition. It is thought that the clinical correlate of this type of anular tear is the self-limiting syndrome of primary or nonspecific back pain with or without radiation. This is the so-called stage of dysfunction described by Kirkaldy-Willis. It is usually self-limited. However, in some instances, there is a pattern of persistent back pain with a gradual evolution toward the pathology to be described subsequently. The anular tear and deterioration is probably the initial anatomic abnormality that begins the sequence of the herniated disc.

If there is continued or recurrent application of eccentric or torsional loading there may be progressive end plate separation. There is structural failure and weakening of the outer anulus. The circumfer-

ential anular tears coalesce to become radial tears. Further anular weakening allows progressive migration of nuclear material toward the periphery of the anulus without rupture of inner anular fibers or distinct change in the external border of the disc. The next step in the evolution of disc herniation is further migration of nuclear material into the outer anulus with deformation of the outer border of the disc (Fig. 2-10). The nuclear material and residual anulus are usually "contained" beneath the posterior longitudinal ligament.

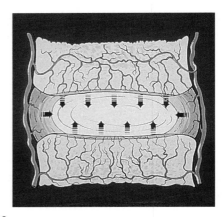

Fig. 2-8
Nutrition of disc is via diffusion through end plate. *(From Selby DK, Saal JS: The degenerative cascade: anatomy and pathophysiology of the lumbar spine, Camp International, Inc. Used with permission.)*

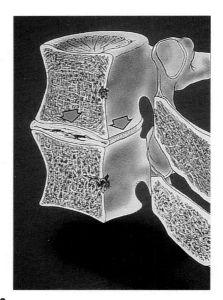

Fig. 2-9
Repetitive microtrauma leads to disruption of anulus, loss of water content, and progressive narrowing of disc space. *(From Selby DK, Saal JS: The degenerative cascade: anatomy and pathophysiology of the lumbar spine, Camp International, Inc. Used with permission.)*

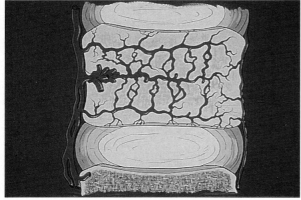

Fig. 2-7
Venous drainage of anterior part of motion segment. *(From Selby DK, Saal JS: The degenerative cascade: anatomy and pathophysiology of the lumbar spine, Camp International, Inc. Used with permission.)*

When the anulus fails there is protrusion of the nuclear material through the confines of the anulus—disc herniation (Fig. 2-11). If the herniation is lateral there may be direct compression of the exiting nerve root (Fig. 2-12). Depending on the type of herniation, nuclear material may migrate superiorly or inferiorly or track along the lateral recess. The mechanism of nerve root injury in this situation is mechanical, but there are chemical or inflammatory factors that are also important in producing clinical symptoms. It is also clear that in many cases significant injury and pain can occur in the absence of frank neural compression. Back pain and nonspecific leg pain can be due to mechanical distortion of the outer anulus, posterior longitudinal ligament, or dura as well. It is hypothesized that chemical irritation of these structures can also cause back or leg pain.

Herniation can also occur anteriorly. It is unclear whether anterior herniations are clinically relevant. They may be associated with nonspecific low-back pain. Anterior herniations are thought to be less common than posterior herniations because of the greater thickness of the anterior anulus and the nature of force distribution in the lumbar spine.

As previously stated, the initial event of degeneration of the motion segment is anular damage and separation of the cartilaginous end plate. The latter results in loss of the nutritional supply to the disc, which in turn begins a sequence of proteoglycan breakdown that then leads to loss of water content of the disc. There is loss of disc height and eventual deterioration of mechanical competence of the disc. As the repetitive forces that led to the disruption of the nutritional supply continue, there is continued loss of the normal stiffness of the anulus fibrosis. Disorganization of the nuclear matrix and progressive separation of layers of the anulus result in prolapse of the degenerative anulus. Transfer of axial loading to the posterior elements gradually occurs in association with disc degeneration.

Instability Phase of Degeneration

Progressive loss of mechanical competence of the trijoint complex results in excessive joint motion, which probably occurs in all planes (Fig. 2-13). This is the instability phase that follows the dysfunction phase. In addition to increased joint motion there is decreased resistance of the trijoint complex to shear forces. Pain may be generated by traction and dy-

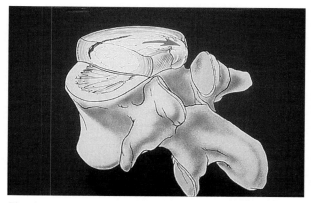

Fig. 2-11

Herniated nucleus pulposus. *(From Selby DK, Saal JS: The degenerative cascade: anatomy and pathophysiology of the lumbar spine, Camp International, Inc. Used with permission.)*

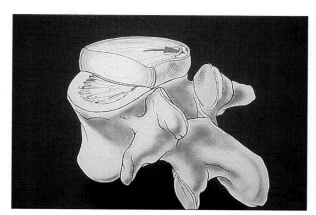

Fig. 2-10

Structural failure of anulus with migration of nucleus pulposus. *(From Selby DK, Saal JS: The degenerative cascade: anatomy and pathophysiology of the lumbar spine, Camp International, Inc. Used with permission.)*

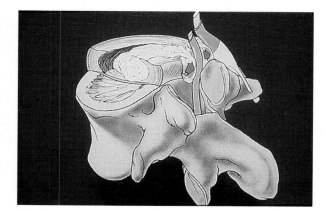

Fig. 2-12

Herniated nucleus pulposus with direct nerve-root compression. *(From Selby DK, Saal JS: The degenerative cascade: anatomy and pathophysiology of the lumbar spine, Camp International, Inc. Used with permission.)*

namic compression of soft-tissue structures. Further tearing of the anulus may also be part of this instability phase.

With progressive loss of disc height there is narrowing of the neural foramen in the cephalad-caudad direction ("up-down" stenosis). However the dimensions of the neural foramen and central canal are dynamic (Fig. 2-14). The foramen opens with lumbar flexion and closes with extension.

Direct compression and mechanical deformation of the nerve root leads to ischemia and traction-induced injury. The presence of exposed nuclear material within the epidural space stimulates an inflammatory response at the level of the nerve root, which appears to cause further ischemia. Damage caused by inflammatory mediators is an additional mechanism of nerve injury due to disc protrusion. There may be associated changes in the nerve root, such as epineural thickening and loss of vascularity. The nerve displays the ability to respond to very gradual deformation without significant functional compromise. As the lateral canals narrow, the nerve roots undergo a process of gradual ischemia. The nerve root loses mobility because of adhesions that develop in the nerve root sheath. An abrupt change in the dimensions of the canal or application of a traction force to the nerve is often the precipitating factor in clinical radiulopathy in the setting of lateral canal stenosis.

Progressive Degeneration of the Motion Segment

Over time dynamic lateral entrapment leads to fixed stenosis. Wolff's law predicts the growth of bone (osteophytes) to stabilize the trijoint complex. The dimensions of the central canal are also significantly reduced by hypertrophy of the inferior facet especially if there is associated thickening and subsequent bulging of the ligamentum flavum. Hypertrophy of the superior articular facet narrows the lateral canal. The mechanical incompetence of the instability phase is resolved by the proliferation of bone and the settling of the disc space with narrowing of the neural canals with compression of neural elements as the result of the bone growth and subsequent stabilization process (Fig. 2-15).

Zygapophyseal (Facet) Joint

The facet joint plays a significant role in the structural degenerative cascade. The facet joint or zygapophyseal joint is a diarthrodial joint that can go through all the changes that occur in the hip or

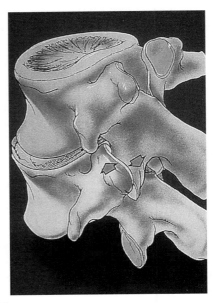

Fig. 2-13
Progressive loss of mechanical competence of the trijoint complex (disc and two facet joints) leads to excessive joint motion, with symptoms generated in part by traction and dynamic compression of soft-tissue structures and neural elements. *(From Selby DK, Saal JS: The degenerative cascade: anatomy and pathophysiology of the lumbar spine, Camp International, Inc. Used with permission.)*

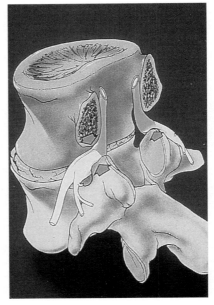

Fig. 2-14
Stenosis of neural foramen may gradually occur due to loss of disc height. Initially stenosis is dynamic. *(From Selby DK, Saal JS: The degenerative cascade: anatomy and pathophysiology of the lumbar spine, Camp International, Inc. Used with permission.)*

knee (Fig. 2-16). The facet joint has articular cartilage, subchondral cartilage, a capsule, and even a small meniscus. There is synovium lining the capsule.

The first stage of facet degeneration appears to be synovitis. This is the stage of dysfunction. Patients present with nonspecific low-back pain. They may be extension-sensitive. Many patients respond to nonsteroidal antiinflammatory medications.

The synovitis or dysfunction phase is followed by progressive destruction of the cartilaginous articular surface. If there is progression there may be subluxation or dislocation of the facet meniscus. Possibly this is the lesion that responds well to manipulation. As cartilaginous destruction continues and there is simultaneous narrowing of the disc space, capsular laxity occurs with accompanying subluxation. The facet joint enters the phase of instability (Fig. 2-17). If there is severe breakdown, the integrity of the joint is lost and there may be progression to degenerative spondylolisthesis.

Facet instability can be a pain generator by two methods. There may be narrowing and motion in the recess that can traumatize the ventral ramus and cause sciatica. Stretching and tearing of the richly innervated capsule can cause back pain with or without referred leg pain. Pain transmission occurs via the medial branch or the dorsal ramus.

The end consequence of degeneration and instability of the facet joint is also osteophyte for-

mation and bony overgrowth of the joint in an attempt to stabilize. Again, new bone will form in accordance with Wolff's law. The facets increase in size as they bear more and more weight in response to the degeneration of the anterior column. This is the phase of fixed deformity. Progressive osteophytosis may contribute to significant narrowing of the neural canals and lead to the symptoms of spinal stenosis. Osteophyte formation of the inferior articular facet will narrow the central canal.

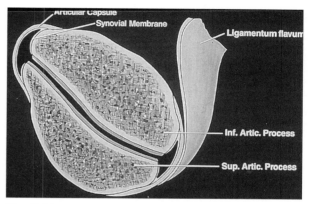

Fig. 2-16

Facet joint or zygapophyseal joint is true diarthrodial joint, which degenerates in fashion similar to hip or knee. *(From Selby DK, Saal JS: The degenerative cascade: anatomy and pathophysiology of the lumbar spine, Camp International, Inc. Used with permission.)*

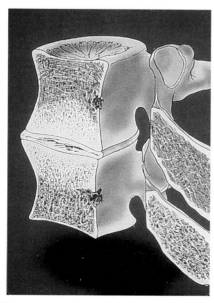

Fig. 2-15

As osteophyte formation occurs in association with loss of disc height, fixed neural forminal stenosis occurs. *(From Selby DK, Saal JS: The degenerative cascade: anatomy and pathophysiology of the lumbar spine, Camp International, Inc. Used with permission.)*

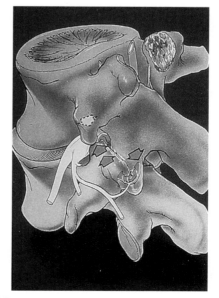

Fig. 2-17

Facet degeneration and instability can cause neural trauma and sciatica as well as pain due to stretching and tearing of facet-joint capsule. *(From Selby DK, Saal JS: The degenerative cascade: anatomy and pathophysiology of the lumbar spine, Camp International, Inc. Used with permission.)*

Enlargement of the superior articular facet will narrow the exit zone of the foramen causing lateral stenosis.

The "K-W" Degenerative Process

Kirkaldy-Willis defines three stages of the degenerative process (Fig. 2-18)—dysfunction; instability; and fixed deformity. The stage of dysfunction would be clinically manifested as nonspecific low-back pain. Exact diagnosis may be difficult, and treatment tends to be symptom-based, with recovery often occurring spontaneously. The phase of instability is a natural sequelae of loss of disc height and capsular laxity. Symptoms may occur from nociceptive stimuli to both dorsal and ventral rami. Fixed deformity is the end result of a mechanism of stabilization and new bone formation. This stage includes multilevel spondylosis and stenosis.

Internal Disc Disruption

Is is not clear where in the degenerative cascade the syndrome of "internal disc disruption" lies. The clinical constellation is primary low-back pain with or without nonspecific lower-extremity referral via the dorsal ramus. The condition usually results from traumatic axial loading, such as a fall landing on the buttocks. Separation of the cartilaginous end plate and acute nutritional loss results in intensified rapid internal degeneration/disruption of the intervertebral disc. Inflammation, immune mechanisms and and micro-instability have all been implicated singularly or in combination as playing roles in pain generation.

Although the internal anatomy of the disc is unremarkable radiographically, discographic patterns of disorganization of the nuclear matrix and loss of delineation between nucleus and anulus is characteristic. There are, however, other patterns representative of this "umbrella" diagnosis. They include discrete anular fissures with attenuation of the anuls and leakage of dye. The natural history and exact pathogenesis of internal disc disruption has not yet been satisfactorily defined.

THE CERVICAL SPINE

John A. Handal
Jeffrey Knapp
Steven Poletti

The seemingly ubiquitous nature of cervical pain is clearly accepted by physicians attending these pa-

tients. The problem is that the cervical pain syndrome is, like other pain syndromes, a multifaceted problem. Cervical pain, as with the rest of the spinal pain syndromes, is a psychologic perception of a physical event. Therefore, we physicians must study our patients and their problems with great precision. A clear and comprehensive understanding of the physical and psychologic nature of the patient's pain is necessary to bring about an anatomic diagnosis and resolution of the cervical pain syndrome.

In the diagnosis and treatment of the physical event, the cervical pain syndrome, we must understand the epidemiology and the forces that shape the natural history of the cervical motion segment. It is these events that must be understood, that is, the cascade of events causing the degradation of the cervical motion segment.

The fate of the cervical motion segment is most common—an early and multisegment degeneration. However, it is not the quiescent, asymptomatic degradation of the motion segment that we treat as physicians. It is the painful degeneration of the motion segment that is the etiology of the cervical pain syndrome.

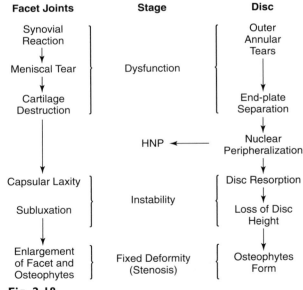

THE DEGENERATIVE CASCADE

Facet Joints	Stage	Disc
Synovial Reaction ↓ Meniscal Tear ↓ Cartilage Destruction	Dysfunction	Outer Annular Tears ↓ End-plate Separation ↓ Nuclear Peripheralization
	HNP ←	
Capsular Laxity ↓ Subluxation	Instability	Disc Resorption ↓ Loss of Disc Height
Enlargement of Facet and Osteophytes	Fixed Deformity (Stenosis)	Osteophytes Form

Fig. 2-18

Kirkaldy-Willis's stages of degenerative process. (*From Selby DK, Saal JS: The degenerative cascade: anatomy and pathophysiology of the lumbar spine, Camp International, Inc. Used with permission.*)

Natural History

To understand the natural history of the cervical motion, one must begin at the beginning. Although similar to the lumbar motion segment, cervical motion segments differs importantly in structure and motion.

The cervical vertebra is of mesodermal origin. During the transition from the embryonic phase to the fetal phase, three ossification centers appear to form the vertebral body in the adult.[18] These are the vertebral body ossification center and the two centers for the neural arches (Fig. 2-19). The disc, a remnant of the notochord, develops in direct relation to the caudad vertebral body ossification center. The ossification centers of the neural arches form the uncus. The uncus, because of its position in the neural arch, lies lateral and posterior to the body and the disc. However, the uncus is cephalad to the body and in the same transverse plane as the disc. The uncus is a vertical structure with a concavity on its medial surface. As such, the uncus is anatomically positioned as a restraint to rotation and lateral bending.[8] At birth, the disc is distinctly separate from the uncus by an inner anulus and lateral to the inner anulus by a loose fibrous tissue. This loose fibrous tissue will be absorbed in the second decade of life. There is a small cleft remaining. This cleft, the joint of Luschka, is medially bordered by the true disc anulus and, otherwise, by an outer anulus (Fig. 2-20).

The disc then has two anuli. The inner anulus surrounds the nucleus pulposus. The outer anulus surrounds the inner anular nuclear complex and the uncovertebral joints of Luschka. Therefore, with respect to the cervical spine, we must expand our concept of the cervical disc to include the uncinate process in the joints of Luschka. Hence, the concept of "the greater disc."

Epidemiology

The prevalence of neck pain is difficult to determine in reviewing the literature. Most large epidemiologic studies focus on back pain and do not differentiate between cervical, thoracic, and lumbar pain. Symptoms of neck pain can be difficult to differentiate from pain secondary to shoulder pathology. Despite these difficulties, several authors have attempted to determine the prevalence of neck pain.

Horal reported that neck pain affected almost 40% of the population during their lives.[9] In Hult's study of 1193 male workers, ages 25 to 59 years, a history of stiff neck or brachialgia occurred in 51%.[10] The incidence was about the same in those doing light and heavy work. The symptoms were frequently benign, and only 5.4% had been incapacitated for work as a result of the symptoms.[10]

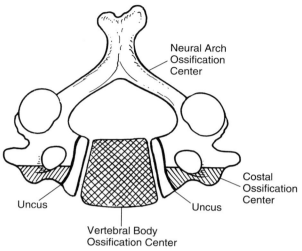

Fig. 2-19

Three ossification centers of cervical vertebra. Uncus arises from neural ossification center. Vertebral body middle arises from central ossification center. Costal center is placed more laterally.

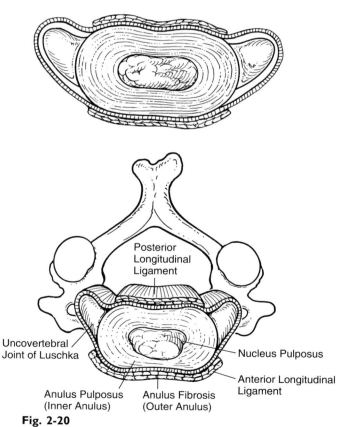

Fig. 2-20

Normal cervical disc.

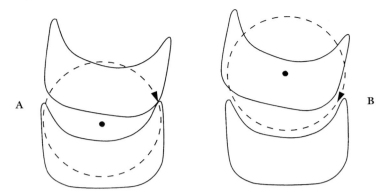

Fig. 2-21

A, Lateral flexion in typical lumbar disc. With axis of rotation in disc, uncinate would impinge. **B,** Lateral flexion in cervical vertebra with axis of rotation in cephalad vertebra; smooth uncinate gliding occurs.

Kelsey et al. studied acute prolapsed cervical discs.[11] Individuals in their 30s were the group most frequently affected with the cervical disc prolapse. The male:female ratio was 1.4:1. The levels most frequently affected were C6-C7 and C5-C6.[11] Other than age and sex, the most important risk factors were cigarette smoking, frequent diving from a board, and lifting heavy objects.

Kondo et al. studied cervical disc herniations in Rochester, Minnesota.[13] The annual incidence was 6.5% per 100,000 for men, and 4.6% for women. The incidence was highest between the ages of 45 and 54. The level most frequently affected was C5-C6. Gore et al. determined the prevalence of degenerative changes in the cervical spine in a group of 200 symptomatic men and women.[7] By age 60 to 65, 95% of men and 70% of women had at least one degenerative change on their radiograph. C5-C6 and C6-C7 had more-severe degenerative changes and more frequent degenerative changes than other levels. Holt found a strong correlation between cervical brachial symptoms and increasing severity of degenerative changes.[10]

Motion

The motion of the cervical spine in the biped is responsible for disc degeneration along with the forces that create that motion. It is then the determinants of motion, forces and restraints that are important to note.

The motions of the cervical spine include flexion, extension, side-bending, and rotation. Rotation plays an important role in disc degeneration.[3] As such, rotation is important in the cascade of degeneration of the cervical motion segment.

In the normal lumbar disc, its instant axis of rotation is located in the middle column portion of the disc. In the cervical spine the access of rotation is above the disc.[5] With the axis of rotation in the disc, the presence of an uncinate process would be an obstruction to motion. With cranial displacement of the access then, an uncinate motion occurs unobstructed (Fig. 2-21). Therefore, control of rotation in the cervical motion segment is a function not only of the disc, but also of the uncinate. The uncus, because of its role in guiding cervical motion, will respond to the stresses placed on it in the course of motion segment degeneration. These stresses will ultimately cause disc degeneration and subsequent uncus hypertrophy, osteophytosis, and degeneration of the outer anulus and ultimately of the entire motion segment.

The cervical facet joints play a lesser role in rotation. Facet rotation appears to be true rotation in the transverse plane. There is forward flexion of the contralateral facet over the inferior facet below. There is retraction on the ipsilateral side. However, in the frontal view these facets appear to be in lateral flexion. The lateral flexion of the facet joints result in rotation. This is not because of facet orientation. It is the position of the uncus that is controlling rotation, and not the cervical facet joints.

In summary, rotational movements and rotational forces have three main structural restraints in the cervical spine. Primarily, the disc determines the pattern of motion, secondarily the uncus and finally the facet joints. Given this basic mechanism, motion segment degeneration should begin in the disc. With progressive degeneration, bony changes in the uncus occur and finally change in the facet. Although cervical degeneration is a whole motion segment phenomenon, this model allows a clarified view of the motion segment's degenerative cascade.

Degenerative Cascade

So far we have discussed the cervical motion segments and the development, anatomy, motions, restraints, and forces that shape its fate. The "degenerative cascade" was first described by Kirkaldy-Willis. In his book[12] he described three phases of degeneration—dysfunction, instability, and stabilization. This concept is certainly applicable to the cervical spine with some redefinition. Normal cervical motion segments will proceed through four phases of degeneration—dysfunction, discogenic, spondylosis, and stabilization. It is worth remembering that these phases represent a conceptual view. Cervical degeneration is a spectrum of disease. It is most often multilevel and occurs early in life. Therefore, at a given time, different motion segments in the same cervical spine may be in different phases of degeneration.

Dysfunction

Dysfunction occurs in the face of few and minor pathologic changes. The patients will complain of axial neck pain—a dull, aching-type muscular pain. It is located along the axial skeleton. The patients can have scapular or interscapular, neck, posterior-auricular, and posterior-occipital pain. Patients may often have an area of point tenderness (trigger point). Patients will often describe a crick in their neck. Peculiar to scapular and interscapular pain is the description of a "stabbing" or "hot poker" feeling in the paraspinal and scapular muscles. Posterior-occipital pain is often and mistakenly described as a migraine headache.

Dysfunction is usually the product of rotational strain. This can result in facet synovitis, muscular sprain, and minor disc anular tears. Dysfunction, as with most complaints of axial neck pain, are self-limited. It is worth noting that approximately 80% of patients presenting with axial neck pain improve in time regardless of radiographic findings.[6] Treatment of dysfunction phase patients in nonoperative. Treatment is usually directed toward the posterior elements—the facets and the muscles. Nonsteroidal anti-inflammatory drugs and physical therapy are mainstays of treatment. Facet-joint injections with steroids have a role in resistant and recurrent dysfunction. The prevalence of primary facet pain is approximately 26%.[1]

Discogenic Phase

The next two phases are dominated by the disc. Disc pathology is of two types; first, anular tears (internal disc disruption); second, anular tear with herniation (herniated nucleus pulposus). The normal disc has, as has been described, compartments and spaces about it. In brief, these spaces are the nucleus, uncovertebral joints of Luschka, the sublongitudinal ligament space, and epidural space. Therefore, with respect to anular (ligament) tears, there are three potential types of tears; first, the inner anulus surrounding the nucleus may tear; second, the outer anulus surrounding the nucleus and uncovertebral joints may tear; and third, the posterior-longitudinal ligament separating the epidural space from the disc may tear. Equally then, anular tears with herniation are of three types—anular herniations, subligamentous herniations (disc protrusion), and herniations in the epidural space (free fragment HNPs). The posterior elements show concurrent involvement with anterior element (the disc) degeneration. The facet changes are noted as capsular laxity/tears. Thinning of the facet-joint cartilage can be associated.

The discogenic phase is dominated by disc pathology. Symptoms of this phase are predominantly of axial neck pain. This axial neck pain is more aptly described as cervicothoracic dorsalgia. Although similar in nature to dysfunctional pain, it can be more severe, recurrent, and even intractable. Radiculopathies seen in this phase are usually self-limited and respond to nonoperative means.[6] Intractable radiculopathies are commonly associated with free fragment herniations. Although less common in the cervical spine, noncompressive or chemical radiculopathies can occur. Radiography in these phases shows few, if any, abnormalities. Malalignment of the vertebral column secondary to muscular spasm and, perhaps, some early interspace narrowing can be seen. As this is the phase of the disc, then directly inspecting the disc is mandatory as part of the clinical assessment. The direct inspection is carried out through two studies only—MRI and discography. Other tests, for example, CT, myelography and CT-enhanced myelography, only visualize the canal and outer contours of the disc. These studies (CT, myelography) can only direct inferences about disc pathology. Much is missed by not inspecting the guilty party directly.

Painful degeneration of the disc has a benign natural history. Most patients will improve through nonoperative means. Surgical treatment can be undertaken after an accurate assessment of the patient and the pain generator has been clearly identified. Tests such as MRI, and especially discography, should rule out more surgery than it rules in. This is because multilevel painful degeneration of the disc most commonly occurs early in life.

Spondylosis

Cervical spondylosis is the product of disc degeneration. How this disc degeneration comes about is a matter of some discussion and importance. The work of several authors[3,14,19] can give us some important insights. However, to place cervical spondylosis in its proper orthopedic perspective, we must view the greater disc (nucleus, inner anulus, outer anulus, joints of Luschka, and posterolongitudinal ligament) wholly as a specialized ligament. Like any other ligament, it connects and couples the motion of two bones. In the case of lower cervical spine, it is the two vertebra of the motion segments that are connected and coupled by this specialized ligament (the greater disc). In in vitro experimentation with torsional forces,[3] Farfan et al. have shown us two things. First, torsional forces on the normal motion segment, within normal limits of motion can cause an anular unraveling (anular degeneration). Second, as anular delamination progresses, eventually with torsional forces, anular tear with nuclear herniation can occur. The in vitro reproduction of these two pathologic events within the normal limits of motion has given rise to the concept of spondylosis as a wear-and-tear process. That is, the constant loading and unloading of the spine within its normal limits of motion can give rise to disc degeneration and spondylosis.[19]

Oda et al.,[15] in looking at the natural history of the cervical disc, have reported progressive calcification of the end plate to occur. Calcification was seen in the cartilage end plates beginning at the age of 20 years. By age 40 years, 70% of end plates had calcification or bone formation within them. At age 70 years, end-plate bone formation was seen in 93% of specimens. This calcification is coincidental with the disappearance of the cartilage growth layer. Simply, the cartilage is not being regenerated. Consequently, calcification of cartilage debris and vascular invasion occurs—hence, end-plate degeneration.

The end plates have important roles in the disc anulus attachment and nuclear nutrition. As the end plate degenerates, these functions are impaired. Wada et al.[19] have shown in vitro that repetitive loading in flexion-extension caused anular delamination, anular tears, and early osteophyte formation. It is the

impaired function of this ligament (the greater disc) that gives the clinical entity of spondylosis. Interestingly, Miyamoto et al.[14] hypothesized spondylosis to be a problem of instability. These investigators have shown the acceleration of disc degeneration and the occurrence of spondylosis (osteophytosis) by removing the supraspinous and interspinous ligaments and detaching the posterior musculature of the cervical spine.

Viewing spondylosis as an instability sheds light on the clinical presentation of this entity. That is, instability pain for the most part is axial (neck, posterior occiput, and interscapular) pain. Radiculopathy can be an associated symptom with spondylosis. With hypertrophy of the uncinate and settling of the interspace, a fixed nerve root compression can occur. Associated in this phase, and less common, is degenerative spondylolisthesis. However, the predominant symptom in most patients with symptomatic spondylosis is that of axial pain. Although patients with painful spondylosis do mostly respond to nonoperative care, a significant percentage, approximately one third will not. Surgical outcome in these patients depends wholly on the measure. Wiberg[20] reported 94% improvement of radicular symptoms after anterior fusion. However, only 45% of patients had improvement in their axial neck pain. This is not an unusual experience among surgeons. Before surgery is undertaken, the surgeon must clearly listen to the patient's complaints. He must understand and differentiate the components of axial and radicular pain. Equally, the patient must be made to understand the limits of surgical intervention.

Stabilization

The instability of spondylosis gives way eventually to the final phase of degeneration, stabilization. During the phase of stabilization three concurrent events converge within the motion segment. These are loss of motion segment height, loss of cervical lordosis, and hypertrophy of the spinal elements. It is the convergence of these three events that can give rise to the clinical entity seen during stabilization, cervical stenosis.

The osteophytosis of the spondylosis phase is a progressive attempt by the vertebral end plate to stabilize the motion segment. The osteophytosis begins with hypertrophy of the uncinate and the anterior and posterior edges of the vertebral end plate. This reactive hyperostosis can progress to a coalescence of the uncinate spur and the osteophytic lip of the posterior end plate. This coalescence is called a "spondylitis bar" (see Fig. 2-22). With further growth of the vertebral end plate comes expansion of the vertebral body. In an attempt to stabilize the motion segment, the space available for the cord (the canal) is progressively being encroached on (Fig. 2-22). In this phase, the posterior elements play a more obvious role both radiographically and clinically. The instability of spondylosis causes facet-joint cartilage destruction. Facet capsule tears will fibrose. This combination of instability, failure of the joint capsule, and end-plate hypertrophy results in facet arthrosis. The arthritic facet enlarges to stabilize itself, and periarticular fibrosis is enhanced. The enlarged and stabilized facet joint expands into the lateral recess of the canal and the foramina. This anterior (uncinate) posterior (facet) encroachment on the foramina can cause a stenotic monoradiculopathy. In this case weakness, neurogenic claudification, fatigue, and numbness are common symptoms.

Secondary changes also occur in the other posterior elements. Lamina hypertrophy and thickening of the ligamentum flavum occurs. As these two elements are positioned centrally, they decrease the space available for the cord.

As the anterior posterior diameter of the canal decreases, the anterior elements (disc and vertebral body) tend to flatten the cord. The cord, because of its ligamentous attachments to the spine will not "float" posteriorly. The concurrent hypertrophy of the central posterior elements (ligamentum, flavum, and lamina) will also act to exacerbate central cord entrapment through loss of interspace height.

One of the earliest changes to occur in spondylosis is loss of motion segment height. This tends to be progressive until stabilization. A second and more subtle event takes place later in spondylosis, loss of motion segment lordosis. The loss of height and lordosis can further decrease the space available for cord and exiting nerve roots.

With progressive loss of height, the posterior longitudinal ligament is effectively lengthened. This enhances the instability of spondylosis. A reactive spondylolytic bar forms underneath the buckled longitudinal ligament and permanently tents the cord anteriorly. This is the origin of cord flattening. With loss of height, the ligamentum flavum also buckles toward the canal. In an attempt to stabilize, the ligamentum flavum hypertrophies. The sumatation is a pincer effect on the cord (Fig. 2-23).

The loss of lordosis associated with loss of height places the motion segment into a relative position of flexion. Flexion reduces the anteroposterior diameter of the dura by 2 to 3 mm in the normal cervical spine. Further, the cord changes length (approximately 2.8 cm) from full extension to full flexion. Therefore, in extension the cord diameter is greatest. This increase in cord diameter is related to cord folding. Flexion has the effect of placing tension on

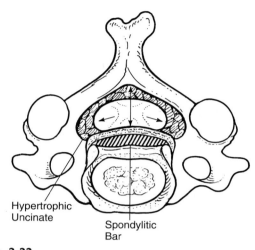

Fig. 2-22

Spondylitic phase: Hypertrophic uncinate fuses with end-plate osteophyte to form spondylitic bar. With progressive hypertrophy of spondylitic bar, cord begins to flatten because of posterior displacement by bar.

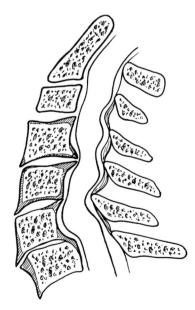

Fig. 2-23

Motion segment degeneration at multiple levels. Spondylitic bars impinge cord anteriorly. Ligamentum flavum hypertrophy and vertical settling (vertical instability) impinge cord posteriorly. Ligament failure and subluxation decrease space available for cord.

Table 2-1
Summary of cervical degenerative cascade

Phase	Symptoms	Anterior Column Pathology (Disc)	Posterior Column Pathology (Facet)
Dysfunction	Neck pain	Normal Small anular tears	Facet synovitis Muscular sprain

Discogenic	Axial cervical pain
	  Neck pain
	  Posterior occiput pain
	  Scapular/interscapular pain
	  Radiculopathy
		Anular tears
		  (internal disc disruption)
		
		Anular tear and HNP
			Capsular laxity
			Capsular tares
			Pseudosubluxation

Spondylosis	Axial cervical pain Spondylitic radiculopathy	Anular degeneration Osteophytosis Loss of disc height Loss of lordosis End-plate sclerosis Uncinate hypertrophy Spondylolytic bars	Subluxation Loss of cartilage end plate Facet osteophytosis
Stabilization	Stenotic radicular syndrome Radiculopathy syndrome Myelopathy syndrome Myeloradiculopathy syndrome Vascular syndrome Anterior stretch syndrome	Increase vertebral body diameter Decr AP canal dia. Foraminal stenosis Flattening of cord Vascular infarction of cord	Facet arthrosis Ligamentum flavum hypertrophy Posterior cord impingement

the cord. With flexion, the cord anteroposterior diameter is decreased and the cord is stretched across the anterior elements. Cord compression of the anterior and lateral columns is then worsened by the presence of a spondylolytic bar, flexion, and loss of lordosis.

The clinical syndrome of cervical spondylytic myelopathy, in the phase of stabilization, is the result of stenosis. There are five basic syndromes of cervical spondylolytic myelopathy. First, lateral cord and root compression present as nerve root symptoms. Pain, numbness, and neurologic deficit in a nerve root distribution are the hallmarks of the lateral cord or spondylotic radicular syndrome. Second, the myelopathic syndrome is characterized by numbness, gait abnormalities, and bilateral upper-extremity weakness. This is caused by the central cord compression. Third, a myeloradicular syndrome is a combination of symptoms produced by central cord and root compression. The myeloradicular syndrome is characterized by gait abnormalities, bilateral lower extremity involvement, and unilateral upper-extremity deficits.

Fourth, the vascular syndrome is the least common. As the zone of ischemia is not predictable from vascular events, so too is the clinical presentation more diffuse. That is, sensory and motor deficits are of variable patterns making level localization difficult. Fifth, the anterior syndrome presents as upper extremity weakness without pain. There is no lower extremity involvement. Ohwada et al. explain this anterior column compression by tenting of the cord over the anterior elements during flexion causing only localized anterior column pathology.

Summary

The degenerative cascade of the cervical motion segment is a spectrum. Degeneration of the cervical motion segment has been divided into four phases—dysfunction, discogenic, spondylosis, and stabilization (Table 2-1). An understanding of these phases allows the physician a clearer perspective of the cervical pain syndrome.

References

1. Aprill CN, Dwyer A, Bogduk N: Cervical zygapophyseal joint pain patterns. II. A clinical evaluation, *Spine* 15:458, 1990.
2. Breig A: *Adverse mechanical tension in the central nervous system,* New York, 1978, John Wiley & Sons.
3. Faran H, Cossette J, Robertson G, et al.: The effects of torsion in the lumbar intervertebral joint: the role of torsion in production of disc degeneration, *J Bone Joint Surg* 52A:468, 1970.
4. Ferguson RT, Caplan LR: Cervical spondylotic myelopathy, *Neurol Clin* 3:383, 1985.
5. Gertzbein S, Seligman J, Holtby R, et al.: Centrode patterns and segmental instability in degenerative disc disease, *Spine* 10:257, 1985.
6. Gore DH, Sepic SB, Gardner GM, et al.: Neck pain: a long term follow-up of 205 patients, *Spine* 12:1, 1988.
7. Gore DH, Sepic SB, Gardner GM: Roentgenographic findings of the cervical spine in asymptomatic people, *Spine* 11:521, 1986.
8. Hall MC: *Luschka's joint.* Springfield, IL, 1965, Charles C Thomas, p 1.
9. Horal J: The clinical appearance of low back disorders in the city of Gothenburg, Sweden, *Acta Orthop Scand Suppl* 118:1, 1969.
10. Hult L: Cervical, dorsal and lumbar spinal syndromes, *Acta Orthop Scand Suppl* 17:1, 1954.
11. Kelsey JL, Ostfeld AM: Demographic characteristics of persons with acute herniated lumbar intervertebral disc, *J Chronic Dis* 28:37, 1975.
12. Kirkaldy-Willis WH: *Managing low back pain,* ed 2, New York, 1988, Churchill Livingstone, p 117.
13. Kondo K, Molgaard CA, Kurland LT, Onofric BM: Protruded intervertebral cervical disc, *Minn Med* 64:751, 1981.
14. Miyamoto S, Yonenobu K, Ono K: Experimental cervical spondylosis in the mouse, *Spine* 16(suppl): 495, 1991.
15. Oda J, Tanaba H, Tsyzuki N: Intervertebral disc changes with aging of human cervical vertebra from the neonate to the eighties, *Spine* 13:1205, 1988.
16. Ohwada T, Miik, Tachibana S, Yada, K: The overstretch syndrome: a new cervical myelopathy caused by the stretch mechanism of the spinal cord, Presented at the annual meeting of the Cervical Spine Research Society, Key Biscayne, FL, November 30 to December 3, 1988.
17. Penning L: *Functional pathology of the cervical spine,* Baltimore, 1968, Williams and Wilkins.
18. Sherk HH, Parke WW: *Development anatomy. The cervical spine,* The cervical spine research society editorial committee: ed 2, Philadelphia, 1989, J.B. Lippincott, p 1.
19. Wada E, Elsara S, Saito, Ono K: Experimental spondylosis in the rabbit: Spine: overuse could accelerate the spondylosis, *Spine* 17(suppl):1, 1992.
20. Wiberg J: Cervical disc defects: results of surgical treatment of cervical vertebral radiculopathy, *Tidsskr Nor Laegeforen* 112:876, 1992.

APPLIED NEUROPHYSIOLOGY OF PAIN

Jerome A. Schofferman

In order to understand why the structural abnormalities of the degenerative cascade cause pain, the clinician needs a working knowledge of the neurophysiology of pain. Pain can be a puzzle. It is fascinating to consider why some patients with structural disorders report severe pain while others with seemingly similar structural pathology have only minimal pain and dysfunction.[2]

Pain is defined by the International Society for the Study of Pain as, "An unpleasant sensory and emotional experience associated with actual or potential tissue damage or described in terms of such damage."[6]

Definitions and Explanations of Essential Terms[6,7]

Allodynia: Pain due to a stimulus that does not normally cause pain.

Descending modulation: The inhibition or facilitation of pain due to centrally acting descending systems. The best studied is the opioid mediated analgesia system (OMAS), which acts via the action of enkephalins and β-endorphin. Serotonin and norepinephrine play roles, although each may act via different circuitry. The diffuse noxious inhibitory control (DNIC) system appears to be an OMAS system activated by environmental stimuli such as pain and perhaps stress. The DNIC is activated by noxious stimuli anywhere in the body and inhibits nociceptive transmission in the dorsal horn.[3]

Gate control: The inhibition of the response of dorsal horn cells to nociceptive input due to coincident activation of large diameter, low threshold mechanoreceptors. This modulation of nociceptive input occurs rapidly. Components of the "gate" include myelinated nerve endings of both $A\beta$ (major?, sensory) and $A\delta$ (minor, nociceptive) fibers. The $A\beta$ and/or $A\delta$ input activates interneurons to produce presynaptic enkephalinergic inhibition of primary afferent nociceptive transmission. There is also descending modulation that occurs at the dorsal horn that is primarily OMAS.[7]

Hyperalgesia: Increased response to a stimulus that is normally painful. Primary hyperalgesia: production of pain in an area of skin damage by less intense stimuli that produce pain in normal skin.

Secondary hyperalgesia: Same as above except outside the area of skin damage.

Neuropathic pain: Pain arising from nerve injury or functional abnormality of the nervous system. Pain may originate in peripheral nerves, nerve roots, and central nervous system.

Nociceptor: A receptor (nerve) preferentially sensitive to a noxious stimulus or to a stimulus that would become noxious if prolonged.

Referred Pain: Pain felt in a site remote from its origin. The "convergence-projection" theory is widely accepted. Nociceptive primary afferent fibers that innervate visceral organs enter the same spinal segment as the nociceptive somatic afferents innervating the body region to which pain from that organ is referred. The two afferents enter the same rostral projection paths, and the message that arrives in the brain could be due to stimulation at either site. Because the somatic site is activated so much more frequently than the somatic site, the brain misinterprets the message and perceives the pain at the somatic site. *Example:* leg pain referred from facet joint or anulus.[1]

Sensitization: Lowered threshold, increased sensitivity and prolonged response (afterdischarge) to repetitive stimulation observed in certain high-threshold polymodal nociceptors. Locally released chemicals thought to be involved in this mechanism include potassium, lactic and other acids, serotonin, histamine, bradykinin, and prostaglandins.[7]

Overview

Most patients seen by spine specialists have pain as the chief symptom. Pain is a complex experience that involves peripheral nociception, neuropathic problems, and the psychologic status of the individual. It is not adequate to understand only the anatomy and biomechanics of the motion segment without a working knowledge of applied pain neurophysiology as well. Armed with basic information, the clinician will be better able to understand the patient's symptoms and response to therapy and will have more satisfaction when seeing patients with complex problems.

In brief, Aδ and/or C nociceptors are stimulated by mechanical, thermal, and/or chemical stimuli (transduction).[1,3,6] These nociceptors are present in the anulus, facet, posterior longitudinal ligament, and other structures. There is afferent conduction (transmission) to the dorsal horn of the spinal cord. Here transmission is modulated (gate control system). The signal is modified (modulation) by other afferent stimuli arriving at the dorsal horn via Aβ fibers (mechanoreceptors) and/or by descending modulation primarily mediated by the endogenous opioid system. The message travels cephalad by several routes to the brain, where further modulation may occur at opiate receptors in the brain and spinal cord. Pain perception is strongly influenced as well by the unique psychologic template of each individual. The sum of the inhibitory and facilitory influences comprise the final perception, which is the experience of pain.

Primary Afferents[1]

For the purposes of this discussion, the important primary afferent nerves are the Aβ, Aδ, and C fibers.

Aβ fibers are larger, myelinated, and conduct rapidly. They are sensitive to nonnociceptive mechanical and thermal stimuli.

Aδ fibers are smaller, thinly myelinated and conduct at 4 to 30 m/sec. There are three types: (1) stimulated by nociceptive mechanical forces; (2) stimulated by both mechanical and heat; and (3) stimulated by cold. Stimulation of Aδ nociceptors is thought to be responsible for "first pain," which is often sharp in quality. Aδ fibers are blocked by compression.

C fibers are unmyelinated fibers that conduct slowly (less than 2.5 m/sec). There are three types of C fiber nociceptors: (1) responds to mechanical stimuli; (2) responds to mechanical, chemical, and heat stimuli (called "polymodal nociceptors"); and (3) responds to cold. C fibers produce "second pain," which is often dull or burning in quality. C fibers are blocked by local anesthetics.

The spinal motion segment is rich in primary afferents. There are both myelinated and unmyelinated afferents. The anulus, facet joint capsules, ligaments (posterior longitudinal ligament), and cartilaginous end plates are all innervated with primary afferents that may be sensitive to mechanical or chemical stimulation or sensitization. Undoubtedly some of these afferents are nociceptive.

Chemical Milieu[1]

There are multiple chemicals involved in pain transduction, transmission, and modulation (Table 2-2). Some are active at peripheral nerve endings, others in the dorsal root ganglion (DRG), dorsal horn, ascending pathways, descending modulating system, and/or the brain. Peripheral nerves are not merely inactive conduits. Nerves themselves liberate chemical mediators in response to damage.

Table 2-2
Chemicals involved in pain transduction

Substance	Source	Produces Pain in Humans?	Effect on Primary Afferent
Potassium	Damaged cells	+ +	Activate
Serotonin	Platelets	+ +	Activate
Bradykinin	Plasma kininogen	+ + +	Activate
Histamine	Mast cells	+ / −	Activate
Prostaglandins	Arachidonic acid from damaged cells	+ / −	Sensitize
Leukotrienes	Same as above	+ / −	Sensitize
Substance P	Primary afferent	+ / −	Sensitize

Modified from Fields H: Pain, San Francisco, 1987, McGraw-Hill.

Substance P and calcitonin gene–related peptide (CGRP) are both produced in skin afferent nociceptive terminals.

Skin damage releases potassium, bradykinin, serotonin, histamine, prostaglandins, and leukotrienes, all of which are able to sensitize nociceptors.

Endogenous opioids include enkephalins, β-endorphin, and dynorphin.

Norepinephrine is present in the spinal cord and brain.

Dorsal Root Ganglion

The DRG contains the cell bodies of primary afferent nociceptors. It is also a rich source of nociceptive chemicals. It is an active site of nociception, not a passive anatomic site. It is mechanically sensitive and is rich in chemicals active in pain transduction, transmission, and modulation.

Dorsal Horn

The dorsal horn is the first and a major site of nociceptive modulation. It is arranged in a laminar fashion into 10 layers.[5] Layers 1 (marginal layer) and 2 make up the substania gelatinosa. Layers 1, 2, and 5 are the major sites of afferent nociceptor input and the principle sites of pain modulation. The first "gating" occurs at the dorsal horn.

Wall theorizes that in many of the prolonged painful conditions the cells of the dorsal horn transform from normal into a pathologic state of allodynia manifested by increased excitability and pain transmission not only from nociceptive input but also due to stimulation from normal low-threshold afferents that would not produce pain in the normal dorsal horn.[5]

Ascending Pathways

Second order neurons project rostrally in the contralateral neospinothalamic (acute pain; sensory, spatial and qualitative aspects) and paleo(reticulo)spinothalamic (chronic pain; motivational-affective) tracts.

The spinal cord is rich in opiate receptors (μ, δ, κ) and opioid-mediated analgesia (endogenous and exogenous) occurs in part at the spinal cord level.

Brain and Descending Modulating Systems

Obviously, the brain is the final destination of afferent transmission. As discussed by Fields and Basbaum,[3] it is extremely interesting and challenging to try and explain the phenomenon that patients with apparently similar structural abnormalities perceive vastly different amounts of pain. Part of this variability is explained by the CNS network for pain control. It appears as if there are both pain-inhibitory systems and pain-facilitating systems.

Wall and Melzack proposed in 1965 that there were supraspinal influences on the "gate."[6] The discovery of stimulation-produced analgesia (SPA) strongly supported this concept.[4] SPA has been demonstrated in animals and humans. It can be induced by stimulation of the PAG and RVM. The PAG receives input afferents from the frontal cortex and hypothalamus and in turn projects neurons to the RVM. Both PAG and RVM are rich in opioid peptides and produce analgesia when stimulated.

Psychologic factors also play a role. Fields has advanced the concept of environmentally induced antinociception that subserves stress-induced analgesia.[4] On-cells, which facilitate pain transmission, and off-cells, which inhibit pain transmission, are well described and are found in the medulla. How psychologic states contribute to analgesia or increased pain is not completely clear.

References

1. Fields H: *Pain,* San Francisco, 1987, McGraw-Hill.
2. Fields HL: Sources of variability in the sensation of pain, *Pain* 33:195, 1988.
3. Fields HL, Basbaum AI: *Endogenous pain control mechanisms,* In Wall PD, Melzack R, editors: *Textbook of pain,* New York, 1989, Churchill Livingstone, p 206.
4. Morgan MM, Fields HL: Activity of nociceptive modulatory neurons in the rostral ventromedial medulla associated with volume expansion-induced antinociception, *Pain* 52:1, 1993.
5. Wall PD: *The dorsal horn.* In Wall PD, Melzack R, editors: *Textbook of pain,* New York, 1989, Churchill Livingstone, p 102.
6. Wall PD, Melzack R, editors: *Textbook of pain,* New York, 1989, Churchill Livingstone.
7. Wilson P: Anatomy and physiology of pain. Presented at the American Academy of Pain Medicine meeting, San Diego, CA, February 1993.

Chapter 3
The Socioeconomic Cascade
Arthur H. White

Low-back pain is extremely common, poorly understood, and frequently overtreated or inadequately treated. Low-back pain in workers' compensation patients carries with it an inextricable combination of employment discord, pain behavior, deconditioning, drug abuse, litigation, and miscommunication.

Back pain is having a major influence on the social structure of the United States today. Estimates of the cost to our society are as high as 50 billion dollars annually. The medical care given for low-back pain in the United States may be inefficient, redundant, and in many cases unnecessary. Even so, the cost for the medical aspects of treatment are only one third of the total cost. The other two thirds consist of socioeconomic factors that include disability payments, legal fees, lack of productivity, administrative costs, and other hidden costs to our society.

It is therefore important for physicians treating back pain to realize that when they are treating a workers' compensation back injury they must understand the socioeconomic cascade. Otherwise, they may be treating the wrong disease process with the wrong tools.

There are social forces at work. After a workers' compensation patient is out of work for over 6 months there is only a 50% likelihood of him/her returning to work. After 1 year, there is a 25% likelihood, and after 2 years, no likelihood of returning to work.[9] Although the incidence of low-back pain has remained relatively static, the increase in disability due to low-back pain has increased 14 times the rate of population growth. The direct cost has similarly increased from 10 to over 15 billion dollars. The indirect costs may be as high as 75 to 100 billion dollars annually.

There may be too much spine surgery being done in the United States today. It is well known that in the United States spine surgery for herniated discs is several times greater than in other countries, such as Sweden.

In the workers' compensation arena 10% to 25% of the patients are costing 90% of the dollars. This implies that certain patients develop bad habits, are provided inadequate care, and have multiple surgeries.

With such a common disorder (80% lifetime prevalence of low-back pain for the U.S. population); with excessive or unnecessary surgery being performed (2% of adults in the United States have surgery for a ruptured disc; approximately 5% to 10% of patients with back and leg pain require surgery); with our workers' compensation system, which does not motivate the patient to return to work; and with frequent adversarial relationships between employees and employers, there is great need for those treating low-back disorders to understand the socioeconomic cascade.

Definition

The socioeconomic cascade is a series of social, economic, and emotional steps through which a back-injured patient passes. These steps transform an otherwise minor and curable injury into a significantly disabling disease (Fig. 3-1).

Setting the Stage

The stage for the socioeconomic cascade is set when the patient is dissatisfied with his/her job and is physically or socially debilitated. The patient blames the job for causing the injury but takes no responsibility for his/her participation in the problem. Through miscommunication between the physicians, employers, insurance companies, and attorneys, the patient falls into a spiral of frustration, anger, inactivity, and further debilitation. He/she may also become depressed, and drug- or alcohol-dependent.[1]

The factors that contribute to the patient's being trapped in the socioeconomic cascade have been sci-

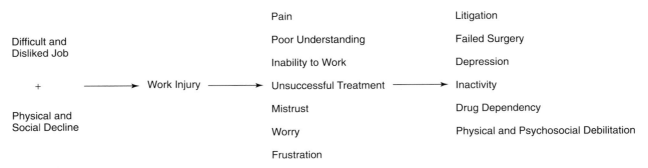

Fig. 3-1
Socioeconomic cascade.

entifically demonstrated.[2,5] The patient's physical conditioning may have declined over the past 10 to 20 years. They have gained weight, become stiff, and lost endurance and the ability to do their job physically. They may have also developed social patterns of excessive smoking and drinking, possibly drug abuse, and may have acquaintances with similarly unhealthy lifestyles. Most do not like their job.

The stage is also set by our society. In the United States, our system of workers' compensation rewards the worker when he/she is unable to perform his/her job. Few if any of the states differentiate between an injured worker who cannot do his/her job because of physical illness, and one who cannot do his/her job because of vaguely defined pain. Most workers' compensation back injuries are considered soft-tissue injuries, which are poorly defined and misunderstood. The socioeconomic cascade may quickly convert these soft-tissue injuries into socioeconomic problems. In such circumstances the patient is disabled not because of an actual physical injury but because of the complex socioeconomic interrelationships defined in this chapter. Patients are therefore receiving compensation benefits for nonstructural conditions. The patient does not understand the difference, nor does the attorney, employer, and frequently not even the physician. Many studies have verified that it is this social situation that is responsible for workers' compensation injuries taking two to four times longer to resolve, costing many times more than non-workers'-compensation injuries, and creating a multi-billion-dollar industry that is a complete waste. It is a socially created disease process created through lack of communication and education.[4,6]

The Injury

We do not know the exact etiology of low-back pain in most workers' compensation cases. Many clinicians feel that it emanates from muscles and ligaments or that it is the beginning of degenerative disc disease or degenerative facet arthritis. Ninety percent of such injuries spontaneously resolve in 4 to 6 weeks. Those that continue, however, whether for physical or psychosocial reasons, are responsible for 80% to 90% of the monetary expenditures for low-back pain in the United States today.

There are, of course, occasional significant definable back injuries in the workers' compensation arena. Spinal fractures, herniated discs, and spinal stenosis can develop secondary to work injuries, which results in significant structural disease and disability. Such conditions in the non-workers'-compensation patient are curable with normal medical means, which occasionally includes surgery. It is the socioeconomic cascade that complicates structural conditions and leads to the consternation and turmoil outlined in this chapter.[3]

Deconditioning

In addition to the injury itself, deconditioning and debilitation may also be present. Other chapters in this book define the parameters of social and physical deconditioning (see Chapter 35). Suffice it to say here that weakness, stiffness, and lack of endurance can be at a pathologic and disease level, and the patient may not have the resilience to overcome or compensate for even a minor injury. Such a deconditioning process can accelerate in the face of a new injury. A feedback process may result that leads to increased pain from the injury with increased debilitation, which in turn increases pain and psychologic problems (see Chapter 36)

The Cascade Players

The players in the socioeconomic cascade are the medical professionals, the employer, the insurance company, and the attorneys. There may be many other ancillary players, but these are the major contributors. None of these players really has the best interest of the patient at heart. They each have their own jobs to do and in general do not have a good understanding of what the others are doing. They do not realize that their ignorance or lethargy may contribute to the socioeconomic cascade.

The Medical Specialist

Some medical specialists treating workers' compensation back injuries are not well versed in the intricacies of the socioeconomic cascade. They are usually highly involved in treating fractures and other types of workers' compensation injuries. A back injury is just another musculoskeletal injury and is treated as such. This generally includes treating the acute phase with pain control, allowing the condition to heal, and sending the patient back to work. Unfortunately, with patients involved in the socioeconomic cascade, pain control does not work in the same fashion as it does with a fracture, contusion, or laceration. The pain continues despite ice, traction, electricity, or any other modality. The patient becomes disillusioned with the medical practitioner, and the medical practitioner becomes disillusioned with the patient. It is frequently assumed that the patient is malingering because he/she continues to have pain beyond what is "normally expected." There is something about soft-tissue injuries or underlying disc disease that seems to promote more long-range pain than would be anticipated in other types of musculoskeletal injuries. It is therefore not long before the patient and the medical provider develop a negative attitude toward one another. The patient either seeks other medical help or the medical provider begins to pressure the patient to return to work. If the patient finds that he/she cannot return to work, he/she begins looking for an attorney or another physician who understands his/her situation. The equally frustrated physician may prescribe medication such as muscle relaxants and narcotic analgesics, which can become habituating as well as decrease the patient's emotional reserve. Other temporizing measures such as acupuncture, traction, biofeedback, and manipulation may be used to control the patient's pain and quell his/her concerns. These measures, however, do not alter the underlying structural or socioeconomic considerations.

At times specific workers' compensation programs are prescribed. These are usually in the form of work hardening (see Chapter 32). If such programs do not take into consideration the degree of the patient's socioeconomic and emotional involvement, they will not only be a waste of time and money, but add to the patient's frustration. There are many programs that do take into consideration all the socioeconomic ramifications outlined here. These will be discussed later in this chapter. Patient treatment organizations have become a common means of properly dealing with the early phases of industrial back injuries. These will be discussed later in this chapter. Chronic phases are treated by functional restoration programs (see Chapter 32).

The Employer

Employers are understandably concerned with maintaining a successful business. Workers' compensation injuries greatly interfere with successful business. Insurance premiums rise and productivity falls when employees are away from work with injuries. Retraining, ergonomic changes, and light work are expensive additions to a business effort (see Chapter 31). We have heretofore buried our heads in the sand, transferred the responsibility of workers' compensation injuries to insurance companies, and gone about our business. Such an approach has clearly not worked. Lethargy and lack of change in the workplace has contributed to the burgeoning cost of workers' compensation injuries. However, there is still much we and the employer can do to help solve the industrial dilemma.

The Insurance Company

The cost of workers' compensation insurance has traditionally been passed on to the employer. Although some insurance companies have made attempts at developing prevention programs and reducing costs by better case management, such cost-saving activities on the part of both insurance companies and employers have been meager. For the past 20 years self-insured organizations such as Southern Pacific Railway and Safeway have been much more aggressive in controlling costs. Since the insurance industry is in the business to make money, they need to find physicians who will help them in their business efforts. This requires close communication between the physician and the insurance companies so that the business can better predict what their costs are going to be, how much to keep in reserve, and how much to invest for profit. Insurance companies do not spend their money on high-level case managers and employees with good communication skills and/or concern themselves with whether the injured worker is confused, frustrated, or having financial difficulties. In fact, many clinicians feel that insurance companies purposefully make communication and financial disability payments difficult in order to force the injured worker to go back to work or make an early settlement. This in turn increases the worker's anger, driving him/her to obtain the assistance of an attorney, increasing the communication difficulties between patient, insurance company, and physician.

The Attorney

One frequently sees advertisements on television or in the newspapers for lawyers who specialize in workers' compensation cases. Rightly or wrongly, guiding these injured patients through the legal, social, medical, and economic complexities is a lucrative business. Such administrative and legal activities account for more than half of the expense in dealing with these cases.[8] Attorneys and administrators of businesses that manage workers' compensation cases receive payment according to the size of the settlement or the length of time that the case remains open. There is, therefore, a potential benefit for some individuals to prolong the case, encouraging the worker to receive more medical care, more surgeries, and more consultations, and second and third opinions. Depositions and trials provide many hours of lucrative work for attorneys and businesses and even physicians. Some physicians make their living doing consultations on workers' compensation patients. There are "qualified" medical examiners, "independent" medical examiners, and "agreed-on" medical examiners. There are rules for the selection of each of these types of examiners and how much they get paid. Some of them have waiting lists of as long as a year. Patients can fall into the trap of disability and deconditioning while they are waiting for yet another consultation and examination.

Ultimately, cases are settled. The patient rarely receives enough compensation to offset the monetary losses. Much of the settlement goes to the attorneys and the unpaid bills of myriad care givers. The patient is either unable to obtain further work or is retrained for a job that is considerably less remunerative than the one he/she formerly held, and that led to his/her injury.

The Result

After the stage is set, the injury occurs, and the cascade players have all played their part, the loser is the patient. Although society as a whole suffers and insurance premiums rise and productivity falls, the only individual who experiences personal suffering and great financial loss is the patient. The following steps of the socioeconomic cascade occur as a part of the pathologic disease process.

1. The unmotivated, deconditioned patient has a soft-tissue injury at work.

2. Time and medical care bring neither relief to the patient nor a return to work.

3. The employer loses productivity, has to replace the injured employee and develops a suspicious and negative attitude toward the injured employee.

4. The patient becomes frustrated by inadequate medical care and lack of support at work.

5. The patient suffers financially and has either been placed on drugs or begins using alcohol excessively.

6. The insurance company and/or physician begin to lean on the patient to return to work even though the patient knows he/she cannot.

7. The patient becomes depressed, inactive, and further deconditioned.

8. The insurance company and the physician begin to withdraw from the patient.

9. The patient becomes frantic and begins searching for someone who understands his/her situation.

10. Attorneys and other physicians are consulted.

11. Breakdown of physical condition, emotional reserve, financial status, communication, and support systems leaves the patient hopelessly exhausted and disabled.

Solving the Socioeconomic Dilemma

The socioeconomic dilemma as outlined in this chapter has been recognized by some individuals, organizations, and companies.[2,4,10] As early as 1970, some self-insured companies with forward-looking medical directors realized that they had great financial losses due to low-back pain. One such organization is the Southern Pacific Railway Company. They set into effect a system that confronted many of the sources of the dilemma. In 1976 they developed educational and training programs for the employees at greatest risk. They demonstrated a 7-million-dollar reduction in cost after their prevention program had been in place for 1 year. They developed treatment programs for patients with chronic problems who had been out of work for many months or years. This included evaluations by the highest-level spine specialists they could find. They developed an inpatient multidisciplinary diagnostic and treatment program that included what is currently considered functional restoration (see Chapters 18 and 32).

Another self-insured, forward-looking organization is Safeway. They developed a prevention program for their employees at risk that included a videotape presentation on lifting and acute low-back care. They introduced early-return-to-work programs and identified and treated the patient with potentially chronic back pain before detrimental habits developed.

Currently, the greatest hope for a solution to the socioeconomic cascade is the development of managed care, management service organizations, and patient treatment organizations such as Intracorp, CCN, private health care service, and many others. Through coordinated tracking and monitoring of workers' compensation patients, these organizations are able to identify patients who are excessively costly or medically poorly managed. They select medical providers who can do the job more effectively and inexpensively.

Other organizations such as the National Back Injury Network take an even more active role in the clinical medical treatment of patients by insisting on the use of specific medical algorithms. They monitor the medical care given, the time frames for predictable results, as well as the cost for and satisfaction of the patient.

Several organizations such as the Quebec Task Force on Spinal Disorders,[7] the agency for health care policy and reform have analyzed the literature and developed guidelines for treatment of low-back pain. Algorithms of care have been developed by these organizations and have been accepted by many industrial and management organizations. Since it is well known that 10% to 25% of low-back pain cases produce 90% to 93% of the costs,[10] the algorithms of diagnosis and treatment are aimed at identifying the patients at the greatest risk and those who may incur the greatest expense. It is also well known that acute episodes of low-back pain spontaneously resolve by 6 weeks 80% to 90% of the time. Expensive intervention during the first 6 weeks is therefore discouraged in these algorithms. Close observation is encouraged so that patients who do not have spontaneous resolution of their problems can be identified before the socioeconomic cascade can occur.

A relatively well accepted standard primary care algorithm for acute cases of low-back pain is found in Fig. 3-2. For the first 6 weeks, general education and exercise is recommended, with close documentation of progressive improvement in function. Patients should be seen at least on a weekly basis with a documented report that the patients are in fact im-

proving in their activity level, decreasing their pain, and anticipating return to work by 6 weeks. Some forms of conservative care such as manipulation, medications, and other alternative care measures may be used if it can be demonstrated that they advance the date of recovery and are not unreasonably expensive.

At 6 weeks, or at any time before then, if the patient demonstrates a lack of improvement or the danger signs of becoming a chronic pain patient, he/she is referred to a secondary care program with spinal specialists who can identify and treat the more severe forms of structural pathology (see Chapters 2, 5, and 17).

The secondary care level treatment algorithm is demonstrated in Fig. 3-3. If the disability and danger signs of chronic pain are only mild, the patient may receive only education and training with good communication between employers, physicians, and insurance carriers. As the disability and danger signs increase, formalized programs may be necessary, such as work hardening or functional restoration (see

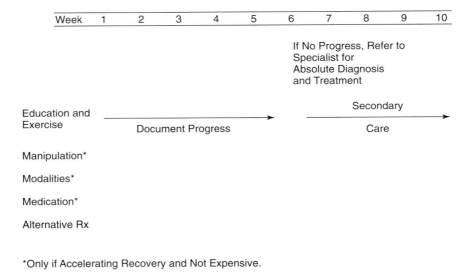

Fig. 3-2
Primary care. Nonspecific low-back pain.

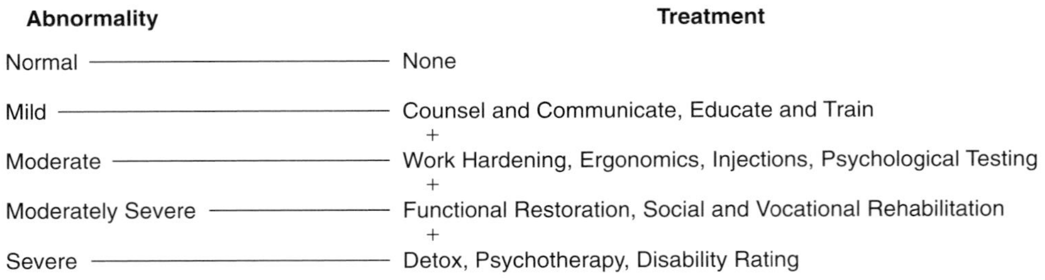

Abnormality		Treatment
Normal ———————————	None	
Mild ———————————	Counsel and Communicate, Educate and Train	
	+	
Moderate ———————————	Work Hardening, Ergonomics, Injections, Psychological Testing	
	+	
Moderately Severe ———————————	Functional Restoration, Social and Vocational Rehabilitation	
	+	
Severe ———————————	Detox, Psychotherapy, Disability Rating	

Fig. 3-3
Socioeconomic cascade. Secondary care and tertiary care.

Chapter 32). Changes in the ergonomics of the job or vocational rehabilitation may be necessary (see Chapter 31). If high level psychologic problems or drug dependencies have already developed, formal programs of detoxification and psychosocial and physical rehabilitation may be necessary (see Chapter 37). These latter more difficult cases are usually referred to a tertiary care program as demonstrated in Fig. 3-4.

With the introduction of these types of algorithms and timeframes, patient treatment organizations have been able to reduce the average lost work days per injury from 72 days as the industry average to 21 lost work days when managed well. These networks have trained hundreds of physicians and therapists in the use of these algorithms, and communication and reporting systems nationwide. More of these programs are anticipated to develop in the future and ultimately to solve the socioeconomic cascade dilemma during the first 6 weeks after injury.

In the meantime, there are many patients who have been out of work for years, have had multiple surgeries, and are deeply entrenched in the socioeconomic cascade. These kinds of cases are being identified by patient treatment organizations and referred to tertiary-care facilities where the complexities of their case can be unraveled, treated, and ultimately brought to an economic and fair closure.

The Future

We are passing through the final stages of a century-long socioeconomic spine care dilemma. Our society developed guidelines to protect the injured worker. Although well-intentioned, these guidelines did not take into consideration that low-back pain is part of a normal aging process and that individuals who are dissatisfied with their jobs are not going to be motivated to continue working with low-back pain. Self-employed farmers and businessmen have continued working with low-back pain for centuries. The structure of our workers' compensation system has allowed such individuals to cease working and still receive reasonable compensation. Our system has also allowed the medical care, legal, and labor organizational structure to confuse an otherwise simple issue of aging back pain and job dissatisfaction.

This approach to the problem is now being challenged. Private enterprise and big business have set into motion systems that are overcoming confusion and miscommunication. The medical care system is being forced to become efficient and economical in its health care delivery. The legal system is being forced out of its participation in the socioeconomic cascade. Employers are being encouraged to reconfigure the workplace and make alternative work available.

This solution to the socioeconomic cascade has occurred in many areas of the United States. It will spread throughout the country over the next 10 years and hopefully eliminate the socioeconomic cascade. This savings of tens of billions of dollars can then be applied to areas of health care, education, and training that will make us a healthier nation. The socioeconomic cascade has been an unfortunate waste of our national resources.

References

1. Cats-Baril WL, Frymoyer JW: Identifying patients at risk of becoming disabled because of low back pain, *Spine* 16:605, 1991.
2. Deyo RA, Diehl AK: Psychosocial predictors of disability in patients with low back pain, *J Rheumatol* 15:1557, 1988.

	Secondary Care					Tertiary Care								
Week	6	7	8	9	10	11	12	13	14	15	16	17	18	19	20

Secondary Care	Tertiary Care
Specific Training	Detox
Document Progress	Functional Restoration
Medication	Surgery
Injections	Disability Rating
Psychological Test and Treat	Social and Vocational Rehabilitation
Industrial Evaluate, Counsel and Communicate	Psychotherapy
Work Hardening	Pain Program

Fig. 3-4
Treatment.

3. Deyo RA, et al.: Morbidity and mortality in association with operations on the lumbar spine, *J Bone Joint Surg* 74:536, 1992.

4. Kelsey JL, White AA: Epidemiology and impact of low back pain. *Spine* 5:133, 1980.

5. McNeill TW, Sinkora G, Leavitt F: Psychologic classification of low back pain patients, *Spine* 11:955, 1986.

6. Nachemson AL: Newest knowledge on low back pain, *Clin Orthop* 279:8, 1992.

7. Quebec Task Force on Spinal Disorders: Scientific approach to assessment and management of activity-related spinal disorders: a monograph for clinicians, *Spine* 12:S1, 1987.

8. Spengler DM, et al.: Back injuries in industry: overview and cost analysis, *Spine* 11:241, 1986.

9. Waddell G: A new clinical model for the treatment of low back pain, *Spine* 12:632, 1987.

10. Webster BS, Snook SH: The cost of compensable low back pain, *J Occup Med* 32:13, 1990.

Chapter 4
The Psychologic Cascade
David J. Anderson

Despite the high prevalence of back and neck complaints in the general population, the average person pays little attention to this part of the body until back or neck pain develops. Although most people recovery quickly, some do not. Those who do not often find their entire lifestyle coming to a grinding halt. While medical care is focused on the discovery of the peripheral stimulus and its treatment, it is often true that the greatest contributions to chronic spine pain and disability are psychologic factors.[2,3,4,6-8] The scope of stressors assaulting the psychologic equilibrium of the spine-injured patient is truly vast. Spine pain can so inhibit function that it causes dramatic changes in self-image and self-esteem. These changes increase exponentially with the chronicity of illness, incomplete physical diagnosis, and inadequate treatment. Other compounding variables include the patient's fears of potential future damage, conflicting medical information, adversarial relationships with care givers, incompatible goals with the medicolegal system, family disruption, financial devastation, occupational uncertainty, loss of social context, prior psychologic problems, and chemical dependency.

Background

In the literature on the psychology of back pain many attempts are made to describe methods for predicting which individuals are at significant risk for failure to respond to conservative and/or surgical care. Most studies of the interrelationships between low-back pain and psychologic factors emphasize either behavioral aspects, compensation payments, secondary gain, or depression.[1-3,6-8,13] These approaches describe the psychologic and[10,12] behavioral results of unremitting back pain. They do not discuss the natural course of the psychologic challenges and changes (the cascade) present during the progressive illness and subsequent recovery from chronic disabling lumbar spine pain. Rather, the focus has been on the patient's personality, family structure and dynamics, work history, litigation, and other factors, with little mention of the psychologic challenges presented to the patient by this particular physical disturbance. The outcome of this approach has been a collection of data about the patient, but no increased understanding of how the patient became that way. Indeed, the approaches are like attempting to predict the outcome of a disease by laboratory tests and x-ray studies, without ever having examined the unique pathophysiology of the specific illness itself. Without such a context the data is clinically superficial.

Sources of the Cascade

Before describing the psychologic cascade that helps to power the "dis-ease" of spine pain it is essential to appreciate the unique position that the lumbar spine has in the human experience. It is the lumbosacral spine that provides the base of support for the human species' upright posture that in part makes our species unique. It is this very upright posture, and all the activity it allows, that contributes to and is threatened by the back pain.

The transition from recumbent to upright position occurs between 10 and 14 months of life. This developmental period is marked by a surge of independence and autonomy. The world is much more within the toddler's grasp than it ever was previously. Unremitting back pain threatens to recreate a state of dependence that few individuals have experienced since the time before they first stood. In addition, this preupright period was one without language. Correspondingly spine pain threatens the patient with a dependency experience that may seem beyond words and beyond verbal communication.

Even the words about the spine that are available in everyday metaphoric language are disparaging. When someone is accused of being "spineless" it is to suggest a cowardly avoidance of responsibility. People are urged to have "more backbone" when being admonished to be more decisive and more independent. We "break our backs" when we work diligently under burdensome circumstances, especially when it involves a martyred sense of duty. We "bend over backward" when inordinate and flexible generosity is required by another's insistent demands. Thus, when someone is disabled by back pain, an ominous threat of potentially humiliating, indescribable dependency that does not allow him/her to stand up for himself (have backbone), work hard (break his/her back), or have flexibility in the face of everyday demands (bend over backward). It is apparent from everyday language that the spine allows the human being far more than just upright posture.

The Cascade

By studying the processes of adjustment, assimilation, and adaptation to spine pain that patients apply with varying degrees of success, one is able to discern a recurrent pattern of affective and cognitive challenges presented to the patient with chronic disabling spine pain (Fig. 4-1). The entire cascade encompasses an inexorable loss of some aspects of the patient's preinjury identity and way of life. Just how much loss and the degree of disruption is highly variable, but the cascade spares few if any patients. Until a new way of being and doing that incorporates the injured spine is discovered and implemented, the patient remains at risk for relapse or remains stuck in one of the first phases of the cascade. If a patient circumvents the process and attempts to return to his/her former life, the recovery may be short-lived. The pain may return with greater intensity.

The large majority of patients who have an acute back injury never see the cascade. The injury is like the usual sprain, bump, bruise, or fracture: a period of acute pain followed by steady progressive resolution and return to the previous level of functioning. These individuals may have some transient anxiety that is assuaged by the autonomous and constructive healing forces of the body. For the unfortunate individuals whose injury does not follow the familiar course of recovery, a far more uncertain, disruptive, and demanding psychologic cascade follows. The cascade has three distinct phases, as discussed below.

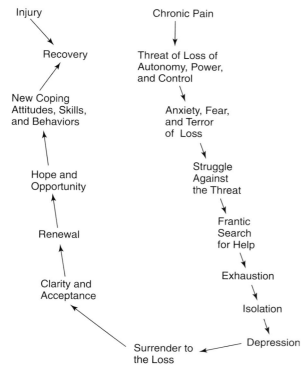

Fig. 4-1

The psychologic cascade.

Phase 1—The Threat

The first phase is the one in which clinicians find most patients. It occurs after the reality of the chronic state of torment becomes evident. The injury is not acute and self-limited, but chronic and relentless. The pain is not going to go away on its own. A battle has become a war without any evident resolution. Usual patterns of coping are not sufficient to put life into its familiar order. For the patient the phase is marked by an omnipresent feeling of threat. The patient is threatened with a state of profound helplessness and consequential loss of autonomy, control, and power by mysterious, destructive, and invisible forces well beyond his/her control. The physical condition may literally bring the patient to his/her knees. The patient's entire external material and emotional life can be under threat of dissolution by an overwhelming pain. The feelings of persecution, victimization, humiliation, and terrifying vulnerability that accompany this phase are aggravated by the absence of an accurate diagnosis. Without a name the suffering feels unauthentic. Without a name some patients fear that the pain is imaginary and could mean that they are going insane.

Anxiety, Fear, and Terror of Loss

During the first part of this phase the patient begins to feel increasingly apprehensive and anxious. Previously automatic and simple activities have become a source of increased pain leading the patient to become increasingly vigilant about the pain. To the extent that the pain is unpredictable, the apprehension grows more rapidly. Unless medical treatment is effective the anxiety increases, with a sleep disturbance emerging. The lack of restorative sleep, particularly deep delta-wave (stage 4) sleep, compounds the worn, frayed, and fatigued state of the patient.

Struggle against the Loss/ Search for Help

Patients attempt to defend themselves against the feelings of anxiety, fear, and terror of loss with a myriad of methods. Repeated attempts are made by individuals to extract themselves from this state using all the coping skills they know, but often these attempts lead only to further frustration and increased pain. Most commonly there is a denial of the seriousness of the problem (e.g., premature return to work or to vigorous recreational activities), narcotic and sedative use, and/or an insistence on surgery as a magical solution to avoid the frightening and mysterious unknown of the continued threat. Buffeted by helplessness and humiliation, the patient struggles to assert some kind of sense of individual power, competency, and real existence in a world that has become increasingly limited and restricted. The patient cajoles, intimidates, pleads, bargains, and uses various and sundry ways of including guilt in care givers so that they will somehow slay the pain monster and remove the threat of loss. The repeated request is made to take away the pain so that preinjury life can be resuscitated and the dreaded loss will not occur. This phase is riddled with feelings of rage, persecution, self-doubt, helplessness, social isolation, and embarrassment because of the loss of autonomy and function.

Exhaustion/Isolation

Physically the struggle has taken its toll with disturbed sleep, appetite, weight loss or gain, and/or loss of sexual interest and energy. The anxiety, apprehension, and sleep disturbance eventually have marked effects on the patient. The patient becomes progressively socially withdrawn as attempts to maintain previous activities are disrupted by the pain. Often substance dependency emerges as the only source of comfort for the pain and becomes an additional problem for the patient and physician. Inevitable social isolation (i.e., "No one knows the trouble I've seen!") occurs despite any and all attempts to empathize. The pain and suffering are so personal that no one can really understand. The spouse, family members, and friends may increasingly have only superficial interactions with the patient to avoid the alien and dreary world that surrounds the patient with chronic pain. In other cases, the family, through its efforts to bring comfort and understanding to the afflicted family member may become unwitting participants in an entrenched chronic pain syndrome. In this state the patient becomes a caricature of the patient with acute pain. Family members hover in attendance on the patient, ready to assist the patient at a moment's notice. Such an arrangement can become a rigid fortress against the further loss of autonomy by everyone in the family. Often even the most skillful and experienced professional attempts to intervene are thwarted.

Depression

As this phase grinds on increasing symptoms of depression emerge.[5,11] For patients with a personal or family history of depression this pain-related depression often emerges more quickly than in those who have no such history. The loss of mental, emotional, and physical energy and stamina leads to a deepening state of hopelessness, powerlessness, apathy, indifference, and despair of recovery.

For the care giver this phase can be the most taxing because of the uncertainty as to whether the patient will ever recover. The care giver can feel frustrated, angry, and quietly wishes to get rid of the patient. The patient's family is frequently in crisis at this time and it is frequently from them the panicked telephone calls are received. "Doctor, *you* must *do* something." Surgery at this time is frequently only temporarily restorative. Psychiatric evaluation can be extremely helpful at this time. The patient, the family, and the physician are disappointed, frustrated, and exasperated with the stalemate. A different perspective can be very valuable and can allow the second phase of the cascade to emerge.

Phase 2—The Pit

The second phase is usually brief relative to the first and third phases. It can last for a few moments or for up to a month. It is marked by a profound state of pervasive passivity and dependency by the patient. The patient has surrendered to the pull of forces beyond his/her control and allowed his/her previous life to collapse without hope of any return. The struggle is over, the defeat, the loss, the death of the former existence is certain. The patient will often describe the state as "hitting bottom." Sometimes the demands of surgery and the intensive physical and emotional care that the patient receives allows the patient to enter this phase.

Surrender—Giving In without Giving Up

Superficially, this phase of the cascade appears to be a profound depression or giving up by the patient. In fact it is very important to make the distinction between the states that are part of the first phase and the true giving in of the second phase.

A physical analogy can help to make the distinction. Many people have had the experience of attempting to wrestle their fingers free from a finger puzzle. This puzzle is a rube of woven straw in which one places one's index fingers into each end. The greater the effort one exerts to pull out the more the tube collapses around the finger and prevents the escape. The finger puzzle has little inherent power, only the power given to it by the force used to get out. The first phase of the cascade is when the person is trapped in the puzzle and is struggling to get out by pulling harder and harder, to no avail. When exhaustion sets in the person is depressed, and can no longer struggle. This patient has submitted to the illusionary power of the finger puzzle and has not moved into the second phase. Such an individual is only waiting for another chance for someone to conquer the pain or for surgery (i.e., cut the finger puzzle off). The patient who has moved into the second phase has surrendered (given in without giving up) and will not fight again. He/she has realized that he/she must work with the painful back and no longer regard it as a dangerous adversary. In the finger puzzle analogy the trapped person is no longer pulling to get out but has noticed the source of the puzzle's strength in his/her struggle against it.

Clarity and Acceptance

Paradoxically, from the vantage point of surrender, the patient perceives the formerly threatening circumstances with clarity, hope, and opportunity. Disordered priorities and distorted perceptions of pain and physical limitations are reexamined. During this phase it can be very valuable for the patient to discus these realizations with someone in order to affirm this new pain perspective. The pain puzzle once completely threatening has become solvable.

Phase 3—Renewal

Hope and Opportunity

At this point the third phase begins. With collapse of the old pain attitudes and the acceptance that a more gradual if not gentle solution must be tried, patients are more receptive to alternatives and begin to try them, tentatively and cautiously. Gradually a new sense of purpose and direction emerges. The pain is frequently still present but it is less of a tormenting enemy and more of a persistent reminder that new ways must be tried. The future is brighter, with some hope of a return to being functional and of value to themselves, their family, and society. Flare-ups, impatience with the tediously slow pace of recovery, vocational uncertainty, and unraveling family support all threaten the survival of the emergence of a new life.

It is at this point that clinicians frequently release the patient from care and expect that they can manage the rest of the recovery on their own. Most patients can sustain the recovery. For those who have had to become markedly different—with new work and leisure patterns—sometimes family members, rather than being enthusiastic about the recovery, are disappointed that the old person has not returned and may actually reject the new priorities and perspectives to which the patient has adapted.

Summary

For some patients, passage through the cascade has to be repeated several times. Fortunately, for most patients the subsequent passages are not nearly as grueling as the initial one, and with each experience the harsh reality that the spine is not going to be the same becomes acceptable and a new lifestyle is found. For many, the process is not necessarily noticeable to anyone but the most intimate loved ones. Nonetheless, without the acceptance of the loss and the openness to alternatives, return to the previous existence is time-limited and renewed pain often results.

Disabling lumbar pain brings to the patient and his/her family strenuous and demanding psychologic challenges. To intercede effectively the clinician must appreciate the inevitability of this cascade and work with the patient to accept the losses necessary to have a sustained recovery. Though sometimes these losses are relatively minor, for many patients the losses are as profound as a natural calamity and are resisted greatly. Thorough evaluation of the patient can often help to differentiate which patient will have the greatest difficulty assimilating and accommodating to these losses.

References

1. Burdette BH, Gale EN: Pain as a learned response: a review of behavioral factors in chronic pain, *J Am Dent Assoc* 116:881, 1988.
2. Dvorak J, Valach L, Fuhrimann P, Heim E: The outcome of surgery for lumbar disc herniation: a 4-17 years' follow-up with emphasis on psychosocial aspects, *Spine* 13:1423, 1988.
3. Dzioba RB, Doxey NC: A prospective investigation into the orthopaedic and psychologic predictors of outcome of first lumbar surgery following industrial injury, *Spine* 9:614, 1984.
4. Feuerstein M, Dobkin P: Biobehavioral assessment of chronic pain, *Pain Manage*, July/August:152, 1988.
5. France RD, Skott A, Krishnan K, et al.: Subtypes of depression in patients with chronic pain, *South Med J* 81:485, 1988.
6. Frymoyer JW, Cats-Baril W: Predictors of low back pain disability, *Clin Orthop Relat Res* 221:89, 1987.
7. Frymoyer JW, Pope MH, Clements JH, et al.: Risk factors in low-back pain, *Joint Surg* 65:213, 1983.
8. Frymoyer JW, Rosen JC, Clements J, Pope MH: Psychologic factors in low-back pain disability, *Clin Orthop Relat Res* 195:178, 1985.
9. Hendler N: Depression caused by chronic pain, *J Clin Psychiatry* 45:30, 1984.

10. Hurme M, Alaranta H: Factors predicting the result for surgery for lumbar intervertebral disc herniation, *Spine* 12:933, 1987.

11. Krishnan K, France RD, Houpt JL: Chronic low back pain and depression, *Psychosomatics* 26:299, 1985.

12. Polatin PB, Kinney RG, Gatchel RJ, et al.: Psychiatric illness and chronic low-back pain: the mind and the spine—which goes first? *Spine* 18:66-71, 1993.

13. Ressor KA, Craig KD: Medically incongruent chronic back pain: physical limitations, suffering and ineffective coping, *Pain* 32:35, 1988.

Chapter 5

Diagnostic Decision Making
Jerome A. Schofferman

Acute Anulus Tear

Painful Degenerative Disc Disease

Herniated Nucleus Pulposus

Internal Disc Disruption

Facet Syndrome

Spinal Stenosis

Instability/Spondylolisthesis

Nonspecific Low Back Pain

  sprain/strain
  psychologic factors
  deconditioning syndrome
  medical causes of low back pain
  seronegative spondyloarthropathies

It is extremely valuable to consider spinal disorders in terms of the structural degenerative cascade because a meaningful clinical correlation exists between the structural changes of the spine and clinical signs and symptoms. The diagnoses listed in the box below are the most common lumbar spine problems we see in practice and should be familiar to all spine clinicians. The conditions are not mutually exclusive. Often, patients suffer from more than one diagnosis, and it is incumbent upon the clinician to determine which structural problems are clinically meaningful and which are innocent bystanders. Structural changes occur along a continuum, and many nonstructural variables can determine when a structural derangement becomes symptomatic.

Differential Diagnosis of Low Back Pain

- Anulus tear
- Painful degenerative disc
- Herniated disc
- Internal disc disruption
- Facet syndrome
- Spinal stenosis Central Intervertebral

- Spondylolisthesis
- Instability
- Spondyloarthropathies
- Psychological illness with LBP
- Medical illness causing LBP
- Deconditioning syndrome
- Nonspecific LBP/strain/sprain

Acute Anulus Tear

Acute anulus tear is, in my opinion, the most common cause of acute low back pain (LBP). Acute LBP is often called muscle strain or sprain or myofascial LBP. A definitive diagnosis is not usually possible at this stage, although definitive diagnosis is not very important if the patient recovers quickly. However, the distinction may be useful when considering secondary prevention, particularly with respect to motivating or educating the patient, and in light of the high incidence of the recurrence of LBP. Furthermore, if the pain does not improve in a few weeks, it is a disadvantage to call the condition a chronic sprain or strain.

The mechanism of injury for an anulus tear is usually flexion with or without torsion, often under loading conditions. The patient may state the pain began when he or she was bending over to lift. Some

patients say they felt or heard a "pop." Lower back pain that often radiates to one or both gluteal regions is present. Pain may be quite severe at first, but generally eases over a few days. Pain is increased by bending forward, sitting, or twisting. Standing may or may not be painful, and walking is often preferred. Although there is no nerve root compression there may be pain referred to one or both legs. Patients may complain of leg weakness, which is probably due to pain inhibition, or numbness despite no sensory loss on examination.

Physical examination is nonspecific. Muscle spasm may be visible or palpable, and a list or shift may be present. Range-of-motion (ROM) testing may show restriction, especially in flexion. Press-ups may ease LBP and centralize leg pain. There is no neurologic loss, even in patients who complain of numbness or weakness. Straight leg raise (SLR) may be limited owing to hamstring tightness or LBP, but there is no true sciatica.

Treatment for acute anulus tear is nonspecific. Ice is helpful. Press-ups may relieve pain although occasionally they worsen the pain. Patients are instructed to do 10 slow press-ups every few hours and to apply ice afterwards. Bed rest may provide symptom relief but should be limited to 2 or 3 days, since longer periods do not change long-term outcome and may lead to abnormal pain behavior and deconditioning.[10]

Many patients respond to nonsteroidal antiinflammatory drugs (NSAIDs). Relief may be due either to their analgesic effect, antiinflammatory effect, or both. If the patient is not responding to NSAIDs, oral or epidural corticosteroids are very useful. One empiric regimen I find useful and simple is prednisone, 10-mg tablets in divided doses, 4 per day for 4 days, 3 per day for 3 days, 2 per day for 2 days, and then 1 per day for 1 day—a total of 30 pills over 10 days. Therapeutic epidural injections may be extremely useful and are discussed in Chapter 22. Rarely, a short course of low-potency opioids may be necessary.

It is generally recommended that the patient be referred for physical therapy (PT) as soon as possible. However, it must be recognized that no data prove the efficacy of any early intervention with regard to long-term outcome. In fact, a recent randomized, controlled study comparing exercise provided by a physical therapist, to placebo PT (low-energy ultrasound), to no treatment except analgesics and support by a general practitioner found no difference between groups in terms of duration of pain, recurrences, or return to work.[11] Initially, PT may consist of modalities for control of pain and muscle spasm. Patients may respond to shift correction and press-ups using McKenzie techniques. An active exercise and body-mechanics training program should be started as soon as possible after the onset of pain. Early PT anecdotally appears to lead to more rapid resolution of pain and the early initiation of restoration of function, and also serves as an entry point into the back-care system to begin a secondary prevention program to decrease the chances of reinjury.

The natural history of acute LBP is reasonably well known.[11,38] Most patients feel much better by 2 weeks. However, it may take up to 12 weeks for complete resolution of symptoms. Unfortunately, recurrences are common.[38] At 1-year follow-up of new-onset LBP patients, 69% report LBP in the previous month.[38] It is not necessary to obtain plain x-ray films, MRI, or CT scan before 6 to 8 weeks unless there are unusual aspects to the problem.

Painful Degenerative Disc Disease

The prevalence of symptomatic degenerative disc disease (DDD) is unknown. In MRI studies of asymptomatic people, the prevalence of disc degeneration is increased with age, but degenerated discs may or may not be painful.[2]

Perhaps 10% of patients do not recover from an episode of LBP. Recurrence is frequent. It may be that anulus injuries do not heal adequately and evolve into painful degenerated discs. The usual mechanism of DDD is thought to be chronic, recurrent, or cumulative trauma. Each micro or macro trauma may or may not have produced symptoms.

The disc becomes dessicated. Narrowing of the intervertebral disc space usually occurs. Presumably, noxious inflammatory chemicals are produced. Nociceptors in the outer anulus or dorsal-root ganglion are stimulated and produce pain.

Clinically, patients complain of chronic LBP often punctuated by acute exacerbations. Pain is often referred to one or both gluteal regions. Nonspecific leg pain may be present as well. Pain is aggravated by activities that load the disc, such as sitting, prolonged standing, bending, or lifting, or with activities such as mowing a lawn or vacuuming.

Physical examination is nonspecific. Posture is usually normal, but in advanced cases there may be loss of lumbar lordosis. Motor loss, sensory loss, or reflex changes do not occur unless the process has advanced to produce spinal stenosis. The straight leg raise and/or the prone knee bend may cause LBP or leg pain owing to muscle tightness.

X-ray studies are not usually necessary at the onset of treatment but are valuable if the patient is not responding. Narrowing of one or more disc spaces, osteophyte formation and, when advanced, degenerative spondylolisthesis or scoliosis may be present.

Treatment requires a functional restoration approach and consists of muscle strengthening and training in body mechanics. Most patients with painful DDD have weak trunk extensor muscles and weak upper and lower abdominal muscles, all of which must be strengthened. Specific techniques are discussed in Chapters 25 and 35.[32] Theoretically, these techniques can "offload" the spine and place some of the burden on the musculature, thereby improving symptoms. Anecdotally, a rigid orthosis may help. In severe disabling cases in which all conservative measures have failed, fusion may be considered, although efficacy data are lacking.

Herniated Nucleus Pulposus

Herniated nucleus pulposus (HNP) is the condition best known and understood by clinicians and the lay public alike. It may be less well appreciated that HNP can produce a wide array of symptoms and signs, depending on the acuity, size, and location of the herniation. It has been established that in addition to nerve-root compression, pain from HNP can arise from stimulation of nociceptors in the anulus or posterior longitudinal ligament.

The mechanism for the causes of disc herniation is similar to that of an anulus tear. The patient usually suffers a flexion-type biomechanical injury with or without load (lifting) and often with some degree of torsion. Again, patients may recall hearing or feeling a "pop." Pain may occur immediately, or the onset of pain may be delayed. In many patients pain develops insidiously. In fact, more than half of patients with HNP do not identify a specific precipitant. Many patients who develop HNP have had several prior episodes of LBP.

Most patients with HNP have some degree of LBP, though it may be mild. Lower back pain may be central or unilateral, often with referral to one or both gluteal regions. Leg pain is common and may be the result of nerve root compression or nerve root irritation, or may be referred from the disc itself. If the HNP is midline, LBP is more likely to dominate the clinical picture. If the HNP is paracentral and causes nerve root entrapment, leg pain is more likely to predominate. Very large herniations can cause functional or dynamic spinal stenosis and/or cauda equina syndrome.

The LBP of HNP can result from mechanical or chemical stimulation of the nociceptors in the wall of the anulus, the posterior longitudinal ligament, or the dura.[25] Patients state that pain is increased by sitting or bending forward. Standing often increases pain, but walking often relieves it. The response of the leg pain of HNP depends on whether it is referred pain or the result of nerve root compression. Referred leg pain usually follows a parallel course to the LBP. The more the back pain increases with certain activities, the more leg pain produced. When leg pain is due to direct compression, it is usually increased by flexion or prolonged sitting or standing, and is frequently increased by walking, particularly uphill.

Physical examination is variable. In the acute situation muscle spasm is usually visible or palpable, and a list may be present. Range of motion is quite restricted in flexion and moderately restricted in extension. Palpation is not specific. Neurologic examination again depends on the location and size if the HNP. If there is nerve root compression, there may be motor loss, dermatomal sensory loss, and possibly loss of or decreased reflexes. The SLR may be positive—producing true sciatica—but in central HNP the SLR is often negative.

If HNP is suspected but there is no motor loss, diagnostic studies may be deferred for several weeks. If the patient is improving rapidly, studies may not be necessary. If the patient has motor loss or is not responding to treatment after 6 to 8 weeks, MRI or CT scan is indicated to define the problem accurately.

Treatment depends on the clinical picture. The only urgent situation is acute cauda equina syndrome, which requires surgery. Other presentations are not emergent. If frank motor loss is present, the patient must be followed carefully; however, surgery may not be necessary if recovery occurs over the following several weeks.[40]

Many treatment alternatives are available. Unfortunately, most have not been evaluated in randomized, controlled studies. Bed rest has been tested for nonspecific LBP but not for sciatica.[8] It appears reasonable to offer 2 to 3 days of bed rest for HNP with severe pain. Longer periods do not affect overall outcome. Ice also reduces pain in many patients.

Medications can be useful. Nonsteroidal antiinflammatory drugs in high doses have been shown to be useful for symptom reduction but do not alter the long-term course.[14] Oral steroids may be used if the response to NSAIDs is poor. There is controversy regarding epidural corticosteroid use[14] (see Chapter 22). If the patient is in severe pain and is basically house- or bed-bound, an epidural injection of corticosteroid is frequently effective in decreasing pain and allowing the patient to begin PT. In a prospective descriptive study with no control group, epidural and/or selective nerve-root injection was shown to be helpful in patients with sciatica owing to HNP of over 4 months duration who had failed to respond to other conservative care.[4] Physical therapy is useful as both primary treatment and secondary prevention. Modalities may be appropriate for pain relief for 1 to 2 weeks but do not alter outcome. An aggressive dynamic lumbar stabilization program must be instituted.

Most patients improve considerably over 6 to 12 weeks.[12,40] They can gradually be progressed into more active PT and returned to full activities. Patients who fail to improve after 6 to 12 weeks may require more aggressive intervention. If the patient has significantly more leg pain than LBP, the patient may be a candidate for a minimally invasive procedure. These include arthroscopic microdiscectomy (AMD), automated percutaneous discectomy (APD),[30] or chymopapain chemonucleolysis.[16] In other instances open surgery may be indicated.

The natural history of HNP is well demonstrated in the classic study published by Weber in 1983.[40] In a randomized, prospective study he compared operative to nonoperative treatment of patients with documented HNP who failed to respond to conservative care while in the hospital (Table 5-1). However, it is not always appreciated that in the Weber

Table 5-1

Outcome of LBP and radiculopathy at 4 and 10 years with conservative care and operative care

	4 Years		10 Years	
	Conservative	Operative	Conservative	Operative
LOW BACK PAIN				
No pain	26/66	35/60	37/66	42/60
Some pain	17/66	15/60	12/66	8/60
Considerable pain	6/66	6/60	0	0
RADICULOPATHY				
No pain	31/66	43/60	48/66	53/60
Some pain	13/66	8/60	1/66	1/60
Considerable pain	5/66	5/60	0	0

study two groups of patients were not randomized. The first was patients with severe pain, sudden onset, or progressive motor weakness, or those with bowel or bladder paresis. The second was patients with moderate symptoms who were improving with bed rest, PT, and medication. In addition, 17 of the 66 patients in the original conservative care group required surgery.

Nonetheless, valuable insight about the natural history of HNP can be inferred from Weber's study. It is clear that at 1 year the surgical group did better. At 4 years the surgical group did better, but the results were not statistically significant. There was little difference between groups at 10 years. In both operative- and nonoperative-care groups about two thirds of the patients were doing good or fair. The table summarizes the Weber results with respect to LBP and to radiculopathy.

Frymoyer has offered the following conclusions regarding the Weber study: Patients who have an unequivocal diagnosis of HNP with sciatica and fulfill AAOS criteria for surgery are best treated operatively.[13] These patients *can* be treated conservatively, but at least 25% will require surgery within the first year. Patients treated conservatively will not fare as well as those operated upon for at least the first year. In addition, it appears that at 4 years a trend is present suggesting that the surgical patients do better.

In our clinic, we attempt to treat all patients initially with aggressive conservative care, which includes stabilization training often supplemented with spinal injections or oral medications. Patients are followed closely. A decision to operate is not made before approximately 8 weeks in the usual situation. If the patient has radiculopathy far in excess of LBP, MRI shows HNP with nerve root compression and no significant intervertebral canal stenosis, and psychologic factors are minimal, we will often use AMD as our initial treatment. Open surgical discectomy is performed if the patient does not meet criteria for AMD or fails to benefit from AMD.

Internal Disc Disruption

Internal disc disruption (IDD) may be one of the most frustrating spinal conditions to treat.[6] The diagnosis is controversial. There is disagreement whether IDD actually exists, and where, or even if, it fits on a continuum from normal disc to clearly degenerated disc. Because nonspecific LBP is so common there are the dangers of overdiagnosis of IDD and overtreatment, especially surgical. Most spine specialists would define IDD as a painful disc

in the presence of normal MRI, CT scan, myelogram, and plain x-ray studies. The diagnosis is made by provocative discography during which severe concordant pain is produced at low volumes of injection. The morphology is abnormal and shows anular tears. It has not been established whether it is best to call the condition IDD or painful DDD if MRI reveals only degeneration. The natural history has not been studied but it appears that patients have long and frustrating illnesses.

Internal disc disruption is seen most often in younger women. Patients often describe an acute injury of a lumbar flexion type, often with associated lifting. A fall with axial loading of the spine is commonly reported. Internal disc disruption may occur after a motor vehicle accident.

Patients complain of LBP and may report nonspecific referred leg pain as well. Sitting intolerance is the most common problem. Walking is limited in some patients but others find walking to be their best activity. Patients become depressed and anxious as time goes by without a diagnosis. Some clinicians have implied that psychologic changes are part of the condition. Often, patients have seen several physicians before a diagnosis is made. They have received multiple diagnoses and some have been labeled as having a somatoform pain disorder.

Physical examination is nonspecific. Patients show some limitation in forward bending. Spasm is not usually present. There are no neurologic changes. When IDD is suspected, palpation of the lumbar spine through the abdomen may produce concordant LBP.

Aggressive conservative care is very important. Pain relief is variable, however, and IDD does not respond as well as HNP or other common forms of back pain. However, many patients can achieve significant functional improvement despite ongoing pain, although high levels of strength and dynamic body mechanic skills are necessary.

Several retrospective surveys have implied that interbody fusion can be helpful in 75% of classic cases, although no prospective controlled data are available.[1,15,27] Most physicians have used anterior interbody fusion with or without posterior-lateral fusion. However, posterior-lumbar interbody fusion can also be successful.[37] Great caution should be exercised not to operate on patients in whom the diagnosis is atypical or equivocal. Many of these patients have coexisting psychologic problems. It is imperative to ensure that the psychologic issues are not the driving force for the pain and disability before surgery is considered.

Facet Syndrome

Controversy exists regarding whether facet syndrome is a distinct clinical entity and whether facet joint injections are useful for diagnosis or treatment.[5,19,26,35] The issue is discussed in detail in Chapter 21. Recent data estimates that facet joint pain is the primary problem in 15-20% of patients with nonspecific LBP. There is no meaningful correlation between the radiologic appearance of the joints and whether or not they are painful.

Clinically, it has been thought that the typical history of facet syndrome was that of nonspecific LBP that radiated into one or both gluteal regions. Proximal leg pain is often present as well. Pain is aggravated by prolonged standing and often increases during transitions from lying to sitting or sitting to standing. On physical examination pain is increased by extension in the standing or prone position. Pain is even further increased by extension in standing with rotation. Neurologic examination is normal.

However, it has recently been stated that there is no typical history for the diagnosis of facet syndrome except that midline LBP alone is unusual.[7] Likewise, there are no typical physical findings.[7] The diagnosis is made by injection with installation of local anesthetic either into the facet joint itself, with concordant pain and then relief of pain, or around the medial branch of the dorsal ramus of the spinal nerve, with significant pain relief.[19,24,26]

Treatment once again is aggressive lumbar training to teach the patient to unload the facet joints during all activities. Patients who fail to improve with PT may obtain short-term relief with facet joint injections. If repeated facet joint injections provide short-term relief, diagnostic medial branch blocks may be considered. If a patient obtains relief with medial branch blocks, medial branch rhizotomy using cryotherapy or radiofrequency needle techniques can be successful in 55% of patients.[35]

Spinal Stenosis

Stenosis can affect the central canals, the intervertebral canals, or both.[22,29] The classic history is that of long-standing mild to moderate LBP that may be constant or intermittent (consistent with DDD), which progresses to pain in one or both legs that is produced by walking and relieved by rest (neurogenic claudication). The LBP may or may not still be present. Many clinicians believe spinal stenosis can cause LBP as well as leg pain, but this issue is controversial. Typically, there is minimal or no pain while sitting or lying. Other patients complain that their leg(s) feel dead, asleep, or heavy and may have paresthesias, dysesthesias, or weakness, all of which typically worsen with walking. When the patient stops walking, pain gradually diminishes, although more slowly than is so with arterial claudication. The distribution of pain depends on the nerve root(s) involved. Many patients have the positive "shopping cart symptom." In the supermarket they do fine while walking the aisles leaning on the cart but experience increased pain while standing in the checkout line.

With advanced central stenosis, physical examination frequently shows loss of the lumbar lordosis. Flexion in standing is normal or slightly reduced. Extension in both prone and standing positions is markedly reduced. The knee-to-chest position is usually comfortable. Straight leg raise is usually limited only by hamstring tightness. Prone knee bend is positive if L3 nerve root involvement is present. Hip examination may be abnormal if there is concomitant degenerative hip disease. The occurrence of motor, reflex, and sensation deficits depends on the degree of nerve root or cauda equina involvement.

Radiologic examination is diagnostic. In an elderly patient in whom spinal stenosis is suspected, multiplanar CT scan yields the best diagnostic information, although high quality MRI will make the diagnosis as well. Some clinicians prefer a CT scan enhanced by intrathecal contrast. We use diagnostic nerve root injection to try to confirm that stenosis visualized on a scan is causing the pain. If pain is relieved, and especially if there is a prolonged steroid effect, the diagnosis is confirmed.

Treatment varies according to the particular patient. The physician must take into consideration age, concomitant medical conditions, and degree of pain and disability. In some patients the stenosis stabilizes and the patient can learn to adapt.[29] In some elderly patients epidural corticosteroid injections provide excellent relief. If this relief is sustained for months, it is reasonable to treat these patients with three or four epidural corticosteroid injections per year. In some elderly patients with a predominance of leg pain and for whom surgery is a considerable risk, percutaneous spinal cord stimulation has been effective.[36] Some patients are able to learn to maintain their spine in enough flexion bias during daily activity to improve their symptoms greatly. Others may benefit from a rigid lumbar orthosis. If the lowest motion segment is involved, a leg extension is preferred, but is poorly tolerated. In patients who do not respond to conservative measures, surgery is necessary.[21,22,29] About two thirds of patients obtain good relief that appears to be sustained.

Instability/Spondylolisthesis

There is no question that spondylolisthesis can be a painful clinical entity, but there is no consensus regarding what structure(s) cause the pain.[41] Pain may arise from the disc at the level of the slip (shearing effect?), the level above or below, secondary spinal stenosis, facet joint(s), or possibly a spondylolytic defect itself. Pain from any of these structural defects can be provoked or exacerbated by the instability that is present. The diagnosis of spondylolisthesis is readily made by conventional radiological techniques.

Clinically, spondylolisthesis manifests quite differently in the young than in the elderly patient, and in fact they are quite different clinical problems. In the young patient with spondylolisthesis the pain may originate from the bone defect itself. In these cases, simple fusion has a high degree of success. In the adult with spondylolisthesis, the source of pain is most commonly spinal stenosis or a degenerated disc. The instability increases the dynamic component of the stenosis and shearing forces may increase the stimulation of intradiscal nociceptors.

The term *instability* is used in many different ways, and this has led to confusion. Many textbooks and papers consider segmental instability to be a synonym for DDD or spondylosis. However, true mechanical instability is a term best reserved to refer to abnormal translation of a motion segment with flexion versus extension or side bending. Plain x-ray studies or CT scan may show gas in the disc space (vacuum phenomenon), which in the absence of infection implies instability.

Nonspecific Low Back Pain

Sprain/Strain

Perhaps the most common diagnoses made in patients with LBP are low back sprain or low back strain. These are nonspecific diagnoses that may be appropriate for patients who develop LBP after minor trauma and who recover in a few days to 2 weeks. Physical examination reveals muscle tenderness and/or spasm with restricted range of motion. The neurologic examination is normal. It is inappropriate to continue to use these diagnoses if pain continues beyond several weeks and other diagnoses should be considered. There are no data to show that a syndrome of chronic strain or sprain exists.

If the cause of LBP is not known, it is more reasonable to use the term *nonspecific LBP*, which implies that a definitive diagnosis has not been reached.

The evaluation may be in progress. If a structural diagnosis cannot be made by MRI, CT scan, plain x-ray studies, or other testing, the diagnosis of nonspecific LBP may be best. However, in most instances structural disease will be discovered. It is necessary that the examiner be confident that structural disease found is in fact the source of the pain.

Psychologic Factors

The interrelationship between psychologic factors and pain is well known. There are instances when psychologic processes or illness antedate the spinal disorder and other instances when the spine pain leads to secondary psychologic problems.[31] Some degree of psychologic issues exists in every patient with spine pain, but the degree to which these issues affect the pain and disability vary greatly. In the acute setting a patient may experience anxiety about the injury, the pain, or the future. In the chronic setting, psychologic factors may be the major obstacle to recovery. We believe that in *most* cases, *severely disabling* LBP is a psychologic problem that usually has some structural component, rather than a structural problem that happens to have a psychologic component.

The vocabulary regarding the psychologic aspects of chronic pain is still evolving. Although it is clear that most patients who complain of pain of spinal origin have some nociceptive input, it is equally clear that there is a group of patients whose pain and level of disability appear far out of proportion to the structural pathology and out of proportion to other patients with similar structural lesions. It is in this group that psychologic factors may be dominant.

Psychologic illness may predate the spinal problem.[29] The pain may be a component of the psychologic illness, or may exacerbate it. The *DSM-III-R* describes a group of illnesses lumped under the category of "somatoform pain disorder." These include somatization disorder, conversion disorder, somatoform pain disorder, and hypochondriasis. In each, the symptoms suggest some physical disorder but the evaluation fails to disclose a physical problem of sufficient magnitude to account for the symptoms. There must be evidence of a psychologic illness, not merely a diagnosis of psychologic illness by exclusion.

Substance abuse disorder is common in patients with chronic pain. In most instances the substance abuse disorder was present before the pain or injury, but in others it occurs as a consequence.[29] Persons who abuse alcohol or other psychoactive substances, including opioid analgesics or sedative hypnotics, are predisposed to injury by virtue of intoxication. In addition, addictive patients may relapse if exposed to psychoactive drugs.

Some patients have a psychologic predisposition toward chronic pain. They have been referred to as "pain-prone."[10,33,34] Often, these patients have suffered severe psychologic trauma during childhood that predisposes them to develop chronic pain after injury. We have identified five childhood risk factors, and have found the prevalence of three or more risk factors to be very high in patients who failed to respond to back surgery and in patients with chronic refractory spine pain. The childhood developmental risk factors are physical abuse, sexual abuse, abandonment, neglect, and having chemically dependent parent(s).

Many patients with chronic pain suffer from depression. In some instances the depression is the cause of the pain, or at least drives the pain so that it is greatly exacerbated. However, more often the unremitting pain causes a secondary or reactive depression. Some patients suffer from dysthymia, a disorder in which the patient suffers from depressed mood almost continuously for 2 or more years. Dysthymia differs from major depression in that it is less severe and of greater duration.

Another *DSM-III-R* category pertinent to pain is called "psychological factors affecting physical condition." In this illness, psychologically meaningful stimuli initiate or exacerbate the physical disorder. There must be a demonstrable structural disorder present for this psychologic diagnosis to be made.

Still another psychologic illness is post-traumatic stress disorder. Patients suffering with this disorder have recurrent dreams, intrusive thoughts, and nightmares, in addition to the chronic pain syndrome. Some patients suffer from an adjustment disorder with either depressed or anxious mood. This form of psychologic disorder occurs within 3 months of an identifiable stress that is followed by symptoms of depression or anxiety out of proportion to that which is expected from the stress. Again, this psychologic disorder may augment pain and disability.

Another form of psychologically driven pain disorder is so-called "secondary gain." In behavioral psychology it is well known that certain behaviors can be encouraged and others extinguished by the positive or negative rewards for the behavior. It is less clear that pain can be enhanced or reduced in a similar manner.

Pain can provide an unconscious excuse for avoiding unpleasant parts of life, such as a hated job, an unpleasant boss, undesired travel, and so on. Pain can also serve to provide things missing in life, such as attention from a spouse, respect from friends or relatives, and an enhanced social life, even if it is only visits to the bed or chairside by friends or visits to the doctor's office. These secondary gains can provide powerful reinforcement to abnormal pain behavior and possibly to pain itself. There are also financial secondary gains, such as disability payments.

Psychologically driven pain is not a diagnosis of exclusion but is a diagnosis that has well-defined characteristics that must be met. However, there are signs on physical examination for which there is no biomechanical or structural explanation that might suggest that psychologic factors are playing a part. These include ratchet-like movements during ROM testing or during manual muscle testing, straight leg raising of only 10 or 15 degrees, frequent grimaces or crying out during the examination, and bizarre gait patterns, among others. Waddell et al. have described five signs, the presence of three or more of which may suggest psychologic elaboration[39]

Some patients are malingering, although this is not common. The prevalence of schizophrenia, delusional disorder, or bipolar disorder does not appear to be increased in patients with psychologic LBP.

Deconditioning Syndrome

Many patients with pain of spinal origin become less active, thereby losing strength in their muscles through disuse. Abdominal muscles, lumbar and cervicothoracic paraspinal muscles, and quadriceps muscle appear most susceptible. These are the very muscles that are most important for supporting the trunk during activity. In addition, many patients suffer significant loss of aerobic capacity.

Inflamed structures hurt. An anulus tear or a facet joint with arthritis and inflammation can be compared to an abrasion. If a person repeatedly irritates and reinflames the lesion, inflammation continues, healing cannot occur, and pain continues. Good muscle strength allows the patient to use the spine in an anatomically correct manner and thereby stop stressing the torn anulus or inflamed facet joint to allow the inflamed abrasion to heal.

Overused muscles hurt and are often tender. When a patient attempts to compensate for structural damage or attempts to maintain good posture, he or she must depend on musculature for compensation. The muscles must work harder and for longer periods and are often stressed beyond their capacity. Blood flow is decreased by the chronic contraction and venous outflow is decreased as well. Lactate and other waste products accumulate. When the muscles are strengthened by a spine-safe exercise program they are able to work harder and sustain contraction longer with less pain.

Weak muscles cannot protect the spine. A spine with structural pathology may be likened to an aluminum pipe with a dent. If the pipe is stressed and restressed, the dent will crack and the pipe will leak. It is difficult to fix a thin pipe, and so the best repair is external reinforcement. Tape is wrapped around the pipe. This analogy applies to the spine. The muscles are the tape. Strong muscles that can function through a dynamic range can minimize the stimulation of nociceptors in the structurally abnormal segment and thereby decrease pain. Further details are described elsewhere in this text.

Tight muscles may hurt. Lack of flexibility makes it difficult for a person to practice good spinal body mechanics. Muscles may remain tight because they are overworked in relationship to their strength, or understretched muscles may feel tight in response to repeated or continuous overcontraction.

Medical Causes of Low Back Pain

It has been estimated that in 10% of patients back pain is a symptom of a systemic disease.[3] In our experience this is a very high estimate, but it does serve as an alert to the practitioner to consider medical problems as a cause of LBP. Most often medical causes of LBP occur in the elderly population. Except for compression fractures of osteopenia or cancer, medical causes of LBP do not usually have a traumatic onset. As opposed to mechanical causes of LBP, in which a comfortable position can usually be discovered, patients with medical LBP may not have a position of comfort.

Patients with fever may have infection or malignancy. There may be discitis, osteomyelitis, or soft tissue abscess. A history of infection elsewhere in the body (particularly the urinary tract), alcoholism, intravenous drug use, recent surgery, or recent invasive procedure of the spine or elsewhere may suggest infection of the vertebrae or disc space. Most patients with spinal infection are somewhat anemic and have an elevated sedimentation rate, C-reactive protein, and/or white blood cell count, but there are many exceptions. Malignancy is the most feared cause of spinal pain. Metastatic disease to the spine must be suspected in any patient with a past history of malignancy, no matter how remote. Some of these patients have pain that at first may resemble nonspecific back pain. It increases with activity and diminishes with rest. However, often the pain increases and becomes constant, no longer changing dramatically with activity level.

Compression fractures may cause localized severe pain. Compression fractures can be seen in any disease that causes osteopenia. Malignancy can cause compression fracture. Occasionally, hemoglobinopathy can weaken bone matrix sufficient to cause fracture after minimal trauma.

There are many potential visceral causes for LBP, although they are not common in our experience. Infiltrative, inflammatory, infections, and obstructive problems can occur to viscera in the chest, abdomen, pelvis, or retroperitoneum. Most often the visceral nature of the symptoms is obvious, particularly with syndromes of colicky pain.

Pain in the region of the thoracic spine can be the result of aortic dissection or angina pectoris. Pancreatic cancer can occasionally present as LBP. Back pain can arise from diseases of the prostate, pelvis, kidney, pancreas, colon, duodenum, and blood vessels. Low back pain owing to obstruction of a ureter, duct of the gallbladder, or bowel should be clear from the history and the appearance of the patient.

Seronegative Spondyloarthropathies

Seronegative spondyloarthropathies are always considered when young patients present with LBP. However, the prevalence of these conditions in a pain clinic is actually low.[31] Spondyloarthropathies take many forms. Ankylosing spondylitis, psoriatic arthritis, and sacroiliitis associated with inflammatory bowel disease are the rheumatic diseases that might present with back pain, but this presentation is not common. Reiter's syndrome and Behçet's syndrome rarely can present with LBP.

The prevalence of ankylosing spondylitis is estimated at 197 cases per 100,000 men and 73 cases per 100,000 women. The illness usually presents between the ages of 18 and 25, with a range of 15 to 40 years. It rarely begins earlier or later in life. Onset is insidious. Low back pain or gluteal pain is the initial presenting symptom in 65% of patients. Typically, the pain increases with rest and improves with activity. Pain and stiffness are most pronounced in the morning or after periods of inactivity. Fatigue may be present.

Physical examination varies with disease severity. There may be sacroiliac tenderness, but this is totally nonspecific. Sacroiliac maneuvers may be positive. In advanced cases there may be limitation of lumbar range of motion, decreased thoracic chest-wall expansion, or thoracic kyphosis. Other joints may be involved, particularly the hips and shoulders, with pain and decreased range of motion. Peripheral joint involvement with true synovitis occurs in 40% of patients. Heel pain occurs in 10%. Eye involvement occurs in 25% of patients at some time in the course of illness, and cardiac involvement with aortic insufficiency or conduction delays may be seen in 5% to 10% of patients at some time in the illness.

Laboratory findings include an elevated sedimentation rate in 90% of patients and the presence of HLA-B27 antigen in more than 85% of patients with ankylosing spondylitis, 50% of patients with seronegative spondyloarthropathy associated with inflammatory bowel disease, and 50% of patients with sacroiliitis of psoriasis. A mild normocytic normochromic anemia or mild thrombocytosis may be present.

Radiographic features become more common and more severe as the disease progresses. Changes of the sacroiliac joints are the earliest to occur, and if plain x-ray studies are not revealing, MRI or CT scan may reveal characteristic changes. In the spine squaring of the anterior aspect of the vertebral bodies and loss of the usual concavity will be noted. Syndesmophytes are common later in the process, and osteoporosis may occur.

References

1. Blumenthal SL and others: The role of anterior lumbar fusion for internal disc disruption, *Spine* 5:566-569, 1988.
2. Boden SD and others: Abnormal magnetic resonance scans of the lumbar spine in asymptomatic subjects, *J Bone Joint Surg (Am)* 72:403-408, 1990.
3. Borenstein D: Approach to the diagnosis and management of medical low back pain. *Semin Spine Surg* 2:80-85, 1990.
4. Bush D and others: The natural history of sciatica associated with disc pathology, *Spine* 17:1205-1212, 1992.
5. Carette S and others: A controlled trial of corticosteroid injections into facet joints for chronic low back pain, *N Engl J Med* 325:1002-1007, 1991.
6. Crock H: A reappraisal of intervertebral disc lesions, *Med J Aust* 1:983-989, 1970.
7. Derby R: Personal communication.
8. Deyo RA, Diehl AK, Rosenthal M: How many days of bed rest for acute low back pain?, *N Engl J Med* 315:1064-1070, 1986.
9. Dworkin RH, Caligor E: Psychiatric diagnosis and chronic pain: *DSM-III-R* and beyond, *J Pain Symptom Manage* 3:87-97, 1988.
10. Engel G: Psychogenic pain and the pain prone patient, *Am J Med* 54:899-918, 1959.
11. Fass A and others: A randomized, placebo controlled trial of exercise therapy in patients with acute low back pain. Presented at the 20th annual meeting of the International Society for the Study of the Lumbar Spine, Marseilles, France, June 15-19, 1993.
12. Fraser RD: Chymopapain for the treatment of intervertebral disc herniation: a preliminary report of a double blind study, *Spine* 7:608-612, 1982.
13. Frymoyer JW: Back pain and sciatica, *N Engl J Med* 318:291-300, 1988.
14. Frymoyer JW: *Surgical indications for lumbar disc herniation.* In Weinstein JN, editor *Clinical efficacy and outcome in the diagnosis and treatment of low back pain,* New York, 1992, Raven Press, pp 117-124.
15. Gill K, Blumenthal SL: Functional results after anterior lumbar fusion at L5-S1 in patients with normal and abnormal MRI scans, *Spine* 17:940-942, 1992.
16. Gogan WJ, Fraser RD: Chymopapain: a 10 year, double blind study, *Spine* 17:388-394, 1992.
17. Grobler LJ and others: Etiology of spondylolisthesis: assessment of the role played by lumbar facet joint morphology, *Spine* 18:80-90, 1993.
18. Haglund MM, Schumacher JM, Loeser JD: Spinal stenosis: an annotated bibliography, *Pain* 35:1-37, 1988.
19. Helbig T, Lee CK: The lumbar facet syndrome, *Spine* 13:61-64, 1988.
20. Hochberg MC: Ankylosing spondylitis, *Semin Spine Surg* 2:86-94, 1990.
21. Johnsson KE, Uden A, Rosen I: The effect of decompression on the natural course of spinal stenosis: a comparison of surgically treated and untreated patients, *Spine* 16:615-619, 1991.
22. Lee CK, Rausschning W, Glenn W: Lateral lumbar spinal canal stenosis: classification, pathologic anatomy and surgical decompression, *Spine* 13:313-320, 1988.
23. Liang MH, Fortin PR: *Efficacy of nonoperative care for low back pain.* In Weinstein JN, editor: *Clinical efficacy and outcome in the diagnosis and treatment of low back pain,* New York, 1992, Raven Press, pp 47-56.
24. Marks R: Distribution of pain provoked from lumbar facet joints and related structures during diagnostic spinal infiltration, *Pain* 39:37-40, 1989.
25. Mooney V: Where is the pain coming from?, *Spine* 12:754-759, 1987.
26. Moran R, O'Connell D, Walsh MG: The diagnostic value of facet joint injections, *Spine* 13:1407-1410, 1988.
27. Newman MH, Grinstead GL: Anterior lumbar interbody fusion for internal disc disruption, *Spine* 17:831-837, 1992.
28. O'Connor M, Glynn CJ: Prevalence of HLA-B27 in patients with back pain attending a pain clinic, *Pain* 44:147-149, 1991.
29. Onel D, Sari H, Donmez C: Lumbar spinal stenosis: clinical/radiologic therapeutic evaluation in 145 patients, *Spine* 18:291-298, 1993.
30. Onik G and others: Automated percutaneous discectomy: a prospective multi-institutional study, *Neurosurgery* 26:228-232, 1990.
31. Polatin PB and others: Psychiatric illness and chronic low-back pain: the mind and the spine—which goes first?, *Spine* 18:66-71, 1993.
32. Robison R: The new back school prescription: stabilization training Part I, *State Art Rev Occup Med* 7:17-32, 1992.

33. Schofferman J and others: Childhood psychological trauma correlates with unsuccessful lumbar spine surgery, *Spine* 17S:S138-S144, 1992.

34. Schofferman J and others: Childhood psychological trauma and chronic low back pain, *North American Spine Society,* Boston, 1992, submitted for publication (abstract).

35. Silvers HR. Lumbar percutaneous facet rhizotomy, *Spine* 15:36-40, 1990.

36. Szabo C: Unpublished observation.

37. Vessa P, Lee C: Internal disc derangements: the results of surgical treatment by disc excision and posterior lumbar interbody fusion (PLIF), *North American Spine Society,* Boston, 1992 (abstract).

38. Von Kroff M and others: Back pain in primary care: outcomes at 1 year, *Spine* 18:855-862, 1993.

39. Waddell G and others: Nonorganic physical signs in low-back pain, *Spine* 5:117-125, 1980.

40. Weber H: Lumbar disc herniation: a controlled, prospective study with ten years of observation, *Spine* 8:131-140, 1983.

41. Weinstein JN, Rydevik. The pain of spondylolisthesis. *Semin Spine Surg* 1:100-105, 1989.

Chapter 6
Lumbar Spine Disorders: Taking and Interpreting the History

Jerome A. Schofferman

The history may be the most important part of the evaluation of the patient with pain of spinal origin. Taking a history is both an art and a science. Often attributed to Osler, it is still true today that "It is more important to know about the patient who has the disease than it is to know about the disease the patient has."

The science of taking the history is to obtain the necessary information to make a structural diagnosis.[9,11,35] Much of this information can be gained from any text on the spine.[9] However, the art of taking the history is to obtain sufficient information to establish a working structural diagnosis and gain some insight into any psychologic or socioeconomic factors that may be present, while at the same time establishing rapport and instilling confidence.[39,43] While taking the history, the examiner will get a feeling about the patient that might suggest how best to plan further diagnosis and therapy. Some patients need long explanations. Others just want to do what the doctor recommends. It is important during this history-taking period to get a feel about how to proceed.

Taking the history actually begins the treatment process and serves many important functions, including

- Establishing a differential diagnosis for the structural disorder
- Guiding the focus and interpretation of the physical examination
- Establishing rapport with the patient
- Developing a psychologic profile
- Developing a socioeconomic profile
- Planning further diagnostic investigations
- Initiating treatment
- Assessing progress and outcome

Interpreting the history to make a diagnosis requires a knowledge of the three major cascades: the degenerative structural cascade and its clinical correlations, the psychological cascade, and the socioeconomic cascade. Armed with the knowledge of what can go wrong structurally, psychologically, and socioeconomically, the clinician can gain invaluable information by beginning with an open-ended, unstructured history and finishing with structured, directive questions to fill in the gaps. When appropriate, the verbal history may be supplemented with questionnaires and pain drawings.

An open-ended history will provide much more information than a directed interview.[39] The clinician may begin by asking such questions as "tell me about your problem" (not "tell me about your pain"). Open-ended inquiry allows the patient the opportunity to discuss problems in the order of importance to the patient. What the patient says may not be as important as the way he or she says it. The tone and direction of the discussion may disclose contributing psychologic and socioeconomic issues. The open-ended format will provide most of the information required, but directed questions will be necessary to complete the data base. During the interview, part of the physical examination may be performed by observing the patient's posture, pain behavior, and movement.

Most clinicians are familiar and comfortable with taking a history. However, merely accumulating data is not enough. The clinician must know how to interpret the information as well. The goal of this chapter is to provide the questions necessary for gathering information as well as clues for interpretation. The format of this chapter assumes the reader is familiar with the information contained elsewhere in this text (see Chapter 5). At the conclusion of the history, the clinician should be able to arrive at a realistic differential diagnosis, which in turn will lead to planning testing and treatment in a cost- and time-efficient manner.

Obtaining a thorough history does not end after the initial visit. The history continues to evolve and may even change over the course of subsequent visits as symptoms and issues become clarified. The history will often be supplemented with information obtained from family members, other physicians, medical records, claims adjusters, and other interested parties.

Most patients seen in spine centers present with a complaint of pain. However, others complain of weakness, numbness, paresthesias, loss of some function, and even changes in bowel, bladder, or sexual ability.[13,20] If such symptoms are present, the clinician must not presume that the patient has only a spine problem. Diagnoses such as multiple sclerosis, amyotrophic lateral sclerosis, and cancer must be considered while taking the history.

Location of Pain

Each patient must be viewed as a whole, with each painful region addressed. However, in patients with back *and* leg pain, it is best to obtain a separate description of each pain. Determining the percentage of back pain versus the percentage of leg pain is important. Much of the information about the long-term outcome of disc herniation relates to changes in sciatic symptoms rather than back pain. Data regarding the long-term outcome of low-back pain (LBP) for most spinal disorders is much less clear. Generally, patients who have a predominance of leg pain secondary to herniated nucleus pulposus (HNP) may be candidates for minimally invasive procedures such as arthroscopic microdiscectomy, automated percutaneous nucleotomy, or microscopic discectomy, while patients who have more LBP than leg pain are not.

Patients with degenerative lumbar scoliosis who have mostly leg pain may have foraminal stenosis as the major pain-producing lesion despite multiple degenerative discs. In refractory spine problems, spinal cord stimulation may be an option for leg pain but not for LBP. Conversely, patients with painful degenerative disc disease (DDD) or HNP who have mostly LBP might require fusion for successful surgical outcome.

Pain in the abdomen or pelvis is occasionally due to lumbar spine disorders and may sometimes be part of the symptom complex of internal disc disruption (IDD). However, abdominal pain can be referred to the lower quadrants from a thoracolumbar disc herniation and to either upper quadrant from a low thoracic disc herniation.

In most instances, spinal pain syndromes are referred distally, not proximally, from their site of origin. Perhaps the most common site of pain referral from the lumbar spine is the area of the posterior iliac crest or the midgluteal area in the sacroiliac region. Often, patients with pain in this area have been diagnosed as having sacroiliac joint problems; that the pain is referred may be overlooked. Discs or facet joints as cephalad as L1 can refer pain to the sacroiliac area.

Most spine clinicians supplement the verbal history regarding the location of pain with a drawing or diagram. Pain drawings have many uses: establishing a baseline reference image, following changes in pain distribution over time and in response to treatment, establishing a differential diagnosis, quantifying pain, and perhaps gaining some psychological insight about the patient.[6,16,24,42]

In 1976 Ransford and associates proposed that the pain drawing could be a useful screening tool for psychologic abnormalities in patients with LBP.[30] They showed a significant correlation between an abnormal drawing and elevations of subscales Hys and D of the Minnesota Multiphasic Personality Inventory (MMPI). Some authors have reported similar findings, but others have not been able to demonstrate these correlations.[16,42] Some patients with strikingly abnormal nonanatomic drawings have definite structural pathology and no psychologic problems, while other patients with drawings that look very anatomic have no significant structural abnormalities but do have marked psychologic problems. The pain drawing cannot currently be recommended as a screening tool for psychologic distress because of the high false-positive and false-negative results.[16,42]

Margolis and associates found a high correlation between the amount of body surface area (BSA) included in a pain drawing and high penalty point scores described by Ransford and associates.[24,30] They proposed a technique to quantify the total BSA indicated in a pain drawing. It may be that patients who show a very high surface area of pain are suffering from higher degrees of psychologic distress.[1,24] Although this hypothesis is not widely accepted, their technique may find value in following individual patients over time.

Pain in the low back can be secondary to many structural causes. The exact location of the back pain is probably not very useful diagnostically. Low-back pain "flows downhill." Therefore, the source of LBP can be almost any single or multiple structures cephalad to the location of the pain.

Much can be learned from the nuances of leg pain. Pain in the leg may be true radicular pain, which implies nerve root compression, or it may be referred leg pain, which is nonspecific.[26] In turn, referred leg pain can arise from the disc anulus, ligaments, the facet joint, or other structures. Surprisingly, even sensations of numbness or tingling do not reliably differentiate radicular from referred symptoms. Numbness, weakness, and cramps can also be referred. Referred leg pain without nerve root compromise has been shown to occur in 56% of patients with LBP of 2 or more years' duration.[26] Referred numbness occurs in 50%, cramps in 22%, sharp pains in 15%, and subjective weakness in 10% of patients with LBP.[26]

Leg pain can also be secondary to arterial disease, peripheral neuropathy, joint disease, bone disease, or even herpes zoster. Pain that occurs in a "stocking" distribution suggests peripheral neuropathy. It is the purpose of the history to attempt to sort out these problems.

Obtain an accurate picture of the distribution of leg pain. Ask the patient to show where the pain is and what route it takes. Pain confined to one dermatome is usually radicular. Nonspecific pain, circumferential pain, or pain in multiple dermatomes tends to be referred pain. The location of the dermatome may provide information regarding the location of the lesion, and provides clues to which extraspinal sources of pain may be involved. L3 pain involves the groin and anteromedial thigh. However, pain in this distribution may indicate hip disease as either the sole cause or a coexisting cause of pain. L4 pain involves the anterior thigh and medial calf and may extend to the medial aspect of the foot. L5 pain involves the lateral thigh, lateral and possibly medial calf, and the great toe. S1 nerve involvement is felt in the posterior thigh, posterior calf, and lateral aspect of the foot and heel.

Quantification of Pain

It is necessary to quantify each patient's pain: it is the only way to determine whether a patient is improving. Quantifying pain means to measure change in an individual patient's pain over time—not to compare one patient's pain to another.

Pain is of course, a totally subjective experience, but there are well established ways to quantify it. Different scales for patients with chronic pain have a high degree of correlation, and the choice of how to quantify the pain will depend on the patient population, the clinical setting, and the needs of the clinician.[18,20,31] Measuring instruments include the McGill Pain Questionnaire (MPQ), visual analog scale (VAS), verbal analog scale, verbal or written descriptive scale, 101-point numerical rating scale (NRS-101), 10-point numerical rating scale (NRS-10), 11-point box scale, among others. More-sophisticated scales may be necessary for research, while simpler scales will suffice for following an individual patient over time. The clinician should become familiar with one or two rating scales.[41]

The visual analog scale is commonly used to quantify pain.[18,19,28,31,41] The patient is presented with a 10-cm uncalibrated line that is anchored with phrases such as "no pain" at one end and "worst pain imaginable" at the other. The patient is asked to place a mark at a place on the line that best represents his or her degree of pain. The distance between the "no pain" anchor and the patient's mark is measured, and represents the pain intensity.

A verbal numerical scale (VNS) is also useful. The patient is asked to rate verbally the pain from 0 to 10. The VNS has been compared with the VAS. The correlation is excellent, although the VNS showed a slight tendency to rate pain higher.[28] The verbal numerical scale is linear and reproducible, correlates well with the VAS, and is readily accepted by patients. It is easy to use in both the ambulatory and the postoperative setting because it does not require patient coordination and has no visual or motor components.

The use of an ordinal analog scale, also called the 11-point numerical rating scale (NRS-11,) is another popular technique. The patient is asked by questionnaire to rate his or her pain from 0 to 10, where 0 represents "no pain" and 10 is the "worst pain imaginable." The patient writes the number on the questionnaire. Obviously, no scoring is necessary. The number chosen is recorded in the medical record. The NRS-11 is easy for the patient to use and understand and appears reliable and reproducible.[28] The NRS-101 is similar except the patient is asked to choose a number from 0 to 100.[18,19]

Descriptive scales offer the patient options such as "absent, mild, moderate, severe, and agonizing," and the patient is asked to choose the word or phrase that best describes the pain. These scales may be slightly less sensitive than numerical scales.[18,19] They can be quantified by assigning a numerical score to each descriptive item. However, correlation is excellent between a 10-item verbal descriptor scale and the VAS.[7] Interestingly, when the VAS was compared with a 10-item verbal descriptor scale for the affective component pain, differences were noted at the higher extremes of experimental pain intensity.[7] It is not possible to state which scale more accurately reflects the meaning of pain to the patient.

At Memorial Sloan–Kettering Cancer Center clinicians have successfully used a VAS for both the sensory and the affective component of pain in the cancer setting.[10] They compared VAS scales for pain intensity, mood, and pain relief with standard measures, including the McGill Pain Questionnaire (MPQ) and the Zung Anxiety Scale, and found excellent correlation.

The MPQ has been used extensively to quantify pain and is generally considered to be the gold standard against which other pain-measurement instruments are measured.[27,31] Seventy-eight adjectives that describe various aspects of the pain experience are arranged into 20 subclasses, within which each word is assigned a rank value score. The word in each category signifying the least pain has a value of 1, the next word has a value of 2, and so on. The Pain Rating Index (PRI) is the total point value of all the words chosen.

The test can be scored in many different ways depending on the needs of the clinician. For most clinical and research situations, the PRI that gives the total score is most valuable and represents the global pain intensity.[27,31] The MPQ also produces scores for four dimensions of the pain experience. These are the sensory (temporal, spatial, punctate pressure, incisive pressure, constrictive pressure, traction pressure, thermal, brightness, dullness)—(items 1 to 10); affective (tension, autonomic, fear, punishment)—(items 11 to 15); evaluative (intensity)—(item 16); and miscellaneous(items 17 to 20). The affective subscore of the MPQ may be a measure of pain-related emotional distress independent of the intensity or quality of the pain. However, there may not be adequate discriminant validity in separating out the 4 dimensions of the MPQ PRI.[33]

The MPQ is easily self-administered by the patient in 4 to 5 minutes and takes less than 1 minute to score by hand. It is reliable, valid, and very sensitive to changes over time with treatment.

The North American Spine Society (NASS) has chosen to use a verbal descriptor item checklist that allows quantification of the sensory component of the pain. The NASS has elected to score axial pain separately from extremity pain. The choice was made because the method is easy for patients to use, reliable, reproducible, and easily scored. (See the two questionnaires that appear at the end of this chapter.)

Quality of Pain

The quality of the leg pain is often useful diagnostically. Pain described as burning suggests a neurologic source. Legs described as dead may suggest central spinal stenosis. Paresthesias, dysesthesias, and lancinating pains are often neurogenic. Numbness may be particularly interesting. Many patients describe numbness in an extremity. However, when tested, sensation is normal. This type of numbness is commonly a referred sensation. Allodynia is a sensation of pain from a stimulus that is not usually painful. Examples include pain induced by light touch, even from a sheet.

Biomechanics of Pain

It is useful to determine the effects of different postures, movements, and activities on LBP and leg pain as a means of diagnosing their source. Most mechanical sources of spinal pain are effected by changes in position or posture and are altered perhaps in different ways by different movements. Intradiscal pressures vary according to position, which of course has an important effect on discogenic sources of pain.[29] Sitting increases lumbar flexion, which may widen the intraspinal canal, which also effects pain, particularly of stenotic origin. If pain is not influenced mechanically a medical or psychologic cause might be suspected. This is particularly true if the patient states that pain is not decreased by rest.

The effect of sitting on a patient's pain is useful in arriving at a working diagnosis. Sitting increases intradiscal pressure, unloads facet joints, and reverses the lumbar lordosis, thereby widening the central or intervertebral canals. Accordingly, sitting intolerance is seen in pain of discogenic origin but sitting relieves the pain of spinal stenosis. Sitting can be expected to worsen the pain of anulus tear, HNP, IDD, and painful DDD. Prolonged sitting will worsen the pain of instability as well. Pain of facet origin may be unchanged. Pain of spinal stenosis is usually improved.

Many patients make the transition from sitting to standing with poor body mechanics. Most people bend forward at the waist, which increases pain of discogenic sources, facet sources, and instability, but does not change other pains in a distinctive–enough fashion to be diagnostic. Standing increases intradiscal pressure less than sitting does, and also may cause some degree of extension.[29] Therefore, standing will initially lessen the pain of discogenic source but prolonged standing eventually increases pain. Static standing usually increases the pain of spinal stenosis, instability, facet syndrome, and spondyloarthropathy.

The effect walking has on LBP and leg pain is important and may be complemented by learning the different effects of walking on a level surface versus uphill versus downhill. Walking produces less intradiscal pressure than standing.[29] However, some people walk flexed, which increases intradiscal pressure while opening the intervertebral and central spinal canals. Therefore, walking may initially improve the LBP of HNP, anulus tear, IDD, and probably facet syndrome. However, long walks will result in increased LBP in almost all spinal conditions. Walking will often produce claudication leg pain in spinal stenosis. Walking uphill (which causes lumbar flexion and increased intradiscal pressure) may not cause leg pain in stenosis but will worsen leg pain in HNP, anular disease, or instability. Some patients with spinal stenosis relate that they can walk longer if leaning on a shopping cart, which puts them in lumbar flexion. Walking downhill causes lumbar extension and therefore may worsen facet pain spinal stenosis, or instability. It may relieve pain of HNP.

Lying supine lowers intradiscal pressure.[29] Pain from most causes decreases. However, in some patients lying supine decreases lumbar lordosis and increases LBP of discogenic origin. In others, lying supine increases lordosis and increases the pain of spinal stenosis. Lying prone usually worsens pain of spinal stenosis and may worsen pain of facet origin, instability, or larger disc herniations.

The effects of usual activities of daily living may help suggest the diagnosis. Leaning forward at the sink to brush teeth or hair or to wash dishes may increase pain of discogenic source or instability, while lifting a leg on a stool may provide relief of discogenic pain. The effect on pain of shopping in the supermarket provides useful information. Patients, particularly the elderly, may report that they feel OK while walking the aisles leaning on the cart but feel a marked increase in pain while standing still in the checkout line. Many of these patients have spinal stenosis.

Onset of Pain

Some patients are able to report a specific event or trauma that started the spine problem. Others cannot be precise or report a gradual onset and progression of the spine pain. In fact, in one study 70% of patients were unable to identify a specific injury to account for the onset of their pain.[9]

In patients with sudden onset of pain, details of the event may allow the practitioner to develop a picture of the biomechanics of the injury and thereby shed light upon the etiology of the pain. Ask the patient to describe the injury. Was the patient bent over at the waist, lifting? Bent lifting is likely to put high pressures on the posterior anulus and cause an anular tear or disc herniation. Adding rotation further increases the likelihood of anular pathology and may also cause facet injury. The typical history of the patient who bends over to take a box out of a car trunk and has the sudden onset of LBP almost certainly has torn an anulus with or without frank herniation. The gymnast who has the onset of LBP after doing a series of back bends may have injured a facet joint.

Patients who are injured in motor vehicle accidents (MVA) are sitting in slight flexion when impact occurs. The most likely structures to be injured are the disc and facet joints. Internal disc disruption may result. If the passenger is turned to look at the driver, torsional stress is increased, making the anulus and facets even more susceptible to injury.

Patients who fall from even a low height and land directly on their buttocks may injure a disc and IDD can occur. Coccyx pain after such a fall may arise from the sacrococcygeal joint trauma but is more likely to be referred from other structures.

A history of recurrent episodes of LBP that resolve, subsequently followed by an episode that persists, strongly suggests one or more painful degenerative discs. Patients who describe constant LBP or multiple episodes of LBP who then develop the new onset of true radicular leg pain are likely to have spinal stenosis of either the central or intervertebral canal or disc herniation.

Review of Systems

There are many reasons to obtain a good review of symptoms (ROS). The ROS may reveal potential medical causes of the spinal pain.[3] It will yield information regarding the patient's general health, which may be necessary to design a treatment program. Medical illnesses may interfere with treatment. A patient with poor cardiovascular or pulmonary function may have to go very slowly in physical therapy, and concomitant cardiac rehabilitation may be needed. One might defer epidural or systemic steroids in a patient with diabetes.

It is useful to begin the ROS with a general inquiry about the patient's own perception of his or her state of health. Ask about any known medical problems and the current treatments.

All patients should be asked if they have fever associated with LBP. The presence of fever may suggest a serious underlying cause such as osteomyelitis, cancer, pyelonephritis, and even bacterial endocarditis.[3,14]

Some of the diseases that may include LBP are ulcerative colitis, psoriasis, and ankylosing spondylitis, all of which can be associated with sacroiliitis.[17] Ankylosing spondylitis can cause cervical and lumbar pain, ankylosis, and deformity. Advanced rheumatoid arthritis can affect the cervical spine.

Degenerative arthritis of this hips or knees may induce gait changes that can increase the pain of lumbar DDD. A patient with known osteoporosis is especially susceptible to compression fracture as a cause of pain. Ask patients whether they have had a change in height and whether or not they feel "humped over." The sudden onset of LBP in an elderly patient after minimal trauma, such as stepping hard off of a curb or lifting a package, might suggest compression fracture.

Infection is an uncommon cause of primary LBP.[38] Again, fever is a hallmark. Spinal infection can be seen after urinary tract infection, especially if the urinary tract has undergone instrumentation. Infection may follow discography, intraspinal or perispinal injections, or surgery. Epidural abscess can occur. Inquire about a history of infection elsewhere in the body and any treatment for that infection. Ask about fever, chills, unexplained weight loss, or low energy and severe fatigue as clues to the presence of infection. If infection is suspected, be sure to ask directly about a history of intravenous drug use, and look for track marks on the arms.

Cancer is the cause of LBP dreaded most by both clinicians and patients. In most cases in which cancer is the cause of LBP, it is metastatic and the patient is known to have or have had a primary malignancy elsewhere. Carcinomas of the breast, lung, and prostate often metastasize to the spine. Multiple myeloma may present with spinal pain. Asking about unexplained weight loss, unexplained fevers, and a feeling about general quality of health will usually provide clues that something is wrong besides a mechanical cause of pain.

Patients with a history of dyspepsia or documented ulcer can develop LBP.[32] Duodenal ulcer may penetrate into the retroperitoneum and cause LBP. Pain is usually more severe than that seen in patients with musculoskeletal causes of LBP, and the patient may be writhing in acute pain. In addition, a history of ulcer may contraindicate the use of non-steroidal antiinflammatory drugs (NSAIDs).

The presence of associated symptoms may help delineate the cause of the pain and suggest diagnostic and treatment alternatives. If the patient states that one leg or foot often feels colder than the other, or that the leg or foot turns blue or dusky, this may suggest a sympathetically maintained neuropathic pain or an arterial cause of the leg pain. These symptoms might suggest that a sympathetic block, intravenous phentolamine test, or arterial studies be performed, depending on the findings of the examination.

A history of alcohol overuse suggests many diagnostic alternatives. Alcohol use may predispose patients to injury from falls, MVA, or workplace injuries. Alcohol is a risk factor for osteoporosis, which in turn can lead to compression fracture after an otherwise minimal trauma, again more likely in one who is alcohol-impaired. Alcoholics have lowered immunity, poor wound healing, and are less likely to follow therapy instructions. Alcohol may cause pancreatitis.

Ask the patient if he or she drinks alcohol for pain relief. If the clinician wishes to gain further information about a possible diagnosis of alcoholism, it is very quick and easy to give the four-question CAGE questionnaire.[8] CAGE is an eponym for the first letter of the key word of each question (see box). A positive response to two or more questions strongly correlates with a diagnosis of alcoholism.

CAGE Questionnaire[8]

> - Have you ever felt you ought to **C**ut down on your drinking?
> - Have you ever felt **A**nnoyed if someone comments on your drinking?
> - Have you ever felt bad or **G**uilty about your drinking?
> - Have you ever had an "**E**ye opener" first thing in the morning to steady your nerves or to get rid of a hangover?

Cigarette smoking predisposes the patient to multiple sources of spinal pain. Cigarette smokers have a small but statistically significant increased occurrence of disc degeneration.[2] Smoking also is a risk factor for osteoporosis and its inherent problems of fracture and pain. Obviously, smokers are at higher risk for cancer of the lung and other organs. Smokers can develop atherosclerosis, coronary artery disease, or peripheral arterial disease, any of which can cause pain that can mimic the pain arising from the lumbar spine.

A sexual history should be obtained. Erectile difficulties occur in a larger-than-expected number of patients with LBP.[14] Rarely are these problems neurologic. In fact, erectile difficulties may be secondary to pain, psychologic issues, alcohol overuse, or medications.

Psychologic Aspects Of Pain

It is essential to gain some degree of psychologic insight about the patient in the initial interview since it is so well-established that psychologic issues are critical to recovery from painful disorders of the spine. Some patients are reluctant to discuss psychologic issues initially. Our society is culturally biased against psychologic problems versus structural ones. Insurers also are less inclined to reimburse for psychologic treatment than for structural treatment. However, psychologic issues are very important in spinal problems and in many studies are the only things that predict outcome.[15,40]

It is best to begin psychologic inquiry with some open-ended questions such as "How is your mood?" or "How is your pain affecting you?" The very fact that the clinician is inquiring suggests to the patient that he or she is interested, and gives the patient the impression that it is important to discuss these issues. Other patients respond to an inquiry about "stress." Almost all patients can recognize the role stress plays in their pain.

Ask the patient about sleep. Does the patient have difficulty falling asleep? Does the patient wake frequently? After a night's sleep does the patient feel restored? Many patients with chronic pain have sleep disturbance. It may be secondary to pain but also may be a symptom of depression. Patients with pain and sleep disturbance often benefit from low doses of sedating antidepressants.

Ask the patient directly if he or she feels depressed. If so, ask for elaboration. Ask if the patient feels cranky and irritable. Ask directly about the other vegetative symptoms of depression, including loss of libido, weight change, and energy level.

Ask the patient about the perceived level of stress. Try to determine the sources of stress. Are they financial? Are they due to the work environment, from co-workers or supervisors? Are there family problems? Does the patient feel these stressors were present before the spine problem or have they occurred since? Many patients tend to use the spine pain as a "black hole" that sucks up the blame for all the patient's problems. Patients may feel that if the spine pain went away, all the other problems in life would also disappear. Unfortunately, this is rarely the case.

It is also useful to obtain a picture of the patient's childhood and development. The correlation is high between multiple childhood psychologic traumas (see box) and chronic refractory LBP and failed back surgery syndrome.[34,36] The major developmental risk factors share the common aspect of rendering the adult more vulnerable to pain. It may be beyond the scope of the initial interview to make theses inquiries, but it becomes increasingly important if patients are not responding to treatment as expected or if surgery is contemplated.

Childhood Psychological Risk Factors[36]

- Physical abuse
- Sexual abuse
- Abandonment
- Neglect
- Chemical dependence in primary care-giver(s)

Vocational History

A vocational history is important in any patient, whether or not the spine injury occurred at work. A work history will shed light about the cumulative trauma the spine has experienced. Patients who were not injured while working may still be receiving or applying for disability payments or Social Security benefits. A large body of information suggests that disability issues may have a negative impact on outcome, although there are reports to the contrary.[23]

Many variables affect the outcome of treatment of the injured worker. Many authors attribute the poor results to the secondary gains of the system. However, it is also important to consider that patients injured on the job and receiving worker's compensation are more likely to have jobs that require heavy physical exertion.[23] Researchers often fail to take into account that a patient's return to work is in part dependent on the physical demands of the job, and is not just a psychosocial issue.[5,23]

It is impossible to be sure in an individual patient how much the worker's compensation system is contributing to the pain and disability. Statistically, injured workers tend to take longer to recover from injuries than patients with similar injuries who were not injured on the job.[12,23] The longer an injured worker remains off work, the lower the chances of that worker ever returning to work.[4,21,22] When treating an injured worker it is very helpful to return the patient to some form of light duty as soon as possible.[4,5] Outcomes from both operative and nonoperative care tend to be better in patients who are not injured workers. However, there are many individual exceptions to this generality and therefore the clinician should approach each patient fresh and without preconceived ideas. On the other hand, the clinician must be aware of the potential delays in recovery seen in the injured worker population.

If the patient was injured while working, obtaining additional information is necessary. Much of this may be obtained by questionnaire supplemented with direct questioning. Ask the patient to describe the injury. The importance of the mechanism of injury in terms of determining pathophysiology has been discussed earlier in this chapter. In addition, does the worker perceive the injury to be due to faulty equipment or the negligence of another worker?[5,12]

Determine the patient's current work status. Is the patient currently working, and if so, is it the usual job? If the patient is not working, is the job still available? If the patient is not working, is it because of the spine problem or other health problems or is the patient retired due to age or other reasons not related to health?

Ask specifically about the job demands with respect to the number of hours spent sitting, standing, and walking. Determine the worker's perspective of the amount of weight lifted and carried occasionally and frequently as well as the maximum weight lifted.

Was the patient doing the usual and customary job at the time of injury, or were the activities unusual? Many workers report they were injured doing something that was not part of their usual routine.[25] How long has the injured worker been at the current job? Patients who are injured at a new job seem to do poorly compared with established workers.[21] Determine the date and time of injury and the exact circumstances under which the injury occurred. Does the patient have an attorney? How does the patient perceive the relationship with the insurance company?

Important insights that may contribute to outcome can be gained by learning more about how the patient perceives the job, the working environment, and the relationship with supervisors and employers.[22] Does the patient perceive the work as physically demanding? Does the patient feel he or she is required to do work that is too heavy for his or her lifting capacity? This is a risk factor for prolonged disability.[5,12] Is the work stressful to the employee and if so, in what ways? Does the patient like the work? Does the patient like his or her co-workers and the immediate supervisor? Patients who like their jobs and who like their supervisors and colleagues return to work with a higher frequency.[22] Does the patient hope to return to the same job and, if this is not possible, would the patient like to return to the same employer in a different capacity? Have there been many injuries to co-workers and does the patient feel the company has not paid attention to this fact? Does the patient believe that the fault for the current problem is his or her own, the employer's, a co-worker's, another person's, or nobody's fault? Patients who place blame on the employer or a co-worker are less likely to return to work.[22]

Has the patient had a previous work injury? Did the patient recover? If so, obtain an estimate of the percentage recovery and if there was a permanent disability and a permanent disability rating. Is the current spine problem part of the prior injury or is it totally new? Did the patient receive vocational rehabilitation or other training for a new job? Is the patient receiving disability payments? Obtain a work history of prior jobs and how long the patient was at each position. Were there restrictions set on the patient (preexisting disability) before the injury in terms of the job?

Determine the worker's pre-injury status in terms of job abilities, social activities, and sports capacities. Elaborate upon prior injuries whether or not they were work-related. Did the patient recover fully from these injuries or was there some residual pain and/or disability?

It is useful to determine whether the patient is experiencing financial difficulties as a result of the spinal injury. Interestingly, patients who are experiencing financial difficulty tend to do less well.[21]

Motor Vehicle Accident

Patients who suffer LBP or neck pain as a result of a MVA present special problems related to potential litigation and the (inaccurate) impression that litigation delays recovery.[34] However, the clinical history is otherwise essentially the same as for patients with other causes of LBP.

It is best clinically to evaluate the current complaint with the usual history performed in any patient with spinal pain. However, it then is necessary to learn about the MVA, the time course of pain problems, and any interval treatment and its results.

Determine the date and time of the MVA, the types of vehicles involved, whether or not the patient was wearing a shoulder-lap restraint, where the patient was seated in the vehicle, and a description of the accident. It is probably useful to obtain an estimate from the patient of the forces and speeds involved although, with the exception of speeds above 55 mph and below 5 mph, the correlation between the speeds of the vehicles and the amount of injury done to the patient is only modest.

Determine whether the patient struck his or her head. Did the patient lose consciousness? Did the chest or head strike the steering wheel? Did an airbag inflate?

Where did the patient receive initial emergency care? What were the initial symptoms when seen in the emergency department and what symptoms occurred subsequently? In addition to the spine problem, did other injuries occur? What type of treatment was rendered and was follow-up care arranged? Frequently, the onset of neck pain or LBP is delayed, making it necessary to describe the onset of the current pain. Which doctor is currently treating the patient? What interval-treatment has ensued since the MVA? Is the patient the same, better, or worse? Try to quantify the change. What tests have been performed?

Did the patient have prior problems with either the cervical, thoracic, or lumbar spine? When did these problems occur and what was the mechanism of injury? What was the time course of the prior problem and the degree of resolution? Although this information may not be necessary to treat the current problem, if the clinician is going to testify, it is useful to obtain documentation of prior injuries and their outcome from old medical records, as this will undoubtedly be a point of contention in litigation and settlement.

Is there litigation? What stage is it in? Did the patient have a job at the time of the MVA? Was there any time lost from work and if so, how much time, why was the patient unable to work, and was the time off work at the instructions of the physician, another person, or the decision of the patient? Are there other forms of disability insurance potentially serving as a secondary gain?

Past Medical History

The past medical history only occasionally helps determine the cause of LBP. Patients may forget to report remote history of trauma or of a cancer that has been treated. I am also occasionally surprised by patients who don't mention a spine surgery that was done 10 years earlier until I ask about the scar on their back!

Family History

A few familial disorders that affect the spine are hereditary. Isthmic spondylolisthesis, Scheuermann's disease, and spinal stenosis in patients with achondroplasia are familial. There may be a familial tendency toward spondylolysis. There are families in which early osteoporosis seems to occur. Breast cancer can run in families.

The family psychologic history may be helpful. If one or both parents had a painful and/or disabling illness when the patient was a child, there may be learned abnormal illness behavior. A history of alcoholism or other chemical dependence in a parent or other essential caregiver may indicate a difficult childhood development with subsequent pain-prone personality disorder.

Conclusion

Experienced clinicians have learned that the history is the most important part of the evaluation of the patient with lumbar spinal disorders. Despite advances in imaging technology, diagnostic spinal injections, and electrodiagnostics, the history provides the information that directs all other aspects of diagnosis and treatment. A good history is worth a thousand pictures.

North American Spine Society Back Pain Questionnaire-Baseline Medical History, Expectations and Outcomes*

(Draft of one of several modules. Reproduced with permission of North American Spine Society © 1993.)

1. HOW LONG AGO did your *current* episode begin?

    1 Less than 2 weeks ago   4 3 months to less than 6 months ago

    2 2 weeks to less than 8 weeks ago   5 6 to 12 months ago

    3 8 weeks to less than 3 months ago   6 More than 12 months ago

2. HOW did your *current* episode begin?

    0 Suddenly

    1 Gradually

3. Have you had back symptoms before your current episode?

    0 No (IF NO, GO TO QUESTION 6)

    1 Yes, one episode

    2 Yes, two or more episodes

Answer #4–5 about your PAST back symptoms.

---

4. Did you receive Worker's Compensation for your PAST back symptoms?

    1 No   0 Yes

5. How much work did you miss because of your worst prior episode?

    0 None   3 More than 4 weeks to 12 weeks

    1 1 day to 2 weeks   4 More than 12 weeks to 24 weeks

    2 More than 2 weeks to 4 weeks   5 More than 24 weeks

---

6. Have you had previous back surgery?

    0 No (If NO, go to question 13)

    1 Yes: How many surgeries? # _____

North American Spine Society Back Pain Questionnaire-Baseline Medical History, Expectations and Outcomes—cont'd

Answer #7–8 about your PAST back surgeries.

7. After your most recent surgery, did you return to work?

   0 No

   1 Yes, with limitations

   2 Yes, with no limitations

   7 Never stopped working

   8 Did not work: _____ Homemaker

   _____ Student

   _____ Retired

   _____ Other

8. After your most recent surgery, did you return to full function?

   0 No   1 Yes

There will be several questions about leg and back pain in this questionnaire. When we say LEG, we mean your thigh, calf, ankle, and foot. When we say BACK, we mean your low back and buttocks.

9. Which hurts you more, your legs or back?

   1 Legs hurt much more

   2 Legs hurt somewhat more

   3 Legs and back hurt about the same

   4 Back hurts somewhat more

   5 Back hurts much more

Please answer every question in the box below .

In the PAST WEEK. how often have you suffered:	None of the time	A little of the time	Some of the time	A good bit of the time	Most of the time	All the time
10. low back and/or buttock pain	1	2	3	4	5	6
11. leg pain	1	2	3	4	5	6
12. numbness or tingling in leg and/or foot	1	2	3	4	5	6
13. weakness in leg and/or foot (such as difficulty lifting foot)	1	2	3	4	5	6

Please answer every question in the box below.

In the PAST WEEK, how bothersome have these symptoms been?	Not at all bothersome	Slightly bothersome	Somewhat bothersome	Moderately bothersome	Very bothersome	Extremely bothersome
14. low back and or buttock pain	1	2	3	4	5	6
15. leg pain	1	2	3	4	5	6
16. numbness/tingling in leg and or foot	1	2	3	4	5	6
17. weakness in leg and/or foot (such as difficulty lifting foot)	1	2	3	4	5	6

North American Spine Society Back Pain Questionnaire-Baseline Medical History, Expectations and Outcomes—cont'd

In the LAST WEEK, please tell us HOW PAIN HAS AFFECTED YOUR ABILITY TO PERFORM the following daily activities. Mark the ONE statement that best describes your average ability.

18. Getting Dressed (in the LAST WEEK)

1   I can dress myself without pain.

2   I can dress myself without increasing pain.

3   I can dress myself but pain increases.

4   I can dress myself but with significant pain.

5   I can dress myself but with very severe pain.

6   I cannot dress myself.

19. Lifting (in the LAST WEEK)

1   I can lift heavy objects without pain.

2   I can lift heavy objects but it is painful.

3   Pain prevents me from lifting heavy objects off the floor but I can manage if they are on a table.

4   Pain prevents me from lifting heavy objects but I can manage light to medium objects if they are on a table.

5   I can lift only light objects.

6   I cannot lift anything.

20. Walking (in the LAST WEEK)

1   Pain does not prevent me from walking.

2   Pain prevents me from walking more than 1 hour.

3   Pain prevents me from walking more than 30 minutes.

4   Pain prevents me from walking more than 10 minutes.

5   I can only walk a few steps at a time.

6   I am unable to walk.

21. Sitting (in the LAST WEEK)

1   I can sit in any chair as long as I like.

2   I can only sit in a special chair for as long as I like.

3   Pain prevents me sitting more than 1 hour.

4   Pain prevents me from sitting more than 30 minutes.

5   Pain prevents me from sitting more than a few minutes.

6   Pain prevents me from sitting at all.

22. Standing (in the LAST WEEK)

1   I can stand as long as I want.

2   I can stand as long as I want but it gives me pain.

3   Pain prevents me from standing for more than 1 hour.

4   Pain prevents me from standing for more than 30 minutes

5   Pain prevents me from standing for more than 10 minutes.

6   Pain prevents me from standing at all.

23. Sleeping (in the LAST WEEK)

1   I sleep well.

2   Pain occasionally interrupts my sleep.

3   Pain interrupts my sleep half of the time.

4   Pain often interrupts my sleep.

5   Pain always interrupts my sleep.

6   I never sleep well.

24. Social and Recreational Life (in the LAST WEEK)

1   My social and recreational life is unchanged.

2   My social and recreational life is unchanged but it increases pain.

3   My social and recreational life is unchanged but it severely increases pain.

4   Pain has restricted my social and recreational life.

North American Spine Society Back Pain Questionnaire-Baseline Medical History, Expectations and Outcomes—cont'd

    5   Pain has severely restricted my social and recreational life

    6   I have essentially no social and recreational life because of pain.

25. Traveling (in the LAST WEEK)

    1   I can travel anywhere.

    2   I can travel anywhere but it gives me pain.

    3   Pain is bad but I can manage to travel over 2 hours.

    4   Pain restricts me to trips of less than 1 hour.

    5   Pain restricts me to trips of less than 30 minutes.

    6   Pain prevents me from traveling.

26. Sex Life (in the LAST WEEK)

    1   My sex life is unchanged.

    2   My sex life is unchanged but causes some extra pain.

    3   My sex life is nearly unchanged but is very painful.

    4   My sex life is severely restricted by pain.

    5   My sex life is nearly absent because of pain.

    6   Pain prevents any sex life at all.

Please answer every question in the box below.

HOW OFTEN do you need to use the following assistive devices?	Never	Sometimes	About half the time	Often	All the time
27. One or two canes	1	2	3	4	5
28. One or two crutches	1	2	3	4	5
29. Walker	1	2	3	4	5
30. Wheelchair	1	2	3	4	5

31. Which health care providers have you used for your current back condition? (CIRCLE ALL THAT APPLY)

    A Acupuncturist   I Osteopath

    B Chiropractor   J Orthopaedic surgeon

    C Emergency room   K Pain Clinic

    D General practitioner   L Physical Therapist

    E Immediate care clinic   M Rheumatologist

    F Internist   N Work Hardening Clinic

    G Massage Therapist   O Other: _____

    H Neurosurgeon   P None of the above

32. During the LAST WEEK, how often have you taken narcotic medication such as codeine, Demerol, Percodan, or Vicodin for your back and/or leg pain?

    1   3 or more times a day   4 Once a week

    2   Once or twice a day   5 Not at all

    3   Once every couple of days

33. During the LAST WEEK, how often have you taken non-narcotic medication such as aspirin, Motrin, or Tylenol for your back and/or leg pain?

    1   3 or more times a day   4 Once a week

    2   Once or twice a day   5 Not at all

    3   Once every couple of days

34. Have you used alcoholic beverages (beer, wine, liquor) to relieve your current back or leg pain?

   0 No

   1 Yes, once in a while

   2 Yes, often

35. If you had to spend the rest of your life with your *back condition as it is right now,* how would you feel about it?

   1 Extremely dissatisfied

   2 Very dissatisfied

   3 Somewhat dissatisfied

   4 Neutral

   5 Somewhat satisfied

   6 Very satisfied

   7 Extremely satisfied

What expectations do you have for your treatment at this office?

As a result of my treatment, I expect	not likely	slightly likely	somewhat likely	very likely	extremely likely
36. Complete pain relief	1	2	3	4	5
37. Moderate pain relief	1	2	3	4	5
38. To be able to do more everyday household or yard activities	1	2	3	4	5
39. To be able to sleep more comfortably	1	2	3	4	5
40. To be able to go back to my usual job	1	2	3	4	5
41. To be able to do more sports, go biking, or go for long walks	1	2	3	4	5

42. What other results do you expect from your treatment? Please describe:

_____

_____

_____

How important are the following treatment outcomes for you?

How important is...	not important	slightly important	somewhat important	very important	extremely important
43. Pain relief	1	2	3	4	5
44. To be able to do more everyday household or yard activities	1	2	3	4	5
45. To be able to sleep more comfortably	1	2	3	4	5
46. To be able to go back to my usual job	1	2	3	4	5
47. To be able to do more sports. go biking. or go for long walks	1	2	3	4	5
48. Other (see your answer to #42 above): _____	1	2	3	4	5

North American Spine Society Back Pain Questionnaire-Baseline Medical History, Expectations and Outcomes—cont'd

Following are some questions about your general health.

49. In general would you say your health is:

    1 Excellent

    2 Very Good

    3 Good

    4 Fair

    5 Poor

    6 Terrible

50. Have you ever had any of the following conditions?
    (CIRCLE ALL THAT APPLY)

    A Diabetes

    B Heart Disease

    C Stroke

    D Arthritis other than in your back

    E Asthma or other lung disease

    F Depression

    G High Blood Pressure (hypertension)

    H Colitis

    I Psoriasis

    J None of the above

51. Do you currently smoke cigarettes?

    0 I have never smoked

    1 Yes

    2 No, I quit in the last 6 months

    3 No, I quit more than 6 months ago

52. Has the treatment for your back condition met your expectations so far?

    1 Yes, totally

    2 Yes, almost totally

    3 Yes, quite a bit

    4 More or less

    5 No, not quite

    6 No, far from it

    7 No, not at all

53. Would you have the same treatment again if you had the same condition?

    1 Definitely not

    2 Probably not

    3 Not sure

    4 Probably yes

    5 Definitely yes

54. If you had back pain, how has your back pain been affected by the treatment?

    (CHECK ONLY ONE STATEMENT)

    1 I did not have back pain to start with.

    2 The pain is totally gone.

    3 The pain is much better than before treatment.

    4 The pain is somewhat better than before treatment.

    5 The pain is about the same as before treatment.

    6 The pain is somewhat worse than before treatment.

    7 The pain is much worse than before treatment.

55. If you had leg pain, how has your leg pain been affected by the treatment?

    (CHECK ONLY ONE STATEMENT)

    1 I did not have leg pain to start with.

    2 The pain is totally gone.

    3 The pain is much better than before treatment.

    4 The pain is somewhat better than before treatment.

North American Spine Society Back Pain Questionnaire-Baseline Medical History, Expectations and Outcomes—cont'd

5 The pain is about the same as before treatment.

6 The pain is somewhat worse than before treatment.

7 The pain is much worse than before treatment.

The following questions are about how you feel and how things have been with you during the last week. For each question. please indicate the one answer that comes closest to the way you have been feeling. Please, CIRCLE ONE ANSWER ON EACH LINE.

How much of the time during the LAST WEEK	All of the time	Most of the time	A good bit the time	Some of the time	Little of the time	None of the time
56. Have you been a very nervous person?	1	2	3	4	5	6
57. Have you felt so down in the dumps nothing could cheer you up?	1	2	3	4	5	6
58. Have you felt calm and peaceful?	1	2	3	4	5	6
59. Have you felt downhearted and blue?	1	2	3	4	5	6
60. Have you been a happy person?	1	2	3	4	5	6

North American Spine Society Back Pain Questionnaire-Baseline Medical Employment History, and Work Status.*

(Draft of one of several modules. Reproduced with permission of North American Spine Society © 1993.)

1. How many jobs have you had in the last 3 years?

    0 None

    1 1 or 2

    2 3 or more

2. Which statements describe your current employment situation? *CIRCLE ALL THAT APPLY*

    A Currently working

    B On paid leave

    C On unpaid leave

    D Unemployed

    E Homemaker

    F Student

    G Retired (not due to health)

    H Disabled and/or retired because of my back problems

    I Disabled due to a health problem not related to my back

    J Other, please specify: _____

3. Are you self-employed?

    0 No   1 Yes

4. If NOT WORKING now, how long has it been since you stopped?

    1 Less than 1 week ago

    2 1 week to less than 3 months ago

    3 3 months to less than 6 months ago

    4 6 months to less than 12 months ago

    5 1 to 2 years ago

    6 More than 2 years ago

    8 Currently working

    9 Never employed

North American Spine Society Back Pain Questionnaire-Baseline Medical Employment History, and Work Status—cont'd

5. What is your primary occupation? If you are not working now, what was your primary occupation? (Please be as specific as possible)

   Occupation: _____

6. Is your current job the same one you had when your current back symptoms started?

   1 Yes, exact same job

   2 Yes, but job was modified or hours reduced because of my back

   3 No, I have changed jobs because of my back symptoms

   4 No, I have changed jobs but for reasons unrelated to my back

   5 Not working now

7. How long have you worked at your current job?

   0 less than 6 months

   1 6 to 12 months

   2 more than 12 months

   3 not working now

Please answer each of the following questions about your current job (or the one you plan to go back to if on leave). CIRCLE ONE ANSWER ON EACH LINE.

	All of the time	Most of the time	A good bit the time	Some of the time	Little of the time	None of the time
8. How much sitting does your work involve?	1	2	3	4	5	6
9. How much standing or walking does your work involve?	1	2	3	4	5	6
10. How often do you lift 25 lbs. on the job?	1	2	3	4	5	6
11. How often do you lift 50 lbs. on the job?	1	2	3	4	5	6

Please answer each of the following questions about your current job (or the one you plan to go back to if on leave):

	Extremely	Very much	Quite a bit	Somewhat	A little	Not at all
12. Is your current work physically demanding?	1	2	3	4	5	6
13. Is your work stressful to you?	1	2	3	4	5	6
14. How much do you like your job?	1	2	3	4	5	6
15. How much do you like your co-workers?	1	2	3	4	5	6
16. How much do you like your supervisor?	1	2	3	4	5	6

North American Spine Society Back Pain Questionnaire-Baseline Medical Employment History, and Work Status—cont'd

17. Other than your salary, what other sources of income does your household receive?
    CIRCLE ALL THAT APPLY:

    A Another person's salary

    B State Support

    C Social Security

    D Disability

    E Other (Investments, Retirement Plan, etc.)

    F No other source of income

18. Are you experiencing financial difficulties because of your back condition?

    0 None at all

    1 Only a little

    2 Some

    3 A lot

Please answer the questions in the box, or check below if none applies.

Are you on or planning to apply for any of the following programs?	Already on it	Applied for it	Planning to apply for it
19. Social Security	1	2	3
20. Disability	1	2	3
21. Workers Compensation	1	2	3
22. Other (please specify): _____	1	2	3

☐ Check here if none of the above applies.

23. Do you think the fault for your current back condition is: (CIRCLE ALL THAT APPLY)

    A Yours?

    B Your employer's?

    C A co-worker's?

    D Another person's?

    E Nobody's?

24. Have you hired a lawyer because of your back condition?

    0 No, I have not hired a lawyer.

    1 Yes, I have and the case is in litigation.

    2 Yes, I have and the case has been settled.

Thank you for your help. Please take a moment to go over the questionnaire to make sure you have not missed any pages or questions. Then return it to the person who gave it to you or in the envelope provided.

References

1. Almay BG: Clinical characteristics of patients with idiopathic pain syndromes. Depressive symptomatology and patient pain drawings, *Pain* 29:335-346, 1987.

2. Battie MC and others: Smoking and lumbar intervertebral disc degeneration: an MRI study of identical twins, *Spine* 16:1015-1020, 1991.

3. Borenstein D: Approach to the diagnosis and management of medical low back pain, *Semin Spine Surg* 2:80-85, 1990.

4. Catchlove R, Cohen K: Effects on a directive return to work approach in the treatment of workman's compensation patients with chronic pain, *Pain* 14:181-191, 1982.

5. Cats-baril WL, Frymoyer JW: Demographic factors associated with the prevalence of disability in the general population, *Spine* 16:671-674, 1991.

6. Dennis MD, Oocchio PO, Wiltse LL: The topographical pain representation and its correlation with MMPI scores, *Orthopedics* 5:432-434, 1981.

7. Duncan GH, Buchnell C, Lavigne GJ: Comparison of verbal and visual analogue scales for measuring the intensity and unpleasantness of experimental pain, *Pain* 37:295-303, 1989.

8. Ewing JA: Detecting alcoholism: the CAGE questionnaire, *JAMA* 252:1905-1907, 1984.

9. Fairbank JC and others: *History taking and physical examination: identification of syndromes of back pain.* In Weinstein JN, Wiesel SW, editors: *The lumbar spine,* Philadelphia, 1990, WB Saunders, pp 88-106.

10. Fishman B and others: The Memorial pain assessment card: a valid instrument for the evaluation of cancer pain, *Cancer* 60:1151-1158, 1987.

11. Frymoyer J: Back pain and sciatica, *N Engl J Med* 318:291-299, 1988.

12. Frymoyer JW: Predicting disability from low back pain, *Clin Orthop* 279:102-109, 1992.

13. Gibson S, Kimmel PL: Genitourinary diseases affecting the spine, *Semin Spine Surg* 2:145-149, 1990.

14. Hadler NM: Regional back pain, *N Engl J Med* 315:1090-1092, 1986.

15. Herron LD and others: The differential utility of the Minnesota Multiphasic Personality Inventory: a predictor of outcome in lumbar laminectomy for disc herniation versus spinal stenosis. *Spine* 11:847-849, 1986.

16. Hildebrandt J and others: The use of pain drawings in screening for psychological involvement in complaints of low-back pain, *Spine* 13:681-685, 1988.

17. Hochberg MC: Ankylosing spondylitis, *Semin Spine Surg* 2:86-94, 1990.

18. Jensen MP, Karoly P, Braver S: The measurement of clinical pain intensity: a comparison of six methods, *Pain* 27:117-126, 1986.

19. Jensen MP and others: The subjective experience of acute pain: an assessment of the utility of 10 indices. *Clin J Pain* 5:153-159, 1989.

20. LaBan MM, Burk RD, Johnson EW. Sexual impotence in men having low back syndrome, *Arch Phys Med Rehab* 9:715-723, 1966.

21. Lancourt J, Kettelhut M: Predicting return to work for lower back pain patients receiving worker's compensation, *Spine* 17:629-640, 1992.

22. Lancourt J, Lancourt V: The employer-employee interaction: can it be measured? does it affect return to work in patients receiving care under the worker's compensation system? Presented at the Seventh Annual Meeting of the North American Spine Society, Boston, July 9-11, 1992.

23. Leavitt F: The physical exertion factor in compensable work injuries: a hidden flaw in previous research, *Spine* 17:307-310, 1992.

24. Margolis RB, Tait RC, Krause SJ: A rating system for use with patient pain drawings, *Pain* 24:57- 65, 1986.

25. McCoy CE and others: Work related injury. Presented at the Seventh Annual Meeting of the North American Spine Society, Boston, July 9-11, 1992.

26. Mellin G, Hurri H: Referred limb symptoms in chronic low back pain, *J Spinal Disorders* 3:52-58, 1990.

27. Melzack R: The McGill Pain Questionnaire: major properties and scoring methods, *Pain* 1:277-299, 1975.

28. Murphy DF and others: Measurement of pain: a comparison of the visual analogue with a nonvisual analogue scale, *Clin J Pain* 3:197-199, 1988.

29. Nachemson AL: Disc pressure measurements, *Spine* 6:93-97, 1981.

30. Ransford AO, Cairns D, Mooney V: The pain drawing as an aid to the psychological evaluation of patients with low-back pain, *Spine* 1:127-134, 1976.

31. Reading AE: *Testing pain mechanisms in persons in pain.* In Wall PD, Melzack R, editors: *Textbook of pain,* London, 1989, Churchill-Livingstone.

32. Roberts IM: Gastrointestinal disorders presenting with back pain, *Semin Spine Surg* 2:141-144, 1990.

33. Salovy P and others: Reporting chronic pain episodes on health surveys, *Vital Health Stat* 6(6), 1992.

34. Schofferman J, Wasserman S: Successful treatment of low back pain and/or neck pain due to a motor vehicle accident, *Spine* 19:1007-1010, 1994.

35. Schofferman J, Zucherman J: History and physical examination, *Spine State Art Rev* 1:13-20, 1986.

36. Schofferman J and others: Childhood psychological trauma and chronic refractory low back pain, *Clin J Pain* 9:260-265, 1993.

37. Schofferman J and others: Childhood psychological trauma correlates with unsuccessful spine surgery, *Spine* 17(suppl):S138-S144, 1992.

38. Schofferman L and others: Occult infections causing persistent low-back pain, *Spine* 14:417-419, 1989.

39. Smith RC, Hoppe RB: The patient's story: integrating the patient and physician-centered approaches to interviewing, *Ann Intern Med* 115:470-477, 1991.

40. Spengler DM and others: Elective discectomy for herniation of a lumbar disc: additional experience with an objective method, *J Bone Joint Surg* 72A:230-237, 1990.

41. Sriwataka K and others: Studies with different types of visual analog scales for measurement of pain, *Clin Pharmacol Ther* 34:234-239, 1983.

42. von Baeyer CL and others: Invalid use of pain drawings in psychological screening of back pain patients, *Pain* 16:103-107, 1983.

43. Zinn WM: Transference phenomena in medical practice: being whom the patient needs, *Ann Intern Med* 113:293-298, 1990.

Chapter 7
Physical Examination
Jerome A. Schofferman

The physical examination is essential in establishing the clinical diagnosis, planning diagnostic testing, and initiating treatment of patients with lumbar spine disorders.[17] The examination may provide information that can lead to a structural diagnosis and also may provide insights about the psychologic status of the patient.[21,22] It is important to recognize, however, that interobserver reliability regarding some components of the physical examination is poor, even when it is performed by experienced clinicians.[14]

There is no correct order in which to perform the examination.[8] However, each examiner should develop an efficient, thorough routine, to avoid omitting any important parts of the examination or needlessly duplicating others. Based on the history, certain components of the examination may require extra emphasis. Appropriate tests of motor function, reflexes, sensation, and root tension are performed in each position. Table 7-1 presents one possible sequence for a full examination. The examination need not be completed in a single session. The examination, like the history, evolves and changes over time as the patient's condition changes.

Observation

The examination begins when the patient enters the office or the physician enters the examining room. Some patients will be sitting; others will be standing, perhaps even pacing.

Observe the patient's behavior throughout the history-taking and the examination. Most patients manifest some degree of pain behavior. It is the judgment of the clinician whether or not the pain behavior is appropriate for the structural disease or is abnormal or inappropriate.[15] For example, patients who are writhing in pain rarely have a mechanical cause of pain but may be suffering from a serious visceral disorder or have significant psychological overlay.[10]

Some patients who have seen many practitioners feel they have not been taken seriously and may consciously or unconsciously manifest abnormal pain behavior in the examining room.[15] No data prove that abnormal pain behavior in the examining room correlates positively or negatively with structural pathology. It has been shown that there is no correlation between the presence of Waddell signs on examination and either return to activity or resolution of pain.[3,21] However, abnormal pain behavior that occurs in the patient's daily life may be an impediment to recovery and must be addressed as part of the overall treatment plan. It is useful to record the type and degree of pain behavior in the medical record.[15]

Table 7-1

Possible sequence for physical examination (modified from Frymoyer[8])

Position	Examination
Standing	Inspection: Skin, deformity, spasm
	ROM
	Gait and walking posture
	Functional motor examination: toe raises, heel-walking, squats
Sitting	Posture
	Motor: Hip flexors; hip ab- and ad-duction; toe dorsiflexion, ankle dorsiflexion, and plantar flexion; foot inversion and eversion; knee flexion and extension
	DTR
	Sensation
	SLR
	Plantar responses
Lying supine	Motor (if not completed sitting)
	Measurements: Muscle circumference, leg length
	SLR and confirmatory tests
	Abdominal palpation
	Pulses
	DTR (if not completed sitting)
	Hip tenderness and ROM
	Sensation (if not completed sitting)
Lying prone	PKB and/or femoral stretch
	Palpation
	Sacroiliac joints
	Motor: Gluteus maximus, hamstring
	Sensation: Perineum (lateral decubitus)
	Rectal examination (lateral decubitus)
Other	General observations

Key: ROM = range of motion; DTR = deep tendon reflex; SLR = straight leg raise; PKB = prone knee bend.

Many types of pain behavior might occur during the physical examination. Verbalizations such as cries of pain, moans, groans, or sighs can generally be considered abnormal.[15] Requesting assistance from family or the clinician during the examination is not usually physiologic. Grimaces or other abnormal facial expressions are pain behaviors. Many patients change positions frequently but do not remark about it or exaggerate the change. This is usually appropriate. Walking with very unusual postures or with guarded and careful steps must be considered in the context of other findings. The use of a self-procured cane, crutches, walker, or wheelchair all reflect some degree of abnormal pain behavior.

Observations about posture shed light on muscle strength, posture at home, pathoanatomy, and response to physical therapy. Observe the sitting posture. Patients who sit comfortably may have spinal stenosis especially if they are elderly or have had many operations. Does the patient sit straight with good lumbar lordosis or is the patient sitting slumped, which both reverses the lumbar lordosis and increases intradiscal pressure? Is any kyphosis or abnormal lumbar lordosis postural or fixed? The patient can correct with cues a postural kyphosis or lordosis but not a structural deformity. If the patient corrects poor posture, is it maintained during the rest of the examination or does the patient revert to poor posture? In patients who revert to poor posture, is it learned abnormal posture and/or muscle weakness due to deconditioning as the cause? This patient will definetly need aggressive physical therapy.

Ask the patient to walk around the room or preferably down the hall. Is the gait antalgic? Is an abnormal gait secondary to increased leg or back pain with weight bearing, degenerative joint disease of the hip, and/or is there spasticity from upper motor neuron disease? Part of the motor examination (discussed in a later section) may be performed at this time.

Observe the patient getting in and out of a chair and on and off the examination table. When getting out of a chair, most people bend at the waist and go into some degree of lumbar flexion. There may also be increased stresses across the facet joints. Any of these forces can increase low back pain (LBP). It is instructive to teach the patient to perform the sit-to-stand transition correctly, bracing with the abdominal muscles, sliding forward, and then standing up straight without bending. If a proper transition is less painful, diagnostic information is gained. Watching the patient get on or off the examination table demonstrates the ability to perform a complex maneuver and tells the examiner much about what the patient has or has not learned in any prior physical therapy and body-mechanics training.

Inspection

Skin

Inspection of the skin can occasionally provide clues to the origin of spinal pain. The patient should be fully undressed but gowned to allow inspection of the skin of the entire body. Look specifically for psoriatic lesions, which may be most pronounced at the elbows or knees. In subtle cases, only the scalp or fingernails may be involved. Psoriasis may be a clue to seronegative spondyloarthropathy and sacroiliitis.

Look for vesicles in a single dermatome distribution. Occasionally herpes zoster (shingles) can present as dermatomal radicular pain.

Café au lait spots or pedunculated skin tags (neurofibromata) may be markers for neurofibromatosis, a disease that can have intraspinal tumors. An unusual patch of hair over the lumbar area may be a clue to a bone defect such as diastematomyelia or spina bifida occulta. Port wine staining or unusual birth marks may also be a clue to spina bifida.

Inspect the skin for evidence of infection. Localized abscess or cellulitis can lead to discitis or even epidural abscess. Track marks, which suggest intravenous drug use, may also be a marker of subtle spine infection or drug seeking.

Posture

Observe the standing posture. Those who wait in the examining room standing rather than sitting may have discogenic pathology, which causes sitting intolerance. Standing often causes more pain in patients with spinal stenosis, especially if instability is present. Is there visible muscle spasm?

Is the patient listing? A list is a lumbar curvature present in the standing position that is gone when the patient is lying.[13] It is secondary to muscle spasm and can be extreme enough to cause postural scoliosis, occasionally referred to as "sciatic scoliosis" or even "defense scoliosis." It often means acute annulus tear or herniated disc, especially with the history of acute-onset LBP. Degenerative or idiopathic scoliosis is more visible with the patient standing or bending forward and does not abate when the patient is prone.

Observe the lumbar lordosis. Fixed reversal in an elderly person suggests long-standing degenerative disc disease (DDD) and probably spinal stenosis. Increased lordosis can aggravate the lumbar facet joints.

Is there kyphosis? In young men, increased thoracic kyphosis may suggest Scheuermann's disease. There may be a compensatory increased lumbar lordosis as discussed above. In older individuals increased thoracic kyphosis may suggest multiple old compression fractures, and new-onset back pain may signal a new fracture.

Look for lumbar scars from prior lumbar or other surgeries. Is there obvious atrophy? The presence of fasciculation may suggest upper motor neuron disease.

Many clinicians advocate measuring leg length. There are various ways to measure leg length; the technique is not standardized. There are few studies using standard techniques to evaluate the role of leg length discrepancy as an etiologic factor for LBP. In one study, which used a highly accurate leg-length measuring device in patients with and without LBP, leg-length discrepancy was not a cause for chronic LBP.[9] Two patients had leg-length discrepancies of greater than 5 cm in the control group, neither of whom had LBP.

Range of Motion

The patient is asked to stand facing away from the examiner. The entire spine should be exposed. Ask the patient to bend forward and try to touch his or her toes while keeping the knees straight. Is the motion smooth and physiologic, or ratchety, reflecting abnormal pain behavior? The return from flexion should be smooth and proceed cephalad to caudally. A hitch may reflect facet pain or unstable spondylolisthesis, or may be abnormal pain behavior.

In addition to observing range of motion (ROM), it is extremely useful to determine the effect of bending on the pain. Discogenic pain is usually worsened by flexion, even more so by repetitive flexion. Pain of spinal stenosis does not change or decreases.

Opinions abound regarding the optimal way to measure ROM. The distance may be measured in inches with respect to an anatomic reference point such as the knees, ankles, or toes. The range might be stated as a percentage of reduction from normal. Range of motion may be recorded in degrees, either using a goniometer or a specially-designed device. However, we believe the ROM need only be an approximate measure because it is very dependent on effort, motivation, and pain.

Restrictions to forward flexion are most commonly indicative of discogenic pain. Observe for deviation to the right or left while the patient is bending.

The effect of flexion on the lumbar lordosis should be observed. Patients with discogenic pain from an annulus tear, herniated disc, or painful disc may demonstrate poor reversal of the lumbar lordosis. However, patients with spinal stenosis may show excellent reversal or fixed loss of lordosis.

Ask the patient to bend backwards, keeping his or her knees and hips locked. It is useful for the examiner to prevent hip extension and control pelvic motion to visualize only lumbar extension. Decreased extension in standing is not specific. It may suggest a facet source if there is concordant pain reproduction. Extension is often quite limited in spinal stenosis. Extension in standing that produces concordant ipsilateral or bilateral leg pain is quite suggestive of spinal stenosis of the central and/or intervertebral canals.

Side bending is also performed. Observe for restricted ROM and particularly for asymmetry bending right compared with bending left.

The Waddell trunk rotation test can be performed at this time.[22] The patient places his or her hands on the hips as the examiner guides axial rotation at the hips. This test does not cause lumbar rotation until at least 30 degrees; therefore, LBP produced early in this maneuver suggests a possible functional overlay.

Motor Examination

Different parts of the motor examination are performed with the patient standing, sitting, and prone. Strength is graded on a standard 0 to 5 scale, as shown in Table 7-2.

The causes for apparent weakness during manual muscle testing are many, including true neurologic deficits, muscle disease, pain inhibition, psychologic problems, or malingering. Motor weakness secondary to neurologic abnormality or muscle disease is usually smooth. Weakness secondary to pain inhibition is either a sudden release of power (give-away weakness) or stepwise release (cogwheel or ratchety). When an area is painful and/or tender, pain may be increased when the area is moved or when the patient is asked to resist pressure. The patient is initially able to maintain resistance but then may "give up" because of the pain, and sudden muscle release occurs. Psychologically based weakness is often a stepwise release.[2] Feigned weakness is usually a stepwise release (cogwheel), but there may be sudden release.

Table 7-2
Grading of muscle strength

Strength	Grade
No evidence of contractility	0
Slight contractility but no movement	1
Full ROM with gravity eliminated	2
Full ROM against gravity	3
Full ROM against gravity with some resistance	4
Full ROM against gravity with full resistance	5

Key: ROM = range of motion.

Keep in mind the innervation of the various muscles being tested to look for inconsistencies when different muscles with the same innervation are being tested, and to compare motor weakness with reflex or sensory changes (Table 7-3). It is remarkable that there is still a lack of agreement about muscle innervation from text to text. Table 7-3 presents a clinically useful consensus. Muscle testing is done both by manual muscle testing and by functional testing.

Ask the patient to perform unilateral toe raises (S1) first on one side and then the other, while standing and perhaps holding a counter top for balance. Test the least painful leg first. Ask the patient to do 10 repetitions on each side and observe for differences in ability; then ask the patient about the perceptions of effort on each side. If there is any question of subtle weakness, it may be productive to ask the patient to self-test at home by doing the maximum number of toe raises possible on one side, and compare it with the other, and report the results at the next visit. Have the patient do unilateral leg squats to test functionally the quadriceps (L4 > L3) and hip flexor complex (L3, L2). Again, compare side to side.

Trendelenburg's test can conveniently be performed next to test gluteus medius strength (L5).[11] The patient stands on both feet facing away from the examiner, who observes the respective heights of the posterior superior iliac crests. Ask the patient to stand on one leg. With normal strength the gluteus

medius of the weight-bearing leg contracts, elevating the pelvis of the leg that has been lifted. If the pelvis over the unsupported leg descends or even remains in position, there is weakness on the side of the weight-bearing leg.

Ask the patient to walk across the room normally and then repeat, walking on the heels with feet slightly inverted. This may detect subtle weakness in the ankle dorsiflexors (L5 and L4).

There are several manual muscle tests of the muscle that control the foot. The L5, L4, and S1 nerves are primarily involved. With the patient in the seated position test extensor hallucis longus (L5) by asking the patient to dorsiflex the great toe against resistance of one thumb. Test extensor digitorum longus, which controls dorsiflexion strength of the remaining four toes (L5). Ask the patient to dorsiflex one ankle without resistance. Observe for inversion during dorsiflexion, which may indicate L5 weakness with intact tibialis anterior (L4 >> L5). Then test pure dorsiflexion against resistance, which is a measure of L4 and L5 function. The test of the tibialis anterior (L4 >> L5) is best performed by grasping the patient's foot on its medial aspect and attempting to push the patient's foot into eversion and plantar flexion.

Test the strength of peroneus longus and brevis (S1) by grasping the heel with one hand and asking the patient to externally rotate against the resistance of the other hand. Test ankle plantar flexion (S1) against resistance of one hand. Test knee extension

Table 7-3
Clinical muscle testing of lumbar nerve roots

Nerve	Muscle	Motor Test
S1	Peroneus longus, brevis	Foot eversion
	Gastrocnemius (S1 > S2)	Ankle plantar flexion (toe raises)
	Gluteus maximus	Hip extension
L5	Hamstrings (L5 >> S1)	Knee flexion
	Gluteus medius	Hip abduction
	Extensor hallucis longus	Great toe dorsiflexion (distal phalanx)
	Extensor digitorum longus	Other toes dorsiflexion
	Tibialis anterior	Ankle dorsiflexion
L4	Tibialis anterior (L4 > L5)	Ankle dorsiflexion (and inversion)
L4 > L3, L2	Quadriceps	Knee extension
L2, L3, L4	Adductor longus	Hip adduction
	Secondary hip adductors	
L1, L2, L3	Iliopsoas	Hip flexion

(L4) and knee flexion (L5 and S1). It is easy to next test hip flexors (iliopsoas, L1, L2, L3) in the seated position and to follow this with the gluteus medius, the primary hip abductors (L5), and hip adductors (L2, L3, L4).

When the patient is supine, repeat muscle testing of the accessible muscles if it is necessary to confirm findings.

When the patient is prone, the hamstring (L5 >> S1) and gluteus maximus (S1) muscles can easily be tested. To test the hamstring ask the patient to flex the knee to 90 degrees and to hold that position against the examiner's attempt to bring the ankle down to the table. To test the gluteus maximus ask the patient to raise the thigh from the table against the examiner's resistance by a hand placed on the posterior thigh. Palpate the gluteus during the test for bulk and tone. Prone knee bend and sacroiliac joint testing can be done next, while the patient lies prone.

Deep Tendon Reflexes

Reflex testing includes an evaluation of normal reflexes and testing for the presence of pathologic reflexes. Reflexes may be graded in several ways, but it is best for clinical communication to grade simply as absent, decreased, normal, or increased.

It is easiest to test the Achilles reflex (S1) with the patient sitting. Gently dorsiflex the foot and then strike the Achilles tendon, this will normally induce plantar flexion of the foot. If the reflex is decreased, augmentation is done by asking the patient to gently plantar flex at the ankle against the resistance of the examiner's hand and then strike the tendon again. Alternatively, the reflex can be reinforced by asking the patient to interlock the fingers of both hands and pull apart as the tendon is struck.

The patellar reflex is predominantly L4, although there is some contribution from both L3 and L2. It is easiest to obtain the reflex with the patient lying supine. Support the knee in slight flexion using your forearm or your own bent knee on the table. Strike the infrapatellar tendon to elicit the reflex. Alternatively, the patellar reflex can be tested with the patient seated, although false-negative results may be more common in this position.

The L5 may be elicited by testing the tibialis posterior tendon. However, this reflex is absent in a high percentage of normal individuals. Thus, it is not a clinically useful test and is often omitted.

Test for clonus at each ankle. It is important to distinguish between one or two beats of clonus, which is seen commonly, versus stained clonus, which is usually pathologic. Many patients develop

hyperreflexia and clonus from causes other than disease of the central nervous system; examples include anxiety, medications, or drug withdrawal. Hyperreflexia and clonus may also be a normal variant. However, it is safest to assume that sustained clonus present on repeat examination is pathologic, until evaluation proves otherwise.

Test the plantar response. With the patient either seated or supine, run a sharp edge such as a key or the metal end of a reflex hammer from the calcaneus along the lateral aspect of the plantar surface of the foot, and observe the toes. A normal response is withdrawal of the whole foot or no reaction. An abnormal response is dorsiflexion of the great toe and fanning out and plantar flexion of the other toes. An abnormal test usually indicates upper motor neuron disease.

Nerve Root Tension Signs

Straight Leg Raise

The SLR is often poorly understood. The test is best performed twice on each leg, once with the patient sitting and again with the patient supine. The SLR is meant to test for sciatic-nerve irritation or compression from herniated nucleus pulposis (HNP) and is only rarely positive in other causes of sciatica.

Bear in mind that a normal SLR does not preclude the diagnosis of HNP. The response to SLR is generally believed to be due in part to the location of the HNP.[18,19] In a recent cadaver study, it has been shown that SLR causes nerve roots to move distally 0.5 to 5 mm, but the nerve roots also move laterally toward the bone and therefore move into a posterolateral HNP and potentially away from a central HNP.[18] Therefore, a midline HNP may not cause sciatica during SLR and the test will be negative. There is also strain of 2% to 4%. We believe that a positive SLR test in HNP is due to both strain and motion of the roots. The L4 nerve root moves less than L5 and S1 during supine SLR. Other authors believe that the location of the HNP does not correlate with whether or not the SLR is positive, and that perhaps inflammation is more important than compression for a positive test to occur.[19]

There are two ways to perform the SLR when the patient is supine. One is to have the contralateral leg fully extended lifting the ipsilateral leg. The second is to have the contralateral leg flexed at the hip and knee with the sole of the foot flat on the examining table. The results of the SLR test performed in the latter position most closely mimic results obtained when the test is performed in the sitting position.

In either the sitting or the supine position with the contralateral hip and knee flexed, sciatic pain will occur at an angle 10 to 20 degrees greater than when the contralateral leg is straight. This is a physiologic difference and not psychologic as is often thought. For consistency the examiner should perform the test the same way each time and record the position of the other leg.

If the patient has a history of unilateral leg pain, it is best to test the nonpainful leg first. A classic positive test is the production of pain in the ipsilateral thigh and/or calf when the leg is elevated to an angle of 20 to 60 degrees. Production of LBP is not considered a positive test but should be noted. Pain provoked before 20 degrees is often considered nonphysiologic, and pain provoked beyond 60 degrees is nonspecific. Pain provoked in the contralateral thigh and/or calf is a positive *crossed* SLR test and usually indicates a high degree of nerve-root irritation secondary to a large HNP. A positive crossed SLR associated with a poor response to conservative care.[13]

The SLR is also performed with the patient sitting on the edge of the examining table. A leg is grasped at the ankle by the examiner and slowly elevated while asking the patient to report any sensations that occur. The results obtained when the patient is sitting can be compared with those obtained with the patient supine. A patient may attempt to shift into lumbar extension near end-range of the SLR by leaning backward to use the arms for support, forming a tripod. This is considered a positive "flip test," which confirms nerve-root tension; it does not signify abnormal pain behavior.[8]

Obviously it is important to differentiate sciatica during SLR from hamstring tightness. In a classically positive test, sciatica is produced at about 45 degrees on one side while the other side has full range. In hamstring tightness, leg pain occurs at about the same angle on each leg and pain is confined to the posterior thigh and does not go below the knee.

Several tests can be used to confirm the findings of the classic SLR. One recommendation is to lower the leg several degrees to the angle just below where the patient experienced sciatica. Then dorsiflex the foot. A positive test is indicated by the reproduction of sciatica with foot dorsiflexion.

The bowstring test may be used as a confirmatory SLR test. It is performed with the patient either supine (usual) or sitting with the knee flexed to 70 degrees. The examiner places pressure in the midline of the popliteal fossa using digital compression. Production of pain in the thigh or calf of a typical sciatic type indicates a positive test.

The Lasegue maneuver is another confirmatory SLR test. The patient is supine with hip and knee flexed to 90 degrees. The knee is then slowly extended until sciatica is produced. Because both knee and hip joints are involved, this test is less valuable than the classic SLR.

Femoral Stretch Test

The classic femoral stretch test is done with the patient prone with the knees straight. The clinician grasps the leg and lifts it upward, perpendicular to the examining table, while keeping the knee straight and inquiring about any sensations produced. A positive test is the production of ipsilateral anterior thigh or groin pain in the leg and indicates irritation and/or compression of the L2 and/or L3 and/or L4 nerve roots. However, this test also causes pelvic rotation, increased lumbar lordosis, and hip extension, and may stress the sacroiliac joint. Therefore, LBP provoked during this test may arise from a facet joint, leg pain could be induced in spinal stenosis, and groin pain may reflect hip disease.

Prone Knee Bend

Some clinicians prefer the prone knee bend to the femoral stretch test. The examiner's hand is placed on the buttock to keep it in place. The hip remains in the extended position while the knee is flexed. A positive test is the production of ipsilateral anterior thigh pain. The left and right sides are compared. Quadriceps tightness may mimic a positive test but in this instance the left and right sides will be approximately symmetrical. It has been reported that production of sciatica during the prone knee bend is diagnostic of L4/L5 HNP.[4]

Bent Knee Pull

A variation of the above tests is called the "bent knee pull."[12] This test is done with the patient lying half prone at a 45 degree angle to the examination table. A positive test is reproduction of concordant anterior thigh or groin pain. However as with prone knee bend production of LBP is not specific and can have multiple sources. The bent knee pull also stresses the hip, knee, and SI joint which can cause confusion.

Sensory Examination

The sensory examination is performed for several reasons: to look for dermatomal sensory loss; to screen the lower sacral nerve roots; to look for peripheral neuropathy, sensory nerve entrapment syndromes, and neuropathic pain; and possibly to screen for psychologic problems. Sensation may be normal, decreased, or increased. Changes in sensation are completely subjective. In addition, sensory examination is very technique-dependent. The light touch of one examiner may be the deep pressure of another. Even under ideal conditions with the ideal patient and an expert clinician, sensory examination is not exact. Many patients complain of numbness but have normal sensation on examination.

The area of skin and subcutaneous tissue innervated by a spinal nerve is called a dermatome. However, dermatomes overlap and borders are not distinct. In addition, injury to a nociceptor can sensitize adjacent nociceptors and produce hyperalgesia or hyperesthesia in adjacent receptor fields.[7]

It is important to communicate the findings of the sensory examination using proper terminology.[1] The examiner may choose to describe the findings in a more descriptive fashion such as, "Decreased sensation to light touch over the lateral surface of the dorsum of the left foot." Current definitions of painful sensations as proposed by the International Association for the Study of Pain are presented in Table 7-4.

Light touch is performed using either fingertips of wisps of cotton. A clean pin that has not been used to examine other patients can be used to test superficial pain sensation. A pinwheel should not be used unless it is sterilized between patients, because of the potential risk of transmission of HIV or hepatitis viruses. Vibratory sense and proprioception should be tested if there is any suspicion of upper motor neuron disease from the history or other aspects of the examination. Temperature sensation can be checked with an alcohol swab.

The dermatomal sensory distribution is shown in Table 7-5. Perianal innervation is arranged in concentric rings. The innermost ring is S5, surrounded by S4, then S3, then S2. The penis and scrotum receive sensory innervation from S2 and S3.

There are also several peripheral neuropathic syndromes that mimic lumbar spine disorders. With peripheral neuropathy, the sensory abnormality has the distribution of a stocking. Often there is concomitant involvement of the hands in the distribution of a glove. There are painful neuropathies that can involve the lateral femoral cutaneous nerve and produce painful dysesthesia and numbness over a broad oval area of the lateral thigh in a nondermatomal distribution. The medial femoral cutaneous nerve syndrome (meralgia paresthetica) involves an area over the anteromedial thigh. The diagnosis is made by mapping out an area of hypoesthesia or allodynia or in the distribution of the appropriate cutaneous nerve.

Palpation

Palpation of the spine is occasionally useful in establishing a diagnosis. Most patients expect that the examiner will feel the spine, and if this part of the examination is not done, some patients may feel the examination was incomplete.

Table 7-4
Sensory examination: definitions of terms[1]

Term	Definition
Allodynia	Pain produced by a stimulus that does not normally cause pain
Anesthesia dolorosa	Pain in an area that is anesthetic
Dysesthesia	An *unpleasant* abnormal sensation—may be spontaneous or provoked
Hyperalgesia	Increased response to a stimulus that is normally painful
Hyperesthesia	Increased sensitivity to stimulation
Hypoalgesia	Diminished sensitivity to noxious stimulation
Hypoesthesia	Diminished sensitivity to stimulation
Paresthesia	A *not unpleasant* abnormal sensation, provoked or spontaneous
Trigger point	A hypersensitive tender area in muscle or connective tissue

Table 7-5
Sensory examination: dermatomal distribution

Nerve Root	Sensory Distribution
S1	Lateral foot
	Posterior-lateral calf
	Posterior thigh
L5	Dorsum of the foot, middle two thirds
	Volar aspect of the foot, lateral to the great toe
	Lower leg, lateral to the tibial sharp crest
	Lateral thigh
L4	Medial foot
	Lower leg, medial to the tibial sharp crest
	Distal anterior thigh
L3	Anteromedial thigh, middle one third

Palpate the muscles for tenderness and spasm. Referred pain can produce tender areas; direct tenderness is not definitive for locating the source of pain.

The spinous processes are readily palpable. Tenderness may identify the most painful motion segment but is nonspecific. The facet joints and laminae are not palpable directly owing to the interposed muscles and fasciae.[6] It is useful to try to palpate the lumbar spine via the abdominal approach if IDD is suspected. Many patients with IDD get reproduction of their usual LBP during palpation of the lumbar spine via the abdomen.

Brief palpation of the abdomen should be a part of the examination in most cases and is described below under the section on systemic examination. With respect to the lumbar spine, the lower lumbar disc spaces may be felt in thin individuals. The umbilicus is located approximately at the L3/4 disc space. It is often possible to feel the L4 and L5 disc spaces. Reproduction of concordant LBP during palpation may help suggest internal disc disruption.

The greater trochanter should be palpated for tenderness. If there is tenderness, and is it concordant with the patients's usual pain or is it discordant? If the pain is concordant, injection of the bursa with local anesthetic and corticosteroids should be considered to distinguish referred LBP versus greater trochanteric bursitis.

Other Joints

Many patients who have lumbar spine disorders complain of "pain in my hip." In fact they mean gluteal pain, which is a classic site for pain referred from the lumbar spine. Conversely, many patients initially think they have spinal problems when in fact pain arises from the hip joint. Therefore, it is important to evaluate the hip in all patients with LBP, especially if leg or groin pain is part of the complaint.

This hip should be put through a ROM examination while the patient is supine. The joint should be stressed through the FABER maneuver of hip flexion at 90 degrees, abduction, and external rotation. There should be unrestricted ROM and no pain. If concordant leg or groin pain is provoked, hip pathology must be considered.

The role of the sacroiliac joint (SI) in the production of lumbar pain is controversial. McCombe and associates found tests of the SI joint to be unreliable.[14] The Maitland test if frequently used to test for SI joint dysfunction.[14] The patient is asked to lie on the side with the upper hip flexed to 90 degrees and the lower hip extended. The clinician faces the patient and puts one hand on the anterior superior iliac crest and the heel of the other hand on the ischial tuberosity. The hands are pushed in opposite directions to cause rotation of the hemipelvis. Production of concordant pain is considered a positive test.

The SI joints can be compressed by the examiner placing one hand on each anterior superior iliac crest and pushing medially. A positive test is reproduction of concordant pain in the region of the SI joint.

The Gainslen's test is performed with the patient supine and with both legs drawn up to the knee-chest position. The patient is moved to the edge of the examining table so that one half of the buttock is on the table and the other half is off. The patient then allows the unsupported leg to slowly drop from the table while the supported leg remains with the hip flexed. Concordant pain in the SI region is considered a positive test.[11]

Systemic Examination

Palpation of the peripheral pulses is necessary in all patients who complain of extremity pain. This is particularly true in the elderly or in patients who have a history of coronary artery disease or stroke. Arterial claudication can mimic neurogenic claudication on first appraisal, but a detailed history will usually serve to differentiate the two. Feel the femoral pulses and auscultate for bruit. Palpate the popliteal, dorsalis pedis, and posterior tibial pulses. Check the capillary filling of the nail beds. If all of these are normal, it is unlikely that extremity pain is due to arterial insufficiency.

Examination of the abdomen is necessary if anything in the history suggests a visceral cause for LBP. Observe for distention, which is common after thoracolumbar compression fracture. Palpate for tenderness, mass, or organomegaly. Bowel sounds should be normal. An intrabdominal bruit may mean renal artery stenosis, which in turn may cause the examiner to consider aneurysm as the source of the LBP. Also palpate for a pulsatile mass, which could indicate an abdominal aneurysm.

The rectal examination is important to check for sphincter tone if there is any history of difficulty voiding or incontinence of urine or stool. Check for a mass, which might be colon cancer. In men the prostate should be felt for tumor. Intrapelvic pathology in women might be discovered during rectal examination.

Miscellaneous Tests

Press-ups

Press-ups are performed in patients with LBP for several reasons. Press-ups are formally part of an entire diagnostic and therapeutic regime proposed by McKenzie. In addition, this maneuver may be useful in patients with LBP that radiates to the buttocks, thigh, or calf who are suspected of having pain of discogenic origin. In situations in which there is an anular tear, bulge, or small HNP, press-ups may improve the pain. In patients with HNP with distal referral, pain that recedes from its distal or peripheral location to a proximal more localized site (centralization) during press-ups strongly correlates with successful conservative care.[5] Conversely, failure to centralize with press-ups may be an early predictor of the need for surgery for HNP.[5] In addition, centralization during press-ups implies that physical therapy should emphasize extension bias rather than flexion. Press-ups may increase the LBP of spinal stenosis and facet joints.

Thomas Test

The *Thomas Test* is used to identify hip flexion contractures.[11] The patient lies supine with hips and knees slightly flexed. The patient is asked to flatten the spine against the examining table and then to extend a leg straight. The inability to extend the leg fully without arching the thoracolumbar spine indicates a fixed hip flexion contracture.

Waddell Signs

Waddell has described five groups of signs that can be elicited during the physical examination that he believed were nonorganic in origin. These are discussed in more detail below. If three or more signs were present, it might indicate a patient who requires psychologic assessment.[21,22] The groups of signs that may suggest a functional component to the pain and disability are (1) superficial and nonanatomic *tenderness;* (2) *simulation tests* (axial loading and pelvis rotation); (3) *distraction* tests (SLR while the patient is distracted); (4) nonorganic *regional disturbances;* and (5) *overreaction.* Waddell found three or more signs to be present in 12% to 50% of patients in four different study groups. The prevalence was higher in patients with failed back surgery and in patients attending a problem-back clinic than in patients being seen for the first time. The evaluation, structural pathology, or psychologic abnormalities in the patients are not discussed.[22]

He believes that tenderness present over a wide area of skin in the lumbar region is nonorganic. Deep tenderness felt over a wide area was also felt to be nonorganic. The simulation tests are meant to trick the patient into thinking a particular structure is being examined and tested when in fact it is not. The first simulation text is axial loading, produced by pushing down on the patient's head. If LBP is produced it is considered nonorganic. The other simulation test is rotation. The patient stands with feet together and is rotated by the examiner at the pelvis, not the lumbar spine. Low-back pain produced is felt to be nonorganic, but leg pain may be secondary to root irritation and is discounted. Distraction tests are those that attempt to verify a positive physical finding from the usual examination when the patient is distracted. He recommends the SLR be done with the patient sitting and compared with the supine SLR. The examiner may seem to be examining the knee or doing a plantar response test while flexing the hip to 90 degrees and straightening the knee. This "incidental" SLR is compared with the formal SLR for gross discrepancy. Regional disturbances include nondermatomal sensory loss (which must be carefully distinguished from multiple dermatomal involvement) or weakness that is ratchety, collapsing, or cogwheel, especially if multiple muscles with differing innervation are involved. Lastly, overreaction during examination is abnormal, although Waddell admits to considerable cultural variations and states "it is very easy to introduce observer bias or to provoke this type of response unconsciously."[21,22]

Of all the signs, the highest correlation was with overreaction. Waddell admits this is the single finding which is most influenced by the subjectivity of the examiner. He also showed there was no correlation between the presence of these signs and patients involved in the worker's compensation system or personal injury litigation.

In this study, some subgroups underwent MMPI testing. The correlation was poor between an abnormal MMPI and the presence of multiple nonorganic signs. It must also be noted that this study was reported in 1980, before MRI or CT scanning was clinically available. There is no evidence presented in the paper regarding the presence or absence of lumbar disc pathology. There was no consistent evaluation of the patients presented.

Bradish and associates studied 120 patients with LBP of less than 6 months' duration.[3] They found no correlation between the presence of three or more Waddell signs and return to work. Other researchers have found the correlation to be significant.[20]

It may be useful to check for Waddell signs, but there is little evidence that their presence or absence can be used to direct treatment or predict outcome.

Conclusion

Successful diagnosis and treatment of a patient with spinal pain is like completing a puzzle. Each part of the evaluation is a piece of the puzzle. The physical examination has a major role in determining the etiology of the patient's pain and planning the course of further evaluation and treatment. A thorough examination also helps to build patient confidence. Therefore, all clinicians should be well versed in the physical examination and its interpretation.

References

1. Bonica JJ: *Definitions and taxonomy of pain*. In *The management of pain*, Philadelphia, 1990, Lea & Febiger, pp 18-27.
2. Borenstein DG, Weisel SW: *Low back pain: medical diagnosis and comprehensive management*, Philadelphia, 1989, W.B. Saunders.
3. Bradish CF, and others: Do nonorganic signs help to predict the return to activity of patients with low-back pain?, *Spine* 13:557-580, 1988.
4. Christodoulides AN: Ipsilateral sciatica on femoral nerve stretch test is pathognomonic of an L4/5 disc protrusion, *J Bone Joint Surg* 71/B:88-89, 1989.
5. Donelson R, Silva G, Murphy K: Centralization phenomenon: its usefulness in evaluating and treating referred pain, *Spine* 15:211-213, 1990.
6. Fairbank JC, Hall H: *History taking and physical examination: identification of syndromes of back pain*. In Weinstein JN, Wiesel SW, editors: *The lumbar spine*, Philadelphia, 1990, W.B. Saunders, pp 88-106.
7. Fields H: *Pain*. New York, 1987, McGraw-Hill.
8. Frymoyer JW, Haldeman S: *Evaluation of the worker with low back pain*. In Pope MH and others: *Occupational low back pain*. Chicago, 1991, C.V. Mosby, pp 151-182.
9. Grundy PF, Roberts CJ: Does unequal leg length cause back pain?: a case control study, *Lancet* 1:256-258, 1984.
10. Hadler NM: Regional back pain, *N Engl J Med* 315:1090-1092, 1986.
11. Hoppenfeld S: *Physical examination of the spine and extremities*, Norwalk, CT, 1976, Appleton & Lange.
12. Jabre JF, Bryan RW: Bent-knee pulling in the diagnosis of upper lumbar root lesions, *Arch Neurol* 39:669-670, 1982.
13. Khuffash B, Porter RW: Cross leg pain and trunk list, *Spine* 14:602-603, 1989.
14. McCombe PF and others: Reproducibility of physical signs in low-back pain, *Spine* 14:908-918, 1989.
15. Richards JS and others: Assessing pain behavior: the UAB Pain Behavior Scale, *Pain* 14:393-398, 1982.
16. Salovy P and others: Reporting chronic pain episodes on health surveys, *Vital Health Stat* 6(6), 1992.
17. Schofferman J, Zucherman J: History and physical examination, *Spine state Art Rev* 1:13-20, 1986.
18. Smith SA and others: Straight leg raising: anatomical effects on the spinal nerve root with and without fusion, *Spine* 18:992-999, 1993.
19. Thelander U and others: Straight leg raising test versus radiologic size, shape, and position of lumbar disc hernias, *Spine* 17:395-398, 1992.
20. Vallfors B: Acute, subacute and chronic low back pain: clinical symptoms, absenteeism and working environment, *Scand J Rehabil Med* 11:1-98, 1985.
21. Waddell G and others: Nonorganic physical signs in low-back pain, *Spine* 5:117-125, 1980.
22. Waddel G and others: Objective clinical evaluation of physical impairment in chronic low back pain, *Spine* 17:617-628, 1992.

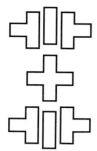

PART II

Basic Science

Chapter 8
Anatomy, Biochemistry, and Physiology of Low-Back Pain

Mamoru Kawakami
Kenichi Chatani
James N. Weinstein

Despite the high prevalence of the problem, the causes of low-back pain remain obscure in many instances. For the past 50 years much of the focus has been on the herniated intervertebral disc. Other potential sources of low-back pain include the nerve roots (including the spinal nerves and dorsal-root ganglion), the lumbar facet joints, and surrounding ligaments and tendons. When and how are the tissues involved in the generation of low-back pain and sciatica? And by what mechanisms are these structures painful? This chapter will attempt to explain with anatomical, neurochemical, and neurophysiologic reasons for the generation and perception of low-back pain.

Disc

Anatomy

Clinically, the concept of "disc pain" is well accepted. However, the inciting events and anatomic pathways by which this pain is generated and modulated remain in part hypothetical. In order for any structure to be a source of pain, it must be innervated. The presence of nerve fibers in the anulus of the intervertebral disc and in the adjacent ligaments has been demonstrated by many authors. Most have identified free nerve endings in the anterior and posterior longitudinal ligaments and in the superficial layers of the anulus fibrosus. Nociceptors have not been identified in the inner regions of the anulus fibrosus or nucleus pulposus.

Innervation of the Intervertebral Disc and Peridiscal Ligaments

The union of branching nerve fascicles from the distal pole of the dorsal-root ganglion (DRG) form the initial part of the spinal nerve, and/or the dorsal section of gray autonomic communicating ramus, the sinovertebral nerve (SVN, nerve of Luschka or ramus meningeus nervorum spinalium) at each vertebral level. The SVN innervates the ventral aspect of the dural sac, posterior longitudinal ligament, annulus fibrosus, blood vessels of the ventral compartment of the spinal canal and vertebral bodies. Branches of the SVN are seen in several structures related to the spinal canal. The inferiorly directed branch (descending branch) ramifies over the dorsum of the disc and posterior longitudinal ligament at the level of nerve entry into the canal. The longer superior branch (ascending branch) courses along the lateral margin of the posterior longitudinal ligament to reach the disc of the nextmost cephalad level and

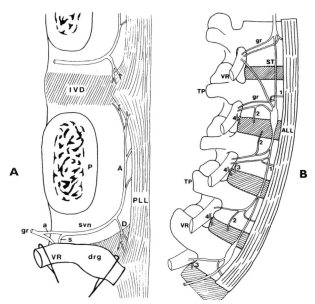

Fig. 8-1

Innervation of lumbar spine. **A,** Left lumbar sinovertebral nerve (*SVN*). **B,** Types of nerves innervating anterior and lateral aspects of lumbar vertebral column. *1* = branch to anterior longitudinal ligament; *2* = branches to lateral aspect of intervertebral disc; *3* = branches to intervertebral disc from gray rami; *4* = branches to intervertebral disc from ventral rami; *a* = autonomic root; *A* = ascending branches; *ALL* = anterior longitudinal ligament; *D* = descending branches; *drg* = dorsal-root ganglion; *gr* = gray rami communicantes; *IVD* = intervertebral disc; *P* = pedicle of vertebra; *PLL* = posterior longitudinal ligament; *s* = somatic root; *ST* = sympathetic trunk; *TP* = transverse process; *VR* = ventral ramus. *(From Bogduk N: The innervation of the lumbar spine, Spine 8:286, 1983.)*

overlaps the innervation of the SVN descending branch of the segment above (Fig. 8-1, *A*).[13] The inability to localize the pain of an offending disc may be related to the rather generous distribution of a single SVN and the poor cerebral representation. The lateral and anterior posrtion of the anulus fibrosis are not innervated by the SVN, but rather by nerve fibers from both ventral rami and gray rami communicans (Fig. 8-1, *B*). It remains controversial whether the annulus itself is innervated. Hirsh[52] and Jackson et al.[60] found nerve endings in the posterior longitudinal ligament and only on the dorsal aspect of the most superficial layer of the anulus. Roofe,[114] Wiberg,[148] Ikari,[58] Pedersen et al.,[111] Stilwell,[133] and Parke[108] failed to demonstrate nerve endings in the anulus. Hirsch and Schajowicz[51] postulated that the fissuring of the pathologic disc permits the invasion of granulation tissue, followed by an ingrowth of nociceptive opinion into these metaplastic regions. Shinohara[129] supported their opinion and demonstrated that with degenerative tissues are seen fibroblastic tissue that later receives an ingrowth of nerve endings.

However, this concept has fallen into disfavor since Malinsky,[84] Bogduk et al.,[15] and Yoshizawa et al.[155] have published accounts demonstrating nerve endings in the external third of the annulus in cadaveric specimens and half that depth in surgically removed specimens. Mendel et al.[92] found receptors resembling Pacinian corpuscles and Golgi tendon organs in the posterolateral region of the upper third of the human cervical disc. Discs may be supplied with both nerve endings and mechanoreceptors. Immunohistochemical methodology has permitted a new look at neural elements in spinal tissues. This method can easily demonstrate which of the neurotransmitters or neuromodulators are present within a nerve. Weinstein et al.[146] identified substance P, calcitonin gene–related peptide (CGRP) and vasoactive intestinal polypeptide (VIP) (all chemicals related to pain perception) immunoreactive nerves among the outer annular fibers of the rat disc (see Plate L). Coppes et al.[21] showed evidence of penetration of immunohistochemically demonstrative nerves into deeper parts of degenerated discs. The posterior longitudinal ligament is highly innervated with both complex encapsulated nerve endings and numerous poorly myelinated free nerve endings. Many of the smaller fibers are postganglionic efferents from the thoracolumbar autonomic ganglia that mediate the smooth muscle control of the various vascular elements within the spinal canal. A number of the large fibers are involved in proprioceptive functions. However, it appears that the smaller nerve fibers that make up the greater bulk of the SVN afferents associated with the simple, nonencapsulated or free nerve endings are generally regarded as nociceptive. The anterior longitudinal ligament is supplied by gray rami communicantes or a branch from the sympathetic chain. Immunohistochemical studies have demonstrated substance P, encephalin, dopamine β-hydroxylase and choline acetyltransferase immunoreactive nerve fibers among the anterior and posterior longitudinal ligaments surgically removed in human cervical and lumbar spine (Fig. 8-2).[65] Grönblad et al.[48] also found abundant neurofilament triple protein, CGRP, substance P immunoreactive nerves in the peripheral of human anterior and posterior longitudinal ligament. Nociceptors are the peripheral terminal endings of sensory neurons that are selectively responsive to potentially or overtly harmful injuries. Stimulation of nociceptors can cause pain in humans and cause affective painlike responses in an-

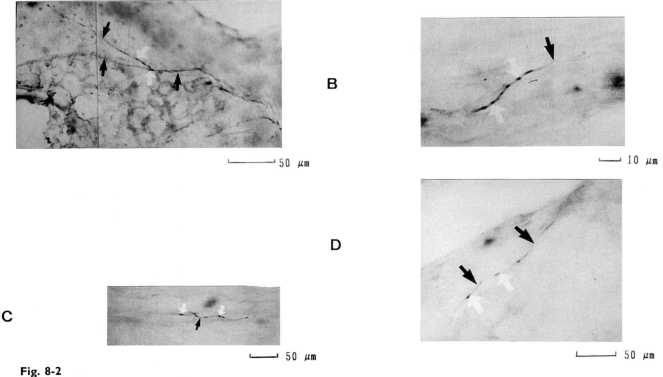

Fig. 8-2
Immunohistochemical demonstrations of immunoreactive nerve fibers in anterior and posterior longitudinal ligaments of human spine. **A,** Substance P. **B,** Methionine encephalin. **C,** Dopamine E-hydroxylase. **D,** Choline acetyltransferase. *(From Kawakami M: Histochemical and immunohistochemical demonstrations of nerve fibers on human perispinal soft tissue, J Wakayama Med Soc 40:621, 1989 [in Japanese].)*

imals. These nerves are likely to be involved in the perception of discogenic back pain and may become sensitized when disc tissue is injured. This is supported by the observations of Kuslich et al.[70] that stimulation to the central anulus and posterior longitudinal ligament produced central-back pain during surgery on the lumbar spine using local anesthesia. Disc protrusion or mechanical deformation may elevate and therefore stimulate these highly innervated connective tissues that contribute in part to the perception of low-back pain.

Biochemistry

Aging Versus Degeneration

The major structural components of intervertebral discs are proteoglycan, collagen, and water, which comprise up to 90% to 95% of the volume of a normal disc. Many authors have described biochemical changes with aging and degeneration in intervertebral discs.[*] In summary, as age and degeneration advance, the total proteoglycan content decreases, the keratan sulfate:chondroitin sulfate ratio increases, and the aggregation ratio decreases. The decrease in proteoglycan content results in the loss of water, and these changes are most remarkable in the nucleus pulposus. There is an alteration in the array of collagen subtypes; type II collagen is replaced by type I, and type III collagen appears. Irreducible cross linking in collagen accumulates with age. The intervertebral disc undergoes the most marked age-related changes in composition and structure of all connective tissue. Although the changes occur earlier and to a greater extent in intervertebral discs than in other organs, if the changes occur uniformly in an age-matched population and are asymptomatic, then they should not be regarded as pathologic. Many previous attempts to differentiate aging changes from degenerative changes have proven difficult. However, it is important to understand the difference between aging changes and pathologic changes that are related to low-back pain.

Some studies have described observations concerning differences between aging changes and pathologic changes. The difference in degrading enzyme patterns between normal intervertebral discs and prolapsed discs has been reported.[101] In normal discs, the major collagenolytic activity is against type II collagen and 1α, 2α, 3α-collagen. There is little

enzyme activity toward type I collagen and virtually none toward elastin. This enzyme's pattern is not variable with aging. In prolapsed discs, on the other hand, there are elastinolytic activity and more collagenolytic activity against type I collagen than aging type II collagen or 1α, 2α, 3α-collagen. Unfortunately, however, it is uncertain whether this alternation of enzyme patterns in prolapsed discs is the cause or the result. Intervertebral discs at a level of spondylolisthesis have lower rates of proteoglycan synthesis than those of other discs in the same spine. No differences in proteoglycan synthesis rates related to disc level are evident for the other spinal disorders.[9] However, it is uncertain whether these changes in spondylolisthesis represent the cause or the effect. "Isolated disc resorption"[23,62,140] should be distinguished from aging changes because it generally occurs at only one disc level, and the heights of other discs remain almost intact.[14] To explain isolated disc resorption, it has been proposed that a trigger such as an end-plate fracture activates endogenous proteolytic enzymes. These enzymes are normally present in the disc[86,91,98,99,124] but are ordinarily inhibited by proteinase inhibitors.[91] Another hypothesis in that following an end-plate fracture the nucleus pulposus elicits an autoimmune response.[14]

Facet

Anatomy

Adjacent vertebral arches are joined together by a superior and inferior articular process to form the facet joint, which allows a gliding type of motion. At various levels, facet orientation helps to limit the mechanical range of the motion segment. With aging, the anterior aspect of concave surfaces of facet joints becomes thickened. Cells hypertrophy, and vertical cartilage fibrillation and sclerotic changes that suggest compressive loads are noted in the anterior medial aspect. In the posterior two thirds of the joint, the cartilage appears to split parallel to the cartilage-bone interface, which forms a meniscus-like structure. Ultimately, there may be denuding of articular surfaces in the posterior aspect, whereas vertical fibrillation, thickening of the cartilage, and sclerotic changes, suggesting continued vertical stress loading, may continue in the anterior medial aspect.[138] The formation of osteophytes occurs at the joint margins at the attachment of the ligamentum flavum or the capsule.

The facet joints are very important biomechanically. Adams and Hutton[1,2] demonstrated that the facet joints take between 16% and 20% of the com-

*References 3, 4, 30, 44, 49, 82, and 139.

pressive load in the spine. These same facets are relatively unloaded in sitting.[1] Yang and King[153] noted that excessive facet loads caused the inferior facet to "bottom out" on the pars and then to begin to pivot about the pars to stretch the joint capsule. Thus, the facet joint does not itself take the increasing loads, but rather the capsule and the skeletal structures of the pars take them. The facet capsules are primarily loaded in flexion and in rotation, whereas facet joints themselves are the primary resistors against rotational or torsional force.[2]

There is a major disagreement about whether the facet joints participate with the disc in tolerating the stresses of function. Lewin[78] found that facet joint arthritis occurred occasionally independently of the disc degeneration. Videman et al.[141] noted that in 20 percent of cadaver discograms, which were normal by discography, degenerative changes were noted in the facet joints from narrowing of the disc

space. Stress to the facet joints may be completely independent of structural overload to the lumbar disc.[94] On the other hand, only in extension do the facets share significant compressive loads with the discs.[2] There appears to be a close correlation between intervertebral disc height, facet loads, and degenerative change.[42] The work of Jackson[61] demonstrated that in rotation, the facet joints protect the disc from torsional forces to which the disc is very susceptible while in active extension, the facets can function as a fulcrum to help unload the spinal column, thereby decreasing disc protrusions and perhaps pain.

The grow anatomic distribution of nerve supply to the facet joint was clearly described by Oudenhoven (Fig. 8-3).[106] The facet joint is innervated by the medial branch of the dorsal ramus from three levels: the direct branch to facet exiting the intervertebral foramen at the same level as the facet joint, as-

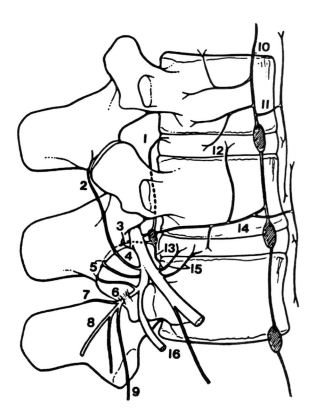

Fig. 8-3

Neuroanatomic definition of lumbar motion segment. *1* = ascending branch of sinovertebral nerve; *2* = ascending facet branch; *3* = sinovertebral to facet; *4* = direct branch to facet; *5* = branches to multifidus; *6* = medial branch of posterior primary ramus; *7* = local facet branch; *8* = descending facet branch; *9* = branch to sacroiliac; *10* = sympathetic chain; *11* = branch under anterior longitudinal ligament; *12* = branches from gray ramus to disc; *13* = sinovertebral to disc; *14* = gray ramus communicans; *15* = branches from anterior primary ramus to disc; *16* = lateral branch of posterior primary ramus. *(From Mooney V: Facet syndrome. In Weinstein JN, Wiesel SW, editors: The lumbar spine, Philadelphia, 1990, W.B. Saunders Co., p 422.)*

cending facet branch exiting the foramen one level below the facet joint and descending facet branch exiting the foramen one level above the facet joint. Thus, complete denervation of one segment may require all three levels to destroy the multiple innervation.[94] It is possible for an autonomic nerve supply to travel with the segmental innervation of facet joints.[13] The fibrous capsule of the facet joint contains encapsulated, unencapsulated, and free nerve endings. Some investigators have demonstrated immunoreactive nerve fibers for substance P,[6,41,65] CGRP,[6] and VIP,[6] all of which have been proposed as mediators or modulators of nociception; and dopamine β-hydroxylase and choline acetyltransferase,[65] which are representative of the sympathetic and cholinergic nervous systems, respectively. Encephalin has been identified in surgically removed human facet joint capsules.[65] Electrophysiologic studies[152] also suggest a presence of nociceptive nerves. Giles and Taylor[40] reported nerves in capsular tissue and synovial folds using silver and gold impregnation. Grönblad et al.[47] observed nerves, which were mainly perivascular, in the synovial folds and nerves with no topographic relationship to blood vessels very near fat tissue. They may be mechanosensitive in nature. Most of these nerves did not demonstrate immunoreactivity to substance P, CGRP, or galanin. Grönblad et al.[47] suggested that plical folds contain nerves involved in vasoregulation but not in sensory innervation. Beaman et al.[10] found substance P nerve fibers within subchondral bone of degenerative lumbar facet joints but not control facet joints. Thus, it appears that the facet joints are sufficiently innervated to create noxious stimuli and may be a source of spine-related symptoms.

Biochemistry

With aging, the deterioration mode of the articular surfaces of the facet joints may be expressed as osteoarthritis. Traditionally osteoarthritis is thought to be directly related to biomechanical factors.[37] Subjective loading, however, is only one factor related to collagen fatigue and secondary subchondral fractures, both of which are accelerated during aging and/or osteoarthritis. The chemical and biologic events involved, however, are less well understood.

As previously stated, nerve fibers that contain neuropeptides (i.e., substance P, CGRP, VIP, etc.) exist in and around the facet joints and capsules. Neuropeptides are transported to peripheral endings of nociceptive afferents as a result of noxious chemical or physical stimulation and can influence the inflammatory process.[109] Substance P is believed to act directly on the blood vessels to produce plasma extravasation and indirectly to produce vascular dilatation by release histamine. Antihistamines and substance P antibodies block the flare induced by histamine; however, it seems that substance P antagonists do not affect the flare produced by capsaicin, suggesting that the final vasodilator is not histamine. CGRP is colocalized with substance P and is a potent vasodilator.[74] CGRP has also been implicated as a mediator in early stages of arthritis.[68] Neuropeptides are also known to stimulate the release from mast cells of leukotrienes and other factors that attract and stimulate polymorphonuclear leukocytes and monocytes.[110] Substance P is released into joint tissues and stimulates proliferation of rheumatoid synovial sites and their release of prostaglandin E_2 and collagenase, thereby implicating this peptide in the pathogenesis of rheumatoid arthritis.[81] Substance P levels are higher in joints with more severe arthritis, and infusion of the neuropeptide into joints with mild disease has been shown to accelerate the degenerative process.[75] When acute inflammation is induced, afferent receptors that are normally silent during joint motion become responsive to previously innocuous stimuli, including motion in the normal range. A similar sensitizing effect is produced by intraarticular infusion of prostaglandins or bradykinin,[100,123] providing further evidence that local sensitization is at least partly responsible for the pain felt in arthritis or inflamed joints.

Thus, these chemicals and inflammatory and immunologic alterations have been directly linked to proteolytic and collagenolytic enzymes known to cause cartilage matrix degradation and osteoarthritis. In the injury and repair cascade, the matrix calls attempt to increase synthesis by increasing cellular proliferation.[113] To help explain the interactions of biomechanics and biochemistry that effect a biologic response, the "degenerative (aging) spiral" hypothesis may be helpful (Fig. 8-4).[145] This model is as follows: The release of neuropeptides from the dorsal-root ganglion, induced by environmental and structural factors (i.e., vibrations), mediates a progressive degeneration of the functional spinal unit structures by stimulating the synthesis of inflammatory agents (e.g., cytokines, prostaglandin E_2), and degradative enzymes (e.g., proteases, collagenase). As a direct or indirect result of these chemical interactions secondary changes in mechanical properties occur that then perpetuate this "degenerative or aging spiral."

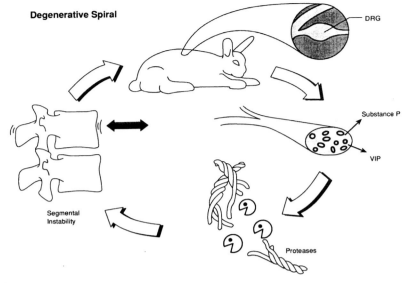

Fig. 8-4

In "degenerative spiral," functional spinal unit may undergo degeneration as result of interaction of mechanical and chemical stimuli seen in injured or environmentally stimulated functional spinal unit. *(From Weinstein JN:* Anatomy and neurophysiologic mechanism of spinal pain. *In Frymoyer JW, et al., editors:* The adult spine: principles and practice, *New York, 1991, Raven Press, p 593.)*

Facet Pain

In 1911 Goldthwait first stated that the apophyseal joints were responsible for low-back pain and instability.[42] Since the phrase *facet syndrome* was first introduced by Ghormley in 1933,[39] many studies followed showing that the facet joint can be a significant cause of low-back pain.[28,93,126] Lewis and Kellgren,[76] Lewin et al.,[77] and Hirsh[52] demonstrated that typical low-back pain, as well as radiation of pain into the posterior thigh, can be induced by injecting hypertonic saline into the facet joint capsules. Facet joint pain may have an inflammatory component and is sometimes treated with a local injection of corticosteroids and/or anesthetic. Cavanaugh and colleagues[17,18,152] have studied the neurophysiology of the lumbar facet joint by using experimental inflammation models. The results of their studies indicated that (1) The facet joint capsule contains low- and high-threshold mechanoreceptors, the low-threshold receptors being probable proprioceptors and the high-threshold probable nociceptors. (2) The surrounding deep back musculotendinous units contain the same type of receptors. (3) Neurons of these spinal tissues are chemosensitive. (4) Loading the spine activates low-threshold units, high threshold units and phasic units. (5) Spine loading or mechanical stimulation does not maintain the discharge of putative nociceptors but chemical mediators do maintain this in the posterior elements in this model.[18] These investigations suggest that facet joint pathology plays an important role in low-back pain.

The clinical picture of facet syndrome is variable. According to provocation studies for patients with low-back pain[93] and volunteers who had no history of back pain,[89] there seems to be no specific pain pattern that would clearly identify the facet joint over other potential sources of noxious neural stimulation. Namely, the pattern of pain was an unreliable predictor of anatomic location.[94] Although Lippitt[80] has proposed diagnostic criteria for facet syndrome, only 66% in this clear group of patients responded at all. Therefore, it is difficult for clinicians to decide whether the patient has pure facet initiated pain. Jackson[60] reported that the facet was not a common or clear source of significant pain, and the facet syndrome is not a reliable clinical diagnosis, based on a review of the literature and his clinical studies.

These neuroanatomic, biochemical, neurophysiologic, and pathologic changes suggest that any incidence of pain in back and leg without radiculopathy can be emerging from a deranged facet joint. However, the role of the facet joints in the production of low-back pain clinically remains obscure.

Referred Pain

The intervertebral disc and/or the facet joint may be the primary source in the production of low-back, buttock, and leg pain. Why do the disc and facet

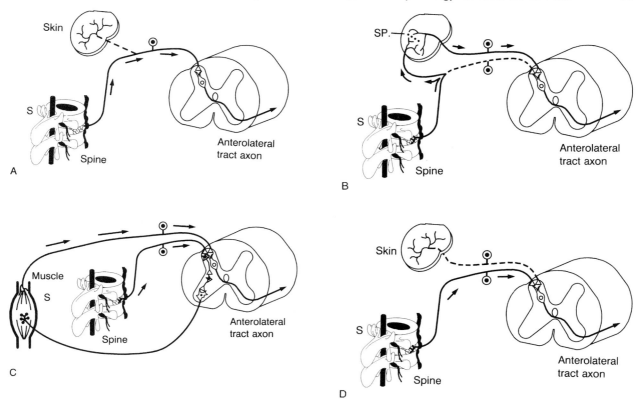

Fig. 8-5

Theories of referred pain. **A,** Branched primary afferent. Single primary afferent branches to supply both deep structure stimulated and structure in which pain is perceived. **B,** Referred pain caused by antidromic activation of receptors at distant secondary site. **C,** Referred pain resulting from reflex muscle contraction that causes activation of distant secondary site. **D,** Convergence-projection theory. Visceral afferent nociceptors converge on same pain projection neurons as afferents from somatic structures in which pain is perceived. *(From Fields HL: Theories of the mechanism of referred pain. In Fields HL, editor: Pain, San Francisco, 1987, McGraw-Hill Book Co., p 89.)*

joint cause low-back pain? The phenomenon of referred pain is defined as pain experienced at a site remote from its source. Hirsh et al.[50] reported that hypertonic saline injected into the disc produced severe pain, "identical to real lumbago," that could not be localized but that was described as a deep aching across the low back. Greenbard et al.[46] demonstrated that of patients whose lateral annulus was mechanically probed under epidural anesthesia. 71% had some pain and 30% had significant pain by this procedure. Kuslich et al.[70] used progressive regional anesthesia in 193 consecutive patients undergoing decompression surgery for herniated disc or lumbar spinal stenosis. Significant pain was reported by 30% of patients on stimulation of the central lateral annulus and by 15% on central anulus stimulation with blunt surgical instruments or electrical current of low voltage. Using injection of hypertonic saline into muscle and the region around joints and periosteum, extensive maps have been constructed showing the consistent segmental pattern of pain referral for these structures.[59,67] Steindler and Luck[132]

did offer direct evidence that referred pain could come from the facet joint using local anesthetic injection and relief of back pain.

Theories of the Mechanism of Referred Pain[33]

Branched Primary Afferent

In order to explain how the segmental convergence of primary afferents results in the mislocalization of sensory input from deep structures, Sinclair et al.[130] advocated that a single primary afferent fiber branch supplied two structures—one visceral and one somatic (Fig. 8-5, *A*). Since in referred pain there is no nociceptive input from the painful site, the brain has referred the sensation to the unstimulated site or structure. Impulses elicited in the branch of the nociceptor innervating the stimulated structure could antidromically invade the other branch, which innervates the unstimulated structure (Fig. 8-5, *B*). The nociceptors in that structure could be sensitized by the chemicals released by the antidromic impulses in the branch. Those sensitized nociceptors could then respond to innocuous stimuli, and pain would be produced. Two premises are needed to prove this theory. (1) Is there anatomically a primary afferent fiber to supply both visceral and somatic tissues? Laurberg and Sorensen[73] found that approximately 1% of cervical DRG cells had two branches supplying both the diaphragm and the shoulder. Also, Alles and Dom[5] demonstrated morphologically that peripheral sensory nerve fibers supplied both the arm skin and the pericardium. (2) Can the antidromic impulses cause the release of nociceptive substances? The DRG cells produce a variety of neuropeptides. Substance P, neurokinins A and B, CGRP, somatostatin, VIP, bombesin, etc. are contained in the DRG cells. These neurotransmitters are transported by the axonal flow, stored at the spinal cord and distal nerve endings. They act as transmitters or modulators, which are released from the endings in the spinal cord by the impulse. Those related to peripheral nerve endings by the antidromic impulses result in focal vasodilation and edema.

Reflex Activation of Nociceptors (Fig. 8-5 C)

Input from visceral nociceptors is known to produce a powerful and sustained reflex muscle contraction[76] and often leads to the development of a secondary source of nociceptive input from the contracting muscles. Noxious input can also elicit a significant increase in sympathetic outflow. Sympathetic efferent activity can produce pain. The noxious input can reflexively induce sympathetic activity that in turn activates or sensitizes peripheral nociceptors. The reflex activation of somatic motor and sympathetic outflow may sustain and intensify pain.

Perceptual Projection (Fig. 8-5, D)

At present, the most widely accepted explanation of referred pain is the "convergence-projection" theory of Ruch.[115] This theory is based on a hypothesis that nociceptive primary afferent fibers innervating visceral organs enter the same spinal segment as the nociceptive somatic afferents innervating the body region to which pain from that organ is referred. In support of this theory, spinothalamic tract cells have been identified that receive convergent input from both visceral structures and cutaneous nociceptors.[19] Furthermore, there is evidence for a specific segmental relationship between the visceral and somatic nociceptive input that converges on spinal neurons.[34] Because of the protected location of the viscera, the spinothalamic neuron is more frequently activated by somatic stimulation during activities of daily living and consequently over time the brain comes to associate activity in that spinothalamic tract cell with somatic stimulation. Subsequently, when visceral afferents activate the spinothalamic tract cell, the brain misinterprets the message and localizes the course of activity as the somatic structure. According to the convergence-projection theory, the mislocalization of sensations arising from stimulation of deep structures results from both their sparse innervation and the fact that their afferent innervation converges onto sensory projection neurons that also receive input from segmentally related somatic structures.

Pain Pathways and Modulation

Nerve Root

Compression of nerve roots is thought to be responsible for a number of neurophysiologic changes. These include the biomechanics of nerve and nerve-root injury, intraneural blood-flow alterations, increased vascular permeability leading to intraneural edema, effects on axonal transport, inflammation accompanied by demyelination, and atrophy with wallerian degeneration followed by regeneration (see box below).[144]

Neurophysiologic Changes after Compression of Nerve Roots

- Biomechanics of nerve-root injury
- Intraneural blood-flow alterations
- Increased vascular permeability
- Effects on axonal transport
- Inflammation accompanied by demyelination
- Atrophy with wallerian degeneration accompanied by regeneration

The nerve roots in the thecal sac, unlike a peripheral nerve, generally lack epineurium and perineurium, yet under tensile loading exhibit both elasticity and tensile strength.[136] The mechanical properties of a human spinal nerve root are different depending on its location within the central canal and/or the lateral intervertebral foramen. Ultimate loads are approximately five times higher for foraminal segments of spinal nerve roots than or the intrathecal portion of the same nerve roots under tensile loading.[71] The ligaments of Hoffmann connect the anterior dura to the posterior longitudinal ligament and vertebral periosteum, acting as a tether to nerve roots. Disc herniation or other types of anterior compression may produce significant nerve-root impingement without compression of the nerve root against the posterior elements.[131]

Evans[29] demonstrated that pain may be related to radicular ischemia as the reduction of oxygen intake in patients with neurogenic claudication exacerbates the symptoms. However, studies on the intrinsic vasculature of the nerve root suggest that the venous side of the system may be the more vulnerable to the spatial restriction of the spinal canal.[108,142] In the pig lumbosacral spine microscopy of the nerve roots has shown that compression of the nerve roots at very low pressures (about 5 to 10 mm Hg) induces pronounced acute changes on the intraneural microcirculation in terms of venous congestion.[104] Total ischemia in the compressed nerve-root segments was induced at about 130 mm Hg, which correlated well with the mean arterial blood pressure of the experimental animal. LaBan[72] noted that patients with diminished right ventricular activity and spinal stenosis may eventually have neurogenic pain even in static or recumbent positions. He attributed this to increased external pressure on the already sensitized roots by engorgement of the epidural venous sinuses. Madsen and Heros[83] showed that "arterialization" of spinal veins by abnormal arteriovenous shunts in the region of the conus medullaris exacerbated the neurogenic pain in patients with spinal stenosis. They suggested that dilated epidural veins and direct increased resistance to radicular circulation by venous hypertension might contribute to the manifestations of neurogenic claudication.

Because nerve roots lack a well-developed endoneural blood-nerve barrier, they are hypothetically more susceptible to compression injury than peripheral nerves, with increased risk of endoneural edema formation. Intraneural edema, seen on fluorescence microscopy by extravasation of albumin labeled with Evans blue, was induced after compression at 50 mm Hg for 10 minutes. When the pressure was applied slowly, however, the intraneural edema formation was less pronounced.[103] In the cauda equina, however, edema in the nerve roots may not necessarily lead to increased endoneural fluid pressure and secondary ischemia as in peripheral nerves because of the absence of a perineural diffusion barrier in the nerve roots.[118,120]

Axoplasmic transport is an energy-dependent process that can be blocked by either ischemia or compression. Analysis of the transport of tritium-labeled methylglucose to the nerve-root tissue during graded compression showed that solute transport

was reduced about 45% when compressed at 10 mm Hg.[102] Compression of nerve at 30 mm Hg and above can block axoplasmic transport.[24] Compression at 100 mm Hg for 2 hours impaired nerve impulse conduction of sensory nerve roots by 75%. This was greater than was seen in the motor nerve roots, which were impaired by 55%. Motor recovery was seen to be more rapid and more complete than sensory recovery after release of pressure.[112] If the distance between two compression sites was increased from one vertebral segment to two vertebral segments, the reduction of muscle action potential amplitude was further enhanced.[105] Chronic blockade of axoplasmic transport may lead to wallerian degeneration of a distal axon. Nerve injury may also interfere with transport of neurotrophic factors from the periphery to the cell body and may produce chromatolysis and/or death of cell body.[45] Thus, interference with axoplasmic transport may produce degeneration both centrally and peripherally.

Inflammation of the nerve-root tissue is a significant factor that has to be present in order for mechanical nerve-root deformation to induce radiating pain. Myelograms[53] and computer-assisted tomographic (CAT, or CT) scans[149] showed that spinal nerve-root compression need not cause leg pain in all circumstances. CT scans following sciatic pain relief after chemonucleolysis demonstrate that pain abatement can occur despite continued mechanical compression.[16] Greenbard et al.[46] reported that compressed inflamed nerve roots in patients undergoing laminectomy and disc excision under epidural anesthesia were very sensitive to mechanical manipulation. Kuslich et al.[70] reported similar findings in patients with back pain undergoing progressive local anesthesia. Stimulation of stretched, compressed, or swollen nerve roots caused significant pain in 90% of 167 patients. Only 9% of cases of normal nerve-root stimulation produced significant pain. It seems, therefore, that the nature of inflammation in or around nerve roots is likely to be characterized by edema, inflammatory cell reaction, and local demyelination.[116] Breakdown products from degenerating nucleus pulposus tissue might leak into the epidural space and induce a "chemical radiculitis" along the nerve root.[87,88] Furthermore, degenerating disc material may produce an acidic environment that may, in part, promote adhesion formations around the nerve root.[95] Application of normal, nondegenerated, autologous nucleus pulposus induced a local inflammatory reaction when applied epidurally in dogs.[90] "Chemical radiculitis" may be significant in the pathophysiology of nerve-root pain. "Radiculitis" may be initiated by directly irritating effects of proteoglycans from the disc[87] and/or by an autoimmune reaction from exposure to disc tissues.[12,38]

In an electrophysiologic study in anesthetized cats, Janig and Koltzenburg[63] reported 14 mechanosensitive units with conduction velocities in the C-fiber range whose receptive fields were to sacral dorsal roots and whose afferent projections were to sacral dorsal roots in the same level. These findings demonstrate a pain pathway through excitation of nervi nervorum on ventral roots and suggest this as a possible mechanism of radicular pain.

The functional changes induced may be either loss of nerve function, seen as sensory deficits and muscle weakness, or a state of hyperexcitability of the nerve tissue; the latter phenomenon may increase nerve activity in terms of pain or paresthesia (Fig. 8-6).[117]

Compression of roots or ganglia was associated with increased amounts of connective tissue around the Schwann cells, signs of axonal and myelin degeneration, and proliferation of Schwann cells. More proximal lesions are associated with more profound degeneration of the cell body, and lesions central to the DRG do not have a regenerative potential equivalent to that of lesions peripheral to the ganglion.[134,135] Therefore, an injury proximal to the DRG may produce serious and less reversible neurologic injury than an analogous injury in the periphery.[144]

Dorsal-root Ganglion

Anatomic studies focused on compression of the DRG indicate that it plays a significant role as a modulator of low-back pain.[79] The epineurally located receptors, such as nervi nervorum, appear to respond in a similar way to cutaneous nociceptors in the peripheral nervous system.[125] Therefore, the epineurium of the dorsal-root ganglion may be directly activated by compression or mechanical stimulation of these receptors. Neurophysiologic findings[26,56] suggested that the elevated excitability of the dorsal-root ganglion is a design compromise. It contributes to reliable afferent impulse propagation past the ganglion but makes the system a likely site of ectopic impulse generation, which can lead to dysesthesia and pain. Devor and Wall[27] reported that spontaneous dorsal-root ganglion firing increased substantially the repetitive stimulation of neighboring axons, a phenomenon that could contribute to sensory abnormalities, including spatial effects such as referred pain and temporal effects, such as aftersensation and wind-up. The failure of C fibers to exhibit cross-excitation limits is significant in pain states. The venous and arterial vascular supply of the dorsal-root ganglion must play a significant role in its function. Bergmann and Alexander[11] suggest that the aging and concomitant vascular changes of the dorsal-root ganglion are associated with degeneration and changes in vibratory sensation. Yoshizawa et al.[154] have shown that mechanical compression of the extradural nerve root disturbs the blood flow in the distal side of the compression and provokes a reduction of the blood flow to a certain extent, not only in the distal part of the nerve root but also in the DRG, suggesting that clinical symptoms derived from the DRG may exist even when it is not compressed directly. Rydevik et al.[119] suggest that it may be a "vascular phenomenon,"

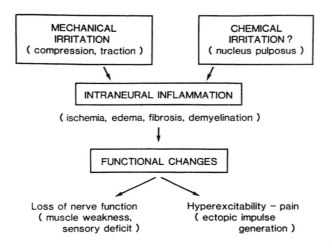

Fig. 8-6

Proposed sequence of events leading to intraneural tissue reaction. Functional changes in compressed nerve roots include loss of nerve function, seen as sensory deficits and/or muscle weakness, and hypersensitivity of the nerve tissue, which may be related to pain. *(From Rydevik B, Garfin S: Spinal nerve root compression. In Szabo RM, editor: Nerve compression syndromes: diagnosis and treatment, New York, 1989, Slack Medical Publishers, p 247.)*

Plate 1-1

Anulus fibrosis of rat disc demonstrating **A**, substance P; **B**, calcitonin gene-related peptide (CGRP); and **C**, vasoactive intestinal polypeptide (VIP), by immunohistochemical staining. (From Weinstein J., Claverie W., Gibson S: The pain of discography, *Spine* 13:1344, 1988.)

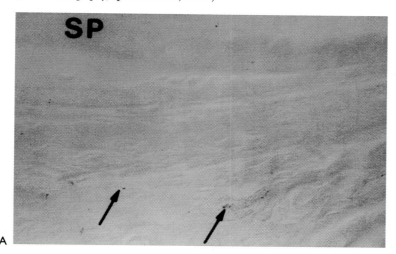

A

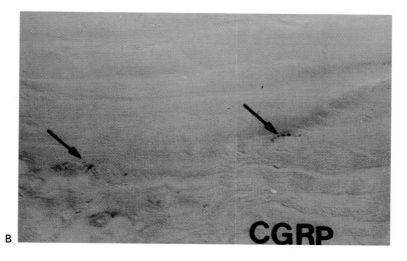

B

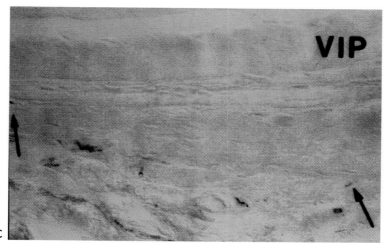

C

wherein the well-vascularized dorsal-root ganglion compromised by a herniated disc or spinal stenosis can cause increased intraneural pressures suggestive of a compartment syndrome. The spinal stenosis model of Delamarter et al. demonstrated that neurogenic claudication appears to begin with venous congestion of the nerve roots and dorsal-root ganglion distal to the induced construction.[25] Secondary to vascular compression cellular degeneration occurs that alters the chemical and neurophysiologic response of the nerve and nerve roots.

The neurogenic and nonneurogenic mediators play a fundamental role in the perception and modulation of pain.[144] The interrelationships between the neurogenic and nonneurogenic mediators in the injury and repair process are important to keep in mind when considering the degenerative spiral of osteoarthritis.[145] Tissue injury activates nerve endings, which send messages and cause release of neurogenic mediators, such as substance P, CGRP, etc. These chemical mediators act centrally within the spinal cord and peripherally in conjunction with polymorphonuclear leukocytes and mast cells to further the inflammatory process (Fig. 8-7). Therefore, the two systems work synergistically in the injury and repair process.

Pain originating in the lumbar spine typically arises from mechanical and/or chemical irritation or primary sensory neurons. The site of activation may involve not only the peripheral terminal endings of these neurons and tissues continued in the anulus of the intervertebral disc, facet joint capsule and meninges, but also a mechanical or chemical irritation to the DRG or the cell bodies within the DRG.[151] Some of the endogenous chemical substances, particularly inflammatory mediators, can excite primarily or decrease the threshold in excitability of primary sensory neurons.

The DRG contains large cells that are thought to be responsible for the myelinated fibers and many small cells that are thought to be responsible for the unmyelinated C fibers, as well as finely myelinated A-delta fibers. It has been known that a large number of primary afferent neurons with small and intermediate diameters produce neuropeptides such as substance P and somatostatin.[55] Anatomic studies of neuropeptides in dorsal-root ganglion cells have found VIP, cholecystokinin, neurotensin, CGRP, substance P, somatostatin, dynorphin, enkephalin, angiotensin II, and bombesin-gastric relating peptide.[122] Most immunoreactive substances, such as neuropeptides resembling substance P (approximately 80%), are produced within dorsal-root ganglion cell bodies of primary afferent neurons. However, only 20% of these substances are transported along dorsal-root afferent fibers to terminals located in lamina I and II in the most dorsal part of the dorsal horn, whereas 80% are transported peripherally.[8] Substance P probably acts as a neuromodulator of pain signals at synapses in the region of the substantia gelatinosa, where pain perception is first integrated in the spinal cord.[85,96,97] Somatostatin is released after thermal noxious stimulation[137] and may also play a role in nociceptor transmission and inflammation. In addition to substance P and somatostatin, it is probably that a cholecystokinin-like

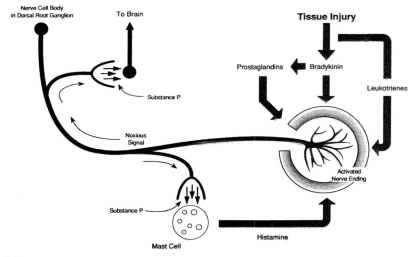

Fig. 8-7

Interaction between peripheral tissue injury and repair and central neurogenic components. This scheme demonstrates how neurogenic mediators can affect nonneurogenic mediators through stimulation of polymorphonuclear leukocytes and mast cells by neurogenic mediators, such as substance P. *(From Weinstein JN: Anatomy and neurophysiologic mechanism of spinal pain. In Frymoyer JW, et al., editors: The adult spine: principles and practice, New York, 1991, Raven Press, p 593.)*

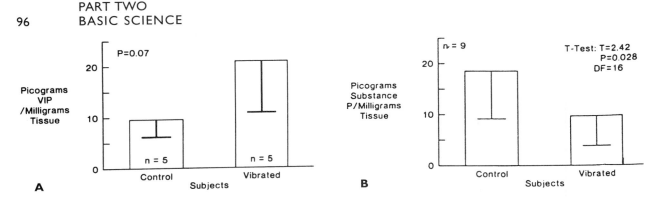

Fig. 8-8

Quantitation of immunoactive vasoactive intestinal polypeptide (VIP) (*A*), and substance P (*B*) on the dorsal-root ganglion from control and low-frequency-vibrated rabbits by radioimmunoassay. There was a significant difference across treatments. *(From Weinstein J, Pope M, Schmidt R, et al.: Effects of low frequency vibration on the dorsal root ganglion, Neuro-Orthop 4:24, 1987 [A] and Weinstein J: Mechanisms of spinal pain: the dorsal root ganglion and its role as a mediator of low-back pain, Spine 11:999, 1986 [B].)*

molecule, VIP, CGRP, gastrin-releasing peptide, dynorphin, enkephalin, and galanin are neuropeptides produced by primarily afferent neurons (see box below). Shehab and Atkinson[127] showed that VIP increases in dorsal-root ganglion and areas of the dorsal horn of the spinal cord from which other neuropeptides are depleted following peripheral axotomy of the sciatic nerve. VIP is a neuropeptide that plays a role in reorganization of the nervous system following injury and that has been shown to affect bone mineralization.[54] Peripheral terminals with CGRP-like immunoreactivity are found in tissues in which sensory stimulation is usually painful,[69] suggesting a role for this peptide in nociceptive processing. The functional role of most neuropeptides still remains unclear.

Neuropeptides in the Dorsal-root Ganglion

- Substance P
- Somatostatin
- Enkephalin
- Vasoactive intestinal polypeptide (VIP)
- Calcitonin gene–related peptide (CGRP)
- Cholecystokinin
- Neurotensin
- Dynorphin
- Angiotensin II
- Galanin
- Bombesin-gastric relating peptide
- Gastrin-releasing peptide

How do these neurotransmitters or neuromodulators in the dorsal-root ganglion and/or spinal cord vary in clinical situations, such as vibration, discography, or mechanical nerve-root compression? The effect of low-frequency vibration on the dorsal-root ganglion transmitters is essential to the understanding of vibration as a source of back pain. An animal model was used to gain a more basic understanding of the cause (vibration)-and-effect (back pain) relationship. The localized decrease in substance P and increased VIP seen following frequency vibration are compatible with results following peripheral injury (Fig. 8-8).[143,147] Depletion of substance P results from decreased synthesis and/or increased axonal transport as a direct result of stimulation. Thus, peptides released from the dorsal-root ganglion, when exposed to whole-body vibration, may have more than just pain-modulating effects. The degenerative changes manifested by low-frequency vibration may result directly or indirectly from DRG stimulation and the release of these neuropeptides.

Why is an abnormal discogram painful in one patient and not in another? Because the center of the normal disc is aneural, the condition of "internal disc disruption,"[22] theoretically, should not be painful. The mechanism for pain production, however, may be the irritation of sensory nerve endings in the annulus, posterior longitudinal ligament, etc. by chemical substances, or mechanical irritation caused by peripheral annular tears and secondary fibrovascular ingrowth associated with nociceptive fibers. A variety of endogenous chemical irritants are found in nonneural tissues, including intervertebral disc, all of which have pain-producing capabilities. These nonneurogenic inflammatory mediators include bradykinin, serotonin, histamine, acetylcholine,

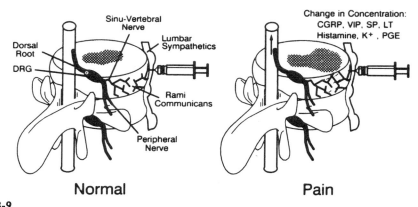

Fig. 8-9

Discography in normal nonsensitized and abnormal sensitized discs. It is thought that sensitization of abnormal disc allows chemical alterations to occur and thereby may be responsible for perception of pain and/or furthering the degenerative process. *(From Weinstein JN: Anatomy and neurophysiologic mechanism of spinal pain. In Frymoyer JW, et al., editors: The adult spine: principles and practice, New York, 1991, Raven Press, p 593.)*

prostaglandins E_1 and E_2, and leukotrienes.[32,64,151] It has been reported that levels of phospholipase A_2 activity are extraordinarily high in symptomatic lumbar disc herniations.[121] This enzyme is one rate-limiting step in the liberation of arachidonic acid from cell membranes and therefore may play an important role in the inflammatory process.[31,35] It has been demonstrated that phospholipase A_2 extracted from human lumbar disc has powerful inflammatory activity in vivo.[36]

A study was performed to investigate the changes in substance P and VIP, found in the dorsal root ganglion following discography in normal and abnormal canine lumbar intervertebral discs. The data suggest that discography elevated the dorsal-root ganglion concentrations of substance P and VIP and that local anesthesia injected into the disc reduces substance P concentration to a greater degree than it affects VIP. It appears that, in the normal animal disc exposed to discography plus anesthesia, substance P and VIP in the dorsal-root ganglion were similarly affected. However, in the injured or sensitized disc, substance P was affected but VIP was not.[146] It may be that various neurochemical changes within the intervertebral disc are expressed by sensitized (injured) anular nociceptors and are in part modulated by the dorsal-root ganglion (Fig. 8-9 and 8-10). Therefore, as hypothesized, the pain response during discography may in part be related to the chemical environment within the intervertebral disc and the sensitized state of its anular nociceptors.

Williams et al.[150] showed an abnormal distribution of substance P and CGRP-like immunoreactivities in right dorsal horn (pain side) of the lumbar

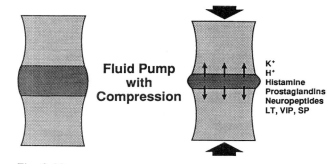

Fig. 8-10

Fluid pump with compression.

spinal cord from a patient with 5 years of severe intractable pain in the right foot. The unusual distribution of CGRP in this case, at the point in the spinal cord corresponding with the perceived origin of pain, together with the anomalous passage of dorsal-root fibers, is striking and suggests that aberrant termination of sensory afferents may have provided the structural framework for the development of a chronic pain syndrome in this patient.

Badalaments et al.[7] showed increased amounts of substance P, as well as substance P immunoreactivity in cell bodies of the dorsal-root ganglia and in the substantia gelatinosa of the spinal dorsal horn 7 days after experimental mechanical stimulation of dorsal-root ganglia and nerve roots. This suggests that substance P may modulate nociception when lumbar nerve roots are stimulated mechanically, Kawakami and Tamaki[66] reported changes in the neurotransmitters associated with pain transmission and regulation in the lumbar spina cord after me-

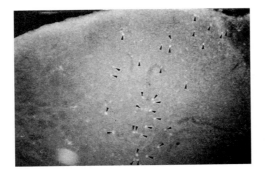

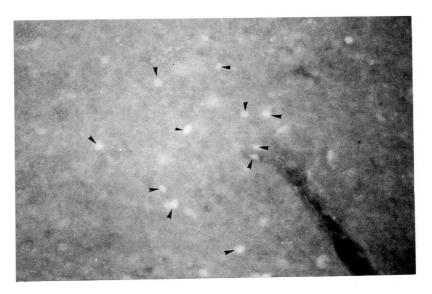

—— 100 μm

Fig. 8-11

c-*Fos*-like immunoreactivity in lumbar spinal cord. c-*Fos* gene expression was shown after mechanical compression of cauda equina.

chanical compression of the cauda equina in rats. Substance P–containing nerve endings were decreased after chronic and continuous compression of the cauda equina. Somatostatin nerve terminals were reduced, and aminergic fibers and serotonin immunoreactivities were enhanced after acute and chronic mechanical compression. In addition, quantitative analysis revealed that the levels of norepinephrine and serotonin, which are concerned with the descending inhibitory pathways, remained elevated after mechanical compression of the cauda equina. Thus, the findings suggest that these neuropeptides and amines have a complicated relationship to pain perception and modulation. Are these changes of neurotransmitters or neuromodulators really concerned with "spinal pain"? It will be difficult to validate this. Further studies into this problem are necessary.

The role of protooncogenes, such as c-*fos*,[128] as "third messengers" in long-term responses of spinal cord cells to noxious stimuli has become a popular topic among neuroscientists involved in pain research. Hunt et al.[57] were the first to demonstrate that in the rat spinal cord the protooncogene c-*fos* is rapidly expressed in appropriate postsynaptic dorsal horn neurons for 24 hours following noxious heating or chemical stimulation of the periphery. Similar results have since been found in response to heating; injection of formalin or carrageenan into skin, joints, and viscera; and electrical stimulation of peripheral C fibers. The total number of cells expressing c-*fos* is found to correlate with "pain behavior."[20] This protein product, c-*fos* protein, can usually be identified by immunohistochemical technique. c-*Fos*-gene expression was also shown in the lumbar spinal cord after acute mechanical compression of the cauda equina (Fig. 8-11) (Kawakami M., et al.: unpublished data). Therefore, c-*fos* gene expression might be used as a marker for research of spinal pain; clearly more work is needed.

Summary

The anatomy, biochemistry, and neurophysiology of each spinal motion segment stimulate many questions. The spine specialist must consider these basic concepts in managing a patients' clinical problems. Without a good understanding of basic cellular functions clinicians are offering their patients a glass half empty. In these times of insufficient research funding on one hand and outside evaluations of our clinical practice on the other, it is more important than ever to combine our clinical and basic resources. Only together can the various spinal disciplines hope to offer more efficacious treatments to our patients.

References

1. Adams MA, Hutton WC: The effect of posture on the role of the apophysial joints in resisting intervertebral compressive forces, *J Bone Joint Surg* 62B:358, 1980.
2. Adams MA, Hutton WC: The mechanical function of the lumbar apophyseal joints, *Spine* 8:327, 1983.
3. Adams P, Eyre DR, Muir H: Biochemical aspects of development and aging of human lumbar intervertebral discs, *Rheumatol Rahabil* 16:22, 1977.
4. Adams P, Muir H: Qualitative changes with age of proteoglycans of human lumbar discs, *Ann Rheum Dis* 35:289, 1976.
5. Alles A, Dom RM: Peripheral sensory nerve fibers that dichotomize to supply the bradium and the pericardium in the rat: a possible morphological explanation for referred cardiac pain? *Brain Res* 342:382, 1985.
6. Ashton IK, Ashton BA, Gibson SJ, et al. Morphological basis for back pain: the demonstration of nerve fibers and neuropeptides in the lumbar facet joint capsule and not in libamentum flavum, *J Orthop Res* 10:72, 1992.
7. Badalaments MA, Dee R, Ghillani R, et al.: Mechanical stimulation of dorsal root ganglia induces increased production of substance P: a mechanism for pain following nerve root compromise? *Spine* 12:552, 1987.
8. Barbut D, Polak JM, Wall PD: Substance P in spinal cord dorsal horn increases following peripheral nerve injury, *Brain Res* 205:289, 1981.
9. Bayliss MT, Johnstone G, O'Brien JP: Proteoglycan synthesis in the human intervertebral disc: variation with age, region and pathology, *Spine* 13:972, 1988.
10. Beaman D, Glover R, Graziano GP, et al.: Substance-P innervation of lumbar facet joints, Presented at the seventh meeting of the North American Spine Society, Boston, July 9-11, 1992.
11. Bergmann L, Alexander L: Vascular supply of spinal ganglia, *Arch Neurol* 46:761, 1941.
12. Bobechko WP, Hirsh C: Auto-immune response to nucleus pulposus in the rabbit, *J Bone Joint Surg* 47B:574, 1965.
13. Bogduk N: The innervation of the lumbar spine, *Spine* 8:286, 1983.
14. Bogduk N, Twomey LT: *Clinical anatomy of the lumbar spine*, ed 2, New York, 1991, Churchill-Livingstone, p 161.
15. Bogduk N, Tynan W, Wilson AS: The nerve supply to the human lumbar intervertebral discs, *J. Anat* 132:39, 1981.
16. Boumphrey FRS, Bell GR, Modic M, et al.: Computed tomography scanning after chymopapain injection for herniated nucleus pulposus: a prospective study, *Clin Orthop* 219:120, 1987.
17. Cavanaugh JM, El-Bony AA, Hardy WH, et al.: Sensory innervation of soft tissues of lumbar spine in the rat, *J Orthop Res* 7:389, 1989.
18. Cavanaugh JM, Weinstein JN: Low back pain: epidemiology, anatomy and neurophysiology, In Wall PD, editors: *Textbook of pain*, pp 441-455, 1992.
19. Cervero F: Visceral nociception: peripheral and central aspects of visceral nociceptive system, *Trans R Soc Lond* (B) 308:325, 1985.
20. Cho HJ, Gogas KR, Levine JD, et al.: Supraspinally immunoreactivity (FLI) and pain behavior by increasing descending inhibitory controls, *Pain Suppl* 5:S270, 1990.
21. Coppes MH, Morani E, Thomeer PT, et al.: Innervation of annulus fibrosis in low back pain, *Lancet* 336:189, 1990 (letter) (Published erratum appears in Lancet 336:324, 1990).
22. Crock HV: Internal disc disruption: a challenge to disc prolapse 50 years on, *Spine* 11:650, 1986.
23. Crock HV: A reappraisal of intervertebral disc lesions, *Med J Aust* 1:983, 1970.
24. Dahlin, LB, Rydevik B, McLean WG, et al: Changes in fast axonal transport during experimental nerve compression at low pressures, *Exp Neurol* 84:29, 1984.
25. Delamarter R, Bohlman H, Dodge L, et al: Experimental lumbar spinal stenosis, *J Bone Joint Surg* 72:110, 1990.
26. Devor M, Obermeyer M: Membrane differentiation in rat dorsal root ganglia and possible consequences for back pain, *Neurosci Lett* 51:341, 1989.
27. Devor M, Wall PD: Cross-excitation in dorsal root ganglion of nerve-injured and intact rats, *J Neurophysiol* 64:1733, 1990.
28. Eisenstein SM, Parry CR: The lumbar facet syndrome: clinical presentation and articular surface changes, *J Bone Joint Surg* 69B:3, 1987.
29. Evans JG: Neurogenic intermittent claudication, *BMJ* 2:985, 1964.
30. Eyre DR, Muir H: Quantitative analysis of type I and type II collagens in human intervertebral discs at various ages, *Biochem Biophys Acta* 492:29, 1977.
31. Farmaey JP: Phospholipases, eicosanoid production and inflammation, *Clin Rheumatol* 1:84, 1982.
32. Ferreira SH: Prostaglandins, aspirin-like drugs and analgesia, *Nature* 240:200, 1972.

33. Fields HL: Theories of the mechanism of referred pain. In Fields HL, editor: *Pain*, San Francisco, 1987, McGraw-Hill Book Co., p 89.

34. Foreman RD, Ohata CA: Effects of coronary occlusion on thoracic spinal neurons receiving viscerosomatic inputs, *Am J Physiol* 238:667, 1980.

35. Franson RC: Isolation and characterization of a phospholipase A2 from an inflammatory exudate, *J Lipid Res* 19:18, 1978.

36. Franson RC, Saal JS, Saal JF: Human disc phospholipase A2 is inflammatory, *Spine* 17:S129, 1992.

37. Frymoyer JW, Moskowitz RW: Spinal degeneration—pathogenesis and medical management. In Frymoyer JW, et al., editors: *The adult spine: principle and practice*, New York, 1991, Raven Press, p 611.

38. Gertzbein SD, Tile M, Gross A, et al.: Auto-immunity in degenerative disc disease of the lumbar spine, *Orthop Clin North Am* 6:67, 1975.

39. Ghormley RK: Low back pain with special reference to the articular facets, with presentation of an operative procedure, *JAMA* 101:1773, 1933.

40. Giles GF, Taylor SR: Human zygapophyseal joint capsule and synovial fold innervation, *Br J Rheumatol* 26:93, 1987.

41. Giles LG, Harey AR: Immunohistochemical demonstration of nociceptors in the capsule and synovial folds of human zygapophyseal joints, *Br J Rheumatol* 26:362, 1987.

42. Goldthwait JE: The lumbosacral articulation: an explanation of many cases of lumbago, sciatica and paraplegia, *Boston Med Surg J* 164:365, 1911.

43. Gotfried Y, Bradford DS, Oegema TR: Facet joint changes after chemonucleolysis-induced disc space narrowing, *Spine* 11:944, 1986.

44. Gower WE, Pedrini V: Age-related variations in proteinpolysaccharides from human nucleus pulposus, anulus fibrosus and costal cartilage, *J Bone Joint Surg* 51A:1154, 1969.

45. Grafstein B: The nerve cell body response to axotomy, *Exp Neurol* 48:32, 1975.

46. Greenbard PE, Brown MD, Pallares VS, et al.: Epidural anesthesia for lumbar spine surgery, *J Spinal Disorder* 1:139, 1988.

47. Grönblad M, Korkala O, Konttinen YT, et al.: Silver impregnation and immunohistochemical study of nerves in lumbar facet joint plical tissue, *Spine* 16:34, 1991.

48. Grönblad M, Weinstein JN, Santavirta S: Immunohistochemical observations on spinal tissue innervation: a review of hypothetical mechanisms of back pain, *Acta Orthop Scand* 62:614, 1991.

49. Hebert CM, Lindberg KA, Jayson MIV, et al.: Changes in the collagen of human intervertebral discs during aging and degenerative disc disease, *J Molec Med* 1:79, 1975.

50. Hirsch C, Ingelmar KUE, Miller N: The anatomic basis for low back pain: Studies on the presence of sensory endings in ligamentous capsular and intervertebral disc structures in the human spine, *Acta Orthop Scand* 33:1, 1963.

51. Hirsch C, Schajowicz S: Studies on structural changes in the lumbar anulus fibrosis, *Acta Orthop Scand* 22:184, 1953.

52. Hirsch C: Studies on the mechanism of low back pain, *Acta Orthop Scand* 20:261, 1951.

53. Hitselberger WE, Witten RM: Abnormal myelograms in asymptomatic patients, *J Neurosurg* 28:204, 1968.

54. Hohmann EL, Elde RP, Rysavy JA, et al.: Innervation of periosteum and bone by sympathetic vasoactive intestinal peptide-containing nerve fibers, *Science* 232:868, 1986.

55. Hökfelt T, Elde R, Johannsos O, et al.: Immunohistochemical evidence for separate populations of somatostatin-containing and substance P-containing primary afferent neurons in the rat, *Neuroscience* 1:131, 1976.

56. Howe JF, Loeser JD, Calvin WH: Mechanosensitivity of dorsal root ganglia and chronically injured axons: a physiological basis for the radicular pain of nerve root compression, *Pain* 3:25, 1977.

57. Hunt SP, Pini A, Evan G: Induction of c-fos-like protein in spinal cord neurons following sensory stimulation, *Nature* 328:632, 1987.

58. Ikari C: A study of the mechanism of low back pain: the neurohistological examination of the disease, *J Bone Joint Surg* 30A:195, 1954 (abstract).

59. Inman VT, Saunders JB: Referred pain from skeletal structures, *J Nerve Ment Dis* 99:660, 1944.

60. Jackson HC, Winkelmann RK, Bickel WH: Nerve endings in the human spinal column and related structures, *J Bone Joint Surg* 48A:1272, 1966.

61. Jackson RP: The facet syndrome: myth or reality? *Clin Orthop* 279:110, 1992.

62. Jaffray D, O'Brien JP: Isolated intervertebral disc resorption: a source of mechanical and inflammatory back pain? *Spine* 11:397, 1986.

63. Janig W, Koltzenburg M: Receptive properties of pial afferents, *Pain* 45:77, 1991.

64. Kanaka R, Schaible HG, Schmidt RF: Activation of fine articular afferent units by bradykinin, *Brain Res* 327:81, 1985.

65. Kawakami M: Histochemical and immunohistochemical demonstrations of nerve fibers on human perispinal soft tissue, *J Wakayama Med Soc* 40:621, 1989 (in Japanese).

66. Kawakami M, Tamaki T: Morphologic and quantitative changes in neurotransmitters in the lumbar spinal cord after acute or chronic mechanical compression of the cauda equina, *Spine* 17(3S):S13, 1992.

67. Kelgren JH: On the distribution of pain arising from deep somatic structures with charts of segmental pain areas, *Clin Sci Mol Med* 4:35, 1939.

68. Konttinen Y, Rees R, Hukkanen M, et al.: Nerves in inflammatory synovium: Immunohistochemical observations on the adjuvant arthritis rat model, *J Rheumatol* 17:1586, 1990.

69. Kruger L, Sternini C, Mantyh CR, et al.: Calcitonin gene-related (CGRP) immunoreactivity and receptor binding sites in relation to specific sensory pathways in the rat, Proc 30th *Int Union Phisiol Sci* 16:328, 1986.

70. Kuslich SD, Ulstrom CL, Michael CJ: The tissue origin of low back pain and sciatica: a report of pain response to tissue stimulation during operation on the lumbar spine using local anaesthesia, *Orthop Clin North Am* 22:181, 1991.

71. Kwan MK, Rydevik BL, Brown R, et al.: Selected biomechanical assessment of lumbosacral spinal nerve roots. Presented at the meeting of the International Society for the Study of the Lumbar Spine, Miami, FL, April 12-16, 1988.

72. LaBan MM: "Vespers curse" night pain: the bane of Hypnos, *Arch Phys Med Rehabil* 65:501, 1984.

73. Laurberg S, Sorensen KE: Cervical dorsal root ganglion cells with collaterals to both shoulder skin and the diaphragm: a fluorescent double labelling study in the rat: a model for referred pain? *Brain Res* 331:160, 1985.

74. Lee Y, Takami K, Kawai Y, et al.: Distribution of calcitonin gene-related peptide in the rat peripheral nervous system with reference to its coexistence with substance P, *Neuroscience* 15:1227, 1985.

75. Levine JD, Clark R, Dever M, et al.: Interneuronal substance P contributes to the severity of experimental arthritis, *Science* 226:547, 1984.

76. Lewis T, Kellgren JH: Observations relating to referred pain, visceromotor reflexes and other associated phenomena, *Clin Sci* 4:47, 1939.

77. Lewin T, Moffet S, Viidik A: The morphology of the lumbar synovial intervertebral joints, *Acta Morphol Neerl Scand* 4:299, 1962.

78. Lewin T: Osteoarthritis of the lumbar synovial joints: a morphologic study, *Acta Orthop Scand Suppl* 73:6, 1964.

79. Lindblom K, Rexed B: Spinal nerve injury in dorsolateral protrusions of lumbar disks, *J Neurosurg* 70A:361, 1948.

80. Lippitt AB: The facet joint and its role in spinal pain: management with facet joint injections, *Spine* 9:746, 1984.

81. Lotz M, Carson DA, Vaughan JH: Substance P activation of rheumatoid synoviocytes: neural pathway in pathogenesis of arthritis, *Science* 235:893, 1987.

82. Lyons G, Eisenstein SM, Sweet MBE: Biochemical changes in intervertebral disc degeneration, *Biochem Biophys Acta* 673:443, 1981.

83. Madsen JR, Heros RC: Spinal arteriovenous malformations and neurogenic claudication, *J Neurosurg* 57:793, 1988.

84. Malinsky J: The ontogenetic development of nerve terminations in the intervertebral discs of man, *Acta Anat* 38:96, 1959.

85. Marks JL: Brain peptides: Is substance P a transmitter of pain signals? *Science* 205:886, 1979.

86. Maroudas A: Nutrition and metabolism of the intervertebral disc. In Ghosh P, editor: The biology of the intervertebral disc, vol 2, Boca Raton, FL, 1988, *CRC Press,* Chapter 9, p 1.

87. Marshall LL, Trethewie ER: Chemical irritation of nerve-root in disc prolapse, *Lancet* 2:320, 1973.

88. Marshall LL, Trethewie ER, Curtain CC: Chemical radiculitis: a clinical, physiological and immunological study, *Clin Orthop* 129:61, 1977.

89. McCall EW, Park WM, O'Brien JP: Induced pain referral from posterior lumbar elements in normal subjects, *Spine* 4:441, 1979.

90. McCarron RF, Wimpee MW, Hudkins PG, et al.: The inflammatory effect of nucleus pulposus: a possible element in the pathogenesis of low-back pain, *Spine* 12:760, 1987.

91. Melrose J, Ghosh P: The noncallagenous proteins of the intervertebral disc. In Ghosh P, editor: The biology of the intervertebral disc, vol 2, Boca Raton, FL, 1988, *CRC Press,* Chapter 8, p 189.

92. Mendel T, Wink C, Zimny M: Neural elements in human cervical intervertebral discs, *Spine* 17:132, 1992.

93. Mooney V: The facet syndrome, *Clin Orthop* 115:149, 1976.

94. Mooney V: Facet syndrome. In Weinstein JN, Wiesel SW, editors: *The lumbar spine,* Philadelphia, 1990, W.B. Saunders Co., p 422.

95. Nachemson A: Intradiscal measurements of pH in patients with lumbar rhizopathies, *Acta Orthop Scand* 40:23, 1969.

96. Naftchi NE, Abrahams SJ, St. Paul H, et al.: Localization and changes of substance P in spinal cord of paraplegic cats, *Brain Res* 153:507, 1978.

97. Naftchi NE, Abrahams SJ, St. Paul H, et al.: Substance P and leucine enkephalin changes in spinal cord of paraplegic rats and cats. In Naftchi NE, editor: *Spinal cord injury,* New York, 1982, Spectrum Publishers, p 85.

98. Naylor A: The biochemical changes in the human intervertebral disc in degeneration and nuclear prolapse, *Orthop Clin North Am* 2:343, 1971.

99. Nalor A: Intervertebral disc prolapse and degeneration: the biochemical and biophysical approach, *Spine* 1:108, 1976.

100. Neugebauer V, Schaible HG: Evidence for a central component in the sensitization of spinal neurons with joint input during development of acute arthritis in cat's knee, *J Neurophyiol* 64:299, 1990.

101. Ng SCS, Weis JB, Quennel R, et al.: Abnormal connective tissue degrading enzyme patterns in prolapsed intervertebral discs, *Spine* 11:695, 1986.

102. Olmarker K, Holm S, Hansson T, et al.: Experimental graded compression of the pig cauda equina: effects of nerve root nutrition, Presented at the meeting of the International Society for the Study of the Lumbar Spine, Dallas, TX, May 29-June 2, 1986.

103. Olmarker K, Rydevik B, Holm S: Intraneural edema formation in spinal nerve roots of the porcine cauda equina induced by graded, experimental compression, *Trans Orthop Res Soc* 13:136, 1988.

104. Olmarker K, Rydevik B, Holm S, et al: Effects of experimental, graded compression on blood flow in spinal nerve roots, *J Orthop Res* 7:817, 1989.

105. Olmarker K, Rydevik B: Single-versus double level nerve root compression: an experimental study on the porcine cauda equina with analyses of nerve impulse conduction properties, *Clin Orthop* 279:35, 1992.

106. Oudenhoven RC: The role of laminectomy, facet rhizotomy and epidural steroids, *Spine* 4:145, 1979.

107. Parke WW: The innervation of connective tissues of the spinal motion segment, Presented at the International Symposium on Percutaneous Lumbar Discectomy, Philadelphia, PA, November 6 and 7, 1987.

108. Parke WW, Watanabe R: The intrinsic vasculature of the lumbosacral spinal nerve roots, *Spine* 10:508, 1985.

109. Payan DG, McGillis JP, Goetzl ET: Neuroimmunology, *Adv Immunol* 39:299, 1986.

110. Payan DG, McGillis JP, Renold FK, et al: Neuropeptide modulation of leukocyte function, Ann N Y *Acad Sci* 496:182, 1987.

111. Pedersen HE, Blunck CFJ, Gardner E: Anatomy of lumbosacral rami and meningeal branches of spinal nerves, *J Bone Joint Surg* 38A:377, 1956.

112. Pedowitz RA, Rydevik BL, Hargens AR, et al.: Motor and sensory nerve root conduction deficit induced by acute graded compression of the pig cauda equina, *Trans Orthop Res Soc* 13:134, 1988.

113. Pedrini-Mille A, Weinstein JN, Found EM, et al.: Stimulation of dorsal root ganglia and degradation of rabbit anulus fibrosus, *Spine* 15:1252, 1990.

114. Roofe PG: Innervation of annulus fibrosis and posterior longitudinal ligament, *Arch Neurol Psychiatry* 44:100, 1940.

115. Ruch TC: *Visceral sensation and referred pain.* In Fulton JF, editor: *Howell's textbook of physiology,* Philadelphia, 1947, W.B. Saunders Co., p 385.

116. Rydevik B, Brown MD, Lundborg G: Pathoanatomy and pathophysiology of nerve root compression, *Spine* 9:7, 1984.

117. Rydevik B, Garfin S: Spinal nerve root compression. In Szabo RM, editor: *Nerve compression syndromes: diagnosis and treatment,* New York, 1989, Slack Medical Publishers, p 247.

118. Rydevik B, Lundborg G, Bagge U: Effects of graded compression on intraneural blood flow: an in vivo study on rabbit tibial nerve, *J Hand Surg* 6:3, 1981.

119. Rydevik BL, Myers RR, Powell HC: Pressure increase in the dorsal root ganglion following mechanical compression, *Spine* 14:574, 1989.

120. Rydevik B, Nordborg C: Changes in nerve function and nerve fibre structure induced by acute, graded compression, *J Neurol Neurosurg Psychiatry* 43:1070, 1980.

121. Saal JS, Franson RC, Dobrow R, et al.: High levels of inflammatory phospholipase A2 activity in lumbar disc herniations, *Spine* 15:674, 1990.

122. Salt TE, Hill RG: Neurotransmitter candidates of somatosensory primary afferent fibers, *Neuroscience* 10:1083, 1983.

123. Schaible HG, Schmidt RF, Willis WD: Spinal mechanisms in arthritis pain. In Schaible HG, Schmidt RF, Vahlettinz C, editors: *Fine afferent nerve fibers and pain,* Weinheim, Federal Republic of Germany, 1987, VCH Publishers, p 399.

124. Sedowfia KA, Tomlinson IW, Weiss JB, et al: Collagenolytic enzyme systems in human intervertebral disc, *Spine* 7:213, 1982.

125. Shantha TR, Evans JA: The relationship of epidural anesthesia to neuromembranes and arachnoid villi, *Anesthesiology* 37:543, 1972.

126. Shealy CN: Facet denervation in the management of back pain and sciatic pain, *Clin Orthop* 115:157, 1976.

127. Shehab SA, Atkinson ME: Vasoactive intestinal peptide increases in areas of the dorsal horn of the spinal cord from which other neuropeptides are depleted following peripheral axotomy, *Exp Brain Res* 62:422, 1986.

128. Sheng M, Greenberg ME: The regulation and function of c-fos and other immediate early genes in the neuron system, *Neuron* 4:477, 1990.

129. Shinohara H: A study on lumbar disc lesions: Significance of histology of free nerve endings in lumbar discs, *J Jpn Orthop Assoc* 44:553, 1970 (in Japanese).

130. Sinclair DC, Weddell G, Feindel WH: Referred pain and associated phenomena, *Brain* 71:184, 1948.

131. Spencer DL, Irwin GS, Miller JA: Anatomy and significance of fixation of the lumbosacral nerve roots in sciatica, *Spine* 8:672, 1983.

132. Steindler A, Luck IV: Differential diagnosis of pain in the low back: Allocation of the source of pain by procaine hydrochloride method, *JAMA,* 110:106, 1938.

133. Stilwell DL Jr: The nerve supply of the vertebral column and its associated structures in the monkey, *Anat Rec* 125:139, 1956.

134. Sunderland S: Avulsion of nerve roots. In Vinken DJ, Bruyn GW, editors: Handbook of clinical neurology, vol 25, Injuries of the spine and spina cord, part I, New York, 1975, *American Elsevier,* p 393.

135. Sunderland S, Bradley KC: Stress-strain phenomena in human peripheral nerve trunks, *Brain* 84:102, 1961.

136. Sunderland S, Bradley KC: Stress-strain phenomena in human spinal nerve roots, *Brain* 84:120, 1961.

137. Takagi H, Kuraishi Y: Substance P, somatostatin and pain transmission, *Metab Dis* 23:33, 1986 (in Japanese).

138. Twomey LT, Taylor JR: *Physical therapy of the low back,* Melbourne, Australia, 1987, Churchill-Livingstone.

139. Urban JPG, McMullin JF: Swelling pressure of the lumbar intervertebral discs: influence of age, spinal level, composition, and degeneration, *Spine* 13:179, 1988.

140. Venner RM, Crock HV: Clinical studies of isolated disc resorption in the lumbar spine, *J Bone Joint Surg* 63B:491, 1981.

141. Videman T, Malmivaara A, Mooney V: The value of axial view in assessing diskograms: an experimental study with cadavers, *Spine* 12:299, 1987.

142. Watanabe R, Parke WW: Vascular and neural pathology of lumbosacral spinal stenosis, *J Neurosurg* 65:64, 1986.

143. Weinstein J: Mechanisms of spinal pain: the dorsal root ganglion and its role as a mediator of low-back pain, *Spine* 11:999, 1986.

144. Weinstein JN: Anatomy and neurophysiologic mechanism of spinal pain. In Frymoyer JW, et al., editors: *The audit spine: principles and practice,* New York, 1991, Raven Press, p 593.

145. Weinstein JN: The role of neurogenic and non-neurogenic mediators as they related to pain in the development of osteoarthritis (a clinical review), *Spine* 17:S356, 1992.

146. Weinstein J, Claverie W, Gibson S: The pain of discography, *Spine* 13:1344, 1988.

147. Weinstein J, Pope M, Schmidt R, et al.: Effects of low frequency vibration on the dorsal root ganglion. *Neuro Orthop* 4:24, 1987.

148. Wiberg G: Back pain in relation to the nerve supply of the intervertebral disc, *Acta Orthop Scand* 19:211, 1947.

149. Wiesel SW, Tsourmas N, Feffer HL, et al.: A study of computer-assisted tomography: 1. The incidence of positive CAT scans in asymptomatic group of patients, *Spine* 9:549, 1984.

150. Williams S, Wells C, Hunt S: Spinal cord neuropeptides in a case of chronic pain. *Lancet* 7:1047, 1988.

151. Wyke B: *Receptor systems in lumbosacral tissues in relation to the production of low back pain.* In White AA, Gordon SL, editors: *American Academy of Orthopedic Surgeons symposium on idiopathic low back pain,* St. Louis, 1982, CV Mosby, p 97.

152. Yamashita T, Cavanaugh JM, El-Bohy AA, et al.: Mechanosensitive afferent units in the lumbar facet joint, *J Bone Joint Surg* 72A:865, 1990.

153. Yang KH, King AI: Mechanism of facet load transmission as a hypothesis for low back pain, *Spine* 9:557, 1984.

154. Yoshizawa H, Kobayashi S, Hachiya Y: Blood supply of nerve roots and dorsal root ganglia, *Orthop Clin North Am* 22:195, 1991.

155. Yoshizawa H, O'Brien JP, Smith WT, et al.: Neuropathology of intervertebral disc removed for low back pain, *J Pathol* 132:95, 1980.

Chapter 9
Neurophysiology of Chronic Idiopathic Back Pain

Ronald C. Kramis
Richard G. Gillette
William J. Roberts

Primary Afferent Divergence and Convergence within the Spinal Cord: Relationship to the Referral Patterns and Diffuseness of Low-Back Pain

clinical implications

Neuronal Plasticity

nociception-induced sensitization of spinal neurons

sensitization and recruitment of nociceptive afferents

clinical implications

Sympathetic Mechanisms and Low-Back Pain

clinical implications

Comments on the Somato/Neuronal vs. Psychogenic Origin of Low-Back Pain that Occurs in the Absence of Identifiable Somatic Pathology

Summary

The usual direct relationship between pathology, nociception, and pain is often distorted or absent in individuals suffering from persistent pain. Frequently, severe pain is reported even though commensurately severe peripheral pathology cannot be demonstrated. Pain may be determined to a greater extent by central neuronal events than by ongoing pathology/nociception in peripheral tissues. These central neuronal events are often thought to be psychologically or psychosocially determined, an orientation discussed more extensively in other chapters of this book. Here, instead, we focus on neurophysiologic events within the dorsal horn of the spinal cord as mechanisms that allow additional/alternative explanations for several of the most perplexing aspects of low-back pain (LBP).

The data and concepts to be presented here have important clinical implications in relation to LBP. They suggest, for example: (1) that severe persistent pain can occur as the result of minimal nociceptive, or even *non*nociceptive, afferent activity and that effective pharmacologic intervention in this type of pain may depend on the development of new compounds that block central neuronal sensitization; (2) that diagnostic procedures based upon the stimulation or blockade of spinal nerves are compromised by both divergence/convergence and sensitization mechanisms within the spinal cord; (3) that peripheral nerve blocks, even during general anesthesia, may be important in preventing persistent iatrogenically induced LBP; (4) that there exists a neurophysiologic basis for sympathetic involvement in LBP, although the extent of this involvement is unknown; and (5) that understanding physiologic mechanisms that mediate the placebo response may offer insights concerning the control of LBP.

The existence of the neurophysiologically based mechanisms to be discussed here does not exclude the potential involvement of more complex, for example, psychosocial, events in LBP. Clearly, ascending and descending pathways within the central nervous system (CNS) allow interaction of spinal and supraspinal events. However, many opportunities for "functional" disorder in the nervous system may exist between the level of the primary afferent and the level of the "supracortical" psychosocial mechanisms. Given the potentially greater ease of intervention at these intermediate levels, it seems important that they not be disregarded by either researchers or clinicians who attempt to understand the mechanisms of persistent idiopathic LBP.

Neurophysiologic evidence clearly indicates that persistent functional changes occur within the spinal cord as the result of nociception and suggests that *abnormal* persistence of these functional changes may contribute to pathologically persistent pain. In particular, this evidence strongly suggests that prior pathology/nociception can induce persistent changes in nociceptive spinal neurons such that these neurons become intensely responsive even to nonnociceptive afferent activity.

The fact that pain-related central neurons can become intensely responsive (i.e., sensitized) to nonnociceptive primary afferent activity may have important implications for understanding, preventing, and treating many "pathologic" pain syndromes, including idiopathic LBP and persistent pain associated with failed back surgery. An often puzzling characteristic of persistent LBP, for example, is its unresponsiveness to antinociceptive treatment modalities.[47] If, as we propose, persistent LBP is often due to nonnociceptive activation of sensitized central pain mechanisms, then the inefficacy of pain interventions addressing nociceptive mechanisms becomes less puzzling.

A recent report by Cooper and others[11] on 70 postlaminectomy patients provides a typical description of the inefficacy of common treatment modalities applied to patients with severe and persistent back pain. Pain symptoms had persisted in these patients "despite the administration of various potent analgesic agents (e.g., buprenorphine, pentazocine, pethidine, and morphine sulfate), nonsteroidal anti-inflammatory agents, psychotropic agents, and carbamazepine. Physical regimes, including physiotherapy, traction, bed rest, plaster jackets, transcutaneous nerve stimulation, and epidural injections, had all previously failed to relieve symptoms." We suspect many patients such as these have developed sensitized central pain mechanisms resulting from prior nociceptive afferent activity, but these mechanisms are now being activated by normal and/or ectopic (e.g., neuromal) nonnociceptive afferent activity. These patients may, indeed, be suffering primarily from nonnociceptive rather than nociceptive pain.

We are currently investigating, via animal experiments, central neuronal mechanisms[17-19] that may mediate both the diffuse localization and referral patterns of LBP. These investigations may ultimately explain the severity and persistence of pain in some patients who demonstrate little or no identifiable pathology.[21] We are also examining the potential involvement of sympathetic mechanisms in LBP. Recent clinical experiments have raised the possibility that unusually strong and persistent placebo response by patients suffering LBP may offer clues about central neuronal mechanisms of persistent pain. Some of our recent data and related concepts are presented below.

Primary Afferent Divergence and Convergence Within the Spinal Cord: Relationship to the Referral Patterns and Diffuseness of Low-Back Pain

Ruch suggested in the early 1940s that referred pain might occur as the result of the convergence of afferent activity from separate tissues onto the same neuron(s) within the CNS. Similarly, the convergence of afferent activity from multiple lumbar tissues onto individual spinal neuron(s) could provide a neural basis for the perceived diffuseness and lack of tissue specificity associated with LBP. This would be particularly likely if, as suggested by our research, there are relatively few "low back" spinal neurons, each receiving input from extensively branched and widely distributed (divergent) lumbar afferent axons.

Animal experiments have allowed us to examine divergence/convergence mechanisms in relation to lumbar structures in three ways: (1) by labeling afferent axons with WGA-HRP and determining the distribution of those axons within the spinal cord; (2) by using c-fos immunohistochemistry to label cells activated by unilateral paraspinal noxious stimulation; and (3) by recording from spinal neurons to determine whether individual neurons do indeed respond to converging input from many separate lumbar and hindlimb tissues. Although we expected evidence of divergence/convergence, we were surprised by its extent, as reflected both by the extensive rostrocaudal and bilateral distribution of labeled primary afferents from individual lumbar tissues and by the responsiveness of individual lumbar neurons to stimulation of multiple spinal, paraspinal, and limb tissues.

Unilateral WGA-HRP injection into single facet joints or multifidus muscles demonstrated an extensive intraspinal projection, both rostrocaudally and bilaterally, by lumbar primary afferents.[18] Examination of dorsal-root ganglia indicated that when individual facet joints or multifidus muscles were injected, the labeled afferents entered the cord at only two segmental levels but they projected within the cord across several segments, for example, from S2 to T13. Assuming a similarly extensive topographic distribution of afferents from each joint/multifidus muscle, one could envisage massive convergence of afferent input from multiple lumbar structures onto neurons innervated by other lumbar structures and onto neurons innervated by afferents from limb tissues.

The presence of afferent terminals in a particular region does not necessarily imply that neurons postsynaptic to the terminals would be activated by them. As the result of tonic inhibitory control or the absence of sufficient summation with input from other synapses, the afferents might be ineffective in eliciting action potentials.[50] C-fos immunohistochemistry allows labeling specifically of neurons that respond to the application of a noxious stimulus. Figure 9-1 shows the bilateral distribution of primary afferent terminals that occurred following unilateral WGA-HRP labeling of lumbar tissues and also shows bilateral c-fos labeling after unilateral stimulation of paraspinal tissues. These findings may partially explain bilateral diffuse LBP resulting from focal, unilateral injury. Our research concerning the extent of the rostrocaudal activation of neurons by focal, unilateral noxious stimulation of spinal/paraspinal tissues is at this point incomplete, but appears to indicate activation of neurons throughout the rostrocaudally extensive region in which terminals were labeled by WGA-HRP.

Although c-fos labelling demonstrates that neurons are active in response to noxious stimulation,

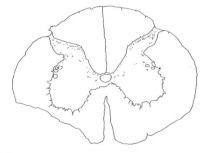
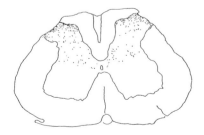

Fig. 9-1

Left, Bilateral distribution of primary afferent terminals is indicated following *unilateral* WGA-HRP labeling of lumbar multifidus muscle. **Right,** A bilateral distribution of c-fos labeled neurons is apparent following *unilateral* noxious stimulation of lumbar deep tissues. Both figures are composites of several lumbar sections; WGA-HRP from cat, c-fos from rat.

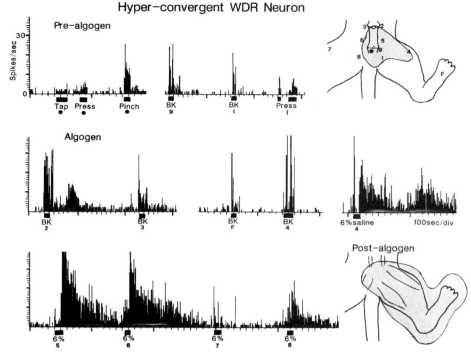

Fig. 9-2

Recordings from a representative "hyperconvergent" lumbar spinal neuron responsive to stimulation of multiple deep tissues and skin. Note the expansion of the cutaneous receptive field (shaded area) that occurred as the result of algogen-induced nociceptive input. In this and all subsequent figures, the neurons were located in the lateral dorsal horn of the cat lumbar spinal cord. Response histograms reflect action potentials/unit of time. Shaded areas in figurines reflect cutaneous receptive fields. BK-bradykinin; 6% hypertonic saline.

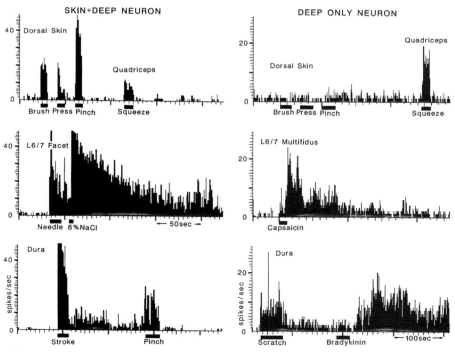

Fig. 9-3

Neurons with dural receptive fields: responses to skin, muscle and joint stimulation.

this cannot be used to determine whether any particular neuron is responsive to afferent input from multiple vs. single tissues. This can be determined using single-cell recording techniques. We used glass micropippettes to record action potentials from individual neurons located in the lateral dorsal horn in cats and rats during stimulation of lumbar and hindlimb tissues. Figures 9-2 to 9-6 show the responses of individual neurons with lumbar receptive fields. (A neuron's receptive field is that area of tissue within which stimulation causes the neuron to generate an action potential, i.e., the neuron "receives" information from that tissue.)

Figure 9-2 shows the responsiveness of a representative "hyperconvergent" neuron that was activated by cutaneous and deep tissue stimulation over the entire leg, including bilateral multifidus muscles, bilateral zygapophyseal joints, bilateral gluteal muscles, and quadriceps. The cell responded to lumbar deep-tissue injection of bradykinin (which activates small diameter, probably nociceptive, muscle afferents) and 6% saline (which activates both nociceptive and nonnociceptive afferents).

Figure 9-3 demonstrates the response of two neurons whose receptive fields included lumbar dura. One neuron responded to both cutaneous and other deep tissues, the other only to other deep tissues. Deep-tissue receptive fields included both paraspinal and proximal leg tissues. The activation of neurons represented in Figs. 9-3 and 9-4 occurred via afferents innervating diverse tissues located in distinct dermatomes/myotomes. Afferent neurons with axons in either the dorsal or ventral rami of the spinal nerves or in meningeal nerves may all converge onto individual spinal neurons.

Clinical Implications

1. These data suggest that the diffuseness of LBP may be, rather than a perplexing oddity, a logical consequence of the extensive divergence and convergence of lumbar primary afferents within the spinal cord. The importance of convergence mechanisms would be enhanced by the presence of relatively few "low back" neurons, as indicated by our studies.

2. The extensive rostrocaudal divergence/convergence of afferent activity implies that afferent activity impinging on individual neurons would enter the cord via many spinal nerves. This organization may defeat diagnostic procedures that attempt to define the locus of deep-tissue pathology by using either stimulation or blockade of spinal nerves.[24,31] As a result of convergence within the spinal cord, stimulation of afferents from normal tissues/nerves may strongly activate the same spinal neurons that are activated by nociceptive input from injured tissue, falsely implicating normal tissues/nerves as the source of pathology and pain. Similarly, blockade of normal tissues/nerves may reduce the total amount of afferent excitation spinal neurons

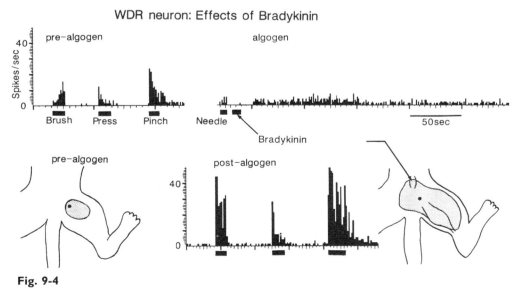

Fig. 9-4

Nociception-induced "sensitization" (increased responsiveness and expansion of receptive-field size) of a wide-dynamic-range (WDR) spinal neuron; algogen injection into lumbar multifidus muscle. Note that after algogen injection the cell became responsive to mechanical stimulation over a larger area, including contralateral tissue and extensive regions of the leg.

receive so that activation of these neurons by input from a pathologic source (and the resulting pain) is considerably reduced. Once again, normal tissues/nerves are falsely implicated as a source of pathology. North[33] has recently provided related clinical evidence. Furthermore, the probability of these diagnostic errors would be greatly increased if central nociceptive neurons had become sensitized as the result of intense or persistent nociception, as discussed in the following section.

3. Patterns of pain that do not correspond well to known distributions of peripheral nerves may occur as the result of divergence/convergence mechanisms within the spinal cord, particularly after normal patterns of neuronal interactions have been altered by the sensitizing effects of prior nociception (see below). Consequently, considerable caution is warranted before attributing unusual pain distributions solely to psychosocial or psychogenic mechanisms.

Neuronal Plasticity

Nociception-Induced Sensitization of Spinal Neurons

It is often tempting to think of the nervous system as a complex, mostly static or "hard-wired" system in which neural plasticity mechanisms operate primarily in relation to "higher order" processes such as associative learning and memory. This temptation must be resisted, however, particularly when considering neuronal mechanisms that mediate nociception and pain. Neurons *at all levels* of the nervous system are dynamic, capable of functional and structural alterations in response to afferent input and changes in tissue environment.

For example, the responsiveness of some nociceptive spinal neurons to subsequent nociceptive and nonnociceptive afferent input has been demonstrated to be altered by input from unmyelinated (c-fiber) nociceptive afferents.[52,54,55] A decade of experiments by many investigators* concerning nociception-induced sensitization of spinal neurons have largely established the following principles:

1. Spinal nociceptive neurons may be categorized as either nociceptive-specific (NS) or wide-dynamic-range (WDR) (multireceptive). Nociceptive-specific neurons are excited by nociceptive afferent activity, but not by activity in nonnociceptive afferents; WDR neurons are activated by both nociceptive and nonnociceptive afferents.

*References 12, 13, 14, 38, 40, 50, and 55.

2. Nociceptive-specific and WDR neurons become sensitized by nociceptive (but *not* nonnociceptive) afferent input. Sensitization is reflected by a more intense response to a given stimulus and by responsiveness to application of that stimulus throughout a larger tissue area.[10] Generally, WDR neurons are more intensely sensitized than are NS neurons.

3. Wide-dynamic-range neurons, once sensitized, may respond as strongly to nonnociceptive afferent input as they had previously responded to some nociceptive inputs. This response characteristic provides a potential basis, at the spinal cord level, for pain secondary to nonnociceptive input.

Some patients with spontaneous pain and/or persistent allodynia have experienced pain relief during a selective pressure/ischemic block of nonnociceptive afferents, as would be expected if nonnociceptive rather than nociceptive afferents were activating central pain mechanisms.[9,34] Electrical stimulation of peripheral nerves innervating allodynic regions produced pain in similar patients at stimulus intensities only sufficient to activate axons from nonnociceptive afferents.[36,37] Similar stimulation of nerves innervating normal contralateral sites did not produce pain.

4. Cross-species evaluations have demonstrated that the activity of WDR neurons has correlated better with psychophysical measures of human pain intensity than has activity in NS neurons.[25,35,46]

5. Central sensitization induced by nociceptive afferent activity persists in the absence of continued nociception.[10,50,53,54] The maximal duration of nociceptively induced central sensitization remains undetermined and is currently an issue of debate.[20]

Most of the animal and clinical experiments supporting the principles listed above have involved superficial tissues of the distal limbs. The relevance of that work to persistent pain associated with deep tissues remains to be determined. However, certain evidence suggests that c-fiber deep-tissue nociceptive afferents may be even more effective than cutaneous afferents in producing central sensitization.[54] We have recently completed initial animal experiments designed to examine sensitization processes in relation to the neurophysiology of the low back.

Figures 9-4 and 9-5 shows the increased response and receptive-field size that are induced by nociceptive activity due to algogen injection in paraspinal deep tissues. Note specifically that following nociceptive input, the response to nonnociceptive afferent input (brushing the skin) exceeded the magnitude of the response to a noxious pinch that occurred prior to algogen injection. This increased respon-

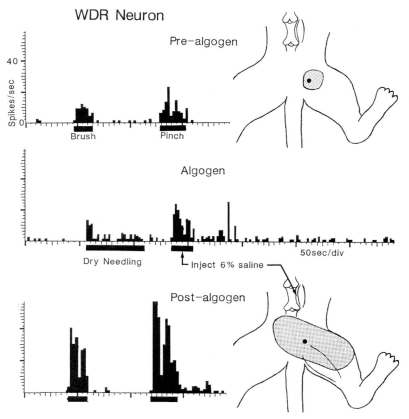

Fig. 9-5

Nociception-induced "sensitization" of a WDR spinal neuron. Note that in this and the previous figure, algogen-induced nociception caused the post-algogen response to nonnoxious touch (brush) to exceed the magnitude of response induced by a noxious stimulus (pinch) prior to the algogen.

siveness may provide the physiologic basis for allodynia, that is, pain in response to activation of nonnociceptive afferents, a definition suggested by Lindblom and Hansson.[28] The increased responsiveness to noxious stimulation (pinch) may represent hyperalgesia, that is, abnormally intense pain in response to a normally painful stimulus. Note that in both figures, nociception caused expansion of the receptive field into contralateral tissue and down the leg, an effect sometimes noted in clinical testing of patients with LBP.

While studying the sensitization of potentially "pain-producing" central neurons, we have also examined, to a limited extent, inhibitory phenomena that may be important in pain suppression rather than pain production. For example, a subset of the dorsal-horn neurons from which we have recorded (approximately 20% of the total) show complex forms of response suppression to paravertebral stimulation.[18] Brief inhibition of cellular discharge (both background and stimulus-evoked) can, in some instances, be obtained by innocuous mechanical stimulation of the superficial (cutaneous) receptive field of these cells. This short-lived phasic response suppression is reminiscent of the effect of spinally mediated inhibition as proposed by Melzack and Wall in their gate-control theory. Additionally, noxious mechanical pressure applied to deep tissues of the back and hip sometimes produced a more longlasting and substantial inhibition, which suggests involvement of additional segmental and suprasegmental inhibitory processes. Thus, it appears that many low-back neurons are subject to powerful inhibitory controls, any of which might be mobilized by the various mechanical and electrical interventions currently used for amelioration of lumbar spine pain.

Relative to the persistence of clinically important pathologic pain, as measured in terms of months and years, the experimentally demonstrated persistence of nociception-induced central sensitization is relatively short-lived (to date, several days maximum). However, noxious stimulation in experimental situations has been very moderate in relation to that which often occurs in the clinical situation. Quite clearly, many questions remain to be answered. Does persistent or intermittently repeated nociception produce increasingly persistent central sensitization? (Do repeated bouts of "acute" LBP lead to "chronic" LBP?[4]) Can central sensitization persist in the complete absence of even minor or intermittent nociception? (Can nonnociceptive pain become entirely independent of nociceptive input, and are some forms of chronic LBP completely refractory to antinociceptive medications?) Are the neural processes involved in sensitization more active and persistent in some individuals than in others and, if so, why? (Many individuals experience acute LBP, but relatively few proceed to chronic LBP. Why?)

Sensitization and Recruitment of Nociceptive Afferents

It is not our intention to suggest that pathologically persistent pain is only of nonnociceptive origin. Clearly persistent pain may occur secondary to normal nociception associated with persisting nonneural tissue pathology.[45] Even in the absence of obvious pathology, nociceptive afferent activity may be persistent due to peripheral neuroplastic mechanisms that result in receptor sensitization,[29,30,39] ectopic firing by peripheral axons or dorsal-root ganglion cells,[7] or the recruitment of "normally silent" unmyelinated afferents by inflammatory processes.[44] Biochemical events associated with lumbar disc herniation may be of particular importance in this latter regard.[42] Persistent nociception, whether in response to continuing tissue pathology or the result of peripheral neuroplastic processes, is extremely important in relation to persistent pain of nonnociceptive origin. Any process which facilitates or maintains nociceptive afferent activity would simultaneously facilitate or maintain the sensitization of spinal WDR nociceptive neurons. This sensitization would increase the probability of the WDRs being activated by non-nociceptive afferent activity and, consequently, would increase the probability of nonnociceptive pain. Clearly, when nociception is persistent, pain at any particular moment would likely involve nociceptive and nonnociceptive components.

As noted already, important questions remain to be answered. Is minimal, though persistent, nociception sufficient to sustain already established intense central sensitization and nonnociceptive pain? At what point might central sensitization secondary to persistent nociception become "fixed" or independent of that nociception? When antinociceptive treatment modalities are only partially effective, is the remaining pain nonnociceptive in origin?

Clinical Implications

1. General anesthesia does not prevent afferent excitation of spinal neurons. Therefore, even when general anesthesia is necessary, concomitant use of peripheral nerve blocks may provide important protection against sensitization of nociceptive spinal neurons and the subsequent development of intractable iatrogenic nonnociceptive pain.[3,26]

2. Stoicism and nontreatment of persistent though tolerable nociceptive pain should be avoided. By sensitizing spinal neurons, minor but persistent nociceptive afferent activity may seriously increase the risk of developing intractable nonnociceptive pain in the event of additional trauma or, perhaps, solely due to the additive effects of persistent nociceptive input. This supposition remains to be experimentally verified, but see Nathan.[32]

3. Effective pain intervention, once sensitization has become established, would seem to depend upon development of methods to reduce central sensitization rather than upon methods to reduce nociception*.

Sympathetic Mechanisms and Low-Back Pain

The characteristics of persistent LBP that occurs in the absence of identifiable tissue pathology often parallel the characteristics of reflex sympathetic dystrophy (RSD).[23] For example, in both: (1) spontaneous pain appears excessive in relation to known pathology or may occur in the absence of identifiable pathology; (2) minor, normally nonnoxious events may elicit severe pain (light touch may produce severe burning pain in patients with RSD; minimal movement may produce severe aching or stabbing pain in patients with LBP); (3) cold allodynia may be a characteristic symptom;[16,28] and (4) analgesic intervention is partially or largely ineffective.[1,11,21]

We have begun to examine potential sympathetic involvement in LBP in two ways: (1) in animal experiments, by investigating the effect of sympathetic trunk stimulation on the activity of spinal nociceptive neurons that respond to noxious stimulation of spinal and paraspinal tissues, and (2) by a double-blind examination of the effect of a systemically administered noradrenergic antagonist (phentolamine) on pain in patients with chronic LBP. (Phentolamine

*References 2, 22, 27, 48, and 53.

is intended to block sympathetic transmitter/receptor binding in peripheral tissues, thus interrupting the "sympathetic efferent/primary afferent/sensitized spinal nociceptive neuron" loop proposed by Roberts[38] to mediate RSD. This clinical investigation is a collaborative effort conducted with, largely by, and using the patients of Dr. Perry Fine at the University of Utah Medical School.[15]

Our neurophysiologic investigations in cats indicate that most WDR and some NS spinal neurons respond to stimulation of the sympathetic trunk (80% and 30% respectively). Analysis of the data suggests that trunk stimulation activates these neurons in two ways: (1) by activation of visceral or paraspinal somatic *afferent* axons projecting via the sympathetic trunk, and (2) by activation of sympathetic *efferent* axons which project to cutaneous and deep tissues of the low back and hind limb.

Our analysis indicates that NS neurons were excited only by stimulation of the somatic *afferents* in the trunk, not a true sympathetic process, and thus NS neurons probably would not be involved in sympathetically mediated LBP. On the other hand, WDR neurons would likely be involved since our current and prior[17,19,40] evidence indicates that these spinal neurons indirectly respond to activation of *sympathetic efferents* via a sympathetic efferent/nonnociceptive afferent/sensitized WDR loop. Thus, at the primary afferent level, sympathetically mediated LBP would be of largely nonnociceptive rather than nociceptive origin and, like RSD, it would be resistant to antinociceptive treatment modalities. (Recent evidence suggests that following trauma some, though relatively few, nociceptive afferents become responsive to sympathetic efferent activity.[8,39,43] Therefore, sympathetically mediated pain may not be entirely nonnociceptive.)

Examples of activity elicited by sympathetic trunk stimulation are shown in Figure 9-6 (right half of figure). Systemic injection of 1.2 mg/kg of the

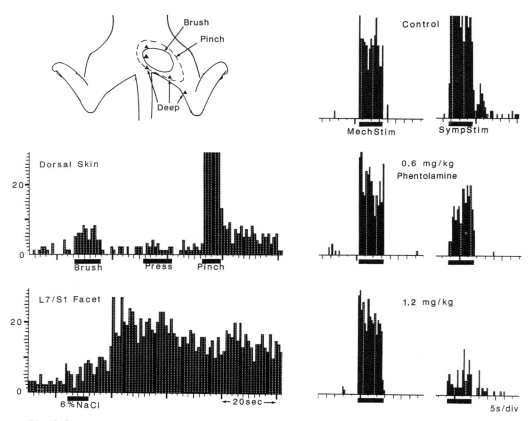

Fig. 9-6

Response to sympathetic trunk stimulation in a "hyper-convergent" low-back neuron is reduced by α-adrenergic blockade with systemic phentolamine (right half of figure). Note that the general responsiveness of the neuron was not reduced, as indicated by continued strong responding to mechanical stimulation of the skin. This neuron was responsive to mechanical or algogen stimulation of deep tissues at all loci indicated by triangles.

α-adrenergic antagonist phentolamine blocked almost all response to truncal stimulation of sympathetic efferents. Other data indicates that the remaining responses were due to activation of afferent axons within the sympathetic trunk. The fact that the neuron's responsiveness to mechanical stimulation was not altered indicates that the phentolamine effect was not due just to a generalized reduced response of the recorded neuron.

Clinical Implications

1. Evidence presented here and in our previous work[19,40] indicates that activity in sympathetic efferents can, via an as yet unproven afferent mechanism, activate nociceptive "low-back" spinal neurons. This data, together with evidence from the RSD literature which indicates that sympathetic intervention can relieve sympathetically maintained pain, would seem to warrant investigation of sympathetic intervention as a diagnostic and perhaps occasional therapeutic tool in relation to LBP.[6]

2. The presence within the sympathetic trunk of somatic and/or visceral afferents that project to low back spinal neurons[17,19] complicates the interpretation of the effects of sympathectomy in relation to LBP. Relief could be attributed to: (1) the transection of sympathetic efferents, as suggested above; (2) the transection of somatic/visceral nociceptive afferents and the relief of normal nociceptive pain; or (3) both of these. (It might be noted that transection of afferents within the trunk may contribute to post-sympathectomy neuralgia via partial deafferentation of both low-back and proximal thigh spinal neurons.[41])

3. Sympathetic involvement in LBP might be more definitively determined by pharmacologic blockade of sympathetic transmitters, as attempted in our phentolamine study with Dr. Fine at the University of Utah Medical School.

Although our phentolamine study with Dr. Fine was intended to examine sympathetic efferent/primary afferent mechanisms in relation to chronic LBP, it has to date provided little evidence concerning sympathetic mechanisms, per se, largely because of unusually intense placebo responses by the patients. The intensity of the placebo response in these patients, as revealed by a double-blind placebo-controlled experimental design, is extremely interesting. To date, seven of eight patients tested with infusions of normal saline demonstrated placebo responses of such strength that essentially no chronic pain was left against which to test the effect of subsequently injected systemic phentolamine. Greater than 50% pain relief persisted for several hours, and in some cases, days, in most of these patients. However, we caution against interpreting these results to be indicative of a psychogenic origin for persistent LBP.

Comments on the Somato/ Neuronal vs. Psychogenic Origin of Low-Back Pain that Occurs in the Absence of Identifiable Somatic Pathology

A psychogenic origin of persistent LBP syndrome is sometimes entertained on the basis of the following characteristics: (1) the occurrence and persistence of LBP, in some patients, in the absence of identifiable or seemingly adequate pathology; (2) its occurrence in response to normally nonnoxious stimulation (e.g., minor movements, deep pressure, or touch); (3) its resistance to pharmacologic antinociceptive intervention; (4) its diffuseness or "distribution" in patterns not restricted to the known distribution of potentially involved peripheral nerves; and sometimes, (5) its relief by treatment with placebo.

Pain relief in response to the administration of a placebo is well known, even when the pain is clearly of somatic origin, and, by itself, a placebo response indicates nothing other than an individual is a placebo-responder. The implication that pain is solely of a higher order CNS (i.e., psychogenic) origin cannot be inferred.[51] As with all painful syndromes, the interpretation of LBP as being psychogenic in origin depends on validly defining other characteristics of the syndrome that would support psychogenicity.

The data and concepts presented in this chapter suggest that in some patients neural mechanisms operating at the primary afferent and spinal neuronal level could mediate the unusual characteristics of persistent LBP listed above, thus suggesting caution before interpreting these characteristics primarily in terms of "higher order" psychogenic processes. On the basis of neurophysiologic and clinical evidence presented or referenced in this chapter, characteristics (1), (2), and (3) above may be interpreted as being secondary to the *persistent sensitization* of spinal nociceptive neurons which, as the result of being sensitized, become unusually responsive to *nonnociceptive* afferent activity.

Concerning characteristic (4), our anatomical and single cell electrophysiologic data clearly indicate the convergence of afferent information from multiple individual nerves (and even from axons projecting separately in the dorsal vs. ventral rami of the spinal nerves) onto individual neurons in the spinal dorsal horn. Thus it would be expected, especially after sensitization of these spinal neurons, that individual neurons would respond to stimulation of many areas or tissues, the separate tissues often being innervated by different peripheral nerves. As the result of this convergence of information, precise localization of the source(s) of afferent activity by additional CNS processing may be (but would not necessarily be) impossible.

Clearly, interpretation of placebo responding by patients with LBP requires careful consideration; additionally, its strength and prevalence in Dr. Fine's population suggests interesting questions. Is *intense* placebo responding *unusually* characteristic of persistent LBP in patients? Is pain of nonnociceptive origin more susceptible to placebo (descending inhibitory?) processes than pain of nociceptive origin? Are spinal and supraspinal pain mechanisms that mediate *persistent* pain considerably different from those that mediate *acute* pain and are they differently affected by the physiological mechanisms which mediate the placebo response?

Finally, in several of Dr. Fine's patients and in a larger group of patients with pathologically persistent limb pain,[49] a "delayed" onset of the placebo response has been noted, the response often beginning no sooner than 30 minutes following administration of the placebo treatment. Does this delayed onset, in conjunction with the extended duration of the response, suggest that placebo mechanisms involve alterations in neuronal biochemistry rather than solely in electrophysiologic activity? Investigation of these questions in both clinical and animal experiments may allow development of procedures to relieve central sensitization and nonnociceptive pain.

Summary

In this chapter, we have discussed research suggesting (1) that the diffuse localization and lack of tissue specificity associated with LBP may be explained by extensive divergence and convergence of afferents from lumbar (and hindlimb) tissues and (2) that *persistent* LBP may, to an undetermined extent, be dependent upon *sensitization* of nociceptive spinal neurons and activation of those neurons by *nonnociceptive* afferents. Parallels were drawn between the neuronal mechanisms of LBP and mechanisms mediating aspects of other "pathologic" pain syndromes, most specifically RSD. Throughout, experimentally demonstrated physiologic mechanisms were offered as potential alternative/additional explanations of symptoms of low-back pain often otherwise considered to be primarily of psychogenic origin.

References

1. Arner S, Meyerson BA: Lack of analgesic effect of opioids on neuropathic forms of pain, *Pain* 33:11, 1988.
2. Arner S and others: Prolonged relief of neuralgia after regional anesthetic blocks. A call for further experimental and systematic clinical studies, *Pain* 43:287, 1990.
3. Bach S, Noreng MF, Tjellden NU: Phantom limb pain in amputees during the first 12 months following limb amputation, after preoperative lumbar epidural blockade, *Pain* 33:297, 1988.
4. Bigos SJ, Battie MC: *The impact of spinal disorder in industry.* In Frymoyer JW, editor: *The adult spine: principles and practice,* New York, 1991, Raven Press.
5. Bonica JJ: *General considerations of acute pain.* In Bonica JJ, editor: *The management of pain,* Philadelphia, 1990, Lea & Febiger.
6. Brena SF and others: Chronic back pain: electromyographic, motion and behavioral assessments following sympathetic nerve blocks and placebos, *Pain* 8:1, 1980.
7. Burchiel KJ: Spontaneous impulse generation in normal and denervated dorsal root ganglia: sensitivity to alpha-adrenergic stimulation and hypoxia, *Exp Neurol* 85:257, 1984.
8. Campbell JN, Meyer RA, Raja SN: Is nociceptor activation by alpha-1 adrenoreceptors the culprit in sympathetically maintained pain?, *Am Pain Soc J* 1:3, 1992.
9. Campbell JN and others: Myelinated afferents signal the hyperalgesia associated with nerve injury, *Pain* 32:89, 1988.
10. Cook AJ and others: Dynamic receptive field plasticity in rat spinal cord dorsal horn following C-primary afferent input, *Nature* 325:151, 1987.
11. Cooper RG and others: The role of epidural fibrosis and defective fibrinolysis in the persistence of postlaminectomy back pain, *Spine* 16:1044, 1991.
12. Devor M: *Central changes mediating neuropathic pain.* In Dubner R, Gebhart GF, Bond MR, editors: *Proceedings of the Fifth world congress on pain,* Amsterdam, 1988, Elsevier.
13. Dubner R: *Neuronal plasticity in the spinal and medullary dorsal horns: a possible role in central pain mechanisms.* In Casey KL, editor: *Pain and central nervous system disease: the central pain syndromes,* New York, 1991, Raven Press, Ltd.
14. Dubner R, Ruda MA: Activity-dependent neuronal plasticity following tissue injury and inflammation, *Trends Neurosci* 15:96, 1992.
15. Fine PG and others: Slowly developing placebo responses confound tests of intravenous phentolamine to determine mechanisms underlying idiopathic chronic low back pain. *Pain* 56:235, 1994.

16. Frost SA and others: *Does hyperalgesia to cooling stimuli characterize patients with sympathetically maintained pain (reflex sympathetic dystrophy)?* In Dubner R, Gebhart GF, Bond MR, editors: *Proceedings of the Fifth World Congress on Pain,* Amsterdam, 1988, Elsevier.

17. Gillette RG, Kramis RC, Roberts WJ: Characterization of spinal somatosensory neurons having receptive fields in lumbar tissues of cats, *Pain* 54:85, 1993.

18. Gillette RG, Kramis RC, Roberts WJ: Spinal projections of cat primary afferent fibers innervating lumbar facet joints and multifidus muscle, *Neurosci Lett* 157:67, 1993.

19. Gillette RG, Kramis RC, Roberts WJ: Sympathetic activation of cat spinal neurons responsive to noxious stimulation of deep tissues in the low back, *Pain,* 56:31, 1994.

20. Gracely RH, Lynch SA, Bennett GJ: Painful neuropathy: altered central processing maintained dynamically by peripheral input, *Pain* 51:175, 1992.

21. Haldeman S: Failure of the pathology model to predict back pain. *Spine* 15:718, 1990.;

22. Hao J-X and others: Baclofen reverses the hypersensitivity of dorsal horn wide dynamic range neurons to mechanical stimulation after transient spinal cord ischemia; implications for a tonic GABAergic inhibitory control of myelinated fiber input, *J Neurophysiol.* 68:392, 1992.

23. Janig W: *Pathophysiological mechanisms operating in reflex sympathetic dystrophy.* In *Advances in Pain Research and Therapy,* vol 20, New York, 1992, Raven Press.

24. Kellgren JH: The anatomical source of back pain, *Rheumatol Rehab* 16:3, 1977.

25. Kenshalo DR Jr, Anton F, Dubner R: The detection and perceived intensity of noxious thermal stimuli in monkey and in human, *J Neurophysiol* 62:429, 1989.

26. Kiss IE, Kilian M: Does opiate premedication influence postoperative analgesia? A prospective study, *Pain* 48:157, 1992.

27. Kristensen JD, Svensson B, Gordh T Jr: The NMDA-receptor antagonist CPP abolishes neurogenic "wind-up pain" after intrathecal administration in humans, *Pain* 51:249, 1992.

28. Lindblom U, Hansson P: *Sensory dysfunction and pain after clinical nerve injury studied by means of graded mechanical and thermal stimulation.* In Besson JM, editor: *Lesions of primary afferent fibers as a tool for the study of clinical pain,* Amsterdam, 1992, Elsevier.

29. McMahon S, Koltzenburg M: The changing role of primary afferent neurones in pain, *Pain* 43:269, 1990.

30. Mense S: Slowly conducting afferent fibers from deep tissues: neurobiological properties and central nervous actions, *Prog Sens Physiol* 6:139, 1986.

31. Mooney V: Where is the pain coming from? *Spine* 12:754, 1987.

32. Nathan PW: Pain and nociception in the clinical context, *Philos Trans R Soc Lond. [Biol]* 308:219, 1985.

33. North RB: *Low back pain: fundamental issues of sensory mechanisms.* Eleventh Annual Scientific Meeting, American Pain Society, Symposia 012, 1992 (abstract).

34. Ochoa J and others: Two mechanical hyperalgesias in human neuropathy, *Soc Neurosci Abst* 15(1):472, 1989.

35. Price DD: *Psychological and neural mechanisms of pain.* New York, 1988, Raven Press.

36. Price DD, Bennett GJ, Rafii A: Psychophysical observations on patients with neuropathic pain relieved by a sympathetic block, *Pain* 36:273, 1989.

37. Price DD, Long S, Huitt C: Sensory testing of pathophysiological mechanisms of pain in patients with reflex sympathetic dystrophy, *Pain* 49:163, 1992.

38. Roberts WJ: A hypothesis on the physiological basis for causalgia and related pains, *Pain* 24:297, 1986.

39. Roberts WJ, Elardo SM: Sympathetic activation of A-delta nociceptors, *Somatosensory Res* 3:33, 1985.

40. Roberts WJ, Foglesong ME: I. Spinal recordings indicate that wide-dynamic-range neurons mediate sympathetically maintained pain, *Pain* 34:289, 1988.

41. Roberts WJ, Kramis RC: *Sympathetic nervous system influence on acute and chronic pain.* In Fields HL, editor: *Pain syndromes in neurology,* London, 1990, Butterworths.

42. Saal JS and others: High levels of inflammatory phospholipase A2 activity in lumbar disc herniations. *Spine* 15:674, 1990.

43. Sato J, Perl ER: Adrenergic excitation of cutaneous pain receptors induced by peripheral nerve injury, *Science* 251:1608, 1991.

44. Schaible H-G, Schmidt RF: Effects of an experimental arthritis on the sensory properties of fine articular afferent units, *J Neurophysiol* 54:1109, 1985.

45. Schofferman L and others: Occult infections causing persistent low-back pain. *Spine* 14:417, 1989.

46. Simone DA and others: Neurogenic hyperalgesia: central neural correlates in response of spinothalamic tract neurons, *J Neurophysiol* 66:228, 1991.

47. Spitzer WO and others: Scientific approach to the assessment and management of activity-related spinal disorders: A monograph for clinicians. Report of the Quebec task force on spinal disorders, *Spine* 12:S1, 1987.

48. Tverskoy M and others: Postoperative pain after inguinal herniorrhaphy with different types of anesthesia, *Anesth Analg* 70:29, 1990.

49. Verdugo R, Ochoa JL: High incidence of placebo responders among chronic neuropathic pain patients, *Ann Neurol* 30:229, 1991.

50. Wall PD: *Recruitment of ineffective synapses after injury.* In Waxman SG, editor: *Adv Neurol* Vol. 47, New York, 1988, Raven Press.

51. White L, Tursky B, Schwartz G, editors: *Placebo: theory, research and mechanisms,* New York, 1985, Guilford Press.

52. Woolf CJ: Evidence for a central component of post injury pain hypersensitivity, *Nature* 306:686, 1983.

53. Woolf CJ, Thompson WN: The induction and maintenance of central sensitization is dependent on N-methyl-D-aspartic acid receptor activation; implications for the treatment of post-injury pain hypersensitivity states, *Pain* 44:293, 1991.

54. Woolf CJ, Wall PD: Relative effectiveness of C primary afferent fibers of different origins in evoking a prolonged facilitation of the flexor reflex in the rat, *J Neurosci* 6:1433, 1986.

55. Woolf CJ, Walters ET: Common patterns of plasticity contributing to nociceptive sensitization in mammals and aplysia, *Trends Neurosci* 14:74, 1991.

Chapter 10
Biomechanics of the Spine
Serge Gracovetsky

Evolution of the Human Spine

The theory of evolution and natural selection implies the survival of the fittest and the elimination of the weak from the pool of genetic information available for the continuation of a species. What is the meaning of "fit for survival"? One can start with the hypothesis that survival means that the animal will not self-annihilate. The implication for the musculoskeletal system is that, at any given time, the level of mechanical stress within the system cannot exceed some ultimate value. Hence, regardless of the task being accomplished, the central nervous system (CNS) will activate appropriate components in such a way as to prevent a breakdown of the structures.

The various parts of the spine have different roles and different mechanical characteristics. An efficient animal will execute a task in such a way that the stress within the spine's diverse components is equalized at its lowest level. It is not unreasonable, therefore, to speculate that the overall level of stress during the execution of a task will be proportional to the ultimate limit of each individual component. For example, if, for an arbitrary task, the stress within the bone reaches two-thirds of its ultimate, then the stress within the ligaments would be expected to reach two-thirds of its own ultimate.

But what is the task for which the spine has been designed? Although there is no way of knowing for sure what that particular task might be, we propose that the most important activity for members of the vertebrate species is locomotion: to get food, to flee from predators, and so on. It is therefore appropriate to examine the stages of development of our ancestors' locomotive ability. In so doing, the spine and its surrounding tissues emerge as the pervasive element, the primary engine of locomotion in animals such as ourselves.

In analyzing the evolution of humanity's fish-like ancestors, it becomes obvious that a fish's spine and its surrounding tissue represent the primary engine the animal uses for locomotion. This fact—that the spine is essential to our ancestors' mobility—seems to have been lost in the present-day analysis of human locomotion. To this day, gait analysis is essentially the analysis of the motion of the legs. The legs are certainly useful, but are they essential? The answer is definitely no. It can be demonstrated that human bipedal gait does not require the presence of any extremities; the primary locomotion function of the spine, so obvious in the fish, was never transferred to our extremities during the long evolutionary journey.

Locomotion is but one of the many tasks that the human spinal engine is expected to perform. The spinal engine may not have been optimally designed for tasks such as weight lifting. The consequences of this are felt in the ever-rising claims for work-related accidents involving the musculoskeletal system.

The spinal engine theory leads to several developments in the study of the spine. The theory reveals certain parameters as indicators of spinal function. These parameters are measurable and demonstrate that there are constant patterns of motion across healthy functioning spines. These data on normal spine motion provide functional, relevant information the clinician can use in the evaluation of the spine.

Development of Knowledge: From Antiquity to the Seventies

Understanding the function of the spine was first attempted through clinical experiments. These experiments were basically conducted or controlled by medical professionals interested in improving their patient's care. No significant advances were made until after the Second World War.

The need to appreciate why fighter pilots injured their spine in emergencies triggered the use of mathematic models. Indeed, in vivo experiments were too dangerous to conduct, so mathematic tools were used to predict the outcome of flying maneuvers for both humans and machine.

This opened the door to considerable benefits, but also abuses. The fifties and sixties saw a flurry of models for describing spinal performance, hastily derived from in vitro experiments of dubious value. A typical protocol consisted of setting a spine or portion of a spine in a mechanical press and deriving some equations to describe the response. As expected, the model was always validated. Indeed, putting a spine in a press tells us how the spine behaves in a press. But is this meaningful for in vivo situations? Other experiments in spinal research used animals. However, installing spinal instrumentation into a swine tells us how the instrumentation behaves in a swine. Does a swine use its spine like a bipedal human?

One would expect that the study of spinal anatomy would precede the development of mathematical models. Regrettably, this has not always been the case. Although mathematical modeling was a highly popular exercise in the 1960s and 1970s, these approaches were invariably based on ill-defined descriptions of the back musculature, such as those found in *Gray's Anatomy*.[26] Surprisingly, few individuals challenged these fuzzy descriptions, and it was not until 1984 that the correct anatomic description of back musculature was finally established by Bogduk.[5]

Debate Over the Role of Muscles in Lifting

The consequence of such errors can be appreciated when considering the role of the spinal musculature as the spine flexes. During the past 50 years, it has been frequently argued in the literature that the back muscles are responsible for lifting loads in the sagittal plane. In 1955, Floyd and Silver studied a series of sagittal lifts performed by 144 individuals.[14] To their great surprise, they noted that the electromyographic activity of the erectores spinae decreased at the time when they are most needed—that is, when the load has just been lifted off the ground. This muscle relaxation phenomenon presented quite a challenge to the schools that promote the role of the lumbar musculature in lifting.

To resolve the difficulty, Bartelink proposed that the internal abdominal pressure would rise and supplement the action of the back muscles.[2] Theoretic and experimental considerations refuted this suggestion,[20,22,23,33]. There is no doubt that the maximum L5-S1 moment those muscles are able to generate is about 250 Nm.[6] This is sufficient to handle 50 kg or so, but not much more. Hence, the question: If the erectores are too small to lift significant loads and do not fire at the very moment they are needed most, then where does the necessary lifting force come from?

To address this problem, models of back musculature were developed, including the posterior ligaments as described by Bogduk.[7] However, these very same ligaments were then disabled by the model's internal logic expressing that ligaments are meant to intervene at the very end of a movement.[41-43] Consequently, the resulting solution does not include any significant ligament contribution during motion. The calculations were performed for small loads (approximately 27 kg), ensuring that the compressive forces on the L5-S1 intervertebral joint remained within the known limits supportable by that joint. Simulating heavy lifting was always avoided as it would have resulted in a calculated compression force exceeding the ultimate vertebrae compressive resistance by an order of three (36 KN vs. a maximum of 12 KN),[25] and the muscle firing density would then have also exceeded any plausible level. The reader will appreciate how embarrassing it would be to argue that weight lifters do routinely destroy their spines during training. This demonstrates that these models are not reasonable representations of heavy lifting.

A solution to this problem—the small size of the erectores and the lack of firing at critical moments in lifting—was proposed in 1977.[22] Briefly, the force necessary to perform a lift is generated by the hip extensors, which are attached to the ilium. This force must then be transmitted from the ilium to the upper extremities where it is required. It was hypothesized that the posterior ligamentous system (PLS), comprising the ligamentum flavum, the capsular ligaments of the facets, and the thick lumbodorsal fascia, is the main structure channeling these forces. Bogduk's[5,7] anatomic studies showed that the lumbodorsal fascia portion of the PLS is capable of such transmission of forces.

Another path is represented by the continuation of the biceps femoris and attached to the ischial tuberosity, itself connected to the sacrum by the sacrotuberous ligament: the whole of which would connect with the erectores spinal aponeurosis, which is itself an extension of the iliocostalis thoracis.[69] This path transmits forces directly to the shoulder girdle where it is needed.

Spinal Coordination

The available data in the literature on weight lifting in the sagittal plane can be explained by the hypothesis that the musculoskeletal system will transfer forces with minimum stress at each spinal level.[21] This force transmission system, discussed earlier, is illustrated in Fig. 10-1. This hypothesis implies that proper force transmission demands a very specific spinal coordination strategy.

As a person moves, lifts loads, and so on, the motion of the spinal segments takes on a specific pattern in order to optimize the transmission of forces and minimize the stress on each segment.[18,19,20,21] "Spinal coordination" is the specific pattern of motion throughout the spine, and between spinal segments (e.g., the relative motions of L4 over L5 during flexion). Coordination may be a protection mechanism ensuring that no spinal component will become overloaded and fail.

Normal individuals exhibit a specific coordination that is remarkably similar from one person to the next. Conversely "abnormal" individuals would be expected to deviate significantly from the normal coordination patterns. Spinal coordination is affected by spinal pathology; therefore, measuring spinal coordination should give us a window on pathology.

It seems reasonable to propose that an injured spinal element cannot be loaded with the same amount of stress it normally withstands. To reduce

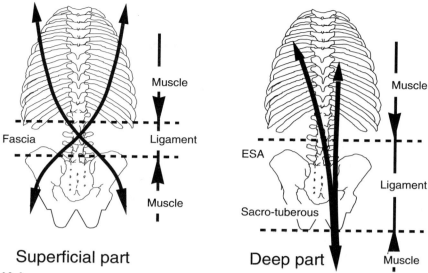

Superficial part   **Deep part**

Fig. 10-1

Handling loads requires the transmission of forces to the shoulders. This diagram illustrates two fundamental force-transmission systems, referred to as the "superficial part" and the "deep part." The superficial part includes the hip extensors (and equivalents attached to the iliac crest), the latissimus dorsi (and equivalents attached from the spinous processes), and the rib cage (attached to the shoulder complex); in between, the ligamentous lumbodorsal fascia is not under muscle control. To tighten this ligament demands a reduction in lordosis. This lordosis reduction is therefore essential in tightening the fascia for transmission of forces. The deep part of the force-transmission system comprises the hamstrings/sacro-tuberous ligament/erectores spinae aponeurosis, and the nonlinear effect of the collagen fibers of overstretched muscles.

the stress on that element (and to some degree overload the healthy elements) requires a change in coordination of the spinal segments. This change in coordination is an important physiologic parameter that may contain information on functional impairment. In fact, for spinal evaluation, the clinician does use information regarding spinal coordination—although perhaps not defined as such. Instinctively the clinician uses his or her own definition of normal patterns of movement as part of a spinal evaluation. Clinicians watch a patient flex his or her spine or walk and take note of any deviation from "normal." A change from normal movement is a change in coordination.

Spinal coordination is an objective measure of physiology, in that it is very difficult to control consciously the motion of two adjacent joints. This is in contrast to range of motion (ROM), which is easy to change. Therefore, spinal coordination should be relatively independent of voluntary control.

The Role of the Spine in Human Locomotion

It is generally believed that the spine is essentially a supporting column linking pelvis to shoulders. As an individual walks or runs, his trunk is believed to be carried passively by his legs. However, this simple

and attractive idea leads to numerous contradictions. For example: why is the spine curved in the form of an S instead of being straight? It would appear that a straight column would support compressive loads better than a curved one, and the curved spine impacted at each heel strike would be at a disadvantage. The argument that spinal lordosis is a transient condition that will be eliminated as a matter of evolutionary improvement contradicts the fact that monkeys have a straight spine and, as far as can be observed, are quadrupeds. The uniqueness of human bipedalism suggests that the unique features of the human spine must be related in a fundamental way to our locomotion process.

This perspective of human locomotion is so ingrained in our culture that, to date, the study of human gait has been essentially an exercise in analyzing the motion of the legs. The rhythmic, alternating trunk motions are considered the result of jostling by the legs[65]; likewise, the associated muscular contractions are assumed to be part of the effort required to keep from falling over—an aspect of the widely held view that locomotion is a precarious process.[54b] The graceful, flowing stride of the Olympic runner has even been described as "essentially a series of collisions with the ground."[44] However, there are substantial mathematic and clinical arguments to reject this rather crude representation of human gait.

In most studies, the head, arm, and trunk are lumped together and not assigned any function essential to the dynamics of walking. Numerous objections to such a representation have been raised. For example, the motion of the shoulders cannot be hampered without disturbing the locomotion process; people with fused spines exhibit gait modifications; 77% of patients with failed fusions are nonetheless satisfied with the results;[75] and if the torso is in a brace or cast, "walking at moderate or higher speeds becomes awkward and the energy requirements as measured by oxygen consumption rise sharply."[31] If the spine is a column, how do we explain vertical displacement of the body's center of gravity during locomotion? Why do we not flex the knees more in order to clear the ground rather than lift the entire trunk? Indeed, Newton's first law encourages the straightest possible trajectory for the center of gravity; yet it is impossible to walk while maintaining the center of gravity in the horizontal plane. Clearly, there must be an evolutionary advantage to our body's close interaction with the gravitational field.

This is not a philosophic argument. Living organisms *do* exploit their environment, either as a source of energy or for other important purposes. For example, pigeons assess the direction of the earth's gravitational field in navigation. The earth's gravitational field is remarkably constant and it seems unrealistic not to exploit it for survival.

Furthermore, from an evolutionary point of view, it is difficult to think of the trunk, arms and head as passive (i.e., nonfunctional) elements in locomotion. It would be a waste of muscular mass not to use them in some essential way, instead of just dragging them about while walking and running.

In the search for an answer, consider the 20-year-old male subject depicted in Fig. 10-2, *A*. He has reduced arms and legs. The X-ray study of his pelvis shown in Fig. 10-2, *B* clearly demonstrates the absence of lower extremities. Therefore, this young man is standing on his ischium. If it is true that legs are necessary for human locomotion, then a person with the anatomy depicted in the figure would not be able to walk.

The fact is that legs are not necessary for human locomotion. The subject shown in the figure walks using the same spinal/pelvic motion as an individual with legs, albeit with a greater amplitude of pelvic axial rotation.[20] The lack of detectable difference in locomotive patterns between a person with legs, and our subject without legs, raises some serious issues of consistency. Quite clearly, the representation of the spine as a passive structure, totally reliant on the

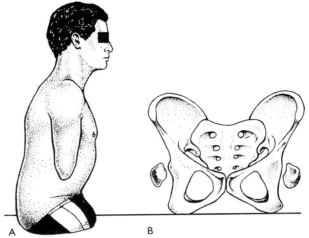

Fig. 10-2

A, Lateral view of a subject with no legs and reduced upper extremities. *B*, Anteroposterior view of the pelvis showing clearly the absence of lower extremities. *(From Gracovetsky S and others: The spinal engine, New York, 1988, Springer Verlag.)*

motion of the legs to carry it, cannot be maintained. A radical change in the perception of the role of the spine must be made. To resolve this and other contradictions, it has been proposed that the spine be considered a sort of engine driving the pelvis.

The basic problem of human bipedal locomotion is that the pelvis must be rotated axially using a muscular system that is more or less parallel to the spine. There are small pelvic muscles that could conceivably contribute to the axial rotation of the pelvis. However, the anatomic arrangement of these muscles does not provide for efficient axial pelvic rotation. Moreover, any torque transmitted by the leg to the pelvis must be canceled by a countertorque at the foot-to-ground interface—when running on our tiptoes we do not transmit torque to the ground. Consequently, the need to conserve angular momentum implies that the leg cannot transmit torque to the pelvis. The question is this: what is driving the pelvis? If it is not driven from below, it must be driven from above.

The theory of the spinal engine is an attempt to explain how the spine participates in our locomotive efforts in conjunction with our natural environment, that is, the earth's gravitational field. According to this theory, the mechanism by which the spine drives the pelvis is the following:

1. The hip extensors contract and the body is lifted in the gravitational field. This can be clearly seen as, for example, a runner's feet leave the ground.
2. During the flight phase, the unloaded spine fires its erectors to rearrange its posture by bending to one side. This requires a relatively small

amount of muscle power, which can be easily supplied by the trunk muscles.

3. The coupled motion of the spine transforms this lateral bend into an axial torque as the legs prepare for landing.

4. Upon heel strike, a substantial pulse propagates through the leg and is shaped by the mechanical responses of knee, hip, and sacroiliac joints. This compressive pulse applied to the intervertebral joint has the effect of enhancing the latter's ability to resist axial torque.

5. At the same time, the descending thorax, arrested by the impact of the heel striking the ground, converts its potential energy into kinetic form. The net effect is to enhance the lateral pull on the spine initiated by the erectores during flight. Through this elaborate sequence of energy transformation, which requires the existence of the earth's gravitational field, the hip extensors flex the spine laterally. In that sense, the hip extensors become lateral spine flexors. The hip extensors are also spine extensors in the sagittal plane via the strong lumbodorsal fascia. Hence, the hip extensors represent the primary source of "economical" power that the spinal engine transforms in the execution of physical activities. The associated trunk muscles "control" the flow of power to and from the extremities, using the gravitational field as temporary storage whenever required.

6. Here again, the coupled motion of the spine transforms this lateral bend into the axial torque needed to rotate the pelvis axially. The power delivered by this torque is enhanced by two factors: by the lordosis and by the joint stiffness that is increased by the compression pulse propagated through the spine at heel strike. Hence, it could also be argued that the hip extensors end up being the primary axial rotators of the spine.

7. From this point on, the legs follow the pelvic motion to enhance the stride.

8. The moving shoulders are derotated by the cervical spine, which acts like a mechanical decoupling device stabilizing the head. This function is opposite to that of the lumbar spine.

This theory explains the need for a runner to use shoes that do not unduly absorb shocks; indeed, the shape of the compressive pulse returned to the spine must be very specific to permit the chemical energy liberated by the hip extensors to be transformed into pelvic motion. An incorrect pulse shape, as is produced when walking on sand, forces the trunk musculature to generate directly the energy needed by the spine to drive the pelvis. This source of energy is inefficient and tires the body rapidly.

The Importance of Lordosis in Locomotion

The coupled motion of the spine is crucial to locomotion because it converts the primitive lateral bend of our fish ancestors into an axial torque. This conversion is possible only because the spine is not straight—that is, it has a curvature, or lordosis. The coupled motion of the spine was first demonstrated by Lovett in 1903.[35] The theory of the spinal engine suggests that the control of lordosis is perhaps the most important feature that makes locomotion possible. Hence, in the event of spinal injury, control of lordosis must be restored.

Understanding the Mechanical Etiology of Spinal Disorders

The spinal-engine theory makes it necessary to change how we look at the mechanical etiology of spine disorders. If we are concerned about the spine viewed as an engine rather than a static supporting column, we need to know how the spine and its components move in space and handle forces. Movement and the handling of forces become the relevant factors in analyzing spine disorders.

The mathematic analysis of flexion/extension reveals that a symmetric spine flexing in the sagittal plane is exposed essentially to pure compressive forces. Yet Virgin[69] demonstrated that the anulus fibrosis is rarely damaged by compression. Numerous other researchers have repeated this experiment with the same results. The calculation made by Shirazi-Adl and associates[60] suggests that when the end plate ruptures, the collagen fibers of the anulus fibrosis are stretched by only about 4%, well below their limit estimated to be 20% to 30%. In short, the anulus cannot be damaged easily by compression and therefore disc prolapse cannot be a consequence of the application of pure compressive forces to the joint. In spite of a considerable body of evidence confirming these conclusions, it is interesting to note the importance assigned to compression injuries in the biomechanical literature.[48] Since anular damage is frequently related to low-back pain (LBP), and pure axial compression cannot damage the disc, another mechanism of injury must exist.

There are many possible loading configurations to which the intervertebral joint can be exposed. At least three appear to be responsible for serious damage when combined in specific ways. They are compression, axial torque, and lateral bending. However, lateral bending may also induce an axial rotation because of the coupled motion of the spine. Hence, it could be argued that there are really only two basic loading configurations responsible for a large number of pathologic observations: axial compression and torsion. In this regard it is interesting to note that Hirsch and Schajowicz[27] reported two distinct early injuries in the anulus as well as at the central portion of the disc, while in the early 1970s, Farfan proposed that the existing data on pathology could be explained by the existence of two families of degenerative patterns.[13] Each behaves in its own clinical manner and responds to its own different type of treatment. Thus, it is not unreasonable to suggest that the mechanical etiology of LBP must comprise at least two basic sequences of pathologic processes.

Compression Injury

The compression injury results in central damage to the disc with an end-plate fracture of varying magnitude, followed by an ingrowth of vascular granulation tissue through the fracture into the disc nucleus. As a result, the avascular nucleus and inner anulus are gradually destroyed. In the early stages, the facet joints are not greatly affected. At a later stage, with continued loss of volume of the nucleus, the disc loses its height and the facet joints dislocate. Arthritic changes appear but are rarely severe. The outer anulus survives and is gradually pushed out from between the end plates (Fig. 10-3, *A*).

Torsion Injury

The other sequence is the so-called torsional injury, which is caused by excessive axial rotation of the spine. This causes peripheral damage to both the discs and facet joints. The anulus is avulsed from the end plate and its laminae separate. However, the central portion of the disc and end plate remain intact. At a later stage, the anulus develops radial fissures, while the nucleus remains relatively untouched. Because the changes in the facet joints are severe, the intervertebral joints may become unstable (Fig. 10-3, *B*).

At the local level, the type of injury is determined by the actual distribution of stress in the components of the lumbar spine. Thus, one of the key factors in determining the final outcome is the geometric arrangement of the individual spinal segments. From the geometric features seen in simple radiographs, it is sometimes possible to locate the particular joint that is at risk. This factor is particularly helpful either when the radiographs of the joints show no in-

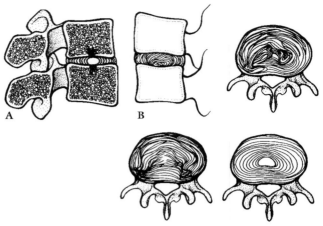

Fig. 10-3

A, The compression injury is characterized by the rupture of the end plate. The nucleus pulposus is injected into the vertebral body (Schmorl's nodes). In the early stages, the anulus and the facets are intact. The injury is inside the joint, and is essentially a rupture of cancellous bone, which heals relatively quickly. **B,** The torsional injury is characterized by damage to the anulus and the facets. In extreme cases, nuclear material can find its way through anular fissures into the canal or the vertbral foramen. The injury lies at the periphery of the joint. Because the injury is essentially a ligamentous one, it takes a long time to repair itself. This type of injury evolves very differently from a compression injury—hence, the importance of early diagnosis to differentiate between the two. *(From Gracovetsky S: The spinal engine, New York, 1988, Springer Verlag.)*

jury or where other indications point to multiple possibilities. In the lumbar spine, the L4-L5 and L5-S1 levels account statistically for approximately 95% of all cases of spinal injury. Of the three remaining joints, problems at L3-L4 appear to be far more common than at the other two higher levels. For example, in a series of 140 cases, five L3-L4 lesions accounted for an overall incidence of 3.5% of injuries.[12] The shape and size of the disc, as well as its location relative to the pelvis, have considerable influence on both the type of injury incurred and its consequences for the anatomy and function of the joint. It is therefore incomprehensible that disc problems are sometimes amalgamated into a single entity.

Many of the observed injuries can be reproduced in the laboratory by subjecting the joint to either excessive compression or torsion—or both. For this reason, these injuries have been described respectively as compression and torsion injuries. This simplification of the mechanical etiology of LBP is not universally accepted, although over the past few years there seems to be a trend toward accepting that torsional injuries are responsible for a wide variety of symptoms related to ligamentous damage. This damage may be to either the anulus fibrosis (causing herniation of the nucleus), the capsular ligament of the facets, or both.

The simple distinction made between axial compression and torsion is attractive but incomplete. The joint is subjected to more complex types of loading. Although some attempts have been made to determine experimentally the effect of axial compression and torsion on a joint bent in the sagittal and coronal planes, much research remains to be done before this issue can be clarified. Yet, there are theoretic and clinical reasons to believe that this is the primary type of loading applied to the spine during locomotion.

To appreciate what other types of forces may act upon the spine, consider that a load is rarely lifted without being carried some distance. The data provided by the NIOSH standards should be accepted with caution because "lift and carry" implies the presence of torsion within the spine. It would be equally logical (or illogical) to argue that torsion alone is responsible for spinal injury. Thus is seems more realistic to consider that both compression and torsion together may contribute to the injury process. Not everyone agrees.

Experiments involving bending (such as hyperflexion) did produce anular damage[1] and were believed to represent a plausible explanation for disc prolapse. There are, however, a number of reasons to be cautious. First, there is no clear-cut relationship between the data collected and an in vivo situation; second, the initial conditions of the discs are unknown. For example, it is conceivable that discs already damaged by torsion were included in the sample. Hence, the prolapse subsequently observed may have been secondary to the combination of the preceding injury and the hyperflexion. In fact, the observed statistical distribution of prolapse may very well reflect the distribution of torsional injuries among the population of discs selected, rather than be the consequence of the particular mode of loading selected. Third, the level of facet asymmetry was not noted, even though it is bound to have an effect as it may result in a net torque being applied to the anulus. Thus it could be argued that Adams and Hutton[1] observed anular failure from a peculiar combination of compression and torsion.

There is an additional problem: failure did not occur until the displacements were abnormally high. Extreme ROM had to be imposed upon the joint before prolapse resulted. Even then, only a fraction of the discs tested actually failed. This type of experiment testifies, to the reluctance of many, that axial torsion may actually have a role to play in the etiology of spine disorders.

For a long time, it has not been understood why some mechanism has not evolved that would prevent the spine from being injured by torsion. There has

to be some fundamental advantage in exposing the spine to such potentially damaging types of forces. This issue is put to rest if we consider that the spine is not a passive structure, but rather an engine capable of driving the pelvis that has adapted to our bipedal mode of locomotion. Torsion thus emerges as perhaps the most important motion of the spine.

However, if torsion is indeed necessary to ensure pelvic rotations, how could any axial torque be generated from the more-or-less longitudinal pull of the erectores? It is conceivable that the obliques could contribute to axial rotation during locomotion; the problem, though, is that they do not.[2a] Somehow the spine converts the primitive lateral bend of our fish-like ancestors into an axial torque. How this is done was discovered by Lovett some 80 years ago.[35] It is the coupled motion of the spine that is the basis for understanding how we walk.

Difficulties in Spinal Assessment

The spinal-engine theory also has implications for spinal assessment. If, for example, the spine is envisioned as some kind of passive structure carried by the legs, then we will measure certain parameters and look for certain signs and symptoms that are essentially manifestations of weaknesses of that passive column. If, however, the spine is viewed as an engine, then it is necessary to review what we measure and how we are measuring, in order to arrive at a diagnosis. Obviously, evaluating the function of an active engine can not possibly be the same as evaluating the function of a passive column. This may explain why common tools used in spinal assessment could not produce the informative data needed by clinicians.

Common Spinal Evaluation Tools Cannot Deliver Complete Information

Many tools are available for spinal evaluation and yet, "according to many experts, the precise diagnosis is unknown in 80 to 90% of patients with disabling low back pain."[62] Not only are diagnoses imprecise, there is often variation in the diagnosis of the same patient. "Frequently, one finds in a medical chart two or three diagnoses, made by different physicians."[61] This suggests that something is wrong with the standard approaches to diagnosing and treating mechanical spine problems. For diagnosis and treatment, and/or rating impairment and disability, physicians must evaluate the spine based on function. "The question of the integrity of the musculo skeletal system revolves around evaluating its function, as defined by dynamic activity . . . such as lifting, bending, standing, sitting, walking, carrying, climbing, and crawling."[37] Therefore, to be valid and/or appropriate for spinal evaluation, a tool must be able to deliver relevant information regarding function.

Physical Examination

There is considerable debate in the literature about the accuracy and reliability of the physical examination.* In particular, it has been found that the physical examination is not independent of the clinician. For example, Nelson and associates[49] identified a high level of observer differences for examination of patients with LBP. The physical examination cannot provide information on detailed spinal motion. As well, the clinician does not generally test the individual under load, which is often necessary to make return-to-work decisions.

Pain Analysis

Pain is an indicator of spinal problems. Generally, it is the pain that prompts the patient to seek medical attention. Rosomoff and associates[57] suggested that chronic intractable benign pain (CIBP) may be evidence of musculoskeletal disease. However, it has been found that pain is not a valid measurement of spinal disability. Waddell[70] found that the correlation coefficient between pain and impairment is 0.27, and between pain and disability is 0.44. Spitzer and associates[61] found that there is often a discrepancy between the level of pain and the actual loss of function. Furthermore, Troup and associates[67] found that a patient's perception of what is or may be painful—thus causing or aggravating LBP—may be unreliable.

Radiology

Radiologic findings are not appropriate for functional evaluation. The correlation between anatomic anomalies (positive radiologic findings) and spinal function is 0.57.[70] This poor correlation is reflected in current legislation. The Americans with Disabilities Act specifically forbids consideration of radiologic impairments in the evaluation of a patient's disability.[11]

Furthermore, Heslin and associates[26a] reported that 80.6% of 7016 x-ray films of asymptomatic males showed one or more anatomic abnormalities. Boden[4] found that MRI demonstrated abnormal scans in 28% of asymptomatic persons. According to Spitzer and co-workers,[61] radiology is of limited value in the first evaluation of the majority of spinal disorders. Spitzer[61] states that there is no reason to take an x-ray during the first two weeks of acute pain—unless there is possible fracture, evidence of cauda equina syndrome, or indication of systemic disease. Pearcy and Tibrewal[53] reported several cases of subjects who had abnormal radiographs, but normal spinal movements.

These studies suggest that there are serious problems with translating radiologic findings into quantifiable indicators of actual functional disability. Nevertheless, "the majority of physicians continue to assume a direct relationship between anatomy and function in most cases, resulting in the greatest single error in low back diagnosis."[38]

Assessment of Function

The goal of a health-care professional is to restore function with a minimal level of pain. Although information on anatomy and pain should have a role in evaluating the patient's condition, it has been suggested that "clinical assessment of disability must concentrate on loss of function rather than pain or anatomy."[28, 47] Therefore, if the focus of spinal evaluation is function, it should be measured directly.

Range of Motion

Range of motion is used to determine spinal function by measuring the amount the trunk can bend. However, studies show ROM is not a valid measure of spinal function. For example, according to Thomas J. Horn[30] "range of motion (ROM) in the lumbar spine cannot distinguish between normal individuals and those with a true impairment due to pathological conditions. Spinal ROM should not be used as an indicator of spinal impairment or disability." In fact, "ROM may over-estimate impairment by up to 38%."[36]

Range-of-motion tests do not consider the allocation of work between the spine and the pelvis. A patient suffering from a stiff lumbar spine may have normal ROM by using more pelvic mobility than normal.[40] As well, ROM is under the voluntary control of the examinee. For a valid measurement, ROM requires examinees to demonstrate their best effort. Any number of factors may cause an examinee not to do this: malingering, symptom exaggeration, or fear of pain.

Using an inclinometer to measure ROM has also been shown not to be a valid measure of function, with results being highly variable, even on successive measures.[32] As well, inclinometer measurements are generally taken with the patient in a static posi-

*References 9, 16, 34, 45, 62, and 71.

tion, but meaningful measures of function assess how well a patient's spine performs in motion.

Functional Capacity Evaluation —Strength Testing

Functional capacity evaluation (FCE) testing methods assume that the level of strength demonstrates the level of function. An example is a "maximum effort" test, which involves lifting a weight from the floor to various heights. The individual determines when he or she has had enough, which marks the end of the exercise.

As with ROM, the degree of effort can profoundly affect strength measurements. According to Reid and co-workers,[56] people with chronic back pain are frequently influenced by depression, fear of reinjury, or pain. Functional capacity evaluation tests of patients with chronic back pain may actually be tests of their pain level and tolerance.[3] Conversely, Mayer and associates[39] found that sufferers of chronic LBP are often capable of providing excellent strength measurements. Strong relationships have been found between force measurements and activity scales, so that one needs to exercise caution in using force measurements as indicators of health.[17]

Strapping the Pelvis in Strength Testing

Isokinetic or isometric testing techniques are designed to restrict the patient's freedom of motion so that trunk muscle strength alone will be recorded. It has been shown that these devices also have problems in evaluating the spine. Chaffin and Anderson[10] found that if the testing position of the trunk is not well chosen, static strength measurement could either overpredict or underpredict the actual strength of a patient. Thorstensson and Arvidson[65] used an isokinetic device called a *dynamometer* for dynamic evaluation of strength, and found no significant difference between a group of injured males and a group of normal individuals.

Back-testing machines stabilize the inferior part of the body by strapping the pelvis. This does not take into consideration basic human anatomy. For instance, the thick lumbodorsal fascia connecting the ilium to the spinous processes inextricably interconnect the spine and pelvis. Therefore, strapping the pelvis to stabilize it makes it impossible to determine the spine's own natural ability to handle forces. Shirazi-Adl and associates[60] concluded that "Pelvic fixation during training and/or evaluation of trunk muscles may be inappropriate and adversely affect the spine performance."

Gross Motion Analysis Systems

Gross motion analysis systems use video cameras to track relatively large markers placed on the patient's back and limbs. This method does not allow for the finer measurements involved in functional analysis of the spine. "They are good for gross joint motion, they are not measuring spinal movement."[54]

Requirements of a Functional Spinal Assessment Tool

The common evaluation tools are not adequate to measure the function of the spine. Objective information and relevant, dynamic functional measurements are required. The key criteria for an ideal evaluation tool for spinal function are one that

- allows unrestrained freedom of movement,
- directly assesses the spine's function in performing specific tasks (such as lifting), and
- is independent of the patient's voluntary control of spinal motion.

The Spinoscope is an optoelectronic device that has been developed to meet these key criteria in spinal evaluation. It uses high-resolution infrared cameras to track the motion of infrared light-emitting markers placed on the skin over the spinous processes and the iliac crests. As the examinee moves freely, the movement of the markers is monitored at a rate of 180 images per second. Bilateral electromyographic data of relevant muscles is simultaneously collected via skin-surface electrodes. From the kinematics of the markers, a computer automatically calculates its best estimate of the motion of the pelvis and the spine. The electromyographic data is used to correlate spinal motion and muscle activity.[24]

The standard testing procedure begins with placing markers (Fig. 10-4, *A*). For the lumbar spine, markers #1 and #9 (positioned over C7 and L4, respectively) are placed first, since these are landmarks for locating the position of the remaining markers vis-à-vis the anatomic structures. Twelve markers in total are affixed to the skin along the spinal column, from C7 to S2, concentrated in the lumbar area. In addition, two markers are placed above the iliac crests, and two reference markers are placed on the backs of the heels.

For the cervical spine, seven markers are located between vertebrae C3 and T3, two more are placed at T4 and T7, as well as four above the iliac crests and the scapulae. In addition, two electromyogram (EMG) surface electrodes are positioned bilaterally above the sternocleidomastoid muscles. The configuration of diodes and EMG electrodes for the Cervical Spinoscope is illustrated in Fig. 10-4, *B*.

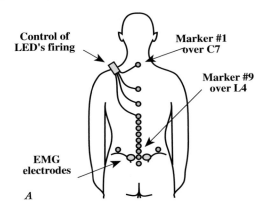

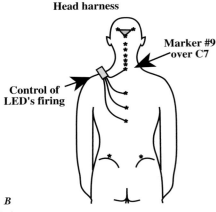

Fig. 10-4

A, Back view of the lumbar-harnessed patient. **B,** Back view of the cervical harnessed patient. Placing markers requires a reasonably precise location of spinous processes of L4 and C7, for proper identification of all neighboring levels. Each of the 16 markers consists of a small infrared light-emitting diode (LED) emitting a brief flash of light under computer control.

Once the markers are placed, the patient stands at a designated place in the testing room, in the field of view of the camera system (Fig. 10-5). The examinee performs a series of movements while the cameras record the motion of the light-emitting diodes (LEDs). The system derives the dynamic three-dimensional coordinates of the markers on the examinee's spine, then calculates specific parameters, the pattern of which represents the measurable spinal coordination. Standard movements are standing still, flexion and recovery from flexion, and lateral bend. These movements or others may then be performed while lifting weights (loaded).

Database for Normal Lumbar Spine Motion

To make clinical decisions using a device such as the Spinoscope, a set of data is required to use as a ref-

erence for judging normality/abnormality in spinal motion.

Forty normal subjects segregated by age, sex, and occupation were selected from hundreds according to strict inclusion/exclusion criteria developed by McGill University and the University of Montreal at the request of the IRSST (Workers' Compensation Board of Quebec). Each subject performed a series of movements consisting of standing still; flexion/recovery from flexion, unloaded and with loads of 11 kg, 23 kg, and 45 kg; and lateral bending (left to right and right to left), unloaded and lifting 4.6 kg.

Normal Flexion/Recovery from Flexion (Movement in the Sagittal Plane)

The Effects of Loading on Spinal Coordination

The flexion and recovery from flexion motions can be decomposed into basic components: the pelvis rotating about the acetabulum, and the unfolding spine. Figure 10-6 shows the effective contribution of the pelvis for recovery from flexion, unloaded and at varying loads. There is no difference ($p = 0.21-0.97$) between unloaded and loaded movements (up to 45 kg) for trunk flexions up to 60 degrees. The same can be said regarding effective lumbar elongation and effective lordosis ($p = 0.32-0.92$).

Figure 10-7 shows the average effective intersegmental mobility (EISM) for the L4-L5 level, unloaded and loaded, in recovery from flexion. For ranges of motion up to 60 degrees, there is a significant difference ($p < 0.0001-0.02$) between unloaded and loaded EISM at L4-L5 and all lower lumbar levels. The EISM increases as the load increases in the lower lumbar levels for any given value of

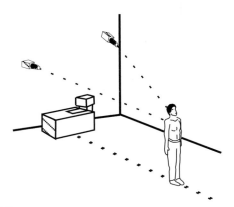

Fig.10-5

Testing room. *(From Gracovetsky, S: The spinal engine, New York, 1988, Springer Verlag.)*

TRUNK returning to erect stance WHILE LIFTING WEIGHT

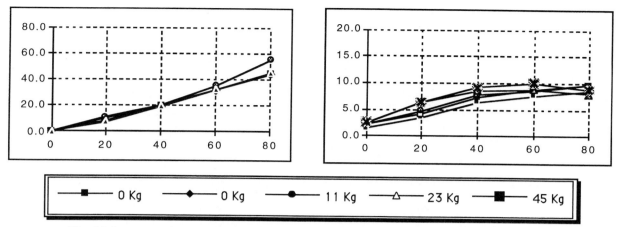

Fig. 10-6

The pelvis motion is derived from the kinematics of markers placed above the iliac crest and the S2 area. As the patient flexes and recovers from flexion in the sagittal plane with various loads, the pelvic plane rotates. The rotation (around the acetabulum) is given as a function of the trunk flexion angle (horizontal axis). Note the relative independence of pelvic motion for loads up to 45 kg. The corresponding standard deviation for the set of 40 normal individuals is given on the right.

trunk flexion. (For all levels, the mean difference between unloaded and loaded EISM is in the order of 1.12° to 2.68°.)

The normative data demonstrate that there is no significant variation in gross spinal coordination (effective lordosis, lumbar elongation, and effective contribution of the pelvis) between unloaded and loaded movements, regardless of ROM (up to 60°) and regardless of load (up to 45 kg). However, when examining the motion at individual levels, spinal co-

ordination (EISM) does vary with load in the lower lumbar levels.

There is a trend with age for the measured parameters: effective contribution of pelvis, effective lordosis, and lumbar elongation. Results for the effective contribution of the pelvis are shown for each age group: "young" (age 19-30 n 1 = 10), "old (age 50-64, n 2 = 11), and "average" (the entire population, $n = 40$) in Fig. 10-8. Note that the effective contribution to motion of the pelvis increases with

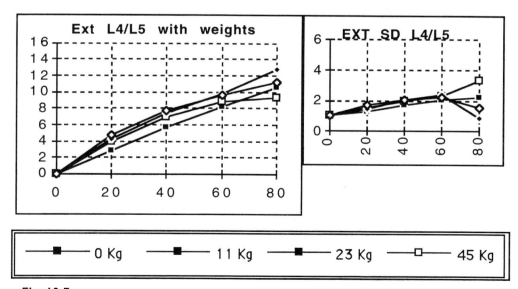

Fig. 10-7

The effective intersegmental mobility at L4-L5 is calculated as a function of the trunk angle for various loads. The corresponding standard deviations are on the right. Note that the motion increases with load; that is, the spine flexes more under load.

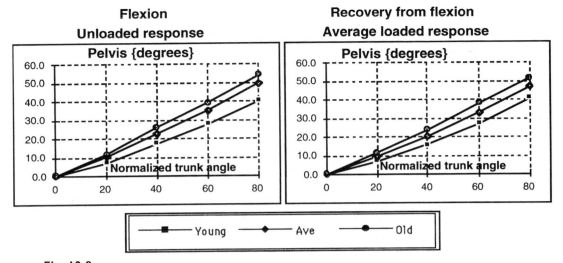

Fig. 10-8

The effects of age on spinal coordination. Older individuals have more pelvic motion, which corresponds to a reduced spinal motion. (The old spine is stiffer on average than the younger one, and the individual compensates by increasing his or her pelvic motion.)

age. This is a consequence of a reduction of the spine contribution. With this reduction, we observe corresponding decreases in the effective lordosis and the lumbar elongation. The age dependency can be expressed such that the older the individual's spine, the more stiff it is.

Figure 10-9 shows the effects of age on EISM for the L4-L5 level. There is a significant difference between age groups for EISM in the lower lumbar levels at all ranges of motion ($p = 0.0043 - 0.0351$). As expected, the older an individual is, the lower the segmental mobility in the lower lumbar spine.

Figure 10-10 compares the L4-L5 EISM for males and females. For EISM at all levels, in recovery from flexion, lifting 45 kg, the only notable dif-

ference between male and female subjects is at small ranges of motion ($20°$) ($p = 0.005 - 0.04$). For large ranges of motion, (e.g., $60°$), there is no significant difference in EISM between male and female ($p = 0.13 - 0.95$).

Normal Lateral Bend (Movement in the Frontal Plane)

The Effects of Loading on Spinal Coordination

The trunk motion in lateral bending projected in the frontal plane can be decomposed into two basic components: the pelvic motion, which can be approxi-

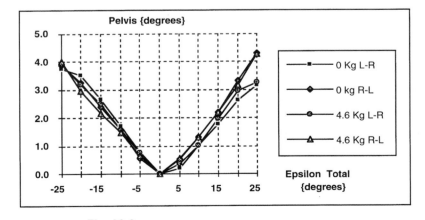

Fig. 10-9

The effects of age on mobility shows a reduction in motion of the spine as one becomes older.

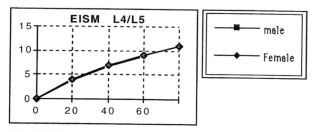

Fig. 10-10

The effects of gender on spinal coordination. Essentially, gender has no impact on coordination.

mated by a rotation around an axis perpendicular to the frontal plane, and the bending of the spine in the frontal plane. Figure 10-11 shows the effective contribution of the pelvis to the motion loaded and unloaded. Note the consistent response whether lifting no weight or 4.6 kg.

Figure 10-12 shows a summary of the results, for which the right and left data, unloaded and loaded, are averaged, then plotted for all assigned lumbar levels. The standard deviation, which is 0 at time = 0 (since both EISM and trunk ROM are normalized), is no longer 0 when the subject returns to the erect stance from either a start to the right or to the left.

Comparison of Left and Right Bending

There is no significant difference in spinal coordination between left and right bending for all ROMs and loads studied ($p = 0.4-0.98$).

Effective intersegmental mobility varies little with age in lateral bend, as illustrated in Fig. 10-13.

Statistical results concerning the difference between spinal coordination parameters for different loads, age groups, or gender, are similar to the re-

sults for the flexion/recovery from flexion movement.

Usefulness of Data from Skin Markers

The preceding section discussed patterns for normal spinal motion to use as reference data in clinical decision making. One concern that arises, however, is the usefulness of data derived from skin markers. The motion of skin markers placed about the lumbar spinous processes has often been compared, with variable degrees of success, with that of the underlying vertebrae. However, the clinician is more interested in knowing whether the motion of skin markers contains information related to pathology of mechanical origin, rather than obtaining a faithful replicate of vertebral motion. This section addresses two questions: (1) Is it possible to use kinematic data from skin markers to differentiate between the normal individual and a patient with LBP? (2) Assuming that we can, is it possible to further separate patients with LBP into two subgroups with specific measurable functional features?

Forty-two patients suffering from nonspecific LBP (exhibiting neither leg pain nor neurologic involvement nor any previous surgery) for a duration greater than three months were selected. These patients underwent a Spinoscope examination, the results of which were compared with the normal database of spinal motion derived from the normal subjects.

The gross trunk angular velocity in the sagittal plane was calculated as the average angular velocity of the 12 spine markers, while the patients lifted a maximum load ranging from 5 to 45 kg.

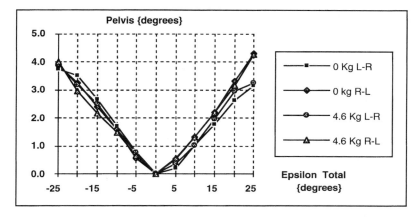

Fig. 10-11

For the range of loads considered, there are no significant changes in pelvic motion.

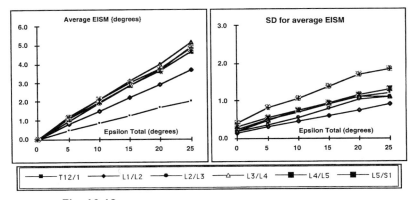

Fig. 10-12

There is no significant difference in right versus left mobility. The difference is between lumbar levels.

The maximum trunk velocity during lifting was recorded as a function of the load lifted. The velocity variation across the load range was measured and divided by the corresponding maximum load range. In addition, the relative variation in EISM of the five lumbar segments for the maximum trunk flexion was calculated. The patients with abnormal results were divided into two groups: those whose EISM variation was significantly lower than normal (2 S.D. from the average normal) and those whose EISM was close to normal.

Unpaired *t*-tests between the group of normal subjects and the two subgroups of abnormal subjects were made since the three sets of measurement belong to different people. The program used is Statsview by Abacus Concepts, Berkeley, CA.

The difference in the ratio of maximum velocity versus load range between the normal group and the subgroup with a reduced EISM is signifi-cant ($p = 0.008$). The difference in the ratio of maximum trunk velocity versus load range between the normal group and the subgroup with normal EISM is not significant ($p = 0.33$). The difference between the two abnormal subgroups is significant ($p = 0.073$). Hence, the clinically homogeneous group of 42 patients with LBP can be separated into two groups with functionally different characteristics of trunk velocity on the basis of their EISM responses.

It has been proposed that patients with a mechanical etiology of their spinal disorders fall into one of two broad groups: those whose predominant injury would be located at the anterior element of the spine (mainly the disc, which will be affected by excessive compression), and those whose predominant injury would be located at the posterior elements of the spine (mainly the facet area and the soft tissues around it, which will be affected by excessive axial rotation). Sagittal lifting increases compression

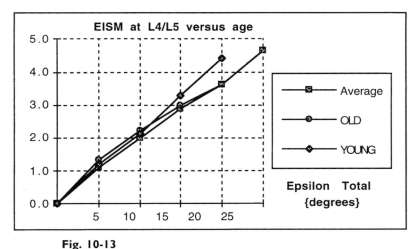

Fig. 10-13

The effects of age on spinal coordination in lateral bending is smaller than that in flexion and recovery from flexion.

on the spine without inducing axial torque (unless the spine is grossly asymmetric). Presumably, the patient with a compression-type injury would exhibit an abnormal EISM under sagittal load, whereas the patient with a rotational type of injury would not. Hence, it could be argued that this technique has distinguished between patients whose injury is sensitive to compression and those who are not.

Irrespective of the merit of this argument, the fact is that the EISM does contain information that clearly impacts on gross behavior, and as such suggests that studying the EISM of the injured is not an academic exercise. The so-called randomness of skin motion may not be as random as generally believed and therefore skin marker kinematics might be informative at the segmental level.

Case Studies—Lumbar Spine

Case 1

Case 1 had a clinically diagnosed disc injury at L5-S1, resolved by interbody fusion (anterior approach). Figure 10-14 depicts the patient's evaluation before and after surgery. His preoperative results show restricted spinal motion, with almost no measurable variation in the lumbosacral angle. After the spinal

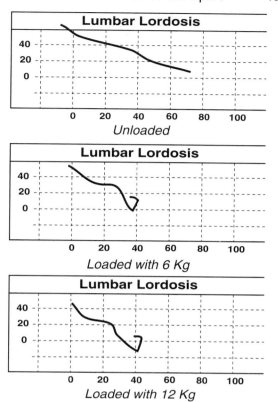

Fig. 10-15

Top, Unloaded response. It is reasonably normal. **Middle,** A load of 6.6 kg is lifted. Note the breakdown at around 20 degrees of trunk flexion. **Bottom,** Load of 11 kg. The same pattern is repeated.

fusion at L5-S1, the mobility of the spine increased, as did the percent elongation of the posterior tissues. This paradoxic result of increased mobility following fusion may be due to the relief of pain at L5-S1, which allowed the section of the spine above L5 to move more freely. The surgical intervention was, therefore, successful in the sense that it improved the ROM of each segment of the spine and, therefore, its functionality.

Case 2

Case 2 demonstrates a breakdown of spinal coordination with increasing load (Fig. 10-15). The lordosis curve shows normal spinal motion when lifting no weight; however, with increasing load, the curve reveals abnormal spinal motion. This patient suffered a low-back injury while lifting. The clinical examination shows 45 degrees trunk flexion, with the Schober test showing only 30% lumbar elongation. Due to the injury, the patient experiences a loss of spinal coordination when loaded. Some conditions only become apparent under conditions of excess loading.

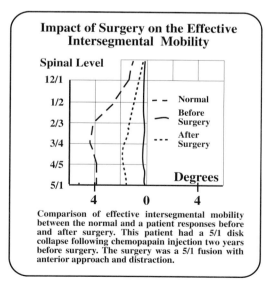

Fig. 10-14

This failed chymopapain injection was salvaged by an L5-S1 fusion using an anterior approach. The preoperative data show no motion throughout the entire lumbar spine, although only L5-S1 was implicated in the chymopapain injection. Postoperative data demonstrate a mobility that is about one third of normal. Since pain decreased by half (as measured by Oswestry questionnaire), it is concluded that this surgery was successful.

Case 3

Case 3 shows symptom exaggeration and/or possible malingering. The examinee tries to manipulate the test by demonstrating a small ROM. However, there is a similar coordination pattern for 30-degree and 80-degree ROM (Fig. 10-16).

Case 4

Case 4 tracks the effectiveness of a conservative therapy treatment program. The patient experiences progress, and then a setback (Fig. 10-17). The data from this patient's first visit showed that almost all of his mobility in flexion/extension came from pelvic motion; his spine motion was negligible. A physical therapy program was initiated, and the data from his second visit, 2 weeks later, demonstrates an improvement in both range of spine motion and lordosis. This pattern of improvement continued until his fourth visit, when he demonstrated a dramatic decrease in performance. In fact, the patient's response returned to the level observed during his first visit and he demonstrates the same injury pattern. This suggests that this

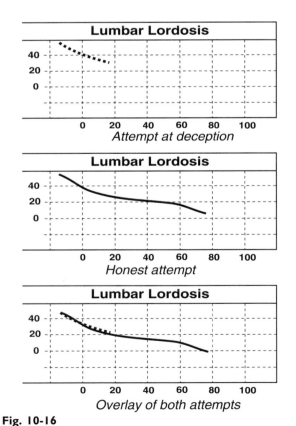

Fig. 10-16

Top, Unloaded response; attempt to deceive. **Middle,** Unloaded response; honest attempt. **Bottom,** Overlay of Top and Middle. The coordination (the slope of the curves) is identical. The range of motion of the two attempts is widely different.

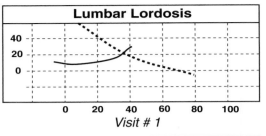

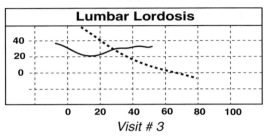

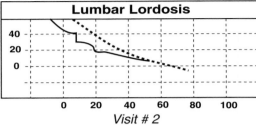

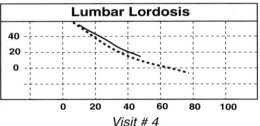

Fig. 10-17

Top, Two days after injury. The lordosis increases when the trunk flexes. Compare with the normal smooth decreases. **Next down,** After 2 weeks of physical therapy, the lordosis demonstrates a more normal response. **Next down,** One month later, the patient has been reinjured and the lordosis pattern exhibits the same abnormal response as that in the Top. **Bottom,** One month later; the patient has fully recovered.

patient's new loss of performance is not secondary to a new injury but a break in the scar tissue that was built up after the first injury.

The ability to detect similarity in injury patterns over several months may be important in insurance cases, in which there is a need to distinguish between new and old injuries.

Case 5

Case 5 compares pre- and postoperative test results (Fig. 10-18). This woman had disc degeneration disease at L4-L5 and L5-S1. The first Spinoscopy was performed one week before her surgery. Figure 10-18 shows preoperative and postoperative effective intersegmental mobility (EISM), and how her EISM compared with the normal pattern.

The Importance of Coupled Motion in the Cervical Spine

There appears to be no clear consensus concerning the exact nature of coupled motion in the cervical spine. This disagreement may perhaps be attributed to the wide variety of techniques used, as well as to the complexity of the analysis.

According to Schultz,[58] the three-dimensional nature of bending and twisting of the spine makes it difficult to describe these configurations; further-more, attempts to correlate changes in motion ranges with various spinal abnormalities have met with mixed success.

Frymoyer and associates[15] suggested that noninvasive methods be developed to analyze coupling motion, referring to the results of earlier work by Panjabi: "The most important attribute of this spinal behavior is the complex coupling which occurs. . . . It is important that these motion characteristics be quantitatively analysed as far as possible."[50]

Pearcy and co-workers[32] also examined the phenomenon of coupled motion in the spine, and concluded: "The complex nature of the intervertebral joints results in coupling movements, such that when a joint flexes it also may exhibit lateral bending or axial rotation at the same time; a full three-dimensional analysis is required to describe these movements."

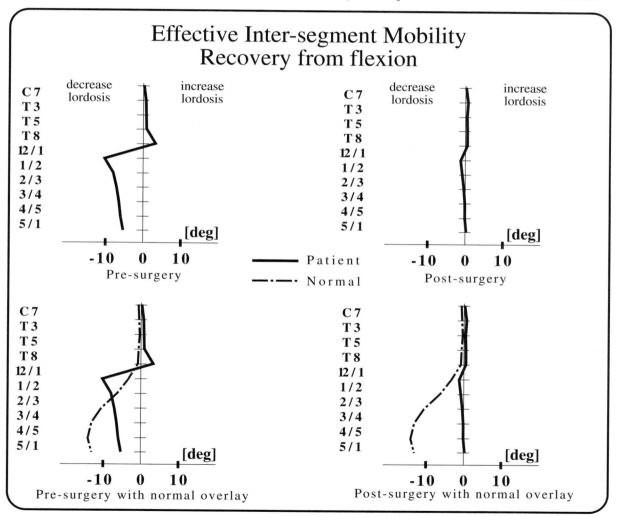

Fig. 10-18

This patient demonstrated a decent function preoperatively. Because of her pain (68% on Oswestry scale) she was fused L4-L5-S1 posteriorly. The postoperative data demonstrates that this woman was trans-formed into a stick. Little or no motion can be demonstrated. Pain was 47% by the Oswestry scale. It can be debated whether the surgery was beneficial.

The nature of coupled motion in the cervical spine may be attributed to the unique arrangement of facets, ligaments, and discs in the region. The geometry of the articulating surfaces and the elastic properties of the ligaments determine the relative motion of the vertebrae; hence, the kinematics of the lower and upper cervical spine are quite different. In lateral bending to the left the spinous processes move to the right, and vice versa for bending to the right. This coupling decreases gradually between C2 and C7, owing to the change in incline of the facet joints.

Reich and Dvorak[55] found that a rotational component is always coupled with a segmental side-bending movement; the cervical articulations are described as "viconvex," or saddle joints. This allows coupled rotation and lateral flexion, as well as flexion extension. As the spine is displaced away from its neutral position, axial rotation and lateral bending occur together.

According to Stokes and co-workers,[63] the literature shows that as the spine is displaced away from its neutral position, axial rotation and lateral bending occur together. However, the coupled motions in the lumbar and cervical spine are known to be different. The arrangement of cervical facets, ligaments, and discs results in a unique type of coupled motion.

Previous Studies of Coupled Motion in the Cervical Spine

Hohl[29] used cineradiography to illustrate cervical coupling as early as 1964. Later, Panjabi and White[51] helped to pioneer three-dimensional mathematic techniques for analyzing biplanar radiography. They represented the displacement of vertebral bodies in terms of translation plus rotation. Euler's angles were introduced to represent the rotational aspect of transformations between moving reference frames.

However, the error in using Euler's angles was considered by them to be unacceptable. Suh[64] considered the distortion associated with radiographic images. He adapted methods developed for surveying and map production to the analysis of x-ray films of the cervical spine, which involved the design of a radiopaque reference frame that would appear on the radiograph together with the subject.

Brown and associates[8] constructed an analogous reference frame to appear in the x-ray films, but this frame enclosed the entire torso, and they used anatomic landmarks to define the spatial orientation

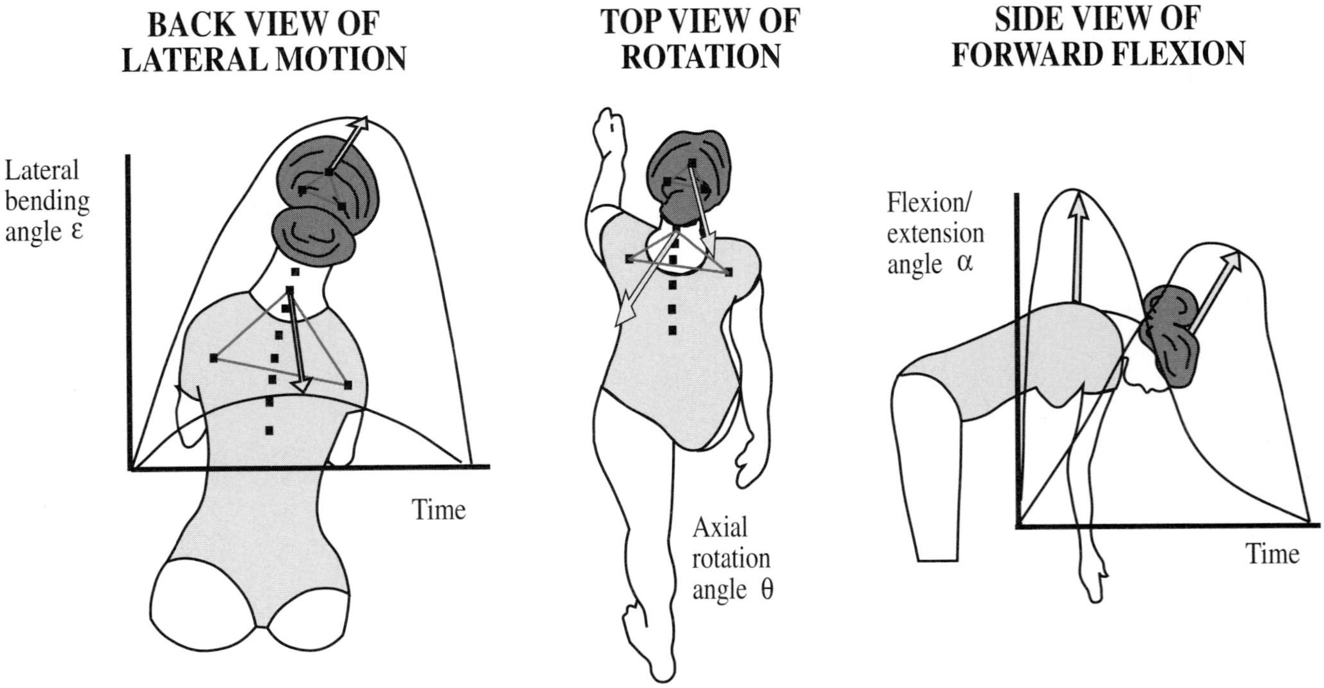

BACK VIEW OF LATERAL MOTION

Lateral bending angle ε

Time

TOP VIEW OF ROTATION

Axial rotation angle θ

SIDE VIEW OF FORWARD FLEXION

Flexion/ extension angle α

Time

Fig. 10-19

Vectors normal to the triangles formed by groups of IREDs on the head, neck, and shoulders. The normal vectors originate from IREDs at the apices of these triangles (on the head, cervical spine, and thoracic spine). Direction angles are derived from projections of these vectors onto the principal planes. Inset shows two normal vectors with their base at the origin, and the angle between them.

of the vertebrae. The orientation of each body was described by a translation vector and three Eulerian angles; the dates were then normalized to ensure a common basis for subsequent evaluation. Several years later, Pearcy and associates,[52] as well as Pearcy and Tibrewal,[53] were among many who elaborated upon these techniques, pointing out that the diagnosis of back pain. . . "requires a knowledge of the pattern of movement in normal individuals to establish what constitutes an abnormal movement and how it is related to pathology."

Mimura and co-workers[46] used biplanar radiographs to determine in vivo ranges of cervical rotational motion. They showed that the direction of lateral bending produced by coupling is dependent on the level. Below C3-C4, lateral bending was in the same direction as rotation. Above C2-C3, it was in the opposite direction.

Plamondon and Gagnon[54a] developed a method for controlling the experimental error involved in using Euler's angles. They used the least-squares method to correct for error in determining anatomic landmarks, and concluded that this method can provide accurate, precise results.

Definitions Used in the Study of Cervical Motion

For the purpose of this study, the subject is prepared with markers placed on the spine and head, as shown in Fig. 10-4, *B*. From the position of the markers, it is possible to define several vectors, characterizing the head motion. Another vector is perpendicular to the plane defined by the two markers on the scapula and another marker (such as T5) along the spine.

As the subject moves, these vectors move. By projecting these vectors in the sagittal plane, we obtain the angular motion of the head in this plane. Projecting the head vector in the frontal plane gives us ϵ and projection in the horizontal plane generates Θ (Fig. 10-19).

Case Study—Cervical Spine

Consider the case of a man sitting on a stool. The patient is asked to move his head forward (flexion), then sideways (right and left lateral bend). The values of α, ϵ, and Θ are shown in Figs. 10-20 and 10-21 as functions of time or relative to each other. Indeed, a normal individual flexing his spine should move only in the sagittal plane with ϵ and Θ being 0. Pathology will force the subject to deviate away

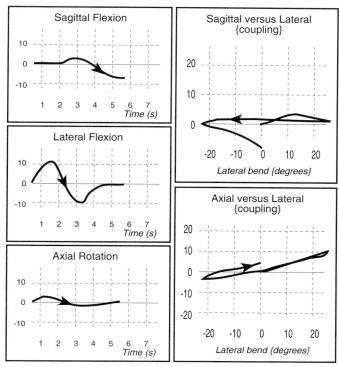

Fig. 10-20
Movement of the head and the shoulder girdle when the patient is asked to bend his head to the left and right sides. *Column A:* The three graphs on the left plot the primary motion (lateral bend) versus time (10 frames = 1 second) in the three planes. The primary motion, indicated by ϵ (xz plane), shows the left then right bend. During this motion, the patient cannot maintain his head in the frontal plane; the head tilts forward as demonstrated by the induced motion in the sagittal plane, α (yz plane). In addition, there is an induced axial rotation, θ (xy plane). *Column B:* The two graphs on the right look at relative motion by plotting the primary movement of lateral bend versus the two induced movements of flexion (LB vs FE) and rotation (LB vs ROT). The coupled motion is clearly visible.

from this ideal plane and the corresponding ϵ and Θ will no longer be 0. The following coupled motion plots highlight these deviations from normality.

Conclusion

The spine can no longer be seen as a static "column," being passively carried away by the leg: the available data suggest that the spine's motion is consistent with the hypothesis that the spine converts the primitive lateral bend of our fish-like ancestors into an axial torque driving the pelvis. The sequence of movements of the various spinal components is not arbitrary and the overall patterns of movement called "spinal coordination" can be explained by the need to execute acquired tasks while the stress within

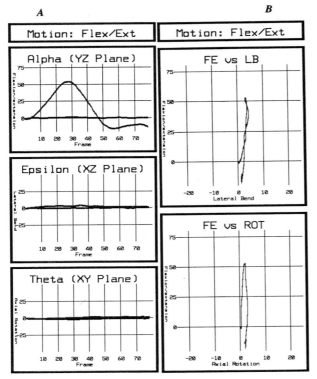

Fig. 10-21

Movement of the head and the shoulder girdle versus time in the sagittal plane. *Column A:* From the graphs on the left, we see that although the primary motion is in the sagittal plane (note the large α variation of the head), there are two other coupled motions: that is, a lateral bend (very small) and axial rotation. *Column B:* The graphs of the three decomposed motions can be replotted to show relative motion, as indicated in the graphs on the right. The primary motion (flexion) is now plotted versus the induced lateral bend (FE vs LB) or versus the induced axial rotation (FE vs ROT). The latter coupled-motion graph indicates that when the subject flexes his head, the head rotates axially to the right by 3 degrees or so.

the spine is equalized at its lowest level. This coordination is remarkably similar across normal, healthy spines; deviation of coordination from the normal contains information on pathology.

References

1. Adams MA, Hutton WC: Prolapsed intervertebral disc: a hyperflexion injury, *Spine* 7(3):184, 1982.
2. Bartelink DL: The role of abdominal pressure in relieving the pressure on the lumbar intervertebral disc, *J Bone Joint Surg (Br)* 39B:718, 1982.
2a. Basmajian JV: *Muscles alive; their functions revealed by electromyography,* ed 4, Baltimore, 1979, Williams and Wilkins.
3. Beimborn DS, Morrissey MC: A review of the literature trunk muscle performance, *Spine* 13(6):665, 1988.
4. Boden SD: Incidence of abnormal lumbar spine magnetic resonance imaging scans in asymptomatic patients: a prospective and blinded investigation. Presented at the American Academy of Orthopaedic Surgeons, New Orleans, 1990.
5. Bogduk N, Macintosh J: The applied anatomy of the thoracolumbar fascia, *Spine* 9:164, 1984.
6. Bogduk N, Macintosh JE, Pearcy MJ: A universal model of the lumbar back muscles in the upright position, *Spine* 17(8):897, 1992.
7. Bogduk N, Towney LT: *Clinical anatomy of the lumbar spine.* New York, 1987, Churchill Livingstone.
8. Brown RH and others: Spinal analysis using a three-dimensional radiographic technique, *J Biomech* 9:355, 1976.
9. Burton AK, Tillotson KM: Prediction of the clinical course of low back trouble using multivariable models, *Spine* 16(1):7, 1991.
10. Chaffin DB, Anderson GBJ: *Mechanical work-capacity evaluation.* In *Occupational mechanics,* Toronto, 1984, John Wiley & Sons.
11. Connolly J: Understanding the ADA, *Clin Manage* 12(2):40, 1992.
12. Farfan HF, Kirkaldy-Willis WH: The present status of spinal fusion in the treatment of lumbar intervertebral joint disorders, *Clin Orthop* 158:198, 1981.
13. Farfan HF and others: The effects on the lumbar intervertebral joints: the role of torsion in the production of disc degeneration, *J Bone Joint Surg [Am]* 52A(3):468, 1970.
14. Floyd WF, Silver PHS: The function of erector spinae muscles in certain movements and postures in man, *J Physiol (Lond)* 129:184, 1955.
15. Frymoyer JW and others: The mechanical and kinematic analysis of the lumbar spine in normal living human subjects in vivo, *J Biomech* 12:165, 1979.
16. Gauvin MG and others: Reliability of clinical measurements of forward bending using the modified fingertip-to-floor method, *Phys Ther* 70:443, 1990.
17. Gomez T and others: Normative Database for trunk range of motion, strength, velocity, and endurance with the Isostation B-200 Lumbar Dynamometer, *Spine* 16:15, 1991.
18. Gracovetsky S: The determination of safe load, *Br J Ind Med* 7:120, 1986.
19. Gracovetsky S: Function of the spine, *J Biomed Eng* 8:217, 1986.
20. Gracovetsky S: *The spinal engine,* New York, 1988, Springer-Verlag Wien.
21. Gracovetsky S, Farfan H: The optimum spine, *Spine* 11(6):543, 1986.
22. Gracovetsky S, Farfan HF, Lamy C: A mathematical model of the lumbar spine using an optimization system to control muscles and ligaments. *Orthop Clin North Am* 8(1):135, 1977.
23. Gracovetsky S, Farfan H, Lamy C: The mechanism of the lumbar spine, *Spine* 6:249, 1981.
24. Gracovetsky S and others: Analysis of spinal and muscular activity during flexion/extension and free lifts, *Spine* 15(12):1333, 1990.
25. Granhed H, Jonson R, Hansson T: The loads on the lumbar spine during extreme weight lifting, *Spine* 12(2):146, 1987.
26. Gray's anatomy, CM Goss, editor, Philadelphia, 1973, Lea & Febiger.

26a. Heslin DJ, Saplys RJ, Brown W: Frequency of asymptomatic abnormalities in the lumbosacral, spine, *Mod Med Can* 42(6): 469, 1987.

27. Hirsh C, Schajowicz F: Studies on the structural changes in the lumbar anulus fibrosus, *Acta Orthop Scand* 22:184, 1953.

28. Hochschuler SH: Diagnostic studies in clinical practice, *Orthop North Am* 14(3):517, 1983.

29. Hohl M: Normal motion in the upper portion of the cervical spine, *J Bone Joint Surg* 46A:1777, 1964.

30. Horn TJ and others: Presentation at the Annual Meeting of the International Society for the study of the lumbar spine, Heidelberg, Germany, 1990.

31. Inman VT: Human locomotion, *Can Med Assoc J* 94:1047, 1966.

32. Keeley J and others: Quantification of lumbar function. Part 5: Reliability of range-of-motion measures in the sagittal plane and an in vivo torso rotation measurement technique, *Spine* 11(1):31, 1986.

33. Krag MH and others: Intraabdominal pressurisation: failure to reduce erector spinae loads during lifting tasks. Conference of the International Society for the Study of the Lumbar Spine, May 29-30, 1986.

34. Lankhorst GJ and others: Objectivity and repeatability of measurements in low back pain, *Scand J Rehab Med* 14:21, 1982.

35. Lovett AW: A contribution to the study of the mechanics of the spine, *Am J Anat* 2:457, 1903.

36. Lowery WD and others: Meeting of the American Academy of Orthopaedic Surgeons, Washington, D.C., 1992.

37. Mayer T, Gatchel M: Functional restoration for spinal disorders: the sports medicine approach, Philadelphia, 1988, Lea & Febiger.

38. Mayer TG and others: Improved physical performance outcomes after functional restoration treatment in patients with chronic low-back pain: versus recent training results, *Spine* 15(12):1321, 1988.

39. Mayer TG and others: Quantification of lumbar function. Part 2: Sagittal plane trunk strength in chronic low back pain patients, *Spine* 10(8):765, 1985.

40. Mayer T and others: Use of noninvasive techniques for quantification of spinal range of motion in normal subjects and chronic low back dysfunction patients, *Spine* 9:588, 1984.

41. McGill SM, Cholewicki J: Lumbar posterior ligament involvement during extremely heavy lifts estimated from fluoroscopic measurements, *J Biomech* 25(1):17, 1992.

42. McGill SM, Norman RW: Effects of an anatomically detailed erector spinae model on L4-L5 disc compression and shear, *J Biomech* 20(6):591, 1987.

43. McGill SM, Norman RW: Partitioning of the L4-L5 dynamic moment into disc, ligamentous, and muscular components during lifting, *Spine* 11:666, 1986.

44. McMahon TA, Greene PR: The influence of track compliance on running, *J Biomech* 12:893, 1979.

45. Merritt JL and others: Measurement of trunk flexibility in normal subjects: reproducibility of three clinical methods, *Mayo Clin Proc* 61:192, 1986.

46. Mimura M and others: Three-dimensional motion analysis of the cervical spine with special reference to the axial rotation, *Spine* 14(12):1135, 1989.

47. Mooney V: Impairment, disability and handicap, *Clin Orthop Rel Res* 221:14, 1987.

48. National Institute for Occupational Safety and Health (NIOSH): *Work practice guide for manual lifting*. Cincinnati, OH, 1981, DHHS (NIOSH) Publication No. 81-122.

49. Nelson MA and others: Reliability and reproducibility of clinical findings in low back pain, *Spine* 4:97, 1979.

50. Panjabi MM: Experimental determination of spinal motion segment behavior, *Orthop Clin North Am* 8:169, 1977.

51. Panjabi M, White, AA: A mathematical approach for three-dimensional analysis of the mechanics of the spine, *J Biomech* 4:203, 1971.

52. Pearcy M, Portek I, Shepherd J: Three-dimensional X-ray analysis of normal movement in the lumbar spine, *Spine* 9:294, 1984.

53. Pearcy MJ, Tibrewal SB: Axial rotation and lateral bending in the normal lumbar spine measured by three-dimensional radiography, *Spine* 9:582, 1984.

54. Pearcy MJ and others: Measurement of human back movements in three dimensions by opto-electronic devices, *Clin Biom* 2:199, 1987.

54a. Plamondon A., Gagnon M: Evaluation of Euler's angles with a least squares method for the study of lumbar spine motion, *J Biomed Eng* 12(2):143, 1990.

54b. Poirier FE: Fossil evidence, ed 2, St. Louis, Mosby.

55. Reich C, Dvorak J: The functional evaluation of craniocervical ligaments in sidebending using x-rays, *Manual Medicine* 2:108, 1986.

56. Reid S, Hazard RG, Genwick JW: Isokinetic trunk strength deficits in people with and without low-back pain: a comparative study with consideration of effort. *J Spine Disord*, 68, 1991.

57. Rosomoff HL and others: Physical findings in patients with chronic intractable benign pain in the neck and/or back, *Pain* 37(3):279, 1989.

58. Schultz AB: Biomechanics of the human spine and trunk. In Skalak R, Chien S, eds.: Handbook of bioengineering, 1987, McGraw-Hill, New York.

59. Shirazi-Adl SA, Shrivastavi SC, Ahmed A: Stress analysis of the lumbar disc-body unit in compression: 3-dimensional non-linear finite element study, *Spine* 9:120, 1984.

60. Shirazi-Adl and others: Towards determination of mechanisms for spinal stability: integration of local spinal and global postural stability, presented at the 39th Annual Meeting of the Orthopaedic Research Society, San Francisco, 1993.

61. Spitzer WO, LeBlanc FE, Dupuis M: Scientific approach to the assessment and management of activity-related spinal disorders, *Spine* 12(7S):SI, 1987.

62. Spratt KR and others: A new approach to the low back physical examination: behavioral assessment of mechanical signs, *Spine* 15:96, 1990.

63. Stokes, IAF, Krag MH, Wider DG: A critique of "the optimum spine," *Spine* 12:511, 1987.

64. Suh, CH: The fundamentals of computer aided x-ray analysis of the spine, *J Biomech* 7:161, 1974.

65. Thorstensson A, Arvidson A: Trunk muscle strength and low back pain, *Scand J Rehab Med* 14:69, 1982.

66. Thurston AJ, Harris JD: Normal kinematics of the lumbar spine and pelvis, *Spine* 8:199, 1983.

67. Troup JDG and others: The perception of back pain and the role of psychophysical tests of lifting capacity, *Spine* 12(7):645, 1987.

68. Van Wingerden JP and others: The Spine-pelvis-leg mechanism, with a study of the sacrotuberous ligament, In Proceedings of the First Interdisciplinary World Congress on Low Back Pain and Its Relation to the Sacroiliac Joint, San Diego, 1992.

69. Virgin W: Experimental investigations into the physical properties of the intervertebral disc, *J Bone Joint Surg (Fr)* 33B(4):607, 1951.

70. Waddell G: Clinical assessment of lumbar impairment, *Clin Orthop Rel Res* 221:110, 1987.

71. Waddell G: Normality and reliability in the clinical assessment of backache, *Br Med J* 284:1519, 1982.

72. White AA, Gordon SL: Synopsis workshop on idiopathic low back pain, *Spine* 7(2):141, 1982.

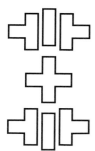

PART III

Diagnostic Measures

Chapter 11
Imaging of the Spine
Betsy A. Holland
Damon C. Sacco

As the variety of therapeutic and surgical approaches to spinal disease has become more complex, so, too, has spinal imaging. Computed tomography and magnetic resonance imaging are the current mainstays of the radiographic evaluation of the spine. Familiarity with the anatomic information provided by each technique is necessary for an understanding of their respective roles in spine imaging. Also important is familiarity with the optimal imaging protocols for both CT and MR because the results of both modalities are limited by the manner in which the studies are performed. Since both CT and MR continue to evolve from a technical standpoint, the diagnostic capabilities of imaging may be expected to expand and imaging algorithms, to change, as the radiographic definition of spinal pathology by both modalities becomes even more precise.

Technical Considerations

Computed Tomography with Multiplanar Reformations

Computed tomography employs an x-ray source to generate cross-sectional images. The cross-sectional images produced are a representation of tissues with varied x-ray attenuation. Attenuation of the x-ray beam is determined by the various tissues' electron density. Spatial and contrast resolution depend on the thickness of the slice, the size of the area to be studied or field of view, and scanning matrix. To produce high-resolution multiplanar CT images (CT/MPR) of the cervical spine, a series of axial images using a slice thickness of 2 mm or less is employed. Following acquisition of the axial images, computerized reformatted sagittal and coronal images are then generated from the set of axial images. The examination is then filmed to delineate optimally either soft-tissue or osseous structures.

For CT/MPR imaging of the thoracic and lumbar spine, 3-mm-thick contiguous or 5-mm-thick sections at 3-mm intervals are generally obtained over the region of interest. Again, following acquisition of the axial images, computerized reformatted images in both the sagittal and coronal planes are obtained.

With the advent of MRI, the use of either intrathecal or intravenous contrast with CT is infrequent. For evaluation of spinal cord abnormalities and arachnoiditis, MRI is the preferred modality, rendering CT with intrathecal contrast unnecessary. Additionally, MRI with intravenous gadolinium-diethylenetriamine pentacetate (Gd-DTPA) has become the study of choice for the evaluation of epidural fibrosis and central nervous system tumors, limiting the use of intravenous contrast-enhanced CT of the spine.

Magnetic Resonance Imaging

In contrast to computed tomography, in which an x-ray source is employed, magnetic resonance (MR) images are generated by placing the patient in a static external magnetic field and then subjecting the patient to repeated short bursts of radio waves of a specific radiofrequency (RF). This frequency (resonant frequency) is dictated by the strength of the applied external magnetic field. In brief, this short burst of RF energy excites the hydrogen nuclei or protons within the body. With termination of the RF pulse, the excited protons relax or release the RF energy they absorbed. RF energy released by the protons is detected by sensitive receiver coils within the instrument. This signal is encoded with information as to its point of origin within the imaging plane. Numerous measurements of RF pulses into the body are made and an image is formed. This characteristic absorption and release of energy is called "nuclear magnetic resonance."

The process of returning from the excited to the equilibrium state, with the release of RF energy, is called "relaxation." The process of relaxation is characterized by two independent time constants, T_1 and T_2. The T_1 relaxation time is also referred to as the longitudinal relaxation time. This reflects the time required for realignment of the protons within the applied magnetic field. The T_2 relaxation time is also referred to as the transverse relaxation time. This reflects the time required for the protons to lose coherence following excitation. The T_1 and T_2 relaxation are intrinsic physical properties of tissue. The MR signal intensity displayed on the images is mainly dependent on the T_1, T_2, and proton density (number of mobile hydrogen ions) of the tissue being evaluated.

The repetition time (TR), represents the time between RF pulses; and the echo time (TE), represents the time between the application of the RF pulse and the time of recording the MR signal. These parameters, T_1 and T_2, are set prior to acquiring the image. By varying the scanning parameters (TR and TE), the relative contributions of the T_1, T_2, and proton density of the tissue will determine image contrast. A T_1-weighted image, which emphasizes the T_1 properties of the tissue, is produced with a short TR (< 1000 msec) and a short TE (< 30 msec). T_1-weighted images are ideal for evaluating structures containing fat, subacute or chronic hemorrhage, or proteinaceous fluid, since these materials have a short T_1, resulting in a high signal on T_1-weighted sequences. The T_1-weighted sequence produces images with high signal-to-noise ratios and provides excellent anatomic detail.

Images with a long TR (> 1500 msec) and a short TE (15 to 30 msec) are referred to as proton-density or spin-density studies. With spin-density images the signal intensity reflects the absolute number of mobile hydrogen ions or protons in the tissue.

A T_2-weighted sequence, which emphasizes the T_2 properties of tissue, requires a long TR (> 1500 msec) and a long TE (> 45 msec). On T_2-weighted studies the signal intensity is related to the state of hydration of the tissue. Any tissue rich in free or extracellular water (e.g., cerebrospinal fluid, cysts, necrotic tissue, fluid collections, intervertebral discs, neoplasms) will demonstrate increased signal intensity.

With MR, any desired imaging plane can be directly acquired. Computerized reformatted images are generally not necessary using MRI data. In addition to direct acquisition of an imaging plane, MRI has the capability of imaging as entire volume of tissue. This data set can then be sectioned into very thin slices (1 to 2 mm thick) along any desired plane of interest. This has proven useful in the evaluation of neural foramina and the posterior articulating facets.

Normal Anatomy and Normal Variations

Cervical Spine

In the sagittal imaging plane, the normal cervical spine has a slightly lordotic curvature. The first cervical vertebral body, the atlas, is an osseous ring comprised of both anterior and posterior arches connected by two lateral masses that articulated with the base of the skull. The C1 vertebra does not have a vertebral body, nor is there a disc space between C1 and C2 vertebrae. The C2 vertebra, the axis, has an osseous extension that extends in a cephalad direction off its vertebral body. This is referred to as the odontoid process or dens. The cervical vertebral bodies become broader and increase in size as you extend caudally from C3 to C7.

The cervical pedicles are short, cylindrical, osseous structures that extend off the posterolateral aspects of the vertebral bodies to the articular pillars, and the paired osseous struts are referred to as the lamina. On an axial image at the level of the pedicles, the spinal canal is completely surrounded by an osseous ring comprised of the vertebral body, the paired lateral pedicles, the articular pillars, and posteriorly the paired laminae. Extending posteriorly off the laminae in the midline is the spinous process.

The transverse foraminae of the cervical spine usually extend from C2 through C6. This is identified as a round or oval defect within the transverse processes of the cervical vertebral bodies. The uncinate processes are best demonstrated on coronal and axial images. These consist of osseous ridges that extend off the lateral margins of the superior end plates of the vertebral body. This articulation is referred to as the uncovertebral joint or the joint of Luschka.

The cervical vertebral bodies are interconnected by the anterior and posterior longitudinal ligaments. The anterior longitudinal ligament extends from the anterior aspect of the foramen magnum caudally to the level of the sacrum. The ligamentous fibers blend with the outer anular fibers of the discs or anulus fibrosus. Along the posterior aspect of the spine is the interspinous ligament, which extends between the spinous processes of the vertebral bodies. The transverse ligament is a fibrous band that extends across the atlas, along the posterior aspect of the odontoid process, to maintain close apposition of the odontoid process with the anterior arch of C1.

Axial images through the cervical cord reveal the cord to be round or elliptical. There is a normal, subtle, enlargement of the cord from approximately the C1 to the C4 level. Eight pairs of spinal nerves arise from the lateral margins of the cord and exit through the intervertebral nerve root canals. The size and morphology of the cervical cord are probably best evaluated on sagittal T_1-weighted images, where the cord is of higher signal intensity than the cerebrospinal fluid (CSF). However, on a high-quality, high-resolution, multiplanar CT scan of the cervical spine, the cord can be identified within the thecal sac as a round or elliptical structure of slightly higher density than the adjacent CSF. Sagittal MR images are also excellent for evaluating the size of the central canal and the morphology of the cord as well.

Directly anterior to the anterior longitudinal ligament is the prevertebral space. This space contains fat and the longus colli and longus capitis muscles. It is contained anteriorly by the prevertebral fascia. The prevertebral space is important, as edema and hemorrhage secondary to cervical trauma collect in this space. This space is directly imaged by both CT and MRI so that even small hematomas or fluid collections can be detected following an acute hyperextension injury.

Thoracic Spine

The thoracic vertebral bodies have a more rectangular configuration. The pedicles extend off the superior half of the vertebral bodies. The thoracic intervertebral disc is narrow with flat adjacent end plates as compared to the lumbar disc and end plates. The neural foraminae have a direct lateral orientation as opposed to the more oblique course of the cervical neural foraminae. On sagittal images the exiting nerve roots reside centrally within the foraminae, with the foraminae being more superior relative to the disc than in the cervical spine.

Because of the normal kyphosis of the thoracic spine, the thoracic cord on axial and sagittal images is typically positioned more anteriorly within the central canal. The central canal is circular and maintains a relatively constant diameter along its length. Anteriorly, the epidural space contains very little fat. The posterior and anterior longitudinal ligaments are relatively thick and easily identified throughout the thoracic spine on MRI. It should be remembered that depending on the level, the thoracic nerve roots must descend two to three vertebral body segments within the thecal sac before leaving the sac and exiting through their corresponding neural foraminae. At the upper thoracic levels the cord segment is typically two levels lower than the corresponding vertebral segment. At the level of the lower thoracic spine the cord segment is typically three levels lower.

Lumbar Spine

On sagittal and coronal images the lumbar vertebral bodies have a rectangular configuration with slight concavity of the end plates toward the intervertebral disc. The pedicles extend posterolaterally from the superior aspect of the vertebral body and form the cranial and caudal walls of the neural foraminae. The lumbar facet joints have a coronal orientation and are formed by the superior and inferior articulating processes. The pars interarticularis bridges or links the inferior and superior facets. The facets are covered with hyaline cartilage, which ranges in thickness from 2 to 4 mm and are enclosed by a fibroelastic capsule. The facets are best evaluated on axial images in which the articulating surfaces are seen on cross section.

Degenerative Change

Disc Degeneration

The intervertebral disc is composed of the nucleus pulposus and the anulus fibrosis, and intimately related as a functional unit to the cartilaginous end plate.[81, 139] The intervertebral disc contains water, collagen, and proteoglycans. The nucleus pulposus is normally well-hydrated, containing approximately 85% to 90% water in the first decade and 70% to 80% water in the adult.[69] Elongated fibrocytes are loosely organized, forming a gelatinous matrix.[117] The nucleus has a higher content of proteoglycans than the disc anulus. The anulus fibrosis contains 75% water in the first decade and 70% to 80% water in the adult.[69, 117] The peripheral anulus is composed primarily of type I collagen, lending tensile strength to the intervertebral disc. The inner anulus is composed primarily of type 2 collagen, which, in conjunction with the nucleus pulposus, provides compressive strength.[1] Type 2 collagen may have a higher water content than type I collagen.[223] The collagenous lamellae are fewer, thinner, and more tightly packed posteriorly than anteriorly.[147] The central depression of the vertebral endplate is covered by hyaline cartilage.

With aging, the volume of the nucleus pulposus diminishes with decreasing hydration and increasing fibrosis.[139] The change in water content is due to an alteration in the relative composition of proteoglycans as well as a decrease in the extent of aggregating proteoglycans.[103, 104] By age 30, ingrowth of fibrous tissue into the nucleus results in an intranuclear cleft.[2, 235] Fibrocartilage, derived from cells in the anulus and end plate, gradually replaces mucoid material within the nucleus. Gradual loss of definition between the nucleus and the inner anular fibers occurs.[127] In the final stages of degeneration, the nucleus is completely replaced by fibrocartilage, indistinguishable from the fibrotic disc anulus. Collagen content of the disc anulus increases. Specifically, type I collagen content increases, particularly posteriorly and type 2 collagen content diminishes.[1, 20, 96] Cartilaginous metaplasia begins in the inner anular fibers, with a change in overall fiber direction from vertical to horizontal. Infolding of fibers of the outer anulus occurs early, with myxoid degeneration of outer anular fibers.[170] Concentric and/or transverse tears in the anulus fibrosis are frequent incidental findings.[35, 233] The peripheral tears are more common posteriorly or posterolaterally, where the anulus lamellae are fewer.[38] The development of a radial tear, particularly a tear extending to the disc nucleus, is one of the major hallmarks of disc degeneration. The degenerated intervertebral disc loses height and overall volume.[117] Herniation of both nuclear material and anulus fibrosis may occur through the tear. With aging, the cartilage end plate may become thinner and may eventually calcify. In advanced disc degeneration, the cartilage end plate is ossified, with fissuring and micro fractures.[117, 139] It should be stressed that disc degeneration and even herniation does not necessarily imply symptomatic back pain.

Degeneration of the intervertebral disc and end plate are commonly seen at autopsy and on imaging studies in asymptomatic patients. At autopsy, 97% of adults over age 49 years demonstrate degenerative change.[114] In the lumbar spine, CT scans are abnormal in 35% of asymptomatic volunteers of all age and in 50% of those 40 years and older. Findings include disc degeneration and herniation, central canal stenosis, and facet joint degenerative change.[224] On MRI, substantial abnormalities are demonstrated in approximately 30% of asymptomatic people of all ages and in 57% of those 60 years and older. Disc degeneration or a bulging intervertebral disc is demonstrated in 35% of subjects between 20 and 39 years old and in nearly 100% of those between 60 and 80 years old. A disc herniation is demonstrated in 20% of those less than 60 years old and in 36% of those 60 years old or older.[12] In the cervical spine, in one study[207], MRI in asymptomatic subjects older than 64 years demonstrated disc space narrowing in 67%, disc herniation in 57%, cord impingement in 26%, and osteophytosis in 37%. In a second cervical spine study,[15] MRI demonstrated abnormalities in 19% of asymptomatic volunteers of all ages. In scans of those less than 40 years old, 14% were abnormal, including disc degeneration in 25% and a disc herniation in 10%. In scans of those over 40 years old, 28% were abnormal, including disc degeneration in 60% and disc herniation in 5%.

Computed Tomographic Findings In Disc Degeneration

Lumbar Spine Computed tomography is accurate in the diagnosis of disc herniation since disc material is relatively hyperdense against the low-density epidural fat.[55,74] Overlapping 5-mm axial sections at 3-mm increments with multiplanar reformations is the optimal protocol. Symmetric, uniform degenerative changes of the disc result in a diffuse anular disc bulge, seen as diffuse peripheral extension of disc material. The margin of the anular bulge is usually smooth in contour but may be asymmetric.[93, 229] The posterior aspect of the intervertebral disc usually assumes a convex margin but may retain a midline concavity. Sagittal reformations or the CT

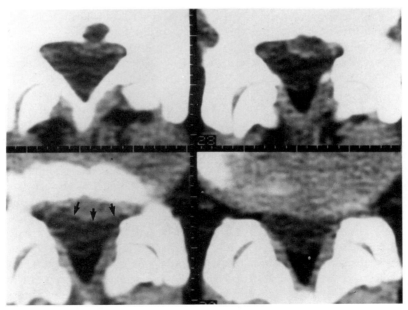

Fig. 11-1
CT of disc protrusion. Note hyperdense left paracentral disc protrusion (*black arrows*) with resultant compression along ventral-lateral aspect of thecal sac.

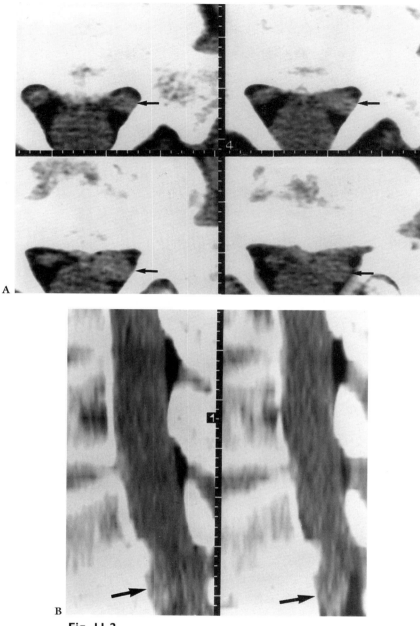

Fig. 11-2

Disc sequestration. **A,** Axial images reveal mass within left ventral-lateral recess at L5-S1 level. There is effacement of left S1
nerve root (*black arrow*). **B,** Sagittal reformatted images demonstrate hyperdense mass caudal to degenerated L5-S1 intervertebral disc space (*black arrow*).

scout radiograph may demonstrate loss of intervertebral disc height. An intradiscal vacuum phenomenon is commonly seen as focal or linear areas of
markedly diminished density within the intervertebral disc.[150]

The main CT finding in disc herniation is focal
peripheral extension of high-density disc material,
partially effacing anterior epidural fat.[230] Because the
posterior longitudinal ligament and the components
of the intervertebral disc cannot be distinguished by
CT, differentiation of a subligamentous disc protrusion from an extrusion that extends through the peripheral anular fibers can be problematic. Disc protrusions are usually less than 5 mm in diameter and
do not have cephalocaudal extension (Fig. 11-1). A
disc sequestration or free fragment appears as a rel-

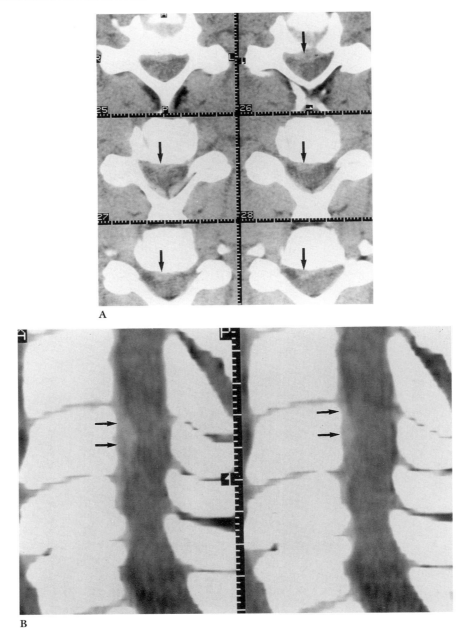

Fig. 11-3

Cervical disc extrusion. **A,** Series of 1.5-mm-thick axial images reveals right paracentral disc extrusion (*black arrow*). **B,** Reformatted sagittal images reveal hyperdense mass extending caudal to C3-C4 disc space (*black arrows*).

atively high density soft-tissue mass that may be remote from the parent disc space (Fig. 11-2). Occasionally sequestrations are nearly isodense with CSF and may be apparent only because of associated mass effect.[42,60,227] Secondary CT findings of disc herniation include thecal-sac or nerve root sheath deformation or compression, nerve root sheath enlargement adjacent to the level of the disc herniation, and if the herniation is lateral, loss of the normal intraforaminal fat.[206,228] End-plate degenerative changes include sclerosis and cortical irregularity

with erosions. Differential diagnosis of disc herniation by CT includes epidural venous plexus, particularly at the L5-S1 level, conjoined nerve root sleeves,[83,206] synovial facet joint cysts,[32,80] and a variety of neoplasms, including neurofibromas[23,64] and epidural lesions such as metastatic disease or lymphoma.

Cervical and Thoracic Spine CT detection of disc herniation in the cervical and thoracic spine requires careful technique since the intervertebral discs are relatively small and of only slightly higher density than CSF (as compared with the very-low-density epidural fat in the lumbar spine). In the cervical spine, sections should be obtained at 1.5-mm increments; in the thoracic spine, at 3-mm increments. Multiplanar reformations should be performed. The sensitivity of CT is increased if scans are performed with intrathecal contrast.[176] Disc herniations appear as focal soft tissue, slightly hyperdense as compared with adjacent cerebrospinal fluid[6,9] (Fig. 11-3). Secondary findings include effacement of the anterior subarachnoid space and cord compression or rotation. Calcified disc herniation, more common in the thoracic spine, may present as a dense epidural mass, sometimes difficult to differentiate from a meningioma.[164,214]

Findings On Magnetic Resonance Imaging in Disc Degeneration

MRI is sensitive to degenerative changes of the intervertebral disc. In one study MRI demonstrated degenerative changes in three times as many motion segments as did contrast CT.[171] Degeneration of the intervertebral disc results in diminished signal intensity on T_1- and T_2-weighted sequences

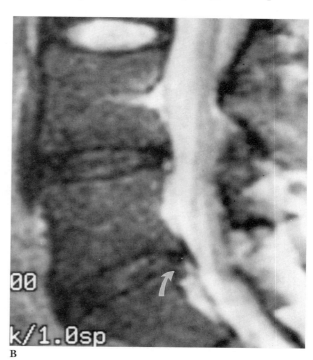

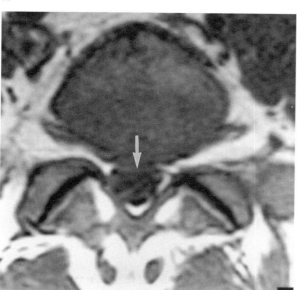

Fig. 11-4

MR findings of disc degeneration and herniation. **A,** Sagittal T_1-weighted sequence reveals posterior bulging of anulus at L4-L5 level with focal protrusion at L5-S1 level (*curved white arrow*). **B,** T_2-weighted sagittal sequence reveals relatively normal disc at L3-L4 level with disc desiccation noted at the L4-L5 and L5-S1 levels. Note posterior anular fissure at the L5-S1 level (*curved white arrow*). **C** Axial T_1-weighted images through L5-S1 intervertebral disc space reveals central posterior anular protrusion (*white arrows*).

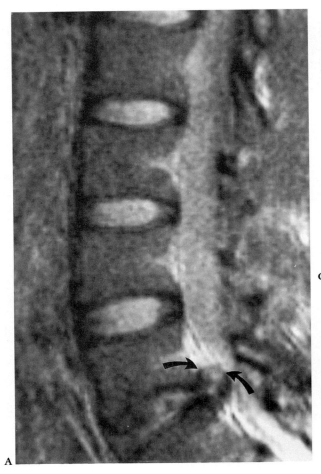

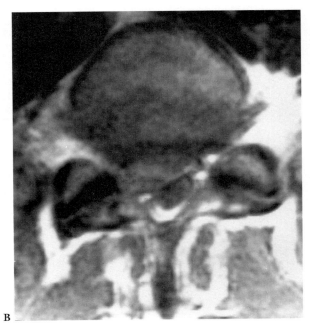

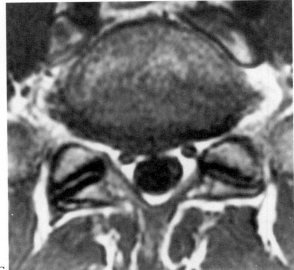

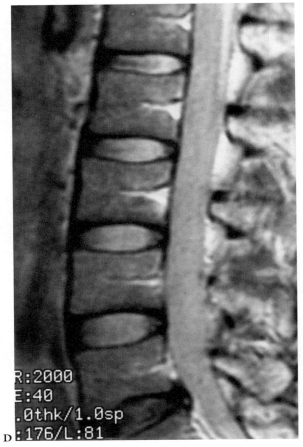

Fig. 11-5.

MRI of disc extrusion. **A,** T_2-weighted sagittal image demonstrates relative loss of signal intensity of L5-S1 intervertebral discs. Note posterior extruded disc material with extension of disc through posterior longitudinal ligament (*curved arrows*). **B,** Axial T_1-weighted image through L5-S1 level demonstrates large extruded disc fragment residing predominantly to right of midline with resultant compression of thecal sac. **C,** Sagittal proton density image of same patient approximately 12 months later. Note marked decrease in size of disc extrusion without previous surgery. **D,** Axial T_1-weighted image of same patient again demonstrates marked reduction of size of disc extrusion without surgical intervention.

(Fig. 11-4). These signal intensity changes are due to diminished water and glycosaminoglycan content and increased collagen content of the intervertebral disc.[172, 178, 223,233] Loss in intervertebral disc height is seen, best appreciated on sagittal images. Bulging of the disc anulus is demonstrated, well seen on both sagittal and axial images. Posterior extension of the disc anulus more than 1.5 mm almost invariably correlates pathologically with radial tears of the disc anulus.[236] In vitro, MRI is capable of demonstrating radial tears of the disc anulus as a region of high signal intensity within the disc anulus (Fig. 11-4, *B*). The sensitivity of MRI is 67% compared with discography.[234] Focal anular enhancement of radial tears may be seen on T_1-weighted sequences after the administration of Gd-DTPA.[158] The enhancement has been attributed to granulation tissue within the tear. A vacuum phenomenon is demonstrated by MRI as an area without signal within the intervertebral disc, best appreciated on T_1-weighted images in the sagittal plane.[71] The findings are less conspicuous than with CT and can be difficult to distinguish from anular calcification and chemical shift artifact.

The contrast sensitivity of MRI, in conjunction with direct multiplanar imaging, frequently allows the identification of the outer anulus and posterior longitudinal ligament complex distinct from the inner anulus-nucleus pulposus. Consequently, a contained herniation or disc protrusion with intact outer anular fibers and posterior longitudinal ligament can be distinguished from a disc extrusion that has extended through the outer anular fibers (subligamentous) or through the posterior longitudinal ligament.[70]

A disc protrusion (see Fig. 11-4) results in focal peripheral extension of the disc anulus. Its shape and location are best seen on axial images. The herniation is usually isointense with the adjacent intervertebral disc. It may be focally of higher signal intensity on T_2-weighted sequences due to an anular fissure (see Fig. 11-4, *B*). The disc protrusion is outlined by a thin line of low signal intensity corresponding to residual outer anular fibers and posterior longitudinal ligament. Disc herniations may be central or lateral, resulting in effacement of epidural or neural foraminal fat.

A disc extrusion is of variable signal intensity with respect to its parent intervertebral disc (Fig. 11-5). The extrusion may be of decreased or increased signal intensity on T_2-weighted sequences. The disc herniation is in contiguity with the intervertebral disc but may extend cephalad or caudad. The posterior longitudinal ligament is usually intact, demonstrated as a line of diminished signal intensity along the margin of the herniation on both T_1-weighted and proton-density sagittal sequences.[70]

A disc sequestration or free fragment is usually hyperintense on T_2-weighted sequences[108] (Fig. 11-6). Consequently, the sequestration may be difficult to identify on T_2-weighted sequences and is most conspicuous on T_1-weighted scans. The high signal intensity of the free fragment is not fully understood but may be related to granulation tissue within the disc fragment[117] or inflammatory reactive changes.[112] Sequestrations usually extend through the posterior longitudinal ligament with disruption of the linear area of diminished signal intensity normally seen peripherally. Migration cephalad or caudad from the intervertebral disc space is common. Sequestrations that have migrated are usually oblong and irregular in appearance, while sequestrations located at the interspace of origin are usually more rounded in configuration.[108] The differential diagnosis may include other epidural processes, including tumors, abscess, or hematoma. These entities can be distinguished by differences in signal intensity characteristics and patterns of contrast enhancement (see below).

Serial MRI scans may demonstrate spontaneous reduction in size of disc herniations (see Fig. 11-5). In a 2-year prospective study,[16] 63% of patients showed a reduction of 30% or more in the size of the herniation and approximately 50% of the patients had a reduction of 70% or more. A small minority (8%) experienced an increase in size of the herniation. The mechanism of herniation reduction may be due to shrinkage associated with dehydration, resorption by granulation tissue, regression by means of anular tears, and fragmentation.[90,100,165]

An important component of the degenerative process of the discovertebral joint is degeneration of the cartilaginous vertebral end plate.[5,139,147,212] The cartilaginous end plate cannot be discretely identified by MRI because of its thinness and chemical shift artifact at the end plate.[70] However, MRI demonstrates the reactive changes within the bone marrow secondary to the degenerative process in the discovertebral joint[39] associated with chronic, repetitive stress. Disruption and fissuring of the end plate with granulation tissue and reactive woven bone result in type I end-plate changes.[121] The adjacent marrow is replaced by vascularized fibrous tissue. Type I end-plate changes are characterized by decreased signal intensity on T_1-weighted sequence and increased signal intensity on T_2-weighted images. Disruption of the end plate with replacement of the hematopoietic elements within the adjacent marrow by fat result in type II changes (Fig. 11-7).

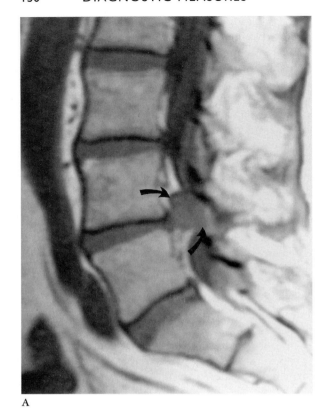

A

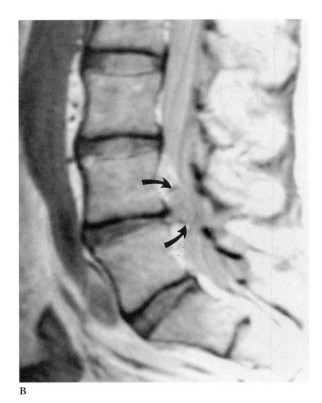

B

Fig. 11-6

MRI of disc sequestration. **A,** T_1-weighted sagittal image demonstrates large sequestered fragment posterior to L4-L5 intervertebral disc space (*curved black arrows*). Note compression of thecal sac with effacement of epidural fat posterior to the L4-L5 intervertebral disc space. **B,** T_2-weighted sagittal images demonstrates the sequestered fragment to be of relatively increased signal intensity (*curved black arrows*).

Type II end-plate changes are consequently nearly isointense with fat, of increased signal intensity on T_1-weighted sequences, and of isointensity or slightly diminished signal intensity on T_2-weighted sequences. Type I changes appear to convert to type II changes over time.[121] Extensive bony sclerosis with thickening of subchondral trabeculae result in type II end-plate changes.[121,189] The type III changes demonstrate decreased signal intensity on both T_1- and T_2-weighted images. The reactive signal intensity changes, regardless of type, may extend into up to one half of the vertebral body.

Cervical and Thoracic Spine In the detection of disc herniations, MRI is at least equivalent to CT myelography in the cervical spine[48,122] and equiva-

lent in the thoracic spine.[159] Because of the relatively small size of cervical and thoracic intervertebral discs and the lack of anterior epidural fat, special attention to scan technique is important. T_1- and T_2-weighted sequences in the sagittal plane should be performed. Thin section volume T_2^* gradient-echo imaging, particularly in the axial plane, is helpful.[215]

The early changes of anular degeneration are less well seen in the intervertebral discs of the cervical and thoracic spine than in the lumbar spine. However, later changes of disc degeneration include diminished signal intensity of the intervertebral disc on T_1- and T_2-weighted sequences, an anular disc bulge, and loss of intervertebral disc height (Fig. 11-8). The anular disc bulge is most conspicuous on T_2 or T_2^*-weighted sequences in which the peripheral margin

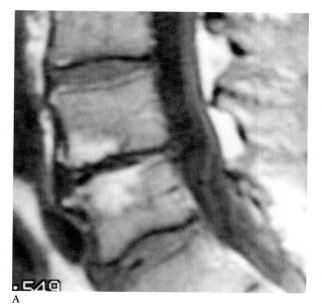 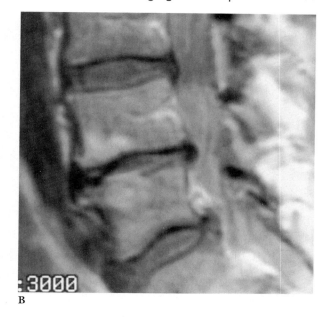

Fig. 11-7

Modic type II changes. **A,** T$_1$-weighted sagittal image demonstrates disc degeneration L4-L5 level with disc space narrowing. Note regions of high signal intensity involving anterior aspects of adjacent end plates. **B,** Proton-density image demonstrates slight relative reduction of signal intensity of end plates adjacent to L4-L5 intervertebral disc. Findings are consistent with fat replacement of hematopoietic marrow.

of the disc is outlined by high-signal-intensity CSF. Vacuum phenomena may be demonstrated as areas of diminished or absent signal intensity within the intervertebral disc.

The anatomy within the intervertebral disc is less well demonstrated in the cervicothoracic spine than in the lumbar spine due to the smaller size of the discs. Specifically, the nucleus pulposus-inner anular fibers cannot be distinguished from the posterior anular fibers. However, the most peripheral outer anular fibers and the posterior longitudinal ligament are seen as a thin rim of diminished signal intensity along the peripheral margin of intervertebral disc. Disc herniations are usually of intermediate signal intensity on both T$_1$- and T$_2$-weighted sequences. Disc extrusions and sequestrations may be of increased signal intensity on T^2* gradient echo images (Fig. 11-9). Densely calcified intervertebral disc herniations, more common in the thoracic spine, are often midline[48,58] and well demonstrated on sagittal scans. However, lateral herniations are best seen on axial images. Additionally, correlation of sagittal and axial images may be necessary to differentiate a disc herniation from a marginal osteophyte. Associated findings in disc herniation include displacement of the dura or nerve root sleeve, effacement of the

anterior subarachnoid space, and spinal cord compression or rotation.

Spinal Stenosis

The role of imaging in the evaluation of spinal stenosis includes the definition of the etiology, site, and degree of stenosis. Central canal stenosis may be developmental or acquired.[7] In developmental stenosis, central canal compromise is due to shortened pedicles attributed to abnormal development of the posterior elements.[149, 217, 218] Acquired spinal stenosis is usually due to degenerative changes including posterior extension of the intervertebral disc anulus, marginal osteophytes,[95,106,130,147] facet joint degenerative changes,[102] and in the lumbar spine, ligamentum flavum hypertrophy.[82,102] A small central canal on a developmental basis is a predisposing factor in the development of acquired stenosis.[50,95,125,130,133]

The sagittal diameter of the central canal is measured from the anterior aspect of the spinolaminar line to the posterior cortex of the middle of the vertebral body or the posterior margin of the intervertebral disc or marginal osteophyte. The former mea-

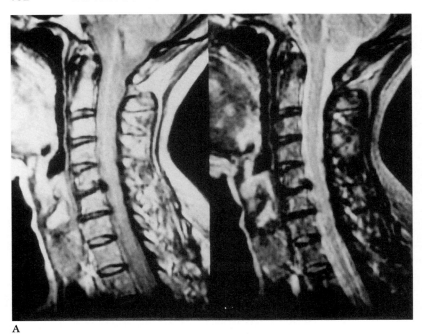

A

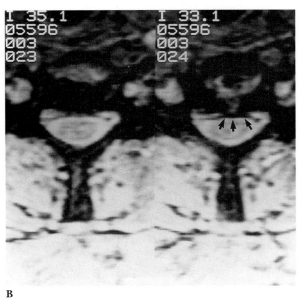

B

Fig. 11-8

MR demonstration of cervical disc protrusion. **A,** Sagittal proton density and T_2-weighted images of cervical spine reveal intervertebral disc space narrowing at C5-C6 level with posterior protrusion and resultant compression of anterior aspect of thecal sac. **B,** Axial gradient echo images through C5-C6 level reveals small central protrusion with effacement of anterior aspect of thecal sac (*small black arrows*).

surement is referred to as the developmental midsagittal diameter; the latter, as the degenerative midsagittal diameter.[45,46] In the cervical spine, from C3 through C6, the normal anteroposterior diameter is 14 to 14.5 mm. A central canal of sagittal diameter less than 12.5 mm is relatively stenotic; less than 10.5 mm, absolutely stenotic.[191] The measurements in the lumbar spine are similar. A central canal with an anteroposterior diameter of less than 12 mm is considered relatively stenotic; of less than 10 mm, absolutely stenotic.[217] However, wide normal anatomic variations limit the utility of simple measurements alone.[163] The general shape and configuration of the central canal should also be considered.

In the evaluation of lumbar stenosis, MRI has been shown to have an accuracy similar to or greater than that of CT. Nearly 100% agreement has been demonstrated between MRI and CT in the diagnosis of spinal stenosis.[171] In one study of spinal stenosis, MRI findings agreed with surgical findings in 77%; CT findings, in 79%; and myelography, in 54%.[120] In a more recent study, MRI had a higher

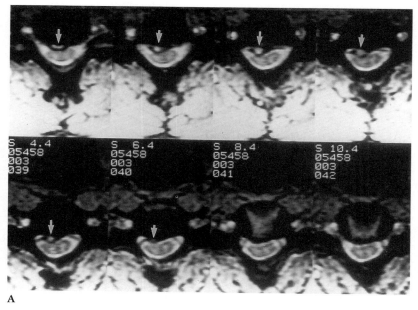

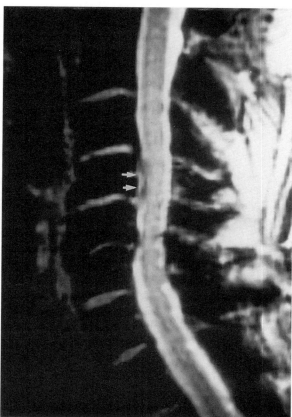

Fig. 11-9
MRI of the cervical disc extrusion. **A,** Series of 1.5-mm thick gradient axial images reveal high signal intensity of extruded disc material (*white arrow*). Extrusion results in compression along right ventral-lateral aspect of thecal sac with effacement of anterior subarachnoid space. **B,** Sagittal gradient echo images of same patient reveal extruded disc to extend cephalad to C4-C5 intervertebral disc space (*white arrows*).

diagnostic accuracy than CT or myelography and provided additional diagnostic information in almost all patients studied.[138] In the evaluation of cervical stenosis, MRI correlates with the surgical findings slightly better than does CT.[24]

Lumbar Spine

The radiographic findings in developmental lumbar spinal stenosis include a central canal diminished in cross-sectional area with thickened, shortened pedi-

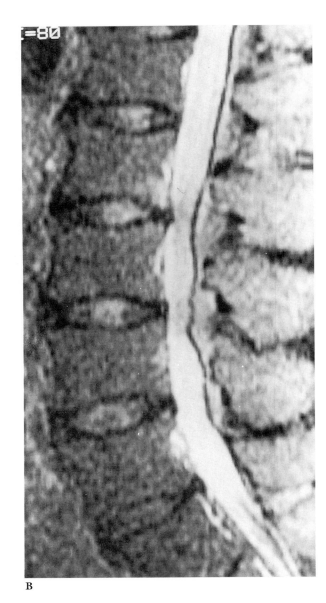

B

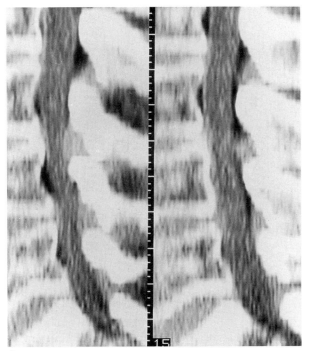

A

Fig. 11-10

CT and MRI of developmental lumbar stenosis. **A,** Reformatted sagittal CT scan of lumbar spine reveals developmental narrowing of central canal from L2 to S1. **B,** Sagittal T$_2$-weighted MRI scan of same patient again reveals diffuse narrow of central canal. There is no evidence of focal disc protrusion.

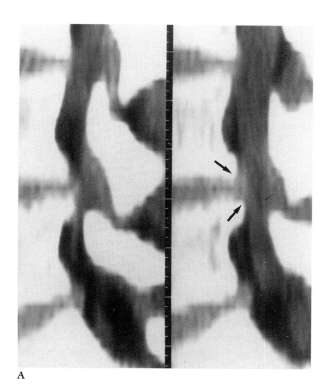

A

Fig. 11-11

CT of acquired central canal stenosis. **A,** Sagittal reformatted CT images demonstrate remodeling and osteophytic ridging off the posterior aspects of the end plates adjacent to L4-L5 intervertebral disc (*black arrows*). There is posterior bulging of anulus as well. **B,** Axial image through same level reveals hypertrophic and degenerative changes involving posterior articulating facets with thickening of ligamentum flavum (*curved black arrows*). There is resultant lateral recess stenosis secondary to osseous encroachment (*small black arrows*).

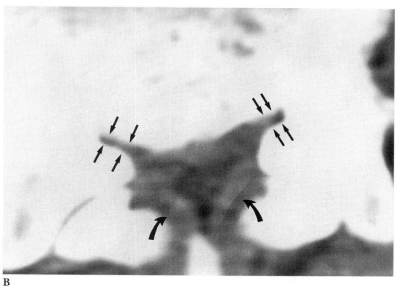

B

cles (Fig. 11-10).[50] In degenerative lumbar spinal stenosis findings may include a disc herniation or an anular disc bulge, flattening or compressing the anterior aspect of the thecal sac (Figs. 11-11 and 11-12). Marginal osteophytes arising from the posterior aspect of the vertebral end plates may also distort the anterior contour of the thecal sac. Osteophytes are well demonstrated on both CT and MRI but are more easily appreciated by CT. On MRI, osteophytes are best demonstrated on proton-density im-

ages (long TR/short T).[72] On axial MRI alone, osteophytes may be difficult to distinguish from disc material, and correlation with sagittal images is essential. The overall quantity of epidural fat surrounding the thecal sac may be reduced.[110] Hypertrophy of the ligamentum flavum may be demonstrated. This may be due to shortening and thickening of the ligament associated with reduction in height of the intervertebral disc spaces.[79] The ligamentum flavum is of higher signal intensity than

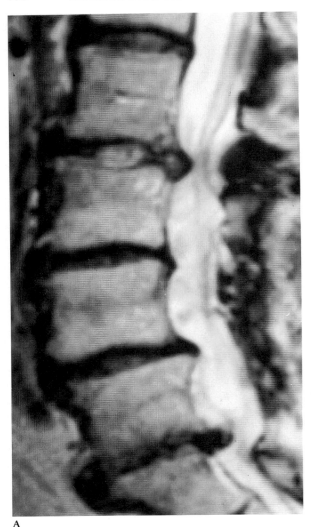

A

Fig. 11-12

MRI of acquired central canal stenosis. **A,** Sagittal T_2-weighted MRI reveals prominent disc protrusions at L2-L3 and L5-S1 levels. There is resultant narrowing of central canal at both levels. **B,** Axial T_1-weighted MRI through L2-L3 intervertebral disc space reveals degenerative changes involving posterior articulating facets with thickening of ligamentum flavum and diffuse anular bulging. Combination of findings results in marked narrowing of central canal (*small black arrows*).

cerebrospinal fluid on T_1-weighted sequences and of slightly higher signal intensity than CSF on proton-density sequences.

Degenerative and hypertrophic changes of the facet joints may compromise the central canal posterolaterally, resulting in a trefoil configuration of the central canal. Of note, this shape is a normal finding at the L5 level in 10% to 20% of the population.[47,52] Radiographic findings in facet joint degenerative changes include osteophyte formation,[31] joint space narrowing, subchondral sclerosis and subchondral cyst formation, and erosive changes. Although MRI is capable of demonstrating hyaline cartilage, thinning of the cartilage within the facet joint cannot be reliably shown because of the variable axial obliquity of the joint, chemical shift artifact, and partial volume averaging.[72] MRI may demonstrate a small amount of fluid within the normal facet joints.[72] Rarely, synovial cysts may form due to herniation of synovium through the facet joint capsule and ligamentum flavum.[221] These cysts, nearly isodense with CSF, may be difficult to distinguish from the thecal sac on CT. On MRI, the cyst compared

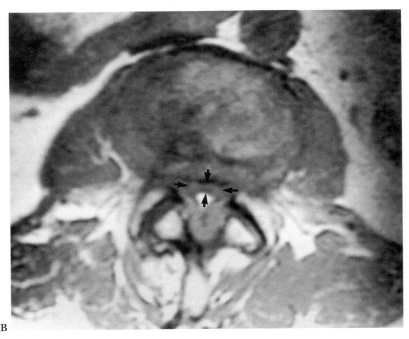

B

with CSF is of slightly higher signal intensity on both T_1- and T_2-weighted sequences.

The lateral recess is formed anteriorly by the posterolateral cortex of the vertebral body, laterally by the medial aspect of the pedicle, and posteriorly by the superior articular process of the facet joint. Stenosis results from degenerative changes of the superior articular facet, including hypertrophic change and osteophyte formation. In the transverse plane, a lateral recess of less than 2 mm in anteroposterior diameter is stenotic; between 2 to 3 mm in anteroposterior diameter, strongly suggestive of stenosis (see Fig. 11-11).[34,94,113] The most common site for stenosis is at the level of the rostral border of the pedicle. The superior articular process is angled forward at this level, rendering this the narrowest portion of the lateral recess and consequently most vulnerable to degenerative stenosis.[34,184]

The radiographic findings in neural foraminal stenosis include posterolateral extension of the intervertebral disc and vertebral end-plate marginal osteophytes, and facet joint hypertrophic changes. A degenerative anterolisthesis may further compromise the neural foramen, resulting in flattening of the foramen in the craniocaudal direction.[51] Loss of normal perineural fat is demonstrated in the axial and sagittal planes. On CT, bone windows most accurately depict stenosis due to facet joint degenerative changes and marginal osteophytes (Fig. 11-13).[148] Stenosis secondary to disc material is best evaluated at soft-tissue windows. On MRI, neural foraminal stenosis is best demonstrated on T_1-weighted sequences[72] (Fig. 11-14). However, the proton-density sequences (long TR/short TE)

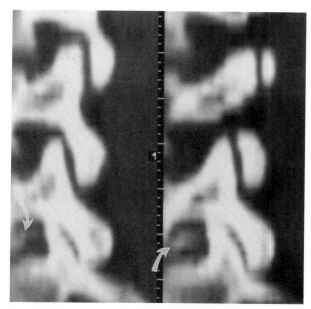

Fig. 11-13

Foraminal stenosis. Reformatted sagittal CT images of lumbar spine reveal osteophytic ridging extending off of inferior end plate of L5 into intervertebral nerve-root canal (*curved white arrow*).

are most useful in distinguishing osteophytes from soft tissue.[72] Osteophytes containing fatty bone marrow with a cortical margin of diminished signal intensity are better demonstrated on MRI than are sclerotic osteophytes. Sclerotic osteophytes, of low signal intensity, cannot always be differentiated from adjacent capsuloligamentous structures, particularly at the posteroinferior aspect of the facet joint.[72]

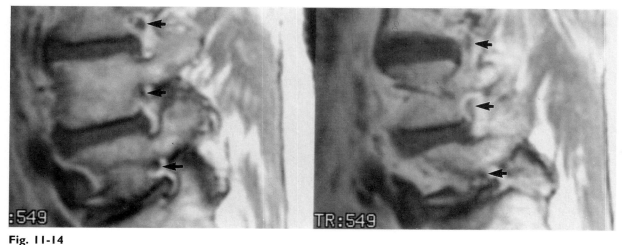

Fig. 11-14

Sagittal T_1-weighted MRI demonstrate foraminal stenosis at L4-L5 and to slightly greater extent at L5-S1 levels. Exiting nerve roots are identified within intervertebral nerve-root canals (*small black arrows*). Note overall reduction of volume of intervertebral nerve root canals with extension of anulus into caudal aspects of intervertebral nerve-root canals, most notably at L5-S1 level.

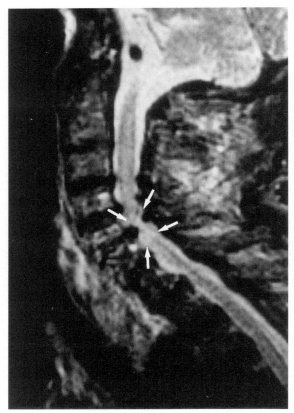

Fig. 11-15
Sagittal gradient echo image of cervical spine reveals central canal stenosis with increased signal intensity of cervical cord (*white arrows*), indicating cord edema secondary to chronic compression.

Cervical Spine

Radiographic findings in acquired cervical central canal stenosis include posterior extension of the disc anulus and marginal osteophytes arising from the posterior aspect of the vertebral endplates. A myelogram CT or MRI demonstrates focal effacement of the anterior cervical subarachnoid space with rotation, flattening, or compression of the cervical cord. Myelopathic symptoms correlate with at least 30% reduction of the cross-sectional area of the cervical cord to a value of about 60 mm by contrast CT.[131] In patients with chronic compressive lesions, increased signal intensity may be demonstrated on T_2-weighted sequences, usually focal at the level of compression (Fig. 11-15). The frequency of this finding correlates with the degree of central canal compromise and the severity of clinical myelopathy. More than 60% of patients demonstrated this finding when

the grade of myelopathy or degree of canal stenosis was moderate or marked.[199] This finding may be due to demyelination and neuronal loss and to compromise of the anterior or spinal artery secondary to chronic compression.[76,125,198] Patients with this finding respond less favorably to both surgical decompression and conservative medical treatment than patients without this finding.[199]

Ossification of the posterior longitudinal ligament (OPLL) may result in central canal stenosis. On CT, OPLL is shown as thick calcification along the posterior aspect of the vertebral bodies in the midline. The calcifications may be continuous, extending over several vertebral bodies, or segmental. On MRI, the ossified lesions are of diminished signal intensity on both T_1- and T_2-weighted sequences.[126] However, in almost half of patients, areas isointense with fat are demonstrated within the ossified lesions attributed to fatty marrow. OPLL is best demonstrated on proton-density sequences and most easily detected in the axial plane.[126]

Radiographic findings in neural foraminal stenosis include posterolateral extension of the disc anulus, end-plate marginal osteophytes, and uncovertebral and facet-joint degenerative changes (Fig. 11-16). On CT, the neural foramen is best demonstrated in the axial and coronal plane. Sagittal reformations are also useful. MRI is less accurate than CT in demonstrating the degree and etiology of neural foraminal stenosis.[24,118,119] The accuracy of MRI is dependent on the type of sequence performed. With current technology, the optimal imaging sequence in the axial plane is contiguous section gradient-refocused three-dimensional Fourier transformation (3DFT) MRI.[211,232] Using this sequence, MRI findings were seen to agree with those of CT in the detection of neural foraminal stenosis and in the determination of the etiology in 76% of the neural foramina.[232] Of the cases in which MRI failed to detect neural foraminal narrowing demonstrated on CT, nearly 100% were due to osseous encroachment. In this study, MRI was more likely to be interpreted as showing foraminal stenosis when CT was normal than for MRI not to demonstrate stenosis when CT was abnormal. Using a 3DFT sequence, magnetic susceptibility artifacts may accentuate or mimic neural foraminal stenosis.[211] In a two-dimensional gradient echo or T_1-weighted sequence with a thicker section thickness, MRI typically underestimates neural foraminal stenosis. Additionally, due to partial volume averaging associated with larger section thickness, even greater difficulty may be encountered in determining the etiology of neural foraminue stenosis.[24,118,119]

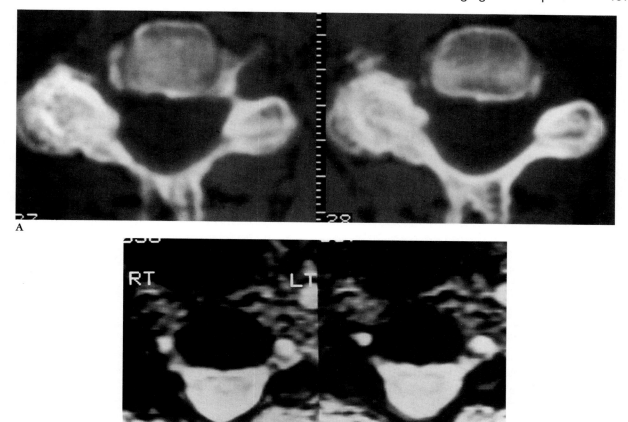

Fig. 11-16
Axial CT and MRI images of neural foraminal stenosis. **A,** CT image reveals rather advanced hypertrophic and degenerative changes involving predominantly right-sided facet. Mild, bilateral, uncinate spurring is also noted. **B,** Axial MRI through this same level does demonstrate stenosis; however, osseous detail is better demonstrated on CT.

Spondylolysis and Spondylolisthesis

The term *spondylolysis* refers to defects involving the pars interarticularis. This is a relatively common deformity occurring in approximately 6% of adults.[162] Spondylolysis occurs more commonly in males and is usually bilateral.[204] Spondylolysis most commonly involves the lumbar spine but can rarely be identified in the cervical spine.

While the spondylitic defects involving the pars can be identified on axial imaging, the sagittal plane is ideal for identifying the pars defects. On sagittal CT images, the pars interarticularis is identified directly cephalad to the intervertebral nerve root canals. With spondylolysis, the fractured ends of the pars are often hypertrophied and sclerotic. Even without subluxation, this may contribute to lateral recess and intervertebral nerve root-canal stenosis.[44] Compression of the thecal sac and stenosis of the lateral recess is best appreciated on axial MR and CT images, while the degree of intervertebral nerve root canal stenosis is best demonstrated on sagittal images.

Computed tomography with reformatted sagittal and coronal images is probably more sensitive than MRI in the detection of spondylolysis. However, the pars defects can frequently be identified with MRI. On sagittal MRI through the region of the pars interarticularis, there is discontinuity of the cortical margins of the pars.[89] This is typically best demonstrated on the proton-density images. Other signs of spondylolysis include separation or distraction of the osseous fragments of the pars interarticularis[89] and a step-off or displacement of the adjacent ends of the pars.[73] The diagnosis of spondylolysis using MRI may be difficult when there is no subluxation and only a linear area of diminished signal intensity is identified in the region of the pars interarticularis. This may represent a thin dense sclerotic pars or perhaps healing of a previous pars defect. However, the possibility of a nondisplaced spondylitic defect often cannot be ruled out. CT is probably more sensitive in detecting thin sclerotic defects in the pars.[204]

Spondylolisthesis, a complication of spondylolysis, is easily detected on MRI. Even small degrees of spondylolisthesis can be determined on sagittal MRI. The sagittal images also allow for direct imaging and evaluation of the degree of associated intervertebral nerve root-canal stenosis.[89]

Other associated complications of spondylolysis include degenerative changes involving adjacent intervertebral discs and facet joints as well as possible central canal stenosis. Both MRI and CT can identify and quantitate the severity of these associated complications.

Postoperative Spine

The failed back surgery syndrome (FBSS) includes a variety of persistent or recurrent symptoms after back surgery. Intractable low-back pain or radicular pain and varying degrees of functional incapacities are characteristic.[23,63] Up to 30% of patients may experience a lack of improvement or recurrent problems after surgery.[29,78] The most common causes of FBSS are recurrent or persistent disc herniation, spinal stenosis (central or lateral), arachnoiditis, and epidural fibrosis.[29,61,141]

Normal Appearances of the Postoperative Spine

The radiographic findings in the postoperative spine depend on the type and extent of the surgical procedure. After microscopic discectomy, focal absence of the ligamentum flavum may be the only abnormality on CT or MRI. After laminotomy and discectomy, a defect along the inferior aspect of the upper lamina and absence of the ligamentum flavum will be demonstrated. Following conventional discectomy, findings may include absence of a lamina and focal absence of the ligamentum flavum, a bilateral laminectomy defect and a medial or partial facetectomy defect. After a foraminotomy, resection of the anterior portion of the superior articular process and/or the posterolateral aspect of the vertebra is demonstrated. These bony postsurgical defects are more easily appreciated on CT than on MRI.

A solid lateral or posterolateral fusion appears as a mass of bone between the transverse processes without evidence of a pseudoarthrosis when examined in multiple planes. The fusion may extend an-

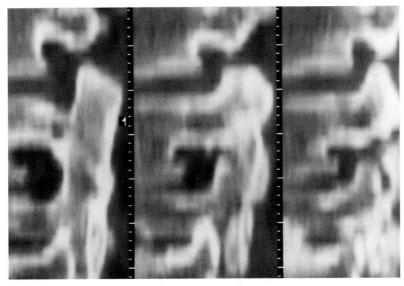

Fig. 11-17
Reformatted sagittal CT scans demonstrate solid posterolateral fusion mass at L4-L5 level.

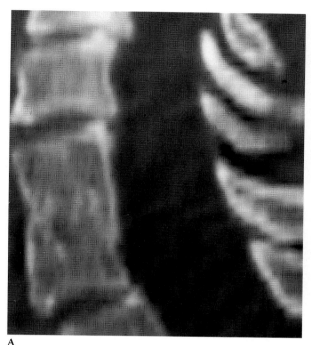

A

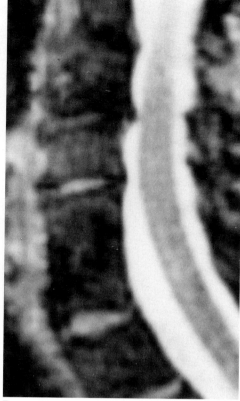

B

Fig. 11-18

CT and MRI of anterior interbody fusion. **A,** Sagittal reformatted CT scan of cervical spine reveals solid osseous mass extending across fused intervertebral disc space. Adjacent endplates are no longer identified. **B,** Sagittal T_2-weighted MRI of same patient reveals isointense marrow extending across intervertebral disc space, indicating longstanding, ossified fusion mass.

teromedially to encompass the facet joints or posteromedially to involve the laminae (Fig. 11-17). On CT, interbody fusion bone grafts or plugs are initially discretely defined within the intervertebral disc space. With fusion, the superior and inferior margins of the bone plug are no longer defined, and are incorporated into the adjacent vertebral end plates[107,177] (Fig. 11-18). On MRI, the signal intensity of grafts immediately after surgery is variable, ranging from hypointense to hyperintense.[155,157] The margins of the grafts are sharply defined, linear, and of diminished signal intensity. The vertebral end plates may be normal in signal intensity or of diminished signal intensity on T_1-weighted sequences and increased signal intensity on T_2-weighted sequences.[151] These signal intensity changes may correspond pathologically to end-plate degenerative changes or marrow edema. Months to years after surgery, the appearance of the normal interbody fusion ranges from a graft at least partially discretely identifiable to loss of definition of the bone plug with isointense marrow traversing the intervertebral disc space (see Fig. 11-18). The marrow of the adjacent vertebral bodies may be normal

in signal intensity or of diminished signal intensity on T_1-weighted sequences.[151]

Soft Tissue

On CT, normal low-density epidural fat is replaced at the surgical site by soft tissue of intermediate density. In the immediate postoperative period, this soft tissue is due to edema. Subsequently, similar-appearing soft tissue is due to epidural fibrosis (Fig. 11-19). The fibrous tissue is nearly isodense with ligamentum flavum and nerve root and slightly hyperdense compared with thecal sac. The fibrosis is lower in density than disc material.[107] CT will demonstrate anterior epidural fibrosis in 75% of postoperative patients.[203] Additionally, after discectomy, gas is seen more commonly within the intervertebral disc than preoperatively.[107]

On MRI, in the immediate postoperative period, extensive soft tissue of intermediate signal intensity on T_1-weighted sequences and high signal intensity on T_2-weighted sequences will be demonstrated, obliterating normal fat planes due to edema.[151] Postoperative fibrosis, developing later, is similar in sig-

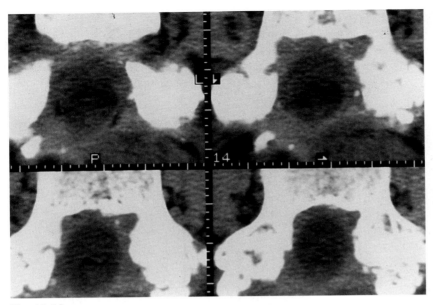

Fig. 11-19

Axial CT images demonstrating epidural fibrosis. Note loss of normal perithecal and perineural fat.

nal intensity. After discectomy, anterior epidural soft tissue is seen in the majority of patients within the first week after surgery (Fig. 11-20).[155] This soft tissue is nearly isointense with intervertebral disc on T_1-weighted sequences and slightly hyperintense on T_2-weighted sequences. Peripheral enhancement may be seen after the administration of contrast material (see Fig. 11-20). The soft tissue may exert mass effect and mimic in size and configuration the resected disc herniation.[13,151,155] The soft tissue diminishes with time, seen in 40% of asymptomatic patients at 3 weeks and in 12% at 3 months.[13] On T_2-weighted sagittal imaging, surgical disruption of the anulus and posterior longitudinal ligament may be seen as a focal area of high signal intensity that resolves by 2 to 6 months after surgery.[151] Additionally, in the first few months after surgery, enhancement of paraspinal muscles and facet joints at the operative level occurs in the majority of patients. At 3 weeks, enhancement of the nerve root at the operative level is demonstrated in 80%, with enhancement tracking cephalad along the intradural portion of the nerve root in 60%. This enhancement, hypothesized to be due to surgical trauma or a reparative process, resolves in the vast majority of asymptomatic patients by 3 months.[13]

Recurrent Disc Herniation Versus Scar

Recurrent or persistent disc herniation is the cause of failed back surgery syndrome in 12% to 16% of patients. Epidural fibrosis is the cause in 6% to 8%.[29] Differentiation of these two entities, not always possible clinically, is important since reoperation for disc herniation has a much better prognosis than repeat surgery for epidural fibrosis.[54,99] Consequently, epidural fibrosis is usually treated conservatively.

By CT, epidural fibrosis is usually of lower density than intervertebral disc. Fibrosis is typically diffuse with irregular contours and results in retraction of adjacent structures. Disc herniations are usually higher in density than fibrosis and more focal, resulting in compression, rather than retraction of adjacent structures. However, the density differences between intervertebral disc and scar can be subtle. Disc material may appear lower in density in small disc fragments or due to partial volume averaging. Anterior fibrosis can have a mass-like configuration with apparent compression of adjacent structures. Additionally, recurrent disc herniation surrounded by fibrosis may have an indeterminate density. Consequently, in the differentiation of fibrosis from disc herniation, CT has a reported accuracy of 43% to 60%.[19,55] Thin section scans obtained during the bolus intravenous administration of high-dose iodinated contrast material increases the accuracy of CT to 65% to 90%.* During and shortly after contrast infusion, epidural fibrosis enhances uniformly. The mechanism of contrast enhancement of fibrosis on CT is most likely due to the intravascular concen-

*References 19, 26, 55, 174, 190, 202, and 220.

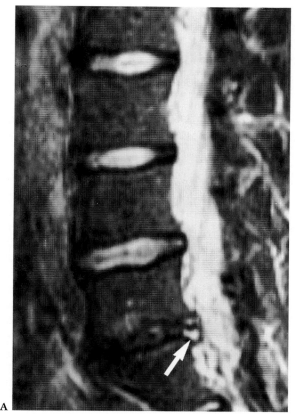

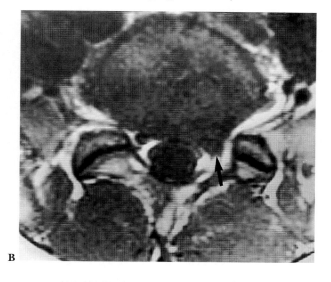

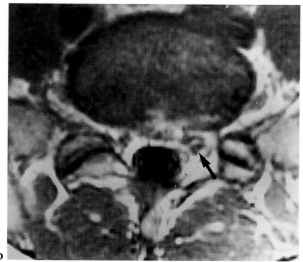

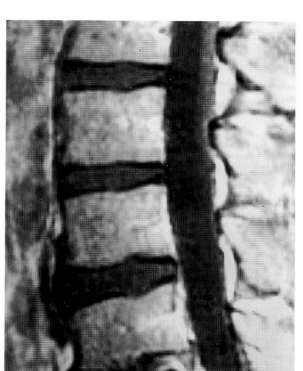

Fig. 11-20

MRI of postoperative granulation tissue. **A,** T$_2$-weighted sagittal image demonstrates area of high signal intensity posterior to operative L5-S1 segment (*white arrow*). **B,** Axial T$_1$-weighted image demonstrates mass of intermediate signal intensity extending predominantly into region of left ventral lateral recess. Exiting left S1 nerve root is poorly defined (*black arrow*). **C,** T$_1$-weighted sagittal image of lumbar spine following infusion of Gd-DTPA reveals enhancement along posterior aspect of L5-S1 anulus. This corresponds with area of high signal intensity noted in *A.* **D,** Axial T$_1$-weighted image through L5-S1 level following infusion of Gd-DTPA reveals enhancement along posterior aspect of anulus. Exiting left-sided nerve root is identified (*black arrow*). These findings are indicative of vascularized granulation tissue.

tration of iodine and dispersion of contrast into the local extracellular space through intercellular gaps.[99,167] Intervertebral disc material does not enhance immediately after contrast infusion, although peripheral enhancement may occur. This peripheral enhancement is thought to be due to a number of factors, including granulation tissue, venous plexus, and vascularized anulus.[55,174] Delayed scans (30 to 60 minutes after contrast administration) may show enhancement of the intervertebral disc itself.[40]

The accuracy of noncontrast MRI in the differentiation of epidural fibrosis from recurrent disc herniation compares favorably to CT, at 80% to 85%.[124,190] The signal intensity of epidural fibrosis varies with its location. On T_1-weighted sequences, anterior epidural fibrosis is usually of low or intermediate signal intensity, nearly isointense with disc mate-rial (Fig. 11-21). On proton-density and T_2-weighted sequences, scar is usually higher in signal intensity than intervertebral disc but lower in signal intensity than CSF.[25,85,190] Epidural fibrosis is usually more linear than mass-like. Disc protrusions are typically lower in signal intensity than fibrosis on T_2-weighted sequences (see Fig. 11-21). An exception is disc extrusions, which may be of high signal intensity on T_2-weighted sequences, similar to that of epidural fibrosis and even CSF. The disc herniation is usually in contiguity with the intervertebral disc and exerts mass effect. Commonly, a hypointense rim surrounds the disc herniation on T_2-weighted images due to a combination of the posterior longitudinal ligament and outer anular fibers surrounding the disc herniation. The intravenous administration of contrast material results in an increased MRI accuracy of 96% to 100% in differentiating scar from disc.[85,154] Scar enhances immediately and homogeneously with maximum enhancement at 5 minutes (see Fig. 11-21).[152] The mechanism of enhancement of fibrosis by Gd-DTPA appears to be similar to that of iodinated contrast, with diffusion of Gd-DTPA into the extravascular space through intercellular gaps in endothelium. As with CT, on MRI, herniated disc material does not enhance on the images obtained immediately after the administration of contrast material. Peripheral enhancement may be seen due to scars along the margin of the disc herniation (Fig. 11-22). On delayed scans, performed 30 to 60 minutes after the administration of contrast material, peridiscal enhancement extending into the disc or diffuse enhancement of the herniated disc may be seen.[152,154] Enhancement of regions of the previous surgical curettage in the posterior aspect of intervertebral discs may occur.[154] The mechanism of de-

layed enhancement of the intervertebral disc is poorly understood but may be related to diffusion via vascularized peridiscal scar or granulation tissue associated with severe degenerative change.[152]

Postoperative Stenosis

The most common cause of FBSS is spinal stenosis.[29,140] The stenosis is more commonly lateral than central.[29,78] The stenosis may have been present preoperatively and not adequately decompressed, or it may result from progression of spondylosis changes. In cases of inadequate stabilization, excessive mobility may lead to hypertrophic change with secondary stenosis. Radiographic findings in central canal stenosis include decreased volume of the central canal and thecal sac compression. The findings in lateral stenosis include decreased volume of the neural foraminae secondary to marginal osteophytes, posterolateral extension of the disc anulus, anterolisthesis, or cephalad migration of the superior articular process with hypertrophic change. Since the etiology of postoperative stenosis is frequently bony, CT with multiplanar reformation is usually more helpful than MRI.

Arachnoiditis

Arachnoiditis is the cause of persistent symptoms after spine surgery in 6% to 16% of patients.[28] Patients with arachnoiditis may be asymptomatic or present with a variety of nonspecific symptoms within the first 18 months after surgery.[183,226] Arachnoidal adhesions associated with spine surgery usually involve only one to two motion segment levels.[21,28,92] The radiographic findings can be anticipated based on the pathologic changes. An inflammatory process results in a fibrinous exudate. The fibrin-coated nerve roots and arachnoid membrane adhere. The adhesions are subsequently collagenized by proliferating fibroblasts.[144,188]

Early radiographic findings include blunted, shallow nerve root sleeves, lack of filling of nerve root sleeves, segmental nerve root fusion, and small irregularities of the thecal sac.[179,186] Subsequently, as the nerve roots adhere to the dura, the thecal sac appears featureless, smoothly marginated, and empty (Fig. 11-23). As the adhesions become more exuberant, multiple irregular intradural masses are seen with irregularity of the contour of the thecal sac (Fig. 11-24). In severe arachnoiditis, a myelographic block may be demonstrated.[105,143,166]

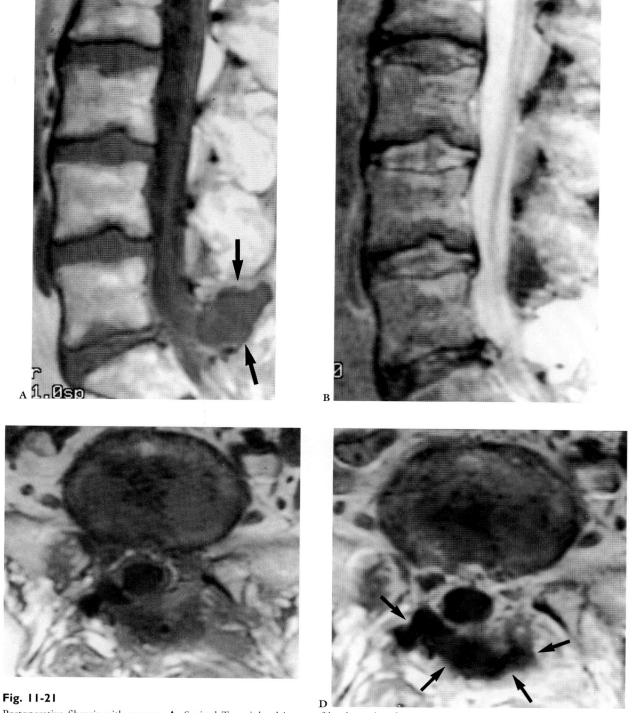

Fig. 11-21

Postoperative fibrosis with seroma. **A,** Sagittal T_1-weighted image of lumbar spine demonstrates isointense mass posterior to L5-S1 intervertebral disc space. In addition, note low signal intensity collection posterior to thecal sac in region of laminectomy defect (*black arrows*). **B,** On T_2-weighted sequence, mass posterior to disc space increased slightly in signal intensity. There is marked increase in signal intensity of mass posterior to thecal sac; appearance is consistent with fluid collection/seroma. **C,** Axial T_1-weighted image demonstrates loss of perithecal fat planes with intermediate to low-density mass posterior to thecal sac. **D,** Following infusion of Gd-DTPA, this axial T_1-weighted image demonstrates enhancement along the posterior aspect of anulus and within epidural space. Findings are consistent with prominent epidural fibrosis. Note lack of enhancement of posterior seroma (*black arrows*).

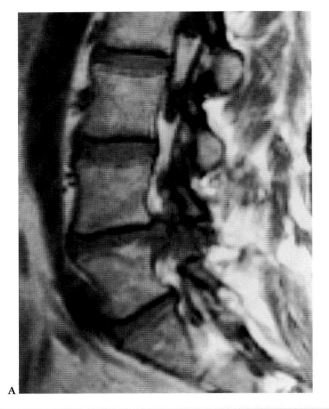

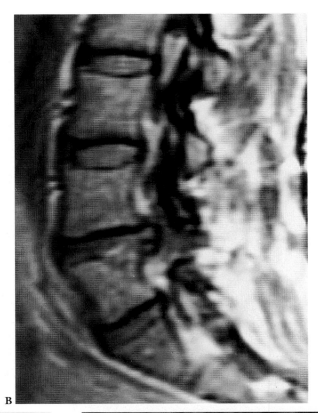

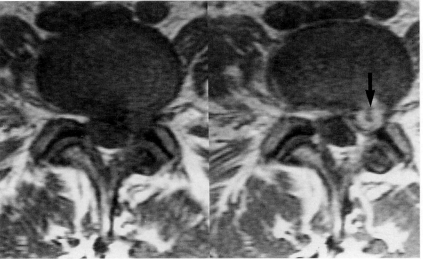

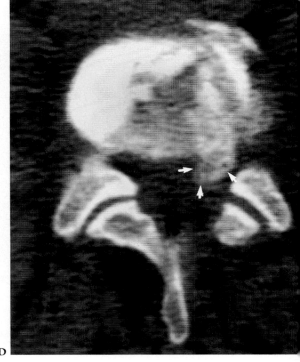

Fig. 11-22

Recurrent disc herniation. **A,** Sagittal T_1-weighted image demonstrates isointense mass posterior to L4-L5 intervertebral disc space. **B,** Sagittal proton-density image again reveals isointense mass posterior to L4-L5 intervertebral disc space. **C,** Axial T_1-weighted images both without (*left image*) and with (*right image*) Gd-DTPA. On nonenhanced image, there is isointense mass extending into left ventral-lateral recess. Following infusion of gadolinium, there is note made of enhancement in this region with central area of low signal intensity (*black arrows*). Appearance is consistent with a recurrent disc herniation and surrounding fibrosis-granulation tissue. **D,** CT scan through this level following discography demonstrates extension of contrast into region of recurrent disc herniation (*small white arrows*).

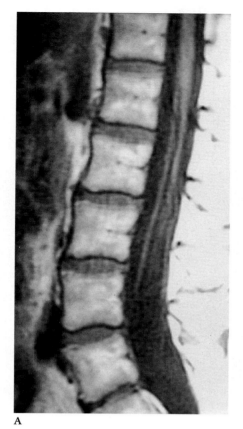

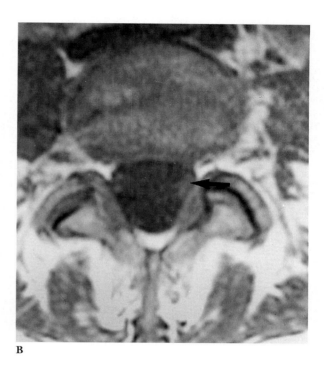

A

B

Fig. 11-23

Arachnoiditis. **A,** Sagittal T_1-weighted MRI reveals irregularity and clumping of nerve roots of cauda equina. **B,** On axial T_1-weighted image, note clumping of nerve roots along left side of thecal sac (*black arrow*).

CT myelography is the most sensitive radiographic method in the detection of arachnoiditis. However, the reported sensitivity of MRI is 92%, with an accuracy of 99% to 100%.[91, 156] T_2-weighted axial images best demonstrate the nerve roots, well-defined against the high-signal-intensity CSF. The findings may be evident on T_1-weighted axial images as well. At the L2 and L3 levels, the nerve root may normally assume a slightly clumped appearance in the dependent portion of the thecal sac. However, at the L4 and L5 levels, the nerve roots are more dispersed, better defined individually, and asymmetric in arrangement.[156] The diagnosis of arachnoiditis should be based on abnormal appearance of the nerve roots on several axial images, not one image alone. After intravenous MR contrast in arachnoiditis, minimal to moderate enhancement of nerve roots is seen in the majority of patients. Contrast enhancement is an inconstant finding, and the degree of enhancement is not related to the degree

of arachnoidal adhesions. Intravenous contrast material does not contribute to the sensitivity of MRI in the detection of arachnoidal adhesions, although it may add to their differentiation from leptomeningeal tumor, which should enhance markedly.[92] MRI is inaccurate in demonstrating the findings of myelographic block in severe arachnoiditis.[92]

Fusion

The assessment of solidity of a fusion is usually adequately accomplished with plain film radiographs, including lateral flexion-extension views. However, the fusion can also be evaluated with thin-section CT with multiplanar reformations through the fusion mass (Fig. 11-25). CT findings of a nonsolid fusion include a fragmentary fusion mass, a pseudoarthrosis of the fusion, and gas within the intervertebral disc space or facet joints, indicating persistent motion and distraction. Although MRI is not useful in the evaluation of the fusion mass itself, an

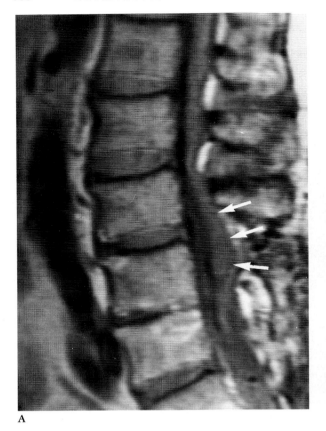

A

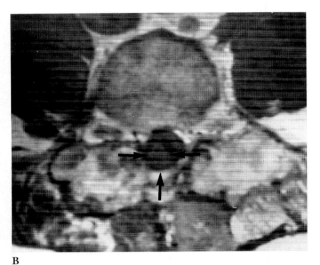

B

Fig. 11-24

"Clumped" arachnoiditis. **A,** Sagittal T_1-weighted image reveals arachnoiditis with rather pronounced clumping of nerve roots of cauda equina (*white arrows*). **B,** Axial T_1-weighted image through area of arachnoiditis demonstrates clumped nerve roots on posterior aspect of thecal sac (*black arrows*).

indirect finding in a nonsolid fusion is diminished signal intensity in the vertebral end plates on T_1-weighted sequences with increased signal intensity on T_2-weighted sequences consistent with persistent marrow reactive change due to motion. In a solid fusion, the end-plate reactive marrow should be replaced by fat of high signal on T_1- and low signal on T_2-weighted sequences.[177] Other complications of spinal fusion are best demonstrated by multiplanar CT, including extrusion of a bony plug or block, fusion overgrowth with secondary spinal stenosis, and acquired spondylolysis after a failed fusion.[22, 62, 141, 161]

Postoperative Discitis

Discitis occurs after surgery with a frequency of 0.75% to 2.8%.[53, 101, 132] Patients present with recurrent pain 7 to 28 days after surgery.[36, 146, 201] Plain film radiographs are abnormal at 4 to 6 weeks

after infection, demonstrating end-plate destruction with loss in intervertebral disc space height.[53, 153] Computed tomography is only slightly more sensitive than plain film radiography, demonstrating end-plate destructive change at an earlier stage. Technetium radionuclide imaging is more sensitive than CT but may be nonspecific.[75] Magnetic resonance imaging is ideally suited for the diagnosis of discitis because of its precise definition of anatomy and its demonstration of small changes in vertebral marrow and disc space water content associated with inflammatory processes.[59] In an experimental study using a rabbit model of discitis MRI was much more sensitive (93% vs. 41%), more accurate (95% vs. 60%), and slightly more specific (97% vs. 93%) than radionuclide imaging.[197]

The findings on MRI in postoperative discitis include (1) signal intensity changes in the vertebral marrow consisting of diminished signal intensity on T_1-weighted sequences and increased signal inten-

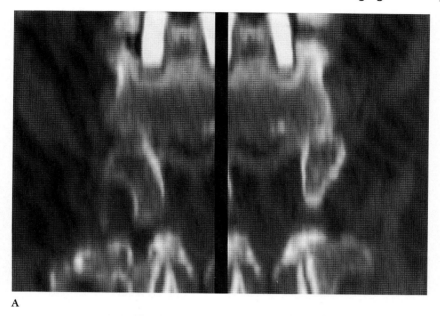

A

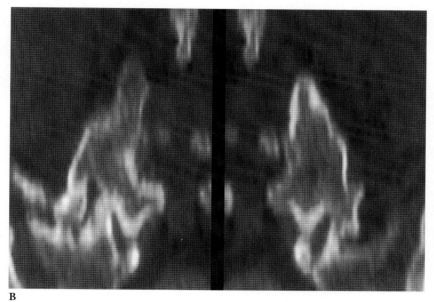

B

Fig. 11-25

Spinal fusion. **A,** Coronal CT reformation shows partially incorporated anterior interbody plugs at L3-4.
B, Coronal CT reformation more posteriorly shows solid posterolateral fusion bilaterally at L4-5; smaller
fusion mass at L5-S1 is not definitely solid.

sity on T_2-weighted sequences involving one third
to one half of the vertebral body; (2) signal intensity changes in the intervertebral disc consisting of
diminished signal intensity on T_1-weighted sequences and increased signal intensity on T_2-
weighted sequences with loss of normal intranuclear
cleft and; (3) contrast enhancement of the adjacent

bone marrow, the posterior disc anulus, and less
commonly, the disc space[14] (Fig. 11-26). MRI scans
in normal postoperative patients may occasionally
demonstrate some of these findings, including vertebral marrow signal intensity changes, increased signal on T_2-weighted sequences either within the disc
space or within the posterior disc anulus, and con-

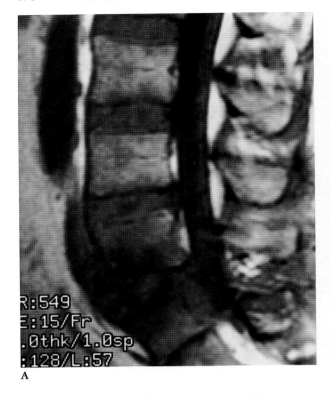

A

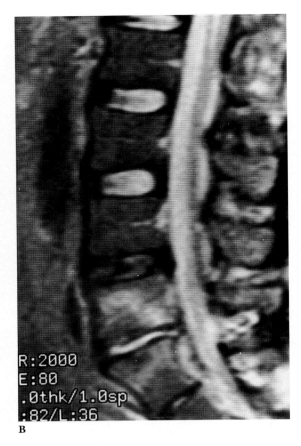

B

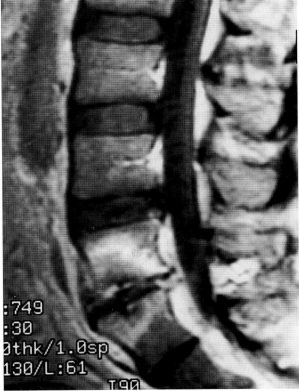

C

Fig. 11-26

MRI of discitis. **A,** Sagittal T_1-weighted image demonstrates poorly defined end plates adjacent to L5-S1 disc. There is more edema with diminished signal intensity involving adjacent marrow spaces. Collection of intermediate signal intensity is noted to extend posterior to intervertebral disc space and S1 vertebral body. **B,** Sagittal T_2-weighted study demonstrates increase in signal intensity of L5-S1 disc with loss of normal internal structures such as intranuclear cleft. Mass of intermediate signal intensity posterior to disc space and S1 vertebral body is now of increased signal intensity. There is increased signal intensity involving adjacent marrow spaces as well. These MR findings are indicative of discitis with adjacent vertebral osteomyelitis. **C,** Sagittal T_1-weighted image following infusion of Gd-DTPA reveals enhancement of adjacent marrow spaces. Note lack of definition of adjacent vertebral body end plates with enhancement along posterior aspect of anulus as well.

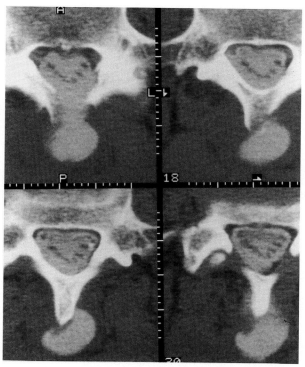

Fig. 11-27

CT scan of lumbar pseudomeningocele. Following infusion of contrast material into subarachnoid space, CT reveals extension of contrast material into collection posterior to thecal sac. Apparent dural tear is demonstrated on upper left image.

trast enhancement of the disc and marrow. However, in a series of asymptomatic postoperative patients, none demonstrated the entire triad of findings. The most reliable finding of postoperative discitis is diminished signal intensity in the vertebral marrow on T_1-weighted sequences with homogeneous enhancement after the administration of contrast material. These bone marrow changes resolve at approximately 2 to 4 months. Disc space enhancement may persist longer.[205]

Pseudomeningocele and Dural Tear

Pseudomeningoceles may form when a small surgical defect in the dura results in herniation of arachnoid membrane through the tear, with development of a sac of CSF.[205] Alternatively, a fibrous membrane may develop around a chronic CSF leak, resulting in a cystic mass.[129] On CT or MRI these lesions appear as a smoothly marginated, rounded mass directly adjacent to the thecal sac (Fig. 11-27). Its contents are usually identical in appearance to CSF, unless the cyst contains blood. The site of the dural

tear is defined only at myelography, followed by CT. The pseudomeningocele will fill with contrast material, resulting in a contrast agent-CSF fluid-fluid layer.

In the immediate postoperative period, both CT and MRI may demonstrate a circumscribed fluid collection in the soft tissues posterior to the spine in the surgical bed (see Fig. 11-21). Most commonly, this represents a seroma, which will resolve spontaneously over the ensuing months. However, if it directly abuts the thecal sac, its radiographic appearance on noncontrast CT or MRI is indistinguishable from a CSF leak. In such cases, if there is clinical suspicion of a dural tear, a CT myelogram is necessary.

Spine Tumors

Tumors of the spinal canal are traditionally categorized as to location: intramedullary, intradural, extramedullary, and extradural. This compartmentalization is useful in the differential diagnosis of a specific lesion and in determining the radiologic approach to a lesion. With the exception of the rare primary bone tumor, MRI is the method of choice in evaluation of tumors of the spinal column.

In intramedullary spinal cord lesions, myelography and CT myelography may demonstrate cord enlargement or contour irregularities. However, contrast resolution within the cord is very low, rendering the findings of myelography nonspecific. However, MRI is capable of demonstrating the anatomy and pathology of the spinal cord in detail. On MRI intramedullary lesions usually result in increased diameter of the spinal cord (Fig. 11-28). The lesions are usually of diminished signal intensity on T_1-weighted sequences and increased signal intensity on T_2-weighted sequences. Hemorrhage or hemosiderin and cystic necrotic components may be demonstrated.[123] Enhancement with Gd-DTPA occurs almost invariably even with low-grade gliomas.[43,128,194] Contrast material improves the assessment of lesion size and configuration, recognition of additional lesions, and differentiation of tumor from areas of necrosis and edema.[128,192,194,195] Additionally, the presence of enhancement is useful in distinguishing a cyst within a tumor from an adjacent nonmalignant cyst and in distinguishing idiopathic syringomyelia from neoplasm.[43,194,213] In evaluating therapeutic response, contrast enhancement is helpful in differentiating residual or recurrent tumor from areas of gliosis or edema.[194] Contrast enhancement may occur in other intramedullary processes, including transverse

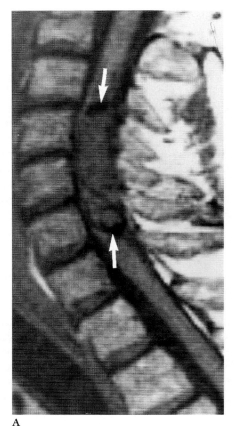

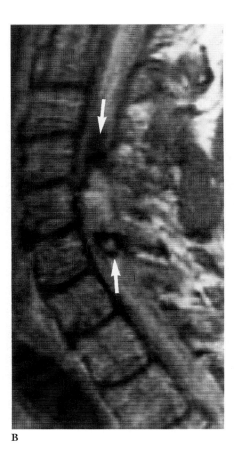

A   B

Fig. 11-28

Cervical cord astrocytoma. **A,** Sagittal T_1-weighted image reveals abnormal morphology of cervical cord with mass of slightly diminished signal intensity involving midcervical cord (*white arrows*). **B,** T_2-weighted sagittal image of same patient now demonstrates mass to be of mixed signal intensity with peripheral areas of diminished signal intensity (*white arrows*). These findings may be related to previous areas of hemorrhage or hemosiderin deposition.

myelitis, multiple sclerosis, cord infarcts, arteriovenous fistulae, and chronic arachnoiditis.

Intradural extramedullary tumors and extradural tumors are more completely demonstrated on MRI than CT.[109,175] These tumors, such as meningiomas and neurofibromas, are usually isointense with the spinal cord on both T_1- and T_2-weighted sequences and enhance intensity with Gd-DTPA, rendering them more conspicuous[77,173] (Fig. 11-29). In the evaluation of leptomeningeal neoplasms such as meningeal metastases, nonenhanced MRI is relatively insensitive in the detection of tumor nodules[97] (Fig. 11-30). However, these nodules enhance prominently, allowing the diagnosis of drop metastases 2 to 3 mm in diameter by enhanced MRI. In addition to nodular enhancement, extensive enhancement of all nerve roots may be seen, corresponding to the myelographic findings of thickened, clumped nerve roots.[193]

The most common extradural or bony neoplastic disease of the spine is metastatic disease, commonly involving bone marrow because of its rich vascularity. The lumbar spine is most commonly affected, followed by the thoracic and cervical spine. The most common primary tumors are breast, prostate, and lung. Radionuclide bone scintigraphy provides a relatively inexpensive, quick method of screening the entire skeleton for metastases. However false-negative findings may occur in aggressive osteolytic metastases.* CT myelography has a sensitivity of 0.95 and a specificity of 0.88 in the evaluation of spinal metastases with spinal cord compression, and 0.49 and 0.88, in the evaluation of spinal metastases with an epidural mass without cord compression.[3] Disadvantages of CT myelography include the relatively limited area that can be scanned, the need for lumbar and possibly cervical puncture, risk of the usu-

*References 30, 65, 84, 86, 187, and 208.

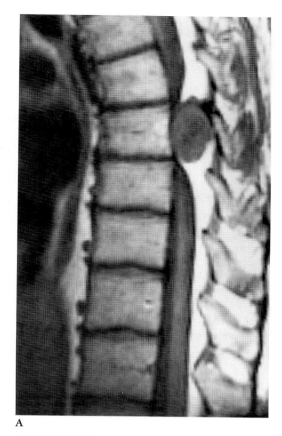

A

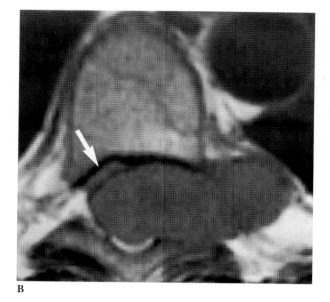

B

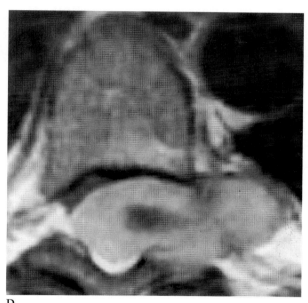

D

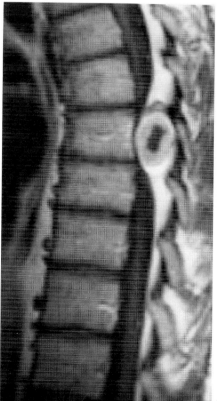

C

Fig. 11-29

Thoracic neurofibroma. **A,** Sagittal T_1-weighted image demonstrates mass of intermediate signal intensity posterior to thecal sac. Note anterior displacement of posterior aspect of thecal sac, indicating the extradural position of neurofibroma. **B,** Axial T_1-weighted image reveals a large mass extending through left-sided intervertebral nerve-root canal. Note compressed cord along right ventral-lateral aspect of mass (*white arrows*). **C,** Sagittal T_1-weighted image following infusion of Gd-DTPA. There is enhancement of mass with central area of diminished signal intensity; this may represent a central area of necrosis. **D,** Corresponding axial T_1-weighted image following infusion of Gd-DTPA. Central area of diminished signal intensity is again noted. Cord and thecal sac are compressed along right ventral-lateral aspect of the mass.

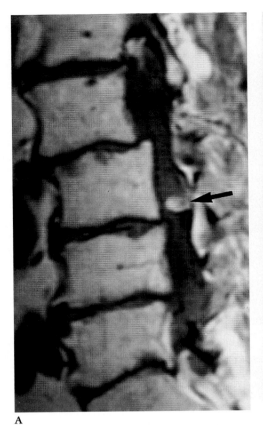

A

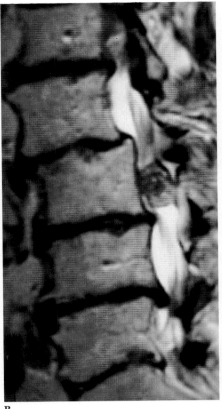

B

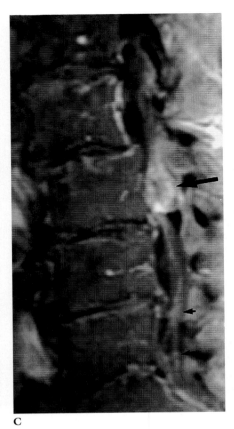

C

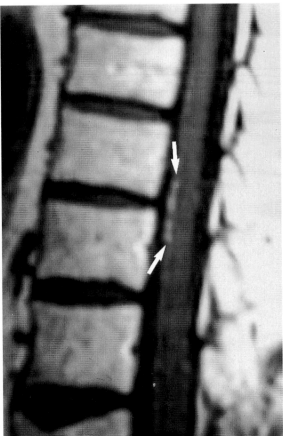

D

Fig. 11-30

Hemorrhagic metastatic lung carcinoma. **A,** Sagittal T_1-weighted images reveal area of increased signal intensity within thecal sac posterior to L3 vertebral body (*black arrow*). **B,** On sagittal T_2-weighted image, there is a mass of mixed signal intensity associated with area of hemorrhage. **C,** Sagittal image of lumbar spine with selective attenuation of signal from fat and following infusion of Gd-DTPA reveals enhancement of above described mass posterior to L3 vertebral body (*black arrow*). There is also subtle enhancement along nerve roots of cauda equina (*small black arrows*). Appearance is consistent with metastatic disease and tumor seeding along nerve roots. **D,** Sagittal T_1-weighted image of thoracic spine following infusion of Gd-DTPA in same patient. Note subtle areas of enhancement along anterior aspect of midthoracic cord (*white arrows*) secondary to metastasis.

ally transient neurologic complications of intrathecal contrast, risk of neurologic deterioration after lumbar puncture in patients with complete subarachnoid block,[87] and inability to image intervening lesions between upper and lower blocks. The sensitivity and specificity of MRI in the evaluation of spinal metastases with cord compression is similar to myelogram CT. However, for extradural metastases without cord compression, the sensitivity and specificity of MRI at 0.73 and 0.90, respectively, is considerably better than CT. Additionally, MRI is far more sensitive than CT in the detection of metastases restricted to bone (0.90 vs. 0.49).[3] With MRI, the need for lumbar puncture and intrathecal contrast is obviated. Furthermore, the whole spine can be screened with T_1-weighted sequences, rapidly permitting detection of additional areas of canal compromise and other osseous spinal metastases.[30]

On MRI, metastatic lesions appear as focal areas of diminished signal intensity or as diffuse homogeneous or inhomogeneous low signal intensity (Fig. 11-31). On T_2-weighted sequences, the lesions are usually of increased signal intensity. However, blastic metastases may be of diminished signal intensity. T_1-weighted sequences and short TI inversion recovery (STIR) sequences demonstrate the lesions to best advantage.[84] Intravenous contrast may result in decreased conspicuity of bone metastases. Enhancement results in an increase in the signal intensity of tumor, decreasing the contrast between low signal intensity tumor and high signal intensity marrow fat.[187] Consequently, after the administration of contrast material, lesions may become isointense, with normal marrow[187, 196] (Fig. 11-31). Enhancement is a nonspecific finding, occurring in degenerative change with edema, bone infarction, and acute benign fractures.[187] Contrast material may be useful in differentiating sites of tumors from edema for biopsy and in distinguishing unusual epidural tumor from disc herniation.[187]

Spinal Infection

The role of imaging in the diagnosis and management of suspected spinal infection includes the detection of disease, differentiation from other pathology including neoplasm, and demonstration of the site and extent of involvement. Additionally, imaging studies are helpful in the identification of the most appropriate site for biopsy, in the determination of the need for surgical decompression, and in the evaluation of therapeutic response.[181]

Infectious Spondylitis

Pyogenic spondylitis is rare, occurring in less than 5% of all patients with pyogenic osteomyelitis.[27] The lumbar spine is most commonly affected, followed

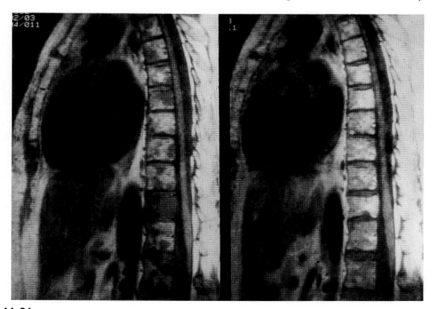

Fig. 11-31

Sagittal T_1-weighted images of the thoracic spine prior to (*left image*) and following (*right image*) infusion of Gd-DTPA. On image obtained without and with gadolinium note multiple focal low signal intensity defects within visualized marrow spaces of the thoracic vertebral bodies. Following infusion of Gd-DTPA, there is enhancement of these lesions, resulting in diminished conspicuity of metastatic lesions.

by the thoracic spine. Modes of infection include direct implantation, contiguous spread, and hematogenous spread.[219] Direct implantation of infection may occur due to trauma, diagnostic procedures such as lumbar puncture or discography, or surgery. Contiguous spread from a paravertebral infection such as a retropharyngeal abscess can occur. Sources of hematogenous spread include the genitourinary tract, the skin, and the respiratory tract (most commonly), with no identifiable source in about 50% of patients.[219] In the adult, venous and, more importantly, arterial channels carry blood-borne pathogens (*Stophylococcus aureus*, *Enterobacter* sp., *Salmonella* sp., anaerobes) to the richly vascularized cancellous bone of the vertebral body.[225] Infection of the intervertebral disc and adjacent vertebral body is caused by subsequent direct extension. In contradistinction, in childhood (less than 20 years old), since the intervertebral disc is highly vascularized, primary infection of the disc is characteristic, with subsequent involvement of adjacent vertebral bodies.[56,169]

The CT findings in pyogenic infection include (1) decreased height of the intervertebral disc on reformatted images; (2) loss of definition of the cortex of the vertebral end plates with subsequent lytic bone destruction; (3) paravertebral soft-tissue infiltration or mass; (4) gas throughout the intervertebral disc space; (5) gas within the vertebral body; (6) new bone formation at 10 to 12 weeks with sclerosis of vertebral endplates* (see Fig. 11-38).

The MRI findings in pyogenic infection include (1) diminished signal intensity of the vertebral bodies on T_1-weighted sequences; (2) increased signal intensity of the vertebral bodies on T_2-weighted or STIR sequences; (3) loss of definition of the cortex of the vertebral end plate; (4) loss of height of the intervertebral disc; (5) abnormal configuration of the intervertebral disc and/or loss of the normal nuclear cleft; (6) variable signal of the intervertebral disc; normal or diminished in signal intensity on T_1-weighted sequences, usually increased in signal intensity on T_2-weighted sequences; (7) enhancement of the vertebral marrow after administration of contrast material with decreased conspicuity of signal intensity abnormalities and variable enhancement of the intervertebral disc; (8) gas within the intervertebral disc; (9) paraspinous and epidural soft-tissue masses.[116,180,209] (see Fig. 11-32). The abnormal signal intensity of the vertebral bodies has been attributed to the infiltration of normal fatty marrow with an inflammatory exudate with variable secondary ischemia. Loss of the normal discal nuclear cleft has been attributed to involvement of the nuclear and fibrous components by infection.[116]

The sensitivity of MRI in the detection of osteomyelitis is 94% to 96%.[33,116,180,209] Its reported specificity is 92%, and accuracy, 94%.[116] These findings are similar to those of combined gallium and bone scans. However, the sensitivity of MRI is markedly superior to that of plain film radiography and CT.[33,116] MRI has a unique role in the assessment of therapeutic response. With successful therapy, the T_2-weighted and STIR sequences demonstrate a decrease in the abnormal high signal intensity. The T_1-weighted sequence shows in-

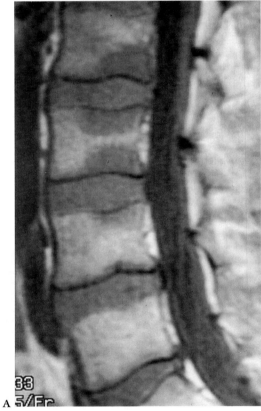

Fig. 11-32

Postdiscography discitis and vertebral osteomyelitis. **A,** T_1-weighted sagittal image of 40-year-old adult male with complaints of low back pain following discography. Focal areas of diminished signal intensity are noted along end plates adjacent to the L2-L3 and L3-L4 intervertebral disc spaces. **B,** Axial CT images obtained shortly after MRI are unremarkable. **C,** Reformatted sagittal CT scan of lumbar spine is essentially normal. **D,** Sagittal T_1-weighted MRI scan of lumbar spine approximately 10 days after initial studies. There is now progressive decreased signal intensity involving the L2, L3, and L4 lumbar vertebral bodies. Findings are consistent with osteomyelitis with osseous edema. **E,** Following infusion of Gd-DTPA, no decrease conspicuity of areas of diminished signal intensity previously noted within L2, L3, and L4 vertebral bodies.

*References 27, 41, 68, 145, 216, and 222.

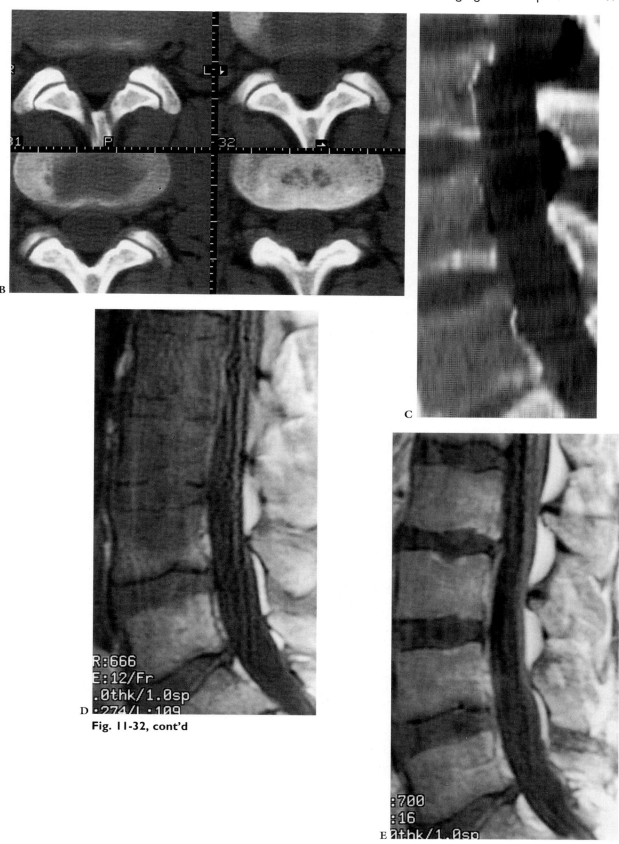

Fig. 11-32, cont'd

creased signal intensity in areas previously of diminished signal intensity, reflecting replacement of cellular marrow by fat.[116,180] Other findings include the beginning of bony fusion and resolution of the paraspinous soft-tissue components of infection.[209]

Tuberculous spondylitis has characteristic radiographic findings. The thoracic spine is the site of predilection. The infection usually involves the vertebral body itself, frequently anteriorly. However, involvement of the posterior elements is also commonly seen (in contradistinction to pyogenic infections). On MRI, the affected vertebral bodies are heterogeneous in signal intensity on T_1-weighted sequences, including areas of increased signal intensity. Also seen is extensive loss of cortical definition. Relative sparing of the intervertebral disc is seen. Vertebral collapse with a gibbus deformity may be seen in later stages. Subligamentous spread of disease results in large anterior and paraspinous masses as well as skip lesions. Intravenous contrast may result in rim enhancement of intraosseous and paraspinal abscesses.[180,182,209,216]

Epidural Abscess

Infection of the epidural space with development of an abscess occurs via hematogenous spread or direct extension from a paravertebral source or a vertebral osteomyelitis. Epidural abscesses may be detected by CT in the lumbar region as a mass of intermediate density, detectable against adjacent low-density epidural fat. However, the demonstration of an epidural abscess in the cervical or thoracic spine requires intrathecal contrast.[17] Intravenous contrast may result in rim enhancement. On MRI, an epidural abscess appears as a mass of low signal intensity on T_1-weighted sequences and increased signal intensity on T_2-weighted sequences (Fig. 11-33). In a majority of cases, the abscess is more inhomogeneous in signal intensity and more difficult to distinguish from thecal sac.[4,136,168] Contrast enhancement results in much improved conspicuity and demonstration of abscess extent.[168,182] Enhancement may be homogeneous, possibly corresponding to the phlegmonous stage of infection with extensive granulation

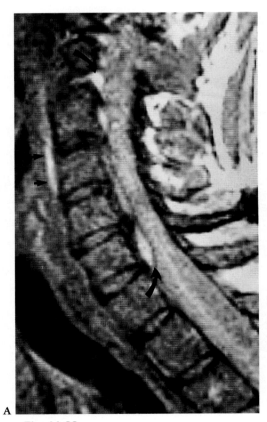

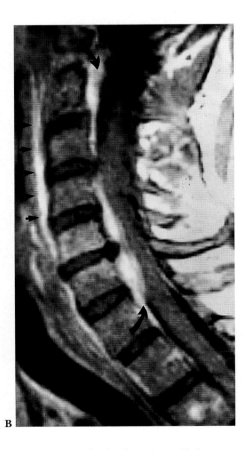

A   B

Fig. 11-33

MRI imaging of epidural abscess. **A,** Sagittal T_2-weighted images, cervical spine in patient with known history of intravenous drug abuse. Note linear area of increased signal intensity anterior to thecal sac extending from C2 to C6-C7 intervertebral disc space and anterior to C2 and C3 vertebral bodies (*small black arrows*). **B,** T_1-weighted image of cervical spine following infusion of Gd-DTPA demonstrates enhancement of epidural abscess (*curved arrows*) and prevertebral abscess (*small black arrows*).

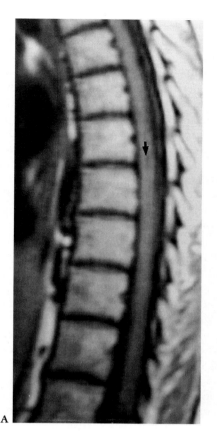

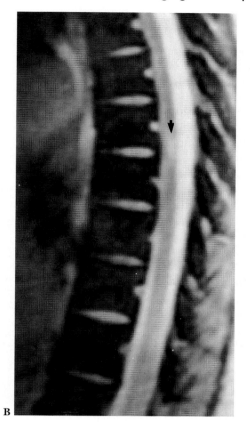

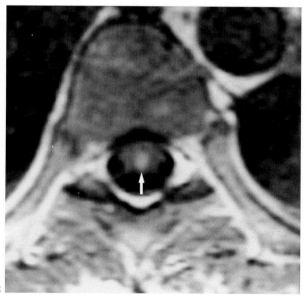

Fig. 11-34

MRI findings of infectious myelitis. **A,** T_1-weighted sagittal image of thoracic spine reveals small subtle area of diminished signal intensity within midthoracic cord (*small black arrow*). **B,** T_2-weighted sagittal image, same patient, demonstrates focal area of increased signal intensity (*small black arrow*) corresponding to area of diminished signal intensity noted on T_1-weighted study. **C,** Axial T_1-weighted MR image following infusion of Gd-DTPA through above lesion demonstrates corresponding area of enhancement within cord (*small white arrow*).

tissue and microabscesses, or peripheral, presumably due to enhancement of a rim of granulation tissue surrounding a necrotic, liquefied abscess.[168]

Infectious Myelitis

Infectious myelitis is usually viral in origin. MRI findings include segments of increased signal intensity within the spinal cord on T_2-weighted sequences. On T_1-weighted sequences, two subsets of findings are seen. In the first set, the cord is enlarged, occasionally with normal intervening skip segments. A subtle increase in signal intensity may be seen, possibly due to petechial hemorrhage. Contrast enhancement is diffuse, peripheral, or speckled. In the second set, the cord may be normal in diameter with faint nodular enhancement (see Fig. 11-34). The MRI findings in infectious myelitis may be indistinguishable from other inflammatory processes, such as multiple sclerosis or acute idiopathic transverse myelitis.[180] Pyogenic or granulomatous intramedullary abscesses result in more focal lesions, with nodular enhancement indistinguishable from neoplasms.[67,180]

Spine Trauma

The role of imaging in spine trauma includes the diagnosis of fractures, demonstration of central canal compromise, assessment of instability including ligamentous disruption, posterior element fractures, facet joint subluxation, and detection of spinal cord injury. From a radiologic standpoint, these abnormalities can be divided into osseous, soft-tissue, and spinal cord injuries.

Computed tomography is the primary imaging method in the evaluation of spine fractures. Thin-section CT with multiplanar reformations demonstrates the location of bone fragments, the diameter of the spinal canal, posterior element fractures, facet joint subluxation, and vertebral malalignment.* Although the osseous resolution of MRI is less than that of CT in the diagnosis of fractures, MRI shows most fractures involving the vertebral body itself (Fig. 11-35). However, MRI demonstrates only 25% to 57% of posterior element fractures (Fig. 11-36).[57,200] CT and MRI provide similar information in the evaluation of vertebral subluxation.[57,210]

The MRI findings in acute vertebral fractures include changes in the signal intensity of the fatty ver-

---

*References 18, 88, 111, 115, 134, 135, and 210.

tebral marrow, alteration in the configuration of the vertebral body, and fracture fragments. Within the first 1 to 3 months after injury, the vertebral marrow is of diminished signal intensity on T_1-weighted sequences and of increased signal intensity on T_2-weighted and STIR sequences (Fig. 11-37). These signal intensity changes, presumably related to marrow edema, render problematic the differentiation of acute benign compression fractures from pathologic compression fractures due to tumor. The signal intensity changes are usually more homogeneous and extensive in neoplastic disease than in benign fractures.[8,237] Secondary findings in neoplastic fractures include pedicle involvement, a paraspinal mass, lack of vertebral fragmentation, and additional vertebral lesions.[237] The marrow in benign compression fractures should regain normal signal intensity in 1 to 3 months[8] (see Fig. 11-37). Consequently, sequential scans may be helpful in cases that are indeterminate acutely.

In the evaluation of soft-tissue, ligamentous, and discal injuries, MRI is more useful than CT.[37,111,115,200,210] Rupture of the anterior longitudinal ligament by MRI is seen as focal discontinuity of the normally linear appearing low signal intensity ligament on T_1-weighted images with focal increased signal intensity on T_2-weighted sequences. Separa-

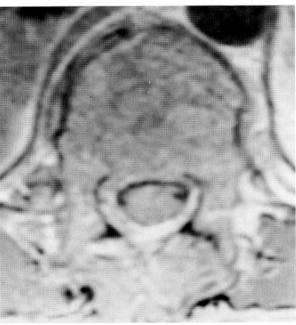

A

Fig. 11-35

Imaging of vertebral body fractures. **A,** Axial CT image through thoracic vertebral body demonstrates comminuted fracture. There is posterior displacement of osseous fragment into region of spinal canal (*black arrows*). **B,** On corresponding T_1-weighted axial MRI, fracture lines are not as well defined. Posterior displacement of osseous fragment is appreciated with effacement of subarachnoid space. However, cord is not compressed.

B

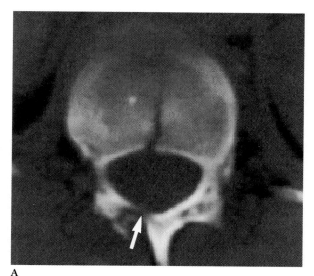

A

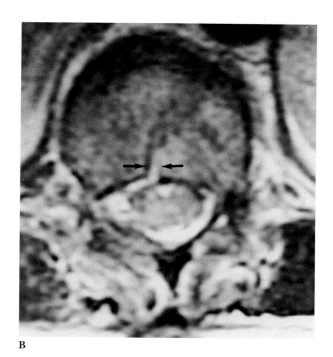

B

Fig. 11-36

Imaging of posterior element fractures. **A,** Axial CT scan of thoracic vertebral body demonstrates sagittal fracture line through vertebral body. Also note fracture through right-sided lamina (*white arrow*). Fracture lines are well defined and osseous fragments are easily identified. **B,** Corresponding axial MRI does demonstrate sagittal fracture line through vertebral body (*black arrow*). However, fracture involving right lamina is less obvious. Note apparent edema and induration in region of right-sided posterior elements secondary to fracture.

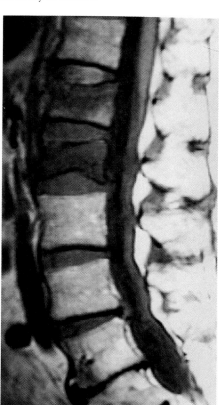

A

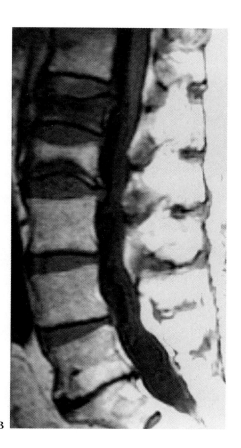

B

Fig. 11-37

MRI evaluation of compression fractures. **A,** Sagittal T_1-weighted MRI scan of lumbar spine reveals compression deformities of L1 and L2 vertebral bodies. Marrow spaces of vertebral bodies are of diminished signal intensity. Appearance is consistent with marrow edema; however, metastatic disease with pathologic fracture could have similar appearance. **B,** Follow-up examination approximately 4 months later demonstrates normal marrow signal intensity within superior portion of the L2 vertebral body. Appearance is consistent with healing of compression fracture. This change would be unlikely with neoplasm.

tion of the disc from the vertebral end plate is demonstrated as increased intradiscal signal intensity paralleling the vertebral endplate on T_2-weighted sequences. The location and extent of acute disc herniations and integrity of the posterior longitudinal ligament can be assessed with MRI. Acute traumatic disc herniation occurs most commonly in the cervical spine. The injured intervertebral disc may be hyperintense on T_2-weighted sequences. In the presence of a concomitant fracture, the disc herniation usually occurs at or immediately above or below the fractured segment.[37,57] The findings on MRI in tears of anterior precervical muscles include increased signal intensity within the muscle and enlargement of the muscle due to hemorrhage and edema.[10,37] MRI is superior to CT in the demonstration of spinal cord injury due to its greater soft-tissue resolution. The findings on MRI in acute spinal cord trauma fall into two main categories depending on the presence or absence of hemorrhage.[98] The nonhemorrhagic pattern is characterized by a normal signal intensity cord on T_1-weighted sequences. Cord enlargement may be seen (Fig. 11-38). This pattern corresponds to cord edema and contusion, which usually resolves over 1 to 3 weeks with significant improvement in neuro-

logic deficit.[37,98] The hemorrhagic pattern of the cord injury is characterized by high signal intensity on T_1-weighted sequences and low signal intensity on T_2-weighted sequences due to deoxyhemoglobin. These hemorrhagic contusions are associated with a lack of recovery of significant neurologic function.[98]

In patients with longstanding spinal trauma, MRI findings may include a normal-appearing cord, cord atrophy, myelomalacia, and syringomyelia[142,185] (Fig. 11-39). The findings in myelomalacia include a focal area of increased signal intensity on T_2-weighted sequences and normal or diminished signal intensity on T_1-weighted sequences. Areas of microcystic change may coalesce, resulting in a cyst within the myelomalacic segment, termed "cystic myelomalacia." The cord may be normal in diameter or expanded in the region of the cyst. The cyst is smoothly marginated and of diminished signal intensity on T_1-weighted sequences and intermediate to increased signal intensity on proton-density sequences.[49,142] At variable times after injury, patients may experience neurologic deterioration, a syndrome known as posttraumatic progressive myelopathy (PTPM).[66] In a series of 94 patients with PTPM, MRI demonstrated a syrinx in 48%, cord atrophy in 43%, and cord compression in 24%. Myelomalacia

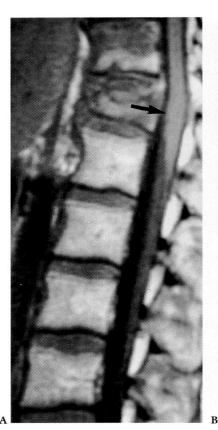

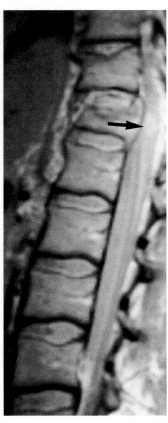

A   B

Fig. 11-38

MRI evaluation of spinal cord. **A,** Sagittal T_1-weighted image of lower thoracic and upper lumbar spine reveals compression fracture involving root of lower thoracic vertebral bodies. There is slight posterior displacement of vertebral body with compression of thecal sac and conus. There is slight enlargement of conus (*black arrows*). **B,** Corresponding proton-density image reveals focal area of high signal within conus medullaris (*black arrows*). Appearance is consistent with area of cord contusion.

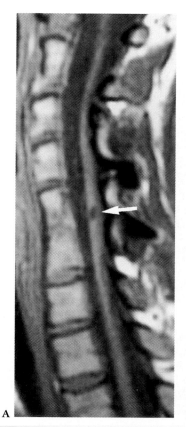
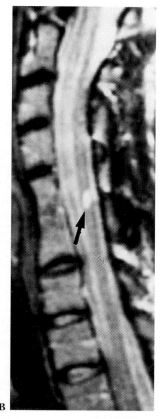

A   **B**

Fig. 11-39

MRI evaluation of posttraumatic myelomalacia. **A,** Sagittal T_1-weighted image of cervical spine reveals anterior interbody fusion at C5-C6 level. Cervical cord appears to be atrophic with focal area of diminished signal intensity within cord, posterior to fused level (*white arrow*). **B,** T_2-weighted sagittal image of the cervical spine again demonstrates atrophy of cervical cord. There is focal area of high signal intensity within cord (*black arrow*), which corresponds to area of diminished signal intensity noted on T_1-weighted examination. Appearance is consistent with focal area of myelomalacia.

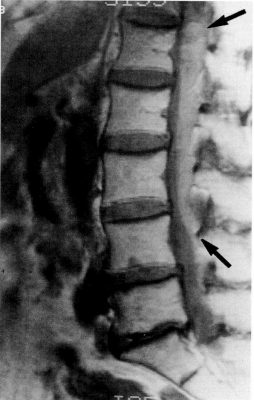
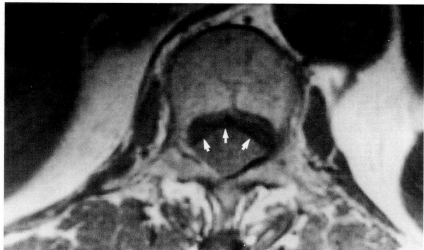

B

A

Fig. 11-40

MRI demonstration of spontaneous epidural hematoma. **A,** Sagittal T_1-weighted MRI scan of lumbar spine in 50-year-old female with history of hypertension demonstrates linear area of increased signal intensity extending from T12 to L4 along the posterior aspect of thecal sac (*black arrows*). **B,** Axial T_1-weighted image through lumbar spine demonstrates area of intermediate signal intensity along posterior aspect of central canal. This results in compression along posterior aspect of thecal sac (*white arrows*).

was seen in 26% and cystic myelomalacia in 15%.[185]

Epidural hemorrhage is relatively uncommon, and may be idiopathic or associated with procedures such as lumbar puncture or predisposing conditions such as anticoagulation, hypertension, or trauma. The etiology of idiopathic or spontaneous epidural hematoma is conjectural, and may be either venous or arterial in origin.[11] CT demonstrates a hyperdense biconvex epidural mass along the bony margins of the spinal canal.[137,160,238] MRI demonstrates an epidural lesion of high or intermediate signal intensity on T_1-weighted sequences[160] (Fig. 11-40). These lesions must be distinguished from synovial cysts, extruded disc material, tumor, and epidural abscess.

References

1. Adams P, Eyre DR, Muir H: Biochemical aspects of development and aging of human lumbar intervertebral discs, *Rheumatol Rehabil* 16:22, 1977.
2. Aguila LA, Piraino DW, Modic MT, et al.: Intranuclear cleft of the intervertebral disc: magnetic resonance imaging, *Radiology* 155:155, 1985.
3. Algra PR, Bloem JL, Tissing H, et al.: Detection of vertebral metastases: comparison between MR imaging and bone scintigraphy. *RadioGraphics,* 11:219, 1991.
4. Angtuaco EJC, McConnell JR, Chaduck WM, et al.: MR imaging of spinal epidural sepsis, AJNR Am *J Neuroradiol* 8:879, 1987.
5. Aoki J, Yamamoto I, Kitamura N, et al.: End plate of the discovertebral joint: Degenerative change in the elderly adult, *Radiology* 164:411, 1987.
6. Arce CA, Dohrmann GJ: Thoracic disc herniation, *Surg Neurol* 23:356, 1985.
7. Arnold CC, Brodsky AE, Chauchoix J, et al.: Lumbar spinal stenosis and nerve root entrapment syndromes: a definition and classification, *Clin Orthop* 115:4, 1975.
8. Baker LL, Goodman SB, Perkash I, et al.: Benign versus pathologic compression fractures of vertebral bodies: assessment with conventional spine-echo, chemical-shift, and STIR MR imaging, *Radiology* 174:495, 1990.
9. Baleriaux D, Noterman J, Ticket L: Recognition of cervical soft disc herniation by contrast-enhanced CT, *AJNR Am J Neuroradiol* 4:607, 1983.
10. Beale SM, Pathria MN, Masaryk TJ: Magnetic resonance imaging of spinal trauma, *Top Magn Reson Imaging* 1(1):53, 1988.
11. Beatty RM, Winston KR: Spontaneous cervical epidural hematoma, *J Neurosurg* 61:143, 1984.
12. Boden SD, Davis DO, Dina TS, et al.: Abnormal magnetic-resonance scans of the lumbar spine in asymptomatic subjects: a prospective investigation, *J Bone Joint Surg* 72A:403, 1990.
13. Boden SD, Davis DO, Dina TS, et al.: Contrast-enhanced MR imaging performed after successful lumbar disc surgery: prospective study, *Radiology* 182:59, 1992.
14. Boden SD, Davis DO, Dina TS, et al.: Postoperative discitis: distinguishing early MR imaging find

ings from normal post-operative disc space changes, *Radiology* 184:765, 1992.
15. Boden SD, McCowin PR, David DO, et al.: Abnormal magnetic-resonance scans of the cervical spine in asymptomatic subjects: a prospective investigation, *J Bone Joint Surg* 72A:1178, 1990.
16. Bozzao A, Gallucci M, Masciocchi C, et al.: Lumbar disc herniation: MR imaging assessment of natural history in patients treated with surgery, *Radiology* 185:135, 1992.
17. Brant-Zawadzi M: *Infections.* In Newton TH, Potts DG, editors: *Computed tomography of the spine and spinal cord,* San Anselmo, CA: 1983, Clavadel Press.
18. Brant-Zawadzki M, Miller EM, Federle MP: CT in the evaluation of spine trauma, *AJR Am J Roentgenol* 136:369, 1981.
19. Braun IF, Hoffman JC Jr, Davis PC, et al.: Contrast enhancement in CT differentiation between recurrent disc herniation and postoperative scar: prospective study, *AJNR Am J Neuroradiol* 6:607, 1985.
20. Brickley-Parson D, Glimcher MJ: Is the chemistry of collagen intervertebral discs as expression of Wolff's law? A study of the lumbar spine, *Spine* 9:148, 1984.
21. Brodsky AE: Cauda equina arachnoiditis: a correlative clinical and roentgenologic study, *Spine* 3:51, 1978.
22. Brodsky AE: Post-laminectomy and post-fusion stenosis of the lumbar spine, *Clin Orthop* 115:130, 1976.
23. Brown HA, Pont ME: Disease of lumbar discs. Ten years of surgical treatment, *J Neurosurg* 20:410, 1963.
24. Brown BM, Schwartz RH, Frank E, Blank NK: Preoperative evaluation of cervical radiculopathy and myelopathy by surface coil—MR imaging, *AJR Am J Roentgenol* 151:1205, 1988.
25. Bundschuh CV, Modic MT, Ross JS, et al.: Epidural fibrosis and recurrent disc herniation in the lumbar spine: MR imaging assessment, *AJNR Am J Neuroradiol* 9:169, 1988.
26. Bundschuh C, Stein L, Slusser JH, et al.: Distinguishing between scar and recurrent herniated disc in postoperative patients: value of contrast-enhanced CT and MR imaging, *AJNR Am J Neuroradiol* 11:949, 1990.
27. Burke DR, Brant-Zawadzki M: CT of pyogenic spine infection, *Neuroradiology* 27:131, 1985.
28. Burton CV: Lumbosacral arachnoiditis, *Spine* 3:24, 1978.
29. Burton CV, Kirkaldy-Willis WH, Young-Hing K, et al.: Causes failure of surgery on the lumbar spine, *Clin Orthop* 157:191, 1981.
30. Carmody RF, Yang PJ, Seeley GW, et al.: Spinal cord compression due to metastatic disease: diagnosis with MR imaging versus myelography, *Radiology* 173:225, 1989.
31. Carrera CF, Haughton VM, Syversten A, Williams AL: Computed tomography of the lumbar facet joints, *Radiology* 134:145, 1980.
32. Casselman ES: Radiologic recognition of symptomatic spinal synovial cysts, *AJNR Am J Neuroradiol* 6:971.

33. Chandrani VP, Beltran J, Monis LS, et al.: Acute experimental osteomyelitis and abscess: detection with MR imaging versus CT, *Radiology* 174:233, 1990.

34. Ciric I, Mikheal MA, Tarkington JA, Vick NA: The lateral recess syndrome: a variant of spinal stenosis, *J Neurosurg* 53:433, 1980.

35. Coventry MB, Ghormley RK, Kernohan JW: The intervertebral disc: its microscopic anatomy and pathology. Part III. Pathologic changes in the intervertebral disc, *J Bone Joint Surg* 27A:460, 1945.

36. Dall BE, Rowe DE, Odette WG, et al.: Postoperative discitis—diagnosis and management, *Clin Orthop* 224:138, 1987.

37. Davis SJ, Teresi LM, Bradley WM, et al.: Cervical spine hyperextension injuries: MR findings, *Radiology* 180:245, 1991.

38. DePalma AF, Rothman RH: *The intervertebral disc*, Philadelphia, 1970, W. B. Saunders Co.

39. de Roos A, Kressel H, Spritzer C, Dalinka M: MR imaging of marrow changes adjacent to end plates in degenerative lumbar disc disease, *AJR Am J Roentgenol* 149:531, 1987.

40. DeSantis M, Crisi G, Folchivici F: Late contrast enhancement in the CT diagnosis of herniated lumbar disc, *Neuroradiology* 26:303, 1984.

41. Digby JM, Kersley JB: Pyogenic nontuberculous spinal infection: an analysis of thirty cases, *J Bone Joint Surg* 61B:47, 1979.

42. Dillon WP, Kaseff LG, Knackstedt VE, et al.: Computed tomography and differential diagnosis of extruded lumbar disc, *J Comput Assist Tomogr* 6:874, 1982.

43. Dillon W, Norman D, Newton TH, et al.: Intradural spinal cord lesions: Gd-DTPA-enhanced MR imaging, *Radiology* 170:229, 1989.

44. Edelson JG, Nathan H: Nerve root compression in spondylolysis, and spondylolisthesis, *J Bone Joint Surg* 66B:596, 1986.

45. Edwards WC, LaRocca SH: The developmental segmental sagittal diameter in combined cervical and lumbar spondylosis, *Spine* 10:42, 1985.

46. Edwards WC, LaRocca SH: The developmental segmental sagittal diameter of the cervical spinal canal in patients with cervical spondylosis, *Spine* 8:20, 1983.

47. Eisenstein S. The trefoil configuration of the lumbar vertebral canal: a study of South African skeletal material, *J Bone Joint Surg* 62B:73, 1980.

48. Enzmann DR: *Degenerative disc disease*. In Enzmann DR, DeLaPaz RL, Rubin JB, editors: *Magnetic resonance of the spine*, St. Louis, 1990, Mosby, P437.

49. Enzmann DR, DeLaPaz RL: *Trauma in magnetic resonance imaging of the spine*. In Enzmann DR, DeLaPaz RL, Rubin JB, editors: St. Louis, 1990, Mosby, P237.

50. Epstein JA, Carras R, Hyman RA, et al.: Cervical myelopathy caused by developmental stenosis of the spinal cord, *J Neurosurg* 51:362, 1979.

51. Epstein JA, Epstein BS, Lavine LS, et al.: Lumbar nerve root compression at the intervertebral foramina caused by arthritis of the posterior facets, *J Neurosurg* 39:362, 1973.

52. Epstein JA, Epstein BS, Lavin L: Nerve root compression associated with narrowing of the lumbar spinal cord, *J Neurol Neurosurg Psychiatry* 25:165, 1962.

53. Fernand R, Lee CK: Postlaminectomy disc space infection: a review of the literature and a report of three cases, *Clin Orthop* 209:215, 1986.

54. Finnegan WJ, Delin JM, Marvel JP, et al.: Results of surgical intervention in the symptomatic multiply-operated back patient, *J Bone Joint Surg* 61A:1077, 1979.

55. Firooznia H, Benjamin V, Kricheff II, et al.: CT of lumbar spine disc herniation: correlation with surgical findings, *AJNR Am J Neuroradiol*, 5:91, 1984.

56. Fischer GW, Popich CA, Sullivan DE, et al.: Diskitis: a prospective diagnosis analysis, *Pediatrics* 62:543, 1978.

57. Flanders AE, Schaefer DM, Doan HT, et al.: Acute cervical spine trauma: correlation of MR imaging findings with degree of neurologic deficit, *Radiology* 177:25, 1990.

58. Francavilla TL, Powers A, Dina T, et al.: MR imaging of thoracic disc herniations, *J Comput Assist Tomogr* 11:1062, 1987.

59. Frank AM, Trappe AE: The role of magnetic resonance imaging (MRI) in the diagnosis of spondylodiscitis, *Neurosurg Rev* 13:279, 1990.

60. Fries JW, Abodeely DA, Vijungco JG, et al.: Computed tomography of herniated and extruded nucleus pulposus, *J Comput Assist Tomogr* 6:874, 1982.

61. Frymoyer JW. Symposium: the role of spine fusion, *Spine* 6:284, 1981.

62. Frymoyer JW, Hanley EN, Howe J, et al.: A comparison of radiographic findings in fusion and nonfusion patients ten or more years following lumbar disc surgery, *Spine* 4:435, 1979.

63. Frymoyer JW, Matteri RE, Hurley EN, et al.: Failed lumbar disc surgery requiring a second operation: a long-term follow up study, *Spine* 3:7, 1978.

64. Gado M, Patel J, Hodges FJ: Lateral disc herniation into the lumbar intervertebral foramen: differential diagnosis, *AJNR Am J Neuroradiol* 4:598, 1983.

65. Galasko CSB: *Detection of skeletal metastases*. In Galasko CSB, editor. *Skeletal metastases*, Stoneham, MA, 1986, Butterworth, P52.

66. Gebarski SS, Maynard FW, Gabrielsen TO, et al.: Post-traumatic progressive myelopathy, *Radiology* 175:379, 1985.

67. Gero B, Sze G, Sharif H: MR imaging of intradural inflammatory diseases of the spine, *AJNR AM J Neuroradiol* 12:1009, 1991.

68. Golimbu C, Firooznia H, Raffi M: CT of osteomyelitis of the spine, *AJR Am J Roentgenol* 142:159, 1984.

69. Gower WE, Pedrini V: Age-related variations in protein polysaccharides from human nucleus pulposus, anular fibrosus, and costal cartilage, *J Bone Joint Surg* 51A:1154, 1969.

70. Grenier N, Gresselle JF, Vital JM, et al.: Normal and disrupted lumbar longitudinal ligaments: correlative MR and anatomic study, *Radiology* 171:197, 1989.

71. Grenier N, Grossman RI, Schiebler ML, et al.: Degenerative lumbar disc disease: pitfalls and usefulness of MR imaging in detection of vacuum phenomenon, *Radiology* 164:861, 1987.

72. Grenier N, Kressel HY, Schiebler ML, et al.: Normal and degenerative posterior spinal structures: MR imaging, *Radiology* 165:517, 1987.

73. Grenier N, Kressel H, Schiebler ML, et al.: Isthmic spondylolysis of the lumbar spine: MR imaging at 1.5T, *Radiology* 170:489, 1989.

74. Gulati A, Weinstein R, Studdard E: CT scan of the spine for herniated discs, *Neuroradiology* 22:57, 1981.

75. Guyer RD, Collier R, Stith WJ, et al.: Discitis after discography, *Spine* 13:1352, 1988.

76. Hashizume Y, Iijima S, Kishimoto H, Yanagi T: Pathology of spinal cord lesions caused by ossification of the posterior longitudinal ligament, *Acta Neuropathol* 63:123, 1984.

77. Haughton VM, Rimm AA, Gzervionke LF, et al.: Sensitivity of Gd-DTPA-enhanced MR imaging of benign extra-axial tumors, *Radiology* 166:829, 1988.

78. Heithoff KB, Burton CV: CT evaluation of the failed back surgery syndrome, *Orthop Clin North Am* 16:417, 1985.

79. Helms CA, Vogler JB: *Spinal stenosis and degenerative lesions.* In Newton TH, Potts DG, editors: *Computed tomography of the spine and spinal cord,* San Anselmo, CA, 1983, Clavadel Press, P251.

80. Hemminghytt D, Daniels DL, Williams AL, et al.: Intraspinal synovial cysts: natural history and diagnosis by CT, *Radiology* 145:375, 1982.

81. Higuchi M, Kaneda K, Abe K: Postnatal histogenesis of the cartilage plate of the spinal column: electron microscopic observations, *Spine* 7:89, 1982.

82. Ho PS, Yu S, Sether LA, et al.: Ligamentum flavum: appearance on sagittal and coronal MR images, *Radiology* 168:469, 1988.

83. Hoddick WK, Helms CA: Bony spinal cord changes that differentiate conjoined nerve roots and differentiation from a herniated nucleus pulposus, *Radiology* 154:119, 1985.

84. Hollis PM, Malis LI, Zappulla RA: Neurological deterioration after lumbar puncture below complete spinal subarachnoid block, *J Neurosurg* 64:253, 1986.

85. Hueftle MG, Modic MT, Ross JS, et al.: Lumbar spine: postoperative MR imaging with Gd-DTPA, *Radiology* 167:817, 1988.

86. Jacobson AF, Stomper PC, Cronin EB, et al.: Bone scans with one or two new abnormalities in cancer patients with no known metastases: reliability of interpretation of initial correlative radiographs, *Radiology* 174:503, 1990.

87. Jahre C, Sze G: Magnetic resonance imaging of spinal metastases, *Top Magn Reson Imaging* 1(1):63, 1988.

88. Jandel SF, Ya Yen L: Computed tomography of spinal fractures, *Radiol Clin North Am* 19(1):69, 1981.

89. Jinkins JR, Matthis RN, Venkatappan S, et al.: Spondylolysis, spondylolisthesis and associated nerve root entrapment in the lumbar spine: MR evaluation, *AJR Am J Roentgenol* 159:799, 1992.

90. Jinkins JR, Whittemore AR, Bradley WG: The autonomic syndrome associated with lumbar disc extrusion, *AJNR Am J Neuroradiol* 10:219, 1989.

91. Johnson CE, Sze G: Benign lumbar arachnoiditis: MR imaging with gadopentetate dimeglumine, *AJNR Am J Neuroradiol* 11:763, 1990.

92. Jorgensen J, Hansen PH, Steenskov V, Ovesen N: A clinical and radiological study of chronic lower spinal arachnoiditis, *Neuroradiology* 9:139, 1975.

93. Kieffer SA, Sherry RG, Wellenstein DE, et al.: Bulging lumbar intervertebral disc: myelographic differentiation from herniated disc with nerve root compression, *AJR Am J Roentgenol* 138:709, 1982.

94. Kirkaldy-Willis WH, Wedge JH, Yong-Hing K, et al.: Lumbar spinal nerve root entrapment, *Clin Orthop* 169:171, 1982.

95. Kirkaldy-Willis WH, Wedge JH, Yong-Hing K, et al.: Pathology and pathogenesis of lumbar spondylosis and stenosis, *Spine* 3:319, 1978.

96. Koehller W, Muehlhaus S, Meier W, Hartmann F: Biochemical properties of human intervertebral discs subjected to axial dynamic compression: influence of age and degeneration, *J Biomech* 19:807, 1986.

97. Krol G, Sze G, Malkin M, et al.: MR of cranial and spinal meningeal carcinomatosis: comparison with CT and myelography, *AJR Am J Roentgenol* 151:583, 1988.

98. Kulkarni MV, Bondurant FJ, Rose SL, et al.: 1.5 Tesla magnetic resonance imaging of acute spinal trauma, *RadioGraphics* 8(6):1059, 1988.

99. Law JD, Lehman RAW, Kirsch WM: Reoperation after lumbar intervertebral disc surgery, *J Neurosurg* 48:259, 1978.

100. Lindblom K, Hultqvist G: Absorption of protruded disc tissue. *J Bone Joint Surg* 32A:557, 1950.

101. Lindholm TS, Pylkkaene P: Discitis following removal of intervertebral disc, *Spine* 7:618, 1982.

102. Lipson SJ: Rheumatoid arthritis of the cervical spine, *Clin Orthop* 182:143, 1984.

103. Lipson SJ, Muir H: Experimental intervertebral disc degeneration: morphological and proteoglycan changes over time, *Arthritis Rheum* 24:12, 1981.

104. Lipson SJ, Muir H: Proteoglycans in experimental intervertebral disc degeneration, *Spine* 6:194, 1984.

105. Lumbardi G, Passerini A, Migliavacca F: Spinal arachnoiditis, *Br J Radiol* 35:314, 1962.

106. MacNab I: Cervical spondylosis, *Clin Orthop Relat Res* 109:69, 1975.

107. Mall JC, Kaiser JA, Heithoff KB, et al.: *Postoperative spine.* In Newton TH,, Potts DG, editors: *Computed tomography of the spine and spinal cord,* San Anselmo, CA, 1983, Clavadel, P187.

108. Masaryk TJ, Ross JS, Modic MT, et al.: High-resolution MR imaging of sequestered lumbar intervertebral discs, *AJR Am J Roentgenol* 150:1155-1162.

109. Mayer PJ, Kulkarni MV, Yeakley JW: Craniocervical manifestations of neurofibromatosis: MR versus CT studies, *J Comput Assist Tomogr* 11:839, 1987.

110. McAfee PC, Ullrich CG, Yuan HA, et al.: Computed tomography in degenerative spinal stenosis, *Clin Orthop* 161:221, 1981.

111. McArdle CB, Crafford MJ, Mirfakhraee M, et al.: Surface coil MR of spinal trauma: preliminary experience, *AJNR Am J Neuroradiol* 7:885, 1986.

112. McCarron RF, Wimpee MW, Hudkins PG, Laros GS: The inflammatory effect of nucleus pulposus: a possible element in the pathogenesis of low-back pain, *Spine* 12:760, 1987.

113. Mikhael MA, Ciric I, Tarkington JA, et al.: Neuroradiologic evaluation of the lateral recess syndrome, *Radiology* 140:97, 1981.

114. Miller JAA, Schmatz C, Schultz AB: Lumbar disc degeneration: Correlation with age, sex, and spine level in 600 autopsy specimens, *Spine* 13:173, 1988.

115. Mirvis SE, Geisler FH, Jelinek JJ, et al.: Acute cervical spinal trauma: evaluation with 1.5T MR imaging, *Radiology* 166:807, 1988.

116. Modic MT, Feiglein DH, Piraino DW, et al.: Vertebral osteomyelitis: assessment using MR, *Radiology* 157:157, 1985.

117. Modic MT, Masaryk TJ, Ross JS, Carter JK: Imaging of degenerative disc disease, *Radiology* 168:177, 1988.

118. Modic MT, Masaryk TJ, Ross JS, et al.: Cervical radiculopathy: value of oblique MR imaging, *Radiology* 163:227, 1987.

119. Modic MT, Masaryk TJ, Mulopulos G, et al.: Cervical radiculopathy: prospective evaluation with surface coil MR imaging, CT with metrizamide, and metrizamide myelography, *Radiology* 161:753, 1986.

120. Modic MT, Masaryk T, Boumphrey F, et al.: Lumbar herniated disc disease and canal stenosis: prospective evaluation by surface coil MR, CT and myelography, *AJR Am J Roentgenol* 147:757, 1986.

121. Modic MT, Steinberg PM, Ross JS, et al.: Degenerative disc disease: assessment of changes in vertebral body marrow with MR imaging, *Radiology* 166:193, 1988.

122. Nakstad PH, Hald JK, Bakke SL, et al.: MRI in cervical disc herniation, *Neuroradiology* 31:382, 1989.

123. Nemoto Y, Inoue Y, Tashiro T, et al.: Intramedullary spinal cord tumors: significance of associated hemorrhage at MR imaging, *Radiology* 182:793, 1992.

124. Norman D, Steven EA, Wing SD, et al.: Quantitative aspects of contrast enhancement in cranial computed tomography, *Radiology* 129:683, 1978.

125. Ogino H, Tada K, Okada K, et al.: Canal diameter, anteroposterior compression ratio, and spondylotic myelopathy of the cervical spine, *Spine* 8:1, 1983.

126. Otake S, Matsuo M, Nishizawa S, et al.: Ossification of the posterior longitudinal ligaments: MR evaluation, *AJNR Am J Neuroradiol* 13:1059, 1992.

127. Panagiotacopulos ND, Pope MH, Krag MH, Block R: Water content in human intervertebral discs, Part I. Measurement by magnetic resonance imaging, *Spine* 12:912, 1987.

128. Parizel PM, Baleriaux D, Rodesch G, et al.: Gd-DTPA-enhanced MR imaging of spinal tumors, *AJNR Am J Neuroradiol* 10:249, 1989.

129. Patronas NJ, Jafer J, Brown F: Pseudomeningoceles diagnosed by metrizamide myelography and computerized tomography, *Surg Neurol* 16:188, 1981.

130. Payne EE, Spillane JD: The cervical spine: an anatomicromicropathological study of 70 specimens (using a special technique) with particular reference to the problem of cervical spondylosis, *Brain* 80:571, 1957.

131. Penning L, Wilmink JT, Van Woerden HH, et al.: CT myelographic findings in degenerative disorders of the cervical spine: clinical significance, *AJR Am J Roentgenol* 146:793, 1986.

132. Pilgaard S: Discitis (closed spaced infection) following removal of lumbar intervertebral disc, *J Bone Joint Surg* 51A:713, 1969.

133. Porter RW, Hibbert CS, Wicks M: The spinal cord in symptomatic lumbar disc lesions, *J Bone Joint Surg* 60B:485, 1978.

134. Post MJ, Green BA, Quencer RM, et al.: Use of computed tomography in spinal trauma, *Radiol Clin North Am* 21:327, 1983.

135. Post MJ, Green BA, Quencer RM, et al.: The value of computed tomography in spinal trauma, *Spine* 7(5):417, 1982.

136. Post MJD, Quencer RM, Montalvo BM, et al.: Spinal infection: evaluation with MR imaging and intraoperative US, *Radiology* 169:765, 1988.

137. Post MJD, Seminer DS, Quencer RM: CT diagnosis of spinal epidural hematoma, *AJNR Am J Neuroradiol* 3:190, 1982.

138. Postacchini F, Amatruda A, Morace GB, Perugia D: Magnetic resonance imaging in the diagnosis of lumbar spinal canal stenosis, *Ital J Orthop Traumatol* 17(3):327, 1991.

139. Pritzer KPH: Aging and degeneration in the lumbar intervertebral disc, *Orthop Clin North Am* 8(1):65, 1977.

140. Quencer RM, Murtah FR, Post MJD, et al.: Postoperative bony stenosis of the lumbar spinal canal: evaluation of 164 symptomatic patients with axial radiography, *AJR Am J Roentgenol* 131:1057, 1978.

141. Quencer RM, Murtagh FR, Post JHD, et al.: Postoperative bony stenosis of the lumbar spine canal: evaluation of 164 symptomatic patients with axial radiography, *AJR Am J Roentgenol* 131:1059, 1978.

142. Quencer RM, Sheldon JJ, Donovan Post MJ, et al.: MRI of the chronically injured cervical spinal cord, *AJR Am J Roentgenol* 147:125, 1986.

143. Quencer RM, Tenner M, Rothman L: The postoperative myelogram, *Radiology* 123:667, 1977.

144. Quiles M, Marchisello P, Tsairis P: Lumbar adhesive arachnoiditis. Etiologic and pathologic aspects, *Spine* 3:45, 1978.

145. Ram PC, Martinez S, Korobkin M, et al.: CT detection of intraosseous gas: a new sign of osteomyelitis, *AJR Am J Roentgenol* 137:721, 1981.

146. Rawlings CE, Wilkings RH, Gallis HA, et al.: Postoperative intervertebral disc space infection, *Neurosurgery* 13:371, 1983.

147. Resnick D: Degenerative diseases of the vertebral column, *Radiology* 156:3, 1985.

148. Risius B, Modic MT, Hardy RW, et al.: Sector computed tomographic spine scanning in the diagnosis of lumbar nerve root entrapment, *Radiology* 143:109, 1982.

149. Robertson GH, Llewellyn HJ, Taveras JM: The narrow lumbar spinal canal syndrome, *Radiology* 107:89, 1973.

150. Rosnick D, Niwayama G, Guerra G, et al.: Spiral vacuum phenomena: anatomical study and review, *Radiology* 139:341, 1981.

151. Ross JS: Magnetic resonance imaging of the postoperative spine, *Top Magn Reson Imaging* 1(1):39, 1988.

152. Ross JS, Delamarter R, Hueftle MG, et al.: Gadolinium-DTPA-enhanced MR imaging of the postoperative lumbar spine: time course and mechanism of enhancement, *AJNR Am J Neuroradiol* 10:37, 1989.

153. Ross PM, Fleming JL: Vertebral body osteomyelitis: Spectrum and natural history: a retrospective analysis of 37 cases, *Clin Orthop* 118:190, 1976.

154. Ross JS, Masaryk TJ, Schrader M, et al.: MR imaging of the postoperative lumbar spine: assessment with gadopentetate dimeglumine, *AJNR Am J Neuroradiol* 11:771, 1990.

155. Ross JS, Masaryk TJ, Modic MT, et al.: Lumbar spine: post-operative assessment with surface coil MR imaging, *Radiology* 164:851, 1987.

156. Ross JS, Masaryk TJ, Modic MT, et al.: MR imaging of lumbar arachnoiditis, *AJNR Am J Neuroradiol* 8:885, 1987.

157. Ross JS, Masaryk TJ, Modic MT: Postoperative cervical spine: MR assessment, *J Comput Assist Tomogr* 11:955, 1987.

158. Ross JS, Masaryk TJ, Modic MT: Tears of the anulus fibrosus: assessment with Gd-DTPA-enhanced MR imaging, *AJNR Am J Neuroradiol* 10:1251, 1989.

159. Ross JS, Perez-Reyes N, Masaryk TJ, et al.: Thoracic disc herniation: MR imaging, *Radiology* 165:511, 1987.

160. Rothfus WE, Chedid MK, Deeb AL, et al.: MR imaging in the diagnosis of spontaneous spinal epidural hematoma. *J Comput Assist Tomogr* 11(5):851, 1987.

161. Rothman RH, Booth R: Failures of spinal fusion, *Orthop Clin North Am* 6:299, 1975.

162. Rothman SLG, Gunn WV: CT with multiplanar reconstruction in 253 cases of lumbar spondylolysis, *AJNR Am J Neuroradiol* 5:81, 1984.

163. Roub LW, Drayer BD. Spinal computed tomography: limitations and applications, *AJR Am J Roentgenol* 133:267, 1979.

164. Ryan RW, Latty JF, Kozic Z: Asymptomatic calcified herniation thoracic discs: CT recognition, *AJNR Am J Neuroradiol* 9:363, 1988.

165. Saal JA, Saal JS, Herzog RJ: The natural history of lumbar intervertebral disc extrusion treated non-operatively, *Spine* 15:683, 1990.

166. Sackett JF, Strother CM: *Lumbar examination.* In Sackett JF, Strother CM, editors: *New techniques in myelography,* Hagerstown, MD, 1979, Harper & Row, P70.

167. Sage MR: Blood brain barrier: phenomenon of increasing importance to the imaging clinician, *AJR Am J Roentgenol* 138:887, 1982.

168. Sandhu FS, Dillon WP: Spinal epidural abscess: Evaluation with contrast-enhanced MR imaging, *AJNR Am J Neuroradiol* 12:1087, 1992.

169. Sartoris DJ, Moskowitz PS, Kaufman RA, et al.: Childhood discitis: computed tomographic findings, *Radiology* 149:701, 1983.

170. Schiebler M, Grenier N, Fallon M, et al.: Normal and degenerated intervertebral disc: in vivo and in vitro MR imaging with histopathologic correlation, *AJR Am J Roentgenol* 157:93, 1991.

171. Schnebel B, Kinston S, Watkins R, Dillin W: Comparison of MRI to contrast CT in the diagnosis of spinal stenosis, *Spine* 14:332, 1989.

172. Schneiderman G, Flannigan B, Kingston S, et al.: Magnetic resonance imaging in the diagnosis of disc degeneration: correlation with discography, *Spine* 12:276, 1987.

173. Schroth G, Thron A, Guhl L, et al.: Magnetic resonance imaging of spinal meningiomas and neurinomas: improvement of imaging by paramagnetic contrast enhancement, *J Neurosurg* 66:695, 1987.

174. Schubiger O, Valavanis A: CT differentiation between recurrent disc herniation and postoperative scar formation: The value of contrast enhancement, *Neuroradiology* 22:251, 1982.

175. Scotti G, Scialfa G, Colombo N, Landoni L: MR imaging of intradural extramedullary tumors of the cervical spine, *J Comput Assist Tomogr* 9:1037, 1985.

176. Scotti G, Scialfa G, Pieralli S, et al.: Myelopathy and radiculopathy due to cervical spondylosis: myelographic-CT correlations, *AJNR Am J Neuroradiol* 4:601, 1983.

177. Seeger JF. *Imaging of the postoperative lumbar spine.* In Latchaw RE, editor: *MR and CT imaging of the head, neck, and spine,* St. Louis, 1991, Mosby, P1159.

178. Sether LA, Yu S, Haughton VM, Fischer ME: Intervertebral disc: normal age-related changes in MR signal intensity, *Radiology* 177:385, 1990.

179. Shapiro R. *Inflammatory lesions.* In Shapiro R, editor: *Myelography,* ed 4, Chicago, 1984, Year Book Medical, P282.

180. Sharif HS: Role of MR imaging in the management of spinal infections, *AJR Am J Roentgenol* 158:1333, 1992.

181. Sharif HS, Aideyan OA, Clark DC, et al.: Brucellar and tuberculous spondylitis: comparative imaging features, *Radiology* 171:419, 1989.

182. Sharif HS, Clark DC, Aabed MY, et al.: Granulomatous spinal infections: MR imaging, *Radiology* 177:101, 1990.

183. Shaw MOM, Russel JA, Grossart KW: The changing pattern of spinal arachnoiditis, *J Neurol Neurosurg Psychiatry* 41:97, 1978.

184. Sheldon JJ, Sersland T, Leborgne J: Computed tomography of lower lumbar vertebral column, *Radiology* 124:113, 1977.

185. Silberstein M, Tress BM, Hennessy O: Delayed neurologic deterioration in the patient with spinal trauma: role of MR imaging, *AJNR Am J Neuroradiol* 13:1373, 1992.

186. Simmons JD, Newton Th: *Arachnoiditis.* In Newton TH, Potts DG, editors: *Computed tomography of the spine and the spinal cord,* San Anselmo, CA, 1983, Clavadel, P223.

187. Smoker WRK, Godersky JC, Knutzon RK, et al.: The role of MR imaging in evaluating metastatic spinal disease, *AJR Am J Roentgenol* 149:1241, 1987.

188. Smolik E, Nash F: Lumbar spinal arachnoiditis: a complication of the intervertebral disc operation, *Ann Surg* 133:490, 1951.

189. Sobel DF, Zyroff J, Thorne RP. Discogenic vertebral sclerosis: MR imaging. *J Comput Assist Tomogr* 11(5):855, 1987.

190. Sotiropoulos S, Chafetz NI, Land P, et al.: Differentiation between postoperative scar and recurrent disc herniation: prospective comparison of MR, CT, and contrast-enhanced CT, *AJNR Am J Neuroradiol* 10:639, 1989.

191. Stanley JH, Schabel SI, Frey GD, Hungerford GD: Quantitative analysis of the cervical spinal canal by computed tomography. *Neuroradiology* 28:139, 1986.

192. Stimac GK, Porter BA, Olson DO, et al.: Gadolinium-DTPA-enhanced MR imaging of spinal neoplasms: preliminary investigation and comparison with unenhanced spin-echo and STIR sequences, *AJNR AM J Neuroradiol* 9:839, 1988.

193. Sze G, Abramson A, Krol G, et al.: Gadolinium-DTPA in the evaluation of intradural extramedullary spinal disease, *AJR Am J Roentgenol* 150:911, 1988.

194. Sze G, Krol G, Zimmerman RD, et al.: Intramedullary disease of the spine: diagnosis using gadolinium-DTPA-enhanced MR imaging, *AJNR Am J Neuroradiol* 9:847, 1988.

195. Sze G, Stimac GK, Bartlett C, et al.: Multicenter study of gadopentetate dimeglumine as an MR contrast agent: evaluation in patients with spinal tumors, *AJNR Am J Neuroradiol* 11:967, 1990.

196. Sze G, Zimmerman RD, Deck MDF: Malignant extradural spinal tumors: MR imaging with Gd-DTPA, *Radiology* 167:217, 1988.

197. Szypryt EP, Hardy JG, Hinton CE, et al.: A comparison between magnetic resonance imaging and scintigraphic bone imaging in the diagnosis of disc space infection in animal model, *Spine* 13:1042, 1988.

198. Takahashi M, Sakamoto Y, Miyawaki M, Bussaka H: Increased MR signal intensity secondary to chronic cervical cord compression, *Neuroradiology* 29:550, 1987.

199. Takahaski M, Yamashita Y, Sakamoto Y, Kojima R: Chronic cervical cord compression: clinical significance of increased signal intensity on MR images, *Radiology* 173:219, 1989.

200. Tarr RW, Drolshagen LF, Kerner TC, et al.: MR imaging of recent spinal trauma, *J Comput Assist Tomogr* 11:412, 1987.

201. Taylor TKF, Grainger WD: Disc space infection as a complication of disc surgery, *J Bone Joint Surg* 55A:435, 1973.

202. Teplick JG, Haskin ME: Intravenous contrast-enhanced CT of the postoperative lumbar spine: improved identification of recurrent disc herniation, scar, arachnoiditis, and discitis, *AJNR Am J Neuroradiol* 5:373, 1984.

203. Teplick JG, Haskin ME: Computed tomography of the postoperative lumbar spine, *AJR Am J Roentgenol* 141:865, 1983.

204. Teplick JG, Laffery PA, Berman A, et al: Diagnosis and evaluation of spondylolisthesis and/or spondylolysis on axial CT, *AJNR Am J Neuroradiol* 7:479, 1986.

205. Teplick JG, Peyster RG, Teplick S, et al.: CT iden-

206. Teplick JG, Teplick SK, Goodman L, et al.: Pitfalls and usual findings in computed tomography of the lumbar spine, *J Comput Assist Tomogr* 6:888, 1982.

207. Teresi LM, Lufkin RB, Reicher MA, et al.: Asymptomatic degenerative disc disease and spondylosis of the cervical spine: MR imaging, *Radiology* 164:83, 1987.

208. Thrall JH, Ellis BI: Skeletal metastases, *Radiol Clin North Am* 25:1155, 1987.

209. Thrush A, Enzmann D: MR imaging of infectious spondylitis, *AJNR Am J Neuroradiol* 11:1171, 1990.

210. Tracy PT, Wright RM, Hanigan WC: Magnetic resonance imaging of spinal injury, *Spine* 14(3):292, 1989.

211. Tsuruda JS, Norman D, Dillon W, et al.: Three-dimensional gradient-recalled MR imaging as a screening tool for the diagnosis of cervical radiculopathy, *AJNR Am J Neuroradiol* 10:1263, 1990.

212. Urban JPG, Holm S, Maroudus A, Nachemson A: Nutrition of the intervertebral disc: an in vivo study of solute transport, *Clin Orthop* 129:101, 1977.

213. Valk J: Gd-DTPA in MR of spinal lesions, *AJNR Am J Neuroradiol* 9:345, 1988.

214. VanDuym FCVA, Van Wiechan PJ: Herniation of calcified nucleus pulposus in the thoracic spine, *J Comput Assist Tomogr* 7:1122, 1983.

215. VanDyke C, Ross JS, Tkach J, et al.: Gradient-echo MR imaging of the cervical spine: evaluation of extradural disease, *AJNR Am J Neuroradiol* 10:627, 1989.

216. Van Lom KJ, Kellerhouse LE, Pathria MN, et al.: Infection versus tumor in the spine: criteria for distinction with CT, *Radiology* 166:851, 1988.

217. Verbiest H: Results of surgical treatment of idiopathy developmental stenosis of the lumbar vertebral canal, *J Bone Joint Surg* 59B:181, 1977.

218. Verbiest H: Pathomorphologic aspects of developmental lumbar stenosis, *Orthop Clin North Am* 6:177, 1975.

219. Waldvogel FA, Vasey H: Osteomyelitis: the past decade, *N Engl J Med* 303:360, 1980.

220. Weiss T, Treisch J, Kazner E, et al.: CT of the postoperative lumbar spine: the value of intravenous contrast, *Neuroradiology* 28:241, 1986.

221. Wener L, Perl SM: *Magnetic resonance imaging of degenerative disease of the spine*. In Latchaw RE, editor: *MRI and CT imaging of the head, neck, and spine*, St. Louis, 1991, Mosby, P1147.

222. Whelan MA, Schonfeld S, Post JD, et al.: Computed tomography of nontuberculous spinal infection, *J Comput Assist Tomogr* 9:280, 1985.

223. White AA, Gordon SL: Synopsis: workshop on idiopathic low-back pain, *Spine* 7:141, 1982.

224. Wiesel SW, Tsourmas N, Feffer HL, et al.: A study of computer-assisted tomography: I. The incidence of positive CAT scans in an asymptomatic group of patients, *Spine* 9:549, 1984.

225. Wiley AM, Trueta J: The vascular anatomy of the spine and its relationship to pyogenic vertebral osteomyelitis, *J Bone Joint Surg* 41B:796, 1959.

226. Wilkinson HA: *Alternative therapies for the failed back syndrome*. In Frymoyer JW, editor: *The adult spine: principles and practice*, New York, 1991, Raven Press, P2069.

tification of post laminectomy pseudomeningocele, *AJNR Am J Neuroradiol* 4:179, 1983.

227. Williams AL, Haughton VM, Daniels DL, et al.: Differential CT diagnosis of extruded nucleus pulposus, *Radiology* 148:141, 1983.

228. Williams AL, Haughton VM, Daniels DL, et al.: CT recognition of lateral lumbar disc herniation, *AJR Am J Roentgenol* 139:345, 1982.

229. Williams AL, Haughton VM, Meyer GA: Computed tomographic appearance of the bulging anulus, *Radiology* 142:403, 1982.

230. Williams AL, Haughton VM, Syversten A: Computed tomography in the diagnosis of herniated nucleus pulposus, *Radiology* 135:95, 1980.

231. Yang WC, Zappulla R, Malis L: Neurilemmoma—lumbar neural foramen, *J Comput Assist Tomogr* 5:904, 1981.

232. Yousem DM, Atlas SW, Goldberg HI, Grossman RI: Degenerative narrowing of the cervical spine neural foramina: evaluation with high-resolution 3DFT gradient-echo MR imaging, *AJNR Am J Neuroradiol* 12:229, 1991.

233. Yu S, Haughton VM, Sether LA, et al.: Criteria for classifying normal and degenerated lumbar intervertebral discs, *Radiology* 170:523, 1989.

234. Yu S, Haughton VM, Sether LA, Wagner M: Comparison of MR and discography in detecting radial tears of the anulus: a post-mortem study, *AJNR Am J Neuroradiol* 10:1077, 1989.

235. Yu S, Haughton VM, Lynch KL, et al.: Fibrous structure in the intervertebral disc: correlation of MR appearance with anatomic section, *AJNR Am J Neuroradiol* 10:1105, 1989.

236. Yu S, Haughton VM, Sether LA, Wagner M: Anulus fibrosus in bulging intervertebral discs, *Radiology* 169:761, 1988.

237. Yuh WTC, Zachar CK, Barloon TJ, et al.: Vertebral compression fractures: distinction between benign and malignant causes with MR imaging, *Radiology* 172:215, 1989.

238. Zilkha A, Irwin GAL, Fagelman D: Computed tomography of spinal epidural hematoma, *AJNR Am J Neuroradiol* 4:1073, 1983.

Chapter 12
Electrodiagnostic Evaluation of Spine Problems

Joel M. Press

Jeffrey L. Young

Electrodiagnostic evaluation is an important tool in the evaluation of the patient with spine problems. Appropriate diagnosis and subsequent treatment of patients with low-back or neck complaints requires a balanced approach to the problem: a thorough history to understand the disability caused by the back or neck pain, a complete physical examination to delineate the site of impairment and potential pain generators, proper imaging studies to reveal structural abnormalities, and appropriate electrodiagnostic studies to evaluate the physiology of the peripheral nervous system. Understanding the usefulness and limitations of the electrophysiologic examination is critical in order to utilize it to its greatest potential in the diagnosis and treatment of spine problems. Electrodiagnostic studies such as electromyography (EMG) are an extension of the clinical examination and should be guided by pertinent information gathered by the history, physical examination, and anatomic or radiologic data. Furthermore, the electrophysiologic information gathered by the examination needs to be interpreted in the light of this clinical picture. It is always important to keep in mind that the electrodiagnostic examination evaluates the physiology of the nerves and muscles studied *at that time*. Some abnormalities might not yet have appeared; others may have resolved and have left to detectable residual deficit. Therefore, the electrodiagnostic impression must be based on the entire clinical picture. A finding of no electrophysiologic abnormality does not necessarily mean that there is not or has not been nerve damage. Conversely, lack of nerve damage does not mean that the patient is free of abnormalities.

This chapter will describe the chronology of electrophysiologic events that occur with nerve injuries, the usefulness and limitations of various aspects of electrophysiologic testing, the sensitivity and speci-ficity of these tests, and common clinical presentations of cervical and lumbar radiculopathies. The purpose of this information will be to provide the clinician with specific indications and limitations of electrodiagnostic studies in the evaluation of patients with spine problems. These indications and limitations will be presented in the final section of the chapter.

Anatomy

The spinal nerves are composed of dorsal and ventral roots (Fig. 12-1). The axons of the ventral root originate primarily from cells in the anterior and lateral gray columns of the cord, whereas those of the dorsal roots originate in the dorsal root ganglia. The dorsal root ganglia are usually situated within the entrance of the bony interverbral foramina.[16,17] This is situated along the distal portion of the dorsal root near the area where the dorsal and ventral roots join to form the spinal nerves. The spinal nerve is formed at about the level of the intervertebral foramina. Disruption of the nerve root by a herniated disc occurs prior to the exit at the intervertebral foramina, and therefore, proximal to the dorsal root ganglia.[52] As a result, the sensory fibers to the periphery are not affected. However, the afferent fibers from the dorsal root ganglia to the spinal cord can be affected, therefore explaining why hypesthesia can be present despite normal sensory studies.

Almost all muscles are innervated by more than one root level. The only exception to this may be the rhomboids, which are thought to be exclusively C5 in origin.[55] Needle EMG is based entirely on finding abnormalities in myotomal distributions. There is still controversy regarding some muscles and their specific nerve root supply, which is complicated and fueled by the natural variability in muscle in-

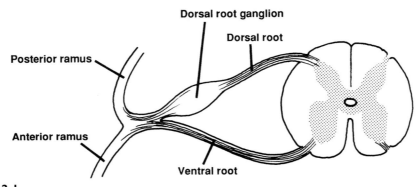

Fig 12-1

Spinal nerve root anatomy. Note that the spinal nerves terminate by dividing into anterior and posterior rami.

nervation.[55] For this reason, when electromyographic studies are performed, a number of muscles with overlapping innervations need to be studied to get the clearest picture of which nerve root is most likely the one affected. Sensory dermatomes overlap to a great extent. Due to the extensive sensory overlap, as well as myofascial pain syndromes and nonneural causes simulating radicular pain, it is difficult to assess sensory symptoms well with standard nerve conduction studies.[49,52] Other studies such as somatosensory evoked potentials, which are discussed in other sections of this book, may improve diagnostic yield.

Chronology/Pathophysiology

In order to use electrophysiologic studies efficiently and effectively in patients with spine problems an understanding of the chronology and pathophysiology of changes that occur with nerve injury, and in particular radiculopathy, is essential. Compression of the nerve tissues may induce structural damage to the nerve fibers, impairment of intraneural blood flow, and formation of intraneural edema as well as axonal transport block.[41] Some electrodiagnostic changes occur from the onset of irritation or damage to a nerve. If the initial injury to the nerve fibers is mild, a focal conduction slowing or block occurs, which can be very transient (neurapraxia) or when more persistent, with focal demyelination.[13-15,40] With this type of injury the sensory or motor deficit may last only hours to days. Electromyographic changes of spontaneous single muscle fiber discharges (e.g., positive waves and fibrillation potentials) or changes in the parameters of the motor unit action potential (MUAPs) never occur since there has not been any axonal loss. Weakness that is not apparent clinically may be recognized electrophysiologically, though, as a reduced recruitment pattern on maximal contraction.[25] However, if weakness is minimal, the recruitment pattern may not be identified as reduced. Then, with minimal contraction, a reduced recruitment interval can be seen. The reduced recruitment interval occurs because there are fewer motor units available, and the first unit will fire more rapidly at the moment the second unit is recruited.

Other electrodiagnostic changes that can be detected from the onset of nerve injury are changes in the H-reflex latency and amplitude of the compound muscle action potential (CMAP). The H-reflex latency is prolonged in S1 radiculopathies from the onset.[52] Opinions regarding what constitutes a significant difference in H-reflex latency from side to side in unilateral radiculopathies varies among authors from 1.0 to 2.0 msec.[4,6,25,44] The reduction in the amplitude of the CMAP over the appropriate muscle group can also be seen early after nerve injury.[25]

With more severe injuries, axonal loss occurs. Typically, sensory abnormalities are prominent, muscle stretch reflexes are reduced or lost, and denervation occurs in the muscles of that myotome.[52] The electrophysiologic hallmark of findings of axonal degeneration are the spontaneous single muscle fiber discharges called "positive sharp waves" and "fibrillation potentials." Positive sharp waves are first noticeable in paraspinal muscles (posterior primary ramus distribution) within 7 to 10 days after loss of axon function.[25] By 14 to 18 days, positive sharp waves can appear in the limb muscles beginning proximally and quickly becoming evident throughout the involved myotome. Soon the positive waves are accompanied by fibrillation potentials.[25,27,35] By 18 to 21 days, all muscles in the involved myotome have abnormalities including positive sharp waves and fibrillation potentials. Positive sharp waves start out as large-amplitude waves of approximately 200 mV that gradually drop in amplitude over many weeks to approximately 100 to 150 mV.[24,42] Fibrillation potentials follow a similar course. With time, if reinnervation of muscle fibers remains incomplete, both positive sharp waves and fibrillation potentials decrease in amplitude to values between 20 and 50 mV. As the nerve root pathology resolves, paraspinal muscles, which are the first muscles to show abnormalities on EMG, are also the first muscles to reinnervate and cease fibrillating. Thereafter, proximal limb muscles follow suit, followed by the more distal muscles.

Most radiculopathies will not show the presence of positive waves and fibrillations within the first 3 weeks of symptoms and, therefore, electrodiagnostic studies are not pursued in the short term. However, if the patient has had previous episodes of radicular symptoms, or prior spinal surgery, it may be useful both diagnostically and from a medical-legal standpoint to perform initial electrodiagnostic studies as soon as possible after the appearance of new symptoms.[47] If positive waves are seen within the first week or two, they can be assumed to have been present prior to the onset of symptoms. New electromyographic abnormalities seen 4 to 6 weeks later can be assumed to represent new findings.

In chronic radiculopathies, fibrillation potentials are typically seen only in distal muscles. If the radiculopathy resolves (does not become chronic) the spontaneous single muscle fiber discharges (positive sharp waves and fibrillation potentials) begin to diminish in 5 to 6 weeks, and disappear in 6 months or less unless the root lesion was severe.[35] Evidence of reinnervation (long duration, large-amplitude polyphasic MUAPs) may be found several weeks after the onset of symptoms, but this does not become readily apparent unless the radiculopathy has been quite severe.[35] Absence of positive waves (i.e., absence of denervation) even though weakness is present portends a good prognosis, assuming there has been sufficient time since the onset of nerve compromise for them to develop.[35]

Specific Electrodiagnostic Studies

There are many specific steps that comprise comprehensive electrodiagnostic evaluation. Each of these will be discussed separately to delineate their usefulness and limitations in evaluating patients with back pain. Specific procedural details of each of these studies will not be discussed in this chapter because they are explained fully in standard electrodiagnostic text books.[25,31]

Nerve-Conduction Studies

Distal peripheral motor and sensory nerve conduction studies are often normal in a single-level radiculopathy. They may be useful though to evaluate the possibility of nerve entrapment or peripheral neuropathy, which may mimic symptoms of radiculopathy. In radiculopathy, if the root lesion is purely demyelinative, there will be no change in the CMAP amplitude following stimulation distal to the lesion. If axonal degeneration occurs at one root level, either reinnervation of the muscles by fibers from the other uninvolved roots may occur, or another root that also innervates the affected muscles is not involved at all, allowing CMAP amplitudes to be only minimally decreased. Also, root compromise is nearly always incomplete, and rarely do the majority of motor fibers degenerate. When considerable axon degeneration does occur, the CMAP amplitude may be reduced. Maximum reduction is reached 7 days post injury,[55] and is easily recognized in the peroneal muscle groups in L5 radiculopathy and in the tibial groups when S1 is involved. A reduction of the CMAP of a specific muscle to 50% or less compared to the uninvolved side is probably significant. In general, the CMAPs are likely to be significantly reduced only in situations in which considerable axonal degeneration has occurred, or especially when multiple nerve roots are acutely involved. In clinical situations in which muscle is very weak, yet the CMAP

is large, a good prognosis for recovery is present. Chronic nerve-root compression, such as occurs with central lumbar stenosis, tends not to cause axonal degeneration until late in the course of progression.

Sensory nerve action potentials and conduction velocities are often normal in radiculopathies. Since the lesion in a herniated disc is almost always proximal to the dorsal-root ganglion, degeneration of peripheral sensory fibers does not occur.[5,7,55] However, in a far lateral lumbar disc herniation, particularly at the L5-S1 level, the dorsal-root ganglion may be injured and cause abnormal sensory studies. In the cervical spine, a disc that herniates into the intervertebral foramina and impinges on the posteriorly located dorsal-root ganglion will cause sensory symptoms and present with electrophysiologic findings on sensory studies. In the cervical spine, rarely, a herniated disc may impinge only on the anterior roots and cause no sensory deficits and a normal sensory nerve action potential, and only motor weakness as the manifestation of the radiculopathy.

H Reflex

The H reflex is the electrophysiologic analog to the ankle muscle stretch reflex. It measures afferent and efferent conduction along mainly the S1 nerve root and is used in localizing nerve-root compromise at that level.[1,4,6,9,34,48] Authors differ as to which component, the distal latency or the amplitude of the response, is the most important in determining S1 root pathology. A latency difference of at least 1.0 to 2.0 msec is significant. H-reflex latency shows a high correlation with S1 nerve-root pain production, as demonstrated by selective nerve root blocks.[42] Amplitude differences of <25% to 50% compared to the uninvolved side or < 1 mV are also significant.[9,54,55] However, since the amplitude of this reflex is sensitive to contraction of the plantar flexor muscles, caution is recommended about accepting a significant finding based solely on amplitude changes.

There are a number of advantages in performing H-reflex studies in patients with spine problems as part of the electrodiagnostic evaluation. H-reflex parameters can become abnormal as soon as root injury occurs and therefore are detectable much earlier than standard EMG.[18] Because the H reflex is able to look at both afferent and efferent pathways, it can give information about the status of sensory fibers that is not available with standard EMG, which evaluates only motor-nerve fibers. H reflexes are also very helpful in distinguishing S1 from L5 radiculopathies. Because these two levels are involved in over 90% of lumbar radiculopathies, H-reflex studies may help put together a clinical picture that is not otherwise clear. If surgery is contemplated, H reflexes may assist in localizing the involved level and help guide the surgical approach.

H reflexes in the forearm, recorded from the flexor carpi radialis (FCR), are found in the overwhelming majority of normal subjects.[9] As with the physiologically similar phasic myotactic reflexes, however, it is important to recognize that symmetrically absent H reflexes are not necessarily abnormal and that the percentage of absent responses increase in the elderly.[53] Nevertheless, FCR H reflexes may be abnormal with C6 or C7 root injury.[43] Upper limits of normal for side-to-side latency differences is 1.0 msec for FCR H reflexes.[21,38]

Certain limitations need to be understood in performing H-reflex studies.[9] They provide direction information only about the segmental level being studied—S1—although by inference they provide information about L5 as well.[18,44] The H reflex is sometimes normal in persons with proven S1 radiculopathies, presumably because of incomplete root involvement with sparing of the fibers over which the reflex is mediated.[53] H-reflex studies give no information about chronic versus acute radiculopathies, nor do they correlate with the severity of the radiculopathy. H-reflex studies, once unelecitable, may remain so indefinitely.[55] H-reflex studies reveal nothing about etiology of the S1 root pathology, and, in fact, do not even specifically localize the lesion to the root because they can be abnormal in peripheral neuropathies (often bilaterally), tibial or sciatic nerve injuries, lumbosacral plexus, spinal cord, and even central nervous system (CNS) disorders. Therefore, evaluation of other peripheral nerves via standard nerve-conduction studies may be helpful if the clinician warrants. Furthermore, patient relaxation is important because mild muscle contraction of the antagonist muscles will inhibit the H reflex.[18,27]

In conclusion, the H reflex may be part of an electrodiagnostic study in patients with low back and leg complaints in whom you are considering a possible S1 nerve injury, or in a patient with arm pain in whom you suspect a C6 or C7 root injury. When electromyographic abnormalities on needle examination are limited to the paraspinal muscles, a prolonged H reflex suggests an S1 or a C6 or C7 radiculopathy. H-reflex studies are especially important when EMG abnormalities are inconclusive. They may be very helpful in making a diagnosis early in the course of nerve irritation in a patient with radicular symptoms before needle electromyographic findings are present.

F Wave

The F wave is a late muscle potential that results from the backfiring of antidromicaly and supramaximally activated anterior horn cells.[9,36,42,58] F-wave studies have been shown by some to be useful in the diagnosis of lumbar nerve-root lesions when the side-to-side minimal latency is > 2.0 msec.[12,48] Like H reflexes, F-wave abnormalities occur immediately after injury to a nerve root. In one study, F-wave abnormalities were found to be the only abnormality in up to 15% of patients with radiculopathy.[11] Other studies have found that the F waves are most often abnormal when other abnormalities are also present and are rarely the only abnormality noted.[48,55] Unlike the H reflex, the F wave can be elicited at many spinal levels and from any muscle.

There are a number of limitations of the F wave in evaluating patients with spine problems. First, F-wave studies, like needle EMG, assess only motor fibers, not sensory fibers.[18] Second, only a small population of all the fibers of an axon are evaluated, and if these are not involved the study will be normal. Third, F-wave studies, like the H reflex, look at the entire pathway of the nerve, and small focal abnormalities tend to be obscured by the longer segments. Fourth, because the F wave is elicited by stimulating the nerve of the muscle studies, and all muscles receive more than one nerve root innervation, it is not specific for a given nerve root level. Fifth, like the H reflex, the F wave cannot distinguish between acute and chronic changes. Sixth, because there is a range of latencies, 10 to 20 stimuli are required for each nerve studied to determine the shortest and longest latencies. Finally, as with H reflexes, a variety of conditions can injure the nerve pathways at sites other that the nerve root and result in abnormal F waves. In conclusion, F-wave studies can be useful in evaluating radiculopathies and should be utilized as clinical indications dictate.

Needle Examination

The chronology of electrophysiologic changes that occur with nerve injury in the lower extremity have been discussed. The steps in performing a proper needle examination study are well documented.[23] Needle EMG is probably the single most useful electrodiagnostic study in evaluating patients with low-back and neck complaints for evidence of nerve injury. In spite of the fact that EMG only evaluates motor fibers for axonal loss, the diagnostic yield is considerably higher than with other techniques.[3,54,55] Although the needle examination is an excellent way to evaluate limb symptoms associated with neck and back pain, still the studies are not always abnormal even when true nerve injury exists. There are a few explanations based on electrophysiologic grounds. First, there can be weakness in the presence of a normal needle examination owing to neurapraxia or conduction block, in which the nerve is not conducting normally but no axonal injury occurred. Second, if only a few axons degenerate, the lesion could be missed by random sampling of the muscles.[55] Third, the timing of the needle examination will also be important: If the examination is performed more than 4 to 6 months after symptoms have occurred, reinnervation by collateral sprouting has probably halted the occurrence of spontaneous single muscle fiber discharges (positive waves and fibrillations). If performed less than 2 to 3 weeks following onset, spontaneous single muscle fiber discharges have not yet appeared. Therefore, the needle examination done "too early" (i.e., less than 2 to 3 weeks) or "too late" (i.e., more than 40 to 6 months) does not reveal the abnormalities that may be prominent with these time limits.

The needle study is particularly useful in localizing a nerve injury to a specific root level. It is important to sample a variety of muscles in a multisegmental distribution that are innervated by different peripheral nerves. Then, if the abnormalities are confined within a single myotome but fall outside the distribution of a single peripheral nerve, the evidence is strongly in favor of a radiculopathy. However, individual variations in muscle innervation occur, sometimes making exact localization less precise.[56] Clinical experience has shown that certain muscles have higher yields for positive needle examination findings in specific nerve root injuries[35] (Table 12-1).

The needle examination can help differentiate acute from chronic denervation. In an acute radiculopathy, positive waves, fibrillation potentials, and fasciculations are usually present in the affected muscle at rest. Chronic radiculopathy without significant ongoing denervation will show large or giant motor unit potentials with polyphagia and often very small fibrillation potentials or positive waves.

Needle examination of paraspinal muscles in suspected radiculopathies or nerve injury is essential.[10] Paraspinal fibrillation potentials indicate that the lesion is proximal to the posterior primary ramus, eliminating the concern of a possible plexopathy.[8,27,55] Chronologically, paraspinal muscles are also the first muscles to show fibrillation following onset of

radiculopathies in patients with low-back or neck pain. They are the first to stop fibrillation as the patient recovers.[42] Of all patients with positive findings on EMG 3 weeks or more after the onset of symptoms, about 70% will have abnormalities in the distribution of the posterior primary rami (paraspinal muscles) and 90% in the anterior rami distribution.[35] Electromyographic abnormalities appear only in the distribution of the posterior primary rami in 10 to 30% of all cases of lumbar radiculopathy.[24,35] Therefore, evaluating the paraspinal muscles as part of the needle examination is quite important.

There are limitations to the needle examination of the paraspinal muscles. First, fibrillation potentials have been shown to be present in the paraspinal muscles for up to 3 days after lumbar myelography.[50] Similar findings have been noted in the paraspinal muscle after lumbar epidural injections, as well as lumbar selective nerve root blocks in which abnormalities may last for as long as 4 weeks.[42] Second, as paraspinals are the fist muscles to reinnervate, needle electromyographic findings may not be noted because reinnervation has already occurred at the time of the examination. Furthermore, there may be incomplete root involvement which does not affect the posterior ramus.[55] Like other aspects of electrodiagnostic abnormalities, positive sharp waves and fibrillation potentials in paraspinal muscles are indicative only of very proximal nerve or muscle pathology; they are not diagnostic of radiculopathy. Other causes for these changes include metastatic disease affecting the proximal nerve roots, anterior horn cell disease, inflammatory myopathies (e.g., polymyositis), and particularly diabetes mellitus, which can cause widespread fibrillation potentials throughout the paraspinal muscles, especially in the lumbar region.[54] Because of overlapping innervation, questions have been raised about the localizing value of paraspinal electromyographic findings. The specificity of this information is probably enhanced if care is taken to examine the main muscles of the deeper group of intrinsic back muscles—the musculi multifidi.[11] Anatomic data indicate relatively localized innervation by dorsal rami in these muscles.[29] It is more prudent to try to correlate findings in peripheral muscles with paraspinal muscle findings for precise localization of nerve-root injuries. Complete relaxation of the patient can be difficult in the paraspinals, causing misinterpretation of distant motor units as positive waves. Also, nonreproducible trains or burst of positive waves in the paraspinals are usually normal and are generated by the needle passing through an endplate zone.[51]

The significance of positive sharp waves and fibrillation potentials in the paraspinal muscles in pa-

Table 12-1

Specific needle examination findings

Radiculopathy	Electrodiagnostic Clinical Findings	Findings	Comments
L4	P/D in hip to groin and anterior thigh to medial leg and foot; decreased knee MSR; weak knee extensors, ankle dorsiflexors	PSW—anterior tibialis quadriceps	—
L5	P/D in back of thigh and anterior tibial region to first web space on dorsum of foot; weak ankle dorsiflexor, great toe extension; diminished medial hamstring MSR; SLR positive	PSW—anterior tibialis hamstrings, hip abductors, TFL, medial gastrocnemius; peroneal F wave may be abnormal	Need to differentiate from peroneal neuropathy
S1	P/D from hip to posterior thigh and calf to lateral aspect of foot; weak plantar flexors and ankle eversion; diminished ankle MSR; SLR positive	PSW—gluteus maximus, medial hamstrings, lateral gastrocnemius ± sural SNAP	—
C5	P/D over lateral deltoid weal deltoid; ± biceps weakness; decreased biceps MSR	PSW—rhomboids (C5 only) supraspinatus, infraspinatus biceps, deltoid	Consider rotator cuff pathology in DD
C6	P/D over shoulder to lateral forearm and thumb. Weak biceps, wrist extensors. Decreased biceps and pronator MSR	PSW—pronator tens, ECR, brachioradialis biceps; NL deltoids supraspinatus, intraspinatus	May be confused with carpal tunnel syndrome ; common radiculopathy
C7	P/D in index and long fingers; decreased triceps MSR; weak elbow extension, wrist flexion	PSW—triceps, pronator teres, FCR, EDC, ECR, ECU; median FCR H reflex may be abnormal	May be confused with carpal tunnel syndrome
C8	P/D radiating to ulnar aspect of arm into fourth and fifth digit; weak intrinsic of hand	PSW—EDC, first DI, APB; prolonged median and ulnar F waves	DD—ulnar entrapments, TOS

APB = adductor pollicus brevis;
DD = differential diagnosis;
DI = dorsal interossious;
ECR = extensor carpi radialis;
ECU = extensor carpi unaris;
EDC = extensor digitorum communis;
FCR = flexor carpi radialis;
MSR = manual strength response;
NL = normal;
P/D = paraesthesia and/or dysesthesia;
PSW = positive sharp waves and/or fibrillation potentials;
SLR = straight leg raise;
SNAP = sensory nerve action potential;
TFL = tensor fascia lata;
TOS = thoracic outlet syndrome.

tients who have undergone spinal surgery is controversial[25] Recurrent herniation of a lumbar disk, for instance is not common, but when it does occur, it usually occurs at the same level and side as it did originally. Johnson et al. concluded, after reviewing 77 EMGs in 60 patients, that electromyographic abnormalities present at one level at least 3 cm lateral to the scar are probably not related to trauma from surgery and rather are active radiculopathy.[26] They also claimed that inserting needle electrodes 2 to 3 cm from the midline and deeper than 3 cm in the muscle is likely to be at the level of the vertebral body spine of the root innervating that particular muscle.[27] However, See and Kraft showed that in 20 patients who had undergone laminectomy for root compression, electromyographic changes in the paraspinal for periods of up to 41 months postoperatively can occur, even without recurrent radiculopathy.[45] These findings were usually present both 1 and 3 cm lateral from the midline and at multiple vertebral levels. Absence of spontaneous single muscle fiber discharges on needle examination of the paraspinal muscles at the site of the surgical scar decreases the possibility that a radiculopathy is present. In conclusion, positive waves and fibrillations in the paraspinal muscles of patients who have undergone lumbar surgery or other invasive procedures (e.g., recent injections or even recent electrodiagnostic studies) should be correlated with the clinical history, physical findings, and anatomic studies and should never be used alone to diagnose cervical or lumbar radiculopathies.

Although the presence of positive waves and fibrillation potentials confined to a specific myotome is the most reliable electromyographic evidence of acute radiculopathy, analysis of motor unit potentials and their recruitment patterns plays a role in evaluating patients with subacute, chronic, and old resolved radicular syndromes. Abnormal motor-unit recruitment will occur almost immediately after the onset of any nerve injury in which interrupted conduction of nerve impulses occur.[7,25,31] Evaluating radiculopathy by abnormal recruitment intervals or frequencies has been described and felt possibly to be of particular benefit early in the course of the nerve injury before positive sharp waves and fibrillation potentials occur.[7] Johnson and co-workers suggested in early and mild L5 radiculopathy a recruitment interval of 70 to 90 msec in the extensor digitorium longus as compared to the normal interval of 100 to 120 msec was significant.[26,28] However, motor-unit recruitment abnormalities are unlikely to be recognized unless muscle weakness is easily detectible clinically. Mild weakness is accompanied by only mini-

mal alterations in recruitment intervals, which can be difficult to detect, even for experienced electromyographer. Although, the recruitment pattern at maximal contraction is thought to be indicative of the number of active motor unit potentials, Johnson et al. showed this parameter to be a less sensitive finding in patients with radiculopathy than positive sharp waves and fibrillations.[23]

Changes in motor unit size and configuration are seen in patients following the acute phase of radiculopathy. They are due to reinnervation of denervated muscle fibers and include polyphasic potentials, often of long duration and sometimes of large amplitude; but such changes by themselves cannot be considered evidence of ongoing, active nerve degeneration. In radiculopathy, reinnervation occurs by intramuscular collateral sprouting from the distal portions of the remaining viable nerves. There are always many viable nerves supplying any given muscle in monoradiculopathy because muscles are innervated by more than one nerve root. As viable nerves sprout, they begin to reinnervate the denervated muscle fibers. Then, when the nerve discharges, it activates not only its own muscle fibers but some of those belonging to an adjacent denervated nerve fiber. The recorded motor unit potential under such conditions is larger and wider than normal and may be polyphasic. Polyphasicity has long been recognized as one of the electrophysiologic abnormalities found in radiculopathy.[20,32,42,54]

It should be noted that when a muscle fiber is reinervated, it stops fibrillating. Therefore, persistent fibrillations indicate ongoing nerve degeneration, a reflection of chronic radiculopathy. Although it is not uncommon for chronic pain to persist following acute radiculopathy, it is relatively uncommon to find evidence of progressive nerve degeneration. Such findings are more often seen in the chronic, progressive narrow spinal canal syndromes.[35]

In conclusion, the needle examination appears to be the most reliable aspect of the electrodiagnostic examination in patients with neck and low-back complaints and provides the highest yield of abnormalities in radiculopathy.[3,39] Nerve-conduction studies and late responses also yield useful information, which, when taken within the entire context of the patient's complaints, physical findings, and anatomic studies aids in diagnosing nerve injuries in the back and upper and lower extremities.

Single-fiber Electromyography

Single fiber electromyography (SFEMG) is not used in routine electrodiagnostic studies of patients being evaluated for low-back or neck pain. Some reasons for this are the lack of expertise by many electromyographers to do these studies, the amount of time necessary to do the studies, and uncertainty as to what additional information can be gained. SFEMG can be helpful in evaluating patients with low-back complaints, particularly when it is used to evaluate recurrent radiculopathy and to assess the onset and process of reinnervation. The electrophysiologic changes that occur and how the parameters of blocking and jitter are affected are well described elsewhere.[52] It is important to note, however, that useful information is obtainable only if serial studies are performed and compared or if the study is done very soon after a new nerve injury occurs. Depending on the timing of the examination and the availability of comparative SFEMG studies, these types of examinations may allow one to differentiate an acute injury from a chronic one; however, they are rarely used in clinical practice.

Accuracy of Electrodiagnostic Studies

For decades, clinical investigators have been comparing electromyographic results, which reveal the electrophysiologic properties of nerve and muscle, with imaging studies, which delineate anatomic configuration of the tissues.[30,33,57] Surgically "proven" nerve root compromise has also been evaluated.[11,34,56] This concept is based on fallacious reasoning. The misconception that the two can be accurately compared comes from the observed high coincidence of nerve root pathology at the site of an often caused by disc protrusion and other anatomic distortions. However, while it is true that distorted spinal architecture can damage a nerve root, it is also well known that nerve root pathology can be demonstrated in the absence of macroanatomic abnormality. Furthermore, disc protrusion can be seen at postmortem examination in the spine of almost all patients over the age of 40 years, the majority of whom are asymptomatic of radiculopathy.[37]

The EMG supplies the following information: (1) It reveals the presence and to some degree the extent of motor nerve degeneration. This information is provided neither by imaging studies nor by direct observation of the tissues during surgery. In radiculopathy, during the acute or subacute phase of muscle fiber denervation, the observation of fibrillation, that is, the sensitivity of the test, approaches 100% accuracy—there either has been nerve degeneration (fibrillation is present) or there has not. By the time muscle fibers have been reinnervated, EMG must

rely on findings that are sometimes less obvious than fibrillation potentials, but the presence of such findings indicates that nerve degeneration has led to reinnervation of muscle fibers. The specificity for radiculopathy, based on the findings of positive waves and fibrillation potentials is not known; however, it greatly increases when the distribution of the abnormalities is clearly segmental. (2) The EMG allows recognition of the segmental level involved as long as the abnormality is distributed to at least three or four muscles within a single myome. Detection of anatomic abnormality at another level does not alter the location of nerve root pathology.

Some studies have attempted to compare findings on physical examination with those on EMG.[19,33] This is also improper. The EMG is an extension of the physical examination; one does not supplant the other. The presence of absence of electromyographic abnormalities always adds information. At times the EMG reveals abnormality when no neurologic deficits can be found on physical examination. This is particularly true in chronic radiculopathy such as with spinal stenosis.[19,22,46]

Clinical and Electrophysiologic Presentations of Radiculopathies

The most common referral to an electrophysiology laboratory from arm pain, leg pain, or back pain is to evaluate for potential radiculopathy. Patients often present with symptoms of numbness, tingling, dysesthesia, or weakness in various distributions. Although radiculopathy is most commonly due to a herniated disc or degenerative foraminal stenosis, electrophysiologic studies reveal only the presence of nerve root irritation, not the cause of the radiculopathy. Table 12-1 shows some common signs, symptoms, and electrophysiologic findings in common cervical and lumbar radiculopathies, and clinical points to consider when evaluating patients for potential radiculopathy.

Indications for Electrophysiologic Testing in Patients With Back or Neck Pain

The utility of electrodiagnostic testing in a given patient may be estimated following a thorough history and physical examination, by a review of supplemental information (i.e., imaging studies), and through an appreciation for the chronology of the electrophysiologic changes that occur following nerve injury. Some helpful generalizations as to the indications and limitations of electrodiagnostic studies are worthy of review and are discussed below.

Establish and/or Confirm a Clinical Diagnosis

Pain in the upper or lower extremities and back is often referred from pain-sensitive structures other than nerve tissue. This pain may even appear to follow a dermatomal pattern. If there is no electrophysiologic abnormality, the studies give the physician confidence that this is the case, which may help in treating and reassuring the patient. With nerve injury, however, a properly timed EMG can show evidence of the nature, location, and severity of the injury. A thorough electrophysiologic examination may alert the examiner to the possibility of an unsuspected pathologic condition, such as concomitant peripheral neuropathy with radiculopathy, an active common peroneal nerve entrapment superimposed upon a chronic L5 radiculopathy, or carpal tunnel syndrome concomitant with a C6 radiculopathy. In a small percentage of patients the diagnosis of radiculopathy is established by EMG when the diagnosis on clinical grounds seems unlikely.[35]

Localize Nerve Lesions

Signs or symptoms of nerve injuries in the extremities can be from a number of causes, including root lesions (radiculopathy), brachial or lumbosacral plexus lesions (i.e., metastasis, retroperitoneal hematoma), or peripheral-nerve injuries (i.e., carpal tunnel syndrome, ulnar lesions at the elbow, meralgia paresthetica, saphenous nerve entrapment, tarsal tunnel syndrome). Various conduction studies and EMG can evaluate many of these nerve segments to localize the lesion specifically. Occasionally, what may appear clinically as a single-level radiculopathy may in fact be multileveled, or in the case of spinal stenosis, bilateral. Frequently, clinical assessment only predicts a uniradicular lesion, but EMG may reveal involvement of two roots. This has importance in planning an operative approach.[57]

Determine the Extent of Nerve Injury

A properly timed EMG can differentiate a neuropraxic injury (conduction block) from active axonal degeneration. It can also semiquantitatively assess the degree of reversible motor axon damage and the severity of the neuronal deficit. This information may have significant impact on the aggressiveness of treatment for a lumbar radiculopathy. The acuteness or chronicity of the lesion may also be obtained.

Correlate Findings on Anatomic Studies

The existence of nerve root dysfunction cannot be determined or even assumed from diagnostic procedures that determine structural pathology.[18] Electromyography can show if physiologic nerve injury has occurred or is ongoing and if these findings correlate with the symptoms and radiologic studies. This information may have significance as to what type of treatment is instituted (surgical vs. nonsurgical). Furthermore, in presurgical candidates it is useful to know what nerve root levels are most involved in order to plan the most appropriate approach and level. Selective nerve blocks can complement EMG studies in localization of pathology.

Assist in Prognosis

The paucity of positive sharp waves and fibrillation potentials in acute radiculopathy with proper timing of the examination portends an excellent prognosis for return of muscle strength. Comparing the CMAP of a very weak muscle to that of the same muscle on the asymptomatic side gives an idea of the extent of neurapraxia and of potential recovery. A side-to-side amplitude difference of greater than 50% is probably significant. Recovery is prolonged and less complete when more than one root is involved, which may be determined at times only by EMG.[5,57]

Documentation in Medical-legal Situations

Occasionally, documentation of a nerve injury is necessary for medical-legal or worker's compensation situations, even when the clinical diagnosis is well established. The timing of the electrophysiologic examination can give information as to the acuteness or chronicity of the findings as well as establish a base line if repeat testing becomes necessary.

Limitations of Electrophysiologic Tests

The EMG is not a perfect test and should not be done in every patient referred for evaluation of spine problems. Some of the limitations of electrophysiologic testing, and situations in which it may not be necessary to obtain them, are described below.

In the first 2 to 4 weeks after onset of symptoms. In most cases in the clinical situation and examination are strongly suggestive of radiculopathy, treatment can be instituted without an EMG. Many findings may not be seen if the examination is done to early.

If the patient has progressive neurologic deficits the results of the EMG will not be important, as the patient will require emergent care. If a patient is not improving to the extent that is anticipated for that level of care, then an EMG may be useful, but not in the very acute situation.

In unequivocal radiculopathy. When the clinical history and the motor, sensory, and reflex changes are consistent, EMG adds little information and generally is not necessary. However, it may still be required if the patient is not improving with treatment.

When the history and examination are highly inconsistent with acute radiculopathy. If the clinical situation is not clear, some important points need to be considered. When a patient with back or neck pain is being evaluated, acute radiculopathy is unlikely if the pain is confined to the axial skeleton, if it involves both upper or lower limbs, or if it occurs intermittently. If, in addition, there is no detectable neurologic deficit on physical examination, acute radiculopathy is highly improbable and electrodiagnostic studies may not be needed.

When there has been no change in clinical situation in previously studied patients. Many patients have had multiple EMGs in an attempt to determine an etiology for nonsegmental, nondermatomal complaints. When multiple studies have been done, and they have been of high quality, with no change in the clinical signs or symptoms, very little information will be gained with further studies.

The results will not change medical or surgical management. For whatever reasons (e.g., extreme illness, patient refusing surgery), if the results of the studies will in no way change the treatment plan, EMG should probably be avoided.

Barriers to acquiring sufficient information are present. If a patient cannot be moved from a prone to a supine position or if dressings, casts, or stabilizing devices cannot be repositioned or temporarily removed, the information from performing the electrodiagnostic studies may be limited.

Electromyography Evaluation and Report

A thorough, comprehensive eletrophysiologic medicine consultation is an essential component in the overall approach to the evaluation and treatment of patients with spine problems. The evaluation must include a thorough history and physical examination preceding the appropriate electrodiagnostic studies.[2]

The electrophysiologic report should include a number of important pieces of data for the referring physician. First, the electrophysiologic findings should be correlated with any physical findings noted or discrepancies identified. Inconsistencies may have as much importance in the clinical treatment of the patient as consistent results, if not more. Second, the degree of certainty or "hardness" of the finding needs to be conveyed to the referring physician. A diagnosis of an S1 radiculopathy by H-reflex changes only will carry different weight compared to abundant spontaneous discharges in an S1 myotomal distribution. Third, the diagnosis that have been excluded can be as important as those confirmed. Fourth, information should be noted about potential diagnoses that are suggested by the clinical examination but not by the electrophysiologic study. Fifth, significant concomitant pathology noted (e.g., carpal tunnel syndrome superimposed on a cervical radiculopathy) should be mentioned. Sixth, any change from previous studies may be useful information. Seventh, the degree of acuteness or chronicity of the lesions identified needs to be stated. Finally, prognosis, when possible, is critical information for treating patients. This is particularly important when electromyography shows only neurapraxic changes in contrast to significant axonal degeneration.

Summary

The effectiveness and reliability of the electrodiagnostic examination in detecting pathology in patients with spine problems is high but must always be understood in light of its capabilities and limitations. Indiscriminate use of this or any testing procedure should be avoided. Electrodiagnostic studies are very examiner-dependent and, when possible, should be performed by a physician who is a specialist in electrodiagnostic medicine. Ideally, this physician is involved in the diagnosis and treatment of the patient studied. Electrodiagnostic studies evaluate nerve physiology in a certain chronologic sequence, but do not measure pain. Suggested guidelines have been given for possible situations in which an EMG may or may not be helpful in treating patients with spine problems, which in turn leads to better care.

References

1. Aiello I, Rosati G, Serra G, et al. The diagnostic valve of H-index in S1 root compression, *J Neurol Neurosurg Psychiatry* 44:171, 1981.

2. American Association of Electrodiagnostic Medicine: Guidelines in Electrodiagnostic medicine, *Muscle Nerve* 15:229, 1992.

3. Aminoff MJ, Goodin DS, Parry GJ, et al.: Electrophysiologic evaluation of lumbosacral radiculopathies: electromyography, late responses, and so

matosensory evoked potentials, *Neurology* 35:1514, 1985.

4. Baylan SP, Yu J, Grant AE: H-reflex latency in relation to ankle jerk, eletromyographic, myelographic, and surgical findings in back pain patients, *Electromyogr Clin Neurophysiol* 21:201, 1981.

5. Benecke R, Conrad B: The distal sensory nerve action potential as a diagnostic tool for the differentiation of lesions in dorsal roots and peripheral nerves, *J Neurol* 223:231, 1989.

6. Braddom RL, Johnson EW: Standardization of H-reflex and diagnostic use in S1 radiculopathy, *Arch Phys Med Rehabil* 55:161, 1974.

7. Eisen A: Electrodiagnosis of radiculopathy. In Aminott MJ, editor: Symposium on electrodiagnosis, *Neurol Clin* 3:495, 1985.

8. Eisen A, Schamer D, Melmed C: An electrophysiological method for examining lumbosacral root compression, *Can J Neurol Sci* 2:117, 1977.

9. Fisher MA: AAEM Minimonograph #13: H reflexes and F waves physiology and clinical indications, *Muscle Nerve* 15:1223, 1992.

10. Fisher MA, Kaur D, Houchins J: Electrodiagnostic examination, back pain and entrapment of posterior rami, *Electromyogr Clin Neurophysiol* 25:183, 1985.

11. Fisher MA, Shivde AJ, Teixera C, et al.: Clinical and electrophysiological appraisal of the significance of radicular injury in back pain, *J Neurol Neorsurg Psychiatry* 41:303, 1978.

12. Fisher MA, Shivde AJ, Teixera C, et al.: The F-response: A clinically useful physiological parameter for the evaluation of radicular injury, *Electromyogr Clin Neurophysiol* 19:65, 1979.

13. Fowler T, Danta G, Gilliatt R: Recovery of nerve conduction after a pneumatic tourniquet: Observations on the hind limb of the baboon, *J Neurol Neurosurg Psychiatry* 35:638, 1972.

14. Gilliatt R: *Acute compression block.* In Sumner A, editor: *The patho physiology of peripheral nerve disease,* Philadelphia, 1980, WB Saunders, p 287.

15. Gilliatt R: *Recent advances in the pathophysiology of nerve conduction.* In Desmedt J, editor: *Developments in electromyography and clinical neurophysiology,* vol 2, Basel, 1983, S Karger, p 2.

16. Glantz RH, Haldeman S: *Other diagnostic studies: electrodiagnostic.* In Frymoyer JW, editor: *The adult spine: principles and practice,* New York, 1991, Raven Press, Ltd, p 541.

17. Goss CM, editor: *Gray's anatomy of the human body,* ed 29, Philadelphia, 1973, Lea & Febiger, 1466.

18. Haldeman S: The electrodiagnostic evaluation at nerve root function, *Spine* 9(1):41, 1984.

19. Hall S, Bartlesen JD, Onotrio BM, et al.: Clinical features, diagnostic procedures and results of surgical treatment in 68 patients, *Ann Intern Med* 103:271, 1985.

20. Hoover BB, Caldwell JW, Krusen EM, et al.: Valve of polyphasic potentials in diagnosis of lumbar root lesions, *Arch Phys Med Rehabil* 51:546, 1970.

21. Jabre JF: Surface recording of the H-reflex of the flexor carpi radialis, *Muscle Nerve* 4:435, 1981.

22. Jacobson RE: Lumbar stenosis: an electromyographic evaluation, *Clin Orthop Relat Res* 115:68, 1976.

23. Johnson EW: *The EMG examination.* In Johnson EW, editor: *Practical electromyography.* Baltimore, 1988, Williams & Wilkins, p 1.

24. Johnson EW: *Electrodiagnosis of radiculopathy: Advanced concepts in evaluation of focal neuropathy.* Course of the American Association Electromyography and Electrodiagnosis, Las Vegas, Nevada, Jan. 1985.

25. Johnson EW: *Electrodiagnosis of radiculopathy.* In Johnson EW, editor: *Practical Electromyography.* Baltimore, 1988, Williams & Wilkins, p 229.

26. Johnson EW, Burkhart JA, Earl WC: Electromyography in postlaminectomy patients, *Arch Phys Med Rehabil* 53:407, 1972.

27. Johnson EW, Melvin JL: Value of electromyography in lumbar radiculopathy, *Arch Phys Med Rehabil* 52:239, 1971.

28. Johnson EW, Stocklin R, LaBan MM: Use of electrodiagnostic examination in a university hospital, *Arch Phys Med Rehabil* 46:573, 1965.

29. Jonsson B: Morphology, innervation, and electromyographic study of the erector spinae, *Arch Phys Med Rehabil* 50:638, 1969.

30. Khatri BO, Barvah J, McQuillen MP: Correlation of electromyography with computed tomography in evaluation of lower back pain, *Arch Neurol* 41:594, 1984.

31. Kimura J: *Electrodiagnosis in diseases of muscle and nerve,* Philadelphia, 1985, FA Davis.

32. Lajoie WJ: Nerve root compression: correlation of electromyographic, myelographic and surgical findings, *Arch Phys Med Rehabil* 53:390, 1972.

33. Lane ME, Tamhankar MN, Demopoulos JJ: Discogenic radiculopathy: use of electromyography in multidisciplinary management, *NY State J Med* 32, 1978.

34. Leyshon A, Kriwan EOG, Wynn PCG: Electrical studies in the diagnosis of compression at the lumbar root, *J Bone Joint Surg* 63B:71, 1981.

35. MacLean IC: *Acute radialopathy.* Presented at EMG and neurophysiology: a high intensity review. Chicago, April 6, 1989.

36. Mayladeny JW, McDougall DB: Electrophysiological studies of nerve and reflex activity in normal man. Identification of certain reflexes in EMG and conduction velocity of peripheral nerve function, *Bull Johns Hopkins Hosp* 86:265, 1950.

37. McCrae DL: Asymptomatic intervertebral disc protrusions, *Acta Radiol* 46:9, 1956.

38. Ongerboer de Visser BW, Schimsheimer RJ, Hart AAM: The H reflex of the flexor carpi radialis muscle: a study in controls and radiation-induced brachial plexus lesions, *J Neurol Neurosurg Psychiatry* 47:1098, 1984.

39. Rodriguez AA, Kanis L, Rodriguez AA, et al.: Somatosensory evoked potentials from dermatomal stimulation as an indicator of L5 and S1 radiculopathy, *Arch Phys Med Rehabil* 68:366, 1987.

40. Rudge P, Ochoa J, Gilliatt R: Acute peripheral nerve compression in the baboon, *J Neurol Sci* 23:403, 1974.

41. Rydevik B, Braun MD, Lundborg G: Pasthoanatomy and pathophysiology of nerve root compression, *Spine* 9:7, 1984.

42. Saal JA: Electrophysiologic evaluation of lumbar pain: establishing the rationale for therapeutic management, *Spine State Art Rev* 1:21, 1986.

43. Schimsheimer RJ, Ongerboer BW, Visser DE, Kemp B: The flexor carpi radialis H-reflex in lesion of the sixth and seventh cervical nerve roots, *J Neurol Neurosurg Psychiatry* 48:445, 1985.

44. Schuchmann JA: H-reflex latency in radiculopathy, *Arch Phys Med Rehabil* 59:185, 1978.

45. See DH, Kraft GH: Electromyography in paraspinal muscles following surgery for root compression, *Arch Phys Med Rehabil* 56:80, 1975.

46. Seppalainen AM, Alaranta H, Solni J: Electromyography in the diagnosis of lumbar spinal stenosis, *Electromyogr Clin Neurophysiol* 21:55, 1981.

47. Spindler HA, Felsenthal G: Electrodiagnostic evaluation of acute and chronic radiculopathy, *Phys Med Rehab Clin North Am* 1(1):53, 1990.

48. Tonzola RF, Ackil AA, Shahani BT, Young RR: Usefulness of electrophysiological studies in the diagnosis of lumbosacral root disease, *Ann Neurol* 9:305, 1981.

49. Travell JG, Simons DG: *Myofascial pain and dysfunction: the trigger point manual,* Baltimore, 1983, Williams & Wilkins.

50. Weber RJ, Weingarden SI: EMG abnormalities following myelography, *Arch Neurol* 36:588, 1979.

51. Weichers DO: Electromyographic insertional activity in normal limb muscles, *Arch Phys Med Rehabil* 60:359, 1979.

52. Weichers DO: Radiculopathies. *Phys Med Rehab State Art Rev* 3:713, 1989.

53. Weintraub JR, Madalin K, Wong M, et al.: Achilles tendon reflex and the H response, *Muscle Nerve* 11:972, 1988.

54. Wilbourne AT: *The value and limitations of electromyographic examination in the diagnosis of lumbosacral radiculopathy.* In Hary RW, editor: *Lumbar disc disease,* New York, 1982, Raven Press, p 65.

55. Wilbourne AJ, Aminoff MJ: The electrophysiologic examination in patients with radiculopathies and nerve, *Muscle Nerve* 11:1099, 1988.

56. Young A, Getty CMJ, Jackson A, et al.: Variations in the pattern of muscle innervation by the L5 and S1 nerve roots, *Spine* 8(6):616, 1983.

57. Young A, Wynn PCB: The assessment and management of the failed back, Part I, *Int Disabil Stud* 9:21, 1987.

58. Young RR, Shahani BJ: Clinical value and limitation of F-nerve determination, *Muscle Nerve* 13:248, 1978.

Chapter 13
Somatosensory and Motor Evoked Potentials
Erwin G. Gonzalez

History

Somatosensory Evoked Potential

    stimulation and recording techniques
    anatomic and physiologic basis
    clinical interpretation
    indications
    functional versus organic sensory complaints
    intraoperative monitoring

Motor Evoked Responses

    stimulation technique
    anatomic and physiologic basis
    clinical interpretation
    clinical indications

Conclusion

Somatosensory evoked potential (SEP) and motor evoked potential (MEP) are integral parts of clinical neurophysiology. Their applications reflect the widely expanding field of electrodiagnostic medicine. These procedures provide a window to examine portions of the nervous system that are currently unexplored by standard electromyography (EMG) and nerve conduction velocity (NCV) studies.

History

Dawson[21] recorded the first clinical SEP by photographic superimposition of individual responses obtained in the scalp of a patient with myoclonic epilepsy. Serendipitously, the large SEP amplitude that is characteristically found in this disease facilitated the recording. Initial attempts to record SEPs were hampered by instrument limitations. Over the past decade, however, major strides have been made in the use and availability of microprocessors. This heralded the advent of sophisticated electronic averagers and low-noise amplifier systems. These technologic developments led to the widespread use of evoked responses for research and clinical purposes, including radicular and spinal sydromes.

In addition to the sophisticated exploration of the afferent limb, neurophysiologists have now begun to examine the previously untapped efferent limb of the central loop. Electrical stimulation of the unexposed motor cortex became possible when Gualtierotti and Paterson[58] tried the technique in 1954. Very little enthusiasm was generated, and clinical interest rapidly waned because the procedure was intensely painful. Almost 30 years elapsed before Merton and Morton[86] would refine the technique. The pioneering works by Cowan et al.,[17] Mills et al.,[88] and Levy[80] on cortical electrical stimulation had barely penetrated the clinical community, when a new technique of transcranial stimulation (TCS) via magnetic stimulation was described by Barker et al.,[10] which rapidly overshadowed electrical TCS. In the United States, the use of magnetic TCS has not reached the same level of application as SEPs because of the Food and Drug Administration's classification of the technique as "experimental."

Somatosensory Evoked Potential

Stimulation and Recording Techniques

Nomenclature

When an appropriate peripheral nerve or dermatome is stimulated, SEP is generated along the neuroaxis and in specific topographic areas of the cortex. These potentials are made up of various wave components that occur at different time latencies. The wave forms are labeled according to polarity and latency. In most instances, the mean latency of a particular wave is used to identify the potential, no matter when the component wave actually occurs. Thus, a positive (downward) potential with a mean latency of 38 msec is identified as P38, although, the actual latency may occur at 37 or 40 msec. A negative (upward) wave, known as N45 may appear sooner or later than 45 msec. For this reason, some laboratories simply identify the components based on their sequence of appearance, such as P1, N1, P2, N2 (Fig. 13-1).

Types of Recording

The configuration of the SEP depends on whether the recording is obtained with unipolar (far-field) or

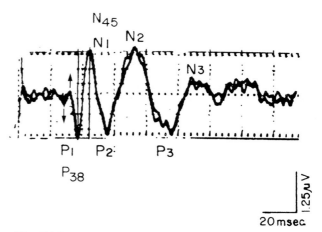

Fig. 13-1

Typical example of a normal tibial nerve cortical SEP. Components are identified according to polarity and mean latency. For individual examinations, absolute latency is reported. Thus, P38 may in fact be P37, while N45 could be N46. As an alternative, components are labeled according to polarity and their sequence of appearance—e.g., P1, N1, P2, N2. *(From Gonzalez EG, Hajdu M, Bruno R, Keim H, Brand L: Lumbar spinal stenosis: an analysis of pre- and postoperative somatosensory evoked potentials,* Arch Phys Med Rehabil *66:11, 1985, with permission.)*

bipolar referential (near-field) technique.[74,75] In the former, the active recording electrode is placed at the scalp or spine, while the reference electrode is situated at a distant site, such as the knee or shoulder. In the latter, both recording and reference electrodes are located in close proximity to one another. A change in the recording montage may result in reversal of a particular wave's polarity, and although the latency remains constant, the generator site of the wave may not necessarily be the same. For purposes of discussion, this section will deal only with short latency potentials; that is, latencies under 25 msec and 45 msec when stimulating the arm and leg, respectively. Short latency potentials are more stable and less affected by state of wakefulness and light anesthesia.[1,56] These are the potentials currently of interest in clinical SEP examination.

Recording Electrodes

A variety of recording electrodes can be used to record SEPs. Gold or silver-silver chloride electroencepholographic (EEG) cup electrodes are preferred to platinum needle or clip EEG electrodes because of their lower impedance. Needle and clip electrodes on the other hand are quicker to place and secure, and are the preferred electrodes in the intraoperative setting. To achieve impedance of less than 5000 ohms, the scalp and skin in all electrode sites are abraded with commercially available gel preparation.

Stimulation Sites

Almost any nerve or dermatome can be stimulated. For upper extremity examination, mixed nerves like the median, ulnar, and radial nerves at the wrist are often used because they yield more consistent wave forms.[114,118,119] Pure sensory fibers can also be used to examine specific segments, as for instance, the forefinger for C6, the middle finger for C7, and the pinky for C8.[28,30-32] In the lower extremity, mixed nerves such as the posterior tibial and peroneal nerves can be stimulated at the ankle or knee. Segmental cutaneous nerve stimulation can be easily performed using the sural (S1), superficial peroneal (L5), and saphenous (L4) nerves at the ankle, the saphenous nerve (L3) at the knee and lateral femoral cutaneous nerve (L2) at the thigh.[30-32] The lower sacral roots can be evaluated by pudendal nerve stimulation at the penis or clitoris.[60] Dermatomes at the lateral aspect of the foot (S1), the first web space (L5), superomedial aspect of the ankle (L4), medial aspect of the knee (L3), and anteromedial aspect of the thigh (L2) are easily accessible.[31,32,34,70] Table 13-1 summarizes the different stimulation sites and the normal latencies following segmental sensory examination,[28] while Fig. 13-2 illustrates the signature areas for dermatomal stimulation.

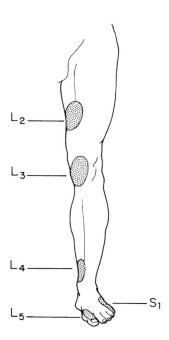

Fig. 13-2
Signature areas for placement of stimulating electrodes in dermatomal segmental SEP determinations in lumbosacral radiculopathy.

Table 13-1
Segmental Sensory Stimulation*

Cutaneous Nerve	Stimulation Site	Segment	Normal Values†
Musculocutaneous	Forearm	C5	17.4 ± 1.2
Median	Thumb	C6	22.5 ± 1.1
Median	Fingers 2-3	C7	21.2 ± 1.2
Ulnar	Finger 5	C8	22.5 ± 1.1
Lateral femoral	Thigh	L2	31.8 ± 1.8
Saphenous	Knee	L3	37.6 ± 2.0
Saphenous	Ankle	L4	43.4 ± 2.2
Superficial peroneal	Above ankle	L5	39.3 ± 1.8
Sural	Ankle	S1	42.1 ± 1.4

*From Eisen A, et al.: Evaluation of radiculopathies by segmental stimulation and somatosensory evoked potentials, *Can J Neurol Sci* 10: 178-182, 1983.
†In msec (N19/P38).

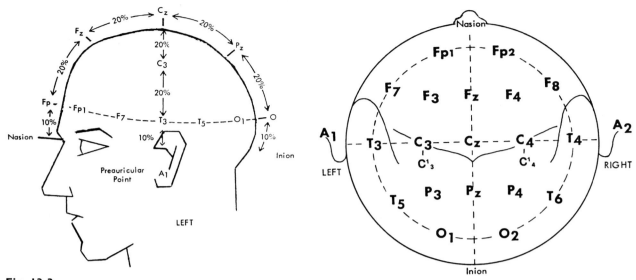

Fig. 13-3

The 10-20 EEG system *(From Rinzler G: The 10-20 System Booklet: Diagrams.)*

Surface stimulating electrodes are placed with the cathode proximal to the anode. Wherever the site of stimulation, the intensity is usually three to four times the sensory threshold, or one to two times the motor threshold. The intensity of stimulation ranges from 10 to 15 mA for constant current, or 80 to 120 V for constant voltage stimulation. The pulse duration is kept at 0.1 to 0.2 msec, and delivered at a rate of 3 to 4 Hz. In contrast to cortical SEP, spinal SEP latencies and amplitudes are not altered with stimulation rates of up to 10 Hz. For cortical recordings, however, the optimal compromise between expediency and attenuation of amplitude is 5 Hz.[98,117-119] The analysis time spans from 60 to 80 msec, but the time acquisition should be extended up to 200 msec before a judgment is made regarding the absense of any identifiable SEP. It is suggested that 250 to 1000 stimuli be averaged to acquire clearly defined wave forms, and that each trial should be replicated in order to ensure that the wave forms are reproducible.

Montage

The recording montage and stimulation sites may vary according to the specific components of interest. Nomenclature based on the international EEG 10/20 system will be used to describe electrode placement (Fig. 13-3).

The American Association of Electrodiagnostic Medicine recommends a four-channel montage to conduct lower extremity examination,[5] consisting of (1) Cz′ to Fpz′; (2) T12S (spine) to 4 cm rostral to T12S; (3) L3S to 4 cm rostral to L3S; and (4) popliteal fossa to medial surface of the knee. Figure 13-4 illustrates tibial nerve SEP recordings obtained following the above configuration.

Anatomic and Physiologic Basis

Somatosensory evoked potential is primarily mediated via large diameter peripheral sensory fibers and the dorsal column-lemniscal pathways.[6,7,15,45,61] There is evidence from animal studies that extralemniscal activity may also play a role, particularly if the stimulus is sufficiently intense.[84]

With mixed nerve stimulation, group I muscle afferent nerves are depolarized, which results in a faster, shorter-latency SEP, as compared to stimulation of a slower group II cutaneous nerve.[15] Whether excitation of C and delta fibers also produce an SEP is subject to speculation.[4,114]

There is much less certainty about the generator sources of lower-extremity-nerve SEP as compared to the upper extremity. When recording electrodes are placed over the lower spine, two distinct potentials are recorded. One represents a propagated volley that increases in recorded latency from caudal to rostral. This wave represents the afferent volley in the cauda equina at caudal lumbar sites and the gracile tract rostrally.[38,109-113] This wave is attenuated with bipolar recording. A second potential, N22, is seen that remains constant in latency although the maximum amplitude is over the T10-L1 spinal area, which coincides with the termination of the conus medullaris at L1 or L2 (see Fig. 13-4, *B*).

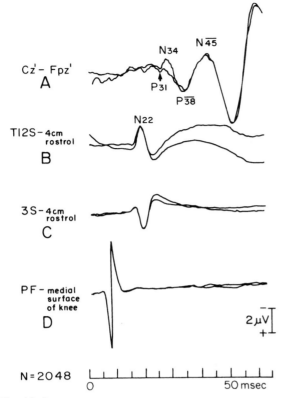

Fig. 13-4

Four-channel recording following tibial nerve stimulation at the ankle. **A,** Bipolar recording using standard scalp recording sites, Cz′ to Fpz′. Note that first identifiable wave occurs at P38. Small negative potential preceding P38 could be barely made out at N34. **B,** Spinal SEP recorded over the twelfth thoracic spine (T12S) referenced 4 cm rostrally. **C,** Spinal SEP recorded over the third lumbar spine (L3S) referenced 4 cm rostrally. **D,** Peripheral sensory recording over the popliteal fossa (PF). *(From Guidelines for somatosensory evoked potentials, Rochester, MN, 1984, American Association of Electrodiagnostic Medicine.)*

N22 provides a direct measure of dorsal-root integrity[38,111] and probably represents postsynaptic activity in the gray matter of the lumbar cord and is analogous to the N13 following median-nerve stimulation.[39]

P31 and N34 are two widely distributed scalp responses that are barely visible with bipolar recording (see Fig. 13-1). The precise sources of these wavelets are not known, but their similarity to P14 and N18 after median-nerve stimulation infer that they also reflect caudal medial lemniscus and subcortical postsynaptic activity in the thalamus and/or brainstem.[23,85]

The cortical components in a Cz′ to Fpz′ configuration results in virtual cancellation of all earlier wave forms, and P38 is the first readily visible potential (see Fig. 13-3, *A*). In most subjects, when the recording electrode is placed lateral to Cz, the

maximum amplitude is paradoxically ipsilateral to the side of stimulation. Some authors explain the phenomenon as the electrical reflection of the leg and foot primary sensory cortex, which is located in the mesial aspect of the postcentral gyrus within the interhemispheric fissure.[20,48,109] Although there are some investigators who contend that the earlier N34 reflects the somatosensory cortex,[24,28] it is generally believed that P38 represents activation of several regions within the primary sensory area for the leg and foot.[54,117]

Clinical Interpretation

Several pitfalls plague the clinician in interpreting SEPs. Because of the variation in techniques, it is necessary for each laboratory to establish its own normal values. Responses are evaluated by analyzing the absolute latency of the various components. Latency depends not only on limb length, height, and type of nerve stimulated, but also on temperature, state of wakefulness, type of recording, frequency band-pass setting, etc.* A positive correlation between height and SEP latency has been demonstrated[3,53] and should be taken into consideration (Fig. 13-5). To minimize the effect of temperature, ambient temperature must be kept between 20° C and 22° C. While short-latency SEPs are relatively unaffected by state of wakefulness, they nevertheless drop in amplitude and prolong their latencies during sleep.[38] This is significant since patients often doze off during the test and because some laboratories administer sedatives, such as diazepam, prior to SEP examination.[100]

Selecting the appropriate filter settings is often a juggling act. A common setting used is 30 to 3000 Hz. The low filter setting is a key element in reducing the background noise and enhancing reproducibility of the evoked response. Lowering the low filter setting to 1 Hz results in unacceptable SEP variability, while increasing it to 75 Hz markedly reduces the amplitude.[103]

Caution must be exercised when interpreting results in the pediatric and geriatric age groups, realizing that adult ranges may not be reached until about 8 to 12 years of age[25,89] and because values tend to be prolonged in the elderly.[25]

Deviation in latency or interpeak values by more than 3 standard deviations from the norm or 95% confidence interval related to height[99] is regarded as abnormal. A less stringent criteria results in an unacceptable percentage of false positive results.[7,8]

*References 3, 24, 25, 28, 35, 38, 49, 68, 89, and 103.

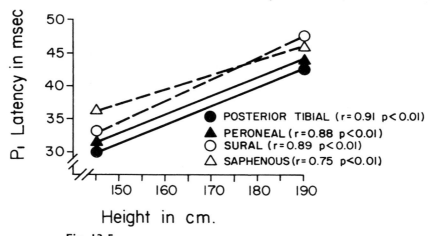

Fig. 13-5

Cortical SEPs as a function of height. The tibial, peroneal, sural, and saphenous nerves were stimulated at the ankle, and SEPs were recorded using Cz′ to Fz′ montage. *(From Gonzalez EG, Hajdu M, Bruno R, et al.: Lumbar spinal stenosis: an analysis of pre- and post-operative somatosensory evoked potentials, Arch Phys Med Rehabil 66:11, 1985, with permission.)*

Moreover, side-to-side difference in amplitude of more than 50% is also often considered abnormal, although such variation may occasionally occur even among normal individuals.[6] Wave form morphology is more subjective and more difficult to substantiate. To quantitate dispersion of SEPs, the fast Fourier transform technique has been employed.[28]

Indications

Although several studies have reported the use of SEP in many disease states, the fact remains that SEPs are never pathognomonic of any specific disease.

Radiculopathy

Eisen and Aminoff[30] have suggested several indications for using SEPs in evaluating peripheral nerve pathology: (1) to measure nerve conduction in anatomic sites not routinely accessible to routine studies; (2) to document axonal continuity in the absence of sensory nerve action potential; (3) to evaluate plexopathies; and (4) to evaluate radiculopathies, particularly when sensory signs or symptoms predominate. The last indication is the topic of discussion in this chapter.

To ensure that an abnormal SEP is not due to central nervous system (CNS) pathology, central conduction time (CCT) should be determined.[30] CCT can be obtained by subtracting cortical SEP latencies from the cervical or lumbar spinal potential, which should not exceed 7.5 msec in the arm and

22.5 msec in the leg. It is likewise important to rule out peripheral neuropathy by clinical and standard electrodiagnostic tests before attributing SEP abnormalities to spinal nerve root pathology.

While new imaging techniques have greatly facilitated the anatomic localization of root lesions, they remain inadequate in defining the physiologic changes that ensue, nor do they provide information regarding severity or prognosis. For these reasons, various electrophysiologic examinations are used in their conjunction.

Electromyography (EMG) and nerve-conduction velocity (NCV) studies are the standard electrophysiologic examinations in radiculopathy.[67] The presence of fibrillations or positive waves in the paraspinal muscles are the only definitive means of delineating radicular involvement in a specific myotome. However, it takes 7 days or more for these potentials to appear, and they are notably absent in neuropraxia. The interpretation of EMG recruitment pattern is subjective at best, and its computerized analysis awaits refinement.

Radiculopathy implies pathology proximal to the dorsal root ganglion, and therefore, the conventional sensory conduction velocities are unaffected. The amplitude of M response has been used by some to define severity,[67] but routine motor-nerve conduction velocities are likewise unrevealing. The use of F waves[73] and H reflex[12] have initially been heralded as major breakthroughs, but these techniques have fallen short of their initial promise. F waves require supramaximal stimulation of mixed nerves, which re-

which results in multisegmental activation, thus masking pathology in a single root. Consequently, F waves are frequently normal in radiculopathy. H reflex on the other hand is limited to the gastrosoleus (S1 sensory root), although it could be facilitated in other muscles by voluntary contraction.[33] These factors contribute to the reported 25% to 50% false negative EMG/NCV examinations despite definitive radiologic or clinical findings.[9,77,115]

The predominant presenting signs and symptoms in radiculopathy are sensory in nature. In these circumstances, type Ia afferent and type II cutaneous fibers are most likely affected.[53] This is a perfect rationale why SEPs have been employed by several investigators in evaluating radiculopathies.*

Several methods have been advanced in exploring the best technique to unravel the causative pathologic root(s). For the same reasons that F waves have a low yield, mixed nerve stimulation to elicit an SEP is often unproductive.[36,42,120] It is conceivable that patients with altered position and vibration senses or altered two-point discrimination can present with abnormal mixed nerve SEP. However, these presentations would be unusual in early root compression.[32] Despite this limitation, Noterman and Vlek[91] found that tibial and deep peroneal, along with saphenous and sural nerve SEPs correlated well with surgical findings in 66% of cases. Keim et al.[72] found tibial-nerve SEP as a useful screen among patients with spinal stenosis. In a study of tibial nerve SEPs, Knutsson et al.[77] reported that a restitution of SEPs occurred after autotraction in four of five patients with low or abolished SEP. Cassvan and Sook Park[16] reported a 71% diagnostic yield using the peroneal nerve, while Feinsod et al.[40] reported that all 76 patients in their series with myelographically proved disc herniation at varying levels from L3-S1 showed abnormal peroneal SEP. These reports are contestable, realizing that the SEPs obtained after mixed nerve stimulation are derived from several segments, unless profound compression at several roots exists.

Segmental studies that include cutaneous nerve, dermatomal and motor point stimulation appear to be most promising.[29,32,34,69,83] The simplest technique consists of stimulating cutaneous nerves. However, recording of spinal SEP following cutaneous-nerve stimulation has been hampered by technical difficulties. The only spinal SEP parameter that can be measured with consistency is the latency,

which frequently tends to be absent in 50% of normal subjects.[99] Additionally, spinal SEP may remain normal, particularly in the lower extremity because of the long distance that must be traversed by the afferent pathway from point of stimulation to the recording site. In this situation, the normally conducting distal segment could potentially cancel out the slowing in the spinal nerve root, which is comparatively a very short segment.[6,7] For these reasons spinal SEPs are not used in isolation. With meticulous cutaneous-nerve stimulation technique, the quality of cortical and spinal SEPs are comparable to those obtained after mixed-nerve stimulation, although their latencies are longer and their amplitudes are lower.[32] As reported by Seyal et al.,[113] the combination of cortical and spinal SEPs increased the yield to 41%, in contrast to cortical SEPs alone, which has a reported low yield of 20%. The disappointing results reported in this particular study may have been skewed by the authors' criteria for scalp latency abnormality, which required absolute latency exceeding the 99% prediction interval on the height-latency curve, or an interleg latency difference exceeding the 99% prediction interval rather than the 95% confidence interval.[41] Perlik et al.[99] on the other hand, found scalp SEPs to be useful in detecting radiculopathy in 21 of 27 patients with clinical and computed tomography (CT) evidence of root injury. These investigators argued for using the criteria of a 95% tolerance limit to define abnormality, which provides a normal range for individual values and also considers population distribution as well as normal limits for a given sample size. In other studies, Eisen et al.[29,32,34] reported a 57% yield using cortical SEPs following cutaneous-nerve stimulation by using the criteria of latency exceeding 3 standard deviations along with a 50% reduction in amplitude, when the involved side is compared to SEP evoked by stimulation of a contralateral homologous nerve, or an ipsilateral nerve representative of a segment above or below the one in question.

The ability of dermatomal SEP to pinpoint specific nerve-root involvement, particularly in lumbosacral radiculopathy has been hailed as a major stride in the clinical application of SEP.[54,55] But there are also drawbacks to the technique, which requires the application of large stimulating electrode strips over "signature areas" (see Fig. 13-2). Pulses of up to 2.5 times sensory threshold are required to excite the cutaneous afferent nerves. Although the resultant evoked responses following dermatomal stimulation are relatively consistent, the wave forms are usually smaller and more dispersed than either mixed- or cutaneous-nerve stimulation. The main

---

*References 16, 29, 32, 34, 36, 40, 41, 53 to 55, 62, 79, 91, 106, 107, 112, and 113.

advantage of the technique is its potential to examine just about any dermatome. Proponents believe this method to be an advantageous, noninvasive and repeatable diagnostic and prognostic tool, particularly in situations in which clinical and anatomic information are inconclusive.[54,55,70,79,107] In a study of 38 patients with disc herniation, Scarff et al.[107] stimulated the medial aspect of the first toe (L5) and the fifth toe (S1), and reported the technique to confirm 92% of cases. Green et al.[54,55] likewise found a high correlation (90%) between dermatomal SEP and the side of complaint among patients with low-back pain. Saal et al.[106] studied the value of dermatomal SEPs for upper lumbar radiculopathy and demonstrated a high positive predictive value, suggesting a strong correlation between SEP with anatomic abnormalities noted on CT, magnetic resonance imaging (MRI), and discograms. Other investigators, however, remain skeptical.[8,108] In an attempt to prevent any ambiguity, Aminoff et al.[9] restricted their selection to 19 subjects with definitive clinical and radiographic evidence of unilateral L5 and/or S1 radiculopathy. In this particular series, the dermatomal SEPs correctly localized the lesion in only five cases. Dermatomal SEPs correctly lateralized the lesion in only one case, but pinpointed the lesion incorrectly at an adjacent root. Furthermore, Aminoff et al.[9] found misleading information in 10 cases, in which 9 were interpreted as being normal, and 1 abnormality was detected on the wrong side. The controversy regarding dermatomal SEPs probably lies in the types of patients selected for the various reports and the criteria used by the different investigators in defining abnormality. It is quite feasible that further refinement of technique and interpretation will enhance the usefulness of this method.

The disparate involvement between the early and late cortical SEPs in radicular syndromes has been observed by Gonzalez and Hajdu.[50] In many instances, the early potentials tend to be prolonged, or sometimes absent, while the later waves fall within normal limits. This behavior is akin to those found in tourniquet paralysis, pointing to the possible roles played by both ischemia and compression.

In a recent development, Tsuji, Murai, and Yarita[116] used magnetic stimulation at the thoracic and lumbar regions, as well as the gluteal fold and ankle to obtain SEPs. The technique proved useful in evaluating the spinal roots and rostral SEP pathways in an effective and expeditious fashion, as compared to standard electrical stimulation. The authors offered the magnetic stimulation as a noninvasive alternative to electrical stimulation of the spinal cord, cauda equina, and sciatic nerve, which are often dif-ficult to perform. The disadvantage of the method is the restriction of the number of stimuli that can be delivered because the magnetic coil heats excessively if stimulation is delivered more than 64 times.

Another variation of employing SEPs in radiculopathy requires the transmission of a stimulus of at least 1.0-msec duration through a needle electrode inserted in the motor point. This activates type Ia muscle afferents and produces consistently reproducible evoked potentials. While the method has the potential to be helpful in evaluating radiculopathies, like mixed-nerve stimulation, it cannot isolate a single nerve root.[30]

Functional versus Organic Sensory Complaints

To establish whether a sensory complaint has an organic basis is a frequent dilemma in clinical practice. The medicolegal implications are self-evident. For the most part, a normal SEP and peripheral sensory examination would indicate that sensory symptoms have no pathologic basis. This conclusion, however, should be weighed carefully, for indeed, there are exceptions to the rule. One such example is the presence of normal SEPs in pure sensory stroke secondary to lacunar infarcts.[102]

Intraoperative Monitoring

A delicate balance is needed to provide maximum decompression while preserving neural integrity during spinal surgery. SEP monitoring has been employed for this purpose to predict neurologic outcome and to minimize postoperative morbidity. SEP provides electrophysiologic monitoring under anesthesia and has been used in lieu of a crude examination in a lightly anesthetized patient.[56,57]

Various intraoperative SEP techniques have been described in the past, employing either cortical SEP, spinal SEP, or both.* The experiences learned from scoliosis surgery have spilled over to surgeries intended to decompress spinal nerve roots. The SEP aquisition parameters during preoperative and intraoperative periods are held constant, with a few exceptions. For instance, needle electrodes are preferred to surface cup electrodes to facilitate quick placement in the intraoperative setting. To improve spinal recordings, several permutations have been advanced. Nordwall et al.[90] used Kirshner wire in the lumbar spine, while Jones and Small[68] utilized epidural recordings. Lueders et al.[82] reported a sim-

*References 14, 37, 51, 52, 56, and 92 to 94.

ple technique to obtain spinal SEPs that required the insertion of a needle electrode only in the interspinous ligament. Stimulation employing a constant current is preferred over constant voltage in order to overcome the fluctuating skin resistance at the stimulation site.

Various operating room equipment and machineries interfere with SEPs. Perhaps the most important precautionary measures to observe are the careful insertion of all electrodes and the isolation of the SEP equipment from all other power sources.[51,52,56]

A balanced anesthesia consisting of nitrous oxide/oxygen, thiopenthane, pancuronium, D-tubocurarine, are the agents of choice.[37,51,95] Halogenated agents are reported to be incompatible with intraoperative SEPs[56] but there are reports to the contrary, indicating that controlled doses of halothane, enflurane and isoflurane are compatible with intraoperative monitoring.[51,52,95] Bolus injections of any medication are avoided during critical periods of monitoring.[51,52,56] Hypotension is often induced during spinal surgery in order to reduce blood loss, despite its attenuating effect on SEP amplitude.[57] Gonzalez et al.[52] found that SEP values obtained during the period of hypotension provided the best baseline information with which subsequent periods can be compared. The surgeon is cautioned if SEP latency is prolonged by more than 8% to 10% of base line and/or when amplitude decrement approaches 50%.[51,52] Based on their experience in more than 2000 cases, Meyer et al.[87] established a protocol to minimize the risk of neurologic sequelae in case of SEP deterioration, such as increasing the inspired oxygen, elevating the mean blood pressure, ceasing further inhalation agents, discontinuing instrumentation or distraction, and irrigating the wound with warm saline and hydrogen peroxide. If SEPs fail to return, dexamethasone 50 to 100 mg intravenous push is administered, all hardware is removed, and reevaluation is done over a 60-minute period. Out of 184 cases monitored by Harper et al.,[63] postoperative neurologic deficits developed in 4 patients, 2 of whom demonstrated evidence of lumbar radiculopathy that were not detected by SEP monitoring. These authors emphasized the importance of stimulating each leg individually as well as simultaneously and to continue the monitoring until skin closure.

It is often believed that SEP is carried primarily through the posterior columns, and despite injury to the anterior portion of the cord, SEP is most likely preserved. However, there is evidence that the entire transverse diameter of the spinal cord will be infarcted if vascular injury occurs distal to the feeder,

and therefore results in abnormal SEP.[37] The debate continues whether SEP is the appropriate response to monitor. Indeed, there are reports of false negative monitoring,[46,79] but a number of clinical studies continue to demonstrate its usefulness.*

Owing to the perceived deficiencies of SEP monitoring, attention has gradually shifted toward monitoring the motor tracts. New variations have evolved in recent years. Levy[80] introduced the use of transcortical electrical stimulation, and techniques are being explored utilizing magnetic stimulation.[26,27,44,76,101]

A more recent application of intraoperative monitoring is in decompressive spinal surgery for spinal stenosis.[43,59] A recent analysis of intraoperative predecompression and postdecompression SEP values among spinal stenosis patients by Hajdu et al.[59] showed a statistically significant improvement in the decompressed nerves. Monitoring under these circumstances provides the surgeon some guidance as to the adequacy of decompression or may unfold a previously unrecognized pathology. The same sentiments are shared by Gepstein and Brown,[43] who concluded that intraoperative SEP testing is valuable in determining the adequacy of lumbar nerve root decompression and for prediction of successful relief of symptoms. Preoperative and postoperative SEPs were analyzed by Gonzalez et al.[53] in a group of 20 patients with spinal stenosis and found significant improvement in latencies and amplitudes of the involved nerves. The immediate relief of root compression and the subsequent increase in available numbers of functioning large-diameter myelinated fibers, conversion from conduction block to normal conduction and improved axoplasmic flow were hypothesized as mechanisms for the quick reversal of pathologic findings. Figure 13-6 typifies preoperative and postoperative SEP findings in a patient with multiple-level spinal stenosis.

Motor Evoked Responses

The electrical, thermal, and magnetic energies following TCS are known to be less than, if not comparable to electroconvulsive therapy and MRI. To date, no case of seizure has been reported in the literature. Goddard et al.[47] have indicated that such kindling is unlikely if the stimulus is less than 3 Hz. In TCS, the maximum rate is no greater than 0.3 Hz. Apart from transient headaches and memory lapse, no adverse effects have been reported.[13,18,64,104] Using a pendulum model, Katz et al.[71] showed that

---

*References 14, 37, 51, 52, 56, 92, and 93.

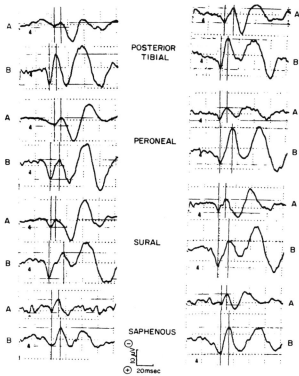

Fig. 13-6

Cortical SEP recordings preoperative (*A*) and postoperative (*B*) in a 46-year-old woman, 161 cm in height, with 2-year history of back pain and radiculopathy at the right L4, L5, S1. Note 10-day postoperative improvement in SEP latencies and amplitudes. The recordings were enhanced 4 times. *(From Gonzalez EG, Hajdu M, Bruno R, et al.: Lumbar spinal stenosis: an analysis of pre- and post-operative somatosensory evoked potentials, Arch Phys Med Rehabil 66:11, 1985, with permission.)*

only a minuscule amount of energy is imparted onto metallic fixation devices by the magnetic coil, but no significant paraspinal activity could be detected among healthy volunteers. However, it is prudent to consider the following as contraindications: individuals with known seizures, history of unconsciousness after head injury, cranial surgery, and those with implanted biomedical devices.[31]

Stimulation Technique

In magnetic stimulation, a high-energy capacitor bank is charged from a high-voltage source through a copper coil, which produces a brief magnetic field pulse. Unlike an electrical field, a magnetic field penetrates biologic structures without significant attenuation and the field travels in an anular fashion, with the highest intensity under the coil's circumference.[104]

In all types of TCS, surface electrodes are placed

over a target muscle to record the MEP. It has been observed that placement of the active recording electrode over the motor end plate with the reference electrode at a distant site resulted in higher-amplitude MEPs.[31]

The locations of optimal cortical sites for TCS correlate well with the "motor strip." Thus, Rossini[104] found the lowest threshold for eliciting MEP in the hand on the contralateral side, lateral to the vertex, and slightly frontal to the line connecting the earlobes. Stimulation of the vertex on the other hand results in bilateral MEPs in the lower extremities. The best method to apply the magnetic coil is still subject to conjecture.[31] Cervical[19] and lumbar[11] spinal stimulation, as well as peripheral nerves are achieved with relative ease using magnetic stimulation.

Anatomic and Physiologic Basis

The simplistic notion that a single TCS shock causes a synchronous depolarization of groups of cortical motor neurons, which in turn produces a single efferent volley that is propagated down their axons to spinal motor neurons, depolarizing the α motor neurons and after a short synaptic delay results in the eventual activation of the muscle, is attractive but highly unlikely. It is doubtful that only the pyramidal tracts are activated.[121]

A robust MEP amplitude results following different maneuvers that apparently lower the excitability threshold, such as voluntary contraction of the target muscle shortly prior or during TCS, nonspecific maneuvers such as sticking out the tongue, counting aloud, and postural facilitation.[2,31,66,96,97,104,105] This phenomenon may be due to facilitation of a large population of spinal motor neurons through group I afferent activity from muscles and tendons in addition to the enhanced firing of descending corticospinal tracts.[104]

MEPs in the hand are larger in amplitude than the leg or foot muscles. The deeper location of the lower-extremity homunculus in the interhemispheric fissure could explain the discrepancy. The relative abundance of pyramidal-tract fibers in the cervical cord as compared to the rest of the spinal cord is an added explanation.[78]

MEP latency to magnetic stimulation has been observed to be longer as compared to electrical stimulation.[18,22,88] It is possible that the extra delay is consumed in the central motor pathways. Another hypothesis suggests that magnetic stimulation excites the corticospinal neurons transynaptically, whereas electrical stimulation excites them directly.[22]

Clinical Interpretation

Like SEPs, several factors are considered to determine normal versus abnormal responses. No single normative values are universally applicable because of differing techniques. As with SEPs, there is positive correlation between arm length and height and MEP latency.[31] Side-to-side comparison may be more difficult to apply in TCS MEP than with SEPs. It has been observed that side-to-side difference in latencies commonly occurs even among healthy subjects and statistically significant amplitude difference has been reported, particularly in the lower extremity.[31,104] However, it may be a safe assumption that a 50% amplitude difference can be considered abnormal. To avert such a variable, the amplitude can be expressed as a percentage of maximum peripheral M response, which is almost never less than 20%. A value less than 10% is considered abnormal.[31]

Clinical Indications

Measurements of MEPs using magnetic TCS among 268 patients with cervical spine disorders was performed by Dvorak et al.[27] Their data suggest that the method has a high sensitivity in detecting compression of the neural structure, particularly among those with degenerative changes. They also found a high incidence of abnormal central conduction times among patients with whiplash injuries despite absence of major motor deficit. The same group of researchers previously established their normative data after cervical spine and plexus stimulation in the axillary region.[26] They hailed the technique as a major advance in spinal cord diagnostics and motor-root compression in the intervertebral foramen or canal. Application to lumbosacral radiculopathy is forthcoming.

Transcranial electrical stimulation holds promise in intraoperative monitoring. Levy[81] has reviewed his extensive experience in employing the technique during spinal procedures. He found that peripheral nerve or electromyographic responses were substantially more sensitive than the spinal cord responses to injury and hypotension. Reversal of abnormalities did not result in any deficit, but their failure to recover could warn of postoperative motor defect. Kitagawa et al.[76] recorded MEP from epidural electrodes and found the technique to be a satisfactory predictor of outcome in a small group of patients undergoing cervical spinal surgery. In addition to epidural recording, Preston et al.[101] improved on the method by adding MEP recordings subpially and obtained larger, more consistent amplitudes. For now, the use of magnetic stimulation in the operating room should be performed under research protocol.

The use of magnetic stimulation to evaluate the peripheral nervous system is enticing, particularly because of the relative ease with which proximal and deeply situated nerves can be stimulated.[31] The restricted focusing of the currently available magnetic coils, however, limits its usefulness for stimulating peripheral nerves. Its main domain in peripheral nervous system evaluation may rest in its ability to evaluate the proximal segments of peripheral motor nerves including spinal nerve roots through TCS and spinal stimulation.

Conclusion

A new era in electroneurophysiology has emerged. The boundaries have all but vanished with new methods and improved techniques. The ultimate utility of evoked potentials in radicular syndromes still awaits refinement, but they are likely to be invaluable in the very near future. Currently, it offers new electrophysiologic venues to explore inaccessible portions of the nervous system.

References

1. Abrahamson HA, Allison T, Goff WR, Rossner BS: Effects of thiopenthal on human cerebral somatic evoked potential, *Anesthesiology* 24:650, 1963.
2. Ackerman H, Scholz E, Koehler W, et al.: Influence of posture and voluntary background muscle action potentials from anterior tibial and soleus muscle following transcranial magnetic stimulation, *Electroencephalogr Clin Neurophysiol* 81:71, 1991.
3. Alonso JA, Hajdu M, Gonzalez EG, et al.: Cortical somatosensory evoked potentials: effects of positional changes, *Arch Phys Med Rehabil* 70:194, 1989.
4. Alpsan D: The effect of selective activation of different peripheral nerve fiber groups on the somatosensory evoked potentials in the cat, *Electroencephalogr Clin Neurophysiol* 51:589, 1981.
5. American Association of Electrodiagnostic Medicine: *Guidelines for somatosensory evoked potentials*, Rochester MN, 1984, American Association of Electrodiagnostic Medicine.
6. Aminoff MJ: The use of somatosensory evoked potentials in the evaluation of the central nervous system, *Neurol Clin* 6:809, 1988.
7. Aminoff MJ: Use of somatosensory evoked potentials to evaluate the peripheral nervous system, *J Clin Neurophysiol* 4(2):135, 1987.
8. Aminoff MJ, Goodin DS, Barbaro NM, et al.: Dermatomal somatosensory evoked potentials in unilateral lumbosacral radiculopathy, *Ann Neurol* 17:171, 1985.

9. Aminoff MJ, Goodin DS, Parry GJ, et al.: Electrophysiological evaluation of lumbosacral radiculopathies: electromyography, late responses, and somatosensory evoked potentials, *Neurology* 35:1514, 1985.

10. Barker AT, Jalinour R, Freeston IL: Non-invasive magnetic stimulation of the human motor cortex, *Lancet* 1:1106, 1985.

11. Booth KR, Streletz LJ, Raab VE, et al.: Motor evoked potential and central motor conduction: studies of transcranial magnetic stimulation with recording from the leg, *Electroencephalogr Clin Neurophysiol* 81:57, 1991.

12. Braddom RL, Johnson EW: Standardization of H reflex and diagnostic use in S1 radiculopathy, *Arch Phys Med Rehabil* 55:161, 1966.

13. Bridgers S, Delaney R: Transcranial magnetic stimulation: an assessment of cognitive and other cerebral effects, *Neurology* 39:417, 1989.

14. Brown RH, Nash CL: Current status of spinal cord monitoring, *Spine* 4:466, 1979.

15. Burke D, Skuse NF, Lethlean AK: Cutaneous and muscle afferent components of cerebral potential evoked by electrical stimulation of human peripheral nerves, *Electroencephalogr Clin Neurophysiol* 51:579, 1981.

16. Cassvan A, Sook Park Y: Cortical somatosensory evoked potentials following peroneal nerve stimulation in lumbosacral radiculopathies, *Electromyogr Clin Neurophysiol* 23:393, 1983.

17. Cowan JMA, Dick JPR, Day BL, et al.: Abnormalities in central motor pathway conduction in multiple sclerosis, *Lancet* 2:304, 1984.

18. Cracco RQ: Evaluation of conduction in control motor pathways: technique, pathophysiology, and clinical interpretation, *Neurosurgery* 20:199, 1987.

19. Cres D, Chiappa KH, Gominak S, et al.: Cervical magnetic stimulation, *Neurology* 40:1751, 1990.

20. Cruse R, Klem G, Lesser RP, et al.: Paradoxical lateralization of cortical potentials evoked by stimulation of posterior tibial nerve, *Arch Neurol* 39:222, 1982.

21. Dawson GD: Investigations in a patient subject to myoclonic seizures after sensory stimulation, *J Neurol Neurosurg Psychiatry* 10:141, 1947.

22. Day BL, Thompson PD, Dick JP, et al.: Different sites of action of electrical and magnetic stimulation of the human brain, *Neurosci Lett* 75:101, 1987.

23. Desmedt JE, Cheron G: Non-cephalic reference recording of early somatosensory potentials to finger stimulation in adult or aging normal man: Differentiation of widespread N18 and contralateral N20 from the prerolandic P22 and N30 components, *Electroencephalogr Clin Neurophysiol* 52:553, 1981.

24. Dorfman LJ: Indirect estimation of spinal cord conduction velocity in man, *Electroencephalogr Clin Neurophysiol* 42:26, 1977.

25. Dorfman LJ, Bosley TM: Age-related changes in peripheral and central nerve conduction in man, *Neurology* 29:38, 1979.

26. Dvorak J, Herdmann J, Theiler R: Magnetic transcranial brain stimulation: painless evaluation of central motor pathways, normal values and clinical application in spinal cord diagnostics: upper extremities, *Spine* 15:155, 1990.

27. Dvorak J, Herdmann J, Janssen B, et al.: Motor evoked potentials in patients with cervical spine disorders, *Spine* 15(10):1013, 1990.

28. Eisen A: The somatosensory evoked potentials, *Can J Neurol Sci* 9:65, 1982.

29. Eisen A: Electrodiagnosis of radiculopathies, *Neurol Clin* 3:495, 1985.

30. Eisen A, Aminoff MJ: *Somatosensory evoked potentials,* In Aminoff MJ, editor: *Electrodiagnosis in clinical neurology,* ed 2, New York, 1986, Churchill-Livingstone, p 532.

31. Eisen AS, Shtybel W: Clinical experience with transcranial magnetic stimulation, *Muscle Nerve* 13:995, 1990.

32. Eisen A, Hoirch M, Moll A: Evaluation of radiculopathies by segmental stimulation and somatosensory evoked potentials, *Can J Neurol Sci* 10(3):178, 1983.

33. Eisen A, Hoirch M, White J, et al.: Sensory group Ia proximal conduction velocity, *Muscle Nerve* 7:636, 1984.

34. Eisen A: The use of somatosensory evoked potentials for the evaluation of the peripheral nervous system, *Neurol Clin* 6:825, 1988.

35. Eisen A, Roberts K, Low M, et al.: Questions regarding the sequential neural generator theory of the somatosensory evoked potential raised by digital filtering, *Electroencephalogr Clin Neurophysiol* 63:384, 1986.

36. El Negamy E, Sedgwick EM: Delayed cervical somatosensory potentials in cervical spondylosis, *J Neurol Neurosurg Psychiatry* 42:238, 1979.

37. Engler GL, Spielholz NI, Bernhard WN, et al.: Somatosensory evoked potentials during Harrington instrumentation for scoliosis, *J Bone Joint Surg* 60A:528, 1978.

38. Emerson RG: Anatomical physiologic basis of posterior tibial nerve somatosensory evoked potentials, *Neurol Clin* 6:735, 1988.

39. Emerson RG, Seyal M, Pedley TA: Somatosensory evoked potentials following median nerve stimulation, 1. The cervical components, *Brain* 107:169, 1984.

40. Feinsod M, Blau D, Findler G, et al.: Somatosensory evoked potential to peroneal nerve stimulation in patients with herniated lumbar discs, *Neurosurgery* 11:506, 1982.

41. Fischer MA: SSEPs in lumbar radialopathy, *Neurology* 40:287, 1990.

42. Ganes T: Somatosensory conduction times and peripheral cervical and cortical evoked potentials in patients with cervical spondylosis, *J Neurol Neurosurg Psychiatry* 43:683, 1980.

43. Gepstein R, Brown M: Somatosensory-evoked potentials in lumbar nerve root decompression, *Clin Orthop Relat Res* 245:69, 1989.

44. Gianutsos J, Eberstein A, Ma D, et al.: A non-invasive technique to assess completeness of spinal cord lesions in humans, *Exp Neurol* 98:34, 1987.

45. Giblin DR: SEP in healthy subjects and in patients with lesions of the nervous system, *Ann N Y Acad Sci* 122:93, 1964.

46. Ginsburg HH, Shetter AG, Raudzens PA: Postoperative paraplegia with preserved intraoperative somatosensory evoked potentials, *J Neurosurg* 63:296, 1985.

47. Goddard GV, McIntyre DC, Leech CK: A permanent change in brain function resulting from daily electrical stimulation, *Exp Neurol* 25:295, 1969.

48. Goff WR, Allison T, Vaughan HG Jr: *The functional neuroanatomy of event-related potentials,* In Callaway E, Tueting P, Koslow SH, editors: *Event-related brain potentials in man,* New York, 1978, Academic Press, p 1.

49. Gonzalez EG, Berman WS, Hajdu M: Influence of height and type of lower extremity nerve tested on P1 somatosensory evoked potential latency, *Arch Phys Med Rehabil* 64:502, 1983.

50. Gonzalez EG, Hajdu M: Disparate involvement of short and long latency somatosensory evoked potentials in nerve root decompression, *Arch Phys Med Rehabil* 64:494, 1983.

51. Gonzalez EG, Hajdu M, Keim HA, et al.: Intraoperative somatosensory evoked potential monitoring, *Orthop Rev* 13:47, 1984.

52. Gonzalez EG, Hajdu M, Keim HA, et al.: Quantification of intraoperative somatosensory evoked potential, *Arch Phys Med Rehabil* 65:721, 1984.

53. Gonzalez EG, Hajdu M, Bruno R, et al.: Lumbar spinal stenosis: analysis of pre- and postoperative somatosensory evoked potentials, *Arch Phys Med Rehabil* 66:11, 1985.

54. Green J, Gildenmeister R, Hazelwood C: Dermatomally stimulated somatosensory cerebral evoked potentials in the clinical diagnosis of lumbar disc disease, *Clin Electroencephalogr* 14:152, 1983.

55. Green J, Hamm A, Benfante P, et al.: Clinical effectiveness of dermatomal evoked cerebrally recorded somatosensory responses, *Clin Electroencephalogr* 19(1):14, 1988.

56. Grundy BL: Monitoring of sensory evoked potentials during neurosurgical operations: methods and applications, *Neurosurgery* 11:556, 1982.

57. Grundy BL, Nash CL, Brown RH: Deliberate hypotension for scoliosis surgery, *Anesthesiology* 51:578, 1979.

58. Gualtierotti J, Paterson AS: Electrical stimulation of the unexposed cerebral cortex, *J Physiol* 125:278, 1954.

59. Hajdu M, Gonzalez EG, Michelsen C: Somatosensory evoked potential as an intraoperative measure of lumbar nerve root decompression, *Arch Phys Med Rehabil* 67:618, 1986.

60. Haldeman S, Bradley WE, Bhatia N, et al.: Pudendal evoked responses, *Arch Neurol* 39:280, 1982.

61. Halliday AM: Changes in the form of cerebral evoked responses in man associated with various lesions of the nervous system, *Electroencephalogr Clin Neurophysiol* 25:178, 1967.

62. Hallstrom YT, Lindblom U, Meyerson BA: Distribution of lumbar spinal evoked potentials and their correlation with stimulation-induced paresthesiae, *Electroencephalogr Clin Neurophysiol* 80:126, 1991.

63. Harper CM Jr, Daube JR, Litchy WJ, et al.: Lumbar radiculopathy after spinal fusion for scoliosis, *Muscle Nerve* 11:386, 1988.

64. Hess CW, Mills KR, Murray MF: Responses in small hand muscles from magnetic stimulation of the human brain, *J Physiol* 388:397, 1987.

65. Hess CW, Mills KR, Murray NM, et al.: Magnetic brain stimulation: central motor conduction studies in multiple sclerosis, *Ann Neurol* 22:744, 1987.

66. Hufnagel A, Jaeger MN, Elger CE: Transcranial magnetic stimulation: specific and non-specific facilitation of magnetic motor evoked potentials, *J Neurol* 237:416, 1990.

67. Johnson EW, Melvin JL: Value of electromyography in lumbar radiculopathy, *Arch Phys Med Rehabil* 52:239, 1971.

68. Jones SJ, Small DG: Spinal and subcortical evoked potentials following stimulation of posterior tibial nerve in man, *Electroencephalogr Clin Neurophysiol* 44:299, 1978.

69. Jorg G, Dullberg W, Koeppen S: *Diagnostic value of segmental somatosensory evoked potentials in cases with chronic progressive para- or tetraspastic syndromes.* In Courjon J, Mauguiere F, Revol M, editors: *Clinical applications of evoked potentials in neurology,* New York, 1982, Raven Press, p 347.

70. Katifi HA, Segwich EM: Evaluation of the dermatomal somatosensory evoked potential in the diagnosis of lumbo-sacral root compression, *J Neurol Neurosurg Psychiatry* 50:1204, 1987.

71. Katz RT, Vanden Berg C, Weinberger D, et al.: Magnetoelectric stimulation of human motor cortex: normal values and potential safety issues in spinal cord injury, *Arch Phys Med Rehabil* 71:597, 1990.

72. Keim H, Hajdu M, Gonzalez EG: Somatosensory evoked potential as a diagnostic aid in the diagnosis and intraoperative management of spinal stenosis, *Spine* 10:338, 1985.

73. Kimura J: F-wave velocity in the central segment of the median and ulnar nerves: a study in normal subjects and in patients with Charcot-Marie-Tooth disease, *Neurology* 24:539, 1974.

74. Kimura J, Mitsudome A, Beck DO: Field distribution of anitdromically activated digital nerve potentials: model for far field recording, *Neurology* 33:1164, 1983.

75. Kimura J, Mitsudome A, Yamada T: Stationary peaks from a moving source in a far field recording, *Electroencephalogr Clin Neurophysiol* 58:351, 1984.

76. Kitagama H, Itoh T, Takano H, et al.: Motor evoked potential monitoring during upper cervical spine surgery, *Spine* 14:1078, 1989.

77. Knutsson E, Skoglund CR, Natchev E: Changes in voluntary muscle strength, somatosensory transmission and skin temperature concomitant with pain relief during autotraction in patients with lumbar and sacral root lesions, *Pain* 33:173, 1988.

78. Lassek AM: The human pyramidal tract. II, A numerical investigation of the Betz cells of the motor area, *Arch Neurol Psychiatry* 44:718, 1940.

79. Lesser RP, Raudzens P, Luders H, et al.: Postoperative neurological deficits may occur despite unchanged intraoperative somatosensory evoked potentials, *Ann Neurol* 19:22, 1986.

80. Levy WJ: Spinal evoked potentials from the motor tracts, *J Neurosurg* 58:38, 1983.

81. Levy WJ: Clinical experience with motor and cerebellar evoked potential monitoring, *Neurosurgery* 20:169, 1987.

82. Lueders H, Gurd A, Hahn J, et al.: New technique for intraoperative monitoring of spinal cord function: multichannel recording of spinal cord and subcortical evoked potentials, *Spine* 7:110, 1982.

83. Lueders H, Lesser RP, Hahn J, et al.: Cortical somatosensory evoked potentials in response to hand stimulation, *J Neurosurg* 58:885, 1983.

84. Martin HF, Katz S, Blackburn JG: Effects of spinal cord lesion on somatic evoked potentials altered by interactions between afferent inputs, *Electroencephalogr Clin Neurophysiol* 50:186, 1980.

85. Mauguiere F, Desmedt JE, Courjon J: Neural generators of N18 and P14 far-field somatosensory evoked potentials studied in patients with lesions of thalamus or thalamocortical radiations, *Electroencephalogr Clin Neurophysiol* 56:283, 1983.

86. Merton PA, Morton HB: Stimulation of the cerebral cortex in the intact human subject, *Nature* 285:227, 1980.

87. Meyer PR Jr, Cotler H, Gireesan GT: Operative neurological complications resulting from thoracic and lumbar spine internal fixation, *Clin Orthop Relat Res* 237:125, 1988.

88. Mills KR, Murray NM, Hess CW: Magnetic and electrical transcranial brain stimulation: physiological mechanisms and clinical applications, *Neurosurgery* 20:164, 1987.

89. Mutoh K, Hojo H, Mikawa H: Maturation study of short latency somatosensory evoked potentials after posterior tibial nerve stimulation in infants and children, *Clin Electroencephalogr* 20:91, 1989.

90. Nordwall A, Axelgaard J, Harado Y, et al.: Spinal cord monitoring using evoked potentials recorded from vertebral bone in cat, *Spine* 4:486, 1979.

91. Noterman SLH, Vlek NMT: Cortical and spinal somatosensory evoked potentials in patients suffering from lumbosacral disc prolapse, *Electromyogr Clin Neurophysiol* 28:33, 1988.

92. Nuwer MR: Use of somatosensory evoked potentials for intraoperative monitoring of cerebral and spinal cord function, *Neurol Clin* 6:881, 1988.

93. Nuwer MR: *Evoked potential monitoring in the operating room,* New York, 1986, Raven Press.

94. Nuwer M, Dawson E: Intraoperative evoked potential monitoring of the spinal cord: a restricted filter, scalp method during Harrington instrumentation for scoliosis, *Clin Orthop* 183:42, 1984.

95. Pathak CS, Amaddio MD, Scoles PV, et al.: Effects of halothane, enflurane, and isoflurane in nitrous oxide on multilevel somatosensory evoked potentials, *Anesthesiology* 70:207, 1989.

96. Patton HD, Amassian VE: Single and multiple unit analysis of cortical stage of pyramidal tract activation, *J Neurophysiol* 17:345, 1954.

97. Patton HD, Amassian VE: *The pyramidal tract: its excitation and functions,* In Field J, editor: *Handbook of physiology-neurophysiology,* Washington, DC, 1960, American Physiological Society, p 237.

98. Pelosi L, Balbi P, Caruso G: The effect of stimulus frequency on spinal and scalp somatosensory evoked potentials to stimulation of nerves in the lower limb, *Electroencephalogr Clin Neurophysiol* 41:149, 1990.

99. Perlik S, Fisher MA, Patel DV, et al.: On the usefulness of somatosensory evoked responses for the evaluation of lower back pain, *Arch Neurol* 43:907, 1986.

100. Pfeiffer FE, Peterson L, Daube JR: Diazepan improves recording of lumbar and neck somatosensory evoked potentials, *Muscle Nerve* 12:473, 1989.

101. Preston B, Zgur T, Polenc VV: Epidural and subpial cortico-spinal potentials evoked by transcutaneous motor cortex stimulation during spinal cord surgery, *Electroencephalogr Clin Neurophysiol* 41:348, 1990.

102. Robinson RL, Richey ET, Kase CS: Somatosensory evoked potentials in pure sensory stroke and related conditions, *Stroke* 16:818, 1985.

103. Rossini PM, Cracco RQ, Cracco JB, et al.: Short latency somatosensory evoked potentials to peroneal nerve stimulation: scalp topography and effect of different frequency filters, *Electroencephalogr Clin Neurophysiol* 52:540, 1981.

104. Rossini PM: The anatomic and physiologic bases of motor-evoked potentials, *Neurol Clin* 6:751, 1988.

105. Rossini PM, Zarola F, Stalberg E, et al.: Pre-movement facilitation of motor evoked potentials in man during transcranial stimulation of the central motor pathways, *Brain Res* 458:20, 1988.

106. Saal JA, Firtch W, Assl JS, et al.: The value of somatosensory evoked potential, testing for upper lumbar radiculopathy: a correlation of electrophysiologic and anatomic data, *Spine Suppl* 17(6):133, 1992.

107. Scarff TB, Dallmann DE, Toleikis JR, et al.: Dermatomal somatosensory evoked potentials in the diagnosis of lumbar root entrapment, *Neurosurgery* 32:489, 1981.

108. Schmid UD, Hess CW, Ludin H-P: Somatosensory evoked potentials following nerve and segmental stimulation do not confirm cervical radiculopathy with sensory deficit, *J Neurol Neurosurg Psychiatry* 51:182, 1988.

109. Seyal M, Emerson RG, Pedley TA: Spinal and early scalp-recorded components of the somatosensory evoked potential following stimulation of the posterior tibial nerve, *Electroencephalogr Clin Neurophysiol* 55:320, 1983.

110. Seyal M, et al.: SSEP in lumbar radiculopathy, *Neurology* 40:386, 1990.

111. Seyal M, Gabor AJ: The human posterior tibial somatosensory evoked potential: synapse dependent and synapse independent spinal components, *Electroencephalogr Clin Neurophysiol* 62:323, 1985.

112. Seyal M, Palma GA, Sandhu LS, et al.: Spinal somatosensory evoked potentials following segmental sensory stimulation: a direct measure of dorsal root function, *Electroencephalogr Clin Neurophysiol* 69:390, 1988.

113. Seyal M, Sandhu LS, Mack YP: Spinal segmental somatosensory evoked potentials in lumbosacral radiculopathies, *Neurology* 39:801, 1989.

114. Simpson RK, Blackburn JG, Martin HS, et al.: Peripheral nerve fiber and spinal cord pathway contributions to the somatosensory evoked potentials, *Exp Neurol* 73:700, 1981.

115. Tonzola RF, Ackil AA, Shahani BT, et al.: Usefulness of electrophysiological studies in the diagnosis of lumbosacral root disease, *Ann Neurol* 9(3):305, 1981.

116. Tsuji S, Murai Y, Yarita M: Somatosensory potentials evoked by magnetic stimulation of lumbar roots cauda equina and leg nerves, *Ann Neurol* 24(4):568, 1988.

117. Tsumoto T, Hirose N, Nonaka S, et al.: Analysis of somatosensory evoked potentials to lateral popliteal nerve stimulation in man, *Electroencephalogr Clin Neurophysiol* 33:379, 1972.

118. Yamada T: The anatomic and physiologic bases of median nerve somatosensory evoked potentials, *Neurol Clin* 6:705, 1988.

119. Yamada T, Kimura J, Young S, et al.: Somatosensory evoked potentials elicited by bilateral stimulation of the median nerve and its clinical application, *Neurology* 28:218, 1978.

120. Yiannikas C, Shahani BT, Young RR: Short latency somatosensory evoked potential from radial, median, ulnar and peroneal nerve stimulation in the assessment of cervical spondylosis, *Arch Neurol* 43:1264, 1986.

121. Young RR, Cracco RQ: Clinical neurophysiology of conduction in control motor pathways, *Ann Neurol* 18:606, 1985.

Chapter 14

Discography

Nikolai Bogduk
Charles Aprill
Richard Derby

The term *discography* conveys different meanings to different people. Originally and classically it referred to a procedure in which contrast medium was instilled into the nucleus pulposus of an intervertebral disc in order to demonstrate its internal morphology. In contemporary practice, *discography* refers to provocation discography, the cardinal component of which is the reproduction of pain on injecting contrast medium or normal saline into the disc. Additional variants are analgesic discography, which aims to relieve disc pain by infiltrating the disc with local anesthetic, and CT discography in which the internal morphology of the disc is demonstrated by scanning the disc after instillation of contrast medium into the nucleus pulposus.

Historical Background

Lumbar Discography

Discography was developed in the late 1940s as a technique for diagnosing lumbar intervertebral disc herniation.[75-78] Previously, myelography had been the only means of confirming a suspected disc herniation, but myelography showed only the space-occupying effect of the lesion; it did not demonstrate the lesion itself. Discography was intended to show the internal structure of the disc and to demonstrate prolapses directly.

Early authorities embraced discography as a technique in the pursuit of disc herniation.* In this regard, some found it superior to oil-contrast myelography,[28,42,134] but others disagreed and thought that lumbar discography should be reserved for the investigation of unusual or atypical cases.[59,94]

As discography was used more, it was found to reveal more about the morphology of lumbar discs than just the presence or absence of herniation. Various grades of so-called degeneration were recognized, including degeneration with and without protrusion short of frank prolapse.†

Another agenda also arose. The pioneers of lumbar discography had noted that during discography patients commonly reported reproduction of their accustomed pain[53,75,76]; this was the experience of those who followed. Some emphasized the reproduction only of radicular pain,[134] in keeping with the then prevailing view that nerve root irritation was the leading, if not the only, mechanism by which lumbar discs could become symptomatic. Others, however, noted that back pain, not just radicular pain

*References 19, 25, 28, 33, 42, 43, 99, 126, 133, and 134.
†References 19, 28, 33, 39, 42, 59, 67, 126, 132, 133 and 134.

was reproduced by discography, which suggested that the disc itself could be the source of pain.[19,39,42,67,132]

The notion of primary disc pain had been espoused by authorities as eminent as Inman and Saunders as early as 1947[62]; and Falconer et al.,[38] Wiberg,[130] and later, Hirsch et al.[54] reported that probing the back of a lumbar disc at operation under local anesthesia reproduced back pain. However, the notion of primary disc pain ran contrary to then conventional, anatomical wisdom that held that the disc did not have a nerve supply and, therefore, could not be a primary source of pain—a view that continued to be espoused until the 1980s.[10] Nevertheless, several early investigators sought to establish correlations between disc morphology and reproduction of back pain.

Friedman and Goldner[42] and Feinberg[39] reported that discographically normal discs were rarely painful, but degenerative discs with posterior bulges and discs with epidural leaks on discography were virtually always painful.

An obvious issue was whether abnormal discs occurred in subjects with no pain; this was addressed by Massie and Stevens,[82] who reported their findings on discography in 52 normal subjects and 570 patients with back pain. They found that abnormal discs did occur in asymptomatic subjects, but they occurred far more commonly in patients. Moreover, abnormal discs were relatively more common in patients with advancing age. However, in asymptomatic subjects, abnormal discs were rarely painful on provocation discography. In patients, although more than one disc might appear abnormal morphologically, usually only one was found to be symptomatic on provocation discography. Accordingly, Massie and Stevens[82] emphasized the role of discography in distinguishing a symptomatic disc from similarly degenerated ones on the basis of pain reproduction.

After this seemingly productive phase in the study of intrinsic disc pain, controversy erupted. A disparaging review appeared that addressed the shortcomings of discography versus myelography in revealing frank disc prolapse[117]; but it ignored pain reproduction as the mainstay of lumbar discography. Then came the now infamous study of Holt, in which he studied allegedly asymptomatic, volunteer prisoners, and found a 37% false positive rate for pain reproduction.[57] Wilson and McCarty[132] elected to ignore pain reproduction; they thought that the morphologic picture must be definitive and concluded that discography had only a limited role in the diagnosis of lumbar disc protrusion.

For a while the literature was supportive of discography. Some surgeons and radiologists reported it as a useful aid in planning spinal arthrodesis—to identify normal discs and thereby plan the extent of fusion, or to avoid fusion in patients with abnormal discs at multiple levels.* Others emphasized the value of lumbar discography in evaluating patients with mechanical back pain and no neurologic signs[97,98] or when myelography was equivocal or negative.[18,89]

Vehement controversy erupted again in 1986 in correspondence to leading journals. In the *Journal of Neurosurgery,* prompted by some event in New Orleans, Clifford[20] sought to discredit discography, claiming that there was little, if any, use for discography given the availability of water-soluble myelography, CT, MRI, and EMG. Strangely, he overlooked the paradox that the investigative techniques he listed were all designed to identify nerve-root entrapment, whereas discography was designed to identify painful lumbar discs—a totally different phenomenon. In reply, Shapiro[108] emphasized the role of CT as the primary imaging technique for patients with herniated lumbar discs. Again the notion of intrinsic disc pain was ignored. Discographers rallied to the defense of discography, emphasizing its role in establishing the source of discogenic pain, not the location of a herniation.[101]

Shapiro's remarks were reiterated in the journal *Radiology,*[109] where Scullin,[107] also referring to events in New Orleans, mounted a scathing attack on discography. In support, he referred to the study of Holt[57] and to the essay of Bosacco.[15] Bosacco's essay criticized discography but as a test of disc morphology not as a test of discogenic pain. Again, discographers rallied, emphasizing the importance of pain-reproduction.[6,34,90]

Unperturbed by this correspondence in the United States, British investigators persevered with discography and found it to be a useful predictor of surgical outcome. Of patients undergoing interbody fusion for low-back pain, 89% derived significant relief when discography had revealed disc disease and pain reproduction, whereas only 52% derived relief when the disc exhibited morphologic changes but no pain reproduction.[26] Meanwhile, American investigators formally demonstrated the value of provocation discography and how symptomatic discs could not be identified by x-ray or myelography.[50] Others advocated that for optimal yield, discography should be performed when the patient was experiencing maximal pain.[86]

*References 18, 27, 31, 48, 52, 97, and 121.

Continuing controversy in the United States (largely in the form of unpublished remarks and debates) prompted the Executive Committee of the North American Spine Society to issue in 1988 a position statement on discography, emphasizing the pain response as the most important part of the procedure.[35]

By this time pathologists and anatomists had established that the lumbar discs were indeed innervated.[13,135] Moreover, reviews of the literature established that this had been known since 1959, but had somehow been ignored or suppressed.[9,10] There was no longer a defense that lumbar discs could not hurt because they lacked a nerve supply.

Dissection and histologic studies using classic techniques established that nerve endings occurred throughout the outer third of the anulus fibrosus and that the source of these endings were branches of the sinovertebral nerves, the gray rami communicantes and the lumbar ventral rami.[13,49,80,135] These studies were extended by histochemical studies in human and animal material to show that nerves in discs contain peptides such as calcitonin gene-related peptide (CGRP), vasoactive intestinal peptide, and substance P, which are characteristic of nociceptive nerve fibers.[70,71,128]

Some investigators have postulated that the innervation of discs is only adventitious, occurring only as a result of ingrowth of granulation tissue after disc injury[123]; but this theory has been explicitly studied and denied[135] and is incompatible with the observations that fetal and infant human discs are well innervated.[49,80]

These anatomic data, however, did little to dissuade opponents of discography, who relied on Holt's adverse proclamations.[57] This prompted a thorough review of Holt's study, which was summarily refuted on methodologic grounds.[111] Furthermore, Holt's study was replicated in a stringently designed and executed study. Walsh et al.[127] studied a selection of normal volunteers and patients with low-back pain. The discographer was blinded as to the status of the subject, injection pressures were monitored manometrically, and patient responses were recorded on videotape and assessed independently by two external observers. It emerged that normal discs in asymptomatic volunteers do not hurt and resisted injection. Only abnormal discs in patients were painful. This established that lumbar discography is a highly specific procedure for symptomatic lumbar discs.

The next epoch in the evolution of lumbar discography was the advent of CT discography.[85,124] At best, plain radiographs obtained during discography could reveal organized (normal) dispersal of contrast medium, disorganized (abnormal) patterns, or leakage of contrast medium out of the disc. The use of CT to provide an axial view of the disc revealed the radial dispersal of contrast medium, from which it emerged that seemingly disorganized patterns evident on lateral and anteroposterior plain films were more organized than had been realized. In abnormal discs, rather than spreading haphazardly, the contrast medium dispersed outward along radial fissures and circumferentially around the anulus fibrosus. The irregular pattern seen in lateral radiographs arose because of superimposition of regular, radial, and circumferential tracts of contrast medium.

On the basis of CT discographic findings, a new concept arose—that of anular disruption. The emphasis lay not on the extent of disc degeneration as such, but on the extent to which the anulus fibrosus was disrupted. Sachs et al.[106] developed the Dallas discogram scale, in which anular disruption was graded on a 4-point scale. Grade 0 described contrast medium contained wholly within a regular nucleus pulposus. Grades 1 to 3 described extension of contrast medium along radial fissures into the inner third, middle third, and outer third of the anulus fibrosus respectively (Fig. 14-1).

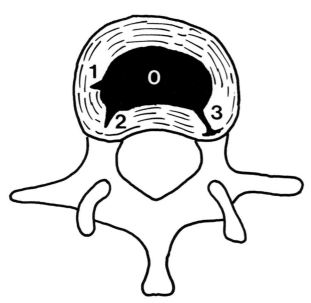

Fig. 14-1.

Dallas discogram scale.[120] Grade 0: disruption, if any, is confined to nucleus pulposus. Grade 1: disruption extends into inner third of anulus fibrosus. Grade 2: disruption extends as far as inner two thirds of anulus. Grade 3: disruption extends into outer third of anulus fibrosus and may spread circumferentially between laminae of collagen.

Subsequently, Vanharanta et al.[120] found that pain reproduction on discography correlated with the extent of anular disruption. Grade 0 and grade 1 disruptions were rarely painful, but 75% of grade 3 disruptions were associated with exact or similar pain reproduction; conversely, 77% of discs with exact or similar pain reproduction exhibited grade 3 anular disruptions. Grade 2 disruptions were less regularly associated with pain reproduction.

These correlations, in turn, correlated with the distribution of nerve endings in the anulus fibrosus—the inner third is never innervated, the outer third is regularly innervated, and the middle third may or may not be innervated. For the first time in the history of the study of low-back pain, firm correlations had been established between the innervation of a structure, pain reproduction from it, and a demonstrable lesion.

These experimental studies corroborated what had previously been declared on clinical grounds. Crock[29] maintained that the hitherto elusive and radiologically "invisible" cause of many cases of low-back pain was "internal disc disruption"—a condition in which a lumbar disc could become painful as a result of internal disruption of its architecture, but with no external features; the contour of the disc remained normal, or essentially so, and consequently, the disc appeared normal on CT and myelography, but nonetheless was painful. The only means of establishing the diagnosis was by provocation discography. The studies of Vanharanta et al.[120] extended this proclamation by revealing the internal architecture of the disc and revealing the responsible lesion.

Also converging to this same end point were the studies of Farfan et al.,[36,37] who described so-called compression injuries of the disc. These investigators maintained that end-plate fractures could trigger an abnormal inflammatory response that eventually disrupted first the integrity of the nucleus pulposus and subsequently the anulus fibrosus, in a radial fashion. These concepts provide the basis for a model of the pathogenesis of internal disc disruption and anular disruption.[11]

Pathology

Despite any prevailing traditional wisdom in this regard, when compressed, intervertebral discs do not fail by prolapsing. In biomechanical experiments it is exceedingly difficult to induce disc failure by prolapse. Even if a channel is cut into the anulus fibrosus the nucleus fails to herniate.[16] A normal nucleus is intrinsically cohesive and resists herniation. Even in specimens with partially herniated discs, comple-

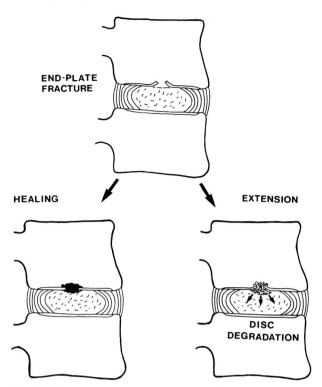

END-PLATE
FRACTURE

HEALING

EXTENSION

DISC
DEGRADATION

Fig. 14-2.
Model of pathogenesis of internal disc disruption. Excessive compression force may result in fracture of vertebral end plate. This lesion may heal and be of no consequence, but on the other hand it may initiate a process of disc degradation affecting nucleus pulposus near fracture site but gradually extending into the rest of the nucleus.

tion of the prolapse rarely occurs even after repeated flexion and compression.[2]

When compressed, intervertebral discs typically fail by fracture of a vertebral end plate.* Under natural conditions, such injuries can be sustained as a result of a heavy fall[36,37] or as a result of excessive, strenuous activity of the back muscles.[11]

An end-plate fracture is of itself not symptomatic and may pass unnoticed. Furthermore, an end-plate fracture may heal and cause no further problems (Fig. 14-2). However, it is possible for an end-plate fracture to set in motion a series of sequelae that manifest as pain and a variety of end stages.

The matrix of the nucleus pulposus has not been studied according to contemporary standards of immunology, but available evidence suggests that the matrix does have antigenic properties. Prolapsed nuclear material elicits an inflammatory response if it enters the epidural space[84] or the vertebral spongiosa in the case of traumatic Schmorl's nodes.[83] Patients with prolapsed discs exhibit changes in lymphocyte

migration and antibody profiles consistent with an antigenic response.† Biochemically, the proteoglycans of the nucleus pulposus are similar to those of the vitreous humor, and it is well known that in penetrating injuries of the eye, exposed lens protein can sensitize lymphocytes to the extent that if they reach the intact eye they can exert a destructive inflammation: the condition of sympathetic ophthalmia.

By the same token, proteoglycans of the nucleus pulposus are essentially foreign to the body. Throughout its entire development the nucleus pulposus lacks a blood supply and is never exposed to the circulation. Consequently, in a disc that suffers an end-plate fracture, proteoglycans may for the first time be exposed to the body's immune system, triggering an inflammatory response.

The consequence of this inflammatory response is a progressive degradation of the nuclear matrix. As this degradation progresses the biophysical properties of the nucleus change. The nucleus is less able to bind water, whereupon during weight-bearing the bracing effect of the nucleus on the anulus fibrosus is reduced and the anulus fibrosus is left to bear weight alone. In time, the anulus fibrosus may creep under compression, with buckling and bulging of the anulus fibrosus and narrowing of the disc space (Fig. 14-3). This condition has been described clinically as isolated disc resorption,[122] which may become symptomatic as a result of foraminal stenosis or canal stenosis; but isolated disc resorption is only one possible end stage of disc degradation.

Nuclear degradation may progress to involve erosion of the anulus fibrosus along radial fissures; a condition now referred to as "internal disc disruption"[29] (see Fig. 14-3). This name specifies that the disc is abnormal, but abnormal internally. It is the nucleus and inner anulus that are disrupted, while the outer perimeter of the disc remains intact and normal in contour. There is no element of disc bulge or herniation.

If a radial fissure completely erodes the anulus, the stage may be set for disc prolapse. The fissure provides a channel through the anulus, while degradation of the nuclear matrix destroys its intrinsic cohesiveness and renders the nucleus expressible. A compression load on the disc may succeed in herniating nuclear material into the vertebral canal, where it irritates or compresses nerve roots.

This model stipulates that disc herniation does not occur in normal discs. For herniation to occur there must have been antecedent injury to denature the nucleus and render it expressible and to produce

*References 2, 17, 61, 64, 100, 102, and 103.

†References 8, 32, 44, 45, 46, and 81.

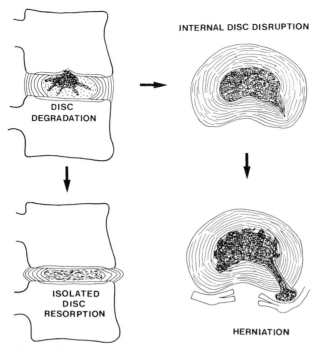

Fig. 14-3.

Disc degradation spreads to involve all of nucleus pulposus. If anulus fibrosus remains relatively intact, disc narrows because of loss in water-binding capacity of nucleus, resulting in condition of isolated disc resorption. On the other hand, disc degradation may spread radially into anulus fibrosus, causing a fissure. External appearance of disc remains normal; pathologic process remains wholly within disc, and condition of disc is described as internal disc disruption. If remaining fibers of anulus fibrosus are breached, nuclear herniation may follow internal disc disruption.

a channel through the anulus fibrosus. However, disc herniation is but an extreme possible end stage of internal disc disruption; hence its relative rarity. However, prior to and without herniating, a disrupted disc can be symptomatic.

A disc with internal disc disruption confined to the nucleus pulposus and inner anulus has no means of being symptomatic. Nerve endings are absent from these portions of the disc, and chemical processes affecting the nucleus pulposus are not detected by the nervous system. Meanwhile, the outer anulus is sufficiently intact to subserve the mechanical functions of the disc. However, as a radial fissure reaches the middle and outer thirds of the anulus fibrosus it encounters nerve endings, and the stage is set for chemical nociception.

Nerve endings in the anulus fibrosus may become exposed to enzymes and breakdown products involved in the degradative process of the disc. Furthermore, there is evidence that inflammatory cells penetrate the anulus fibrosus of disrupted discs,[63]

whereupon inflammatory chemical mediators may trigger nociceptive nerve endings.

The middle third of the anulus fibrosus may or may not be innervated, but the outer third is regularly innervated. Therefore, the probability of the disc becoming painful increases the further the radial fissure extends into the anulus.

Apart from being stimulated chemically, nociceptors in the anulus fibrosus may be activated mechanically. In this regard the nociceptors involved are not those in the disrupted portion of the anulus but those in the intact, remaining portions. Under normal circumstances all the collagen fibers in a given sector of a disc share the everyday loads applied to it. If 30% of these fibers were to be destroyed, the remainder would continue to face the same total load imposed on the disc and would increase their individual stress by 43%. If two thirds of the anulus were disrupted by a radial fissure, the remaining one third would be exposed to 3 times their accustomed stress. At some point along this scale, the remaining and innervated outer fibers would be so excessively strained by normal activities of daily living that they would become symptomatic.

Coupling both the chemical and mechanical transduction processes, it is possible that inflammatory chemicals could sensitize the nerve endings in the anulus fibrosus, rendering them activated at mechanical thresholds lower than would be anticipated if only the mechanical process operated.

From a theoretical perspective, therefore, the clinical features of internal disc disruption would be as follows.[29] Constant deep aching pain would be present due to the chemical nociception, and would be aggravated by any movement that mechanically stressed the affected disc; but conspicuously lacking would be any neurologic signs, because the lesion does not involve nerve root irritation or compression. Because the outer perimeter of the disc is intact, CT scans and myelography would be normal. The likelihood of symptoms increases the greater the erosion of the anulus fibrosus, but by the same token the condition may be present for some time but remain asymptomatic for as long as the disruption is confined to the nucleus and inner anulus.

It is this condition that can be diagnosed by CT discography. The provocation phase of discography reveals whether the disc is symptomatic. Instilling contrast medium marks the internal structure of the disc, which can be clearly visualized by CT, and the degree of internal disruption can be graded according to the extent of the contrast medium, using the Dallas discogram scale[106] (see Fig. 14-1) or a more extensive scale developed by Bernard.[7]

Although CT discography provides images of the lesion responsible for the patient's pain in internal disc disruption, this facility is not a prescription for CT discography in all cases of low-back pain. Clinical management may not require visualization of the disease process, particularly if conservative measures are to be undertaken, and postdiscography CT adds little more information to what can be inferred from discography alone.[4]

The usefulness of CT discography is twofold. First, in an academic arena, when undertaken in research it serves to demonstrate unequivocally the presence and nature of genuine lesions in patients with otherwise unexplained pain and in whom investigations such as myelography and CT reveal nothing of consequence. Secondly, CT discography may be undertaken to corroborate discography if there is a need to demonstrate the lesion either for the satisfaction of the patient, the physician, or perhaps a court in medicolegal proceedings.

Cervical Discography

The first use of cervical discography has been attributed by Cloward[24] to George Smith,[113,114] but it was Ralph Cloward who pioneered the procedure.[21-24] From the outset, Smith[113,114] emphasized reproduction of the patient's pain as the key feature of cervical discography; so did Cloward,[22] who described two sorts of pain encountered during discography: discogenic pain that arose from the disc itself and neurogenic pain that occurred when pressure was transmitted through a herniated disc fragment onto a nerve root or the dura mater of the spinal cord. Discogenic pain was said to be dull and aching in quality and was perceived over the lower cervical and thoracic spinous processes when cervical discs were stimulated in the midline, or over the scapula when the disc was stimulated anterolaterally. Neurogenic pain was typically lancinating in quality.

At operation, under direct vision, Cloward[23] stimulated cervical discs mechanically and electrically to verify that discogenic pain stemmed from the disc and was not due to irritation of adjacent structures. He argued that disc pain must be mediated by sinovertebral nerves, but commented that in the cervical region these nerves were "so small as to defy ordinary anatomical methods."[23]

Subsequent, anatomic studies demonstrated the cervical sinovertebral nerves and their role in innervating the cervical discs,[14,49,87] thereby providing the anatomic substrate for Cloward's experimental observations and inferences. The cervical discs receive an innervation posteriorly from the sinovertebral nerves, laterally from the vertebral nerve, and anteriorly from the cervical sympathetic trunks,[14,49] a pattern analogous to that of the lumbar discs.

Although pain reproduction remained the cardinal component of cervical discography, the procedure was soon confounded by attempts to identify abnormal morphologic patterns in symptomatic discs.[24,116] Investigators interpreted various forms of "extravasation" of contrast medium from the injected disc as indicative of disc "pathology."[116] However, others soon reported that there was no good correlation between disc morphology and the reproduction of pain.[69,88,115] Fissuring of the disc seemed to be no more than an age change.[115]

As for lumbar discography, Holt[56] reported that pain reproduction and fissuring were features of cervical discs in normal volunteers, and therefore, cervical discography had no diagnostic value.

Later investigators bypassed pain reproduction and disc morphology as absolute entities and emphasized instead that the role of cervical discography was to discriminate between painful and nonpainful discs in a given patient.[110] As a complement to this role, Roth[105] introduced analgesic discography the rationale for which was that once a putatively painful disc was identified, the pain it caused could and should be relieved by injecting local anesthetic into the disc.

The purpose of this form of precision diagnosis was to determine which disc should be operated on; this has continued to be the main role of cervical discography.[55] The studies of Kikuchi et al.[68] bear testimony to this. By localizing a symptomatic disc by provocation discography and by establishing that the discogenic pain could be relieved by appropriate nerve root blocks, these investigators found that their operation results were improved. At 1-year follow-up, 80% of their patients were pain-free, as compared to 40% when discography was not used.[68]

Pathology

In stark contrast to what is known about the pathology of painful lumbar discs, there is no data on the pathology of painful cervical discs. Cervical discs are embryologically and morphologically different from lumbar discs, and there is no evidence that they suffer from internal disc disruption. Consequently, the model advanced for the pain of lumbar discs cannot be applied to the neck.

Circumstantial evidence favors the notion that when cervical discs are injured the pathology involves tears of the anterior anulus fibrosus—so-called rim lesions of the anulus,[30,118] or avulsion of the end plate from the vertebral body.[66] However, there is no clinical evidence correlating either the reproduction or relief of pain to the presence of such lesions. The pathology of painful cervical discs remains elusive.

Techniques

Prior to any discographic procedure the clinician should explain to the patient the nature of the procedure, its risks and complications, and what to expect. It is critical that the patient be able to recognize and report if and when the accustomed pain is reproduced, and he or she must be able to distinguish this pain from any other pain felt. Unless the patient is able to make this distinction, the procedure has no value. In this regard, it is an advantage to have a trained observer as an independent witness to monitor the patient's pain response while the operator concentrates on the technical aspects of the procedure.

At best, discography is uncomfortable; at worst, it can be very painful. For this reason it is recommended that patients be sedated. Midazolam, 3.5 to 5.0 mg should be administered intravenously slowly over 3 minutes, and titrated by patient response to establish a level of sedation in which the patient remains clearly conversant and responsive yet tolerant of the procedural discomfort. The advantage of midazolam is that it frequently leaves the patient amnestic for the events immediately following administration of the drug. In older patients, a dose of 2.5 mg may suffice. In the experience of the authors, respiratory depression has not been encountered with this protocol, but nevertheless, the procedure must be performed in a facility capable of ventilatory support.

Discography can be performed in any radiography suite suitable for myelography. C-arm fluoroscopy is necessary to expedite cervical discography but is not essential for lumbar discography. The procedures require 3.5-in. and 6-in. spinal needles, and separate, 3-ml syringes loaded with normal saline, 1% lignocaine, 0.5% bupivacaine, and nonionic, contrast medium.

Lumbar Disc Puncture

The patient lies in a prone position on a fluoroscopy table, and a wide area of the skin of the back is prepped and draped, as for any aseptic procedure, from the costal margin to the midbuttock and from the midline to the flank on the side selected for puncture. As a rule the side to be punctured is that opposite the patient's dominant pain. This is to eliminate any confusion between reproducing the patient's accustomed pain and the pain of penetrating the outer anulus fibrosus. If there is any evidence or suspicion of congenital or postoperative anomalies of the vertebral column or the nerve roots on either side, that side should be avoided for disc puncture; otherwise, extreme care should be exercised in negotiating any anatomic anomaly.

The technique to be described here is a lateral (extrapedicular) approach, and is a modification of the technique described by Troisier.[119] For the lumbosacral disc, a modification of the technique of Laredo[73] is used. Other techniques are available, such as the posterior, midline approach[76,89,131] and the posterolateral approach,[33,67] but both incur the unnecessary side effects and complications of dural puncture.

Once the side to be punctured has been selected, the patient is rolled into the lateral decubitus position with the selected side up. The downside arm is stretched over the head so that the patient lies on his or her chest along the midaxillary line; a pillow is placed between the head and the outstretched arm. If required, a folded towel is placed under the patient's flank to prevent side bending of the lumbar spine. The patient is then rolled forward into an oblique, prone position with the upper leg flexed at the hip and the knee. By varying the degree of flexion, the patient can be rolled backward to a lateral position or forward into a more prone position.

The technique for disc puncture at typical lumbar levels is straightforward and relies on direct visualization of the surrounding anatomy. For the lumbosacral level extra considerations pertain.

To obtain the optimal angle of approach for typical lumbar levels, the patient is rotated until the superior articular process of the vertebra below the disc to be punctured projects midway between the anterior and posterior margins of the superior end plate of the disc to be punctured. A 3.5-in., 25-gauge needle is then directed perpendicularly toward the anterior margin of the superior articular process until it contacts this process (Fig. 14-4). It is then used to anesthetise the future needle track. Between 3 and 5 ml of 1% lignocaine is injected while withdrawing this needle.

Subsequently, a 6-in. (25- or 22-gauge) spinal needle is inserted along the former track aiming toward the center of the target disc, but with the objective of first striking the outer anulus fibrosus. If bony obstruction is encountered, the patient is rolled into the lateral position to ascertain whether the needle has contacted the superior articular process or the verte-

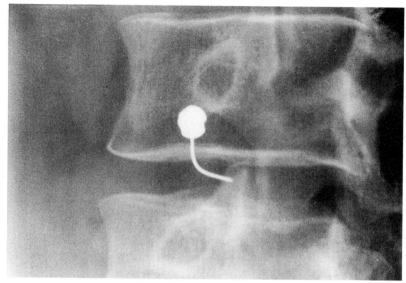

Fig. 14-4

Radiogram of guide needle in position against superior articular
process of L4 in preparation for puncture of L3-L4 intervertebral
disc.

bral body. If necessary, the needle is withdrawn
slightly and its trajectory modified appropriately.

Contact with the anulus fibrosus is characterized
by the perception by the operator of firm but resilient resistance, and usually by the experience by
the patient of a momentary, sharp, or sudden aching
sensation in the back or the buttock. Thereafter, the
needle is advanced into the substance of the disc,
aiming to have its tip reach the center of the disc.
Its position must be monitored and checked in both
the sagittal and frontal planes (Fig. 14-5).

Puncture of the lumbosacral disc is challenging.
With the patient in the lateral decubitus position,
the lumbosacral angle is observed and a line depict-
ing this angle is projected back to the skin surface.
This represents the transverse level at which skin
puncture will be made. The patient is then rolled to
a prone or slightly prone oblique position. A point
along the transverse level is selected that will allow
the passage of a needle medial to the iliac crest and
adjacent to the lateral margin of the superior articular process of the sacrum. A 25-gauge, 3.5-in. spinal

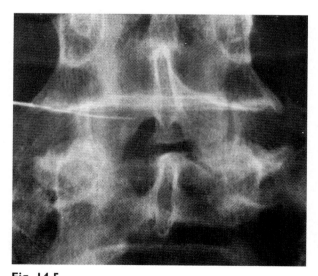 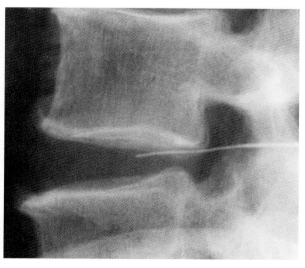

Fig. 14-5
Posterior and lateral views of needle correctly located in the center of L4-L5 disc.

needle is then directed from the selected point cau-dally and medially toward the superior articular process. This needle should not be overinserted lest it injure the L5 ventral ramus. In most patients, the needle need be advanced only 2.5 to 3 in. to reach the superior articular process.

The patient is then rolled into the lateral position and its location is checked. Note is taken whether the cephalocaudad orientation of the needle is cor-rectly in line with the transverse axis of the disc space. Any changes in depth or orientation of the needle are made at this time in order to place its tip against the superior articular process. Once proper position has been established, 5 ml of 1% lignocaine is in-jected as the needle is slowly withdrawn. This anes-thetizes the back muscles and thoracolumbar fascia that are penetrated by the subsequent needle.

Disc puncture at the lumbosacral level requires a double-needle technique. A guide needle is required because the procedure needle will be precurved to reach the nucleus of the disc; in many patients, a single needle cannot be directed straight into the center of the L5-S1 disc. For less-experienced op-erators a 18-gauge guide needle is recommended. A 20-gauge guide needle is less traumatic but re-quires considerable finesse to control its position with precision. Larger needles are required in mus-cular or obese patients.

The guide needle is introduced so that its tip lies immediately adjacent to the anterolateral aspect of the superior articular process of the sacrum (Fig. 14-6). The procedure needle is precurved by hand. Its tip should not be handled directly, but should be wrapped in sterile gauze. The distal 2 to 3 cm of the needle should be bent in a direction opposite to that in which the bevel faces. The degree of curve is determined by the operator on the basis of how much deflection is required in the patient at hand for the needle to gain the center of the target disc.

The procedure needle is passed through the guide needle while the guide needle is held firmly in po-sition to prevent it from being pushed into the radic-ular canal. The inner needle is advanced until its tip emerges from the guide needle. At this stage the ori-entation of the bevels should be checked. That of the guide needle should face medially; that of the procedure needle should face laterally.

With the patient in the oblique position, the in-ner needle is advanced slightly under direct fluoro-scopic vision. As it emerges, the guide needle is si-multaneously retracted slightly. This unsheathes the procedure needle, which bows medially. Its bevel and its curve direct it toward the center of the disc space (Fig. 14-7). Once the needle encounters the anulus

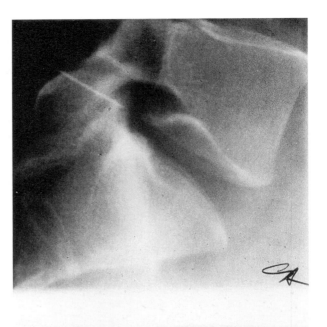

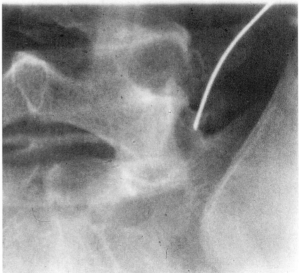

Fig. 14-6.
Lateral and posterior views of guide needle in preliminary posi-tion against superior articular process of S1. (Same patient as Figs. 14-7 to 14-9.)

fibrosus it penetrates easily. Its position must be checked and confirmed in both the sagittal and frontal planes (Fig. 14-8).

If the inner needle fails to curve medially it will not pass to the center of the disc; it may strike the L5 ventral ramus. To avoid this, its course must be monitored. If it fails to curve medially, it should be removed and its curvature accentuated.

normal discs.[64] Therefore, provided small-gauge needles and a small syringe are used, the procedure of disc injection is mechanically safe.

As fluid is instilled into the nucleus, the end plates of the disc bulge and the disc space increases in height. This distraction of the vertebral bodies can be observed on fluoroscopy. In a normal disc, firm terminal resistance is encountered as the nucleus

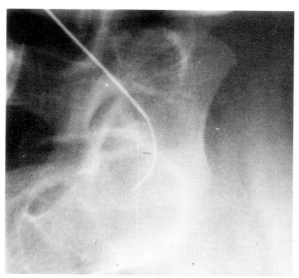

Fig. 14-7
Oblique view of procedure needle having been advanced through guide needle into L5-S1 disc. (Same patient as Figs. 14-6, 14-8, and 14-9.)

Should the procedure needle meet with bony obstruction, the patient should be turned to the lateral position to determine whether the superior articular process or the vertebral body has been encountered. If the vertebral body has been encountered, the course of the needle can be corrected by withdrawing it slightly and rotating the needle appropriately. If the needle is blocked by the superior articular process, the inner needle is retracted into the guide needle and the pair are advanced slightly to pass the process, whereafter the inner needle is continued toward the disc as described above.

Lumbar Discography

Once the tip of needle has been properly placed in the center of the nucleus pulposus, a 3-ml syringe containing contrast medium is attached to it. Injection into the nucleus is accomplished by gradually increasing thumb pressure on the syringe (Fig. 14-9).

A normal disc accepts a limited volume of fluid, ranging from 1.5 to 2.5 ml. The intrinsic disc pressure is the pressure required to start the flow of contrast medium into the nucleus, and in a normal disc has been recorded as 400 to 500 kPa using 22- or 25-gauge needles and a 3-ml Luer-lock syringe.[127] The maximum pressure induced by a hand-held syringe is greater than intrinsic disc pressure but is well below the bursting pressure of both normal and ab-

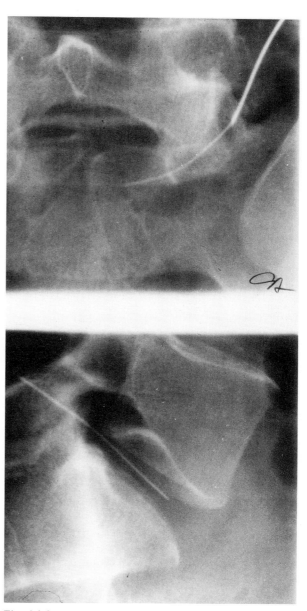

Fig. 14-8
Posterior and lateral views of needle in correct position in center of L5-S1 disc. (Same patient as Figs. 14-6, 14-7, and 14-9.)

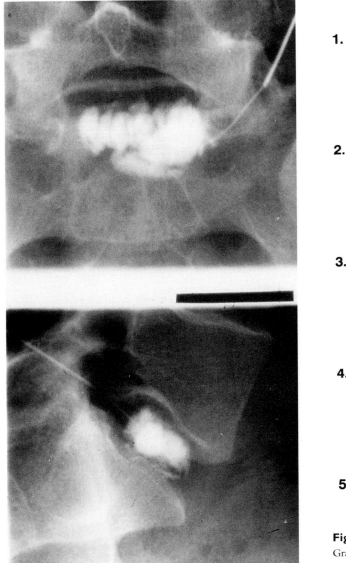

Fig. 14-9

Posterior and lateral views of discogram of L5-S1 disc. (Same patient as Figs. 14-6 to 14-8.)

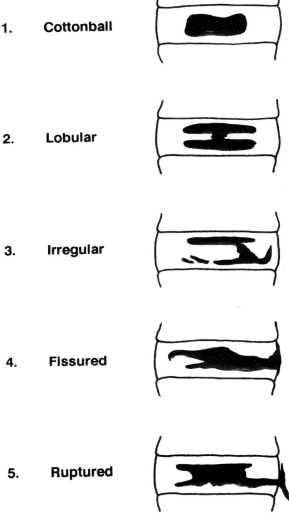

1. **Cottonball**

2. **Lobular**

3. **Irregular**

4. **Fissured**

5. **Ruptured**

Fig. 14-10

Grading system of Adams et al.[1] for lumbar discograms.

opacifies; the plunger of the syringe may recoil if pressure is released.

If firm resistance to injection is encountered before the nucleus opacifies, the needle may be embedded in the cartilage of a vertebral end plate or may not have reached the nucleus and be still in the anulus. Its position should be checked by fluoroscopy. If any nonnuclear location is identified, the needle should be manipulated into the nucleus or withdrawn and reinserted accurately into the nucleus.

If there is little or no resistance to injection of 1 ml of contrast medium, its flow should be monitored throughout by fluoroscopy. Filling of venous structures or free spill into the epidural space is easily recognized.

The appearance of the normal nucleus following the injection of contrast medium is unmistakable. The contrast medium assumes a globular pattern or a bilobed ("hamburger") pattern. Otherwise, a variety of patterns occur in abnormal discs[1] (Fig. 14-10). Contrast medium may extend into radial fissures of various lengths but remain contained within the disc, or it may escape into the epidural spaces through a torn anulus. In some cases, the contrast medium may escape through a defect in the vertebral end plate.[60,83] However, none of these patterns alone is indicative of whether the disc is painful; that can be ascertained only by the patient's subjective response to disc injection.

Cervical Disc Puncture

The patient lies on the fluoroscopy table in a supine position. Neck extension is delayed until the commencement of the procedure lest the patient's pain be unduly and unnecessarily aggravated. Extension is achieved by elevating the upper trunk and placing a triangular sponge between the shoulders; the head is gently lowered and rested on a small supporting sponge, and the chin is extended.

C-arm fluoroscopy can be used to obtain both anteroposterior (through-table) and lateral (cross-table) views. Alternatively, if a myelography table is being used, the C-arm can be positioned for cross-table views and the fixed, vertical imaging of the fluoroscopy table can be used for frontal views. The latter obviates having to swing the C-arm between the two positions.

The skin of the anterior and anterolateral neck is prepared as for an aseptic procedure, from the mandible to the supraclavicular region. Sterile drapes are applied, with their margins overlapping the sternocleidomastoid muscles. A right-sided approach is used because the esophagus lies to the left in the lower neck, and it should be avoided. The disc level to be studied is identified by fluoroscopy. Pressure is applied with the index and middle fingers to the space between the trachea and the medial border of the sternocleidomastoid. Firm but gentle pressure will displace the visceral structures to the left. Below C4, the right common carotid artery, and above C4 the internal carotid artery are palpated; they should lie lateral to the intended path of the needle. The fingers are insinuated until they encounter the anterior surface of the vertebral column.

The needle entry point should be medial to the medial border of the sternocleidomastoid, and not through that muscle. The declination of the sternocleidomastoid ensures that at C3-C4, the puncture point lies more laterally and will avoid the pharynx, whereas at C7-T1 it will be more medial and will avoid the apex of the lung.

A 3.5-in. spinal needle (22- or 25-gauge) is used for the procedure. It is directed through the skin and toward the superior aspect of the vertebral body immediately below the disc to be studied. Contact with this bony structure determines the depth of the vertebral column. On retracting and redirecting the needle cephalad it is advanced onto the anterolateral surface of the target disc. On contact with the anulus, the patient will experience transient pain. The needle is advanced into the substance of the disc under direct fluoroscopic visualization. All movements of the needle should be slow and deliberate. Frontal and sagittal views of the needle should be obtained once its tip has been advanced to the apparent center of the disc (Fig. 14-11).

Cervical Discography

Once the tip of the needle has been correctly placed in the center of the disc, the syringe containing normal saline is attached. Pressure on the syringe is increased slowly until the intrinsic disc pressure is exceeded. Volumes as small as 0.2 ml will cause visible separation of the vertebrae, which should be monitored on fluoroscopy. Pain response should be recorded at the time of this distention. The volume that the disc accepts should be noted.

A normal cervical disc offers firm resistance and accepts less than 0.5 ml of solution with little discomfort at the time of distention. If the disc is painless and discometrically normal, contrast medium is next instilled to opacify the nucleus and to verify and record correct placement of the needle.

If injection of saline provokes a pain response, the location of the pain and its intensity should be recorded. Thereafter, 0.5 ml of 1% lignocaine is injected into the disc to relieve the evoked pain. Contrast medium is then injected to determine the internal morphology of the disc, and anteroposterior and lateral radiographs are obtained (Fig. 14-12). Contrast medium sufficient to opacify the nucleus and to note any lateral or posterior escape of the medium from the confines of the disc should be injected, and no more.

Pain Response

When a disc is stressed by the infiltration of contrast medium, the patient must be asked if he/she perceives any pain and if that pain is similar to, identical to, or different from the accustomed pain. Meanwhile, the opportunity must be taken to corroborate the response by monitoring physical accompaniments such as guarding, bracing, withdrawal, grimacing, and verbalizing. If possible, the patient should rate the evoked pain on a verbal analog scale.

A convincing, positive response to disc stimulation is one in which the patient reports exact or similar reproduction of pain on stimulation of a given disc but provided that stressing one or two adjacent

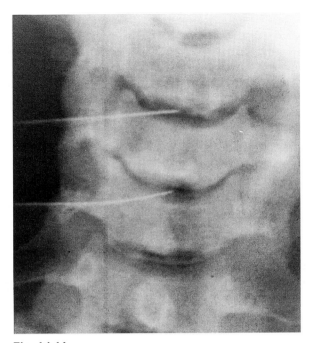
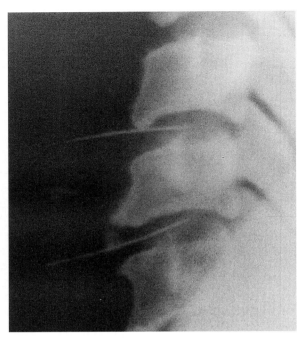

Fig. 14-11

Anterior and lateral radiograms of needles correctly in center of C4-C5 and C5-C6 intervertebral discs.

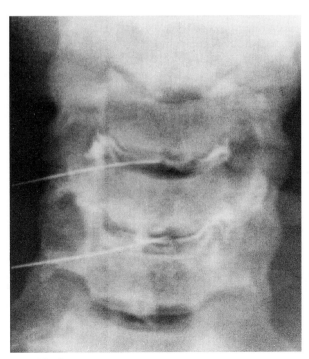
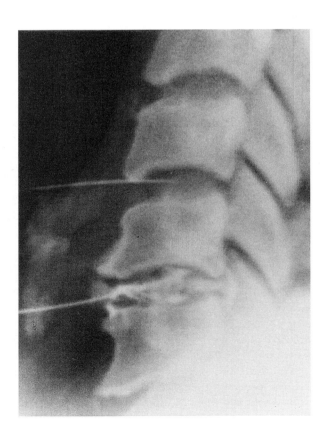

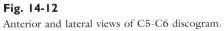

Fig. 14-12

Anterior and lateral views of C5-C6 discogram.

discs is painless or evokes pain totally foreign to the patient's previous experience. Any other pattern of response cannot be held to be reliably indicative that the disc stimulated is the source of the patient's pain.

It may be possible for a patient to have two symptomatic discs, but under those circumstances, it is still mandatory to identify an adjacent disc that is asymptomatic. Without an asymptomatic, "control" disc, there is no evidence that the patient can discriminate between a symptomatic and an asymptomatic disc; and there is no evidence that what they are reporting as disc pain is not simply the pain of needles felt in the back or the neck, or that they are simply complying with the operator's expectation that there should be pain.

Once a painful disc has been identified in the course of discography, and once all discographic radiographs have been taken, 0.5 ml of bupivacaine can be injected into the disc in an effort to obtain prolonged relief of pain from that disc. Should the patient's accustomed pain be relieved by this action, the duration of relief should be monitored and recorded by the patient. Relief of accustomed pain for a period consistent with the expected duration of action of the local anesthetic agent used constitutes strong evidence that the disc in question is the source of pain.

Indications

The single purpose of discography is to obtain information. The morphology of a disc is not diagnostic; it does not indicate whether a given disc is responsible for a patient's pain. However, it is reassuring if a disc proven to be symptomatic on other grounds also happens to be morphologically abnormal.

The cardinal information obtained from discography is whether the patient's pain is reproduced. There is no alternative or superior means of determining if a disc is the source of a patient's pain. Conceptually, discography is an extension of clinical examination, tantamount to palpating for tenderness. It is only the inaccessibility of a disc to palpation that renders the use of needles necessary. In this regard, however, it is critical that the criteria for a painful disc be rigorously satisfied; internal control observations are mandatory; a disc cannot be deemed the source of a patient's pain if stimulating other discs or other structures in the same region similarly reproduces the patient's pain.

Discography is not warranted if there is no desire to establish an anatomic diagnosis, as is the practice when nonspecific therapies or work-hardening are used to manage the patient's problem.

Discography may be warranted for medicolegal purposes to establish a definitive diagnosis even though therapy is not to be directed explicitly at that disc. Otherwise, the prime indication for discography is to establish a diagnosis of discogenic pain when therapy is to be directed at that disc.

A parallel application is to identify normal discs as much as abnormal discs. When a single disc is found to be symptomatic in the presence of adjacent, asymptomatic, and morphologic normal discs, focused surgical therapy can be entertained. A patient with symptomatic or abnormal discs at multiple levels constitutes a greater surgical challenge.

Contraindications

Congenital anomalies of the vertebrae or nerve roots constitute relative contraindications to discography, as do postoperative abnormalities of spinal anatomy. Such conditions require greater care and dexterity to negotiate the abnormal anatomy both to gain access to the target disc and to avoid injury to surrounding structures.

In the case of cervical discography, spinal cord compression constitutes an absolute contraindication to discography. In such cases, the neurologic features are the patients' key problems; and information about whether the disc is painful is immaterial to their management. Moreover, the uncertainty of the relationship between the prolapsed disc and the spinal cord and the resistance of the disc to passage of a needle only invites morbidity.[74]

Complications

Two classes of complications pertain to discography—misplacement of the needle and infection. However, if practiced carefully and meticulously, discography should not cause these complications.

In the case of cervical discography, neural structures are not at risk during the course of the needle to the target disc. However, overzealous insertion of the needle can result in its passage through the disc and into the spinal cord. For this reason, the initial insertion of any needle must be monitored fluoroscopically and be directed, in the first instance, to the vertebral body in order to establish the appropriate depth of insertion. During injection of substances into the disc, the second hand must be used to brace the hub of the needle in order to prevent inadvertent overpenetration of the needle.

Penetration of viscera such as the pharynx and esophagus is not a problem per se, but increases the risk of infection (see below). Pneumothorax is a potential risk with discography at C7-T1. Arterial puncture is a hazard at all levels but the use of fine needles and attention to proper technique with good visualization will limit the occurrence of such complications.

In the case of lumbar discography, striking a ventral ramus is a potential hazard, but is avoided by attention to correct technique, which entails preventing any needle from straying beyond its required and intended course. Fortunately, in a conscious patient, contact with the ventral ramus will be heralded by severe, sharp lancinating pain, which is an indication to withdraw and redirect the needle. Penetration of the intervertebral foramen or the lumbar nerve roots should never be a problem, for the needle should never be allowed to stray behind the midpoint of the target disc.

In the cervical region, epidural abscess, retropharyngeal abscess, and discitis are all possible complications.[51,79,104,125] The organisms introduced may be external or from the pharynx or esophagus if these are penetrated. The reported incidence of cervical discitis is 0.1% to 0.5%.[51,104] The condition is self-limiting but may take several weeks to resolve and is attended by severe, if not excruciating, pain.[51]

Discitis following lumbar discography has been more frequently documented and studied than cervical discitis. When identified, the causative organisms have been *Staphylococcus aureus, Staphylococcus epidermitis,* and *Escherichia coli,*[3,51] suggesting innoculation with surface organisms or misadventure through bowel perforation. Although some authors consider discitis a rare complication of lumbar discography,[18,110,131] others have found an overall rate of 2.3% per patient and 1.3% per disc[40] or 0.1% per patient and 0.05% per disc.[51] The incidence is higher when single, large-gauge needles have been used, and much smaller when double-needle techniques have been used.[40]

Aside from the risk of infection there is no evidence that discography in any way damages the disc.[65]

Persisting Issues

Antibiotics

Following the recognition and publicity of discitis as a potential complication of discography, some proponents have advocated the use of prophylactic antibiotics. The recommended regimen is 1 mg of cefazolin per milliliter of contrast medium, injected into the disc at the time of discography.[95] Animal studies have shown that intradiscal[95] and intravenous[41] antibiotics prevent discitis.

Notwithstanding the alarm about discitis, one of the present authors (C.A.) has managed to avoid discitis in all but 1 case in over 2000 lumbar discograms over a 10-year period. It is therefore suggested that stringent attention to aseptic and expeditious technique are critical to avoiding infection. There should be no delays between withdrawing the procedure needle from its scabbard and introducing it into the patient. With these precautions, the routine use of prophylactic antibiotics may not be necessary. However, physicians uncertain about the asepsis of their facilities or hesitant about their technique would be advised to adopt prophylactic measures.

Validity

The publications of Holt[56,57] cast doubt on the validity of discography. In the case of lumbar discography, these doubts have been dispelled. Lumbar discography is extremely specific; normal lumbar discs do not hurt.[127] What remains unknown, however, is how sensitive lumbar discography is—that is, does provocation discography detect all symptomatic lumbar discs?

The same cannot be said for cervical discography. One study has cast doubt on the validity of cervical discography, inasmuch as cervical discography appears to be falsely positive in 40% of cases.[12] Urgently required are normative studies of cervical discography like those that have been conducted for lumbar discography.[127]

Analgesic discography is an attractive notion insofar as complete relief of pain following infiltration of the disc with local anesthetic constitutes strong evidence that the disc is the actual source of the patient's pain. However, for technical reasons,[10] analgesic discography cannot always be achieved and, indeed, is seldom satisfactorily achieved in clinical practice.[12]

Screening

There is no longer any question that CT can substitute for discography. CT shows only the external contour of the disc—bulges and herniations; it does not reveal the internal architecture of the disc; nor does it establish if the disc is painful. Both criteria need to be satisfied for the diagnosis of internal disc disruption, and both can only be satisfied by discography.

In contrast to CT, magnetic resonance imaging (MRI), when well performed, can reveal the nature of disc structure, and the correlations between MRI and discography are good and positive, although imperfect. Most discs established as symptomatic on the basis of provocation discography exhibit loss of signal intensity on MRI. However, not all discs abnormal on MRI are necessarily symptomatic, and some symptomatic discs appear essentially normal on MRI.[72,136] Explicitly and formally, using provocation discography as the criterion standard for the diagnosis of painful lumbar disc, MRI has a sensitivity of about 80% but a specificity of only 60% (Table 14-1). This renders MRI a reasonable screening test prior to discography. Patients with normal MRI are unlikely to be proven to have a symptomatic disc were they to undergo discography. Patients with abnormal MRI, however, still need to undergo discography, for many will not have a symptomatic disc.

Some discs exhibit a sign on MRI that correlates very highly with discs that exhibit painful, anular fissures.[5] The sign is a zone of high-intensity signal in the anulus fibrosus. Although its prevalence is only about 30%, its specificity is so high that its presence technically obviates the need for discography to confirm internal disc disruption.

Utility

A serious reservation about discography is whether it makes any difference to management and outcome.[92] There is no place for discography if the physician does not want to establish an anatomic diagnosis and if therapy is to be nonspecific. There may be a place for discography to resolve medicolegal disputes. Otherwise, the utility of discography rests on if it can direct therapy to the actual source of pain and if specific treatment of the offending disc results in a good outcome.

Attractive correlations are available between the response to provocation discography and the results of anterior, lumbar, interbody fusion. The likelihood of success with this operation in the treatment of internal disc disruption is 75% to 85% in patients who exhibit a painful disc on provocation, with patterns of internal disruption on discography, and an abnormal MRI.[47,93] The likelihood of success in patients with a painful disc but with a normal MRI is only 50%.[47]

No figures are available correlating the response to discography and the success of other operations such as posterior, lateral, or posterior interbody lumbar fusions. Discography has been used in planning operative procedures to identify the next, normal disc up to which a fusion might be extended, but no comparative data have been published to justify this seemingly accepted application of discography.[91]

In the case of cervical discography, some surgeons are convinced of the utility of discography in determining which disc should be treated with anterior cervical fusion.[68,129] They maintain that at 1-year follow-up, 70% or more of patients have good or excellent results.[68,129] Formal comparison figures are not available, but anecdotal evidence indicates that without discography to guide the operation the results are only 50%.[68]

What has not been explored and which could be of immense value is the negative, predictive value of discography. In some circles, patients with symptomatic discs at multiple segments still undergo surgery, but follow-up has not been reported in such cases. If determined, a correlation between multiple, positive discography and poor outcome would constitute evidence for the utility of discography in advising against operation.

Table 14-1

Contingency table correlating the results of MRI against the results of provocation discography as the criterion standard for a symptomatic lumbar disc*

MRI	Provocation Discography	
	Symptomatic	Asymptomatic
Abnormal	201	153
Normal	50	234

*Based on the pooled data of Osti and Fraser,[96] Horton and Daftari,[58] and Simmons et al.[112] Sensitivity = 0.80; specificity = 0.60; positive predictive value = 0.57; negative predictive value = 0.82.

References

1. Adams MA, Dolan P, Hutton WC: The stages of disc degeneration as revealed by discograms, *J Bone Joint Surg* 68B:36, 1986.
2. Adams MA, Hutton WC: Gradual disc prolapse, *Spine* 10:524, 1985.
3. Agre K, Wilson RR, Brim M, et al.: Chymodiactin post-marketing surveillance: demographic and adverse experience data in 29,075 patients, *Spine* 9:479, 1984.
4. Antti-Poika I, Soini J, Tallroth K, et al.: Clinical relevance of discography combined with CT scanning, *J Bone Joint Surg* 72B:480, 1990.
5. Aprill C, Bogduk N: High intensity zone: a pathognomonic sign of painful lumbar disc on MRI, *Br J Radiol* 65:361, 1992.
6. Bernard TN: Don't discard diskography, *Radiology* 162:285, 1987.
7. Bernard TN: Lumbar discography followed by computed tomography: refining the diagnosis of low-back pain, *Spine* 15:690, 1990.

8. Bobechko WT, Hirsch C: Autoimmune response to nucleus pulposus in the rabbit, *J Bone Joint Surg* 47B:574, 1965.

9. Bogduk N: The innervation of the lumbar spine, *Spine* 8:286, 1983.

10. Bogduk N: *The innervation of intervertebral discs.* In Ghosh P ed: *The biology of the intervertebral disc,* vol 1, Boca Raton, FL, 1988, CRC Press.

11. Bogduk N: The lumbar disc and low back pain. *Neurosurg Clin North Am* 2:791, 1991.

12. Bogduk N, Aprill C: On the nature of neck pain, discography and cervical zygapophysial joint blocks, *Pain* 54:213, 1993.

13. Bogduk N, Tynan W, Wilson AS: The nerve supply to the human lumbar intervertebral discs, *J Anat* 132:39, 1981.

14. Bogduk N, Windsor M, Inglis A: The innervation of the cervical intervertebral discs, *Spine* 13:2, 1989.

15. Bosacco SJ: Lumbar discography: redefining its role with intradiscal therapy, *Orthopedics* 9:399, 1986.

16. Brinckmann P: Injury of the anulus fibrosus and disc protrusions: an in vitro investigation on human lumbar discs, *Spine* 11:149, 1986.

17. Brown T, Hansen RJ, Yorra AJ: Some mechanical tests on the lumbosacral spine with particular reference to the intervertebral discs, *J Bone Joint Surg* 39A:1135, 1957.

18. Brodsky AE, Binder WF: Lumbar discography. Its value in diagnosis and treatment of lumbar disc lesions, *Spine* 4:110, 1979.

19. Butt WP: Lumbar discography, *J Can Assoc Radiol* 14:172, 1963.

20. Clifford JR: Lumbar discography: an outdated procedure, *J Neurosurg* 64:686, 1986.

21. Cloward RB: Cervical diskography: technique, indications and use in diagnosis of rupture cervical disks, *AJR Am J Roentgenol* 79:563, 1958.

22. Cloward RB: Cervical diskography: a contribution to the aetiology and mechanism of neck, shoulder and arm pain, *Ann Surg* 130:1052, 1959.

23. Cloward RB: The clinical significance of the sinu-vertebral nerve of the cervical spine in relation to the cervical disk syndrome, *J Neurol Neurosurg Psychiatry* 23:321, 1960.

24. Cloward RB: Cervical discography, *Acta Radiol Diagn* 1:675, 1963.

25. Cloward RB, Buzaid LL: Discography: technique, indications and evaluation of the normal and abnormal intervertebral disc, *AJR Am J Roentgenol* 68:552, 1952.

26. Colhoun E, McCall IW, Williams L, Cassar Pullicino VN: Provocation discography as a guide to planning operations on the spine, *J Bone Joint Surg* 70B:267, 1988.

27. Collins HR: An evaluation of cervical and lumbar discography, *Clin Orthop* 107:133, 1975.

28. Collis JS, Gardner WJ: Lumbar discography—an analysis of 1,000 cases, *J Neurosurg* 19:452, 1962.

29. Crock HV: Internal disc disruption: a challenge to disc prolapse fifty years on, *Spine* 11:650, 1986.

30. Davis SJ, Teresi LM, Bradley WGJ, et al.: Cervical spine hyperextension injuries: MRI findings, *Radiology,* 180:245, 1991.

31. Doyle T, Tress B, Gillot R: Combined discography and metrizamide myelography in evaluation of confusing low back pain, *Australas Radiol* 29:217, 1985.

32. Elves MW, Bucknill T, Sullivan MF: In vitro inhibition of leucocyte migration in patients with intervertebral disc lesions, *Orthop Clin North Am* 6:59, 1975.

33. Erlacher PR: Nucleography, *J Bone Joint Surg* 34B:204, 1952.

34. Errico TJ: The role of diskography in the 1980s, *Radiology* 162:285, 1987.

35. Executive Committee of the North American Spine Society: Position statement on discography, 13:1343, 1988.

36. Farfan HF: A reorientation in the surgical approach to degenerative lumbar intervertebral joint disease, *Orthop Clin North Am* 8:9, 1977.

37. Farfan HF, Kirkaldy-Willis WH: The present status of spinal fusion in the treatment of lumbar intervertebral joint disorders, *Clin Orthop* 158:198, 1981.

38. Falconer MA, McGeorge M, Begg AC: Observations on the cause and mechanism of symptom-production in sciatica and low-back pain, *J Neurol Neurosurg Psychiatry* 11:13, 1948.

39. Feinberg SB: The place of diskography in radiology as based on 2,320 cases, *AJR Am J Roentgenol* 92:1275, 1964.

40. Fraser RD, Osti AL, Vernon-Roberts B: Discitis after discography, *J Bone Joint Surg* 69B:26, 1987.

41. Fraser RD, Osti AL, Vernon-Roberts B: Iatrogenic discitis: the role of intravenous antibiotics in prevention and treatment: an experimental study, *Spine* 14:1025, 1989.

42. Friedman J, Goldner MZ: Discography in evaluation of lumbar disk lesions, *Radiology* 65:653, 1955.

43. Gardner WJ, Wise RE, Hughes CR, et al.: X-ray visualization of the intervertebral disk with a consideration of the morbidity of disk puncture, *Arch Surg* 64:355, 1952.

44. Gertzbein SD: Degenerative disk disease of the lumbar spine: immunological implications, *Clin Orthop* 129:68, 1977.

45. Gertzbein SD, Tait JH, Devlin SR: The stimulation of lymphocytes by nucleus pulposus in patients with degenerative disk disease of the lumbar spine, *Clin Orthop* 123:149, 1977.

46. Gertzbein SD, Tile M, Gross A, et al.: Autoimmunity in degenerative disc disease of the lumbar spine, *Orthop Clin North Am* 6:67, 1975.

47. Gill K, Blumenthal SL: Functional results after anterior lumbar fusion at L5-S1 in patients with normal and abnormal MRI scans, *Spine* 17:940, 1992.

48. Gresham JL, Miller R: Evaluation of the lumbar spine by diskography and its use in selection of proper treatment of the herniated disk syndrome, *Clin Orthop* 67:29, 1969.

49. Groen GJ, Baljet B, Drukker J: Nerves and nerve plexuses of the human vertebral column, *Am J Anat* 188:282, 1990.

50. Grubb SA, Lipscomb HJ, Guilford WB: The relative value of lumbar roentgenograms, metrizamide myelography, and discography in the assessment of

patients with chronic low-back-syndrome, *Spine* 12:282, 1987.

51. Guyer RD, Collier R, Stith WJ, et al.: Discitis after discography, *Spine* 13:1352, 1988.

52. Hartman JT, Kendrick JI, Larman P: Discography as an aid in evaluation for lumbar and lumbosacral fusion, *Clin Orthop* 81:77, 1977.

53. Hirsch C: An attempt to diagnose the level of a disc lesion clinically by disc puncture, *Acta Orthop Scand* 18:132, 1949.

54. Hirsch C, Ingelmark BE, Miller M: The anatomical basis for low back pain, *Acta Orthop Scand* 33:1, 1963.

55. Hodgkinson A: Neck pain localisation by cervical disc stimulation and treatment by anterior interbody fusion, *J Bone Joint Surg* 52B:789, 1970.

56. Holt EP: The fallacy of cervical discography, *JAMA* 188:799, 1964.

57. Holt EP: The question of lumbar diskography, *J Bone Joint Surg* 50A:720, 1968.

58. Horton, WC, Daftari TK: Which disc as visualized by magnetic resonance imaging is actually a source of pain? A correlation between magnetic resonance imaging and discography, *Spine* 17:S164, 1992.

59. Hsien-Wen S, Yu-Min C, Hsing-T'Ang K, et al.: Lumbar discography: an experimental and clinical study, *Chin Med J* 83:521, 1964.

60. Hsu KY, Zucherman JF, Derby R, et al.: Painful lumbar end-plate disruptions: a significant discographic finding, *Spine* 13:76, 1988.

61. Hutton WC, Adams MA: Can the lumbar spine be crushed in heavy lifting? *Spine* 7:586, 1982.

62. Inman VT, Saunders JBdeCM: Anatomicophysiological aspects of injuries to the intervertebral disc, *J Bone Joint Surg* 29A:461, 1947.

63. Jaffray D, O'Brien JP: Isolated intervertebral disc resorption: a source of mechanical and inflammatory back pain? *Spine* 11:397, 1986.

64. Jayson MIV, Herbert CM, Barks JS: Intervertebral discs: nuclear morphology and bursting pressures, *Ann Rheum Dis* 32:308, 1973.

65. Johnson RG: Does discography injure normal disc? An analysis of repeat discograms, *Spine* 14:424, 1989.

66. Jonsson H, Bring G, Rauschning W, Sahlstedt B: Hidden cervical spine injuries in traffic accident victims with skull fractures, *J Spinal Dis* 4:251, 1991.

67. Keck C: Discography: technique and interpretation, *AMA Arch Surg* 80:580, 1960.

68. Kikuchi S, MacNab I, Moreau P: Localisation of the level of symptomatic cervical disc degeneration, *J Bone Joint Surg* 63B:272, 1981.

69. Klafta LA, Collis JS: The diagnostic inaccuracy of the pain response in cervical discography, *Cleve Clin Q* 36:35, 1969.

70. Konttinen YT, Gronblad M, Antti-Poika I, et al.: Neuroimmunohistochemical analysis of peridiscal nociceptive neural elements, *Spine* 15:383, 1990.

71. Korkala O, Gronblad M, Liesi P, Karaharju E: Immunohistochemical demonstration of nociceptors in the ligamentous structures of the lumbar spine, *Spine* 10:156, 1985.

72. Kornberg M: Discography and magnetic resonance imaging in the diagnosis of lumbar disc disruption, *Spine* 12:1368, 1989.

73. Laredo J, Busson J, Wybier M, Bard M: *Technique of lumbar chemonucleolysis*. In Bard M, Laredo J, editors: *Interventional radiology in bone and joint*, New York, 1988, Springer-Verlag, p 101.

74. Laun A, Lorenz R, Agnoli AL: complications of cervical discography, *J Neurosurg Sci* 25:17, 1981.

75. Lindblom K: Diagnostic disc puncture of intervertebral disks in sciatica, *Acta Orthop Scand* 17:231, 1948.

76. Lindblom K: Technique and results in myelography and disc puncture, *Acta Radiol* 34:321, 1950.

77. Lindblom K: Technique and results of diagnostic disc puncture and injection (discography) in the lumbar region, *Acta Orthop Scand* 20:315, 1951.

78. Lindblom K: Discography of dissecting transosseous ruptures of intervertebral discs in the lumbar region, *Acta Radiol* 36:13, 1951.

79. Lownie SP, Ferguson GG: Spinal subdural empyema complicating cervical discography, *Spine* 14:1415, 1989.

80. Malinsky J: The ontogenetic development of nerve terminations in the intervertebral discs of man, *Acta Anat* 38:96, 1959.

81. Marshall LL, Trethewie ER, Curtain CC: Chemical radiculitis: a clinical, physiological and immunological study, *Clin Orthop* 129:61, 1977.

82. Massie WK, Stevens DB: A critical evaluation of discography, *J Bone Joint Surg* 49A:1243, 1967.

83. McCall IW, Park WM, O'Brien JP, et al.: Acute traumatic intraosseous disc herniation, *Spine* 10:134, 1985.

84. McCarron RF, Wimpee MW, Hudkins PG, et al.: The inflammatory effect of nucleus pulposus: a possible element in the pathogenesis of low-back pain, *Spine* 12:760, 1987.

85. McCutcheon ME: CT scanning of lumbar discography: a useful diagnostic adjunct, *Spine* 11:257, 1986.

86. McFadden JW: The stress lumbar discogram, *Spine* 13:931, 1988.

87. Mendel T, Wink CS, Zimny ML: Neural elements in human cervical intervertebral discs, *Spine* 17:132, 1992.

88. Meyer RR: Cervical diskography: a help or hindrance in evaluating neck, shoulder, arm pain, *Radiology* 90:1208, 1963.

89. Milette PC, Melanson D: A reappraisal of lumbar discography, *J Can Assoc Radiol* 33:176, 1982.

90. Milette PC, Melanson D: Lumbar diskography, *Radiology* 163:828, 1987.

91. Murtagh FR, Arrington JA: Computer tomographically guided discography as a determinant of normal disc level before fusion, *Spine* 17:826, 1992.

92. Nachemson A: Editorial comment: lumbar discography—where are we today? *Spine* 14:555, 1989.

93. Newman MH, Gristead GL: Anterior lumbar interbody fusion for internal disc disruption, *Spine* 17:831, 1992.

94. Nordlander S, Salen EF, Unander-Scharin L: Discography in low back pain and sciatica, *Acta Orthop Scand* 28:90, 1958.

95. Osti OL, Fraser RD, Vernon-Roberts B: Discitis after discography: the role of prophylactic antibiotics, *J Bone Joint Surg* 72B:271, 1990.

96. Osti OL, Fraser RD: MRI and discography of annular tears and intervertebral disc degeneration: a prospective clinical comparison, *J Bone Joint Surg* 74B:431, 1992.

97. Park W: The place of radiology in the investigation of low back pain, *Clin Rheum Dis* 6:93, 1980.

98. Patrick BS: Lumbar discography: a five year study, *Surg Neurol* 1:267, 1973.

99. Peacher WG, Storrs RP: The roentgen diagnosis of herniated disk with particular reference to diskography (nucleography), *AJR Am J Roentgenol,* 1956.

100. Perey O: Fracture of the vertebral end-plate in the lumbar spine, Acta Orthop Scand Suppl 25, 1957.

101. Perkins PG: Lumbar discography, *J Neurosurg* 65:882, 1986.

102. Porter RW, Adams MA, Hutton WC: Physical activity and the strength of the lumbar spine, *Spine* 14:201, 1989.

103. Rolander SD, Blair WE: Deformation and fracture of the lumbar vertebral end plate, *Orthop Clin North Am* 6:75, 1975.

104. Roosen K, Bettag W, Fiebach O: Komplikationen der cervikalen diskographie, *Rofo Fortschr Geb Rontgenstr Neuen Bildgeb Verfahr* 122:520, 1975.

105. Roth DA: Cervical analgesic discography: a new test for the definitive diagnosis of the painful-disk syndrome, *JAMA* 235:1713, 1976.

106. Sachs BL, Vanharanta H, Spivey MA, et al.: The relationship of pain provocation to lumbar disc deterioration as seen by CT/discography, *Spine* 12:287, 1987.

107. Scullin DR: Lumbar diskography, *Radiology* 162:284, 1987.

108. Shapiro R: Lumbar discography: an outdated procedure, *J Neurosurg* 64:686, 1986.

109. Shapiro R: Current status of lumbar diskography, *Radiology* 159:815, 1986.

110. Simmons EH, Segil CM: An evaluation of discography in the localisation of symptomatic levels in discogenic disease of the spine, *Clin Orthop* 108:57, 1975.

111. Simmons JW, Aprill CN, Dwyer AP, Brodsky AE: A reassessment of Holt's data on: "the question of lumbar discography," *Clin Orthop* 237:120, 1988.

112. Simmons JW, Emery SF, McMillin JN, et al.: Awake discography: a comparison study with magnetic resonance imaging, *Spine* 16:S216, 1991.

113. Smith GW, Nichols P: The technic of cervical discography, *Radiology* 68:718, 1957.

114. Smith GW: The normal cervical diskogram, *AJR A J Roentgenol* 81:1006, 1959.

115. Sneider SE, Winslow OP, Pryor JH: Cervical diskography: is it relevant? *JAMA* 185:163, 1963.

116. Stuck RM: Cervical discography, *AJR Am J Roentgenol* 86:975, 1961.

117. Traveras J: Is discography a useful diagnostic procedure? *J Can Assoc Radiol* 19:294, 1967.

118. Taylor JR, Kakulas BA: Neck injuries. *Lancet* 338:1343, 1991.

119. Troisier O: Technique de la discographie extra-dura, *J Radiol* 63:571, 1982.

120. Vanharanta H, Sachs BL, Spivey MA, et al.: The relationship of pain provocation to lumbar disc deterioration as seen by CT/discography, *Spine* 12:295, 1987.

121. Van Niekerk JP de V: Discography simplified. *S Afr Med J* 53:551, 1979.

122. Venner RM, Crock HV: Clinical studies of isolated disc resorption in the lumbar spine, *J Bone Joint Surg* 63B:491, 1981.

123. Vernon-Roberts B: *Age-related and degenerative pathology of intervertebral discs and apophyseal joints.* In Jayson MIV, editor: *The lumbar spine and back pain,* ed 4, Edinburgh, 1992, Churchill-Livingstone, p 17.

124. Videman T, Malmivaara A, Mooney V: The value of the axial view in assessing discograms: an experimental study with cadavers, *Spine* 12:299, 1987.

125. Volgelsang H: Discitis intervertebralis cervicalis nack diskographie, *Neurochirurgia* (Stuttg) 16:80, 1973

126. Walk L: Clinical significance of discography, *Acta Radiol* 46:36, 1956.

127. Walsh TR, Weinstein JN, Spratt KF, et al.: Lumbar discography in normal subjects, *J Bone Joint Surg* 72A:1081, 1990.

128. Weinstein J, Claverie W, Gibson S: The pain of discography, *Spine* 13:1344, 1988.

129. Whitecloud TS, Seago RA: Cervical discogenic syndrome: results of operative intervention in patients with positive discography, *Spine* 12:313, 1987.

130. Wiberg G: Back pain in relation to the nerve supply of intervertebral discs, *Acta Orthop Scand* 19:211, 1949.

131. Wiley JJ, MacNab I, Wortzman G: Lumbar discography and its clinical applications, *Can J Surg* 11:280, 1968.

132. Wilson DH, MacCarty WC: Discography: its role in the diagnosis of lumbar disc protrusion, *J Neurosurg* 31:520, 1969.

133. Wise RE, Garner WJ, Hosier RB: X-ray visualization of the intervertebral disc, *N Engl J Med* 257:6, 1957.

134. Wolkin J, Sachs MD, Hoke GH: Comparative studies of discography and myelography, *Radiology* 64:704, 1955.

135. Yoshizawa H, O'Brien JP, Thomas-Smith W, Trumper M: The neuropathology of intervertebral discs removed for low-back pain, *J Pathol* 132:95, 1980.

136. Zucherman J, Derby R, Hsu K, et al.: Normal magnetic resonance imaging with abnormal discography, *Spine* 13:1355, 1988.

Chapter 15
Diagnostic Tests for the Patient with Work-Related Injuries
Vert Mooney

Barriers to Returning to Work

Disability Evaluation

Diagnostic Testing

> imaging
> diagnostic blockade
> response to treatment

Treatment

Measuring Response to Therapeutic Exercise

Objective Functional Testing

Summary

The implication of this chapter title is that the patient with a work-related injury requires evaluation beyond that which is enumerated in the various other chapters of this book. Thus, the starting point of the discussion is to explore whether there is a difference between the patient with a work-related injury and other patients. The best documentation of the difference emerged from a publication from the Minnesota Department of Labor and Industry summarizing the health care costs for industrial medical care versus private medical care for the year 1989.[14] First of all, it should be no surprise to learn that in this study, 41.2% of Workers' Compensation charges in Minnesota were for back injuries. An additional 17% of the charges were secondary to strains and sprains of other regions, and another 8.8% were secondary to soft tissue contusions. Thus, 67% of the charges were for unverifiable soft tissue injuries. Verifiable injuries, such as fracture (6.2% of the charges) made up a relatively minor portion of Workers' Compensation medical problems. However, more important than the charges for soft tissue injuries is the comparison between these charges and those for private insurance.

This study also compared charges by disease categories billed to private insurance for non-work-related injuries and billed to Workers' Compensation insurance. On the basis of this analysis, it turns out that charges for fracture care, for instance, were about the same. Workers' Compensation charges were about 1.1 times more than Blue Cross charges. However, for nonverifiable diagnostic categories such as back "injuries," the total charges for Workers' Compensation were 2.4 times more than those of private insurance. The same is true for sprains and strains, which were 2.2 times more for Workers' Compensation compared to private insurance. It is quite clear, therefore, that at least for nonverifiable problems such as soft tissue injuries, charges for the insured worker are more than for standard private medical care for the same disease categories.

Is it because the injuries are more severe in the workplace? Not at all. In the case of lower extremity fractures, 50% of privately insured patients had surgery, while 20% of the Workers' Compensation patients required surgery. About the same ratio was true of upper extremity fractures (46.8% of the privately insured patients vs. 16.1% of the Workers' Compensation patients had surgery), and even for the more verifiable back disorders that required surgery (4% of the privately insured patients required surgery, vs. 3.4% of the Workers' Compensation patients). Are these statistics because Workers' Compensation patients get better care in Minnesota? No,

there is no evidence of that. In this study, the same analysis of disease-related group charges was made in the states neighboring Minnesota. The median charges and the ratios were just about the same. There was nothing peculiar about the Minnesota experience. Where does the difference come from? That is the essential question for this chapter.

The answer lies in the limitations of diagnostic tests for soft tissue injuries. There was no discrepancy of costs or treatment expectations for fractures; x-ray studies supplied an objective evaluation. How can we objectively evaluate soft tissue injuries in the patient with a work-related injury? If we could, costs would be controlled and prognosis for recovery would be as secure as for fractures.

In the most extensive recent study on this subject—the Boeing study[2,4]—no physical characteristics were good predictors for Workers' Compensation claims for back injuries. It must be noted that in this study only about 10% of the workers made claims for back injuries. Statistically, the incidence of back pain is much higher; thus, we must assume that only a small portion of individuals with back pain made a claim. In the Boeing study,[2,4] the disgruntled worker (poor reports from supervisor) and poor health habits (smoking, etc.) were significant predictors for claims. The implication is either that the individuals who made claims manufactured complaints or that minor injuries lingered due to habituation of disability.

Barriers to Returning to Work

It must be recognized that there are often major barriers to returning to work based on factors aside from the physical impairment. Disability is the summary of many factors, including impairment, but also must include life realities such as education, age, job market opportunities, etc. When the individual gets too old and lacks the means to rise above the physically demanding job on which he or she was injured, a safety net exists in industrialized societies to offer support to this now ill-qualified individual. The Social Security Disability system allows an individual with a medical diagnosis to achieve lifelong compensation if a medical impairment can be proven after 1 year of inability to return to work. The burden of proof is thrown to the medical profession, who must clearly identify a medical diagnosis as the source of the problem. The impairment must be definable. Of course, that is where the problem of useful diagnostic tests for the industrial soft tissue injury must be solved.

Disability Evaluation

In California, a very sophisticated scheme for rating permanent disabilities is in place.[24] The Schedule for Rating Permanent Disabilities is an 82 page manual published by the state, wherein age and physical demands of the job are used in a formula to rate the injured worker after evaluation by a physician. The physician provides an impairment and disability statement based on historic events and largely subjective physical factors. For instance, the back rating is based on estimated percentage deficits from normal range. Actually this is fair, in that the range of motion of the lumbar spine varies greatly depending on age, sex, and work history. An experienced physician should be able to estimate this. There are expected levels of normal for the rest of the joints, and the percentage deficit is therefore able to be calculated. However, these range deficits are only a small portion of the criteria for physician rating. A work capacity evaluation is necessary wherein the physician must estimate the disability, including various levels of work and/or lifting. There is no requirement actually to test the capacity to work—the physician merely needs to estimate whether the individual can lift 50 lb, etc. In the California scheme, because the system is so complex, professional raters utilize a formula established by the state to come up with the final rating. This is the only state with such a complex system.

The majority of the states use the AMA Guidelines.[7] In the third edition of these guidelines, the only test used for evaluation of the spine is true lumbar sagittal range and lateral bending. The impairment numbers identified from these findings are added to the numbers assigned to diagnostic categories. Additional numbers are added from evaluation of the extremity function, including strength, sensation, and function. The only functional test that is suggested but not necessary for the evaluation of extremity function is the JAMAR isometric grip strength tool. Here, also, expected levels of strength are identified—and deviation from these levels can be calculated as a percentage.

This short discussion of disability evaluation systems is mentioned merely to point out the minimal levels of testing required to establish disability. This testing and evaluation is essentially after the fact. What we really must search for are specific diagnostic tests to establish the physical impairment of the patient with a work-related injury at onset and conclusion of treatment. It must once again be emphasized that we can measure only impairment. Impairment is part of disability—but the other factors of disability such as age, occupation, etc. are unchangeable and uncontrollable. Only the level of physical impairment is controllable on the basis of medical care.

Diagnostic Testing

The answer to the questions posed above as to a specific test for defining the level of soft tissue injury is clear to me. The most important diagnostic test is response to a rational progressive treatment program that uses objective measurement of function as a guide to progress. This will establish the validity of the complaint. If the structural deficit (weak link) is repairable without surgery, the mending will occur.

Imaging

Of course, the major technical advance in defining structural abnormalities in recent years has been the development of MRI. But it is not discriminating. Patients presenting for disability evaluations frequently have had an MRI test within 2 or 3 weeks after injury. They present no evidence of having a progressive neurologic deficit, and there is no evidence that the treatment plan was altered on the basis of MRI findings. In the middle years there is always a "bulging" disc. Statistically, even in the younger years—20s and 30s—disc abnormalities are notable in 20% to 30% of the cases.[5] As the years progress, there are frequent references to minor and progressive degenerative changes—again an anatomic statement, but no evidence that this is a symptomatic source.

Unhappily, the technology of MRI has not progressed to the degree that soft tissue injuries to the muscles, ligaments, or capsular attachments can be defined. Even tears within the disc cannot always be defined. On the other hand, these are the injuries that most likely are the cause of the acute back pain problem. Failure of spontaneous repair allows persistence of pain and progression into chronicity. These are patients for whom no specific physical finding can be assigned. There may be referred pain down the leg, there may be some limitation in range, there may even be muscle spasm and tenderness. However, the repeatability of these findings is quite limited. Rarely are there strong signs of radiculopathy (motor weakness, sensory deficit in an anatomically specific pattern, and straight leg raising with reproducibility of leg pain). These tests should lead into diagnostic studies, but this is a small percentage. MRI is the most sensitive, and the other imaging studies are no more likely to add useful information as to cause.

Verification of the concept that there are no specific tests for low-back pain is one of the summaries from the famous Quebec Task Force Study.[23] In this consensus of opinions from various specialists, after review of the world literature, no specific physical finding could be assessed to identify back disorders without radiculopathy. Only pain location and duration of pain were mechanisms by which classification could be achieved.[23] However, this study did not make any specific recommendation as to how this classification could more clearly elucidate the treatment program or the prognosis. The only recommendation emerging from the study was that exercise was a positive treatment; and there was no evidence that rest or methods such as ultrasound or massage were of benefit.

Diagnostic Blockade

The only specific mechanism by which an injured anatomic structure might be defined would be the use of diagnostic blocks with the assistance of radiographic localization. This subject is discussed in detail in other chapters of this book. There are, of course, advantages to the specificity potentially available from an anatomic localization. Such things as facet blocks, sacroiliac injections, and nerve root blocks do offer some clarification as to anatomic sites serving as a pain generator for nonspecific back pain. For more superficial anatomic locations, the specificity of injections is even more clear, such as in the injection of overuse sites such as the lateral epicondyle of the humerus and its origin of wrist extensor musculature.

Can the patient admit that anything makes them better? The most valuable information gleaned from a specific block is patient response and attitude. For example, if these blocks with their instillation of local anesthetic and steroids cause a significant immediate increase in pain, it is difficult to think that the structural incompetence of the supposed injured site is a major factor in the source of continuing complaints of pain. No improvement even in the short term suggests that the injected site is not the injury site. It suggests the patient may be exaggerating the pain. Overlapping innervation of every anatomic site also makes it difficult to assume that this type of test is foolproof. The distribution of innervation in areas supplied by segmental nerves that are supplying remote areas as well as the injured area may create false localization of anatomic abnormality on the basis of the referred-pain phenomenon. In my own experimentation, it was clear that injection of irritant solutions into the facet joint could cause pain in the buttock and posterior thigh based on this phenomenon of overlapping innervation. In comparing individuals who already had back pain to normal subjects, the amount of stimulus necessary to achieve extension of pain was smaller. Thus, the use of diagnostic blocks, while of help in getting to know the patient better and in identifying specific anatomic sites, have their best role in reducing pain in the short term to allow progression into an appropriate exercise program.[17]

Response to Treatment

Response to treatment, as noted above, is the most significant test available to us to evaluate the severity and validity of work-related soft tissue injuries. Exercise treatment must be measurable, active, and progressive. If no improvement in function occurs after valid effort and increasing "doses" of exercise, the structural deficit either is too severe to be treated conservatively or does not exist. There is no evidence that any of the currently available passive modalities have an effect on the structure relationships in injured soft tissues. Spontaneous repair will be initiated without the benefit of these methods. They may reduce postinjury pain and, therefore, as an accompanying treatment program, should be of benefit. Currently our information suggests that most spontaneous repair of soft tissues should be completed by 6 weeks.[1] Because of this, the Quebec Task Force advised that extensive multispeciality evaluation be focused on the injured worker if repair, and thus pain reduction, has not occurred by 7 weeks.

The need for medication or passive modalities is an additional characteristic in evaluating the response to treatment. Patients for whom we can document an increasing requirement for medication, or an increasing demand for passive physical therapy or chiropractic care are presenting significant diagnostic information. Patients who state that they are no better despite brief benefit from medicine or passive therapy and then ask for more are presenting clear evidence of lack of insight into their problem. In a significant study by Polatin et al.,[19] over 95% of the patients with chronic back pain (most over 6 mo.) that was severe enough to need an intense physical rehabilitation program for low-back disability, had at least one psychiatric diagnosis. Seventy-seven percent had at least two diagnoses. Many of these individuals had histories of significant substance abuse, as well as anxiety and depression. This study points out that a structural problem resolvable by physical treatment does not require additional pain medication. The need for additional medication identifies patients who have factors other than their physical impairment as their source of disability. Chronic low-back pain may result from preexisting emotional disorders.

Treatment

The major treatment for soft tissue work-related injuries is a progressive exercise program that offers increasing load to challenge repair of the injured tissue. The best model for this is the treatment for grades I and II ankle injuries, wherein total disruption of the joint has not occurred. Twenty years ago the standard treatment for this was a plaster cast. However, with improving understanding of the phenomenon of repair, the current treatment for ankle sprains is a removable splint, progressive range-of-motion exercise, and later, muscle strengthening, challenging for range and endurance. Ultimately, documentation of physical performance is necessary before the patient is allowed to return to normal activity. Certainly, an athlete who has had an ankle injury would have to demonstrate return to normal activity in jumping, cutting, and running before returning to competition. Absence of edema and tenderness in the injured area after 1 day of strenuous physical activity are the criteria for return to competition. Persistence of these abnormalities will force the supervising clinician to delay return to normal competitive activity. That is the model for response to treatment.

Some parts of the body are more easily defined than others. The ankle, with its absence of overlying soft tissue or muscle, is relatively easy to define by physical examination. The low back is probably the most difficult to define. Thus, specific testing may be necessary to define functional limitations accurately. Specific testing, to whatever extent possible, must isolate the injured area so that the level of function can most clearly be defined.

What is the relationship between function and painful incompetence of some injured soft tissue? The concept of neurologic inhibition and facilitation is necessary to understand this relationship. We recognize that motor function is based on stimulation of the motor unit. The motor unit is comprised of the anterior horn cell, the axon connecting it with the dependent musculature, and finally, the muscle fibers associated with the synapse of this axon. How does pain vary the functional level? Certainly, willful activity is under the control of the higher central nervous system levels. On the other hand, many factors have an impact on the ability of the anterior horn cell to fire. The balance between facilitory and inhibitory synaptic vesical influence varies the anterior horn cell membrane potential. To fire it must be allowed to come to a critical level. Body position, noxious stimuli emerging from injury in the segmentally innervated area, enthusiasm or lack of it (lassitude) are all factors.[15] Figure 15-1 is a depiction of this phenomenon at work. It emphasizes that to the degree inhibitory influences have an impact on anterior horn cell function, overall motor function of the involved segment is diminished. This concept is the justification for base-line testing of function to evaluate the amount of motor unit inhibition. Testing of motor function at the conclusion of treatment is the best definition of resolution of structural incompetence based on either chemical or mechanical repair processes.

Again, we must focus on neuromotor function tests as the mechanism to demonstrate the hypothesis described above. The lumbar spine is the most difficult anatomic site to examine physically. Muscle strength of the lumbar area is the summation of multiple muscle groups. Overall function of the back can be near normal, even with weak muscle function in the lumbar area, due to the capacity for substitution. The phenomenon of alternative strategies to solve a functional problem is a significant asset of our nervous system. Unfortunately, it also has a potential liability in that habituation to this substitution may be ongoing unless a specific treatment program is initiated. The most specific treatment program to

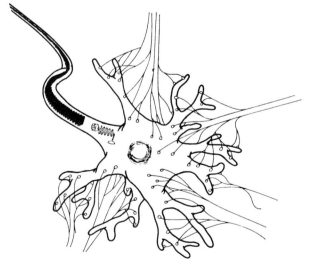

Fig. 15-1

Diagrammatic depiction of anterior horn cell wherein synaptic vesicles are attached to cell membrane. These vesicles vary membrane potential. Potential is lowered by inhibitory vesicles and elevated by facilitory vesicles. If critical potential has occurred, cell will fire in an all-or-none manner.

break the habit of neuromotor substitution for the weak link is an exercise program that specifically isolates the weak link.

Now let us focus on the weak link. If we have a patient who has sustained a work-related back injury, and the problem has not resolved after 6 or 7 weeks, we have to assume that either spontaneous healing of the soft tissue injury has not occurred or that the individual has become habituated to the pain. Of course, it is quite possible that spontaneous healing has not occurred; thus, it is reasonable to develop an exercise program focused on assisting the healing process. All evidence suggests that this must be an active exercise program, wherein increasing physical stresses are applied to the healing soft tissue in an effort to "train" the repair process. These physical stresses must be a gradual overload in order to challenge repair and strengthening. This can be done by instruction in a guided exercise program either done at home or, better, under the supervision of a qualified therapist in a training facility. The training is enhanced by specialized equipment, which can more significantly isolate the weak link.

All facilities do not have specialized equipment. Many do not feel the need for specialized tools to measure function. Therapists at these highly specialized treatment centers certainly can evaluate levels of function based on performance of simple exercises. Certainly, there are an array of appropriate exercises, specially designed for the acute and subacute problems, that have been very effective. McKenzie exercises, stabilization exercises, and generalized calisthenics with aerobic training have been advocated. These all provide a measurable amount of training and thus documentation of the dose of therapeutic exercise. Early in the treatment program, of course, control of pain with manipulation, various methods such as hot packs, cold packs, and various forms of electrical energy have been advocated. Probably these are reasonable in the early phases of treatment, while discomfort is still the major interest of everyone involved—patient, therapist, and funding agency. The use of steroids also is appropriate, especially if specifically directed at presumed sites of reactive inflammation. Here again, however, response to treatment is an appropriate insight as to the nature of the problem. An outline of treatment protocol for low back injuries is presented in the box below. This is used by various managed-care facilities. The emphasis on assessment is clearly a common thread in this type of treatment program.

Special equipment is not a new concept. In the latter part of the past century, specialized equipment was designed by Dr. Gustaf Zander.[11] Dr. Zander

Guidelines for Treatment of Patients with Medical Back Conditions

1. After no more than 2 days of bed rest, a program of progressive exercise should be initiated. Passive methods (e.g., hot packs) should not be used for more than 2 weeks.

2. If more than 2 weeks of treatment are required, there should be an objective, reproducible functional assessment.

3. Total treatment duration should not exceed 6 weeks, and frequency should not exceed three treatments weekly.

4. Diagnostic x-ray examinations may be appropriate initially, but not at intervals during treatment.

5. Specific imaging techniques (e.g., CT scan, MRI, EMG, nerve-conduction studies) are appropriate only when there is deteriorating neurologic function or when progressive exercise therapy has failed.

6. If treatment lasts 6 weeks, the patient should be evaluated by an orthopedic surgeon or neurologist. The evaluation should include measurement of functional status, reassessment of treatment goals, and confirmation of the appropriateness of treatment.

recognized at that time that specialized tools could more appropriately isolate weakened tissues, and on the basis of base-line testing could offer the opportunity to define the dose of progressive therapeutic exercise. The amount of resistance can be easily computed; thus, building on an initial base line, progressive resistance exercises can be prescribed. Compliance and progress, of course, are easily identified (Fig. 15-2).

A confusion developed concerning the benefits of rest for infection; because of incomplete understanding about mechanical inflammation, the false concept that rest was healthy for soft tissue strains emerged. The concept of isolated therapeutic exercise faded from the medical scene in the early decades of this century. Prolonged bed rest was prescribed for everything from heart attacks to postpartum care. Isolated exercise was retired to the gymnasium, where body builders recognized its potential, but in general did not use sophisticated equipment. Barbells and devices for calisthenics were the essential features.

The concept of therapeutic exercise was really not reintroduced into medicine until the urgencies of

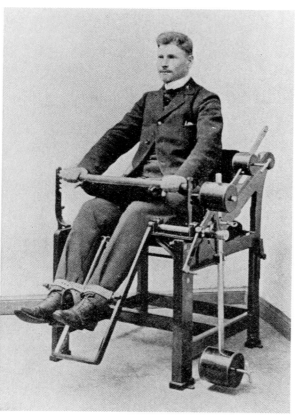

Fig. 15-2

Example of devices designed by Gustaf Zander in the late 1800s to allow medicomechanical treatment. These are predecessors to our current specialized equipment, which define the dose of exercise. (G. Zander's Medico-Mechanical Gymnastic Method, *Rosset, Schwarz, & Co., Wiesbader, 1906*)

the second world war, during which the principles of the weight lifter were brought back into medicine as a mechanism to provide rehabilitation for injured joints.[6] The concept of isolating anatomy to exercise it more efficiently was part of the program. Specialized equipment did not emerge until the invention of the Nautilus by Arthur Jones.[10] This equipment, by innovative design, allowed significant resistance to be spread out through a broad range of the joint activity. This use of special equipment gradually reorganized thinking in exercise treatment. Many variations have occurred since this development in the late 1960s. They all have the potential to measure the dose of therapeutic exercise, build on a base line of measured deficit of function, and allow observation of progress in terms of range, strength, and endurance. Thus, measurement of function and response to treatment has been readily available for several decades. However, range, strength, and endurance of back musculature is the most difficult to measure, and few pieces of equipment specifically isolate this area of the anatomy.

Although many pieces of equipment are available, there are some principles that allow judgment as to which are more useful than others. Exercise that can be performed both in the concentric and the eccentric mode is more likely to be more efficient in strengthening than only concentric exercise. Also, the greater the degree of anatomic isolation, the less opportunity for substitution, and the more efficient and effective the exercise can be.[22] Also, the most accurate testing of muscular performance is in a non-dynamic mode and is better accomplished by measuring isometric strength at various points in the range.[21] The design for the most specific equipment for the lumbar spine is offered in Fig. 15-3. This equipment also has the advantage of being both a testing as well as a training tool, in that once isometric strength at various points in the range has been defined, this leads directly to the definition of deficit and prescription of the dose of therapeutic exercise on the same equipment.

Measuring Response to Therapeutic Exercise

Appropriate response to the training program can, therefore, be specifically measured, and an end point defined, wherein the individual either returns to normal (this assumes, of course, that normative values are known for the strength being tested), or that the individual has reached a plateau in the ability to increase strength.[8] If the individual has documented full effort and indeed increased strength (the normal physiologic response from progressive overload) but still maintains pain complaints, further diagnostic studies are warranted. This individual may have reached maximum medical improvement or permanent and stationary status. However, if the individual is not compliant with the exercise program, it is inappropriate to define him/her as reaching maximum medical improvement.

Noncompliance with the program, of course, is very difficult to establish and becomes a medicolegal label. Is it justified to make this definition? Certainly a test should be available to document lack of compliance very accurately.

It has been thought that compliance could best be documented by noting consistency of maximal effort. This concept has been somewhat threatened by recent publications. In a study by Hazard et al.,[9] it was noted that some subjects were able to produce consistent maximal efforts, and others making full effort produced inconsistent maximal efforts on isokinetic equipment. In fact, in this study, the appearance of efforts such as facial expression was more accurate than curve variability.

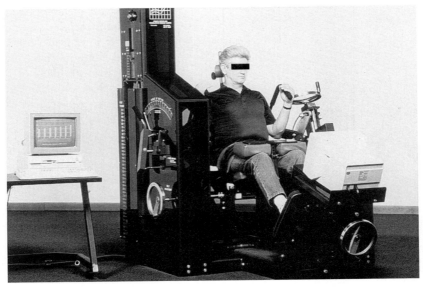

Fig. 15-3

Zander exercise equipment specifically isolates sagittal motion of lumbar spine and measures isometric extensor strength at various points in the range. It also provides variable eccentric resistance, full-range, concentric, and extensory exercise to the lumbar extensors.

Even with the more accurate isometric testing, it is possible to "fake" consistent submaximal effort if the subject is motivated to do so and there is some feedback as to performance. If the test-retest is performed relatively quickly after the first test, fairly reproducible submaximal effort is available if subjects are so motivated.[20] However, if the feedback to the individual willfully trying to mislead the observer is altered, then the deception can be clearly defined and documented. Using isometric strength testing with the results graphically displayed on the screen to both patient and therapist, consistency of effort can be documented by repeatability on various occasions of testing with reference to the crossbars. However, unknown to the subject, the resistance represented by these crossbars can be changed. Thus, although the effort appears consistent, it represents totally different resistance, which is impossible from a physiologic standpoint. The definition of this patient willfully misleading the observer is sufficient to achieve administrative resolution of the case without need for further medical treatment programs.[16]

Objective Functional Testing

Although response to treatment can be the most effective test in identifying soft tissue deficits for the patient with a work-related injury, this does not identify the true functional deficits that prevent this patient from returning to his/her previous job. It has been well documented that no specific test will identify functional capacity with sufficient accuracy that reemployment liability for back injury or predictability of reinjury on returning to work is available.[3] If accurate data are necessary in an effort to assign level of function or identify level of impairment for disability evaluation, objective functional testing must be accomplished. As noted earlier, our standards for functional testing are minimal. Perhaps that is one of the reasons why litigation costs are so high in the area of disability definition. The resistance to having more accurate functional testing is natural. What tool is available? For it to have universal acceptance, it must have relatively minimal expense, it must be sufficiently standardized that it is reproducible, and compliance and effort factor must be sufficiently notable to document an accurate test. The only device that sufficiently qualifies for all these criteria is the JAMAR hand grip. Even range-of-motion testing for the lumbar spine is controversial, and it must be recognized that range of motion is not a true functional test. Is there something on the horizon that has a potential to be a functional capacity test system for the back?

Functional capacity testing of the back should recognize that substitution for the weak link is a normal strategy. Thus, lifting function must be assessed using whole-body performance. Both strength and endurance must be assessed. The first step toward this concept was the development of the PILE (progressive isoinertial lifting evaluation) test by Mayer et al.[13] This used a protocol of lifting weights in a box at a constant rate and with constant increase in resistance until the movement could no longer be performed. Effort was monitored by pulse rate to ensure sufficient work was being accomplished by the test subject so that near-maximum performance could be identified. This particular test used weights that were definable to the observer so that test-retest achievement could be accomplished merely by remembering the amount of weights. The weights lifted from the floor were all equidistant so that there was an inappropriate comparison of tall people versus short people.

An improvement on this test was achieved by Matheson et al., who used blinded weights, a maximum effort, an endurance protocol, and varying heights of weight lifted from the floor or from the knuckle to shoulder in order to allow comparison of individuals of different heights (Fig. 15-4).[12] This PLC (progressive lifting capacity) test did identify

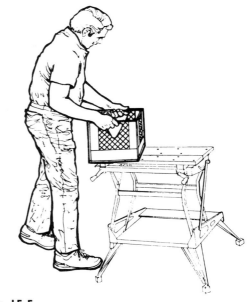

Fig. 15-5

PACT (performance assessment and capacity test) spinal function sort. (*Source:* Pact Spinal Function SDRT, *Matheson, Leonard, 1989*)

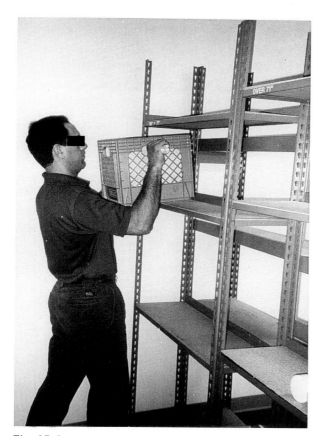

Fig. 15-4

EPIC Progressive Lifting Capacity Test (PLC), which measures functional lifting capacity using weights progressively added to the box. Weights are all same size; thus, individual is unaware of amount of weight lifted.

greater accuracy than its predecessor. However, a significant improvement over purely measuring the functional capacity would be a mechanism by which perception of capacity is also measured. This is accomplished by a 50-page picture book that identifies normal activities of daily living with specific definition of the task (Fig. 15-5).[18] The individual is asked to score whether he/she can accomplish the pictured task or not. Pictured are several tasks that are exact duplications of the lifting capacity test and also exact duplications of efforts under different circumstances. Thus, the validity of the test subject's response can be measured as well. With use of these two tests, a clearer picture of perceived functional capacity and measured functional capacity can be identified. This, coupled with the definition of lumbar impairment based on specific testing and measurement of response of an exercise program, can offer a complete picture of maximal medical improvement or permanent and stationary status.

Traditionally, functional capacity has been measured by various questionnaires of varying length. These require the individual to document deficits in activities of daily living such as walking, sitting, sexual activity, etc. The Oswestry questionnaire probably is the early model for this, but many others have been developed. The balance between duration of the test and sensitivity based on varying and repeated questions has never been achieved, at least through the consensus of individuals using these tests. No one functional test seems to be totally accepted by all.

An important aspect of this question concerning testing is the mental state of the individual being challenged. Certainly, most Workers' Compensation individuals in the acute and subacute phase have a normal mental attitude. My own experience (unpublished data) is that about 5 percent of patients with work-related back injuries willfully mislead observers. On the other hand, once the individual has developed a chronic pain syndrome (perhaps reinforced by ineffective early care), a high level of behavioral problems have emerged. In a study by Polatin et al.[19] noted above, using a structured interview, nearly all patients with back injuries that do not respond to treatment have psychiatric diagnoses, most of which were preexisting. Thus, coming up with a specific test appropriate for all patients is a complex issue. To this point, the gold standard has not emerged.

Summary

The unique diagnostic tests for patients with work-related injuries are ones that identify response to treatment and compliance and attitude. It has been pointed out that the extent of industrial "injury" to soft tissues of the neck or back are essentially undefinable by traditional diagnostic studies. Because of this, treatment for these well-funded patients is more costly than for the patient with a non-work-related injury. A case has been made for the need to document "the dose" of exercise treatment so that objective measurement of response is available. Because compliance and attitude are the key to successful treatment for the majority of industrial injuries, an environment focused on function is basically the best test location. Whether this is called "work hardening," or "functional restoration," objective measurement of function is the key to effective diagnostic testing.

Patient attitude is the only element of concern that may be different in the Workers' Compensation patient versus the private patient. The definitive test for this is the answer to a single question for someone who has had benign pain for over 6 weeks: What is more important to you—to feel better or to function better? How would you answer the question?

References

1. Akeson WH, Woo SL-Y, Amiel D, et al.: *The biology of ligaments*. In Funk FJ, Hunter LY, editors: *Rehabilitation of the injured knee*, St. Louis, 1984, Mosby.

2. Battie MC: The reliability of physical factors as predictors of the occurrence of back pain reports: a prospective study within industry, doctoral thesis, Gothenburg, Sweden, 1989, Gothenburg University.

3. Bigos J, Battie MC, Fisher LD, et al.: A prospective evaluation of pre-employment screening methods for acute industrial back pain, *Spine* 17:922, 1992.

4. Bigos SJ, Battie MC, Spenger DM, et al.: A longitudinal prospective study of industrial back injury reporting, *Clin Orthop* 279:21, 1992.

5. Boden SD, Davis DO, Deena TS, et al.: Abnormal magnetic resonance scans of the lumbar spine in asymptomatic subjects, *J Bone Joint Surg* 72:403, 1990.

6. DeLorme TL: *Progressive resistance exercise*, New York, 1951, Appleton-Century-Croft.

7. Engelberg AL, editor: *Guides to the evaluation of permanent impairment*, ed 3, Chicago, 1988, American Medical Association.

7a. Fairbank JC, Davies JD, Coupa J, Obrien JP: The Oswestry low back disability questionnaire, *Physiotherapy:* 66, 271, 1980.

8. Graves JE, Pollock ML, Foster D, et al.: Effective training frequency and specificity on isometric lumbar eccentric strength, *Spine* 15:504, 1990.

9. Hazard R, Reid S, Fenwick J, Reeves V: Isokinetic trunk and lifting strength measurements: variability as an indicator of effort, *Spine* 13:54, 1988.

10. Jones A: A new exercise tool, *Athlet J* 55:76, 1974.

11. Levertin A, Heiligenthal F, Zander G: *The leading features of Dr. G. Zander's medico-mechanical gymnastic method book.* Wiesbaden, Germany, 1906, Russel, Schwartz and Co.

12. Matheson L, Mooney V, Caiozzo V, et al.: The effect of instructions on isokinetic trunk strength testing variability, reliability, absolute value, and predictive validity, *Spine* 17:914, 1992.

13. Mayer TG, Barenes D, Kishino ND, Nickols G, et al.: Progressive isoinertial lifting evaluation I: a standardized protocol and normative data base, *Spine* 13:993, 1988.

14. Minnesota Department of Labor and Industry: Report to the legislature on health care costs and cost containment in Minnesota workers compensation, March 1990.

15. Mooney V: On the dose of therapeutic exercise, *Orthopaedics* 15:653, 1992.

16. Mooney V, Leggett SH, Holmes BL, Negri S: Strength testing can't identify malingering, *J Workers Comp* 2:55, 1992.

17. Mooney V, Robertson J: The facet syndrome, *Clin Orthop* 115:149, 1976.

18. PACT Spinal Function Sort Epic, Santa Ana, CA, 1991, Leonard Matheson.

19. Polatin PB, Kinney RK, Gatchel RJ, et al.: Psychiatric illness and chronic low back pain: the mind and the spine—which goes first? *Spine* 18:66-1993.

20. Robinson ME, MacMillan M, O'Connor P, Fuller A: Reproducibility of maximal versus submaximal ef-

forts in an isometric lumbar extension task, *J Spinal Disord* 4:444, 1991.

21. Rothstein JM, Lamb RL, Mayhew TP: Clinical uses of isokinetic measurements, *Crit Issues Phys Ther,* 67:1840, 1987.

22. Sapega AA: Muscle performance evaluation in orthopaedic practice: current concepts reviewed, *J Bone Joint Surg* 72A:1562, 1990.

23. Spitzer WO, LeBlanc FE, DePois F, et al.: Scientific approach to the assessment and management of activity related spinal disorders, *Spine* 12:S1, 1987.

24. State of California, Department of Workers' Compensation: Schedule for Rating Permanent Disabilities, Form 302 (Revised 10/91), Sacramento, CA.

Chapter 16
Physical Therapy Approach to Diagnosing the Patient with a Work-Related Injury

Susan Isernhagen

As a diagnostician of spinal conditions, the physician relies on medical tests such as x-ray studies, magnetic imaging, blood tests, electromyography, and others. The medical diagnosis involves structure and pathology. In physical therapy diagnosis, the physical therapist utilizes evaluation of musculoskeletal function and its relation to musculoskeletal pathology.[3,4] This assists the diagnostic process. It is the combination of structural abnormalities with functional implications that provides for optimal treatment of the patient.

Physical therapy evaluation procedures combined with functional outcomes provide a more comprehensive view of the ability and limitations of a patient than does medical diagnosis alone. These are of significance in refining a medical structural diagnosis and in determining case direction.

Physical Therapist's Role in Spinal Function Evaluation

Characteristics of the physical therapy profession that relate to functional diagnosis and case management are specialization in movement science, knowledge of pathology, and whole-body functional evaluation.[9] These are discussed below.

Movement Science Specialization

Physical therapy combines the science of anatomy with the art of analyzing and treating human movement. Since movement is the basis of productive work, the physical therapist is uniquely qualified to utilize movement science skills in evaluating the safety of returning to work and the level of work ability. For analysis of total functional patterns, the physical therapist is well educated in the individual components that comprise movement. For example, the therapist receives intensive education in muscle physiology, kinesiology, neuromuscular patterns, musculoskeletal attributes, and analysis of the body—joint by joint, muscle by muscle, and tendon by tendon. These are the body blocks of productive functional movement.

Knowledge of Pathology

While other professionals also evaluate movement, the physical therapist has comprehensive knowledge of pathologic conditions of the neuromusculoskeletal system that affect movement and capacity. Physical therapists understand the basis of dysfunction, including the principles behind sprain, joint degeneration, overuse syndromes, musculotendinous

problems, disc pathologies, and other specific diagnostic categories. The understanding of the pathology that underlies spinal disorders and how they affect functional work injuries is critical. If only healthy, normal workers needed evaluation, other movement science professionals could be used. However, the pathologic nature of spinal injury necessitates a professional with a strong background in spinal pathologic conditions in order to provide accurate diagnostic evaluation.

Whole-Body Functional Evaluation

The outcome of movement, whether normal or pathologic, is function. In the case of back injury, physical therapists deal with work function, which is a subsection of functional movement of the human body. Function is dependent on adequate physical resources to perform specific tasks. In both activities of daily living evaluation and occupational rehabilitation, work functions can be specifically defined in terms of lifting, carrying, bending, reaching, sitting, squatting, etc. The physical therapist begins with movement patterns, reconciles them with pathologic problems, and integrates them into the outcome—safe work function.[6,7,10,11,15] See the box on the next page for specifics of physical therapy evaluation components.

Physical therapists, like physicians, have specialities. Even within "spine specialization" a manual therapist and industrial therapist have separate competencies and may refer to each other for an application of body "hands on" and "functional" therapeutic interventions.

Teamwork in Diagnosis and Management

Teamwork between physician and physical therapist in back care is crucial. Therapists must understand the medical diagnosis, prognosis, contraindications to certain treatment methods, and other medical conditions. The physician conversely will require information on musculoskeletal abnormalities, neuromuscular dysfunction, aerobic condition, and functional status evaluated by the therapist. These parameters combine medical information needed for comprehensive initial diagnosis.

The quandary of patients with spinal conditions, however, is often one of treatment,[18] not diagnosis. Therefore, the astute, realistic, caring medical practitioner goes beyond discovery of pathology into treatment. Treatment of back pain is currently an expected service. It is not the prevalence, however, that

Physical Therapy
Musculoskeletal/Functional Diagnosis

Structural evaluation components (to be integrated with physician evaluation)

- Range of motion/spinal flexibility
- Joint integrity
- Muscle tone
- Reflex testing
- Muscle testing
- Myofascial components

Treatment (gives prognostic information by determining the extent to which back problems can be resolved and function can be restored)

- Mobilization/manipulation
- Deep-tissue massage
- Modalities
- Stretching
- Strengthening
- Stabilization

---

drives the system, it is the severity. Realistically, it is not even the severity, it is the functional disturbance that is important to the patient. There is not necessarily a similarity among patients with L4-L5 disc problems. One can be in severe pain, a second can have minimal pain but be functionally limited, and a third can be asymptomatic. Diagnosis by the physician is critical as a basis for patient care, but treatment of the patient will require the physical therapist as functional diagnostician.

Ongoing diagnosis is also a dual role. Because spinal structures are not static, the treating therapist and physician must monitor the dynamic spinal status. Most often, a change in structural status is first noted through a change in function. The therapists functional evaluation, therefore, precedes the change in medical status determination. Direct and thorough communication between the physician and the physical therapist and integration of diagnostic and treatment outcomes gives the patient full service. Spinal conditions are understood and evaluated in the context of what the problem means to the patient.

- If the patient has pain and chronic degeneration, as with arthritis or stenosis, physician diagnosis will be informative but physical thera-

pist diagnosis will be meaningful on a daily living or work basis.

- In a client with a work-related injury, physician diagnosis will bring meaning to structural damage, but the physical therapist's diagnosis (through functional evaluation and treatment) will bring about a return to work.
- For the acutely injured patient, the physical therapy diagnosis may occur simultaneously or precede the medical diagnosis, depending on the practitioner first involved in early intervention strategies at the work site.

Algorithmic Methods

Algorithmic care is that which is established by a set of standards organized by time periods or sequences of events. it is an orderly, predesigned plan of care that allows the practitioner to move the patient through evaluation and treatment that has identified beginning and end points as well as decision-tree options.

Regarding spine evaluation and treatment, DeRosa and Porterfield[5] have cogently analyzed extensive research regarding both medical and physical therapy interaction with spinal patients. They suggest an algorithm approach to care that allows scientific diagnostic functional evaluation and treatment patterns to be developed. Currently, insurance companies and workers' compensation systems are also developing spine care algorithms that will be helpful in two ways: (1) development of more efficient and effective diagnostic and treatment methods of spine injured patients based on research, and (2) reduction in number of inappropriate diagnostic tests or ineffective treatments, saving time and money.

One organization that has categorized and synchronized medical and physical therapy diagnosis and treatment is the National Back Injury Network in Charlotte, North Carolina. Ron Basini, President, utilized two committees to develop parallel algorithms. The physician committee, chaired by Arthur White, developed algorithmic diagnostic and treatment care based on diagnosis. The physical therapy committee, chaired by Susan Isernhagen, developed a parallel model for an 8-week algorithm. A condensation of this algorithm is as follows:

Initial Evaluation	Return to Work	
Week 1:	Initial Evaluation	
↓	Activation	→ Return
	Selected modalities	
Weeks 2 to 4:	Reevaluations	
↓	Activation	→ to
	Work-task testing	
Weeks 4 to 8:	Functional-capacity	
	evaluation	→ Work
	Work conditioning	

At all points, a decision to return to work is contemplated. The response to treatment and performance on the appropriate functional test can be utilized for work return as early and safe as possible. If return to work is not accomplished, the next week's treatment plan has been identified. Note the absence of passive modalities after the first week. Note that activation is the driving force. Note also that return-to-work options are evaluated each week.

Functional Evaluations in Physical Therapy Diagnosis

Purpose of Functional Evaluation

The purpose of the functional evaluation is to relate patient pathology to function in order to define or refine (1) *Level or type of the pathology*. For example, Mrs. Roy presented herself in a functional capacity evaluation with a medical diagnosis of L4-L5 disc pathology. During the functional capacity evaluation, extension of the cervical spine created symptoms of pain, dizziness, and tingling of the upper extremities. This led to a secondary diagnosis of cervical disc pathology. (2) *Intensity of the pathology*. For example, Mr. Jones had been diagnosed with lumbar stenosis. Medically, the stenosis significantly encroached on lower lumbar nerve root spaces. Functionally, Mr. Jones showed ability to perform medium-level work (50-lb. maximum). However, flexing and rotating activities of the spine were severely limited. Therefore, he had a motion limitation as a result of the stenosis, but strength capacities remained highly functional. Spinal motion into nonneutral positions appeared to be more severely limiting than compression caused by holding a 50 lb weight. (3) *Ability for the body to overcome the pathology by compensatory movements or actions*. For example, Mr. Jess moved to Minneapolis, where he sought work as a TV cameraman, his former occupation. During a routine medical examination, spondylolisthesis was noted. The company physician felt that the instability might cause future workers' compensation injury. The physical therapy functional testing, however, showed that Mr. Jess had excellent spinal stability in manual materials handling. He utilized strong muscle stabilizers and a locked-in lumbar lordosis during manual materials handling. He was able to perform the essential functions of the job. (4) *Residual function*. For example, it was Mrs. Murphy's third back strain at work. As a nursing assistant, she was again injured while transferring a patient. Her physician found no structural problem, diagnosing her with "recurrent back strain." Her employer asked the physical therapist to do a final "residual function" evaluation as a case-resolution vehicle. The functional determination outlined capabilities in the light-work range, but not suitable for the nursing assistant job. She was still employable at lighter work, even though she could not return to patient handling. In addition to the workers' compensation settlement that followed, the functional diagnosis also clarified her reemployment opportunities.

Preliminary Evaluation

The functional evaluation must begin with a musculoskeletal assessment in order to reestablish the physical parameters relating to the original medical diagnosis, measure additional musculoskeletal parameters in the therapists realm of expertise and identify physical problems that will relate to function observed during the functional evaluation.[6,7,10]

The musculoskeletal evaluation encompasses extremity range of motion and spinal flexibility, manual muscle testing, heart rate, blood pressure, muscle tone, presence of symptoms including numbness and pain, and neurological sign status. The blood pressure and heart rate are of particular importance, as they will be used as additional functional measures and also indicate if test tasks need to be stopped for other than musculoskeletal reasons. The careful functional evaluate will ensure that the evaluee is not placed in a reinjury situation and will ensure that no new problem arises that might involve heart rate or blood pressure.

Once the safety parameters and physical dysfunctions are established through this preliminary evaluation, the actual functional evaluation then begins.

Note: The following tests utilize the skills of either a physical therapist or an occupational therapist.

Work-Task Evaluation

This evaluation is a shortened version of an FCE. It tests critical physical abilities regarding home or work life. For the industrial client, an early return to work is served by this type of evaluation. For example, the worker with a back injury who has received adequate medical treatment for 2 weeks is now ready for an early return to work. The algorithm then triggers medical and return-to-work events. In this case, the treatment algorithm indicates that because it is 2 weeks after injury, a work-task evaluation should be performed. The therapist would select items comparable to the physical components used at work. For example, a warehouse worker would undergo a lifting evaluation. An assembly-line worker would undergo reaching, bending, and static standing tests. A construction worker would perform a combination of climbing, walking over rough ground, lifting, and upper-extremity work.

A work-task test is a short version of an FCE with selected items. Because deconditioning and secondary problems are not in the diagnostic picture, the physical therapy functional evaluation will document abilities and limitations related to the original pathology.

In the above example, if the warehouse worker could lift 50-lb maximum and 30-lb repetitively, he could be placed back at work in full or modified duty, depending on the physical demands of the job. Therapy treatments and further medical care may continue, but the return to work would be effected quickly.

Functional-Capacity Evaluation

The full FCE is performed when the algorithm indicates that there is difficulty in returning the injured worker to work. When the timing of work return, and the levels of physical capacity are in question, this necessitates a full FCE.[6–8,10,11,15] Algorithm methods tend to indicate that after 4 weeks off work this intervention is indicated.

The full FCE is diagnostic in that it will not only analyze the results of the original spinal injury, but it may identify secondary problems such as endurance loss, poor aerobic capacity, secondary weakness or injury, etc. The full FCE format is described in the box opposite and the report format for the employer, physician, worker, and other return to work parties is shown in the box. In the report, information related to diagnosis will be clarified. The following are sample statements relating to both function and diagnosis.

Mr. Brown is limited in kneeling tolerance due to the increase in lumbar lordosis caused by this activity. At 30 seconds into the test, he began to have increased pain in the sciatic distribution, with subsequent muscle spasms in the posterior muscles of the leg. This inability to tolerate extension is consistent with his diagnosis of disc degeneration. It is also consistent with the preliminary evaluation, which indicated loss of lumbar extension, and the test results, which also indicate inability to tolerate lumbar extension in overhead work tests. As a result, lumbar extension beyond neutral should be limited in work and daily living activities. He has been instructed in proper stabilization positioning of the spine so that increased extension does not occur. Functional limitations as noted in the FCE form will be present in kneeling, overhead work, and overhead lifting.

Ms. Day had a lumbar laminectomy 2 years ago. She has continued to have work difficulties. In her FCE, she was able to tol-

ISERNHAGEN WORK SYSTEMS FUNCTIONAL CAPACITY EVALUATION ITEMS

HISTORY

- Musculoskeletal physical (BRIEF)

LIFTS

- Floor to waist
- Waist to overhead
- Horizontal

PUSH/PULL (see Fig. 16-1, A)

- Static
- Dynamic

CARRY

- Front (see Fig. 16-1, B)
- Right-handed
- Left-handed

ELEVATED WORK

- Forward bending tolerance
  Sitting
  Standing
- Unweighted rotation tolerance
  Sitting
  Standing

LOW ACTIVITIES

- Crawl
- Kneel
- Crouch
- Repetitive squat

AMBULATION ACTIVITIES

- Walking
- Stair climbing
- Step-ladder climbing (see Fig. 16-1, C)

STATIC WORK

- Sitting
- Standing

UPPER EXTREMITY FUNCTIONS

- Hand grip
- Coordination

Copyright Isernhagen and Associates, Inc. 1992

Components of a Functional Report

1. Demographic data including spinal diagnosis and all related diagnoses

2. Purpose and type of evaluation

3. History
   - Back/spine injury
   - Work/home activities
   - Symptoms: discomfort, numbness, fatigue
   - Description of functional activities

4. Summary of physical findings
   - Musculoskeletal: range of motion, muscle strength, muscle abnormality
   - Neuromuscular: sensation, reflexes, coordination
   - Cardiovascular: heart rate, blood pressure

5. Client behavior/physical parameters
   - Safety
   - Cooperation
   - Consistency
   - Affective behavior

6. Functional results (all functional items tested)

7. Comparison to work requirements
   - Specific job matching
   - Modified work options

8. Recommendations
   - Return to function
   - Further testing and diagnostic needs
   - Further treatment and rehabilitation

Copyright Isernhagen and Associates, Inc. 1992

---

erate sustained trunk flexion, both in sitting and standing. She was able to do rotation activities with no limitation. In addition, she had full functional extension in overhead work activities. Her limitations relate to inability to stabilize her lumbar spine properly in loaded tasks. In lifting from floor to waist, functional lumbar instability was noted with weights greater than 10 lb. In waist-level lifting, she was able to stabilize more effectively and was able to tolerate 30 lb maximum as long as she was able to control her pace and movement patterns. It is noted that she was slow and guarded in the 30-lb lift, but she remained safe. In lifting at 35 lb, significant lumbar instability was noted and the test was stopped. In summary, her residual functional capacity indicates capability in motion and positional tolerance of spine segments in unloaded work. However, in manual materials handling, she is limited to the designated maximums.

Ms. Frederick reported for her FCE after 8 weeks of being off work with a "lumbosacral strain." Dr. Winter asked that her functional capacities be established before she returned to work in the central supply department of General Hospital.

The preliminary evaluation indicated degenerative changes and crepitus in the right knee. Her history indicated that her right knee has been problematic for the past 5 years. Since that time she has had three back injuries, and it has been noted that she protects her right knee by using her back rather than her legs.

During the FCE, guarding of the right knee (shifting weight to the left and limiting flexion on the right) was noted in all low level activities. In the floor-to-waist lift, she not only exhibited the left weight shift, but she also flexed and rotated her spine to protect the knee. Because spinal safety was compromised in the low level lift, she was not allowed to continue. When the spine position was brought to her attention, she recalled that her back had been in that same bent, rotated position when she was injured. In summary, her knee dysfunction was the limiting factor, not her spine. It is likely that lack of attention to the knee dysfunction has led to the back injuries. Secondary back injuries may often be linked to primary diagnoses elsewhere in the functional chain.

Overall, Ms. Frederick has the ability to return to work in the central supply department with the following modifications: (1) Lower-level storage must be reached by allowing her to sit on a stool and reach forward to get the items rather than to attempt bending and twisting as she has done in the past. Items within her safe functional weight capacities should be placed at waist level or at shoulder level. She will be able to handle the moderate weights in the central supply department as long as they are placed in these safer positions for her. (2) She is referred back to her physician for further diagnosis of the right knee dysfunction. Any remedial rehabilitation should address the whole-body functional activity, including low-back and knee functions.

Work Capacity Evaluation

The work capacity evaluation is similar to a functional capacity evaluation, but the items are specialized to the work setting, rather than generalized as in an FCE.[8]

For example, in a work capacity evaluation, the exact boxes, levels, and weight loads that Ms. Frederick lifts in the central supply department would be replicated in the test. In the case of a truck driver, the truck driver would be asked to ascend and descend steps equal in height to those used in his/her truck, and loading and unloading would replicate the actual work done on the loading dock. A work capacity evaluation for an assembly line worker would include hand and arm activities in the same position done on the assembly line with a repetition factor to measure endurance as well. The work capacity evaluator would not test for tasks not found in the job description. The benefit of a work capacity evaluation in functional diagnostics is that endurance and positional-tolerance testing can be extended into longer periods. Instances where this may be helpful are:

- Repetitive manual materials handling that adds longer-term spinal compression with sequenced loading and unloading. This is particularly helpful with degenerative disc disease, spinal stenosis, patients who have had spinal surgery, and conditions with symptoms radiating into the lower extremity.

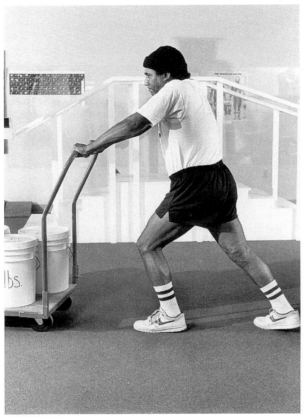

A

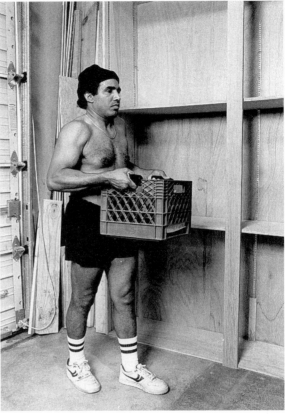

B

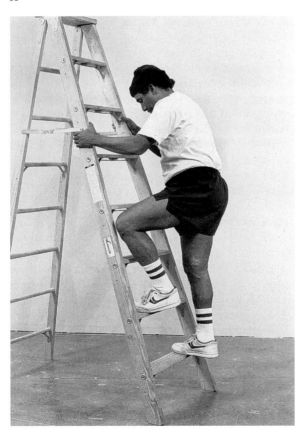

C

Fig. 16-1.

Evaluation components and scoring criteria for functional-capacity testing. **A.** Pushing test evaluates maximum force (strength), distance, coordination, and ability of functional body components to move objects over distance. **B.** Two-handed front carry is evaluated for strength (maximum carrying capacity), endurance (ability to tolerate repetitions and distance), and control. Primary muscles used are biceps, hand grip, and trunk stabilizers. **C.** Step-ladder climbing is utilized in addition to stair climbing to evaluate steps, balance, hand grip, heart response, and endurance as they pertain to ladder-climbing.

- Static sitting tolerances that provoke symptoms necessitating seating adaptation or specific spinal positioning.
- Balance activities that quantify deficits in stability response when base of support is changing or asymmetric movement patterns are required. This identifies any related problems, such as loss of lower-extremity proprioception, spinal muscle weakness, or decreased reflex activity.
- Nonneutral positioning that establishes parameters for tolerable and safe reaching work activity. This defines the specific parameters of movement related to the placement and extent of the pathology.
- Job-specific spine stressors such as transferring patients for nursing personnel and pulling loaded hand carts up curbs for delivery persons.

Issues in Physical Therapy Evaluation and Diagnosis

Normative Data

Normative data has been established in some aspects of physical therapy evaluation. For example, the American Medical Association has identified normal ranges of motion of the spine. However, muscle strength testing is more difficult to normalize and each muscle testing method has its own method of establishing strength performance. At this time strong correlations among strength, range of motion, and function have not been identified.[1,2] Therefore, normative data is limited in scope, and the use of this data would not relate to function or enhance functional diagnosis.

Normative data on FCE items is not available. While there are proprietary tests that purport to have normative data, none has been reviewed, published, or accepted in peer reviewed scientific literature. Therefore, scientific functional normative data is not available today.

The Americans with Disabilities Act indicates that normative data would not be a prudent option on which to base hiring or placement decisions even if it were available. It would not matter where a back-injured patient fell in relationship to the normative range. What would be significant is whether the worker can perform the essential functions of the job. Therefore, the patient, physician, and therapist are most interested in matching the actual functional abilities of the client with safe effective work and daily living activities. Medical and functional diag-

nostics regarding pathology compared to specific work requirements provide establishment of work abilities/limitations.

Therefore, in the diagnosis of lumbar function or dysfunction, normative data may place a person on a longitudinal scale but it cannot give specific work information. Therefore, individualized diagnosis and functional evaluation must take place.[1,2,14,16] The ultimate use of functional diagnostic testing by the therapist, therefore, will be in matching patients to safe activity rather than placing them on an arbitrary and often misleading normative scale.

The Team Approach

The physician's structural diagnosis and the therapist's functional diagnosis must be combined for good medical management. However, for the industrial specialist, the return-to-work process must include other professionals. The psychologist may be a valuable part of the team if emotional factors are present after a spinal injury or if pre-existing psychologic conditions may be interfering with full functional activity after an injury. The medical providers who seek psychologic consultations in the event of psychosocial problems will find case management to be more effective. In these cases, the psychologic diagnosis will be as important as the physical diagnosis for the patient's outcome.[12,13]

In addition, the vocational specialist who will relate the physical functional diagnosis with options for vocational placement will be needed in the more difficult cases. While the physician and therapist may be able to explain the diagnosis, prognosis, and functional work aspects fully, it may be the vocational specialist who actually finds the correct job for the injured worker. Working as a team throughout this planning will be most beneficial for all parties involved.

Summary

Diagnosis of the patient with a work-related injury must be comprehensive, because establishing what is "wrong" is only half the requirement. In order for a patient to have a good result, determining what is "right" with the patient is a critical factor.

Spinal injuries are acknowledged to be difficult and complex to diagnose and manage. The work-injured status of a patient compounds the problem. Diagnosis and management are critical because outcome needs are specific: the patient requires good medical care and requires a positive functional outcome; the employer desires a safe, cost-effective, and timely return of the employee to work; and the insurer wants financial resolution of the problem. The physician must correctly, judiciously, and quickly establish a working structural diagnosis; the physical therapist must add a functional diagnosis.

The combination of the physician and physical therapist roles in diagnosis and management can be powerful. Not only will quality medical management enhance the patient's health, but a functional outcome will result. With the effective methods described, the employer, insurer, and injured worker will all have their needs met.

It is the astute physician or case manager who brings the physical therapist into the team as soon as feasible. With professional cooperation, the result is optimal care of the industrial spine-injured patient.

References

1. Battie MC, Bigos SJ. Industrial back complaints, *Orthop Clin North Am* 22:273, 1991.
2. Bigos SJ, Battie MC: *Surveillance of back problems in industry*. In *Clinical concepts in regional musculoskeletal illness,* New York, 1987, Grune & Stratton, p 299.
3. Canfield J: *Causes of movement dysfunction and physical disability*. In Scully RM, Barnes MR, editors: *Physical therapy,* Philadelphia, 1989, Lippincott, p 130.
4. Canfield JS: *The evaluation process*. In Scully RM, Barnes MR, editors: *Physical therapy,* Philadelphia, 1989, JB Lippincott, p 320.
5. DeRosa C, Porterfield J: A physical therapy model for the treatment of low back pain, *Phys Ther* 72(4):261, 1992.
6. Isernhagen S: *Functional capacity assessment and work hardening perspectives*. In Mayer T, Mooney V, Gatchel R, editors: *Contemporary care for painful spinal disorders,* Philadelphia, 1991, Lea & Febiger.
7. Isernhagen S: *Functional capacity evaluation*. In Isernhagen S, editor: *Work injury: management and prevention,* Gaithersburg, MD, 1988, Aspen Publishers, p 139.
8. Isernhagen S: Isolated testing, functional capacity evaluation and work tolerance testing. *Indust Rehab Q* Spring:7, 1991.
9. Isernhagen S: Physical therapy and occupational rehabilitation, *J Occup Rehab* 1:71, 1991.
10. Isernhagen S: *The role of functional capacity assessment after rehabilitation*. In Bullock M, editor: *Ergonomics—the physiotherapist in the workplace,* London, 1990, Churchill-Livingstone.
11. Key G: *Work capacity analysis*. In Scully M, Barnes M, editors: *Physical therapy,* Philadelphia, 1989, JB Lippincott, p 652.
12. Matheson L: *Symptom magnification syndrome,* Anaheim, CA, 1988, Employment Rehabilitation Institute of California.
13. Mayer T, Gatchel R, Mayer H, et al.: A prospective two year study of functional restoration in industrial low back injury: an objective assessment procedure. *JAMA* 258:1763, 1987.
14. Mellin G, Waddell G: Trunk strength testing with iso machines, *Spine* 18:801, 1993.
15. Miller M: Functional assessments, *Work* 1(3):6, 1991.
16. Newton M, et al.: Trunk strength testing with iso machines, part II. *Spine* 18:812, 1993.
17. Ogden Neimeyer L, Jacobs K: *Work hardening,* Thorofare NJ, 1989, Slack Inc.
18. Smith GM. *The role of the occupational medicine physician in the management of industrial injury*. In Mayer T, Mooney V, Gatchell R, editors: *Contemporary conservative care for painful spinal disorders,* Philadelphia, 1991, Lea & Febiger, p 191.

Chapter 17
Psychiatric Evaluation of the Chronic Spine Pain Patient
David J. Anderson

Goals of the Evaluation

Patient Selection

Selection of the Consultant

Structure of the Evaluation

Psychologic Testing

Specialized Evaluations

Follow-up

Summary

In 1982 the author was asked to join a team of physicians who were evaluating and treating people with spine pain of various etiologies. The principle phenomenon that I was asked to investigate was why some patients with objective structural pathology did not recover as expected despite technically good surgical outcomes. Although some of the failures were explained by the physicians as being due to the patient being "hysterical," many of the patients were viewed as "solid citizens" whose treatment failure perplexed the physicians and lead to extraordinary diagnostic investigations and occasionally to further unsuccessful surgical interventions. My task was to discover the psychological and psychosocial factors that might be contributing to these patients' failure to recover and to develop effective treatment to avert or reverse failure.

Literature on the spine offers many different models of evaluating the psychologic status of patients with spine pain. They are variously based on abnormal psychometric testing, distorted patterns of cognitive functioning, behavioral dysfunction from operant conditioning, unconscious conflict, and pain as a variant of a depression.* In this chapter a concise and straightforward model of evaluation will be presented. This evaluation will serve to expand the clinician's understanding of how well the patient can be expected to do with rigors of the psychologic cascade of disabling lumbar-spine pain.

Goals of the Evaluation

Optimally, the psychiatric evaluation of the patient with spine pain enriches the understanding of the treatment team about the psychologic meaning of illness for the individual patient and improves treatment. Spine disease, in the majority of cases of prolonged disability, is experienced as an intrusive, destructive tormenter that launches a relentless invisible attack on the victim's life. Choices are ultimately made by the patient either to remain a helpless, powerless victim, or to make his/her life work within the limits of the illness. The cases involving workers' compensation and the medicolegal process complicate this set of choices, which are made largely on an unconscious basis.

Surgery is often sought as the relief to suffering, and in many cases it is just that. However, since in American culture surgery often legitimizes spine pain, the push to have surgery may be to make the pain more real. All too often the expectations (by both patient and treating physician) of surgery are unreal-

*References 1, 3, 5 to 7–12, and 14.

istic ones, based on the belief that removal of the pain generator will completely restore the premorbid psychosocial condition. Often, the damage to psyche and social systems are so extensive that by the time surgical correction is effected, the patient has embraced the role of victim. Positive surgical outcome is best predicted by the patient exhibiting an adaptive presurgical style that is already making adjustments to make life liveable, regardless of medical outcome. For other patients, the meaning of spine disease is that of escape from overwhelming responsibility into a role of illness requiring support from the people previously supported by the patient. Others see chronic illness as not merely a crisis, but as an opportunity to change their lives. This attitude can be quite positive, but also can be dangerous if the patient does not resolve the underlying issues at the time of definitive treatment of the physical problems. Again, it is important to understand the unconscious nature of these issues. The patient is not volunteering for illness and is operating at a psychologic level beyond conscious control. Often, a patient who is stuck in the cycle of poor recovery despite effective treatment, in dealing with his/her physician or third party carrier, is blamed for treatment failure, as if he/she willingly and consciously was perpetuating the condition. It is only a very small number of patients who consciously manipulate their treating doctors and insurance carriers in order to receive payment, drugs, disability status, or the sick role.

Patient Selection

Since referring every patient with spine pain for psychiatric evaluation is neither practical nor productive, then knowing when, how, and to whom to refer a spine pain patient is important.[17] Recognizing patients with dramatic emotional symptoms is generally straightforward. Patients with more subtle difficulties can be overlooked by even the most seasoned primary physician.

Certain behavioral indications are reliable signs that psychiatric involvement is warranted. If any of the problems discussed below persist after 12 weeks of treatment, psychiatric involvement is recommended.

Obvious Signs or Complaints of Anxiety and Depression

By including 5 minutes in the initial physical evaluation of the patient to ask how the pain is affecting the patient, his/her work and family life, and leisure activities, critical information can be revealed. Often it can feel to the clinician as if one is opening Pandora's box and that such questions are better left unasked. However, what one does not know about the patient with spine pain can and often does come back to haunt the treating physician.

History of Psychologic Difficulties

If an individual has had any previous difficulties with anxiety, depression, or life crisis, then the probability is fairly high that the spine pain will precipitate another crisis. The patient's current and previous alcohol and prescribed and nonprescribed drug use also needs to be assessed. Studies have shown a much higher prevalence for preexisting psychiatric disturbances in the population of the patients with spine pain than the base rate in the general population.[1]

Excessive Pain Behavior

Many reasons exist for excessive pain behavior (i.e., the data and complaints do not fit). Much of it can be explained by psychologic and psychosocial (including cultural) factors.[18] If such behavior is not readily explained psychologically, then further diagnostic study should be considered to be certain that the physical evaluation is complete.

Excessive or Insufficient Family Involvement

Sometimes the only tip-off that significant psychologic factors are present is in the family's involvement.[2] Spine pain can provoke unusual behavior in both patients and their families so that if one is not at ease with the manner or intensity of family involvement a psychiatric consultation is in order.

Excessive Reliance on Medication

Escalating medication use is often a sign of emotional factors being treated with analgesic or muscle relaxants. Opiate or benzodiazepine dependency can occur before one realizes the underlying emotional difficulties that are fueling the medication escalation.

Inconsolability

Sometimes nothing you say helps, or if it does, not for long. The patient who briefly gets better or does not get better at all despite your best efforts may have psychologic difficulties that overwhelm the efforts of the most seasoned spine physician. Such patients often require intensive psychologic intervention if treatment is to be successful (see Chapter 38 for further details).

The Preoperative Patient

When spine surgery involves a prolonged recovery (longer than 6 weeks) a psychologic assessment is important to evaluate the patient's and his/her support system's capacity to withstand the surgery and the prolonged rehabilitation. Patients often hold unrealistic expectations about their ability to return to full capacity for former spine-intensive activities, both vocational and recreation. The psychiatric evaluation can lay the groundwork for the patient to begin to make the necessary adjustments so that a premature return to these activities does not undermine the recovery.

Severe Intercurrent Stresses

The threat of job loss, financial reversal, marital strain, and chronic illness in a family member are examples of additional disturbances that can interfere with the patient's full participation in any treatment plan. These stresses can easily be overlooked without the more comprehensive picture that a psychiatric evaluation provides.

Selection of the Consultant

On deciding that a psychiatric evaluation would be helpful, the clinician often has difficulty finding someone to perform such an evaluation and the necessary follow-up. The consultant must be an actively involved mental health professional who is at ease as both a consultant and at times a primary care physician. The ability to use psychotropic medications judiciously is extremely helpful in treating the anxiety and depressive symptoms that frequently accompany chronic pain. In addition, the comprehension of the nature of the physical anatomy, pathology, and the nature of various procedures is extremely helpful in establishing oneself as a legitimate part of the multispecialty team. Many psychiatrists do not have the training or interest in the complicated and at times therapeutically challenging circumstances that arise in caring for the patient with spine pain. A psychologist with special interest can acquire much of the understanding that medical training offers the spine psychiatrist, but without this medical background will have difficulty making specific helpful recommendations to the primary physician. The dynamic interaction between the psychologic and physical factors can be both fascinating and frustrating and offers a rich opportunity for a satisfying collaboration for both professionals.

Structure of the Evaluation

The psychiatric interview is the cornerstone on which the psychologic understanding of the patient is developed. The interview should be in the form of a typical psychiatric assessment, with the history focused on the patient's injury, its course of diagnosis and treatment, alterations in the patient's mood, and any specific psychologic symptoms, including elements of posttraumatic stress disorder. A history of medications and their pattern of use is of great importance. Medical history, psychiatric history, social history, and family history must all be carefully assessed. Particular attention to the transient and potentially permanent vocational, marital, financial, and recreational ramifications of the injury should be examined. An objective description of the patient's mental status should then be clearly delineated. Assessment of the patient should integrate all of the above elements. Since the capacity to endure and master the challenges of the psychologic cascade is significantly affected by critical events and traumas during early psychologic stages of development (see Chapter 38) the patient's attachment history must be thoughtfully explored. Often the quality of relatedness during the interview will be a clue to a disturbed capacity for attachment and consolation. The attachment history can be the core of the evaluation from which most of the salient elements are derived. In certain instances, such as medicolegal evaluations, or with patients exhibiting severe psychopathology, a formal DSM-III-R diagnostic assessment should be done.

Psychologic Testing

Psychologic testing is often used by evaluators of patients with chronic spine pain. Various tests have been tried to gain objective data that delineates the degree of psychologic influence in a particular patient with chronic pain. The Minnesota Multiphasic Personality Inventory (MMPI) has been the most widely used and researched psychometric instrument in the field of chronic pain.[11] Despite its popular use and the development of a successor, the MMPI-2, its utility with pain patients is controversial.[13,14,19,20] Recent opinion is that it should be used to reach a conclusion about the severity of the overall distress of the patient rather than more specific judgments about the patient. In addition, the literature on the use of the MMPI to predict outcome of treatment is not strongly supportive.[16] At its best the MMPI requires an experienced and sophisticated interpreter to avoid inappropriate conclusions. In my experience psychometric testing provides a diagnosis or a description of a patient's character style under stress. Unfortunately, this information usually only confirms the impressions of the primary physicians of the patient being "hysterical" or a "psych case,'" and does not suggest a plan for treatment that can be integrated into the medical care.

The opinions of the rest of the multidisciplinary team are very important in the psychiatric assessment. The psychiatrist will spend a few hours with the patient, but the rest of the team has totaled a great deal more exposure to this person. Such things as anxiety level, pain behavior, reactions to testing, frustration tolerance, emotional lability, inconsistence of symptoms, truthfulness, exaggeration of symptoms, ability to follow directions, degree of helplessness, spousal relationship, and relationship with third-party payers may be more directly assessable by the treatment team. It is a mistake for the psychiatric consultant to formulate opinions without the rest of the team's input. The ideal situation is a multidisciplinary conference, but prior to this, informal discussions are helpful.

Once the assessment is completed, a section of recommendations must be made. The recommendations should be numbered, specific, addressed to ideas discussed in the assessment section, and directed toward answers to specific questions from the referring physician.

Specialized Evaluations

More specialized evaluations, such as for hypnotherapy or biofeedback, must share many of the elements of a psychiatric evaluation, unless a recent assessment has been done. Of particular importance is any history of abuse or severe psychological trauma. These types of trauma may play a specific role in the patient's current complex of psychologic symptoms and may point the direction of hypnotherapeutic treatment. One should be aware of these traumas or unusual areas of memory dysfunction that often represent profound levels of repressive psychologic defense.

Assessment of the patient's past experience with hypnosis, biofeedback, meditation, visualization techniques, and relaxation techniques should be directed at understanding what has and has not worked in the past. Often this past hypnotic experience will not be related to pain, but the patient will be expert at achieving trance. When evaluation is complete, a treatment plan using specific approaches, within the context of the overall treatment plan, should be delineated. These approaches should be spelled out and should be geared toward a time-limited approach directed at clear goals and focused on teaching mastery through self-hypnotic techniques. Passivity on the part of the patient should be discouraged.

Follow-up

Follow-up is extremely important after the evaluation of the psychiatric status of the spine-injured patient. Although it may appear to be more of an issue in treatment, one must be willing to use ongoing follow-up as a way to change and refine the psychiatric diagnostic issues. This refining process is extremely important in assessing psychopharmacologic and hypnotherapeutic interventions. It is also important in the patient who initially is assessed as not needing direct psychiatric follow-up. While this may appear to be a contradiction, it actually is quite practical if the evaluating psychiatrist solicits the input of the rest of the treatment team in evaluating the progress of the patient. If predictions of risk and outcome do not appear to be in line with the original assessment, a reformulation or fresh evaluation may be in order. An effective way of managing follow-up for patients who do not require ongoing psychotherapy is for the primary care physician to arrange one afternoon per month to see follow-up patients.

The issues of confidentiality often lead to the isolation of the psychiatric aspects of the case from the physical treatment. The consulting psychiatrist can become the unwitting facilitator of the mind-body split. The consultant needs to expand the traditional boundaries of the therapeutic process to include the larger team and make it clear to the patient that his/her psychologic condition will be carefully interwoven with overall care.

The following example illustrates in several ways the importance of the psychiatric evaluation.

Case Example

The patient is seen during a routine presurgical evaluation prior to laminectomy and discectomy for leg pain and motor weakness. During the initial psychiatric evaluation the patient describes her relationship with her workaholic husband as unsatisfac-

tory and largely nonsupportive. She goes on to describe a sexually abusive father and mother who ignored her daughter's difficulties with her father. The patient has compensated for the lack of attention in her relationship with her husband by conducting a series of affairs and complaining to her friends about her husband. She goes into surgery admitting that she wants to end the relationship, but is frightened of the idea of being a single parent, although that virtually has been her situation for years. Although her motor weakness improves, postoperative pain is severe. In follow-up therapy the patient admits to feeling trapped, much as she did with her father. She has used extramarital relationships to escape her sense of being boxed in, much as she used the relationship with her husband to leave home permanently. It seems clear to her that when her husband ignores her needs, her pain is far worse. The patient is confronted with the idea that she is afraid to live her life without a sense of being trapped and she acknowledges that the next obvious trap is perpetuating her pain.

Summary

As suggested above we know much less than we need to know to comprehend spine pain adequately and to intercede therapeutically. Spine pain quickly becomes a somatopsychic disorder with potentially overwhelming consequences. Many of the consequences are in the form of lost or wasted creative potential, prolonged suspension of a productive living, hardship on family, and extraordinary economics of lost time and medical costs. Psychiatric intervention too often is too little too late, and split off from the main treatment. Well-integrated and timely psychiatric evaluations can help to turn a hopelessly chronic condition into a full recovery.

References

1. Burdette BH, Gale EN: Pain as a learned response: a review of behavioral factors in chronic pain, *J Am Dent Assoc* 116:881, 1988.
2. Dvorak J, Valach L, Fuhrimann P, Heim E: The outcome of surgery for lumbar disc herniation: a 4-17 years' follow-up with emphasis on psychosocial aspects, *Spine* 13:1423, 1988.
3. Dzioba RB, Doxey NC: A prospective investigation into the orthopaedic and psychologic predictors of outcome of first lumbar surgery following industrial injury, *Spine* 9:614, 1984.
4. Feuerstein M, Dobkin P: Biobehavioral assessment of chronic pain, *Pain Manage,* July/August:152, 1988.
5. Frymoyer JW, Cats-Baril W: Predictors of low back pain disability, *Clin Orthop Relat Res* 221:89, 1987.

6. Frymoyer JW, Pope MH, Clements JH, et al.: Risk factors in low-back pain, *J Bone Joint Surg* 65:213, 1983.

7. Frymoyer JW, Rosen JC, Clements J, Pope MH: Psychologic factors in low-back pain disability, *Clin Orthop Relat Res* 195:178, 1985.

8. Hengler N: Depression caused by chronic pain, *J Clin Psychiatry* 45:30, 1987.

9. Hurme M, Alaranta H: Factors predicting the result for surgery for lumbar intervertebral disc herniation, *Spine* 12:933, 1987.

10. Imboden JB: Psychosocial determinants of recovery, *Adv Psychosom Med* 8:142, 1972.

11. Keller LS, Butcher NJ: *Assessment of chronic pain patients with the MMPI-2,* Minneapolis, 1991, University of Minnesota Press.

12. Krishnan K, France RD, Houpt JL: Chronic low back pain and depression, *Psychosomatics* 26:299, 1985.

13. Love AW, Peck CL: The MMPI and psychological factors in low back pain: a review, *Pain* 28:1, 1987.

14. Naliboff BB, Cohen MJ, Yellen AN: Does the MMPI differentiate chronic illness from chronic pain? *Pain* 13:333, 1982.

15. Polatin PB, Kinney RG, Gatchel RJ, et al.: Psychiatric illness and chronic low-back pain: the mind and the spine—which goes first? *Spine* 18:66-71, 1993.

16. Ressor KA, Craig KD: Medically incongruent chronic back pain: physical limitations, suffering and ineffective coping, *Pain* 32:35, 1988.

17. Roistacher SL: Referring pain patients for psychologic evaluation, *Pain* 4:33, 1988.

18. Rook JC, Pesch RN, Keeler EC: Chronic pain and the questionable use of the MMPI, *Arch Phys Med Rehab* 62:373, 1981.

19. Sherrill K, Larson DB: Adult burn patients: the role of religion in recovery, *South Med J* 81:821, 1988.

20. Smythe HA: Problems with the MMPI, *J Rheumatol* 11:417, 1984.

Chapter 18
Multidisciplinary Evaluation

Mark Van Dyke
Gerald P. Keane
Arthur H. White

Definition

No one spinal practitioner can be totally knowledgeable in all medical areas that affect the spine. Back pain is a complex mixture of overlapping cascades. Structural, socioeconomic, and psychological factors are present to some degree in every patient. In a complex patient no single practitioner has the necessary skills to sort them out. Therefore we need help from our subspecialty colleagues who understand other areas of spinal medicine better than we do. The need for a multidisciplinary environment springs from the failure that the solo spinal practitioner has had in adequately diagnosing and treating a large number of spinal patients. These are the patients who are unnecessarily costing 80% of the billions of dollars spent on spine health care today.

The type of multidisciplinary environment that a particular community uses will depend on needs and resources. In a small community with few subspecialists there may be little time or need for a multidisciplinary program. The few difficult to treat patients who do occur in such busy communities are referred to larger centers with formal programs.

In areas where formal programs do not exist, subspecialists refer back and forth to each other for consultations on difficult to treat patients, with one of the professionals assuming the role of the primary care giver. Such a system is certainly not very efficient for the patient or for communication between subspecialists. It can, however, get the job done for patients with mildly to moderately complex cases. When there is extreme complexity such as drug addiction, high psychologic involvement, long-term disability, and multiple failed spinal operations, a formally organized multidisciplinary program is much more successful in both diagnosis and treatment.

There are many varieties of formally structured multidisciplinary programs. The varieties depend on the types of patients referred to that facility as well as subspecialty interests of physicians at that facility. If a program is run mainly by a surgeon there is more likely to be a structural and failed spine surgery type of algorithm used. At facilities run by psychiatrists the structural components of a patient's problem are less of a concern. Anesthesiologists direct programs in which the main focus of diagnosis and treatment is on injection procedures. Other facilities are aimed at rehabilitation, with less concern as to what the structural or psychologic diagnosis is and more interest in returning to functional activities as rapidly as possible.

Although there are all the above variations in philosophies and composition, the major thrust of all multidisciplinary programs should be to find out exactly what is disabling the patient. This includes the structural pathoanatomic diagnosis, the socioeconomic ramifications of the disability, and the psychologic diagnosis and dynamics.

Multidisciplinary Team

The composition of a multidisciplinary program can be divided into administrative and medical.

Administrative Component

The administrative component includes at least one and usually many individuals who are well organized and knowledgeable in systems of data collections, computerization, and communication. Prior to a patient's multidisciplinary evaluation, extensive data need to be collected with regard to the many treatments and surgeries that the patient may have undergone, as well as current symptoms, medications, functional limitations, attitudes, drugs, etc. So as not to duplicate the collection of data by every person who sees the patient, there should be communication among the members of the multidisciplinary team that provides them with the same thorough information prior to their subspecialty evaluation of the patient. As the new subspecialty information is collected it is fed into the data system so that the next person seeing the patient has the complete information regarding the patient's problem.

Medical Component

The medical component of most multidisciplinary programs includes a primary care provider and 3 to 10 other subspecialists who contribute to the final diagnosis. There are ideally two or three physicians who meet on a daily, if not hourly, basis to reassess the evaluation and make decisions with regard to the next step in the evaluation process.

Primary Care Physician

The primary evaluator or primary care giver may be the director of a multidisciplinary program. This person can be any physician from a general practitioner to a neurosurgeon, but is usually someone who has a general knowledge of all spinal subspecialties. Although this may be a surgeon who has taken special interest in the rehabilitation and psychosocial fields, it is more likely to be an occupational medicine physician, a physiatrist, or medical subspecialist. A psychologist, nurse, or clinically oriented paramedic with good communication skills can also fulfill the role as the primary care giver. Communication and coordination are the key.

Physiatrist

The physiatrist may be the leader of the team and is well versed in rehabilitation and electrodiagnostics. Unless there is a neurologist doing the electrodiagnostic testing the physiatrist would be responsible for electromyography and the somatosensory evoked potentials when indicated. The physiatrist, having training in functional disability and rehabilitation, will frequently take charge of the analysis of the patient's physical resources and functional capacity. Many physiatrists who have subspecialized in spinal medicine are trained in diagnostic and therapeutic injection procedures, and many act as the injection specialist on the team if there is not a radiologist, anesthesiologist, or orthopedist occupying that position. Many physiatrists have become interested in occupational medicine and understand the laws and communication methods within the community that are essential to the socioeconomic recovery of the patient. They therefore may become involved in the ergonomics of the workplace, work hardening programs, and directing major rehabilitation facilities and functional restoration and pain programs.

Surgeon

In the past, the surgical expertise of the neurosurgeon and the orthopedic surgeon was very narrowly defined. Today, neurosurgeons are doing what was previously considered orthopedic procedures, including fusions with internal fixation. Orthopedic surgeons are well trained in neurosurgical procedures, including the removal of tumors from the vertebral canal and decompressions of the spinal cord for infections, trauma, and degenerative disease. Most spine surgeons have been trained in all aspects of spinal surgery so that the distinction between the neurosurgeon and the orthopedic surgeon is being blurred.

Although most spinal surgeons are preoccupied with doing surgery, some have elected to become administrators or diagnosticians. In many programs the surgeon's only role is to make decisions regarding surgical treatment. In other programs, however, the surgeon may be responsible for most referrals and becomes involved in the case relatively early on.

There is significant danger in such a situation, in that surgery may be performed prematurely because the momentum of the evaluation drifts toward structural evaluation and surgical intervention in lieu of evaluating the psychosocial parameters.

Many surgeons have become very good occupational medicine physicians, rehabilitations specialists, and diagnosticians. Some prefer to do less surgery and more spinal evaluation. A surgeon may well be the leader of the team.

The surgeon who does surgery for the multidisciplinary team should have a broad training in neurosurgical and orthopedic techniques. He should be familiar with everything from arthroscopic surgery to internal fixation. The "one-trick pony" can be devastating to a medical center, which may get a reputation for doing the same procedure for every condition. This is clearly as antiquated an approach as giving the same medication for every heart condition.

Anesthesiologist

The subspecialty of anesthesiology in the field of spinal medicine has greatly advanced in the past few years. There are anesthesiologists directing pain clinics, spine centers, rehabilitation centers, and multidisciplinary diagnostic centers. Some anesthesiologists have become spine diagnosticians in their own right, having learned the structural, psychologic and social aspects of spinal medicine.

Because the anesthesiologist feels comfortable with heavily sedated or unconscious patients, he or she is much more able to bring patients to a level of comfort and consciousness so they are not traumatized by the procedure itself. Better diagnostic information can be gained and the patient is less apt to fear future blocks if and when they become necessary.

Psychiatrist

Psychiatrists and psychologists run many diagnostic and rehabilitation programs. There is hardly a back pain patient without some psychologic involvement, and many patients have more psychologic and socioeconomic disease than they do structural disease. The psychiatrist is well qualified to deal with the psychosocial issues. The structural aspects are relatively straightforward and easily managed in a psychologically oriented center by the addition of a surgeon, anesthesiologist, or physiatrist.

Few, if any, psychologically oriented programs advocate long-range psychiatric intervention. The current trends are more toward "quick-hit" psychologic intervention, which quickly identifies the psychologic diagnostic aspects and lays out a definitive plan with well-defined goals and time frames.

Although behavioral modification may be part of the therapeutic prescription, it is carried out in most centers with little waste of time, few failures, and a clear economic benefit. Psychiatrists who become involved in this type of program have taken a special interest in spinal patients and back pain. They understand the psychologic ramifications of surgery and help prepare patients for surgery with realistic expectations. They are effective in dealing with the depression, frustrations, and other psychosocial factors that could adversely affect the result of surgery.

Other Team Members

A rheumatologist can be of significant value in a multidisciplinary setting working with patients who develop specific rheumatologic symptoms, fibromyalgia, or fibromyositis.

A spinal radiologist may be a member of the comprehensive team. Radiologists are comfortable reading CT and MRI studies; however, not all radiologists have the same level of expertise. Establish a relationship with a radiologist who has a specialty in spinal evaluations. The conservative-care physician and the radiologist should collaborate on interpreting the studies and deciding what other imaging studies would best help to define the structural abnormalities.

Physician extenders, including nurse practitioners and physician assistants, can be extremely beneficial in treating spinal patients. They can develop an expertise in a specific area of treatment of these patients and provide an important channel for communicating with the patients.

There are many patients who benefit from manual medicine. A multidisciplinary program may have a specialist who does manual medicine techniques. These can be an osteopath, chiropractor, or a physical therapist who has extensive training in manual medicine and practices on a regular basis. These specialists may fill many other roles, such as diagnostician, primary care provider, or director of a multidisciplinary program.

Developing a Treatment Plan

One of the distinct advantages to working in a multidisciplinary setting is the free flow of ideas and opinions that is available daily on an informal basis. Easy access to "curbside" consultations about patients with less complex problems enhances the level of care available to all patients, not just those seen by the formal multidisciplinary team. The multidisciplinary process tends in many ways to be a dynamic one. The patient is often seen for an initial examination by the team members and any prior data are reviewed. The patient's history and physical examination are completed and an initial evaluation plan is undertaken. Members of the team see the patient for an extended period during the first day. At that time team members coordinate what is to be scheduled for the following day, and initial tests and evaluations are completed. Typically, the team members will then meet the following day along with the patient to review the information that has been gained from the first phase of the process. Further steps thought to be necessary are then undertaken to sort out the questions that need to be answered.

A typical example would include a patient who presents with failed back surgery and is seen by many of the team members as outlined above. A scan, perhaps electrodiagnostic testing, and consultations might be obtained on the first day. If there is any doubt as to the underlying nature and source of the symptoms, then diagnostic blocks such as sympathetic block, selective nerve root block, and other tests might then be undertaken. The goal would be to help identify pain generators and sort out the complex nature of the patient's underlying complaints.

As the process is followed through all its phases, team members are actively involved in discussing and looking at the information and sorting through the issues on a test-by-test basis. When all tests have been completed, team members will confer and synthesize and discuss the information in an open fashion. In many cases this leads to considerable debate about not only the interpretation of the test but the issues that this suggests in development of a treatment plan.

Reaching a consensus is not always easy. There is some concern with any patient with a complicated problem that the issues may not resolve themselves in a simple and easily managed treatment plan. It is important, however, for team members to try to develop a consensus of opinion, and if uncertain, usually the most conservative plan is undertaken, with recommendations for more complex or more aggressive intervention to follow depending on the initial results. Although it is important to present to the patient all the information and possibilities that the team has discussed, once a treatment plan has been agreed on, it is also important that this is presented as the consensus and decision of the whole team. Many such patients are often in a quandary themselves, with a great deal of apprehension and uncertainty about what direction they might take. Although it is important to be direct and honest about the treatment options, as long as the treatment plan has been thought through carefully, then it is equally important for the patient to have confidence that the recommended plan has a reasonable potential for success. Leaving the patient with a great deal of doubt in that regard will often undermine any treatment plan, no matter how well thought out. In many cases, what is really developed is a "working plan" that will require monitoring by the assigned primary physician.

When the evaluation process has been completed it is important to identify a team member, usually one of the physicians, who will be responsible for overseeing the implementation of the plan or forwarding the recommendations to the appropriate referral sources. The multidisciplinary team needs to develop a step-by-step process that will lead to a final conclusion. The complications that might arise and their treatment should be outlined. It is important for the patient, and all those involved with the patient's care, to have a final plan of action that will essentially "close the case." The patient should not, after a multidisciplinary type of approach, be left in a long-term dilemma, with no final treatment algorithm.

Establishing a Multidisciplinary Practice

Probably the greatest challenge to putting together and developing a multidisciplinary team is the same challenge of building any type of team, whether in sports, business, or medical treatment. Team members must be chosen for their skills, but also for their ability to cooperate, to respect the abilities of others with different training, and to enjoy and have fun in an atmosphere where team success is placed before individual accomplishments. Developing such an approach takes much mutual respect and an attitude from team leaders that allows everyone to feel their contribution is a valuable one.

Strategic Planning

Strategic planning should basically be coordinated with the long-term goals that have been established.[2] It is often important for the physician to consider bringing in administrators and business people. It would be unfortunate to have an extensive multidisciplinary program that was vertically integrated, but that was a financial disaster. In today's competitive medical marketplace, a multidisciplinary program needs to be as close to breaking even as possible, and certainly, if possible, have an excess of revenue over expenses. Once the business plan is organized, a marketing plan can be developed.

In any community, hospital, clinic, or organized group there are key individuals who are valuable for the success of various programs. It is important to make sure that the key individuals have been brought on board, understand the reason for the program, and are supportive of it. If they are unwilling to support such a program, a multidisciplinary program cannot be established.

It is a good idea to consider having the payers involved. If your primary emphasis is rehabilitation of workers' compensation injuries, then the workers' compensation insurance companies should be involved. If your primary market may be back pain patients in general, then talking to the commercial insurance carriers in your area may be appropriate. Discussing your proposals with them helps to smooth the road when it comes time to generate a bill and expect payment for services rendered. Frequently, the carriers may be able to help you identify needs in your service area.

Organization

Organizational structure needs to be created after you have established your goals and recognized what individual components you plan to include. Is it going to be a group practice, or a portion of a hospital-based clinic with individual practitioners participating under the umbrella of a "spine center"? Or is it going to be an individual doctor who has created a network of various components that form a loose-knit association to provide multidisciplinary spinal evaluations for his/her patients? It may even be a hospital sponsored clinic where all members are employees of the hospital.

It is most important to identify a director who will organize and drive the program forward. This needs to be an individual who will be a product champion. Sometimes the product champion cannot be the director, or chooses not to be, but the product champion must be an individual who believes in the concept and is willing to carry it though. It also helps if the individual has the ability to avoid the political pitfalls that will occur when establishing such a multidisciplinary program. More than likely, this will be an individual who has fairly tough skin. There may be many practitioners who do not believe that such a program is needed. They may fear that it will have a negative impact on their practice.

Implementation

Once you have developed your organizational structure, you have a strategic plan, and you have identified your strengths and weaknesses, the next step is to implement your program. The most important step at this stage of development is to communicate with all the players involved. It is not a good idea for the number one spinal surgeon at your hospital to find out about the program in a flyer mailed to his home. It is important that the medical staff members, if you are working in a hospital area, are informed ahead of time, prior to an announcement made to the public.

There are numerous ways to let the medical community know about your new spine center. One way is to hold a meeting and provide information about your program to the medical staff and/or the public. A second way is to contact the other physicians on staff personally. A third way is to send out a mailing piece.

Good communication among the team members is vital to the success of such a program. The referral sources need to be respected and made part of all communications. The best strategy is to appoint a key contact person in each office who is responsible for seeing that information flows back and forth without difficulty.

It is also best to start small and quietly. Start on a trial basis to make sure that the system works and that all providers agree on communication strategies and/or recommendations for treatment. Lastly, let the referring physician, the payers, and the specialists know how the program is working. If patients complain that they wait too long to see the physician or that the office staff does not appear to understand their situation or do not return phone calls, pass that information along. However, it is also valuable to send positive feedback. If a patient has a good experience, then make sure that the physician and/or the nursing staff hear about it. It is all too easy to provide negative feedback and forget to provide positive feedback.

A key component of any multidisciplinary program is treatment philosophy. If such a system is to work, then the individuals who work in the system ought to agree on the same basic philosophy. That does not mean that they will agree on the exact treatment for all patients, but they ought to approach patients in the same fashion. Although it may be difficult to get all team members to agree on a treatment algorithm, once accomplished, it is an excellent way to move patients through the system.

Education

Educating the Team

It is valuable to stress an ongoing commitment to education. Spinal medicine is rapidly changing. New surgical techniques are being developed and there is more and more documentation about aggressive conservative care being the basis for treatments. Not every new, computerized, automatic measuring and treatment device will do everything that the manufacturer says it will. It is important that you participate in an ongoing educational program to make sure you are aware of the changes that are taking place in spinal medicine. It is also important that the staff be educated. If the staff is more knowledgeable, they can spend more time with the patients, and often, as they become more experienced, they can anticipate patient problems.

Educating the Referring Physician

Referring physicians need to understand the basic treatment philosophy of back pain. Through education you can help the referring physicians understand when it is appropriate to refer. We all would like to see patients from the beginning of their problem. Set up a time frame for referring patients into the network and it can help avoid mistreatment. Also, provide your referring physicians with information about the latest things that you are doing in your clinic that they may want to use in their practice. If you cover a wide geographic region, you may not be able to see patients as quickly as everyone would like. Therefore, it is important that your referring physicians be given the tools to treat patients prior to having them evaluated at the multidisciplinary center.

Educating the Patient

The patient needs to understand his/her back and that treatment of back discomfort is his/her responsibility. Success is dependent on the patient's input and effort throughout the treatment program, whether it is surgery or conservative care. The patient's determination and desire to get better and to accept his/her situation and deal with it as it is presented is probably the single most important factor in determining whether he/she will have a successful outcome. Also, it is important to help patients understand that multiple factors may be involved. Patients may not be psychologically manipulating the system, but those who have inappropriate illness behavior or who have chronic pain because of some underlying childhood trauma not yet resolved should be helped to understand these factors.

Educating the Public

Lastly, we need to educate the public at large—not only the adult public, but also the young. It is important that we start implementing proper back education programs at an early age. People need to understand that proper exercise, proper lifting postures, and proper management of minor injuries can help prevent long-term back disability.

Research

There are significant areas in spinal research that need to be addressed, especially with regard to the outcome of patients with certain diseases and how we can modify the disease process by conservative and/or surgical care. If you are interested in doing such research, there are numerous organizations that will help. These organizations provide continuing education and a format in which you can present your research findings. These include the North American Spine Society, The University of Iowa, and many of the regional spine centers. A group of regional physicians can get together to provide an organization such for educating physicians and developing research and political action. The "Oregon Spine Society," the Dallas "Metraplex Society," the San Francisco "Bay Area Spine Association," and local chapters of the North American Spine Society are examples.

Future Directions

The provision of medical care on a national basis may foster the growth of a multidisciplinary approach to spinal care. Financial incentives are being considered to promote regional centralization of complex treatment methods, to render them more cost effective. Similarly, limits to growth in medical spending will likely lead to alterations in patient access to treatment. Panels of various kinds will likely determine such access in many cases.

One of the greatest challenges faced by those in the field of spinal treatment is the development of more rational and proven protocols for evaluation and treatment based on careful research. The Quebec Task Force[6] has noted that given the complexity of spinal care in its current state for injured workers, any worker who loses 3 months in the course of the first year after an industrial injury should be evaluated by a multidisciplinary team. This recommendation reflects the growing understanding of the magnitude of the problem industrial nations now face in the treatment of back pain.

As we have discussed, there are many issues that need to be resolved. The type of patient who needs this kind of evaluation process is 1 in 100 or less and has a history of prior failed back surgery, multiple medication use, associated significant psychologic factors, and long-term disability that has not been resolved in an appropriate fashion. These patients have complex problems that need to be sorted out by a comprehensive team.

Many areas need to be explored in the future. Only through further research, and in the continued development of new and better methods for a multidisciplinary team approach, can we hope to resolve many of the issues that still remain.

References

1. Doughty C: A multidisciplinary approach to cardiac rehabilitation, *Nurs Stand Spec Suppl* 31(45):13, 1991.
2. Five Year Plan for the Doris Palmer Arthritis Center, Pittsburgh, PA, 1986, St. Margaret Memorial Hospital.
3. Judd FK, Brown DJ: *Paraplegia: the psychosocial approach to rehabilitation of the spinal cord injured patient*, 1988, International Medical Society of Paraplegia.
4. Keith RA: The comprehensive treatment team in rehabilitation, *Arch Phys Med Rehabil* 72:269, 1991.
5. Melvin JL: Status report on interdisciplinary medical rehabilitation, *Arch Phys Med Rehabil* 70:273, 1989.
6. Report of the Quebec Task Force on Spinal Disorders: Scientific approach to the assessment and management of activity-related spinal disorders: a monograph for clinicians, *Spine* 12:538, 1987.
7. Rowlingson JC, Hamill RJ: Organization of a multidisciplinary pain center, *Mt Sinai J Med* 58(3):267, 1991.

Chapter 19
Medical Evaluation of the Spine Patient
George F. Smith

History

pattern of pain

Review of Systems

Physical Examination

Specialized Testing

laboratory studies

Nuclear Medicine Imaging of the Spine (Bone Scans)

The etiology of low-back pain (LBP) in the vast majority of patients is mechanical in nature. It has been estimated that only 1% of patients have a systemic medical illness as the cause for their pain.[53] Unfortunately, the presentations of serious medical illnesses overlap with problems that are benign. The clinician must maintain a high index of suspicion in order to make an early diagnosis of a systemic or medical cause of LBP.

There is often a combination of factors that exist, raising the clinical suspicion for a systemic illness as the cause of LBP. This chapter will help to sort out the clinical clues that assist the physician in separating mechanical from nonmechanical LBP using the history, examination and various diagnostic studies available. It is obvious that the clinician needs to be knowledgeable about the anatomic features of the spine and the neurophysiology of pain and be aware of the various disease processes that can affect the spine.

The medical causes of spinal pain can be divided into five general categories, which are shown in Table 19-1. This table lists the common medical diseases that can commonly affect the spine and correlational data. The type and location of pain produced depends on the effect each disease process has on the spine. For example, the pain of a pathologic fracture will present with sudden onset and may have a positional quality as compared to the pain of metastatic prostate cancer, which may be unremitting.

History

Pattern of Pain

The clinical evaluation is of primary importance in establishing a medical diagnosis. However since in most patients pain is the primary complaint, it is necessary to perform a systematic review of systems and associated factors to assess for nonmechanical causes.

The age and sex of the patient are obvious starting points. For example, an elderly woman may present with either osteoporotic compression fractures or metastatic breast cancer. Elderly men may present with metastatic prostate or lung cancer (in smokers).

The rapidity of the onset of pain provides useful information. However, patients often do not recall the exact onset of symptoms and most commonly there is no clear history of trauma or injury.[11,56,68]

The pain pattern and factors that decrease or exacerbate pain are features that help distinguish mechanical from medical causes. In destructive lesions a focal, insidious, unremitting, and intense pain is common. In inflammatory conditions, early-morning stiffness and ache that persist for longer than 1 hour are characteristic.[10] Infections such as vertebral osteomyelitis typically have constant pain of long duration prior to diagnosis. Acute pain referred from a visceral source is often abrupt in onset and colicky in quality without localized findings of tenderness or spasm of the back. Chronic visceral referred pain may have gradual onset.

In general, a major distinction between mechanical and medical spinal pain is the effect of recumbency. Mechanical pain is generally relieved by rest, whereas medical pain is not. Therefore, pain at rest should provoke inquiry into systemic symptoms such as weight loss or fever. If either is present, infection or tumor should be suspected. It has been thought that nocturnal pain is a particularly helpful clue to an occult neoplasm, but this finding is not consistent.[24]

Pain that radiates to an extremity is a common finding. In clinical practice it is often difficult to differentiate between a referred (sclerotomal) pain pattern and a radicular (dermatomal) one as discs or the facet joints can produce distal pain.[35,43] Patients who present with a predominance of leg pain who do not respond quickly to care should undergo MRI or CT scan to determine if intraspinal pathology is present. Either study may disclose an unsuspected medical cause for pain. In addition, extremity pain may be the result of peripheral-nerve compression such as carpal-tunnel syndrome in rheumatoid arthritis. Also, a paraneoplastic syndrome, the most common of which is a sensory or sensorimotor peripheral neuropathy, can present as extremity pain. This is most commonly seen with carcinomas of the lung, breast, and gastrointestinal tract.[9] In the unusual patient who presents with cauda equina syndrome the most common medical causes are metastatic tumor and epidural abscess.[3,52,55] MRI is the diagnostic study of choice for accurate identification of these lesions.[4,47]

Review of Systems

A complete review of systems is needed in any patient suspected of having nonmechanical back pain. A history of fever, unexplained weight loss, or fatigue may indicate systemic illness but is not specific to differentiate between malignancy, infection, and inflammation. The presence of bitemporal headache, proximal shoulder and neck pain, and visual changes in a patient over 50 may suggest polymyalgia rheumatica. Dyspnea on exertion in a male under 45 with chronic morning low-back ache is suggestive of restrictive lung disease in ankylosing spondylitis. Abdominal pain localized to the epigastrium with upper lumbar radiation can be associated with either pancreatitis, pep-

Table 19-1

Medical categories and diseases causing spinal pain

Category	Onset/Location	Age/Sex	Diagnostic Studies
I. Inflammatory/rheumatologic			
Polymyalgia rheumatica	Gradual Neck, shoulders Temporal headaches	>50 Female > male	ESR > 50 mm/hr Temporal artery biopsy
Ankylosing spondylitis	Gradual LBP, sacroiliitis	20 to 30 Male preponderane	X-rays SI joints HLA-B27 + in 90% bone scan ESR
II. Metabolic			

Osteoporosis	Pain with compression
	  fracture; sudden onset
		>60
		Female
			X-ray for
			  fracture
			Bone density

Paget's disease of spine	Gradual or acute	>40	X-ray Bone scan Alkaline phosphatase
Sickle cell anemia	Acute	Childhood African-Americans	Hemoglobin Blood smear X-ray
III. Infection			
Tuberculosis	Gradual or acute Thoracolumbar Psoas abscess	>40	X-ray, + PPD Biopsy and culture
Spontaneous discitis	Gradual	Children	X-ray MRI ESR, cultures
Vertebral osteomyelitis	Gradual	Adults	X-ray MRI ESR, cultures

tic ulcer disease, cholecystitis, or abdominal aortic aneurysm. Change in bowel habits with or without rectal bleeding may indicate gastrointestinal malignancy or inflammatory bowel disease.

Physical Examination

The physical examination of patients with a suspected medical cause of spinal pain focuses on the structures associated with the area of pain directly or by referral, the neurologic evaluation of those structures, and a general medical examination tailored to but not exclusive for the clues obtained in the history. It is recommended to perform the general physical examination first and to examine the painful area last to assist in maximal patient cooperation.[6]

The presence of fever is associated with infection but may be noted with a neoplasm or inflammatory disorder. The skin should be examined for lesions. Psoriatic patches on elbows or knees may indicate underlying psoriatic arthritis. Café au lait spots are associated with neurofibromatosis. Suspicious nevi (especially in fair-skinned individuals) could prove to be clues to malignant melanoma with metastases to the spine.

Unexplained lymphadenopathy is particularly worrisome and may suggest lymphoma or other malignancy. Cardiopulmonary examination may reveal reduction of chest expansion, murmur of aortic insufficiency, or the rub of pericarditis, any of which might suggest ankylosing spondylitis. Abdominal examination may reveal the pulsatile mass of aortic aneurysm or epigastric tenderness with pancreatitis.

Table 19-1 (Continued)
Medical categories and diseases causing spinal pain

Category	Onset/Location	Age/Sex	Diagnostic Studies
Deep-tissue infection, postoperative	Gradual Surgical area	Adults	MRI CRP Indium or gallium scan, cultures
IV. Tumor			
Metastatic cancer	Acute or gradual	>50 Adults	X-ray CBC, ESR, PSA Biopsy
Multiple myeloma	Acute or gradual	>50	X-ray CBC, ESR, SPEP Serum calcium Biopsy
Primary spinal tumor Extradural (e.g., chordoma)	Gradual	Adults	MRI Biopsy
Intradural (e.g., neurofibroma, ependymoma)	Gradual	Adults	MRI Biopsy
V. Visceral referred pain			
Abdominal aneurysm	Gradual (sudden with leakage, rupture)	Adults Male	X-ray Ultrasound CT scan
Urolithiasis	Acute	Adults	Urinalysis IVP
Pancreatitis	Acute or subacute	Adults	Serum amylase

CBC = complete blood count; CRP = C-reactive protein; ESR = erythrocyte sedimentation rate; IVP = intravenous pyelonephritis; MRI = magnetic resonance imaging; PPD = purified protein derivative; PSA = prostate-specific antigen; SI = sacroiliac; SPEP = serum protein electrophoresis.

Breast masses, prostatic nodularity, or stools positive on the Hemoccult test require further evaluation for malignancy.

The spinal area of pain should be examined for skin changes, temperature differences, soft-tissue masses, and point tenderness over bony prominences to help with the diagnosis of infection.

Specialized Testing

Laboratory Studies

Acute-Phase Reactants: Erythrocyte Sedimentation Rate and C-Reactive Protein

The most commonly used test to help differentiate mechanical from medical spinal pain is the erythrocyte sedimentation rate (ESR). The ESR and C-reactive protein (CRP) become elevated due to hepatic protein production in response to tissue injury. The ESR mirrors the synthesis of fibrinogen, which promotes aggregation of red blood cells (rouleaux formation). The Westergren technique is preferred and measures up to 200 mm/hr.[32] Elevations of the ESR and CRP are nonspecific and may be seen in a variety of disorders, including active rheumatologic disease, malignancy, infection, visceral inflammation, other surgical procedures, pregnancy, myocardial infarction, endocrinopathies, and vaccinations. The ESR is increased by anemia and advancing age, and the upper limit of normal is higher for women. The ESR may be decreased by hemoglobinopathies, corticosteroid use, congestive heart failure, and cachexia.

The ESR and CRP should not be considered general screening tests to rule out systemic illness but has been shown to be a valuable screen when a medical cause for spinal pain is suspected.[54] Waddell[69] has shown a false positive rate of only 6% in those with an ESR over 25 mm/hr. The clinical utility of these tests includes helping to determine the presence or absence of a suspected disease process such as infection or malignancy; to assist in confirming a diagnosis such as temporal arteritis or polymyalgia rheumatica; or in following the activity of disease under treatment such as rheumatoid arthritis or osteomyelitis.[65]

Most patients with an ESR that exceeds 100 mm/hr will have a malignancy, infection, or connective-tissue disease, with infection being most common.[22,74,75] Nearly all patients with cancer and an ESR greater than 100 mm/hr have metastases.[75] Of those cancer patients, a significant number will have myeloma and therefore serum and urine electrophoresis should be obtained.

However, the ESR is not always useful to screen for infection. Patients who have had lumbar spinal fusions have ESRs greater than 100/hr for up to 2 weeks after surgery.[34,64] After simple discectomy, the ESR increases during the first week after surgery to a peak mean of 60 mm/hr and may remain elevated for up to 3 weeks.[39] The conclusion of these recent studies indicates that the ESR is an unreliable marker of infection for up to 3 months after spinal fusion.[64]

CRP is almost always present in quantity in inflammation or infection. Measurement is not affected by anemia or altered serum protein fractions. It is helpful in differentiating the presence of inflammation when the ESR is elevated. Elevation of CRP occurs earlier than ESR and disappears before the ESR returns to normal.[51] Any elevation over 8 μg/dl is considered abnormal.

The CRP can be used as an early indicator of postoperative wound infection in orthopedic procedures. In lumbar discectomy not complicated by infection the return to base line occurs in less than 7 days with discectomy.[41]

Blood Counts and Chemistries

Chronic inflammatory conditions, malignancy, and infections are commonly associated with a normochromic, normocytic anemia that is due to suppression of marrow-producing elements. Mechanical back pain does not produce anemia or other changes in laboratory analysis. A patient with microcytic anemia and chronic back pain should be investigated for chronic blood loss secondary to nonsteroidal antiinflammatory drugs (most common cause) or gastrointestinal ulcer or malignancy.

Abnormalities of the white blood cell count (WBC) are commonly but not invariably seen in infections and malignancy. Leukocytosis up to 20,000/ml due to corticosteroid (oral or epidural) treatment may occur due to demargination. In rheumatologic conditions the WBC may be elevated but is usually normal. In mechanical back pain the WBC is normal.

The most important chemistry studies in evaluating spinal conditions are those reflective of bone metabolism. The serum calcium, phosphorus, and alkaline phosphatase are closely linked to changes in bone. Hypercalcemia with hypophosphatemia is most commonly seen in primary hyperparathyroidism. Hypercalcemia is also associated with metastases to bone, multiple myeloma, or tumors that produce hormone-like substances (i.e., oat-cell carcinoma). Vitamin D deficiency (osteomalacia) is associated with hypocalcemia. Osteoporosis, mechanical spinal pain, and osteoarthritis do not cause changes in these studies except for the elevation of alkaline phosphatase after acute fracture. Elevated alkaline phosphatase levels can be due to increased activity of osteoblasts or disease of the hepatobiliary system and differentiation can be obtained by fractionation of the sample. Increased levels are generally seen in conditions that cause bone destruction and repair such as metabolic bone disease (Paget) and metastatic lesions to bone, with the important exception being myeloma.

Urinalysis is helpful in ruling out referred pain from renal disease in patients with cryptic back pain. The presence of erythrocytes signals infection, urolithiasis, or renal or bladder carcinoma. White blood cells indicate cystitis or pyelonephritis. Proteinuria is indicative of glomerular disease and is most commonly associated with nonsteroidal antiinflammatory drug use in back-pain patients.

Immunologic studies for rheumatologic diseases are occasionally helpful in medical back pain. The HLA-B27 is useful to assist in diagnosing a seronegative spondyloarthropathy. HLA-B27 has a 90% sensitivity and 92% specificity for ankylosing spondylitis but is less helpful in the other inflammatory arthropathies.[36,37] The yield of serologic markers such as rheumatoid factor or antinuclear antibody in cryptic spinal pain is extremely low, as the other rheumatologic diseases do not present with back pain as a primary symptom and false positive results increase with age.[31]

The demonstration that prostate specific antigen (PSA) is a sensitive and specific marker for prostatic carcinoma makes PSA a helpful adjunct in the evaluation of patients with suspected prostatic carcinoma or suspicious lesions to the lumbar spine.[7,49] It is also useful to assess for possible recurrent disease.

Nuclear Medicine Imaging of the Spine (Bone Scans)

The current use of MRI and high-resolution CT scanning has significantly altered the practice of spinal medicine. Initial evaluation of atypical clinical presentations or suspicious x-ray lesions begins with one of these studies, which are discussed elsewhere in this book. Often, unsuspected medical lesions are uncovered in the evaluation of mechanical back pain. However, the lack of specificity of lesions requires the use of other diagnostic tools in many cases.

There are several radioisotopic studies that may be used in the evaluation of skeletal disorders. The most widely used are technetium-99m (^{99m}Tc)-labeled phosphate complexes. These complexes are absorbed onto the surface of hydroxyapatite crystals of bone. New bone formation, which occurs as a reaction to almost every type of injury to bone (neoplasm, infection, inflammation, or trauma) is associated with enhanced affinity for bone tracers. Regional blood flow also modulates the accumulation of these tracers. Certain skeletal disorders have reduced tracer accumulation ("cold" lesions) due to reduced perfusion (aseptic necrosis, radiation injury) or because of osteolysis that is not accompanied by an osteoblastic response (multiple myeloma, eosino-

philic granuloma, or aggressive tumor).[62] Bone scintigraphy reflects regional changes in bone mineral turnover rather than content and therefore will be more sensitive by weeks or months than plain x-ray studies for early bone injury.[38,44] The short half-life (6 hours) and low radiation exposure of γ-rays (150 millirads) of technetium-99m makes it an ideal agent for skeletal examination.[15] The common compounds used are methylene diphosphate (MDP) or ethylene hydroxydiphosphonate (EHDP), which is the more stable.[50]

Images are obtained with a scintillation camera that detects γ-rays. Surveys may include the entire skeleton plus detailed images for regions of clinical suspicion. On intravenous administration, tracer uptake occurs rapidly with an accumulation half-time of 30 minutes and complete uptake at 2 hours.[15,67] Patient imaging is done 3 hours after administration in order to allow most of the tracer that has not localized to the bone to be excreted in the urine. Therefore, a normal image (Fig. 19-1) will show increased uptake at areas of increased mechanical pressure (spine, sacroiliac joints, knees, and ankles); thick bone (calvarium and pelvis); and a bladder filled with 50% of the radionuclide. The normal skeletal distribution of phosphorous compounds features more tracer in trabecular than in cortical bone.[16,23] Poor-quality scans may result from dehydration, obesity, chronic corticosteroid use, increased age, or inadequately prepared materials.[72]

In addition to delayed images, a triple-phase bone scan has been introduced to evaluate inflammatory processes. Initial dynamic images are acquired over the area of concern and then followed by static images obtained over longer periods. The first phase characterizes the blood flow to the area, while the second visualizes the blood pool. These two early phases characterize the degree of inflammation and hyperemia present.

Bone scans are useful in evaluating neoplasms, osteomyelitis, trauma, and metabolic bone disease.[38,44,46] In addition, usefulness has been demonstrated in the diagnosis of rhabdomyolysis and reflex sympathetic dystrophy.[14,25]

In patients with suspected cancer, skeletal scintigraphy that surveys the entire skeleton is the primary screening procedure for metastases to bone.[44] Sensitivity is much greater than roentgenography, which requires a regional loss of 30% to 50% of mineral content to show abnormalities. However, confirmation with appropriate roentgenograms and eventual biopsy should be obtained.

Specific cancers are noteworthy. Prostatic cancer spreads to bone at an early stage. Such metastases

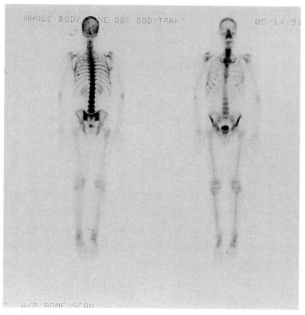

Fig. 19-1
Normal bone scan.

are often asymptomatic, have normal roentgenographic findings, and normal acid phosphatase levels, which makes bone scanning the screening procedure of choice. Metastatic lesions of breast cancer have a profound effect on prognosis, and base-line bone scanning is needed because 20% of patients with stages I and II disease will have bone metastases within a few years. Primary bone tumors such as osteosaroma and Ewing sarcoma produce strikingly abnormal scintigraphic patterns, but standard roentgenograms provide more specific diagnostic information. The exception is osteoid osteoma, which may not be detected on a roentgenogram.[44]

Trauma to bone may be difficult to detect by conventional radiography. In stress fractures or compression fractures of the spine, bone scanning is useful in determining the presence and age of the fracture.[42,57]

Bone scanning is more sensitive than radiography in detection of several metabolic bone diseases, including primary hyperparathyroidism, renal osteodystrophy, and osteomalacia. It is equally sensitive to radiographs for detecting Paget disease. Bone scans are normal in osteoporosis unless compression fracture is present[21] (Fig. 19-2).

Inflammatory arthropathies produce abnormal bone scans due to increased blood flow. In particular, the involvement of the sacroiliac joints is quantifiable in patients with spondyloarthropathies.[28]

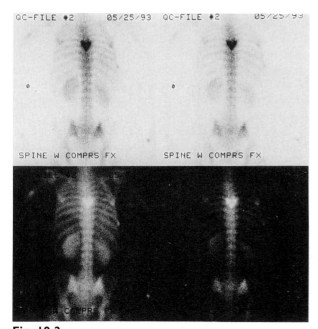

Fig. 19-2
Bone scan illustrating thoracic compression fracture.

The diagnosis of spinal infections is difficult and often delayed, which can result in serious neurologic injury and chronic pain.* Infection may be a complication of spine surgery or can arise from hematogenous spread in patients with infection elsewhere in the body and in intravenous drug use.† Bone scanning is usually abnormal in infection, but occasionally normal scans can occur.[5] Sensitivity precedes that of roentgenograms by days or weeks.[30] However, findings are not specific. Patients who have undergone spinal surgery or skeletal injury may have false positive scans for up to 18 months. Scintigrams are indicated whenever there is doubt regarding the diagnosis of osteomyelitis (normal roentgenogram) or the site of the infection (the sacroiliac joint compared with the lumbar spine in a drug addict).

In acute osteomyelitis, the radionuclide angiogram and blood pool images of the "three-phase" technique shows increased tracer activity in the bone itself and possibly in the surrounding soft tissues. False positive scans may be seen in patients with bone infarct (sickle cell anemia), bone injury, previous surgery (laminectomy or fusion) and with prosthetic implants. In these circumstances, additional scintigraphy with gallium (^{67}Ga) or indium (^{111}In) can be helpful if the diagnosis of osteomyelitis is in doubt.[1,2]

Gallium-67 binds to human polymorphonuclear leukocytes and behaves as a ferric ion analog. Administration is intravenous and the half-life is 78 hours. Excretion during the first 24 hours is by the kidneys and thereafter is through the gastrointestinal tract. Scanning is obtained after 24, 48, and 72 hours to acquire sufficient information. Gallium-67 imaging has been shown to be an accurate and sensitive test for infection of the disc space before changes appear on radiography but is more commonly used in combination with ^{99m}Tc scanning.[8] The sensitivity and specificity for the diagnosis of infection appears adequate but false negative results have been reported.[45,48,59] Gallium-67 has been considered the agent of choice in following the treatment of chronic infections because there is resolution as improvement occurs.[29]

Indium-111-labeled leukocytes can also be used in the evaluation of infections.[33] The technique requires reinfusing autologous leukocytes incubated with indium-111 and scanning at 18 to 24 hours. Indium-111 has shown to be quite promising in diagnosing osteomyelitis and may be the most accurate when combined with technetium-99m scan-

*References 2, 5, 12, 17, 27, 61, and 63.
†References 13, 18, 19, 26, 40, 58, 66, and 71.

ning.[60] However, in the spine studies have shown this not to be a sensitive test, particularly in patients previously treated with antibiotics.[20,70,73]

In summary, for suspected spine infections in the acute setting technetium bone scanning is the primary study. If trauma or previous surgery is present, then indium-tagged white blood cell scanning is preferred if antibiotics have not been used. In the chronic setting, the sensitivity is not high with either gallium or indium scanning, but if either is positive the likelihood of infection is high.

References

1. Al-Sheikh W, Sfakianakis GN, Mnaymneh W, et al.: Subacute and chronic bone infections: diagnosis using In-111, Ga-67, and Tc-99m MDP bone scintigraphy and radiology, *Radiology* 155:501, 1985.
2. Ambrose GB, Neer CS: Vertebral osteomyelitis: a diagnostic problem, *JAMA* 197:101, 1966.
3. Baker AS, Ojeimann RG, Swartz MN, et al.: Spinal epidural abscess, *N Engl J Med* 293:463, 1975.
4. Berns DH, Blaser SI, Modic MT: Magnetic resonance imaging of the spine, *Clin Orthop* 244:78, 1989.
5. Bonefiglio M, Lange TA, Kim YM: Pyogenic vertebral ostemyelitis: disc space infections, *Clin Orthop* 96:234, 1973.
6. Borenstein DG: *Clinical evaluation of low back pain, physical examination.* In Borenstein DG, Wiesel SW, editors: *Low back pain: medical diagnoses and comprehensive management,* Philadelphia, 1989, W.B. Saunders Co.
7. Brawer MK: The diagnosis of prostatic carcinoma, *Cancer* 71:899, 1993.
8. Bruschwein DA, Brown ML, McLeod RA: Gallium scintigraphy in the evaluation of disc-space infections: concise communication, *J Nucl Med* 21:925, 1980.
9. Bunn PA Jr, Minna JD: *Paraneoplastic syndromes in cancer,* In DeVita VT Jr, Hellman S, Rosenburg SA, editors: *Cancer: principles and practice of oncology,* ed 2, Philadelphia, 1985, J.B. Lippincott, p 1797.
10. Calin A, Porta J, Fries JF, Schurman DJ: Clinical history as a screening test for ankylosing spondylitis, *JAMA* 237:2613, 1977.
11. Canadian Back Institute, Unpublished data, 1984.
12. Cloward RB: Metastatic disc infection and osteomyelitis of the cervical spine: surgical treatment, *Spine* 3:194, 1978.
13. Collert S: Osteomyelitis of the spine, *Acta Orthop Scand* 48:283, 1977.
14. Davidoff G, Werner R, Cremer S, et al.: Predictive value of the three-phase technetium bone scan in diagnosis of reflex sympathetic dystrophy syndrome, *Arch Phys Med Rehab* 70:135, 1989.
15. Davis M, Jones A: Comparison of ^{99m}Tc-labeled phosphate agents for skeletal imaging, *Semin Nucl Med* 7:19, 1979.
16. Dibos PE, Wagner HN Jr: Atlas of nuclear medicine. Vol 4. *Bone*. Philadelphia, 1978, W.B. Saunders Co.
17. Eismont FJ, Bohlman JJ, Soni PI, et al.: Pyogenic and fungal vertebral osteomyelitis with paralysis, *J Bone Joint Surg* 65A:19, 1983.
18. El-Gindi S, Aref S, Salama M, Andrew J: Infection of intervertebral discs after operation, *J Bone Joint Surg* 58B:114, 1976.
19. Fernand R, Lee CK: Postlaminectomy disc space infection: a review of the literature and a report of three cases, *Clin Orthop* 209:215, 1986.
20. Fernandez-Ulloa M, Vasavada PJ, Hanslits ML, et al.: Diagnosis of vertebral osteomyelitis: clinical, radiological and scintigraphic features, *Orthopedics* 8:1144, 1985.
21. Fogelman I, Bessent RG, Turner JG, et al: The use of whole-body retention of Tc-99m diphosphonate in the diagnosis of metabolic bone disease, *J Nucl Med* 19:270, 1978.
22. Ford MJ, Innes JA, Parrish FM, et al.: The significance of gross elevation of the erythrocyte sedimentation rate in a general medical unit, *Eur J Clin Invest* 9:191, 1979.
23. Fordham EW: *Osseous nuclear medicine.* In Gottschalk A, Potchen EJ, editors: *Diagnostic nuclear medicine,* Baltimore, 1976, Williams & Wilkins, p 497.
24. Francis KC, Hutter VP: Neoplasms of the spine in the aged, *Clin Orthop* 26:54, 1963.
25. Frymoyer PA, Giammarco R, Farrar FM, Schoreder ET: Technetium Tc-99m medronate bone scanning in rhabdomyolosis, *Arch Intern Med* 145:1991, 1985.
26. Garcia A Jr, Grantham SA: Hematogenous pyogenic vertebral osteomyelitis, *J Bone Joint Surg* 42A:429, 1960.
27. Ghormley RK, Bickel WH, Dickson DD: A study of acute infectious lesions of the intervertebral discs, *South Med J* 33:347, 1940.
28. Goldberg RP, Genant HK, Shimshak R, Shames D: Applications and limitations of quantitative sacroiliac joint scintigraphy, *Radiology* 128:683, 1978.
29. Graham GD, Lundy MM, Frederick RJ, et al.: Predicting the cure of osteomyelitis under treatment: concise communication, *J Nucl Med* 24:110, 1983.
30. Handmaker H: Acute hematogenous osteomyelitis: Has the bone scan betrayed us? *Radiology* 135:787, 1980.
31. Heimer R, Levin FM, Rudd E: Globulins resembling rheumatoid factor in serum of the aged, *Am J Med* 35:175, 1963.
32. International Committee for Standardization in Hematology: Recommendation of measurement of erythrocyte sedimentation rate of human blood, *Am J Clin Pathol* 68:505, 1977.
33. Johnson DG, Coleman RE: *Detection of inflammatory disease using radiolabeled cells.* In Hoffer PB, Potchen EJ, editors: *Diagnostic nuclear medicine,* ed 2. Baltimore, 1988, Williams & Williams, p 1125.
34. Jonsson B, Soderholm R, Stromqvist B: Erythrocyte sedimentation rate after lumbar spine surgery, *Spine* 16:1049, 1991.
35. Kellgren JH: Observations on referred pain arising from deep somatic structures with charts of segmental pain areas, *Clin Sci Mol Med* 4:35, 1939.

36. Khan MA, Khan MK: Diagnostic value of HLA-B27 testing in ankylosing spondylitis and Reiter's syndrome, *Ann Intern Med* 96:70, 1982.

37. Khan MA, Kusher I: *Diagnosis of ankylosing spondylitis*. In Cohen AS, editor: *Progress in clinical rheumatology*, vol 1. New York, 1984, Grune & Stratton, p 145.

38. Kirchner PT, Simon MA: Radioisotopic evaluation of skeletal disease, *J Bone Joint Surg* 63A:673, 1981.

39. Kornberg M: Erythrocyte sedimentation rate following lumbar discectomy. *Spine* 11:799, 1986.

40. Lang EF: Postoperative infection of the intervertebral disk space, *Surg Clin North Am* 48:649, 1968.

41. Larsson S, Thelander U, Friberg S: C-reactive protein levels after elective orthopedic surgery, *Clin Orthop Relat Res* 275:237, 1992.

42. Marty R, Denny J, McKamey MR, Rowley MJ: Bone trauma and related benign disease: assessment by bone scanning, *Semin Nucl Med* 6:107, 1976.

43. McCall IW, Park WM, O'Brien JP: Induced pain referral from posterior lumbar elements in normal subjects, *Spine* 4:441, 1979.

44. McNeil BJ: Value of bone scanning in neoplastic disease, *Semin Nucl Med* 14:277, 1984.

45. Merkel KD, Brown ML, Dewanjee MK, et al.: Comparison of indium-labeled-leukocyte imaging with sequential technetium-gallium scanning in the diagnosis of low grade musculoskeletal sepsis: a prospective study, *J Bone Joint Surg* 67A:465, 1985.

46. Merkel KD, Fitzgerald RH, Brown ML: Scintigraphic evaluation in musculoskeletal sepsis, *Orthop Clin North Am* 15:401, 1984.

47. Modic MT, Planze W, Feiglin DHI, et al.: Magnetic resonance imaging of musculoskeletal infections, *Radiol Clin North Am* 24:247, 1986.

48. Norris S, Ehrlich MG, McKusick J: Early diagnosis of disc space infection using gallium-67, *J Nucl Med* 19:384, 1978.

49. Oesterling JE, Martin SK, Bergstralh EJ: The use of prostate-specific antigen in staging patients with newly diagnosed prostate cancer, *JAMA* 269:57, 1993.

50. Pendergrass H, Porsaid M, Costonovo F: The clinical use of ^{99m}Tc-diphophonate, *Radiology* 109:557, 1973.

51. Petola H, Vahvanen V, Aalto K: Fever, C-reactive protein, and erythrocyte sedimentation rate in monitoring recovery from septic arthritis: a preliminary study, *J Pediatr Orthop* 4:170, 1984.

52. Phillips GE, Jefferson A: Acute spinal epidural abscess: observations from fourteen cases, *Postgrad Med J* 55:712, 1979.

53. Pinals RS: *Approach to the patient with back pain*. In Kelley WN, et al., editors: *Textbook of internal medicine*, Philadelphia, 1989, J.B. Lippincott, p 1063.

54. Rafnsson V, Bengtsson C, Lennartsson J, et al.: Erythrocyte sedimentation rate in a population sample of women, with special reference to its clinical and prognostic significance, *Acta Med Scand* 206:207, 1979.

55. Rodriquez M, Dinapoli RP: Spinal cord compression with special reference to metastatic epidural tumors, *Mayo Clinic Proc* 55:442, 1980.

56. Rowe ML: Low back pain disability in industry: updated position, *J Occup Med* 13:476, 1971.

57. Rupani HD, Holder LE, Espinola DA, Engin SI: Three-phase radionuclide bone imaging in sports medicine, *Radiology* 156:187, 1985.

58. Sapico FL, Montgomerie JZ: Vertebral osteomyelitis in intravenous drug abusers: report of three cases and review of the literature, *Rev Infect Dis* 2:196, 1980.

59. Schauwecker DS, Braunstein EM, Wheat LJ: Diagnostic imaging of osteomyelitis. *Infect Dis Clin North Am* 4:411, 1990.

60. Schauwecker DS, Park HM, Mock BH, et al.: Evaluation of complicating osteomyelitis with Tc-99m MDP, In-111 granulocytes, and Ga-67 citrate, *J Nucl Med* 25:849, 1984.

61. Schofferman L, Schofferman J, Zucherman J, et al.: Occult infections causing persistent low back pain, *Spine* 14:417, 1989.

62. Siegel B, Alazrake N, Davis M, et al.: In Kirchner PT, editor: *Nuclear medicine review syllabus*, New York, 1980, Society of Nuclear Medicine, p 319.

63. Silverthorn KG, Gillespie WJ: Pyogenic spinal osteomyelitis: a review of 61 cases, *N Z Med J* 12:62, 1986.

64. Smith GF, Keaney D, Schofferman J, White AH: *The effect of lumbar fusion with pedicle screws and rods on erythrocyte sedimentation rate*, Presented at the North American Spine Society meeting, July 9-11, 1992, Boston.

65. Sox HC, Liang MH: The erythrocyte sedimentation rate: guidelines for rational use, *Ann Intern Med* 104:515, 1986.

66. Stauffer RN: Pyogenic vertebral osteomyelitis, *Orthop Clin North Am* 6:1015, 1975.

67. Subramanian G, McAfee JF, Blair RJ, Thomas FD: *An evaluation of Tc-99m-labeled phosphate compounds as bone imaging agents*. In Subramanian G, et al., editors: *Radiopharmaceuticals*, New York, 1975, Society of Nuclear Medicine, p 319.

68. Thomas AMC, Fairbank JCT, Pynsent PB, Baker DJ: A computer-based interview system for patients with back pain: a validation study, *Spine* 14:844, 1989.

69. Waddell G: An approach to backache, *Br J Hosp Med* 28:187, 1982.

70. Whalen JL, Brown ML, McLeod R, Fitzgerald RH: Limitations of indium leukocyte imaging for the diagnosis of spine infections, *Spine* 16:193, 1991.

71. Wiesseman GJ, Wood VE, Kroll LL: Pseudomonas vertebral osteomyelitis in heroin addicts, *J Bone Joint Surg* 55A:1416, 1973.

72. Wilson MA: The effect of age on the quality of bone scans using ^{99m}Tc-pyrophosphate, *Radiology* 139:703, 1981.

73. Wukich DK, VanDam BE, Abreu SH: Preoperative indium-labeled white blood cell scintigraphy in suspected osteomyelitis of the axial skeleton, *Spine* 13:1168, 1988.

74. Wyler DJ: Diagnostic implications of markedly elevated erythrocyte sedimentation rate: a reevaluation, *South Med J* 70:1428, 1977.

75. Zacharski LR, Kyle RA: Significance of extreme elevation of erythrocyte sedimentation rate, *JAMA*

Chapter 20
Principles of Assessment of Osteometabolic Bone Disease

Alexander G. Hadjipavlou

Philip N. Lander

Osseous Homeostasis

Pathophysiology of Bone Modeling and Remodeling

Laboratory Investigation of Osteometabolic Bone Diseases

Osseous Homeostasis

Substantial strides in the understanding of osteometabolic bone diseases have been made with the introduction by Frost of the concept of the BMU (basic multicellular unit) and its action on bone envelopes.[21,24] According to Frost[24] bone remodeling is the process of bone turnover (renewal) that combines resorption and reformation* of bone tissue to replace old bone. This process is mediated through the remodeling unit. Activation of the bone BMU leads to the appearance of osteoclasts, producing focal bone resorption. These cells are then supplanted by osteoblasts, which in turn form borne. The BMU pathway therefore consists of a sequence of three unvarying phases: activation, resorption, and lastly, reformation (Fig. 20-1).[34] To date, only a few substances[27] have been identified as BMU stimulators, namely parathormone, thyroxine, adrenal corticoids, and regional trauma. Frost[28] considers the BMU (remodeling unit) to be the osseous analog of the nephron; through this fundamental concept, one can

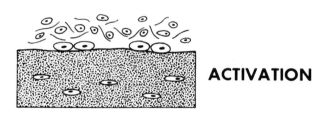

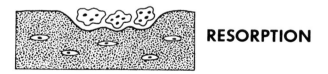

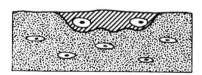

Fig. 20-1

Inviolate sequence of BMU pathway on a bone surface: activation, resorption, and finally formation. *(Adapted from Hadjipavlou A: Osteoporosis: disease, pathophysiology, treatment, Contemp Obstet Gynecol 1:6, 1986.)*

*Formation describes *de novo* formation during skeletal growth.

REMODELING UNIT

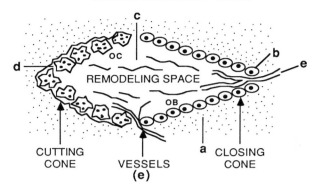

Fig. 20-2

Diagrammatic illustration of structure of complete remodeling unit.

better understand the behavior of bone tissue in normal and abnormal situations. The remodeling unit is the structural assembly that maintains osseous homeostasis and consists of osteoclasts and osteoblasts arranged in a characteristic structural unit (Fig. 20-2) spearheaded by osteoclasts[42] that tunnel through the bone. This region is called the "cutting cone," and in its wake is followed by osteoblasts, producing osteoid tissue, that forms the closing once.[42] The maximal thickness of bone deposited by the BMU seldom exceeds 60 to 80 μ and is called the "Ham constant."[39] The space between the cutting cone and the closing cone is called the "re-modeling space." The osteoblasts in the Haversian system have a linear apposition rate in the closing cone of 1 to 1.5 μ per day, and the osteoclasts have a linear resorption rate in the region of the cutting cone of 40 to 50 μ per day, which means that about 20 to 40 times more osteoblasts than osteoclasts per nucleus have to be created. The speed of the whole remodeling unit is 50 μ per day.[39,40] The duration of the resorption phase is approximately 1 month and the duration of the formation phase is 2 to 3 months. The life span of a remodeling unit is about 4 months in normal situations.[21,23] In osteoporosis, the average length of time for a single lamellar remodeling center (or BMU) to complete its histologic activity is approximately 2.5 years.[23,27,41] The histologic appearance of a remodeling unit eroding a trabecular bone is shown in Fig. 20-3, and a remodeling unit tunneling through cortical bone is shown in Fig. 20-4. From infancy until the third decade of life, the activity of the remodeling unit is accelerated, with formation dominating over resorption, resulting in a net gain

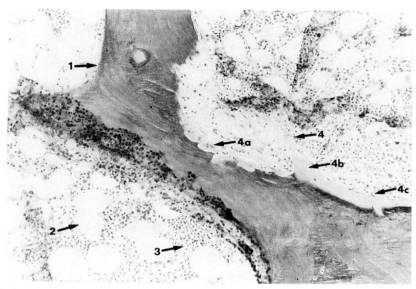

Fig. 20-3

Histology showing structure of active remodeling unit penetrating bone trebeculum. 1 = trabeculum; 2 = marrow fat tissue; 3 = hemopoetic tissue; 4 = remodeling unit; 4a = osteoclasts spearheading the unit form the cutting cone; 4b = osteoid tissue formed by osteoblasts; 4c = in wake of osteoclastic cutting cone. *(From Hadjipavlou A: Osteoporosis: disease, pathophysiology and treatment,* Contemp Obstet Gynecol *1:6, 1986. Courtesy of C. Anderson, M.D.)*

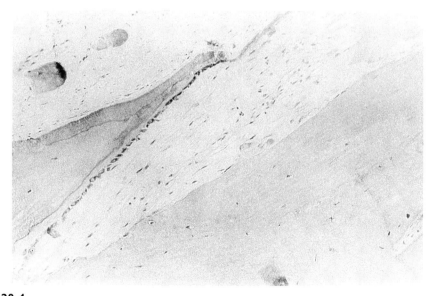

Fig. 20-4

Histologic appearance of active remodeling unit tunneling through cortical bone. Osteoclasts appear first and dig tunnels through bone at daily rate of 20 μ in length and 10 μ in width. When diameter reaches about 200 μ, resorption stops. Osteoblasts appear in the wake of remodeling unit and start laying bone and narrow tunnel by about 2 μ per day until a mature Haversian canal of about 50 μ in diameter is formed.[55] *(From Hadjipavlou A: Osteoporosis: disease, pathophysiology and treatment,* Contemp Obstet Gynecol *1:6, 1986. Courtesy of C. Anderson, M.D.)*

of bone (bone accretion). The turnover of bone is about 50% in the first 2 years of life.[72] After the third decade, bone turnover decreases to about 5% annually, with resorption dominating over formation resulting in a net loss of bone mass.[65] The thickness of new bone deposited per unit time by osteoblasts is called the "appositional rate," which is subdivided into the matrix appositional rate and the mineral appositional rate.

Frost[26] has divided the skeleton into the periosteal, endosteal, trabecular, and Haversian envelopes. Each envelope is controlled by an independent BMU system. Normally, in the periosteal BMU system, reformation by osteoblasts dominates over resorption, leading to bone apposition that may result in cortical bone expansion. In the endosteal envelope, the BMU's resorptive phase dominates over its reformative counterpart, resulting in bone absorption. Normally with age, because there is less periosteal apposition than endosteal absorption, the cortex becomes thinner, leading to so-called age-related bone loss.[40]

Bone modeling refers to the process that determines the size and shape of bone (bone geometry).[25] It is surface phenomenon depending on the amount of bone apposition or absorption at the periosteal and endosteal envelope by the remodeling BMU. This modeling rate is very rapid during childhood and slows considerably after puberty. Throughout life, there is a very slow rate of modeling leading to bone expansion.[11,29,71] Parathyroid hormone thyroxine, vitamin D, and other unknown substances stimulate the osteoprogenitor cells to become bone cells.[27] Although the initial effect of the remodeling unit is osteoclastic bone resorption, Chambers has postulated that cells of osteoblastic lineage are important for the function of osteoclasts. Osteoblastic cells may be able to recruit, localize, activate, regulate, and terminate osteoclastic bone resorption.[8] Osteoclasts by themselves cannot initiate resorption on bone surfaces covered by unmineralized osteoid (Fig. 20-5). Osteoblastic cells appear to initiate osteoclastic resorption by excreting neutral proteases and collagenase that digest the unmineralized surface of bone, thus exposing the osteoclastic resorption-stimulating bone minerals in contact with osteoclasts. Parathyroid hormone (Fig. 20-6) mediates its effect on osteoclasts through the osteoblasts by inducing them to release osteoclastic response–stimulating agents.[8] Interleukin-1, tumor necrosis factor, and lymphotoxin mediate their stimulating effect on osteoclasts through osteoblasts inducing osteoclastic resorption–stimulating activity. Osteoblastic cells are also known to secrete prostaglandins (PGs) of the E series (PGE_1, PGE_2). These may be the agents through which osteoblasts terminate osteoclastic resorption, since both PGE_1 and PGE_2 in nanomolar concentration strongly inhibit osteoclast activity.

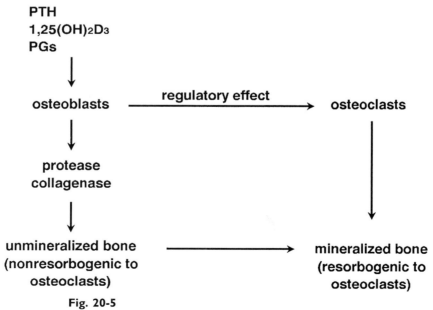

Fig. 20-5

Algorithm for regulatory effects of osteoblasts on osteoclasts. Osteoblasts render bone resorbogenic to osteoclastic action by exposing bone minerals to osteoclasts.

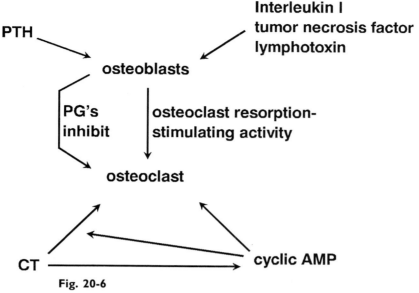

Fig. 20-6

Indirect effects of parathyroid hormone (PTH) on osteoclasts through osteoblasts and direct effect of CT on osteoclasts.

However, in pathologic situations of excessive production of prostaglandins by inflammatory or neoplastic cells, prostaglandins actually promote resorption. In addition to parathyroid hormone, 1,25-dihydroxyvitamin D_3 $((OH)_2D_3)$ and PGs may stimulate osteoblastic cells to produce collagenase, neutral protease, and tissue plasminogen activator, which in turn, by initiating digestion of the unmineralized surface of bone, will render the bone susceptible to resorption by osteoclasts. Bone resorption is stimulated by $1\text{-}25(OH)_2$ D_3 through the additional mechanism by inducing hematopoietic tissue (including spleen cells) to form osteoclasts. Of all the hormones, only calcitonin appears to have a direct osteoclastic effect (inhibition of bone resorption). According to Chambers, calcitonin reduces bone resorption by 50% in isolated mammalian osteoclasts; the remainder of the inhibitory osteoclastic bone resorption influence being exerted through intermediary cells of osteoblastic lineage. Cyclic AMP (cAMP) has been implicated as a second messenger in calcitonin's inhibiting osteoclastic resorption. Agents that may reduce cAMP degradation enhance calcitonin responsiveness. Calcitonin is known to increase cAMP levels in bone.[8] Thus, it is apparent that there is a direct relationship between osteoblasts and osteoclasts. Physiologically, this coordinated effect of osteoclast-induced resorption and osteoblast-induced formation is called "coupling." Dissociation of this coupling is found in pathologic disorders.

Pathophysiology of Bond Modeling and Remodeling

Noncoherent and nontemporal behavior of BMUs in the periosteal and endosteal envelopes gives rise to abnormal bone modeling. Osteopetrosis is characterized by decreased bone absorption in the endosteal envelope, with normal BMU activity in the periosteal envelope,[25] leading to a narrow medullary cavity in the long bones and decreased or absent marrow spaces in the vertebral bodies.

Osteodensity denotes an excess of bone mass and implies that formation dominates over resorption (blastic phase of Paget disease, osteoblastic metastasis, osteopetrosis). *Osteomalacia* is characterized by normal bone mass volume, but decreased mineral content per unit volume. *Osteoporosis* means a reduction in total bone mass and is a heterogenous pathologic condition. *Osteopenia* denotes a decreased volume of mineralized bone tissue and usually is equivalent to osteoporosis, but the terms are not synonymous.

Osteopenia does not necessarily imply disability, and should be distinguished from disease osteoporosis, which combines a bone-deficient skeleton, skeletal biomechanical incompetence, and a causative medical background. In disease osteoporosis, defective BMU repair of accumulated microfractures from everyday loading leads to skeletal failure.[11,25]

In idiopathic osteoporosis, there is excessive endosteal resorption dominating over formation and periosteal bone formation dominating over resorption. This results in femoral expansion and thin cortices with aging.[71] Some studies[54,79] suggest that there is a dissociation between cortical and trabecular osteoporosis in certain groups of patients. Excess corticosteriods produce bone loss by increasing endosteal and trabecular envelope absorption, leading to an increased marrow cavity.[25]

In acromegaly in the younger age group there is excessive periosteal envelope apposition, and, to a lesser degree, endosteal absorption, resulting in think cortices and overall expansion of cortical bone.[25] The mean cortical area of bone mass has been reported to be greater in patients with acromegaly.[15] In Paget's disease, the periosteal and endosteal envelopes display variable activities, giving rise to cortical bone expansion, which may be localized or generalized. Modeling disorders in Paget's disease may lead to bone deformity by the mechanism of centrifugal or centripetal cortical drift.[46]

In high-turnover osteoporosis, there is a dissociation between the speed of the cutting and closing cones of the BMU, resulting in an increased remodeling space.[16] This increased remodeling space results in lack of bone substance. The regional acceleratory phenomenon[25] is an example of high-turnover osteoporosis with an increased remodeling space. About 50% of the local spongiosa can vanish within as short a time as 6 weeks. When the stimulus that triggers increased bone turnover, with its prolonged resorptive phase ceases, BMU activation declines, and the osteoclastic phase is supplanted by an osteoblastic phase, so that the osteopenic condition is reversed. High-turnover osteoporosis, with an increased resorptive phase and a decreased formation phase characterized the osteoporosis of thyrotoxicosis, regional acceleratory phenomenon, migratory osteopenia, Sudeck atrophy, and causalgia. Conceptually, a similar situation may occur in the osteolytic phase of Paget disease. Increased remodeling may result in an osteolytic appearance, with the gaps being filled by new bone in the osteoblastic phase. The behavior of Paget disease is suggestive of an abnormal and uncontrolled BMU birth rate. There are some conditions associated with increased cortical Haversian envelope activity: hyperthyroidism, osteogenesis imperfecta, posttraumatic osteodystrophy, acromegaly, and sometimes hyperparathyroidism.[25] Histomorphometric studies of osteoporosis in hyperthyroidism[50] suggest that this type of osteoporosis is a different entity. The most characteristic findings are loss of trabecular bone and increased cortical porosity. There is an increase in formation of BMUs in the Haversian and endosteal envelopes, producing an excessive number of remodeling units. The length

of the BMU formation phase is also decreased. Trabecular bone loss seems to corelate with the duration of thyrotoxicosis rather than its severity.[52]

Laboratory Investigation of Osteometabolic Bone Diseases

Disturbance in osseous homeostasis can be assessed by investigating remodeling and modeling bone changes. Serum and urinary biochemical and hormonal levels may give some clue, or even determined the factor responsible for abnormal remodeling behavior leading to abnormal osseous structure. The remodeling unit itself can be evaluated by means of biochemical bone markers and radionuclide images. Histomorphometry investigates the various components of bone remodeling activity. Densitometric studies record the net effect of bone remodeling changes, while radiography is the best tool for studying bone modeling changes.

Bone Markers For Bone Metabolism

The biochemical markers for bone metabolism are seen in Table 20-1.[43] All markers for bone reformation are produced by osteoblasts, whereas markers for bone resorption are not solely produced by osteoclasts (tartrate-resistant acid phosphatase), but also are released from bone matrix during the resorption process (hydroxyproline, hydroxylysine, or pyridinium cross links). Through these markers bone turnover can be monitored.

Table 20-1
Biochemical markers for bone metabolism*

Bone Formation	Bone Resorption
Serum alkaline phosphatase	Serum tartrate resistant acid phosphatase
Serum osteocalcin	Urinary hydroxyproline Urinary hydroxylysine
Serum procollagen peptide type one	Pyridinoline (pyridinium cross-links)

*From Kraenzlin ME, et al.: Pharmacia Diagnostic, Clin Symp, 1989.

Bone Formation Markers

Alkaline Phosphatase There are a direct correlation between the level of alkaline phosphatase activity and osteoblastic activity.[32] Bone alkaline phosphatase is found in osteoblasts and mainly in the membranes of osteoblasts.[30] The mode of action of alkaline phosphatase in bone formation and its release into the extracellular fluid is still unknown. Alkaline phosphatase has a biologic half-life ranging from 1.1 to 2.2 days and lacks diurnal variation, therefore it is practical for monitoring overall bone formation, but has little value in monitoring acute changes in bone formation.[57] Alkaline phosphatase, aside from its bone origin is also produced by the liver, intestine, endometrium (placenta), and lungs. The overall serum level of alkaline phosphatase reflects both bone remodeling and liver function. Except during pregnancy and in pathologic conditions, other organs do not contribute to serum levels of alkaline phosphatase activity.[49] Elevated bone alkaline phosphatase can also be differentiated from isoenzymes of other tissues (liver, intestines, placenta) by electrophoresis or by radioimmunoassay. Measurement of skeletal alkaline phosphatase activity as an index of bone formation appears to be more sensitive than measurements of total alkaline phosphatase. It has been shown in patients with osteoporosis that bone alkaline phosphatase is elevated in patients treated with anabolic steroids, whereas there is only a small and insignificant increase in total alkaline phosphatase.[17] Hepatic dysfunction should be ruled out in the presence of elevated alkaline phosphatase levels. Underlying liver disease is unlikely to be present in the face of normal Γ-glutamyltranspeptidase (GGTP) levels, which is a very sensitive enzymatic indicator of liver disease. In widespread Paget disease alkaline phosphatase may reach a record value significantly higher than in any liver or other bone pathologic conditions. In the initial stage of Paget disease, alkaline phosphatase levels fluctuate with an upward trend. After a period of 3 to 6 years it stabilizes for many years in a range characteristic for the individual patient.[81] Although the levels of serum alkaline phosphatase do not help in differentiating osteogenic sarcoma arising in Paget disease of bone,[36] a sudden "explosive rise," as coined by Woodward,[81] may be suggestive of malignant transformation. Apart from Paget disease, elevated alkaline phosphatase can be found in other osteometabolic conditions, such as primary and secondary hyperparathyroidism, osteomalacia, renal rickets, renal osteodystrophy, Gaucher disease, resumption of ambulation following prolonged bed rest, acromegaly, treatment of osteoporosis with fluorides, fracture healing, osteogenic sarcoma, Hodgkin disease of bone, metastatic cancers to bone, and while it may be mildly elevated in thyrotoxicosis.[43,59] Alkaline phosphatase, aside from its bone origin, can also be found elevated in liver diseases (infectious mononucleosis, biliary obstruction, cytomegalic infection, cholangitis, hepatocellu-

lar jaundice, portal cirrhosis, and liver abscess). Other conditions that may contribute to increased alkaline phosphatase are intrahepatic sepsis, ulcerative cholitis, regional enteritis, intraabdominal enteritis, and infection. Milk consumption increases the intestinal coenzyme of alkaline phosphatase in serum, especially in individuals who are blood type O or B, and who are Lewis-positive secretors. Pregnant women have positive placental alkaline phosphatase that appears in the serum during the third trimester.[75]

Osteocalcin Osteocalcin is another biologic bone marker of bone formation, is synthesized by the osteoblastic bone cells,[48] and constitutes about 10% to 20% of total noncollagenous bone proteins.[59] Osteocalcin is also called BGT or Gla protein γ-carboxylglutamic acid-containing protein) and has 49 amino acids and undergoes a vitamin K-dependent posttranslation carboxylation of certain glutamic acid residues[58] and a modification as prothrombin. There is a linear relationship between osteocalcin content and increasing bone density. Circulating osteocalcin is an index of bone formation and not bone resorption.[6] Osteocalcin has a short serum half-life of about 4 minutes, which makes this marker ideal for monitoring acute response of bone formation to challenge. As opposed to alkaline phosphatase, osteocalcin demonstrates a circadian rhythm.[31,56] This disadvantage can be overcome by determination of 24-hour urinary excretion of osteocalcin, giving an integrated value of daily bone turnover rates.[74] This circadian rhythm with the lowest level in the morning and the maximal level during the night as opposed to the constant levels of parathyroid hormone might suggest an even circadian variation of bone formation.[56] Coulton et al.,[10] found that osteocalcin has a lower sensitivity and specificity for measurement of the Paget's disease activity than alkaline phosphatase. However, it seems that this observation may not reflect the same biologic activity as pointed out by Taylor et al.,[74] who found that osteocalcin is a reliable index of bone formation. This difference between the biologic activity of osteocalcin and that of alkaline phosphatase should not be interpreted that osteocalcin has a lower sensitivity and specificity than alkaline phosphatase for measurement of remodeling activity in Paget's disease of bone.[10] According to Davey et al.,[13] serum osteocalcin did not show any response in patients with Paget disease in whom osteosarcoma developed, whereas serum alkaline phosphatase increased rapidly, suggesting that serum osteocalcin does not reflect the same osteoblastic activity as alkaline phosphatase. Serum osteocalcin levels are elevated in osteometabolic diseases characterized by increased bone turnover, such as Paget's disease, hyperparathyroidism, renal osteodystrophy, and perimenopausal osteoporosis. Osteocalcin has been reported in low levels in patients with low bone turnover conditions such as hypoparathyroidism.[48,73]

Procollagen Type 1 Procollagen is a precursor molecule forming the chains for type 1 collagen. These molecules differ from the final molecule by the presence of substantial nonhelical extensions at both the N-terminal and C-terminal ends.[51] Type 1 collagen is the type found in bone and consists of a $2A_1$ and a $1A_2$ chain, coiled around each other, forming a right-handed triple helix. The procollagen is then secreted into the extracellular matrix as an intact molecule and prior to insertion into the existing extracellular matrix the terminal ends are proteolytically removed.[18] Carboxy-terminal extension peptide can be used as an index of total bone formation rate. Low levels of circulating procollagen peptides are found in osteogenesis imperfecta, which is characterized by defective collagen production and also in patients treated with calcitonin or bisphosphonates.[60] High levels of type 1 procollagen peptides are found in patients with Paget disease.[69] Blood immunoassay for C-terminal peptide has been developed to measure the circulating levels of procollagen peptide. This marker merits further study as an index of bone formation during remodeling.

Bone Resorption Markers

Tartrate-resistant Acid Phosphatase Acid phosphatase[75] is a lysosomal enzyme that operates at a low pH. It is present in many tissues, such as bone, platelets, erythrocytes, spleen, and, mainly, prostate. The extraosseous serum acid phosphatase in males is approximately half prostatic and in females, it derives mainly from liver, erythrocytes, and platelets. The likely source of bone acid phosphatase is the osteoclast. Increased serum level of acid phosphatase does not necessarily indicate only prostatic carcinoma but bone reticuloendothelial system diseases as well. Tartrate-resistant acid phosphatase (TR-AcP) activity in serum can be measured by spectrophotometric assay in the presence of sodium tartrate,[47] and it has been used to assess osteoclastic activity. High levels of TR-AcP are found in patients with increased bone turnover, such as Paget disease of bone, and in immobilized patients, in whom resorption dominates over formation. Low levels of TR-AcP are present in patients with low rates of bone turnover, such as in hypoparathyroidism.[47] Serum concentration of TR-AcP is higher in osteoporotic patients. There is a linear correlation between bone mineral concentration (BMC) and serum TR-AcP in patients with osteoporosis suggesting that it can be used as a useful marker for bone loss[14] caused by increased osteoclastic activity and expected to be normal or low in patients with burnout osteoporosis.

Hydroxyproline Urinary hydroxyproline excretion has been found to be an index of bone resorption. Hydroxyproline in the urine derives from bone collagen breakdown. Hydroxyproline, unfortunately, is found in all collagens, not necessarily just in type 1 found in bone. About 10% of urinary hydroxyproline reflects proteolytic processing of collagen and therefore is indicative that some hydroxyproline is formed during the protolytic processing of procollagen. Overall, however, because hydroxyproline in the urine derives mostly from collagen breakdown, it can be used effectively as an indicator of bone resorption.[70] In the osteolytic phase of Paget's disease of bone there is evidence suggesting that hydroxyproline reflects this resorptive phase of bone turnover better than alkaline phosphatase activity.[68] However, urinary excretion of hydroxyproline has no practical use in monitoring postmenopausal or senile patients with osteoporosis. Hydroxyproline levels are measured in a 24-hour urine collection. The patient should be kept on a low-collagen, gelatine-free diet for 3 days before the test. The normal values range between 15 and 43 mg per day or 0.11 to 0.33 mmol per day.

Glycosylated Hydroxylysine Hydroxylysine is produced during collagen synthesis, like hydroxyproline. However, hydroxylysine can undergo further modification by glycolysation, producing galactosyl hydroxylysine (GH) and glucosylgalactosyl hydroxylysine (GGH).[12] The GH is higher in bone than GGH, which is higher in skin. The GGH:GH ratio for bone is 0.15 and for skin is 1.61. It is possible to differentiate bone collagen turnover from other tissue collagens by measuring the urinary ration of GGH:GH.[67] The normal adult ratio of GGH:GH is greater than 1.0. In patients with high bone turnover, such as in Paget disease, this ratio is less than one.[44] Hydroxylysine glycosides, in contrast to hydroxyproline, are not significantly affected by diet, nor are they metabolized prior to urinary excretion; therefore, they are more bone tissue–specific than hydroxyproline. Urinary hydroxylysine glycosides reflect 50% to 100% of collagen breakdown as opposed to 10% to 25% of collagen breakdown for hydroxyproline.[67] The only problem with this bone marker determination is some difficulty with its measurement.

Pyridinium Cross-links (Pyridinoline) Pyridino-line (Pyr) and dioxypyridinoline (D-Pyr) are cross links of collagen molecules present in the extracellular matrix of bone and cartilage and in insignificant amounts in other connective tissues. Dioxypyridinium appears to be specific for bone tissue. Therefore, the urinary excretion of pyridinium and dioxypyridinium can be considered as a very sensitive marker of bone matrix degradation (resorption). Mean adult normal values for urinary pyridinium are measured at 30.8 ± 8 pmol/µmol creatinine and the normal value of D-Pyr is 4.5 ± 1.4 Pmol/µmol creatinine. In women, menopause induces a twofold to threefold increase of pyridinoline, reflecting an increased bone turnover.[76,77] It is also found to be elevated in primary hyperparathyroidism and patients with Paget disease of bone.[61] These markers of bone breakdown represent the first more sensitive and specific substances of bone resorption. It is hoped they will be a valuable tool in the clinical investigation of metabolic bone diseases.

Radionuclide Bone Imaging

The increased bone formation in osteometabolic bone disease enhances the skeleton's affinity for radiophosphate. Therefore, radiophosphate can be used as a tool to investigate osseous metabolic disorders. The methods used are qualitative nucleography, which is not specific, and quantitative scanning, with measurements such as bone:soft tissue ratios or total body retention of radiophosphate, which may be more informative in certain situations.[63] Currently, the principal radiopharmaceuticals used for bone scanning in metabolic bone disorders are 99m technetium = 99m (^{99m}Tc) phosphate compounds [^{99m}Tc]polyphosphate, [^{99m}Tc]pyrophosphate, and [^{99m}Tc]methyldiphosphonate). The amount used for a bone scan is 15 to 20 millicuries (mCi), with a whole-body does of 0.2 cGy. It has a half-life of 6 hours and emits γ-radiation at 140 KeV of γ-ray, which is ideal for γ-camera scintillation imaging. The rate of radiopharmaceutical concentration in bone is related to bone blood flow and to the bone formation phase of the remodeling process by its extraction efficiency (chemisorption: absorption by chemical and physical processes), therefore, it can be used to assess bone turnover (remodeling) activity. Bone chemisorption depends on the rate of bone remodeling in the reformation phase. Technetium-99m is absorbed by both organic (bone mineral)[9] and inorganic bone elements (immature collagen)[62] of newly formed bone during the process of osteogenesis. In a sense, this radionuclide imaging measures bone mineral deposition and collagen pro-

duction (a function of osteoblastic activity). A fourfold increase of bone blood flow can produce a 33% increase of technitium ^{99m}Tc-dioxypyridinium uptake by bone.[66] Rosenthal and Lisbona[63] are of the opinion that both the collagen and minerals are the binding regions for radiopharmaceuticals in metabolic bone diseases, whereas in other conditions such as neoplastic processes and healing fractures, perhaps the binding region is the mineral component of bone. Bone scanning is a very sensitive but relatively nonspecific tool for assessing bone turnover; therefore, one can expect to see more intense activity in areas of increased bone turnover, such as growth plates and epiphyses in children, metaphyses in adults, and high-turnover osteometabolic bone diseases, etc. A 24-hour whole-body radionuclide study is a simple additional step that can quantify and grade the global severity of bone lesions.[35]

The bone scan in osteomalacia may show focal areas of increased uptake scattered in the shoulders, pelvis, and ribs suggestive of insufficiency microfractures, which are not readily demonstrable by radiography (79% on bone scan, 58% on plain radiographs). There is also increased uptake in the mandible, calvarium, axial skeleton, long bones, and costochondral junctions, with faint renal uptake.[63] In renal osteodystrophy, the distribution of radiophosphate is uniform throughout the skeleton, whereas in hyperparathyroidism, there is an increased uptake in the metaphyses of long bones, and the kidney images are absent. Although the incidence of pulmonary calcification in patients with longstanding uremia is 60% to 70%, this is not reflected in the radiophosphate scan because this calcification is not due to apatite crystal formation, but to amorphous microcrystalized compounds with high magnesium and polyphosphate content that do not absorb radiophosphate.[64]

The bone scan in primary hyperparathyroidism demonstrates focal areas of increased uptake found mainly in the peripheral skeleton, rather than being generalized.[45] Diagnostic accuracy is 50%, as compared to 20% accuracy with radiography.[20] In acromegaly there is increased activity in the calvarium, mandible, costochondral junction, long bones, and axial skeleton caused by the increased remodeling process.[63,64] Senile or postmenopausal osteoporosis does not show increased radiotracer uptake by the bones unless there is a recent fracture, whereas slightly increased radionuclide activity is suggestive of old osteopenic fracture. In symptomatic regional migratory osteoporosis the focal abnormalities are seen with radionuclide imaging even before radiographic changes.[4]

Paget disease in the active osteolytic, mixed, and osteoblast phases demonstrates increased uptake on scintigraphy. However, in the inactive osteosclerotic phase there is normal or decreased radionuclide activity related to a metabolically inactive or burned-out phase.[46] Bone scanning is a very useful technique to monitor response to medical antipagetic therapy because it can detect reactivation of the disease up to 20 months before this is detectable with biochemical tests.[33]

Quantitative Radionuclide Scanning

With this method, the bone:soft tissue ratio is seen to be high in osteomalacia, sometimes dramatically so.[63,64] In renal osteodystrophy the ration is very high, even when qualitative scanning is negative.[38] In primary hyperparathyroidism the ratio is not significant, and in osteoporosis it is quite low. A high bone:soft tissue ratio in any osteopenic condition is suggestive of osteomalacia or renal osteodystrophy.

Perfusion Test

Bone blood flow is a good method of assessing pagetic pain and the response to medical antipagetic treatment of uncomplicated pagetic lesions. Usually, this pain is secondary to hyperemia and bone engorgement. The relief of pain with antipagetic therapy coincides with the restoration of bone flood flow to normal. However, end-stage arthritis, insufficiency fractures, etc. are often superimposed and are added contributing pain factors. Therefore, these factors should be excluded by radiographic and clinical means in order for bone flood flow to be meaningful.[3] Radionuclide imaging cannot detect sarcomatous transformation in Paget disease, except when a photon-deficient pagetic lesion is surrounded by increased uptake. In this case, a bond blood flow study may demonstrate localized hypervascularity of the tumor.

Radiogallium Scanning

Abnormal bone formation can also be related to its nonosseous components, such as cells and marrow. Radiogallium can assess not only an inflammatory (infectious and noninfectious) and neoplastic infiltrate in the bone and bone marrow, but also the cellularity of bone in Paget disease. Gallium uptake is dependent on cellular function. Electron microscopic autoradiography demonstrates a high concentration of the gallium (silver grains) over the nuclei of osteoclasts. The cellular mechanism is unknown, but the association of gallium-67 (^{67}Ga) citrate with the nucleus of osteoclasts is unique and different from tumor cells, in which there is a high association of ^{67}Ga citrate with the lysosome fraction within the cytoplasm. Gallium-67 citrate scintigraphy has been used to indicate the extent of bone involvement in patients with Paget disease of bone and is an excellent marker for monitoring the effects of specific therapy.[53]

In one study, radiogallium has been shown to be more sensitive than radiography.[80] Increased radiophosphate activity in Paget disease is due to increased vascularity and chemiabsorption by hydroxyapatite crystals, whereas radiogallium uptake is more dependent on pagetic bone cellularity.

Hormonal and Biochemical Assessment[19,75]

Parathyroid Hormone

Normal parathyroid hormone ranges vary with the laboratory. The C-terminal ranges between 430 and 1860 pg/ml and N-terminal 230 and 630 pg/ml. The total parathormone range is between 20 and 70 mEq/liter. In humans, lowering of plasma calcium by 1.5 mg/dl results in increased parathyroid hormone (PTH), (up to 400 times). Extracellular magnesium may also stimulate PTH secretion through a negative control system. Plasma contains molecules that react with antibodies to both the amino-terminals (N-terminal) and carboxyl-terminals (C-terminal) of parathyroid hormone. The dominant peptide is the C-terminal, which is more easily detected because of a faster clearance of N-terminal (the biologically active portion). Increased values are seen in hyperparathyroidism, ectopic hyperparathyroidism especially associated with renal carcinoma and bronchogenic carcinoma, secondary hyperparathyroidism caused by chronic renal disease (up to 10 times upper limits), and vitamin D deficiency. Decreased values are seen in sarcoidosis even in the presence of renal failure and in surgical hypoparathyroidism after thyroidectomy.

Calcitonin

Basal normal values for serum calcitonin in men are less than 19 pg/ml and in women less than 14 pg/ml. With calcium infusion (2.4 mg of calcium per kg of body weight), the normal values for men are less than 190 pg/ml and for women less than 130 pg/ml. Increased levels of calcitonin are associated with medullary carcinoma of the thyroid, chronic renal failure, Zollinger-Ellison syndrome, pernicious anemia, hyperplasia of the C cells of the thyroid, carcinoid syndrome, pseudohypoparathyroidism, and, occasionally, cancer of the lungs, breast, or pancreas. Decreased levels of calcitonin are observed in osteoporosis and with old age.

Cyclic Adenosine Monophosphate

Increased levels of urinary cAMP are found in primary hyperparathyroidism in more than 90% of patients. Normal values are 3.3 mg per day in 24-hour urine collection.

Vitamin D

Elevated levels of vitamin D are found in primary hyperparathyroidism, vitamin D intoxication, exposure to sunlight, tumoral calcinosis, idiopathic hypercalciuria, sarcoidosis, normal growing children, and pregnant and lactating females. Decreased levels of vitamin D are found in chronic renal failure,

pseudohypoparathyroidism, vitamin D–dependent rickets, postmenopausal osteoporosis, tumor-induced osteomalacia, biliary and portal cirrhosis, steatorrhea, malabsorption, and dietary osteomalacia. Normal values of 1,25-vitamin D_3 are 25 tp 45 pg/ml, and over the age of 65 years, usually lower by 30%. Tables 20-2 and 20-3 list the normal values of gonadal hormone, thyroid hormone, growth hormone, and cortisol.

Bone Biopsy for Histomorphometry

The most precise measurement of bone mass, osteoid tissue, and rates of bone activity can be obtained by dynamic histomorphometry of full-thickness transiliac bone biopsy.[2] The biopsy should be obtained perpendicular to the iliac table with a trephine with an internal diameter between 8 and 10

Table 20-2
Normal values of gonadal hormones

Hormones	Female		Male	
	Serum	Urine	Serum	Urine
Estradiol	pg/ml	μg/day		
Follicular phase	10-90 pg/ml	0-3 μg/day		
Luteal phase	50-240 pg/ml	4-14 μg/day		
Mid-cycle	100-500 pg/ml	4-10 μg/day		
Postmenopausal	10-30 pg/ml	0-4 μg/day		
	ng/ml	μg/g creatinine	ng/ml	μg/g creatinine
Progesterone			0.12-0.3	0.12 + 0.10
Follicular phase	0.02-0.9 ng/ml	1.4 + 1.1		
Luteal phase	6.0-30 ng/ml	7.7 + 4.6		
Pregnancy	15-200 ng/ml	1.5 + 25.7		
Postmenopausal	0.03-0.3 ng/ml			
	IU/ml	IU/day	IU/ml	IU/ml
Follicle-stimulating hormone (FSH)			4-25	4-18
Premenopause	4-30	3-12		
Midcycle peak	10-90			
Postmenopause	40-250			
	mU/ml	U/day	mU/ml	U/day
Luteinizing hormone (LH)			6-23	13-60
Follicular phase	5-30	7.2-23.5		
Luteal phase	3-40			
Mid-cycle	75-150			
Postmenopause	30-200			
Prolactin	ng/ml		ng/ml	
Follicular phase	< 23		< 20	
Luteal phase	5-40			
	pmol/liter	nmol/liter	pmol/liter	nmol/liter
Testosterone	10.8 ± 2.4	37 ± 10	274.1 ± 79.8	19.85 ± 4.68

Table 20-3
Normal values of thyroid hormone, growth hormone, and cortisol

Hormones	Normal Values	
Thyroid hormone		
Free thyroxine	5.0-12.00 (adult)	
index (FTI)	5.5-10.00 (child)	
Free Triiodothyroxine T_3 (FT$_3$)	230-660 pg/dl	3.54-10.16 pmol/liter
Free thyroxine T_4(FT$_4$)	0.8-2.4 ng/dl	10.3-31.0 pmol/liter
Cortisol (hydrocortisol)	5-23 μg/dl	138-635 μmol/liter
Growth hormone	Men, < 5 ng/ml	< 5 μg/liter
	Women, < 10 ng/ml	< 10 μg/liter

mm. It is feasible to carry out the biopsy under local anesthesia if both the internal and external tables are carefully infiltrated. The site of biopsy should be 1 in. posterior to the anterior superior iliac spine and 1 in. inferior to the iliac crest, in order to avoid penetration of the circumflex iliac artery and the lateral femoral cutaneous nerve. In order to assess the non-mineralized and hypermineralized portions of bone, the section for study should be sliced extra thin (0.5 to 1.0 mm) and not decalcified.

Histomorphometry[2,5,7]

Ocular grids such as the planimeter computer system in the microscope or more sophisticated instrumentation allows one to quantify bone tissues obtained at biopsy by measuring the trabecular bone spicules and the number of osteoclasts, osteocytes, osteoblasts, and osteoid tissue. The number of osteoclasts can be used as an index of bone resorption; the amount of bone mass as an index of osteopenia; and the amount of osteoid as an index of osteomalacia. Approximately 20% of the marrow space is occupied by bone (percent bone volume). Normal bone spicules are smooth and measure approximately 200 μm in width. Only 1% of the bone surface shows active osteoclastic resorption. Approximately 0.2 osteoclast is present per square millimeter of bone, and 5% of bone surface shows scalloping. Normally, 20% of the trabecular bone surfaces (trabecular envelope) are covered by osteoid TOS (trabecular osteoid surface), but less than 2% of bone is made up of osteoid TOV (trabecular osteoid volume). The osteoid thickness does not exceed 10 μm. The mineraliza-

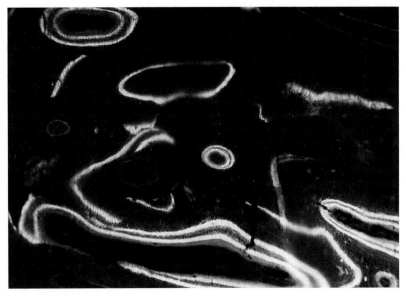

Fig. 20-7
Rate of calcification is calculated by dividing distance between tetracycline labels by interval (in days) between their administration. *(From Hadjipavlou A: Osteoporosis: disease, pathophysiology and treatment,* Contemp Obstet Gynecol 1:6, 1986. Courtesy of C. Anderson, M.D.)

tion front is the basophilic line between surface osteoid and the mineralized bone. Tetracycline is taken up at the mineralizing osteoid, and since tetracycline attaches to the mineralization front and autofluoresces, it can be used as a time-space fluorescent marker to allow measurement of apposition of bone reformation. Therefore, the rate of calcification can be calculated by dividing the distance between the tetracycline labels by the interval in days between their administration (Fig. 2-7). For biopsy study, tetracycline is given orally for 2 to 3 days initially in a dosage of 300 mg twice daily (Declomycin). Since food and dairy products interfere with tetracycline absorption, the tetracycline should be taken at least 1 hour before or 2 hours after meals. Two weeks later this course is repeated and the transiliac bone biopsy is done at least 5 days after completion of the second course. The indices of histomorphometric assessment are summarized in Table 20-4.

Table 20-4
Normal values of histomorphometric assessment*

Terminology	Definition	Volume	Osteoporosis	Osteomalacia	Hyperparathyroidism	Paget disease†
INDICES of BONE MASS						
Trabecular bone volume	Percentage of the medullary cavity occupied by bone	22.5 ± 3.5%	Decrease			Increase
Mean trabecular width	Average width of all trabecular bone spicules	213 ± 65 μm	Decrease	Decrease		
Mean cortical width	Mean thickness of both cortices	909 ± 98 μm	Decrease			Increase
INDICES of OSTEOID						
Trabecular osteoid surface	Percentage of bone surface covered by osteoid	18.9 ± 5.0%		Increase		
Trabecular osteoid volume	Osteoid area expressed as a percentage of trabecular bone area	1.9 ± 0.4%		Increase		
Mean osteoid seam width	Osteoid area divided by the millimeters of bone surface covered by osteoid	9.7 ± 0.4 μm		Increase		
INDICES of RESORPTION						
Trabecular resorptive surface	Percentage of bone surface showing Howship lacunae	5.1 ± 0.6%			Increase	Increase
Osteoclastic resorptive surface	Percentage of bone surface lined by osteoclasts	0.13 ± 0.6%			Increase	Increase
INDICES of MINERALIZATION ACTIVITY						
Calcification rate (apposition)	Distance between middle of all double tetracycline labels divided by number of days between administration of two labels	0.64 ± 0.10 μm/day		Decrease		Increase
Mineralization lag time	Mean osteoid scan width divided by bone formation rate	29.3 ± 3.0 days		Increase		
Bone formation rate	Calcification rate times percentage of trabecular surface labeled	0.44 ± 0.04 μm/day				

*Adapted from Vigorita VJ: *Orthop Clin North Am* 15:613, 1984.
†In Paget disease of bone, these indices may vary according to the phase of the disease activity.

Disturbed Mineralization

All disturbances in mineralization are characterized by an increased amount of osteoid, histologically termed "hyperosteoidosis."[7] Hyperosteoidosis results when the rate of matrix production is greater than the rate of matrix mineralization. There are three basic mechanisms that may lead to hyperosteoidosis: (1) increased rate of bone formation; (2) deficiency of factors necessary for normal mineralization (vitamin D, calcium, etc.), and (3) substances such as aluminum, fluoride, etc. that inhibit osteoid mineralization. The morphology of the interface between bone and osteoid (mineralization front, or osteoid or bone osteoid interface) often provides a clue as to which mechanism is responsible for the hyperosteoidosis. In normal bone formation, the mineralization front is granular, relatively sharp, and parallel to the surface, and the corresponding tetracycline label is thin and well defined.

References

1. Albright F, Reifenstein EC Jr: *The parathyroid gland and metabolic bone disease*, Baltimore, 1948, The Williams and Wilkins Co.
2. Anderson C: *Preparation of calcified tissue for light microscopic histomorphometry*. In Dockos GR, editor: *Method of calcified tissue preparation*, New York, 1984, Elsevier Science Publishers.
3. Boudreau RJ, Lisobona R, Hadjipavlou A: Observations on serial radionuclide blood flow studies in Paget's disease, *J Nucl Med* 24:880, 1983.
4. Bray ST, Partain CL, Teates WB, et al.: The value of bone scan in idiopathic regional migratory osteoporosis, *J Nucl Med* 20:1268, 1979.
5. Bressol C. Courpron P, et al.: *Histomorphometrie des osteopathie endocriniennes: monographie du laboratorie de recherche sur l'histodynamique osseuse*, 1976, Lyon Assn Corp et Med.
6. Brown JP, Delmas PD, Malaval L, et al.: Serum bone GLA-protein: a specific marker for bone fermentation in postmenopause osteoporosis, *Lancet* 1:1901, 1984.
7. Bullough PG, Bansal M, DiCarlo EF: The tissue diagnosis of metabolic bone disease, *Orthop Clin North Am* 21:65, 1990.
8. Chambers TJ: *The regulation of osteoclastic bone resorption*. In Christiansen E, Johansen JS, Riis BJ, Nozhaven A/S, editors: *Osteoporosis; international symposium on osteoporosis*, Denmark 1987, Viborg, Denmark, 1987.
9. Christensen SB, Krogsgaard OW: Localization of ^{99m}Tc-Methylene diphosphate in epipyseal growth plate of rats, *J Nucl Med* 22:237, 1981.
10. Coulton LA, Preston CJ, Couch M, Kanis JA: An evaluation of serum osteocalcin in Paget's disease of bone and its response to diphosphonate treatment, *Athritis Rheum* 31(9):1142, 1988.
11. Courpron P: Bone tissue mechanism underlying osteoporosis, *Orthop Clin North Am* 12:513, 1981.
12. Cunningham LW, Ford JD, Segrest JP: The isolation of identical hydroxylysyl glycosides from hydroxylates of soluble collagen and from human urine, *J Biol Chem* 242:2570, 1967.
13. Davie MW, Worsfold M, Sharp CA: Differential response of serum alkaline phosphatase and serum osteocalcin in Paget's osteosarcoma, *Ann Clin Biochem* 28:194, 1991.
14. De la Piedra C, Torres R, Rapado A, et al.: Serum tartrate-resistant acid phosphatase and bone mineral content in post menopausal osteoporosis, *Calcif Tissue Int* 45(1):58, 1989.
15. Dequeker J: Periosteal and endosteal surface remodeling in pathological conditions, *Invest Radiol* 6:260, 1971.
16. Duncan H, Jarworski FG: *Osteoporosis in practice of medicine*, vol 5, New York, 1979, Harper & Row, p 1.
17. Farley JR, Chestnut CH III, Baylink DJ: Improved method for quantitative determination in serum of alkaline phosphatase of skeletal origin, *Clin Chem* 27:2002, 1981.
18. Fessler LI, Morris NP, Fessler JH: Procollagen: biological scission of amino and carboxyl extension peptides, *Proc Natl Acad Sci U S A* 72:4905, 1975.
19. Fischbach F: *A manual of laboratory diagnostics tests*, Philadelphia, 1992, JB Lippincott Company.
20. Fogelman I, Bessent RG, Beastall GB: Estimation of skeletal involvement in primary hyperparathyroidism, *Ann Intern Med* 92:65, 1980.
21. Frost HM: *Bone remodelling dynamics*, Springfield, IL, 1863, Charles C Thomas.
22. Frost HM: Tetracycline based histological analysis of bone remodeling, *Calcif Tissue Res* 3:211, 1969.
23. Frost HM: Managing the skeletal pain and disability of osteoporosis, *Orthop Clin North Am* 3:561, 1972.
24. Frost HM: The spinal osteoporosis: mechanism of pathogenesis and pathophysiology, *Clin Endocrinol Metab* 2:257, 1973.
25. Frost HM: *Bone remodeling and its relationship to metabolic disease*, Springfield, IL, 1973, Charles C Thomas.
26. Frost HM: *Bone modeling and skeletal modeling errors*, Springfield, IL, Charles C Thomas 1973.
27. Frost HM: The evolution of pathophysiologic knowledge of osteoporosis, *Orthop Clin North Am* 12:475, 1981.
28. Frost HM: Coherence treatment of osteoporosis, *Orthop Clin North Am* 12:649, 1981.
29. Garn SM: The course of bone gain and the phase of bone loss, *Orthop Clin North Am* 3:503, 1972.
30. Gothlin G., Ericson JCE: Fine structural localization of alkaline phosphornonesterase in the fractured callus of the rat, *Isr J Med Sci* 7:488, 1971.
31. Gundberg CM, Markowitz ME, Mizruchi M, et al.: Osteocalcin in human serum: a circadian rhythm, *J Clin Endocrinol Metab* 60:736, 1985.
32. Gutman AB: Serum alkaline phosphatase activity in disease of the skeletal and hepatobiliary system: a consideration of the current status, *Am J Med* 27:875, 1959.
33. Hadjipavlou A, Tsoukas G, Siller T, et al.: Combination drug therapy in treatment of Paget's disease of bone: clinical and metabolic response, *J Bone Joint Surg* 59A:1045, 1977.

34. Hadjipavlou A: Osteoporosis disease: pathophysiogy and treatment, *Contemp Obstet Gynecol* 1:6, 1986.

35. Hadjipavlou A, Lisbona R, Garbuz D, Abitbol JJ: Whole body retention of Tc-99m phosphate in Paget's disease of bone, *Clin Nucl Med* 16(6):435, 1991.

36. Hadjipavlou A, Lander P, Srolovitz H, Enker P: Malignant transformation in Paget's disease of bone, *Cancer* 70:2802, 1992.

37. Hantman DA, Vogel JM, Donaldson CL, et al.: Attempts to prevent disuse osteoporosis by treatment with calcitonin, longitudinal compression and supplementary calcium and phosphate, *J Clin Endocrinol Metab* 36:845, 1973.

38. Holmes W: Qualification of skeletal Tc99M-labeled phosphates to detect metabolic bone disease, *J Nucl Med* 19:330, 1978.

39. Jarworski ZKG: *Three-dimensional view of the gross and microscopic structure of adult human bone*. In Jarworski ZFG, Klosevych S, Cameron E, editors: *Bone morphometry*, Ottawa, 18 = 976, University of Ottawa Press, p 3.

40. Jarworski ZKG: Physiology and pathophysiology of bone remodeling: cellular basis of bone structure in health and in osteoporosis, *Orthop Clin North Am* 12:485, 1981.

41. Jett SWK, Frost HM: Tetracycline based histological measurement of cortical endosteal bone formation in normal and osteoporotic rib, Henry Ford Hosp, editor, *Med Bull* 15:325, 1967.

42. Johnson LC: *Morphological analysis in pathology*. In *Bone biodynamics*, Boston, 1964, Little, Brown and Company, p 543.

43. Kraenzlin ME, Taylor AK, Baylink DJ: *Biochemical markers for bone formation and bone resorption*. In Lindh E, Thorell JI, editors: *Clinical impact of bone and connective tissue markers*, Pharmacia diagnostics clinical symposia 1, New York, 1989, Academic Press.

44. Krane SM, Kantrowitz FG, Byrne M., et al.: Urinary excretion of hydroxylysine and its glycosides: an index of collagen degradation, *J Clin Invest* 59:814, 1977.

45. Krushnamurthy GT, Brockman AS, Blahd WH: Technetium 99m pyrophosphate pharmacokinetics and bone image changes in parathyroid disease, *J Nucl Med* 8:236, 1977.

46. Lander P, Hadjipavlou A: A dynamic classification of Paget's disease, *J Bone Joint Surg* 68B:431, 1986.

47. Lau WKW, Onishi T., Wergedal JE, et al.: Characterization of and assay for human serum tartrate-resistant acid phosphatase activity: a potential assay to assess bone resorption, *Clin Chem* 33:458, 1987.

48. Lian JB, Friedman PA: The vitamin k-dependant synthesis of gamma-carboxyglutamic acid by bone microsomes, *J Biol Chem* 253:6623, 1978.

49. Lum G, Catrou P, Liuzza G, Kokatnur M: Clinical assessment of electrophoretic separation of alkaline phosphatase isoenzymes, *Am J Clin Pathol* 80:682, 1983.

50. Melsen F., Mosekilde L: Morphometric and dynamic studies of bone changes in hyperthyroidism, *Acta Pathol Microbiol Scand* 85:141, 1977.

51. Merry AH, Harwood R, Wooley DE, et al.: Identification and partial characterization of non-collagenous amino- and carboxyl-terminal extension peptides of cartilage procollagen, *Biochem Biophys Res Commun* 71:83, 1976.

52. Meunier PJ, Bianchi GCS, et al.: Bony manifestations of thyrotoxicosis, *Orthop Clin North Am* 3:754, 1972.

53. Mills BG, Masuoka LS, Graham CCJ, Singer FR, Waxman AD: Gallium-67 citrate localization in osteoclast nuclei of Paget's disease of bone, *J Nucl Med* 24(6):1083, 1988.

54. Nordin BEC, Peacock M, Aoro J, et al.: Osteoporosis and osteomalacia, *Clin Endocrinol Metab* 9:177, 1980.

55. Parfitt AM: Quantum concept of bone remodeling and turnover: implications for the pathogenesis of osteoporosis, *Calcif Tissue Int* 28:1, 1979.

56. Pietschann P, Resch H, Woluszczuk W, et al.: A circadian rhythm of serum osteocalcin levels in postmenopausal osteoporosis, *Eur J Clin Invest* 20(3):310, 1990.

57. Posen S, Granstein HS: Turnover rate of skeletal alkaline phospatase in humans, *Clin Chem* 26:153, 1982.

58. Poser JW, Esch FS, Ling NC, Price PA: Isolation and sequence of the vitamin K-dependent protein from human bone, *J Biol Chem* 255:8685, 1980.

59. Price PA, Parthemore JG, Deftos CT: New biochemical marker for bone metabolism, *J Clin Invest* 66:878, 1980.

60. Prockop DJ, Kivirikko KI: Heritable diseases of collagen, *N Engl J Med* 311:376, 1981.

61. Robins SP: Cross-linking of collagen, *Biochem J* 25:167, 1983.

62. Rosenthal L, Kaye M: Observation on the mechanism of ^{99m}Tc-labeled phosphate complex uptake in metabolic disease, *Semin Nucl Med* 6:59, 1976.

63. Rosenthal L, Lisbona R: *Skeletal imaging*, Norwalk, CT, 1984, Appelton-Century-Crofts.

64. Rosenthal L, Lisbona R: *Role of radionuclide imaging in benign bone and joint disease of orthopaedic interest*. In Freeman LM, Weissmann HS, editors: *Nuclear medicine annual* 1980, New York, 1980, Raven Press.

65. Rowland RE: *Resorption and bone physiology*. In Frost HM, editor: *Bone biodynamics*, Boston, 1964, Little, Brown & Co., p 335.

66. Sagar VV, Piccone JM, Charkes ND: Studies of skeletal tracer kinetics III. Tc99m (SN) methylenediphosphonate uptake in canine tibia as a function of blood flow, *J Nucl Med* 20:1257, 1979.

67. Segrest JP, Cunningham LW: Variations in human urinary hydroxylysyl glycoside levels and their relationship to collagen metabolism, *J Clin Invest* 49:1497, 1970.

68. Shapiro JR: *Paget's disease: osteitis deformans. Bone fragility in orthopedics and medicine.* Abstracts of the 12th annual applied bone sciences course, University of Ottawa, Mary 1985.

69. Simon LS, Krane SM, Woztman PD, et al.:Serum levels of the I and III procollagen fragments in Paget's disease of bone, *J Clin Endocrinol Metab* 58:110, 1984.

70. Sjoerdsma A, Udenfriend S, Keiser H, et al.: Hydroxyproline and collagen metabolism: clinical implication, *Ann Intern Med* 63:672, 1965.

71. Smith RW Jr, Walker RR: Femoral expansion in aging women: implications for osteoporosis and fracture, *Science* 145:156, 1964.

72. Steendijk R: Metabolic Bone disease in children, *Clin Orthop Relat Res* 77:247, 1971.

73. Taylor AK, Linkhart SG, Mohan S, Baylink DJ: Development of a new radioimmunoassay for human osteocalcin: evidence for a mid-molecule epitope, *Metabolism* 37:872, 1988.

74. Taylor AK, Linkhart S., Mohan S, et al.: Multiple osteocalcin fragments in human urine and serum as detected by a mid molecule osteocalcin radioimmunoassay, *J Clin Endocrinal Metab* 70(2):467, 1990.

75. Tietz NW: *Clinical guide to laboratory tests,* Philadelphia, 1983, WB Saunders Company.

76. Uebelhart D, Gineyts E, Chapuy MC, Delmas PD: Urinary excretion of pyridinium cross links: a new marker of bone resorption in metabolic bone disease, *Bone Miner* 8:87, 1990.

77. Ueberhart D, Sclemmer A, Johansen JS, et al.: Effect of menopause and hormone replacement therapy on the urinary excretion of pyridium cross links, *Clin Endocrinol Metab* 72(2):367, 1991.

78. Vellenga CJ, Pouwels EHJ, Bijvoet OLM, et al.: Scintigraphic aspects of the recurrence of treated Paget's disease of bone, *J Nucl Med* 22:510, 1981.

79. Vigorita VJ: The tissue pathologic features of metabolic bone disease, *Orthop Clin North Am* 15:613, 1984.

80. Waxman AD, McKee D, Siemsen JE, et al.: Gallium scanning in Paget's disease of bone: effect of calcitonin, *AJR Am J Roentgenol* 134:303, 1980.

81. Woodard HQ: Long term studies of blood chemistry in Paget's disease of bone, *Cancer* 12:1226, 1959.

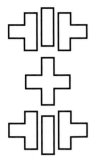

PART IV

Diagnostic and Therapeutic Blocks

Chapter 21

Diagnostic Blocks of Spinal Synovial Joints

Nikolai Bogduk
Charles Aprill
Richard Derby

Various techniques have been developed whereby the zygapophysial joints and other synovial joints of the vertebral column can be anesthetized. In the management of spinal pain these procedures test the diagnostic hypothesis that one or more of the synovial joints in a particular region is the source of the patient's pain. The rationale of these procedures is that if anesthetising a putatively painful joint relieves the patient's pain then that joint can be deemed the source of pain, whereupon treatment can be selectively and exclusively directed at that joint. Moreover, the several diagnostic techniques can be adapted to provide means of treating the symptomatic joint.

Historical Background

Zygapophysial joint blocks were developed first in the context of low-back pain. Claims and beliefs that low-back pain and referred pain could be related to the lumbar zygapophysial joints were raised throughout the first half of the twentieth century. Some early authorities believed that "arthritis" was a common cause of back pain although the pain was "due to strains and not the arthritis per se."[74] Others proclaimed that "an arthritic involvement of the lumbosacral facets may alone cause symptoms of back pain and sciatica,"[6] and treatment at that time was posterior arthrodesis, which reported worked well.[6]

Lumbar Zygapophysial Joint Blocks

The first formal declaration that the lumbar zygapophysial joints in general could be a source of back pain was published by Ghormley,[57] who introduced the oblique view of the lumbar spine to diagnose the problem. This concept was subsequently endorsed by investigators who studied the morphology of the lumbar zygapophysial joints.[7]

The immediate evolution of the concept of lumbar zygapophysial joint pain was hampered by two factors: the preoccupation after 1934 with herniated lumbar intervertebral disc as the leading cause of back pain and sciatica, and the lack of valid techniques whereby zygapophysial joint pain might be diagnosed. Disc herniation consumed virtually all clinical and experimental research interest for some 40 years. Because conventional wisdom maintained that disc disorders were the leading cause of lumbar spine pain problems there was little impetus to pursue alternative models. However, the failure of disc-oriented surgery to deal adequately or comprehensively with all forms of back pain prompted a reawakening of interest in zygapophysial joint pain

and fostered the emergence of two distinct, often competing, approaches to its diagnosis. One approach focused on the nerves to the joints and was distinctly "neurosurgical" in nature; the other focused on the joints themselves and was favored by orthopedic surgeons and radiologists.

Neurosurgical Approach

In the early 1970s, Rees[118,119] proclaimed that the lumbar zygapophysial joints could be a source of back pain, and described an operative technique whereby the presumedly painful joints could allegedly be denervated percutaneously using a scalpel. This inspired Shealy[126-129] to develop an alternative approach in which the joints could be denervated percutaneously using radiofrequency electrodes. Meanwhile, the procedure of Rees was found to be anatomically inaccurate[23,75]; therefore, the results claimed for it could not be attributed to denervation of the lumbar zygapophysial joints.[12,23] In due course, the Shealy procedure similarly was found to be anatomically inaccurate.[19,20] Nevertheless, by then the concept of lumbar zygapophysial joint pain was established in the minds of many clinicians,* but there was a need to refine the accuracy of diagnostic techniques for this condition.

The leading indication for denervating a lumbar zygapophysial joint was declared to be complete relief of pain following anesthetisation of the nerves that supply the joint.[20] The articular branches of lumbar zygapophysial joints, described originally by Pedersen et al.,[111] were found to be too small to serve as explicit target points either for diagnostic blocks or for percutaneous denervation, but the parent trunks of the articular branches—the medial branches of the lumbar dorsal rami—proved eminently suitable for these purposes.[19,20] The medial branches of the lumbar dorsal rami were found to pursue a constant course in relation to bone.[27] The L1-L4 medial branches regularly cross the junction of the root of the transverse process and the root of the superior articular process; the L5 medial branch crosses the ala of the sacrum adjacent to the root of the S1 superior articular process.[16,27] These bony sites could be recognized on fluoroscopy and became the standard target points for local anesthetic blocks of these nerves.[20] By anesthetizing each of the two medial branches that supply a given lumbar zygapophysial joint, that joint could be anesthetized.

*References 9, 30, 31, 39, 43, 47, 51 to 53, 55, 63, 68, 86, 89, 90 to 92, 96 to 99, 103, 105, 107 to 110, 121, 125, 134, 136, 140, and 142.

If complete relief of pain ensued, percutaneous radiofrequency neurotomy of the same nerves could be entertained as a form of treatment.

Arthrologic Approach

Orthopedic surgeons and radiologists were not convinced on the specificity of lumbar medial branch blocks as a diagnostic technique for lumbar zygapophysial joint pain; they developed means of injecting the joints directly. In a landmark study, Mooney and Robertson[101] demonstrated that low-back pain and referred pain could be induced in normal volunteers by injecting hypertonic saline into the lower lumbar zygapophysial joints. Patients with a similar quality and distribution of pain were relieved of their pain when local anesthetic was injected into one or the other of the lower lumbar zygapophysial joints.[101] The aforementioned studies in normal volunteers elaborated earlier observations that had been made by Hirsch et al.[67] and were subsequently replicated by McCall et al.,[94] finally eliminating any remaining skepticism that lumbar zygapophysial joints could not be a source of low-back pain.

Prompted by the studies of Mooney and Robertson[101] radiologists and others developed arthrography of the lumbar zygapophysial joints.* There may have been an expectation that arthrography could reveal morphologic features that were indicative of the joint being abnormal and symptomatic, but no such correlation has ever emerged. Rather, arthrography has become a means of confirming that needles have been inserted accurately into the target joint and that anything injected remains selectively within the joint. Accurate intraarticular placement of a needle allows it to be used to inject local anesthetic for diagnostic purposes or other agents such as corticosteroids for therapeutic purposes.

Cervical Zygapophysial Joint Blocks

The advent of cervical zygapophysial joint blocks lagged behind that of lumbar zygapophysial joint blocks largely because fewer research units addressed neck pain as opposed to low-back pain and because of a seemingly natural reluctance to explore placing needles and injecting substances so close to the cervical spinal cord.

Nevertheless, Sluijter and Koetsveld-Baart[135] devised a technique for blocking the cervical dorsal rami near their origin and described a percutaneous

---

*References 34 to 37, 40, 41, 50, 58, 77, 82, 85, 87, 100, 102, 104, 112, 115, and 116.

radiofrequency technique to coagulate these nerves. Their procedure was later improved by the use of more sophisticated electrodes[134,136] and was adopted by others.[64,65]

Bogduk and Marsland[22] promulgated a neurosurgical approach to cervical zygapophysial joint blocks by devising cervical medial branch blocks, focusing on nerves distal to the target sites used by Sluijter and Koetsveld-Baart.[135] As for the lumbar spine, typical cervical zygapophysial joints could be anesthetized by anesthetizing each of the two medial branches of the cervical dorsal rami that furnished articular branches to the target joint.[15] The C2-C3 zygapophysial joint is innervated by the third occipital nerve and this joint can be anaesthetized by blocking the third occipital nerve.[21]

Okada[106] introduced intraarticular cervical zygapophysial joint blocks using a lateral approach. Dory[42] described a posterior approach based on a pillar view of the cervical zygapophysial joints, and a similar approach was used by Wedel and Wilson[143]; others have followed suit.[44,69,123] Dory[42] advocated that reproduction of pain on injection of contrast medium into the target joint was the diagnostic criterion for cervical zygapophysial joint pain, whereupon corticosteroids could summarily be injected as a form of treatment. Others preferred mixing the corticosteroids with local anesthetic to render the injection less painful.[44,69,143]

Interestingly, however, a sense of diagnosis did not prevail in the early literature on cervical zygapophysial joint pain. Injections of local anesthetic alone to determine whether or not the joint was symptomatic were not advocated; rather, the joints were treated presumptively or on the basis of pain provocation, the diagnosis being justified only retrospectively when the patients reported relief concordant with the therapeutic effect of the steroid.

As with lumbar zygapophysial joint pain, skepticism prevailed concerning the capability of cervical zygapophysial joints to cause pain, but Dwyer et al.[46] demonstrated that in normal volunteers, distention of the cervical zygapophysial joints with contrast medium could induce neck pain and referred pain, with a pattern of distribution of the referred pain being characteristic of the segmental location of the stimulated joint.[5]

Lateral Atlantoaxial Joint Blocks

The lateral atlantoaxial joints have attracted attention by way of two conceptually independent routes. From one perspective, although technically they are not zygapophysial joints, the lateral atlantoaxial joints are the next synovial joints above the series of zygapophysial joints. In this context, McCormick[95] and Bogduk[17] described means of entering the lateral atlantoaxial joint for the purpose of injecting local anesthetic and/or corticosteroid. The lateral atlantoaxial joint does not lend itself to a neurosurgical approach because, unlike the cervical zygapophysial joints, this joint is not supplied by medial branches of the cervical dorsal rami but receives articular branches from the C2 ventral ramus.[14] Before the advent of intraarticular lateral atlantoaxial joint blocks, all that could be done was to block the C2 ganglion,[14] a procedure still used by neurologists and neurosurgeons in the diagnosis of cervicogenic headache,[66,71,93,114] but one that is not particularly selective. When positive, C2 ganglion blocks simply reveal the neurologic segment that mediates the patient's pain. The lateral atlantoaxial joint is but one of several structures innervated by the C2 nerve, and intraarticular blocks are the only way to confirm that the lateral atlantoaxial joint itself is the actual source of pain.

Others have been drawn to the lateral atlantoaxial joint in the pursuit of the source of pain in so-called occipital neuralgia. Several authorities have been disenchanted with a previously traditional concept that occipital pain was indicative of entrapment of the greater occipital nerve.[13,18,45,48,76,130] Others have been critical of the failure to relieve this pain by greater occipital neurectomy.[144] From a theoretical perspective, several authors have proposed that occipital pain could stem from the upper cervical synovial joints.* Ehni and Benner[48] pursued this notion and found that "occipital neuralgia" could be relieved by periarticular blocks of arthritic, lateral atlantoaxial joints, thereby converging to a common site with those who developed intraarticular blocks of this joint.

A logical extension of these developments is whether the atlanto-occipital joints might be a source of pain. However, no blocks have yet formally been described for this joint.

Thoracic Zygapophysial Joint Blocks

The thoracic zygapophysial joints have received little attention, largely because virtually no research units have sought properly to study idiopathic complaints of thoracic pain and because the orientation of thoracic zygapophysial joints does not lend them to either posterior or lateral approaches for intraarticular injections, as have been used for either the

*References 18, 29, 45, 76, 138, and 145.

lumbar or cervical spine. A neurosurgical approach has not been explored for lack of reliable data on the exact course of the medial branches of the thoracic dorsal rami and the pattern of innervation of the thoracic zygapophysial joints.[26] Nevertheless, Wilson[146] described a technique for entering the thoracic zygapophysial joints and reported relief of thoracic posterior spinal pain in a small series of patients following injection of local anesthetic and corticosteroids into these joints.

Sacroiliac Joint Blocks

The popularity of beliefs in whether the sacroiliac joints might be a source of back pain has waxed and waned throughout the twentieth century, but controversies have been fought only on the basis of pronouncement and denial; not on the basis of objective evidence. Among rheumatologists, there has been no fundamental controversy with regard to overtly inflammatory sacroiliac arthropathy, but objective evidence has been lacking with regard to so-called and alleged mechanical disorders of the sacroiliac joint.

In this regard, the sacroiliac joint can be related to the zygapophysial joints; it is a synovial joint, alleged by some to be a source of back pain or referred pain, but one for which no imaging technique has been able to reveal features diagnostic of the joint being symptomatic in the absence of inflammatory changes. Consequently, it has attracted attention as a joint that may be blocked in the pursuit of a diagnosis of low-back pain, but although techniques of blocking the sacroiliac joint are known to and used by the present authors, no formal study has yet appeared in the literature. Sacroiliac joint blocks are the most recent development in the field of precision diagnosis of spinal pain.

Techniques

Zygapophysial joints can be anesthetized by intraarticular blocks or by blocking their nerve supply. The atlantoaxial and the sacroiliac joints are amenable only to intraarticular blocks. Blocks of the sacral dorsal rami have, in the past been advocated to anesthetize the sacroiliac joint, but these nerves supply only the posterior sacroiliac ligament and the interosseous sacroiliac ligament; the joint itself receives a major supply anteriorly from the obturator nerve, superior gluteal nerve and the lumbosacral trunk,[113] which are inaccessible for the purposes of selective nerve blocks.

Would-be operators are advised to familiarize themselves with the details of anatomy that underlie the various techniques described below and to recognize that although analogous, the anatomy of the zygapophysial joints and their nerve supply is not identical in the cervical, lumbar, and thoracic regions. Details of the pertinent anatomy are to be found in various journal articles[14-16,27] and textbooks.[17,25,26]

Intraarticular Lumbar Zygapophysial Joint Blocks

Intraarticular blocks of the lumbar zygapophysial joints are performed under an image intensifier with the patient initially lying prone. The cavity of the target joint needs to be visualized. On the average, upper lumbar zygapophysial joints are oriented in the sagittal plane[25]; therefore, their cavities are usually quite evident on posteroanterior views of a prone patient. Lower lumbar zygapophysial joints and particularly the lumbosacral zygapophysial joints are obliquely oriented on the averaged at about 45 degrees to the sagittal plane, so to visualize them either the patient has to be rotated appropriately and supported in an oblique, prone position, or if C-arm fluoroscopy is being used, the x-ray beam is tilted to bring the joint space into view.

The skin over the target joint is prepared as for an aseptic procedure, and a puncture point is selected over the joint space as seen on fluoroscopy. Some operators may elect to anesthetize the puncture point with an intradermal injection of local anesthetic; others omit this step on the grounds that piercing the skin with a procedure needle is no more harrowing than the intradermal injection designed to render the eventual puncture pain-free.

A 22 or 25 gauge, 90 mm (3.5 in.) spinal needle is used to gain access to the target joint. Needles of wider gauge offer the advantage that they are more readily directed to the target joint through the overlying back muscles, but difficulties may be encountered in penetrating the joint, particularly if it is narrow. Finer needles enter the joint more easily but are apt to stray during penetration of the back muscles. If difficulties are anticipated or encountered using a fine needle, a double-needle technique can be used in which a large gauge needle is introduced into the target joint and a finer needle is passed through the larger needle to penetrate the joint.

The needle is inserted through the puncture point and is directed under periodic, image-intensifier guidance to the back of the target joint. It is worthwhile to rest the needle tip on either the inferior or superior articular process of the joint, for this es-tablishes the critical depth of insertion. Subsequently, the needle needs only to be readjusted slightly to enter the joint space and needs to be inserted just beyond the initial depth.

The primary target site for entering the joint is at the midpoint of the joint cavity. The needle is aimed at this site and the operator then relies on feel to determine if the needle enters the joint. The appropriate feel is one of a loss of resistance, changing from that of firm bone to softer tissue (either the joint capsule or its cartilage), with the needle penetrating a few millimeters deeper than the original depth of the articular processes (Fig. 21-1).

Authorities differ as to exactly how far the needle should be inserted. Penetrating as far as the center of the joint space ensures that the joint has been entered, but this may be excessive, and it may become difficult to inject substances if the needle becomes embedded in articular cartilage. It is sufficient otherwise to have the needle simply penetrate the capsule, entering the joint space deep through the capsule but still peripheral to the margins of the articular cartilages.

Once the needle is believed to be inside the joint space, confirmation is achieved by the injection of a minimal quantity (< 0.3 ml) of contrast medium using a small syringe (2 to 5 ml) to minimize injection pressure. If the needle is inside the joint, an arthrogram will be achieved, smoothly outlining the perimeter of the joint space (Fig. 21-2). On oblique views, a dumbbell-shape is characteristic, in which a

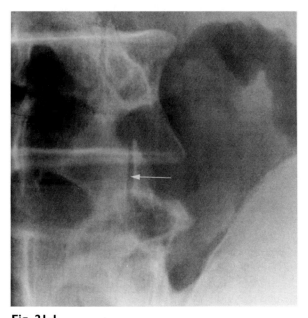

Fig. 21-1

Oblique view of a right L4-L5 zygapophysial joint with the target point for intraarticular injection indicated by *arrow*.

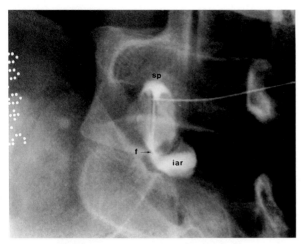

A

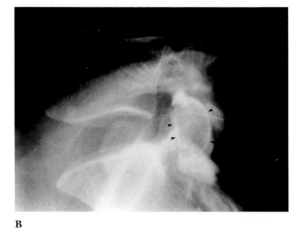

B

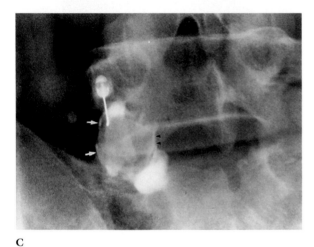

C

Fig. 21-2
A, oblique; **B,** lateral; and **C,** posterior views of L5-S1 zygapophysial joint after injection of contrast medium. In *A,* joint cavity is filled and contrast medium fills superior, subcapsular pockets (*sp*), but inferiorly it escapes through capsular foramen (f) to fill extracapsular, inferior articular recess (*iar*). In *B* and *C,* ventral, dorsal, medial, and lateral perimeters of the joint capsule (***arrowheads***) are outlined by contrast medium.

slender tract of contrast medium outlines the inter-cartilaginous joint space and connects the wider collections of contrast medium in the superior and inferior subcapsular pockets. In lateral views, the circular or discoid silhouette of the joint space is outlined (see Fig. 21-2).

If the injection has not been made into the joint cavity, contrast medium will be seen to spread beyond the vicinity of the joint in a radiating pattern indicative of extension between the fibers of the multifidus muscle.

It is quite normal for contrast medium to spread out of the joint cavity through normal capsular foramina into the extracapsular, superior, and inferior joint recesses (Fig. 21-3). Such extension is not a sign of "extravasation" or joint rupture. Its characteristics are that it lacks a radiating pattern indicative of intramuscular spread, and instead is reminiscent of a lobulated, smooth-edged collection consistent with having outlined the fat deposits in the inferior and superior articular recesses.[81]

Once intraarticular placement has been verified, the

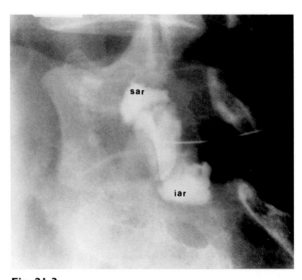

Fig. 21-3
Oblique view of L5-S1 zygapophysial arthrogram showing more extensive escape of contrast medium than in Fig. 21-2, into the superior (*sar*) and inferior (*iar*) articular recesses.

appropriate agent can be injected. This may be local anesthetic, if the procedure is to be a diagnostic block, or corticosteroids, alone or mixed with local anesthetic if the procedure is intended to be therapeutic. To ensure that the joint is not ruptured, not more than 1.0 ml of any agent should be injected. Following injection the needle is summarily withdrawn.

If difficulties are encountered in entering the joint at its midpoint, the needle may be redirected to either the superior or inferior subcapsular pockets. At the superior and inferior poles of the joint, the capsule is lax, leaving subcapsular pockets,[81] which may be entered with the needle without passing between the articular cartilages. The needle should be readjusted to the upper or lower edge of the joint, still contacting the bone of the articular processes, and then finally readjusted so that it passes tangential to the joint margin. It should penetrate just enough to pierce the capsule. Deeper penetration risks having the needle spear the subcapsular pocket and reemerge from the joint ventral to the joint cavity. Once capsule penetration is thought to have occurred, an injection of contrast medium must be made to confirm accurate location. If an arthrogram is achieved, the needle lies correctly in the joint space and may be used to inject diagnostic or therapeutic agents.

Lumbar Medial Branch Blocks

Lumbar medial branch blocks are performed under aseptic conditions and image-intensifier guidance, with the patient lying prone. For the L1-L4 medial branches the target points lie on the dorsal surface of the transverse process immediately below its superior border at its root, where it joins the superior articular process.[17,20] In numerical terms, the L4 medial branch crosses the L5 transverse process; the L3 medial branch crosses the L4 transverse process, and so on (Fig. 21-4). The target point for the L5 medial branch lies at the top of the ala of the sacrum at its junction with the S1 superior articular process.[17,20]

A puncture point on the skin is selected above and lateral to the desired target point, usually above the tip of the target transverse process. This ensures that the needle will be directed forward but medially and slightly caudally onto the target point. The medial inclination allows the needle to pass ventrally to enlarged mammillary processes, which may overhang the target point. The caudad inclination ensures that the injectate is delivered distally onto the target nerve; if the needle is introduced along a rostrad course, the injectate may track toward a spinal nerve and compromise the selectivity of the block.

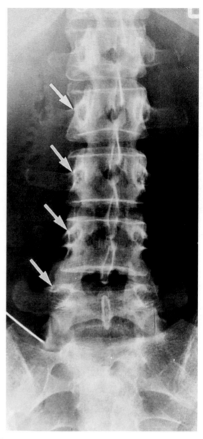

Fig. 21-4
Radiogram of lumbar spine showing target points for lumbar medial branch blocks. Needle is seen in position on the ala of sacrum, in position to block L5 medial branch.

A 22 or 25 gauge, 90 mm (3.5 in.) spinal needle may be used to perform the block. Larger needles are easier to maneuver through the back muscles; finer needles require experience and dexterity to prevent them from diverting from their intended course, but are better tolerated by patients. The needle is introduced through the puncture point and is slowly directed toward the target point using periodic screening to maintain the course. The needle should be directed first to contact the back of the root of the transverse process; this prevents the needle from being inserted too deeply through the intertransverse space, and keeps the needle tip clear of the ventral ramus and spinal nerve. Once located on the back of the transverse process the needle can be readjusted toward the precise target point. Correct location is verified radiographically.

The final phase of introducing a needle onto a lumbar, medial branch can be rendered more expeditious by obtaining an oblique view of the target point. The needle is directed at the anterior end of the "neck," or base, of the superior articular process just above its junction with the transverse process (Fig. 21-5). Once the needle is in correct, final position, local anesthetic may be injected to infiltrate the nerve. A volume of 0.5 ml is sufficient. Extra volume simply spreads beyond the target point. The injection must be made slowly (1.5 ml per minute); more rapid injection simply forces the injectate away from the target point.

Intraarticular Cervical Zygapophysial Joint Blocks

The typical cervical zygapophysial joints (C3-C4 to C6-C7) can be entered using either a posterior or a lateral approach. A posterior approach is impractical for the C7-T1 joint because of its steep slope, and only a lateral approach pertains. The cavity of the C2-C3 zygapophysial joint frequently slopes caudally and medially. Therefore, a lateral approach may be difficult, and a specific oblique approach pertains.

Posterior Intraarticular Blocks

The posterior approach for cervical intraarticular blocks can be performed with the patient in a prone position, or if required, in a sitting position. It involves introducing a 22 or a 25 gauge needle into the target joint from behind along an oblique trajectory that coincides with the plane of the joint. The puncture point lies two or more segments below the target joint and can be selected by project-

ing the plane of the joint as seen in lateral radiographs to a point posteriorly, where it intersects the skin along a parasagittal plane through the midpoint of the target joint.

The needle is passed through the skin and directed upward and ventrally through the posterior neck muscles until it strikes the back of the target joint. It can then be readjusted until it enters the joint cavity. This route of introduction requires repeated, posteroanterior and lateral screening to ensure the needle stays son course. It should not deflect laterally away from joint and especially not medially toward the epidural space and spinal cord.

Repeated posteroanterior screening is used to guide the insertion until the needle strikes the back of the target joint at its midpoint. The needle will usually abut the lip of the superior or interior articular facet. Further adjustment can then be made under lateral screening to guide the needle into the joint, checking finally with posteroanterior screening to ensure that the needle has not strayed medially or laterally.

Once located in the joint the needle can be used to inject contrast medium to obtain an arthrogram and verify accurate placement and then to inject local anesthetic and/or corticosteroid for diagnostic and therapeutic purposes. The capacity of the joint can be gauged from the injection of the contrast medium and is typically less than 1 ml. The joint's capacity should be respected during the injection of local anesthetic of steroid to prevent rupture of the

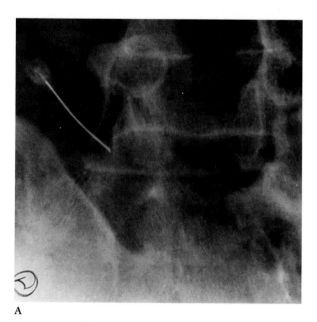

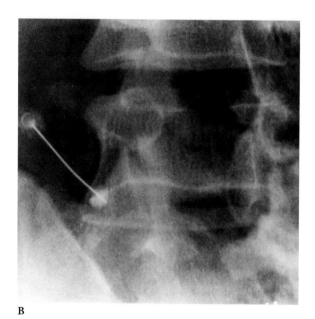

A   B

Fig. 21-5

A, Oblique view of needle in correct position to block L4 medial branch as it crosses root of L5 transverse process at its junction with root of L5 superior articular process. **B,** Same needle after injection of 0.5 ml of contrast medium to demonstrate how injectate remains localized around target nerve.

joint capsule and unwanted spread of the agent into surrounding tissues.

The posterior approach can be streamlined if the x-ray beam can be tilted to obtain a pillar view of the target joint. Once the joint cavity is visualized a needle can be inserted directly in line with the cavity and directed promptly toward its midpoint (Fig. 21-6). Lateral screening is nevertheless still required to check the depth of penetration.

The posterior intraarticular block is a cumbersome procedure because it requires repeated posteroanterior and lateral screening to guide the needle along its course. This can be overcome somewhat by using pillar views, but even then the procedure involves a long course for the needle, during which it is apt to stray. This is particularly so if 25 gauge needles are used. While these needles are easier to introduce into narrow joint spaces, they deflect more readily when passing through the neck muscles. This is less of a problem if 22 gauge needles are used, but then penetration of the joint could become a problem if the joint space is narrow. Either way the procedure still requires repeated screening with the image intensifier to ensure a safe course of the needle until it enters the joint cavity. However, the risks of morbidity are low.

Posteriorly, the needle penetrates only the skin and posterior neck muscles, with the deep cervical artery being the only structure at risk of inadvertent puncture en route, but this poses no risk of morbidity because this vessel supplies no major structures. If the

needle is inserted too deeply or overzealously, it could penetrate the anterior joint capsule. With careful technique and proper screening this should not occur, but the risk is that the vertebral artery or ventral ramus of the spinal nerve lying in front of the joint may be pierced. Since neither structure should be inadvertently injected with contrast medium or local anesthetic, no injection should be made without checking the position of the needle in a lateral view. Similarly, if the needle is overzealously inserted, without checking its course in posteroanterior views, it could deflect into the epidural space or spinal cord. Repeated posteroanterior screening is therefore essential to guard against this possibility.

Lateral Intraarticular Blocks

The lateral approach to the cervical zygapophysial joints is performed with the patient lying on his/her side. The target joint is identified on lateral screening of the neck and a needle is introduced through the skin over the midpoint of the joint. It is advanced deeply, aiming to strike the bone of either the superior or inferior articular process. This provides the operator with a sense of the correct depth of insertion and prevents overinsertion.

A perceptual problem that arises stems from the fact that lateral views demonstrate both joints at any given segment. The object is to identify the image of the target joint, which lies uppermost in the patient. This is achieved immediately after preliminary

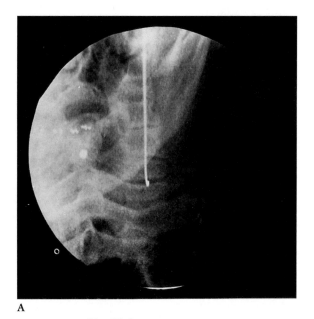

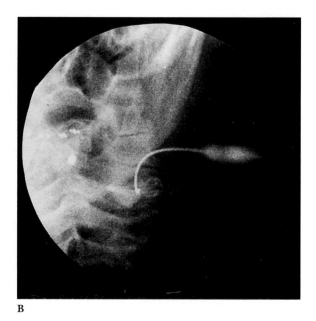

A   B

Fig. 21-6

Pillar view of posterior approach for intraarticular injection into C5-C6 zygapophysial joint. **A,** Before injection of contrast medium. **B,** After contrast medium.

insertion of the needle once it has struck bone. The patient can then be gently rolled ventrally or dorsally, or, if possible, the x-ray beam can be tilted along the transverse plane of the patient. Under these circumstances the inserted needle will move in the same direction as the image of the joint against which it lies, while the opposite joint exhibits a contrary motion. Once the image of the target joint is identified, the needle can be readjusted as required until its tip lies over the cavity of the target joint.

The capsule of the joint is then gently probed until the needle is felt to pierce the capsule and to enter the joint space. Only minimal penetration is required, and this is indicated to the operator by the loss of resistance as the needle pierces the capsule. If desired, insertion can be checked by posteroanterior screening if the x-ray beam can be rotated appropriately, but otherwise insertion can be verified by the presumptive injection of 0.3 ml of contrast medium or less to obtain an arthrogram (Fig. 21-7). Discrete filling of the joint cavity confirms accurate entry into the joint. If the needle has fallen short of the cavity the contrast medium will disperse in a radiating pattern along the lines of the multifidus muscle, which blends with the joint capsule, or along the tendinous fibers of semispinalis capitis that cover the joint. Should this occur, the needle can be readjusted in a renewed effort to enter the joint.

The principal advantage of the lateral approach is that it does not require repeated posteroanterior and lateral screening. Moreover, the course of the needle is short and it is not apt to stray, so a 25 gauge needle can readily be used. During insertion, the risk of morbidity is minimal because only the skin and posterolateral neck muscles are penetrated with no other overlying structure being at risk of puncture. However, penetration must be minimal to prevent the needle passing through the joint into the epidural space or spinal cord.

The lateral approach requires some experience to perceive the feeling of penetration of the joint capsule. However, if the technique is practiced carefully this perception is readily achieved, and the learning phase can be facilitated by adjunctive posteroanterior screening if required, and if available. Otherwise, posteroanterior screening is superfluous. The principal safety factor when using only lateral screening is that the needle must first strike bone during the initial insertion so that the appropriate depth of insertion can be recognized. The needle should not be directed straight at the joint cavity lest it slip through an unexpectedly abundant joint space and into the vertebral canal or its contents.

C2-C3 Intraarticular Blocks

Entering the C2-C3 joint using a lateral approach can be difficult when its cavity slopes downward and medially and is not clearly evident on lateral views. In such cases, the lateral approach can be modified. With the patient still lying in a lateral position, his/her head is rotated to face the table. This will usually bring the cavity of the upper C2-C3 joint into view as it rotates forward of the long axis of the vertebral column. The cavity will become evident from its posterior aspect and can be entered with a needle inserted directly toward the cavity (Fig. 21-8).

An alternative modification can be used if C-arm fluoroscopy is available. Once the target joint is visualized in a conventional lateral view, the C-arm can be tilted slowly along the long axis of the patient, aiming the beam downward and medially. As this is done, the cavity of the caudomedially sloping C2-C3 joint comes into view, whereupon a needle can be directed toward the now apparent joint.

Cervical Medial Branch Blocks

The cervical zygapophysial joints can be anesthetised by blocking the nerves that supply them, which are the medial branches of the cervical dorsal rami. The target points for these nerves, other than the third occipital nerve, are where they cross the waists of the articular pillars—a point proximal to the origin of the articular branches and a point where the nerves have a constant relationship to bone. These points may be reached by needles using either a posterior or a lateral approach.

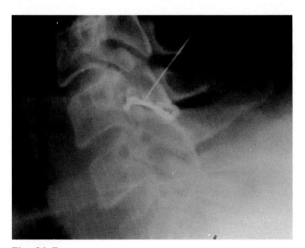

Fig. 21-7
Radiogram illustrating lateral approach for intraarticular injections into cervical zygapophysial joints.

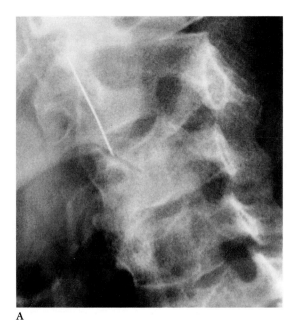

A

Fig. 21-8

A, Lateral radiogram of upper cervical spine rotated to right to reveal cavity of left C2-C3 zygapophysial joint into which a needle has been introduced. **B,** Same joint after injection of contrast medium.

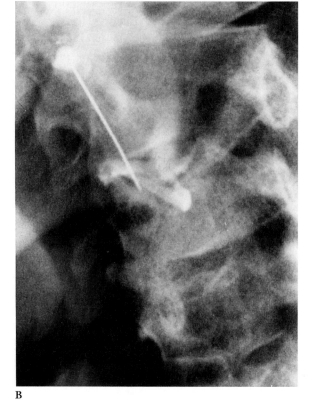

B

Posterior Approach

For the posterior approach, the patient lies prone and a 22 gauge needle is inserted through the skin and posterior neck muscles aiming first for the dorsal aspect of the articular pillar medial to its lateral concavity. Once the needle has struck bone it is readjusted laterally until it just slips off the bone and passes ventrally, tangential to the waist of the articular pillar. This establishes the lateral limit of the bone. The needle is then withdrawn slightly, and readjusted medially until it just rests on bone. Radiologically, its tip should coincide with the concave lateral silhouette of the articular pillar and should lie at the deepest point of this concavity (Fig. 21-9). Here it coincides with the location of the ipsisegmental medial branch. On reaching this point, pain may be evoked as the needle strikes the nerve, but this is not a necessary requirement, for once at the correct target point, the needle lies sufficiently close to the nerve for the purpose of diagnostic blocks.

Once in position, the needle can be used to inject 0.5 ml of a local anesthetic to anesthetize the nerve. To block a given joint, the medial branches above and below the target joint need to be anesthetized. The local anesthetic should be injected very slowly (about 1.5 ml per minute) to prevent it dispersing under pressure away from the target nerve.

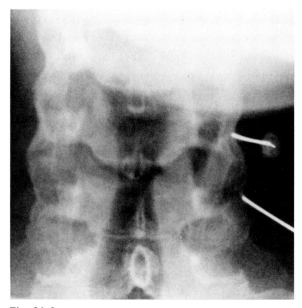

Fig. 21-9

Posterior view of cervical spine showing needles in position for C5-C6 medial branch blocks using posterior approach.

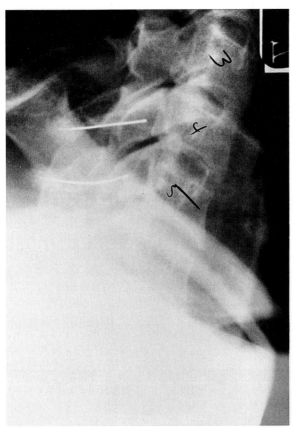

Fig. 21-10
Lateral radiogram of a cervical spine showing needles in correct position for C5 and C6 medial branch blocks using a lateral approach.

Lateral Approach

For the lateral approach, the patient lies on his/her side and a needle is directed through the skin and posterolateral neck muscles toward the midpoint of the silhouette of the articular pillar that the target nerve crosses (Fig. 21-10). To distinguish the uppermost articular pillar from that on the opposite side, the patient may be rolled or the x-ray beam tilted slightly as for the lateral approach to intraarticular blocks (see above). Once the needle has struck bone at the appropriate target point, an injection of local anesthetic can be made.

Other than the general risks attendant to any local injection of anesthetic, neither the lateral nor the posterior approach for cervical medial branch blocks carries any risk of morbidity if carefully performed. The blocks are performed on the external surface of the vertebral column well away from any vital structures. The advantage of the lateral approach is its ease. The target point is clearly visible; minimal tissue penetration is required; and the correct depth of insertion is indicated by bony contact. In contrast,

the posterior approach requires adjustment of the needle onto the very lateral margin of the articular pillar, which is an additional step, but otherwise the technique is quite straightforward.

Third Occipital Nerve Blocks

The target point for third occipital nerve blocks, to anesthetize the C2-C3 zygapophysial joint, is different from that of other cervical medial branches. The third occipital nerve crosses the lateral aspect of the lower half of the C2-C3 zygapophysial joint and winds around its dorsal aspect with articular branches arising from the deep aspect of the nerve.[15,21]

Using a posterior approach, this nerve can be blocked by directing a needle to the lateral margin of the convex silhouette of the C2-C3 joint and slowly infiltrating 0.5 ml of local anesthetic at three points: at the midpoint of the lateral convexity, at the lower end of the convexity, and at a point between these two sites.[21] Multiple injections are required not only to accommodate possible variations in the exact location of the nerve between these points, but also to ensure adequate infiltration of what is a substantially thick nerve compared to other medial branches.

Using a lateral approach, the third occipital nerve can be anesthetized by directing a needle onto the lateral margin of the C2-C3 joint without piercing the joint, and infiltrating local anesthetic at the midpoint of the joint and along its lower half (Fig. 21-11).

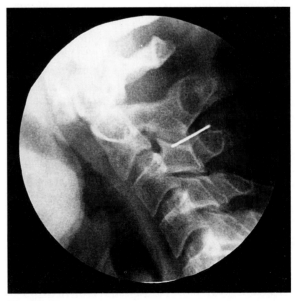

Fig. 21-11
Lateral radiogram of C2-C3 level showing needle in position to execute third occipital nerve block using lateral approach.

Lateral Atlantoaxial Joint Blocks

The lateral atlantoaxial joint lies in a potentially hazardous region, allowing little margin for error during needle insertion. The dural sac and the spinal cord lie close medially; the vertebral artery lies immediately lateral to the joint; the back of the joint is crossed by the C2 ganglion and ventral ramus.

The target point for an intraarticular injection of the lateral atlantoaxial joint is the midpoint of its radiographic silhouette as seen in posteroanterior views. To avoid the dural sac and the vertebral artery, the needle should never stray beyond the middle two quarters of the joint line, and preferably should be directed toward the lateral part of the middle two quarters.

The patient lies prone on the x-ray table with the head supported but the mouth clear to allow breathing and mouth opening. The lateral atlantoaxial joint is identified on posteroanterior screening using an open-mouth view if required. The skin overlying the target joint is prepared, and a puncture point is selected over the joint or just below it. Note should be taken of the location of the posterior arch of the atlas lest this bone overlie the intended course of the needle and obstruct access to the target joint.

A 25 gauge spinal needle is introduced through the puncture point and directed slowly and in small increments (about 5 mm) toward the joint, using repeated screening to ensure that the needle does not stray medially or laterally. It is best to direct the needle initially to the back of the upper or lower articular process in order first to establish the correct initial depth of insertion. If any doubt prevails once bone has been contacted, lateral radiographic view should be taken to confirm the depth of insertion.

During insertion, either the greater occipital nerve or the C2 ganglion or its ventral ramus may be encountered, which will be indicated by the patient feeling a sharp electric shock. Should this occur the needle can be withdrawn and readjusted to assume an alternative course toward the desired target point.

Once the initial depth of insertion has been achieved, the needle is readjusted so that its tip overlies the joint space and fine adjustments are made until the needle is felt to slip into the joint cavity. The needle should not be overinserted lest it emerge from the ventral aspect of the joint near which lies the internal carotid artery. It should be enough just to pierce the joint capsule or to enter at most the posterior quarter of the joint space. The depth of penetration can be established by lateral radiographic views. Once the needle is believed to be in correct position, a minimal volume (< 0.3 ml) of contrast medium can be injected to confirm intraarticular placement (Fig. 21-12). Subsequently, local anesthetic, or a therapeutic agent can be injected, limiting the total volume to less than 1 ml.

Thoracic Zygapophysial Joint Blocks

Intraarticular blocks of the thoracic zygapophysial joints require a unique approach. The thoracic zygapophysial joints cannot be visualized directly, but lie posterior to the thoracic invertebral foramina and therefore between consecutive pedicles, the latter being evident on posteroanterior views of the thoracic spine.

The patient lies prone. A paramedian puncture point is selected adjacent to the tip of the spinous process of the lower vertebra of the two, forming the target joint. A 25 gauge spinal needle is inserted through the puncture point and is directed initially to strike the lamina immediately below the target joint. It is then gradually, in small increments, read-

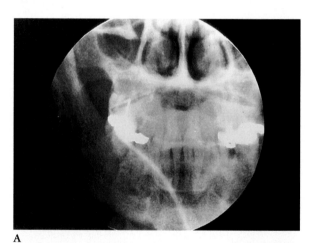

A

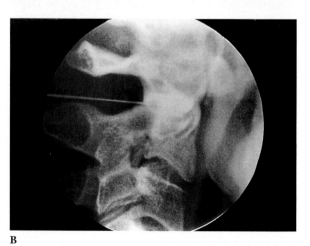

B

Fig. 21-12

A, Posterior and **B,** lateral views of lateral atlantoaxial joint into which needle and contrast medium have been introduced.

justed upward and laterally toward the target joint. The objective is to engage the slight step formed between the edge of the inferior articular process of the upper vertebra and the lamina of the lower vertebra that form the target joint. Accordingly, at each readjustment probing is undertaken for this irregularity. Once the step is located, two options arise. The operator may believe or perceive that the capsule of the target joint has been entered. At this time, a presumptive injection of contrast medium may be made to verify accurate placement. Alternatively, once the step is located an attempt may be made to drive the needle into the target joint, wedging it between the inferior and superior articular processes. This may require several, tedious readjustments and attempts to achieve, but is particularly gratifying once achieved for there is no space other than the zygapophyseal joint over the back of the thoracic vertebra in the plane of the pedicles that can admit a needle. Intraarticular entry is indicated radiographically by an abrupt bend in the needle as it deflects from the plane of the lamina and passes rostrally into the joint.

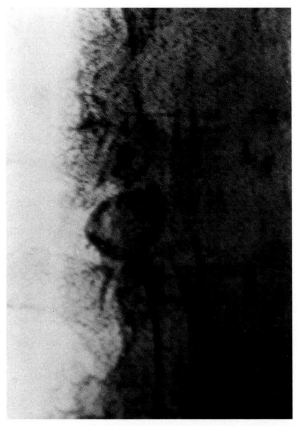

Fig. 21-13
Posterior view of thoracic zygapophysial arthrogram.

Injection of contrast medium to obtain an arthrogram will confirm intraarticular placement (Fig. 21-13). A successful thoracic arthrogram will appear as a circular or discoid blush under posteroanterior screening. Once the needle is in position, a local anesthetic or other agents as desired may be injected into the joint.

Sacroiliac Joint Blocks

For most of its extent, the sacroiliac joint is inaccessible to needles. The joint cavity lies deep to the rough and corrugated interosseous surfaces of the sacrum and ilium, which are connected by the dense, interosseous sacroiliac ligament. Consequently, a direct posterior approach is not possible. However, at its lower end the joint appears below the interosseous ligament and reaches the dorsal surface of the sacrum deep to the gluteus maximus muscle, and along the upper margin of the greater sciatic notch. Here it may be entered with a needle.

With the patient lying prone, the target point is identified and the overlying skin is prepared. A 25-gauge spinal needle is introduced through the skin and gluteus maximus, initially onto the back of the sacrum, to prevent inadvertent entry into the greater sciatic foramen. It is then readjusted toward the lower end of the slit marking the joint space. Once the needle is felt to enter this slit and is wedged between the sacrum and ilium it should be in correct position. Penetration should be just enough to engage the slit. Further penetration risks having the needle emerge from the ventral surface of the joint.

Once the needle is in position, contrast medium is injected to verify accurate placement (Fig. 21-14). The contrast medium should spread rostrally, outlining the joint cavity longitudinally, and in lateral views the contrast medium disperses in an auricular pattern. Subsequently, local anesthetic or other agents may be injected for diagnostic or therapeutic purposes.

Indications

Diagnostic synovial joint blocks can be used to test the diagnostic hypothesis that a patient's pain stems from the target joint. No other indications pertain. The investigator simply must have cause to suspect that the joint in question is the source of pain, but this is largely intuitive and subject to bias. The investigator may choose to believe in the possibility or not. No valid a priori indications have been established.

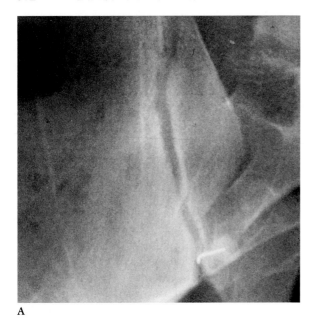

A

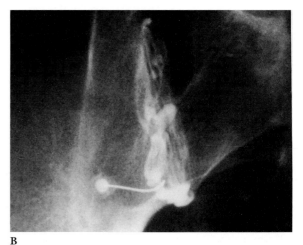

B

Fig. 21-14

Posterior views of sacroiliac arthrogram. **A,** Needle introduced into lower end of joint. **B,** Joint space outlined by injection of contrast medium.

There are no clinical features and no radiographic features that enable an investigator to predict that a given patient suffers zygapophysial joint pain. Some investigators have reported that evidence of degenerative features in CT scans of the joint is predictive,[37,82] but the specificity and sensitivity of these features are poor; normal-looking joints can also be symptomatic.

However, once the decision has been made to investigate for zygapophysial joint pain, certain guidelines pertain. In the case of cervical pain, the level at which to start investigations can be predicted reliably by reference to the patient's major, most constant pain pattern.[5,46] Referred pain to the occiput and head most often stems from C2-C3 or the lateral atlantoaxial joint. Pain from C3-C4 tends to span the entire cervical area but not to extend into either the occiput or the shoulder girdle. Pain in the angle formed by the neck and the top of the shoulder girdle is most often C4-C5 in origin. C5-C6 pain extends over the supraspinous fossa to the acromion, whereas C6-C7 pain characteristically covers the scapula below its spine.

Such rules do not apply for the lumbar spine; there are no valid relationships between the location of referred pain and its segmental source.[94] However, the advantage in the lumbar spine is that most problems involving the low back, the gluteal region, and the thigh stem from L4-L5 or L5-S1; therefore, investigation should be initiated at these levels. Tenderness over the offending joint may be used as a guide but has not been shown to correlate reliably with response to diagnostic blocks.

Pain of thoracolumbar origin tends to be focused over higher lumbar areas with referral to the groin or upper buttock but usually not to the thigh. In such cases investigations could be initiated at the T12-L1 or L1-L2 levels.

No helpful guidelines apply for thoracic pain. Indeed, the pursuit of thoracic zygapophysial joint pain should for the time being be restricted to research units lest patients and health care systems be overloaded with the costs and inconvenience of futile blocks.

No indications have been validated for sacroiliac joint blocks. However, certain features are of possible significance. Sacroiliac joint pain becomes a possibility in patients with low-back pain and referred pain in the lower limb in whom no other source is legitimately evident on the basis of imaging, discography, or lumbar zygapophysial joint blocks. Reproduction of pain on stressing the sacroiliac joint with maneuvers such as those of Patrick or Gaenslen increases suspicion.

Selection of Procedure

The sacroiliac joints, the lateral atlantoaxial joints and the thoracic zygapophysial joints can be investigated only by intraarticular blocks. The cervical and lumbar zygapophysial joints can be investigated either by intraarticular blocks or by medial branch blocks. A choice arises.

As a screening procedure, both cervical and lumbar medial branch blocks are easier and faster to perform than intraarticular blocks and are equally as valid. The penetration and injection of possibly normal joints is, by comparison, not justified as a screening procedure when the diagnosis is still uncertain. If required, a positive response to medial branch blocks can later be confirmed by intraarticular blocks.

The choice of procedure may be dictated by the treatment options. Neurosurgeons seeking to treat zygapophysial joint pain by percutaneous radiofrequency neurotomy have no call to perform intraarticular blocks; blocking the nerves to be coagulated is sufficient. On the other hand, if intraarticular therapy or orthopedic procedures are contemplated, intraarticular blocks become the appropriate diagnostic procedure.

In some situations, gross osteoarthritic changes may preclude entry into the target joint. The joint may nevertheless be anaesthetised using medial branch blocks (Fig. 21-15).

Interpretation

Like any diagnostic procedure that relies on a patient's subjective response, diagnostic joint blocks are prone to false positive responses. Any diagnostic procedure should therefore be designed to ensure that the response offered by the patient is accurate and in accord with the diagnostic hypothesis being tested.

In the case of zygapophysial joint blocks, lateral atlantoaxial joint blocks and sacroiliac joint blocks the hypothesis is that the pain stems from the target joint. Consequently, the pain should be relieved completely if the joint is adequately anesthetized. However, a patient may report a positive response for reasons other than actual relief of pain. The patient may in good faith be wishing for a positive response and suffer a placebo effect. Under these conditions, a single diagnostic block is open to confounding influences. A firm diagnosis is not legitimately possible on the basis of a single block. Some form of control is required to exclude false positive responses lest a mistaken diagnosis be made and lest inappropriate therapy be instituted.

The most stringent form of control would be injections of normal saline, but in most circumstances these might not be ethical. More palatable is a control based on a second, contrasting, and confirmatory block. If, on separate occasions, the same joint is anesthetized on a single-blind or double-blind basis with different local anesthetic agents: one short-acting (e.g., lignocaine) and one long-acting (e.g., bupivacaine), the patient with a genuine joint pain should offer differential responses—short-lived relief and long-lasting relief, respectively—commensurate with the expected duration of action of the local anesthetic used. To identify such patients, it is mandatory that every patient who offers a positive response to the first block should undergo a second confirmatory block using a different local anesthetic agent.

Failure to observe the expected pattern of response is not evidence that the patient is a malingerer. The patient may be a poor witness, or the patient's pain may not constantly emanate from the target joint. In either case, a firm diagnosis cannot be sustained and should not be entertained. If the response to diagnostic blocks is specious, the response to future therapy is unlikely to be lasting. Patients with discordant responses should be reevaluated and not accepted as having an archetypical pain syndrome stemming from the target joint.

Patients may offer a genuine response concordant with the local anesthetic used, and the relief may be definite but not complete. Such patients warrant further investigation because the blocks indicate that the injected joint is a contributor to the patient's pain but not its sole source. Such patients may have pain from more than one synovial joint or from structures in addition to the synovial joints blocked,

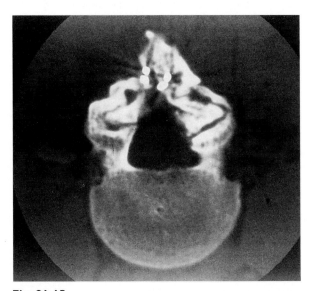

Fig. 21-15
CT scan showing zygapophysial joints with severe osteoarthrosis. Cavities of joints would not be accessible for intraarticular blocks, but pain stemming from them could nonetheless be blocked by anesthetizing the medial branches that innervate them. Target points for medial branch blocks (*arrows*) are unobstructed. *(Courtesy of Dr. Richard North, Department of Neurosurgery, Johns Hopkins Hospital, Baltimore.)*

such as the intervertebral disc. For complete definition of their source of pain these patients require judicious application of joint blocks performed simultaneously at multiple levels or joint blocks performed in combination with provocation and analgesic discography.

Prevailing Controversies

Controversies surrounding the use of diagnostic joint blocks pertain to the specificity of the blocks and their validity, the pathology of synovial joint pain, its clinical features, and its treatment. Each of these fields still needs to be formally addressed. Pure cynicism is insufficient grounds for decrying *ex cathedra* what might otherwise be worthwhile diagnostic procedures; on the other hand, evangelical conviction is inappropriate grounds for sustaining what might be invalid procedures.

Specificity

The specificity of diagnostic blocks is contingent on the agent injected infiltrating the target structure and no other structure that might reasonably be interpreted as an alternative source of pain. Much of the specificity of diagnostic joint blocks stems from their being radiologically controlled. Intraarticular blocks can be confirmed to be intraarticular and selective for the target joint by the injection of contrast medium. The prime caveat is that discrete amounts of local anesthetic be used—less than 1 ml in the case of zygapophysial joints. Larger amounts have been shown to exceed the capacity of zygapophysial joints, with the injectate bursting the joint capsule and tracking through the back muscles or even along the epidural space.[41,102,116] Some volumes that have been used clinically, such as 6 ml,[84] are outrageously inappropriate.

In the case of sacroiliac joints, the maximum tolerable volume appears to be about 3 ml. Thus, provided an operator confirms intraarticular placement arthrographically and uses discrete amounts of local anesthetic there are no grounds for believing the block to be other than target-specific.

In the case of medial branch blocks, injection of contrast medium is not a requisite part of the procedure. Consequently, medial branch blocks are liable to the criticism that more than the target nerve is anesthetized. From a theoretical perspective, this criticism is difficult to sustain, for it is hard to imagine that 0.5 ml of local anaesthetic spreads sufficiently to anesthetize any possibly relevant structure other than the target medial branch. The spinal nerve is nearby, but there have been no reports of patients who have undergone medial branch blocks with 0.5 ml of local anesthetic suffering segmental anesthesia.

In the case of cervical medial branch blocks, formal studies have verified the target-specificity of these blocks[10]; the injectate does not spread to anesthetize any other structure that might reasonably be an alternative source of pain. Such studies have not been performed for lumbar medial branch blocks, and are still required.

Validity

The validity of diagnostic joint blocks has been challenged, although rarely in print, in a variety of ways—most cynically, on the basis that "axiomatically" these joints never hurt and therefore do not warrant investigation; and more respectably, on the basis that placebo studies have not been done.

The first criticism is answered philosophically by the retort that local anesthetic is used simply to test a hypothesis; there is no superior way to identify whether a structure is painful other than by anesthetizing it. That the lumbar and cervical zygapophysial joints can hurt has bene adequately answered by studies in normal volunteers.[46,94,101]

The second criticism is actually meaningless. Formal placebo-controlled studies would establish only the prevalence of placebo responses. They would do no more than warn an investigator of the likelihood of a false positive response. However, such studies would not help an investigator determine in a given case whether the response is genuine. That question can be answered only by performing internal controls in every patient. It is for this reason that the protocol outlined above calls for double blocks to be performed in any and every patient who reports a positive response to the first diagnostic block of any joint.

Pathology

The pathology of spinal synovial joint pain remains unknown. The pathology of so-called mechanical sacroiliac joint pain has not been studied at all, nor has that of thoracic zygapophysial joint pain. The lumbar zygapophysial joints, however, have received some attention.

The lumbar zygapophysial joints are known to be affected by rheumatoid arthritis[72,79,132] and ankylosing spondylitis[8] but rarely in patients without other manifestations of these diseases. Case reports have appeared of lumbar joints being affected by villonodular synovitis[32] and suppurative arthritis,[120,124] but these conditions are rare. The concept of painful subluxations[59,60] has been refuted by radiographic studies.[80]

The evidence for degenerative joint disease being the cause of pain is limited. Symptomatic joints excised at operation have been reported to show changes resembling those of chondromalacia,[49] but no control specimens were studied. In another study, statistically significant correlations were recorded between degenerative changes seen in specimens removed at operation and reproduction of pain on arthrography[28]; however, correlations between morphology and *relief* of pain were not reported.

The lumbar zygapophysial joints are known to be affected by small fractures that are not evident on plain radiography but that can be detected by stereoradiography.[133] However, this technique has not been applied to patients who have undergone diagnostic blocks to determine whether the affected joint was painful. Similarly, although fractures and capsular tears of lumbar zygapophysial joints have been detected in postmortem studies of patients who suffered a traumatic death,[138,141] it could not be established whether these lesions were painful.

Such imaging studies as have been conducted have not established any pathognomonic features of painful lumbar joints. On plain radiographs, osteoarthrosis is equally as prevalent in patients with pain as in patients without pain.[78,88] On CT scans, degenerative joints appear to be symptomatic more often than less affected joints,[37,82] but degenerated joints can be asymptomatic, while essentially normal joints can be painful.

In the cervical spine, osteoarthrosis, as seen on plain radiographs, is equally prevalent in symptomatic and asymptomatic subjects.[54,62] However, there is growing attention to subchondral fractures and fractures of the articular pillar as the cause of pain from cervical synovial joints. These lesions are not evident on plain radiographs[38,56,73,137] and may be missed on conventional CT scans, but they can be demonstrated if pillar-view or high-resolution scanning is performed on the affected joint.[1,2,11,38,137,147] What has not yet been explored is the correlation, if any, between the presence of such findings and the results of diagnostic blocks of the affected joints.

Clinical Features

The addition of lumbar zygapophysial joints to the low-back arena triggered unwarranted skepticism to the effect that zygapophysial joint pain is not a real or worthy phenomenon because it lacks consistent clinical features—that is, if it cannot be diagnosed at the bedside it cannot exist. This skepticism, although never formally printed in the literature, has inspired several nihilistic studies that have denied the existence of zygapophysial joint pain because no consistent clinical features could be found.[70,83,84]

Notwithstanding arguments that might be raised about methodology, these nihilistic studies conspicuously failed to refer to encouraging, although not definitive, positive studies, which suggest certain, putatively significant clinical features.

Fairbank et al.[50] took pains to recruit a sample of 41 patients with pristine low-back pain that was previously uninvestigated and previously untreated. They performed diagnostic intraarticular lumbar zygapophysial joint blocks at levels implicated by overlying tenderness, and then retrospectively compared the clinical features of the patients who responded to diagnostic blocks and those who did not. Although no pathognomonic features were found, several features exhibited statistically significant differences in prevalence. Responders tended to have back pain that was acute in onset, aggravated by sitting and by flexion, and aggravated by straight-leg raises. This pattern suggests a possible clinical profile of patients with zygapophysial joint pain.

Helbig and Lee[61] attempted a prospective study of such a profile. They developed a pretest scoring system in which points were allocated for the presence or absence of certain putatively diagnostic features. These were back pain associated with groin or thigh pain, localized paraspinal tenderness, reproduction of pain with extension-rotation, and significant corresponding radiographic changes. Patients were then subjected to diagnostic intraarticular lumbar zygapophysial joint blocks. It transpired that patients scoring over 40 points in their system all responded to diagnostic blocks. However, some responders also scored much less than this. This system, therefore, was highly specific but poorly sensitive.

Far from denying the existence of an identifiable clinical syndrome for lumbar zygapophysial joint pain, this latter study is encouraging, for it defines a legitimate means of pursuing the question at hand. Sensitivities and specificities can be modified by changing the criteria scored and the weight ascribed to each. Helbig and Lee[61] may have failed to provide more dramatic results simply because they examined insufficient or inappropriate criteria and allocated inappropriate points to each criterion.

The study that stems from this experience is that the clinical features identified by Fairbank et al.[50] should now be investigated prospectively in a large number of patients encompassing individuals with proven zygapophysial joint pain and individuals proven not to have zygapophysial joint pain. Subjecting the data to discriminant analysis should reveal once and for all whether a diagnostic clinical profile exists for patients with zygapophysial joint pain.

Prevalence

Diagnostic joint blocks consume time and health care resources, and they are open to abuse. Notwithstanding the enthusiasm of proponents of diagnostic blocks, a serious issue is the prevalence of the various types of spinal synovial joint pain. If particular conditions are common, then the wholesale application of diagnostic joint blocks is justifiable; but if these conditions are not common, then the nonselective application of expensive, invasive procedures is questionable.

Nothing is known of the prevalence of thoracic zygapophysial joint pain. Estimates of the prevalence of sacroiliac joint pain range from the most common cause of back pain to nonexistence; none of these estimates is based on valid data.

Some figures are available for lumbar zygapophysial joint pain. Estimates from small and probably contrived samples place prevalence at around 16% to 22%,[87,102,116] at around 40%,[77,85] or as high as 75%.[82] Larger and less enthusiastic studies placed this figure as low as 7%.[33,70] A valid figure is urgently required, for if one in four patients with low-back pain could be suffering from zygapophysial joint pain, then the use of zygapophysial joint blocks as a routine procedure is arguably justified; but the same cannot be said if the prevalence is less than 5%. In that event, a better screening procedure needs to be developed. Radionuclide bone scanning has proved unfruitful in this regard,[117] but single photon-emission computed tomography (SPECT) scanning remains a possibility.

The prevalence of cervical zygapophysial joint pain has been studied.[4] In a sample of 318 consecutive patients with chronic posttraumatic neck pain, 128 underwent zygapophysial joint blocks. The prevalence of positive responses in patients investigated for cervical zygapophysial joint pain was 65%, amounting to a prevalence for the sample as a whole of at least 26%. These figures indicate that the cervical zygapophysial joint pain is not uncommon. Consequently, of all the procedures described in this chapter, cervical zygapophysial joint blocks are at present the best and most justified technique on epidemiologic grounds.

It is imperative for the future that similar studies be undertaken for lumbar zygapophysial joint pain,

sacroiliac joint pain, and thoracic zygapophysial joint pain so that their epidemiologic relevance can be determined.

Treatment

Notwithstanding the academic reservations that might be raised with respect to zygapophysial joint blocks and other procedures as diagnostic techniques, the bottom line for clinicians is "Does it make any difference to treatment?" After all, the purpose of precision diagnosis is to direct therapy selectively to the symptomatic joint and effectively.

At present, even if sacroiliac joint pain can be reliably and validly diagnosed, no reliable treatment is available. Corsets, manipulation, and arthrodesis have all been used on a presumptive basis, but not with validated, outstanding, or lasting success. Perhaps outcome might be improved if conventional therapy were to be applied only to patients who responded unequivocally to diagnostic sacroiliac joint blocks. This step would ensure that inappropriate patients did not undergo therapy. On the other hand, sacroiliac joint pain may be a phenomenon whose treatment urgently requires fresh and imaginative reconsideration.

The treatment of zygapophysial joint pain has attracted much greater attention. Two approaches have been used. The orthopedic and radiologic approach has been to treat zygapophysial joint pain with intraarticular steroids. The neurosurgical approach has been to denervate the offending joint. Neither approach has been validated.

Intraarticular steroids were introduced as a presumptive therapy both for lumbar[40,77,82,85,87,104] and for cervical[42,44,69,143] zygapophysial joint pain. However, patients have been treated with intraarticular steroids frequently without a diagnosis of zygapophysial joint pain having first been established. The investigator's suspicion or conviction that the patient had zygapophysial joint pain was the only indication to proceed with therapy. Consequently, in highly selected patients the results appear good; in more randomly selected patients the results are less impressive. More importantly, most of the enthusiasm for intraarticular steroids has been engendered only by uncontrolled trials.

The one carefully designed, double-blind study of intraarticular steroids for lumbar zygapophysial joint pain has produced striking results.[33] Before entering the trial all patients were screened with intraarticular injections of local anesthetic. Only responders entered the trial. Subsequently, comparison of 48 patients treated with intraarticular steroids and 48 patients treated with intraarticular normal saline revealed no clinically significant differences at follow-up 1 month and 6 months later.

This study did not deny the existence of lumbar zygapophysial joint pain. It showed only that intraarticular steroids offer no particular benefit over intraarticular normal saline. Notwithstanding this result, it is notable that in the study an appreciable number of patients reported benefit regardless of the agent used. This may indicate that some other form of intraarticular therapy may prove to be beneficial for lumbar zygapophysial joint pain, but at this stage, intraarticular steroids do not appear to be the definitive answer.

No controlled studies of the value of intraarticular steroids for neck pain have yet been published.

The concept of denervating painful zygapophysial joints is a seductive if not attractive one. The rationale is simple: if anesthetising the nerve to a joint relieves the patient's pain, coagulating the nerves should provide long-lasting relief.

Some investigators have explored the use of phenol injected onto the medial branches of the lumbar dorsal rami.[63,131] The early use of this therapy was attended by modest results[63]; more enthusiastic reports have appeared more recently.[131] However, although long follow-up periods were reported in this latter study, no controls were included.

Surgeons and anesthesiologists have otherwise explored the use of percutaneous radiofrequency denervation in the treatment of zygapophysial joint pain. However, what has polluted and confounded this field and given it a bad name are the poor techniques that have been used. The initial enthusiastic reports of Shealy[126-129] became meaningless once it was demonstrated that the target points he advocated and used for lumbar facet denervation were nowhere near the appropriate nerves.[19,20] Similarly, all the studies that used the Shealy approach are invalid, save only to serve as a warning that good results can be reported even if essentially sham lesions are used in the treatment of back pain.*

Yet, even studies that subsequently used anatomically correct target points must now face scrutiny.† Technical studies have demonstrated that radiofrequency electrodes do not coagulate beyond their tip; they coagulate circumferentially.[24] Consequently, electrodes introduced orthogonally onto a nerve

(the way diagnostic blocks are performed) are very likely to fail to coagulate the nerve adequately. Only short-term (if any) benefits can be expected, which is consistent with the reasonable but limited good results reported at early follow-up and the decay of responses by 1 year.

To achieve thorough coagulation, the electrode must be introduced across or parallel to the target nerve, but to date this correct approach has not been evaluated in clinical trials either open or controlled.

Percutaneous radiofrequency neurotomy remains a plausible means of treatment for both lumbar zygapophysial joint pain and cervical zygapophysial joint pain. The poor results of previous studies can be explained on the basis of technical failure. Consequently, the opportunity exists for resetting this field on a proper scientific foundation. Radiofrequency neurotomy lends itself superbly to double-blind trials. The operator can introduce the electrode with care and conviction but can remain blinded as to whether active or inactive current is passed by an assistant who controls the radiofrequency generator. Such trials should be performed for both lumbar and cervical medial branch neurotomy, so that another potentially sham procedure will not be perpetuated among clinicians in this field.

References

1. Abel MS: Occult traumatic lesions of the cervical vertebrae, *CRC Crit Rev Clin Radiol Nucl Med* 6:469, 1975.
2. Abel MS: The radiology of chronic neck pain: sequelae of occult traumatic lesions, *CRC Crit Rev Diagn Imag* 20:27, 1982.
3. Andersen KH, Mosdal C, Vaernet K: Percutaneous radiofrequency facet denervation in low-back and extremity pain, *Acta Neurochir* 87:48, 1987.
4. Aprill C, Bogduk N: The prevalence of cervical zygapophyseal joint pain: a first approximation, *Spine* 17:744, 1992.
5. Aprill C, Dwyer A, Bogduk N: Cervical zygapophyseal joint pain patterns. II: a clinical evaluation, *Spine* 15:458, 1990.
6. Ayers CE: Lumbo-sacral backache, *N Engl J Med* 200:592, 1929.
7. Badgley CE: The articular facets in relation to low-back pain and sciatic radiation, *J Bone Joint Surg* 23:481, 1941.
8. Ball J: Enthesopathy of rheumatoid and ankylosing spondylitis, *Ann Rheum Dis* 30:213, 1971.
9. Banerjee T, Pittman HH: 1976 Facet rhizotomy: another armamentarium for treatment of low backache, *N C Med J* 37:354, 1976.
10. Barnsley L, Bogduk N: Medial branch blocks are specific for the diagnosis of cervical zygapophysial joint pain, *Reg Anesth* 18:343-350, 1993.

*References 3, 9, 31, 43, 51, 52, 55, 86, 96, 97, 107 to 110, 125, and 142.
†References 64, 65, 105, 115, 122, and 136.

11. Binet EF, Moro JJ, Marangola JP, Hodge CJ: Cervical spine tomography in trauma, *Spine* 2:163, 1977.

12. Bogduk N: 1977 "Rhizolysis" and low back pain, *Med J Aust* 1:504, 1977 (letter).

13. Bogduk N: The anatomy of occipital neuralgia, *Clin Exp Neurol* 17:167, 1980.

14. Bogduk N: Local anaesthetic blocks of the second cervical ganglion: a technique with an application in occipital headache, *Cephalalgia* 1:41, 1981.

15. Bogduk N: The clinical anatomy of the cervical dorsal rami, *Spine* 7:319, 1982.

16. Bogduk N: The innervation of the lumbar spine, *Spine* 8:286, 1983.

17. Bogduk N: *Back pain: zygapophysial blocks and epidural steroids.* In Cousins MJ, Bridenbaugh PO, editors: *Neural blockade in clinical anaesthesia and management of pain*, ed 2, Philadelphia, 1988, JB Lippincott, p 935.

18. Bogduk N: *Greater occipital neuralgia.* In Long DM, editor: *Current therapy in neurological surgery*, ed 2, Philadelphia, 1989, BC Decker, Inc., p 263.

19. Bogduk N, Long DM: The anatomy of the so-called "articular nerves" and their relationship to facet denervation in the treatment of low back pain, *J Neurosurg* 51:172, 1979.

20. Bogduk N, Long DM: Percutaneous lumbar medial branch neurotomy: a modification of facet denervation, *Spine* 5:193, 1980.

21. Bogduk N, Marsland A: On the concept of third occipital headache, *J Neurol Neurosurg Psychiatry* 49:775, 1986.

22. Bogduk N, Marsland A: The cervical zygapophysial joints as a source of neck pain, *Spine* 13:610, 1988.

23. Bogduk N, Colman RRS, Winer CER: An anatomical assessment of the "percutaneous rhizolysis" procedure, *Med J Aust* 1:397, 1977.

24. Bogduk N, Macintosh J, Marsland A: Technical limitations to the efficacy of radiofrequency neurotomy for spinal pain, *Neurosurgery* 20:529, 1987.

25. Bogduk N, Twomey LT: *Clinical anatomy of the lumbar spine*, ed 2, Melbourne, Australia, 1991, Churchill-Livingstone.

26. Bogduk N, Valencia F: *Innervation and pain patterns of the thoracic spine.* In Grant R, editor: *Physical therapy of the neck and thoracic spine*, New York, 1988, Churchill-Livingstone, p 27.

27. Bogduk N, Wilson AS, Tynan W: The human lumbar dorsal rami, *J Anat* 134:383, 1982.

28. Bough B, Thakore J, Davies M, Dowling F: 1990 Degeneration of the lumbar facet joints: arthrography and pathology, *J Bone Joint Surg* 72B:275, 1990.

29. Brain L: Some unsolved problems of cervical spondylosis, *BMJ* 1:771, 1963.

30. Brenner L: Report on a pilot study of percutaneous rhizolysis. *Bull Postgrad Comm Med Univ Sydney* 29:203, 1973.

31. Burton CV: Percutaneous radiofrequency facet denervation, *Appl Neurophysiol* 39:80, 1976/1977.

32. Campbell AJ, Wells IP: Pigmented villonodular synovitis of a lumbar vertebral facet joint, *J Bone Joint Surg* 64A:145, 1982.

33. Carette S, Marcoux S, Truchon R, et al.: A controlled trial of corticosteroid injections into facet joints for chronic low back pain, *N Engl J Med* 325:1002, 1991.

34. Carrera GF: Lumbar facet arthrography and injection in low back pain, *Wisc Med J* 78:35, 1979.

35. Carrera GF: Lumbar facet joint injection in low back pain and sciatica: preliminary results, *Radiology* 137:665, 1980.

36. Carrera GF: Lumbar facet joint injection in low back pain and sciatica: description of technique, *Radiology* 137:661, 1980.

37. Carrera GF, Williams AL: Current concepts in evaluation of the lumbar facet joints, *CRC Crit Rev Diagn Imag* 21:85, 1984.

38. Clark CR, Igram CM, el Khoury GY, Ehara S: Radiographic evaluation of cervical spine injuries, *Spine* 13:742, 1988.

39. Collier BB: Treatment for lumbar sciatic pain in posterior articular lumbar joint pain, *Anaesthesia* 34:202, 1979.

40. Destouet JM, Gilula LA, Murphy WA, Monsees B: Lumbar facet joint injection: indication, technique, clinical correlation, and preliminary results, *Radiology* 145:321, 1982.

41. Dory MA: Arthrography of the lumbar facet joints, *Radiology* 140:23, 1981.

42. Dory MA: Arthrography of the cervical facet joints, *Radiology* 148:379, 1983.

43. Drevet JG, Chirossel JP, Phelip X: Lombalgies-lomboradiculalgies et articulations vertebrales posterieures, *Lyon Med* 245:781, 1981.

44. Dussault RG, Nicolet VM: Cervical facet joint arthrography, *J Can Assoc Radiol* 36:79, 1985.

45. Dugan MC, Locke S, Gallagher JR: Occipital neuralgia in adolescents and young adults, *N Engl J Med* 267:1166, 1962.

46. Dwyer A, Aprill C, Bogduk N: Cervical zygapophyseal joint pain patterns. I: a study in normal volunteers, *Spine* 15:453, 1990.

47. Editorial: Apophyseal joints and back pain, *Lancet* 2:247, 1978.

48. Ehni G, Benner B: Occipital neuralgia and the C1-2 arthrosis syndrome, *J Neurosurg* 61:961, 1984.

49. Eisenstein SM, Parry CR: The lumbar facet arthrosis syndrome, *J Bone Joint Surg* 69B:3, 1987.

50. Fairbank JCT, Park WM, McCall IW, O'Brien JP: Apophyseal injection of local anesthetic as a diagnostic aid in primary low-back pain syndromes, *Spine* 6:598, 1981.

51. Fassio B, Bouvier JP, Ginestie JF: Denervation articulaire posterieure per-cutanee et chirurgicale: sa place dans le traitement des lombalgies, *Rev Chir Orthop* 67(suppl 2):131, 1980.

52. Florez G, Erias J, Ucar S: Percutaneous rhizotomy of the articular nerve of Luschka for low back and sciatic pain, *Acta Neurochir Suppl* 24:67, 1977.

53. Fox JL, Rizzoli HV: Identification of radiologic coordinates for the posterior articular nerve of Luschka in the lumbar spine, *Surg Neurol* 1:343, 1976.

54. Friedenberg ZB, Miller WT: Degenerative disk disease of the cervical spine, *J Bone Joint Surg* 45A:1171, 1963.

55. Fuentes E: La neurotomia apofisaria transcutanea en el tratamento de la lumbalgia cronica. *Rev Med Chile* 106:440, 1978.

56. Gates EM, Benjamin DJ: Studies in cervical trauma. 2. Cervical fractures, *Int Surg* 48:368, 1967.

57. Ghormley RK: Low back pain with special reference to the articular facets, with presentation of an operative procedure, *JAMA* 101:1773, 1933.

58. Glover JR, Arthrography of the joints of the lumbar vertebral arches, *Orthop Clin North Am* 8:37, 1977.

59. Hadley LA: Subluxation of the apophyseal articulations with bony impingement as a cause of back pain, *AJR Am J Roentgenol* 33:209, 1935.

60. Hadley LA: Apophyseal subluxation, *J Bone Joint Surg* 18:428, 1936.

61. Helbig T, Lee CK: The lumbar facet syndrome, *Spine* 13:61, 198.

62. Heller CA, Stanley P, Lewis-Jones B, Heller RF: Value of X-ray examinations of the cervical spine, *BMJ* 287:1276, 1983.

63. Hickey RFJ, Tregonning GD: Denervation of spinal facets for treatment of chronic low back pain, *N Z Med J* 85:96, 1977.

64. Hildebrandt J, Argyrakis A: Die perkutane zervikale Facettdenervation—ein neues Verfahren zur Behandlung chronischer Nacken-Kopfschmerzen, *Manual Med* 21:45, 1983.

65. Hildebrandt J, Argyrakis A: Percutaneous nerve block of the cervical facets—a relatively new method in the treatment of chronic headache and neck pain: pathological-anatomical studies and clinical practice, *Manual Med* 2:48, 1986.

66. Hildebrandt J, Jansen J: Vascular compression of the C2 and C3 roots—yet another cause of chronic intermittent hemicrania? *Cephalalgia* 4:167, 1984.

67. Hirsch D, Ingelmark B, Miller M: The anatomical basis for low back pain, *Acta Orthop Scand* 33:1, 1963.

68. Houston JR: Study of subcutaneous rhizolysis in the treatment of chronic backache. *J R Coll Gen Pract* 25:692, 1975.

69. Hove B, Glydensted C: Cervical analgesia facet joint arthrography, *Neuroradiology* 32:456, 1990.

70. Jackson RP, Jacobs RR, Montesano PX: Facet joint injection in low-back pain: a prospective statistical study, *Spine* 13:966, 1988.

71. Jansen J, Markakis E, Rama B, Hildebrandt J: Hemicranial attacks or permanent hemicrania-asequel of upper cervical root compression, *Cephalalgia* 9:123, 1989.

72. Jayson MIV: Degenerative disease of the spine and back pain, *Clin Rheum Dis* 2:557, 1976.

73. Jónsson H Jr, Bring G, Rauschning W, Sahistedt B: Hidden cervical spine injuries in traffic accident victims with skull fractures, *J Spin Dis* 4:251, 1991.

74. Key JA: Low-back pain as seen in an orthopaedic clinic, *Am J Med Sci* 168:526, 1924.

75. King JS, Lagger R: Sciatica viewed as a referred pain syndrome, *Surg Neurol* 5:46, 1976.

76. Knight G: Post-traumatic occipital headache, *Lancet* 1:6, 1963.

77. Lau LSW, Littlejohn GO, Miller MH: Clinical evaluation of intra-articular injections for lumbar facet joint pain, *Med J Aust* 143:563, 1985.

78. Lawrence JS, Bremner JM, Bier F: Osteoarthrosis: prevalence in the population and relationship between symptoms and X-ray changes, *Ann Rheum Dis* 25:1, 1966.

79. Lawrence JS, Sharp J, Ball J, Bier F: Rheumatoid arthritis of the lumbar spine, *Ann Rheum Dis* 23:205, 1964.

80. Lewin T: Anatomical variations in lumbosacral synovial joints with particular reference to subluxation, *Acta Anat* 71:229, 1968.

81. Lewin T, Moffet B, Viidik A: The morphology of the lumbar synovial intervertebral joints, *Acta Morphol Neerland Scand* 4:299, 1962.

82. Lewinnek GE, Warfield CA: Facet joint degeneration as a cause of low back pain, *Clin Orthop* 213:216, 1986.

83. Lilius G, Harilainen A, Laasonen EM, Myllynen P: Chronic unilateral back pain: predictors of outcome of facet joint injections, *Spine* 15:780, 1990.

84. Lilius G, Laasonen EM, Myllynen P, et al.: Lumbar facet joint syndrome: a randomised clinical trial, *J Bone Joint Surg* 71B:681, 1989.

85. Lippit AB: The facet joint and its role in spine pain: management with facet joint injections, *Spine* 9:746, 1984.

86. Lora J, Long DM: So-called facet denervation in the management of intractable back pain, *Spine* 1:121, 1976.

87. Lynch MC, Taylor JF: Facet joint injection for low back pain, *J Bone Joint Surg* 68B:138, 1986.

88. Magora A, Schwartz TA: Relation between the low back pain syndrome and X-ray findings, *Scand J Rehab Med* 8:115, 1976.

89. Maigne R: Origine dorso-lombaire de certaines lombalgies basses: role des articulations inter-apophysaires et des branches posterieures des nerfs rachidiens, *Rev Rhum* 41:781, 1974.

90. Maigne R: Low back pain of thoracolumbar origin, *Arch Phys Med Rehab* 61:389, 1980.

91. Maigne R: Le syndrome de la charniere dorso-lombaire, *Semin Hop Paris* 57:545, 1981.

92. Maigne R, Le Courre F, Judet H: Lombalgies basses d'origine dorso-lombaires: traitement chirurgicale par excision des capsules articulaires posterieures, *Presse Med* 7:565, 1978.

93. Mayer ET, Herrmann G, Pfaffenrath V, et al.: Functional radiographs of the craniocervical region and the cervical spine: a new computer-aided technique, *Cephalalgia* 5:237, 1985.

94. McCall IW, Park WM, O'Brien JP: Induced pain referral from posterior lumbar elements in normal subjects, *Spine* 4:441, 1979.

95. McCormick CC: Arthrography of the atlanto-axial (C1-C2) joints: technique and results, *J Intervent Radiol* 2:9, 1987.

96. McCulloch JA: Percutaneous radiofrequency lumbar rhizolysis (rhizotomy), *Appl Neurophysiol* 39:87, 1976/1977.

97. McCulloch JA, Organ LW: Percutaneous radiofrequency lumbar rhizolysis (rhizotomy), *Can Med Assoc J* 116:30, 1977.

98. Mehta M: Facet joints and low back pain, *BMJ* 1:1624, 1978 (letter).

99. Mehta M, Sluijter ME: The treatment of chronic back pain, *Anaesthesia* 34:768, 1979.

100. Mooney V: *Facet joint syndrome*. In Jayson MIV, editor: *The lumbar spine and back pain*, ed 3, Edinburgh, 1987, Churchill-Livingstone.

101. Mooney V, Robertson J: The facet syndrome, *Clin Orthop* 115:149, 1976.

102. Moran R, O'Connell D, Walsh MG: The diagnostic value of facet joint injections, *Spine* 12:1407, 1986.

103. Murley AHG: Facet joints and low back pain, *BMJ* 1:1283, 1978 (letter).

104. Murtagh FR: Computed tomography and fluoroscopy guided anaesthesia and steroid injection in facet syndrome, *Spine* 13:686, 1988.

105. Ogsbury JS, Simon RH, Lehman RAW: Facet denervation in the treatment of low back syndrome, *Pain* 3:257, 1977.

106. Okada K: Studies on the cervical facet joints using arthrography of the cervical facet joint, *J Jpn Orthop Assoc* 55:563, 1981.

107. Oudenhoven RC: Articular rhizotomy, *Surg Neurol* 2:275, 1974.

108. Oudenhoven RC: Paraspinal electromyography following facet zhizotomy, *Spine* 2:299, 1977.

109. Oudenhoven RC: The role of laminectomy, facet rhizotomy and epidural steroids, *Spine* 4:145, 1979.

110. Pawl RP: Results in the treatment of low back syndrome from sensory neurolysis of lumbar facets (facet rhizotomy) by thermal coagulation, *Proc Inst Med Chicago* 30:150, 1974.

111. Pedersen HE, Blunck CFJ, Gardner E: The anatomy of lumbosacral posterior rami and meningeal branches of spinal nerves (sinu-vertebral nerves): with an experimental study of their function, *J Bone Joint Surg* 38A:377, 1956.

112. Pheasant HC, Dyck P: Failed lumbar disk surgery: cause, assessment, treatment, *Clin Orthop* 164:93, 1982.

113. Pitkin HC, Pheasant HC: Sacrarthogenetic telalgia I: a study of referred pain, *J Bone Joint Surg* 18:111, 1936.

114. Poletti CE: C2 and C3 dermatomes in man, *Cephalalgia* 11:155, 1991.

115. Rashbaum RF: Radiofrequency facet denervation: a treatment alternative in refractory low back pain with or without leg pain, *Orthop Clin North Am* 14:569, 1983.

116. Raymond J, Dumas J-M: Intra-articular facet block: diagnostic test or therapeutic procedure? *Radiology* 151:333, 1984.

117. Raymond J, Dumas J-M, Lisbona R: Nuclear imaging as a screening test for patients referred for intra-articular facel block, *J Can Assoc Radiol* 35:291, 1984.

118. Rees WES: Multiple bilateral subcutaneous rhizolysis of segmental nerves in the treatment of the intervertebral disc syndrome, *Ann Gen Pract* 16:126, 1971.

119. Rees WES: Multiple bilateral percutaneous rhizolysis, *Med J Aust* 1:536, 1975.

120. Roberts WA: Pyogenic vertebral osteomyelitis of a lumbar facet joint with associated epidural abscess, *Spine* 12:948, 1988.

121. Robertson JA: Facet joints and low back pain, *BMJ* 1:1283, 1978.

122. Rossi U, Pernak J: *Low back pain: the facet syndrome*. In Lipton S, et al., editors: *Advances in pain research and therapy*, vol 13, New York, 1990, Raven Press, p 231.

123. Roy DF, Fleury J, Fontaine SB, Dussault RG: Clinical evaluation of cervical facet joint infiltration, *J Can Assoc Radiol* 39:118, 1988.

124. Rush J, Griffiths J: Suppurative arthritis of a lumbar facet joint, *J Bone Joint Surg* 71B:161, 1989.

125. Schaerer JP: Radiofrequency facet rhizotomy in the treatment of chronic neck and low back pain, *Int Surg* 63:53, 1978.

126. Shealy CN: Facets in back and sciatic pain, *Minn Med* 57:199, 1974.

127. Shealy CN: The role of the spinal facets in back and sciatic pain, *Headache* 14:101, 1974.

128. Shealy CN: Percutaneous radiofrequency denervation of spinal facets, *J Neurosurg* 43:448, 1975.

129. Shealy CN: Facet denervation in the management of back sciatic pain, *Clin Orthop* 115:157, 1976.

130. Sigwald J, Jamet F: *Occipital neuralgia*. In Vinken PJ, Bruyn GW, editors: *Handbook of clinical neurology*, vol 5, New York, 1968, Elsevier, p 368.

131. Silvers HR: Lumbar percutaneous facet rhizotomy, *Spine* 15:36, 1990.

132. Sims-Williams H, Jayson MIV, Baddely H: Rheumatoid involvement of the lumbar spine, *Ann Rheum Dis* 36:524, 1977.

133. Sims-Williams H, Jayson MIV, Baddely H: Small spinal fractures in back patients, *Ann Rheum Dis* 37:262, 1978.

134. Sluijter ME: *Percutaneous thermal lesions in the treatment of back and neck pain: Radionics procedure technique series*, Burlington, MA, 1981, Radionics Inc.

135. Sluijter ME, Koetsveld-Baart CC: Interruption of pain pathways in the treatment of the cervical syndrome, *Anaesthesia* 35:302, 1980.

136. Sluijter ME, Mehta M: *Treatment of chronic back and neck pain by percutaneous thermal lesions*. In Lipton S, Miles J, editors: *Persistent pain: modern methods of treatment*, vol. 3, London, 1981, Academic Press, p 141.

137. Smith GR, Beckly DE, Abel MS: Articular mass fracture: a neglected cause of post traumatic neck pain? *Clin Radiol* 27:335, 1976.

138. Stoddard A: Cervical spondylosis and cervical osteoarthritis, *Manual Med* 8:31, 1970.

139. Taylor JR, Twomey LT, Corker M: Bone and soft tissue injuries in post-mortem lumbar spines, *Paraplegia* 28:119, 1990.

140. Toakley JG: Subcutaneous lumbar "rhizolysis" — an assessment of 200 cases, *Med J Aust* 2:490, 1973.

141. Twomey LT, Taylor JR, Taylor MM: Unsuspected damage to lumbar zygapophyseal (facet) joints after motor vehicle accidents, *Med J Aust* 151:210, 1989.

142. Uyttendaele D, Verhamme J, Vercauteren M: Local block of lumbar facet joints and percutaneous radiofrequency denervation: preliminary results, *Acta Orthop Belg* 47:135, 1981.

143. Wedel DJ, Wilson PR: Cervical facet arthrography, *Reg Anesth* 10:7, 1985.

144. Weinberger LM: Cervico-occipital pain and its surgical treatment, *Am J Surg* 135:243, 1978.

145. Wilkinson M: Symptomatology. In Wilkinson M, editor: *Cervical spondylosis,* ed 2, London, 1971, Heinemann.

146. Wilson PR: Thoracic facet syndrome—a clinical entity? *Pain Supp* 4:S87, 1987.

147. Woodring JH, Goldstein SJ: Fractures of the articular processes of the cervical spine, *AJR Am J Roentgenol* 139:341, 1982.

Chapter 22
Epidural Steroid Injections

Nikolai Bogduk
Charles Aprill
Richard Derby

The term *epidural steroids* applies to a variety of therapeutic and prognostic procedures that involve the injection of a corticosteroid preparation into the epidural space of the vertebral column. The various procedures are distinguished by the route of administration, the specific target site, and the region of the vertebral column addressed. The procedures encompassed are sacral epidural, caudal epidural, lumbar epidural, and cervical epidural steroid injections and transforaminal nerve-root blocks.

Historical Background

The first recorded use of epidural steroid injections was by Robecchi and Capra,[114] who reported the relief of lumbar and sciatic pain in a woman after a periradicular injection of hydrocortisone into the first sacral root. The subsequent literature was initially dominated by reports in the European literature.* The first English-language reports appeared in 1961,[48,53] and a large body of literature followed.†

Sacral Epidural Steroids

The earliest use of epidural steroids was by the sacral, transforaminal route.[87,114] This involved passing a needle through the first dorsal sacral foramen in order to gain access to the first sacral nerve roots. This procedure was popularized largely in the Italian[10,21-24,46,117] and to a lesser extent in the French literature.[49,52,112] Success in relieving sciatic pain was reported, but no controlled studies of this procedure were ever conducted.

Caudal Epidural Steroids

The caudal route of administering epidural steroids involves introducing a needle into the epidural space via the sacral hiatus. This approach requires a substantial volume of fluid to be injected if it is to be relied on to reach the lumbar nerve roots, which lie some 10 cm or more cephalad to the site of injection. The purported attraction of this approach is that it is easily performed and decreases the possible risk of inadvertent dural puncture and, therefore, of inadvertent intrathecal injection.

While agreeing on the route of administration, authors have differed as to exactly what constitutes

*References 9, 10, 21 to 24, 46, 49, 60, 87, 90, 92, 112, 117, and 145.
†References 3 to 8, 11, 13, 15, 17, 18, 20, 25, 29, 31 to 34, 38, 39, 42, 45, 52 to 54, 56 to 58, 62, 63, 66, 67, 71, 73, 76, 81, 90, 93, 96, 100, 101, 113, 115, 118, 121, 124, 125, 129, 132, 133, 137, 139, and 141 to 144.

a caudal epidural injection with respect to the agents injected and their volumes. The majority of investigators have used methylprednisolone or triamcinolone as the corticosteroid, and have mixed it either with substantial volumes of local anesthetic, normal saline, or sterile water (Table 22-1).

No studies have compared the respective values of different total volumes, of different local anesthetics or of the use of local anesthetic versus normal saline or water as the vehicle for introducing the steroid. Local anesthetic has been used as a convenient vehicle to deliver the steroid, with the added advantages that it provides temporary relief of pain, and the onset of numbness or other changes in the appropriate dermatome can be used as an indication that the correct spinal segment has been infiltrated.

Lumbar Epidural Steroids

The lumbar route for administering epidural steroids involves passing a needle through an interlaminar space, usually along the midline through the interspinous ligament or slightly to the side of this ligament. The procedure requires that the needle penetrates the ligamentum flavum to enter the epidural space but to fall short of piercing the dural sac.

Some operators perceive the risk of penetrating the dural sac and the dexterity required to advance a needle precisely into the epidural space as disadvantages of the lumbar epidural approach, for which reasons they prefer the caudal approach; but others contend that this perception is spurious, especially when their training involves extensive and regular experience in performing epidural anesthesia by the lumbar route.

The perceived advantage of the lumbar route is that the needle is directed more closely to the assumed site of pathology, and the drug to be injected is delivered directly to its target. Also, a lesser volume needs to be injected to ensure that the target site is reached. In other words, the lumbar epidural approach is perceived to be more target-specific than the caudal approach.

As with caudal epidural injections, authors have differed as to the volume and constituents of the lumbar epidural injection (Table 22-2), and there is no uniformity as to what constitutes a lumbar epidural steroid injection with respect to what is injected.

The use of large total volumes by many authors seems to fly in the face of the purported advantage of the lumbar route, namely that lesser quantities of injectate are required because the needle is nearer the target site. One can only assume that these operators perceive some sort of reassurance that a

Table 22-I

Preparations used by various authors for caudal epidural injections of steroids

Author	Saline	Local Anesthetic	Steriod	Total Volume
Beyer[9]		Nov 1% 9 ml	PN 10 mg	10 ml
Gardner et al.[48]		Pro 1% 30 ml	HC 125 mg	35 ml
Goebert et al.[53]		Pro 1% 30 ml	HC 125 mg	35 ml
Lindholm and Salenius[90]		Lig 1% 15 ml	PN 50 mg	
Czarski[34]		Nov 1% 10 ml	HC 25 mg	11 ml
Mount[100]		Lig 1% 20 ml	HC 125 mg	
Mount[101]		Lig 1% 20 ml	HC 125 mg	
Beliveau[6]	*		MP 80 mg	42 ml
Breivik et al.[13]		Bup 0.25% 20 ml	MP 80 mg	22 ml
Sharma[121]		Lig 0.5% 40 ml	MP 80 mg + HC 50 mg	43 ml
Yates[144]	47 ml		TC ?	50 ml
		Lig 1% 47 ml	TC ?	50 ml
Gordon[54]	40 ml H₂O	Bup 0.5% 20 ml	HC 50 mg + MP 80 mg	64 ml
White et al.[139]		Bup 0.25% 10 ml	MP 120 mg	13 ml
Matthews et al.[96]		Bup 0.125% 20 ml	MP 80 mg	22 ml
Bush and Hillier[20]	†	Pro 0.5% †	TC 80 mg	25 ml

From Bogduk N, Christophidis N, Cherry D, et al.: Epidural use of steroids in the management of back pain and sciatica of spinal origin: report of the Working Party on Epidural Use of Steroids in the Management of Back Pain, Canberra, Australia, 1993, National Health and Medical Research Council. Used by permission.
*40 ml of procaine 0.5% in normal saline.
†25 ml containing 80 mg of triamcinolone acetonide in normal saline with 0.5% procaine hydrochloride.
Bup = bupivacaine; HC = hydrocortisone; Lig = lignocaine; MP = methylprednisolone; Nov = novocaine; PN = prednisone; Pro = procaine; TC = triamcinolone.

"good dose" of vehicle will ensure that the steroid will get to the desired site, o that the extra volume will "make up for" any dispersal within the epidural space away from the target site. Noticeably, however, the results claimed for small doses (2 ml)[57,58,115,142] are not worse than those following large (10 to 45 ml)* or intermediate volumes (3 to 9 ml).[15,56,73]

Most authors have used only one† or occasionally up to three[5,15,63,115] injections. Some have used up to six injections if they appeared to be of benefit, with the proviso of not using more than three if they

did not appear to be of benefit[73]; only one author describes using up to 10 injections.[66]

Cervical Epidural Steroids

Some physicians have ventured to perform epidural injections in the cervical region, using approaches similar to those of lumbar epidural injections. The procedure, however, has not had widespread appeal because the spinal cord occupies the cervical vertebral canal, and operators are unwilling to risk misadventure involving the spinal cord. Nevertheless, in well-trained hands the procedure can be undertaken safely; and even more safely if radiographic control is used.

*References 5, 8, 18, 38, 62, 63, 67, and 137.
†References 8, 18, 38, 56, 57, 58, 62, 67, 137, 139, and 142.

Table 22-2

Preparations used by various authors for lumbar epidural injections of steroids

Author	Saline	Local Anesthetic	Steriod	Total Volume
Zappala[145]			HC 100 mg	3 ml
Yamazaka[143]			HC 25 mg	
Barry and Kendall[5]	20 ml		MP 80 mg	22 ml
Harley[57]			MP 80 mg	2 ml
Burn and Langdon[18]		Lig 0.75% 40 ml	MP 80 mg + HC 25 mg	43 ml
Swerdlow and Sayle-Creer[133]	3 ml		MP 80 mg	5 ml
Ito[66]			PN 20 mg	?
Winnie et al.[142]			MP 80 mg	2 ml
Warr et al.[137]		Lig 0.75% 40 ml	MP 80 mg + HC 25 mg	43 ml
Jurmand[73]			NS	4 ml
Dilke et al.[39]	10 ml		MP 80 mg	12 ml
Hartman et al.[58]			MP 80 mg	2 ml
D'Hoogue et al.[38]	10 ml		MP 80 mg	12 ml
Snoek et al.[129]			MP 80 mg	2 ml
Brown[15]		Lig 1% 3 ml	MP 120 mg	6 ml
Bullard and Houghton[17]		Cpc 1% 1 ml	DX 8 mg6 ml + MP 200 mg	
Heyse-Moore[62]		Lig 1% 20 ml	MP 80 mg	22 ml
White et al.[139]		Bup 0.25% 5 ml	MP 60 mg	7 ml
Green et al.[56]	6 ml		MP 80 mg	8 ml
Jackson et al.[67]	10 ml		MP 120 mg	13 ml
Berman et al.[8]		Bup 0.5% 10 ml	MP 100 mg	13 ml
Cuckler et al.[33]		Pro 1% 5 ml	MP 80 mg	7 ml
Hickey[63]	7 ml		MP 120 mg	10 ml
Andersen and Mosdal[4]		Lig 1% 18 ml	MP 80 mg	20 ml
Ridley et al.[113]	10 ml		MP 80 mg	12 ml
Rosen[115]			MP 80 mg	2 ml

From Bogduk N, Christophidis N, Cherry D, et al.: Epidural use of steroids in the management of back pain and sciatica of spinal origin: report of the Working Party on Epidural Use of Steroids in the Management of Back Pain, Canberra, Australia, 1993, National Health and Medical Research Council.

Bup = bupivacaine; Cpc = chlorprocaine; DX = dexamethasone; HC = hydrocortisone; MP = methylprednisolone; NS = not specified; PN = prednisone; Pro = procaine.

The literature on cervical epidural steroids, however, is meager compared with that for lumbar and caudal epidural steroids. The procedure was first mentioned anecdotally in 1972,[142] but no further literature appeared until the 1980s.*

Transforaminal Steroids

Developments have occurred among aficionados of lumbar spinal injections to replace conventional approaches for epidural steroid injections. The conventional approach for lumbar epidural steroids does not guarantee that whatever drug is injected will reach the perceived target site. Once a drug is injected into the epidural space, the operator has no control over its dispersal, which is governed by injection pressure, volume injected, and the anatomy of the epidural space. Normal epidural ligaments and epidural scarring may obstruct the passage of injectate to the desired site. Moreover, if one perceives that the cardinal site of pathology is the interface between the back of an intervertebral disc and the front of the dural sac or a nerve-root sleeve, it is somewhat incongruous to rely on an injection delivered to the posterior surface of the dural sac. The operator is totally at the mercy of epidural anatomy and resistance to spread to have the injectate pass around to the front of the dural sac.

To overcome these perceived difficulties, some investigators have taken to delivering drugs not so much to the epidural space as conventionally understood but to the epidural space immediately surrounding the affected nerve root. The procedure is based on described techniques for selective nerve-root blocks with local anesthetics.† The target nerve root is approached with a needle under radiographic (image-intensifier) guidance along an oblique, paravertebral approach not unlike that used for discography.

By targeting the root and not the epidural space the procedure is better concordant with the rationale for epidural steroids, which is to deliver drugs to an afflicted nerve root. Proponents of this procedure maintain that because radiographic guidance is used and because contrast medium reveals where injectate disperses, the procedure is far more accurate than conventional epidural procedures.

Rationale

Epidural steroids were first used in the treatment of lumbar radiculopathy at a time when the use of steroids by injection was becoming fashionable.

When it became apparent that the injection of steroids into joints could relieve certain types of joint pain, investigators turned their use to problems of back pain and sciatica.[87,114] Subsequently, when this form of treatment seemed to work for sciatica, others followed suit and adopted the treatment on empirical grounds.[5,53,90]

Later, and only retrospectively, did investigators search for a rationale for the use of epidural steroids. Given that steroids had strong antiinflammatory effects, it became attractive to believe that lumbosacral radiculopathy might have an inflammatory component. It is notable, however, that this reasoning is retrospective—the inflammation had to be there in order for the steroids to have the effect that they apparently had. To this end various authors* referred to the available literature that indicated that sciatica might be associated with inflammation.†

No direct evidence, however, supported this notion; it was entirely ephemeral and conjectural. No study of epidural steroids had shown (nor has since shown) that, prior to treatment, the patients treated suffered any form of inflammation. The first evidence suggesting inflammation in patients with radiculopathy came in 1981.

Ryan and Taylor[118] performed intrathecal and epidural injections in a series of 70 patients, and obtained samples of cerebrospinal fluid (CSF) during the procedures. On the basis of clinical features they identified two groups of patients: those with "compressive" radiculopathy and those with "irritative" radiculopathy. "Compressive radiculopathy" was characterized by sciatica accompanied by sensory, motor, or reflex disturbances. "Irritative radiculopathy" was characterized by sciatica alone. The responses to intraspinal steroids were far better in the group with "irritative radiculopathy," and better still if the duration of illness was short. Furthermore, it emerged that responders had higher CSF protein levels than nonresponders, particularly in patients with duration of illness of less than 2 weeks. In this latter group, 75% of responders had higher than normal levels of protein whereas only 25% of nonresponders had so.

These observations are concordant with the view that inflammation is a critical component of radicular pain, and that intraspinal steroids are likely to act best when this inflammation is still acute, before the pathology has progressed to nerve-root fibrosis or axonal death.

---

*References 25, 93, 111, 116, 124, and 125.
†References 40, 59, 61, 77, 78, 85, 86, 131, 134, and 138.

*References 8, 13, 15, 20, 39, 53, 54, 56, 58, 62, 121, 133, and 142.
†References 50, 51, 65, 79, 88, 89, 94, 95, 97, 102, 110, and 119.

The bulk of published opinion, the circumstantial evidence, and the little direct evidence that is available, thus favors the view that epidural steroids have a place in the treatment of radicular pain due to nerve-root inflammation. The dilemma remains how to recognize this condition clinically. It is inappropriate for patients to have to undergo CSF sampling as a prelude to epidural steroids. Consequently, the best available clinical ground is the recognition of the quality of radicular pain, which taken together with the physical examination should enable the physician to distinguish this from referred pain (see "indications" below).

A Consideration

In seeking a rationale for the use of epidural steroids, investigators have focused on the known antiinflammatory properties of corticosteroids. It was natural enough to deduce that *if* epidural steroids worked it was because of their antiinflammatory properties and *therefore* the cause of pain was nerve-root inflammation.

Physiologic studies reveal information about the actions of steroids that challenge this logic. It has emerged that methylprednisolone has a direct, reversible action on nociceptive axons that inhibits their activity.[72] In other words, epidural steroids might exert their pain relief not by suppressing inflammation but by blocking nociceptive nerves, like a local anesthetic.

This information opens new grounds for models of spinal pain and its treatment with epidural steroids. The effect of epidural steroids may well be to block branches of the sinuvertebral nerves in the ventral, epidural space that innervate not only the dura mater but also the back of the disc. Consequently, there may be justification for exploring the use of epidural steroids, by a transforaminal route, in the treatment of dural and disc pain. Such use, however, would be totally experimental.

On the other hand, if the action of epidural steroids is to block nociceptive nerves, the entire rationale for their use in inflammatory, radicular pain is thrown into dispute.

Indications

To be consistent with the professed rationale for epidural steroids, they should be used only in the treatment of radicular pain. Fundamental to this indication is the clinical recognition of lumbar radicular pain.

Clinical experiments have shown that radicular pain is characteristic in quality. It is a shooting or lancinating pain that travels down the affected limb or around the trunk wall along bands reminiscent of but not identical to the bands of dermatomes.[98,109,128] Such pain is often associated with paresthesias in a dermatomal distribution, but the pain itself is usually more deep-seated and appears myotomal in distribution. In the limbs the pain typically extends distal to the knee or elbow. In the buttock the pain is usually a deep-seated, cramping one that is especially aggravated by sitting. In the leg the pain is often described as a cramp or vice-like feeling. Sometimes the patient may describe a paresthetic discomfort. The clinical diagnosis is enhanced if signs of nerve-root tension are elicited, most commonly by reproducing the patient's buttock, thigh, or calf pain by straight-leg-raising. To be consistent with the purported rationale for the use of epidural steroids, it is only this type of radicular pain that should be treated.

This guideline precludes the use of epidural steroids for somatic referred pain. In patients with somatic referred pain it is more common for the axial pain, in the back or the neck, to predominate over the referred pain in the limb. Somatic referred pain is perceived deeply and is aching in quality. It is relatively constant in location and usually covers wider areas than the narrow bands of radicular pain. It is unusual for referred pain to extend distal to the knee or elbow. Somatic referred pain does not have a traveling or shooting quality, and signs of nerve-root-tension are not positive; although straight-leg-raising may be restricted, this is because of back pain and not because of reproduction of buttock or leg pain.

In the past, and even currently, somatic referred pain and radicular pain may have been confused, and both described as sciatica. This is neither legitimate nor appropriate. The two types of pain have different causes and different mechanisms. Only radicular pain is compatible with nerve-root inflammation, and for the use of epidural steroids, must be distinguished from somatic referred pain. In this regard, prospective studies have shown that patients with radiculopathy are three times more likely to respond than those with diagnoses such as backache.[3]

There are no empirical, clinical data to support the use of epidural steroids for back pain. Furthermore, it is not consistent, in the first instance, with the perceived rationale for epidural steroids. Nerve-root inflammation has never been shown to cause back pain alone; it is always manifest as pain in the limbs or around the trunk wall.

However, some forms of back pain may involve inflammation at the interface between the back of a herniated or incipiently herniated disc and the ventral surface of the dural sac and nerve-root sleeve.

This belief is engendered by the results of studies[47,120] that found high levels of phospholipase A_2 exuding from lumbar intervertebral discs. Under these circumstances somatic pain could occur as a result of an epiduritis, and as such attracts the use of epidural steroids. However, this perceived pathology is located ventrally in the epidural space, and is not immediately or reliably accessible to conventional lumbar or caudal, epidural injections, which deliver drugs to the epidural space posteriorly or inferiorly. If epiduritis is to be treated by epidural steroids, a transforaminal approach is the most appropriate.

Contradictions

The contraindications for the use of epidural steroids are based on the known and potential technical hazards of epidural injections and the side effects of steroids (see below). Epidural steroids are contraindicated in cases in which congenital anomalies or previous surgery may have altered the normal anatomy of the epidural space; when there is a risk that the steroids may unmask an infection; in patients with a bleeding diathesis in whom the passage of a needle into the epidural space risks puncturing an epidural vein whose bleeding, if not arrested, may result in epidural haematoma; and in patients susceptible to fluid retention and congestive cardiac failure.

Epidural steroids should be used with the knowledge that adrenal function may be suppressed for some 2 to 3 weeks.[19,70] This should be recognized in the event that the patient undergoes surgery in the intervening period or other stressful events that require an adrenal response.

While not constituting contraindications, certain guidelines are available concerning factors that predict poor outcome with the use of lumbar epidural steroids[71]: a large number of previous treatments for pain; a high intake of medications, pain not necessarily increased by activities, pain increased by coughing, unemployment due to pain, pain that does not interfere with activities, normal straight-leg-raising before treatment, and pain not decreased by medication. Also, certain beliefs concerning the efficacy of lumbar epidural steroids are unfounded.[71] Age, duration of pain, pattern and frequency of pain intensity, results of physical examination, and the presence or absence of structural pathology do not predict outcome 2 weeks after treatment; nor is there any relationship between emotional distress and outcome.

Techniques

Epidural injections have conventionally been performed without radiographic control. Details of the techniques used are described in the source litera-ture* and are essentially the same as those for epidural anesthesia.[30] However, in view of the potential complications of epidural injections (see below), the authors advocate radiographically controlled injections. Those techniques are described here.

All procedures are performed under aseptic conditions with rigorous preparation of the skin. Intravenous access should be established beforehand.

Caudal Epidural Steroids

Caudal epidural injections are performed with the patient lying prone. The skin over the sacral hiatus is prepared as for an aseptic procedure. The target point is the sacral hiatus, which must be palpated between the cornua of the sacrum. Using a middle finger, the cornua are located by first finding the coccyx, which is characterized by its ventral mobility under pressure; the finger is then moved cephalad until two bumps are felt at its sides. With the finger still in place, a 22-gauge spinal needle armed with a 5 ml syringe containing 1% or 2% lignocaine is introduced toward the sacral hiatus. As the needle is advanced slowly, the overlying tissues are infiltrated. The needle should encounter the superficial dorsal sacrococcygeal ligament covering the hiatus, which should be infiltrated. The needle is advanced through the ligament and 1 to 2 ml of lignocaine should be injected to infiltrate the hiatus.

Within 5 minutes the region of the sacral hiatus should be fully anesthetised, at which time a 22-gauge spinal needle is advanced through the sacral hiatus into the sacral canal. The needle is advanced slowly with the bevel facing ventrally. The needle should be manipulated to lie in the midline or slightly toward the side of pain. Once the needle is perceived to have entered the sacral canal, a few milliliters of nonionic contrast medium should be injected under fluoroscopic control to verify correct placement.

A localized, dense and poorly spreading injectate indicates that the needle is in the superficial tissues (Fig. 22-1, A). A lateral view will also confirm extrasacral placement, and can be used to guide the needle properly into the epidural space (Fig. 22-1, B) Intravascular injection is readily recognized (Fig. 22-2). If the spread is not satisfactory, the needle should be repositioned and its location once again checked.

Correct placement in the sacral canal will be indicated by free flow of the contrast medium cephalad toward the lumbar region (Fig. 22-3). Once this is the case, the therapeutic agent can be injected.

*References 5, 13, 18, 20, 48, 53, 54, and 57.

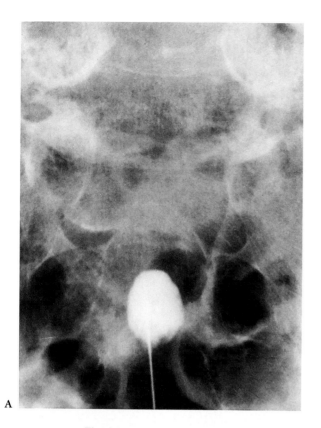

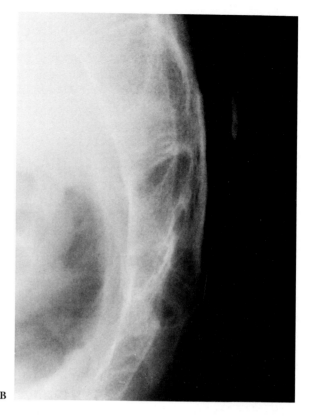

Fig. 22-1

Radiograms of attempted caudal epidural injection of contrast medium in which injection was made dorsal to sacral canal. **A,** Posterior view. **B,** Lateral view.

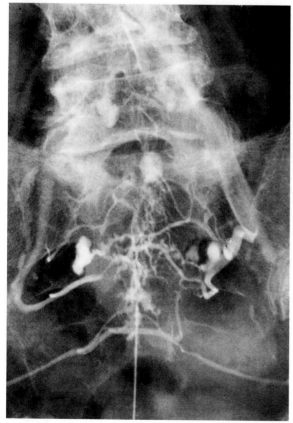

Fig. 22-2

Posterior view of attempted caudal epidural injection that resulted in intravascular injection.

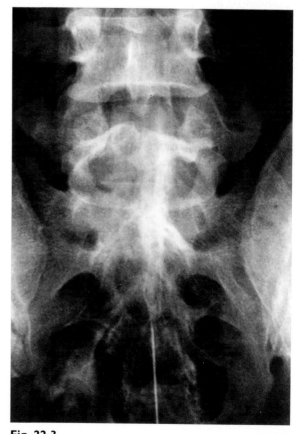

Fig. 22-3

Posterior view of correctly located caudal epidural injection of contrast medium showing free flow through sacral canal as far as L5 level.

This can be 36 mg of betamethasone mixed in 2% lignocaine, with contrast medium added to visualize spread. A volume of 15 ml should be used to reach the L4 segment, 10 ml to reach L5.

Lumbar Epidural Steroids

The injections are performed with the patient lying prone on an x-ray table, over a bolster or a pillow to flex the lumbar spine in order to maximize the height of the interlaminar space. The target space is the one that best corresponds to the segment of origin of the patient's symptoms as determined clinically, and is identified by fluoroscopy.

An entry point is selected within 1 cm from the midline but opposite the midpoint of the spinous process immediately below the target, interlaminar space. A 22-gauge spinal needle is advanced to the upper edge of the lower lamina. One percent lignocaine is injected while the needle is advanced to anesthetize the needle track. Note is taken of the depth of insertion at the point at which the lamina is contacted. This becomes the "critical depth." The spinal needle is withdrawn.

Under fluoroscopic guidance, a short-bevel needle (an 18-gauge Crawford or Tuohy needle) is then advanced to the upper edge of the lamina just lateral to the midline. Once the lamina is contacted, the bevel is turned toward the lamina, and the needle is slowly advanced cephalad and medially until contact is appreciated with the ligamentum flavum. This should occur within millimeters of the "critical depth." Once the bevel is felt to have engaged the ligament, resistance to syringe pressure is tested.

A syringe containing normal saline, contrast medium, or 1% lignocaine without preservative can be used to test resistance. The use of fluid obviates the need for a special, glass syringe, and may allow the dura to be pushed away as the needle passes through the ligament. Loss of resistance to injection is tested intermittently as the needle is slowly advanced through the ligamentum flavum. Entry into the epidural space will be indicated by an abrupt loss of resistance.

Once entry into the epidural space is believed to have been gained, confirmation is required. The syringe may be disconnected; nothing should flow from the needle. The egress of cerebrospinal fluid indicates puncture of the thecal sac, and the procedure should be abandoned. Subsequently, gentle aspiration should be performed; nothing should flow. Finally, 1 to 3 ml of nonionic contrast medium should be injected slowly. The pattern of dispersal of the contrast medium should confirm spread into

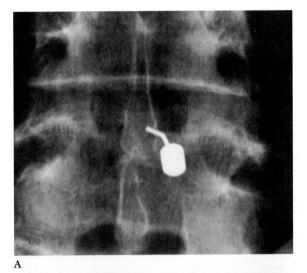

A

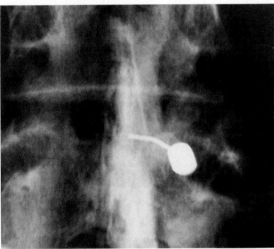

B

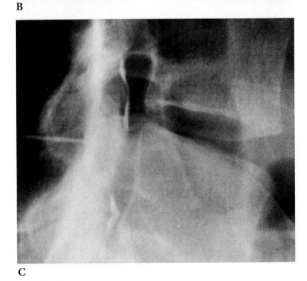

C

Fig. 22-4

Radiograms of lumbar epidural injection at the L4-L5 level. **A**, Posterior view of needle in correct position prior to injection of contrast medium. **B** and **C**, Posterior and lateral views following injection of contrast medium to outline epidural space.

the epidural space (Fig. 22-4) but will indicate intrathecal, subdural, or intravascular placement of the needle if these have not been identified by any of the foregoing measures.

Once correct placement of the needle has been confirmed radiographically, 5 to 10 ml of a solution can be injected. The solution should consist of 80 to 160 mg of depot methylprednisolone or 12 to 24 mg of betamethasone, mixed in 1% or 2% lignocaine or 0.25% bupivacaine.

Cervical Epidural Steroids

Because of the lack of convincing, published data on the efficacy of cervical epidural steroids (see below) and because of the particular hazards of epidural injections at levels occupied by the spinal cord, no description of the technique for this procedure is offered. It should be regarded as an advanced, technical skill restricted to individuals and units properly equipped to handle not only the execution of the procedure but also its complications. Moreover, until its efficacy is properly established it should be performed only in the course of studies designed to obtain data on its efficacy.

Lumbar Transforaminal Steroids

Steroids may be injected around a lumbar nerve root in the course of a lumbar nerve root block. Notwithstanding any diagnostic information that might be obtained as a result of anesthetizing the target nerve, the perceived advantage of adding steroid is that if the nerve root or its dural sheath is inflamed the steroid should have the effect of conferring longer-lasting relief than that afforded by the local anesthetic alone.

The target point for nerve root blocks at lumbar levels is the base of the pedicle immediately above the target nerve—that is, at the 5:30 position on the right and at the 6:30 position on the left, using an analogy with a clock-face (Fig. 22-5). This target point lies at the medial apex of what can be portrayed as a "safe triangle" (Fig. 22-6). The triangle has a base tangential to the pedicle, a side in line with the outer margin of the intervertebral foramen, and a hypotenuse coincident with the upper margin of the spinal nerve and dorsal root ganglion. A needle tip directed into this triangle will therefore lie above and lateral to the nerve and will not incur any other structure or significant risk of morbidity.

To access this target point a 22- or a 25-gauge spinal needle is inserted through the skin and back muscles along an oblique approach. The puncture

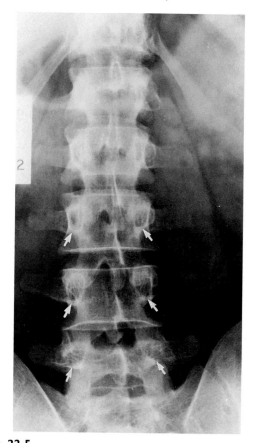

Fig. 22-5
Posterior view of lumbar spine showing target points (*arrows*) for transforaminal steroids.

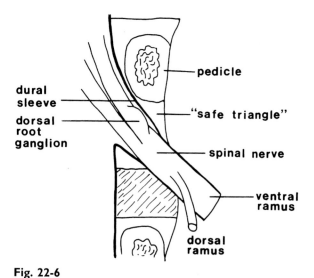

Fig. 22-6
Drawing of right lumbar spinal nerve viewed from rear, with dural sleeve opened, showing relationship of spinal nerve, its roots, and its ventral ramus to pedicle. "Safe triangle" is region where needle may be introduced without striking neural elements or entering dural sleeve.

point is determined by obtaining an oblique view of the target intervertebral foramen such that the apex of the superior articular process of the ipsisegmental zygapophysial joint points directly upward toward the target pedicle. The needle is passed through the skin just above and lateral to this apex. Under repeated fluoroscopic screening, the needle is advanced slowly toward the base of the pedicle until its further advance is arrested by bony contact (Fig. 22-7, *A*). At this stage, its tip should be in correct position which should be confirmed by posteroanterior and lateral views (Fig. 22-7, *B* and *C*). If not, the tip should be readjusted until it assumes correct position.

Once the needle is in correct position, two staged injections are made. The second will be an injection of local anesthetic mixed with corticosteroid. The first will be an injection of contrast medium, the purpose of which is to verify correct placement of the needle but also to determine the volume of injectate that can and should be injected to achieve a block without compromising its selectivity.

One millimeter of contrast medium should be injected slowly under direct visualisation to indicate the direction and extent of spread of any solutions that might subsequently be injected. An appropriate pattern of spread is one in which the contrast medium flows along the surface of the nerve-root complex outlining the bulge of the dorsal-root ganglion and the course of the nerve-root sleeve (Figs. 22-7, *D* and *E*). Centrally, the contrast medium spreads ventral to the nerve-root sleeve curving upward and medially around the pedicle and extending medially into the epidural space. Peripherally, the contrast medium outlines the course of the ventral ramus to greater or lesser extents.

A sufficient volume should be injected to outline the target nerve but not more. The contrast medium should not be allowed to reach the next spinal nerve lest the selectivity of the block be jeopardized. Usually about 1.0 ml is sufficient to outline the target nerve; by 2.0 ml the contrast medium starts to reach the next nerve above. Not more than 2.0 ml of contrast medium should be injected unless the flow is predominantly in a peripheral direction. In that event it is better to readjust the position of the needle slightly to achieve a predominantly central dispersal.

As a precaution against the injection of excessive volumes of contrast medium or subsequent solutions, only 2- or 3-ml syringes should be used. All injections should be performed slowly, at the rate of about 1.0 ml per 20 seconds. The patient should be warned to expect pain during the injection of contrast medium and should be asked to report whether the evoked pain is concordant in quality and distribution with the pain they usually suffer.

During the injection of contrast medium the opportunity is taken to record any pain response offered by the patient. Notes should be taken of the location and appearance of the leading edge of the spreading contrast medium. Pain reproduction can be interpreted in the light of other imaging studies to determine whether it is consistent with the location and nature of the lesion perceived to be responsible for the patient's symptoms. For example, pain reproduction early in the course of the injection, when the contrast medium is still in the intervertebral foramen could be consistent with foraminal stenosis or a far lateral disc herniation. Late reproduction of pain when the contrast medium approaches the disc above could be consistent with the sequestrated fragment from that level.

Failure to outline the nerve-root complex can occur if the injection is intravascular. To reduce the risk of intravenous injection, the patient must be encouraged to breathe normally and not to hold his/her breath. This minimizes the pressure in the epidural venous plexuses and reduces their distension. Distended epidural veins not only increase the risk of vascular injection but also impede the flow of contrast medium into the epidural and periradicular spaces. If inadvertent, intravenous injection does occur, its appearance is obvious; the contrast medium dissipates rapidly into the vessels and is cleared from the field; it does not persist and outline the nerve-root complex. Should intravenous injection occur, the needle should be readjusted slightly and a renewed injection of contrast medium performed.

Once an appropriate dispersal of contrast medium has been established, the syringe containing the contrast medium is replaced with one containing the next agent. This can be local anesthetic alone, for purely diagnostic purposes, or a mixture of local anesthetic and corticosteroid for combined diagnostic and putatively therapeutic purposes. Up to 2 ml of agent should be injected at the same site and at the same rate at which the contrast medium had been injected. Technical success is evident by the onset of numbness in the appropriate dermatome. For this purpose, a long-acting local anesthetic such as 0.5% or 0.75% bupivacaine is recommended. This provides a prolonged period of anesthesia during which the patient can evaluate the effect on his/her symptoms.

The objective of using a steroid preparation is to obtain a more prolonged response. Whereas the local anesthetic component provides an immediate diagnostic effect, the corticosteroid is intended to provide a more sustained, quasitherapeutic effect.

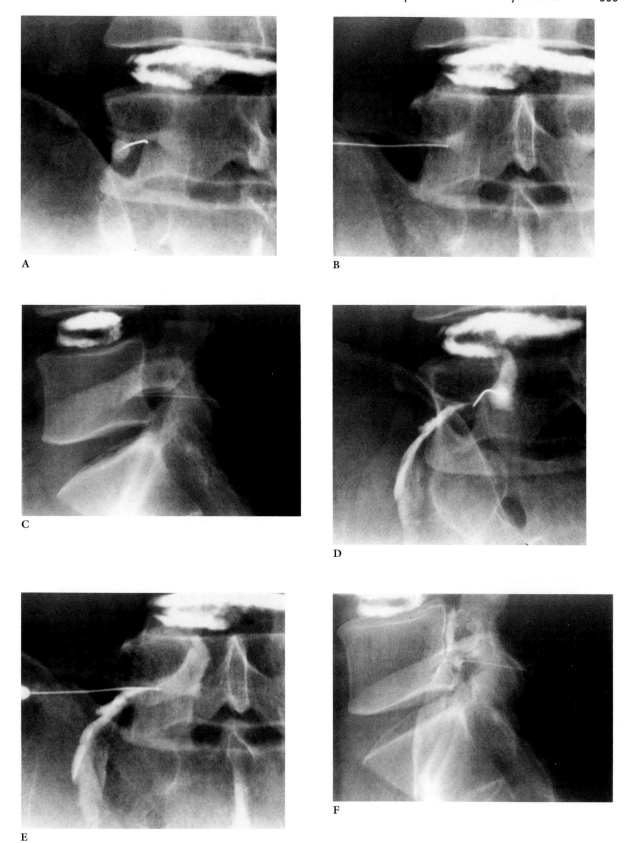

Fig. 22-7

Stages in execution of transforaminal injection at L5-S1 level. **A, B,** and **C,** Oblique, posterior and lateral views of needle in correct position prior to injection of contrast medium. **D, E,** and **F,** Oblique, posterior and lateral views following injection of 1.5 ml of contrast medium.

S1 Transforaminal Steroids

Steroids may be injected onto the S1 nerve root in a manner analogous to that used at lumbar levels, and following the same protocol. The technique is different only because of the anatomy of the sacrum and its foramina.

In a patient lying prone, the sacrum is typically inclined so that the posterior and anterior sacral foramina are not coincident along posteroanterior views. If desired, and if C-arm fluoroscopy is available, the x-ray tube can be tilted in a cephalocaudad direction along the length of the patient to bring the posterior and anterior sacral foramina into view in a coincident pattern, but this is not essential.

The S1 nerve roots course medial to the S1 pedicle before leaving the sacrum through the S1 anterior sacral foramen, which lies below and lateral to the pedicle. The target point for an S1 block lies at the inferior medial corner of the pedicle, and access to this point is obtained through the posterior sacral foramen (Fig. 22-8). On posteroanterior screening, what should be visualized is the S1 pedicle.

A 25- or 22-gauge spinal needle should be inserted through the skin behind the sacrum slightly lateral and below the target point on the S1 pedicle so that the needle passes toward the target point with a slight mediad and cephalad orientation. The objective is to have the tip of the needle rest on the medial end of the caudal surface of the pedicle behind

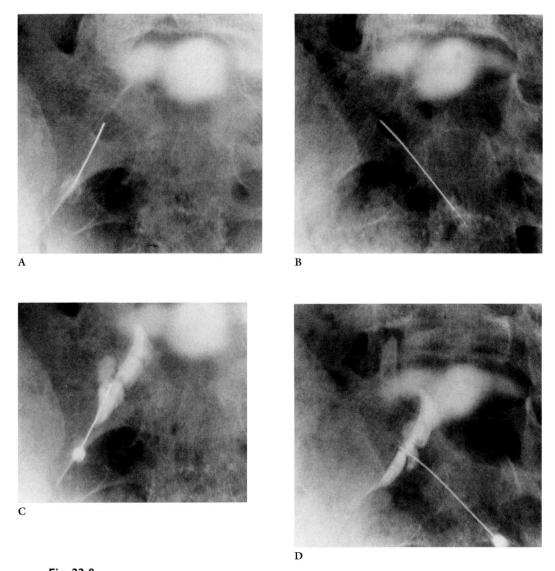

A

B

C

D

Fig. 22-8

Stages in execution of transforaminal injection of steroids at S1. **A** and **B,** Posterior and oblique views of needle in correct position at base of S1 pedicle prior to injection of contrast medium. **C** and **D,** Posterior and oblique views after injection of 1.0 ml contrast medium.

the anterior wall of the sacrum (see Fig. 22-8). To achieve this position, the needle must pass through the posterior sacral foramen but must not leave the sacrum through the anterior sacral foramen.

If the posterior sacral foramen can be visualized, its margin can be negotiated under direct vision. If the posterior sacral foramen cannot be visualized it can nonetheless be negotiated by "feel." By aiming the needle cephalad of the target point, after penetrating the skin, erector spinae aponeurosis and multifidus muscle, the tip will strike the dorsal surface of the sacrum above the S1 posterior sacral foramen. Thereafter, to enter the foramen, the needle need only be readjusted progressively caudad so that it essentially "walks" down the superior wall of the foramen formed by the S1 pedicle. Success in this maneuver will be indicated by progressive increases in the depth of penetration of the needle until it arrives at the target point.

Passage through the anterior sacral foramen is avoided by maintaining contact with the S1 pedicle and by maintaining a medial orientation of the needle so that it is inclined toward the sacral canal. Passage through the anterior sacral foramen will be indicated by loss of resistance, in which case the needle should be withdrawn and replaced in contact with the pedicle.

Once the needle is in position, contrast medium and subsequent agents can be injected following the same protocol as for lumbar nerve root blocks (see Fig. 22-8).

Complications

Each of the techniques for administering epidural steroids is associated with certain side effects and potential complications. Different risks can be attributed to different aspects of the procedure; some relate to the chemistry of the steroid used, some to the local anesthetic used, and others to the act of introducing a needle into the epidural space.

General Risks

As with any needle technique using local anesthetics, epidural steroid injections carry the general risks of infection and allergy to local anesthetic. If local anesthetic is administered into the epidural space, the risk arises from spinal anesthesia and hypotension due to sympathetic blockade. Infection following epidural steroid injection, however, has been rarely recorded and only in case reports[26,41,55,123]; allergies to local anesthetic[53] or to steroid[127] are even more rare. Hypotension has been reported in up to 13% of patients undergoing cervical epidu-

ral steroid injection[25] but in only 2.5% undergoing lumbar injections[8,18] and not at all following caudal injections.[12] Spinal anesthesia has rarely been reported.[53,100] Nausea, vomiting, respiratory insufficiency and facial flushing are common, alarming side effects of cervical epidural steroids.[25,27,124]

Side Effects of Steroids

It is known from several studies that the epidural injection of steroids has an effect of suppressing the secretion of glucocorticoids by the adrenal gland for about 2 to 3 weeks.[19,70] Overt, steroid side effects such as hypercorticism or a cushingoid syndrome ascribed to epidural injections have been recorded only following the frequent administration or the administration of inordinate amounts of steroid.[82,126,130,135]

Technical Risks

The technical risks of epidural steroid injection are those that arise as a result of introducing a needle close to the thecal sac. As such they are not unique to epidural steroid injections but are shared with other spinal procedures such as lumbar puncture and epidural and spinal anesthesia.

Bloody tap[111,140] and nerve-root injury[111] have been encountered, but rarely. More common is dural puncture,* which has an incidence of 1% to 5% following cervical epidural steroids, 5% following lumbar epidural steroids, but only 0.6% following caudal epidural steroids.[12]

Anatomic studies have shown that the lumbar dural sac is frequently triangular in outline and often exhibits a dorsomedian fold.[64] When present, this fold narrows the dorsal, epidural space to 2 mm or less. Consequently, in such cases there is little margin for error in introducing a needle along the midline. Such anatomic irregularities may underlie some of the inadvertent punctures of the dural sac that might occur with the use of otherwise meticulous technique.

Dural puncture, however, is not an event that attracts concern, provided that it is recognized. Dural puncture is associated with known side effects, notably spinal headache. In obstetric practice, the prevalence of spinal headaches due to accidental dural puncture is about 0.4%. Although this complaint is generally believed to be self-limiting,[16] it can persist. Headaches persisting for more than 1 year have been recorded in 0.1% of women who underwent epidural anesthesia.[91] A similar risk would,

*References 5, 6, 8, 18, 27, 39, 52, 57, 66, 73, 111, 113, 133, and 137.

therefore, pertain in the case of inadvertent dural puncture in the course of epidural injection of steroids. Nonetheless, there are established measures available for dealing with spinal headache, which if instituted should lessen the morbidity and duration of symptoms. These include abdominal binders, forced fluid intake, and autologous blood patches.[14]

The major risk of dural puncture is that it goes unrecognized, because then a relatively benign procedure is converted to a potentially hazardous one. If dural puncture occurs and is not recognized, a drug might be delivered into the subarachnoid space. In this location local anesthetic preparations and steroid preparations are potentially neurotoxic, often because of the additives they contain rather than the primary agent itself.[12]

Although dural puncture may not be avoidable, the reigning imperative is that it should be recognized. Even in unskilled but otherwise intelligent and vigilant hands, dural puncture should be obvious. Among other well-established features,[30] the production of cerebrospinal fluid on drawing back or detaching the syringe clearly indicates dural puncture. Under this circumstance the intended epidural injection should not be completed, for the procedure is no longer specifically epidural. To proceed simply courts the unnecessary risk of the undesirable side effects of any intrathecal injection.

Misplaced Needles

Aficionados of epidural steroid injections are usually confident in the accuracy of their technique, but the published literature is sobering in this regard. Despite the best of intentions and despite the best of presumed skills, needles may fail to gain accurate entry into the target space. In this regard the issue is not one of overpenetration and piercing the dural sac, but simply one of not gaining the epidural space.

Studies in which conventional epidural injections have been monitored radiographically have demonstrated that the needle may fail to reach the epidural space in up to 25% of caudal injections[42,139] and in up to 30% of lumbar injections.[99,139] In the case of caudal injections, these incorrect placements included failure to enter the sacral canal and intravascular placement, but dural puncture was never encountered. In the case of lumbar injections[99] the needles fell short of the epidural space or injections were made into the subdural space.

To some operators, well skilled in epidural techniques, these figures appear unduly high,[1,11] but they do serve to illustrate that incorrect needle placement can occur. To avoid performing injections when needles have been incorrectly placed, some authors have advocated that epidural steroid injections are best performed under fluoroscopic control.[42,139]

Exacerbation of Pain

Exacerbation of pain is an enigmatic side effect of epidural steroid injection. Its mechanism is unknown but it is common*; its weighted, mean incidence is 1%.[12] Analysis of the literature indicates that exacerbation of sciatic pain is related to the injection of large volumes of fluid into the epidural space, and it has been suggested that this symptom can be avoided by injecting slowly.[39]

Headache

Headache is a particular troublesome side effect of epidural steroid injections. Although most are transient, some headaches can persist for months or longer. There are few reports of headache following caudal epidural steroids,[6] but many more for lumbar epidural steroids.† The incidence of headache is 4% following caudal injections and about 1% following lumbar injections.[12]

Headache is a complaint known to be associated with epidural anesthesia for childbirth, and is therefore not a complaint unique to epidural steroids.[91] Its mechanism remains obscure. In the context of epidural steroids, it may well be due to unrecognized dural puncture. In this regard, Jurmand[73] found headache in 33 patients in the course of 3544 injections—an incidence of 1%, but these occurred only in the 183 patients who sustained a dural puncture—an incidence of 18%. Headaches could occur following unrecognized dural puncture as a result of CSF leakage or as a result of inadvertent injection of air into the subarachnoid space.[2,74]

Efficacy

All reports on the use of caudal epidural steroids have been favorable with respect to benefit. Uncontrolled studies reported benefits in 33% to 77% of patients.‡ Although encouraging, such reports do not and should not vindicate the use of caudal epidural steroids, because aside from other shortcomings, they offer no control observations. Other studies, however, provide such data.

One study[6] found no difference in outcome between 24 patients treated with caudal injections of

---

*References 18, 39, 48, 52, 57, 66, 100, and 137.
†References 8, 18, 57, 66, 73, and 137.
‡References 48, 53, 90, 100, 101, and 121.

procaine 1% and 80 mg methylprednisolone and 24 patients treated with procaine alone. On the other hand, three studies purported to show superiority of local anesthetic mixed with steroid over local anesthetic alone,[34,96,144] but these reports were marred by lack of sufficient data to enable a critical evaluation of the results.[12]

Two studies have provided sufficient data.[13,20] Both claimed a superiority of steroid and local anesthetic over local anesthetic alone. However, when the data are reanalyzed using chi-square tests and Fisher's exact test for the small numbers involved, the results fail to achieve statistical significance.[12]

The balance of the published evidence thus supports the therapeutic use of caudal epidural steroids but does not vindicate it. There are several enthusiastic, supportive publications and no hostile publications. Open trials claim good results in the treatment of sciatic pain, and the results of controlled trials approach but do not achieve convincing, statistical significance.

The literature on lumbar, epidural steroids is largely supportive of their use, although more negative studies have been published than in the case of caudal epidural steroids. One aspect of uniformity has been that virtually all trials, both open and controlled, have evaluated the use of lumbar epidural steroids in patients with symptoms of sciatica or nerve root pain. Only Jurmand[73] included an additional, large group of patients with simply low-back pain. White et al.[139] studied patients with a variety of carefully defined diagnoses but did not specify how many patients with each diagnosis were treated.

Uncontrolled trials record good results in between 18% and 90% of patients.* In these open trials, better results were obtained in patients with histories shorter than 12 months[18,137] or shorter than 3 months.[8,15,56,57]

In contrast to these favorable, open studies, Andersen and Mosdal[4] abandoned a proposed control trial when only one of 16 patients in a pilot study obtained any relief. Other negative results were obtained in controlled trials.

Snoek et al.[129] studied 51 patients with lumbar root compression with an appropriate neurologic deficit and a concordant myelographic abnormality. They compared the effects of 80 mg methylprednisolone (2 ml) and 2 ml normal saline injected into the epidural space by the lumbar route. They found no significant differences between the two groups with respect to relief of pain and a variety of physical parameters.

In a prospective, randomized, double-blind trial using 73 patients with radicular pain Cuckler et al.[33] found no significant differences in outcome. While heralded as condemning lumbar epidural steroids this latter study was attacked on methodologic grounds.[44,80,84,122,136]

The mainstay of conviction about the efficacy of lumbar epidural steroids is the study of Dilke et al.,[39] which studied 100 patients with unilateral sciatica. Active treatment consisted of a lumbar epidural injection of 40 ml 0.75% lignocaine with 80 mg methylprednisolone and 25 mg hydrocortisone; control treatment was an injection of 1 ml of normal saline into an interspinous ligament. Significantly more patients receiving the active treatment had their pain "clearly relieved." A greater proportion of actively treated patients had no pain at 3 months, took no analgesics, and resumed work at 3 months (Table 22-3). Fewer actively treated patients under-

Table 22-3

Results of Dilke et al.[39] (abridged) comparing outcome measures following lumbar, epidural injection of 40 ml 0.75% lignocaine with 80 mg methylprednisolone or 1 ml of normal saline injected into an interspinous ligament

OUTCOME MEASURE

Pain During Admission

	Clearly Relieved	Intermediate	Clearly Not Relieved
Treated	16	5	14
Control	4	7	25

$\chi^2 = 10.48$, $p < 0.01$

Pain at 3 Mo

	None	Not Severe	Severe	Unknown
Treated	16	24	1	3
Control	8	20	6	4

$\chi^2 = 13.89$, $p < 0.01$

Work at 3 Mo

	Resumed	Not Resumed
Treated	33	3
Control	21	14

χ^2 (with Yates' correction) = 8.1, $p = 0.004$
Fisher's exact test: $p = 0.002$

From Bogduk N, Christophidis N, Cherry D, et al.: Epidural use of steroids in the management of back pain and sciatica of spinal origin: report of the Working Party on Epidural Use of Steroids in the Management of Back Pain, Canberra, Australia, 1993, National Health and Medical Research Council.

*References 8, 15, 18, 38, 52, 56 to 58, 62, 63, 66, 67, 73, 115, 137, and 142.

went subsequent surgery or other nonsurgical treatment but these latter differences were not statistically significant.

The Dilke study[39] has been replicated by Ridley et al.,[113] who purported to show a benefit from epidural steroids, but insufficient data were provided to permit critical analysis and to engender confidence in the reported results.[12] Both these studies reported a statistically significant benefit of lumbar epidural injections to patients with sciatica, but the benefit was of limited duration. Significant effects were evident only at 1 week and at 3 months. Thereafter, the benefit was lost.

This attenuation of effect is typical of single-dose therapy of pain and in the context of epidural steroids has been rigorously documented by White et al.[139] These investigators treated patients with lumbar epidural or caudal epidural injections of steroids and followed them hourly for 8 hours, daily for 2 weeks, and every 2 weeks for 6 months. They found a decay in success rates from 82% on the first day to 7% by 6 months. Only 4 of their 300 patients were free of pain after 2 years.

Of concern is the disparity between the results of Snoek et al.[129] on the one hand and those of Dilke et al.,[39] both of whom compared epidural injections with control injections into an interspinous ligament yet observed different outcomes. Several interpretations arise.

Snoek et al.[129] use only a small injection of methylprednisolone alone, whereas Dilke et al.[39] used methylprednisolone mixed in a large volume of local anesthetic. One might infer that the use of small volumes prevented the drug from dispersing to the appropriate target site. Alternatively, one could infer that the benefit observed by Dilke et al.[39] could be attributed not to the steroid used but to the local anesthetic. Data on which this question might be resolved is mixed.

On one hand, Ridley et al.[113] did not use local anesthetic but used normal saline instead, and found beneficial results. On the other hand, there have been several, uncontrolled reports of the beneficial effects of epidural local anesthetic alone.* Furthermore, in one study, no differences in effect were found when steroid mixed with local anesthetic was compared to local anesthetic alone.[66] In another study[133] the effects of lumbar epidural injections of local anesthetic, saline, and methylprednisolone were compared formally. No significant differences in effect were found between saline alone and lignocaine alone, but the addition of methylprednisolone to lignocaine was found to enhance the results significantly but only in patients with chronic (otherwise unspecified) pain.

This pattern of response was borne out in a study that has infrequently been quoted in the literature. Klenerman et al.[81] conducted a controlled trial of 63 patients with unilateral sciatica in whom the pain had been present for not more than 6 months. The patients were randomly allocated to receive lumbar epidural injections of either 20 ml normal saline, 80 mg methylprednisolone (Depo-medrol) in normal saline made up to 20 ml, 20 ml of 0.25% bupivacaine, or needling an interspinous space with a Touhy needle. Because of the limited numbers of patients enrolled, results could be classified only as "failed" and "not failed," the latter category incorporating patients who were either "improved" or "cured." Assessment at 2 weeks and at 2 months after treatment by an independent physician revealed no significant differences in response among the several forms of treatment (Table 22-4).

These results strongly refute the utility of epidural steroids in acute sciatica. It is clearly evident that although some 75% of patients treated with epidural steroids benefited, similar proportions benefited from each of the other therapies. It is possible that because of the limited numbers of patients in each therapeutic group this study was insufficiently powerful to detect what might have been a small but statistically significant difference between particular forms of therapy, but simultaneously it is unlikely that any difference that may have been missed would be of sufficient magnitude to constitute a clinically significant difference.

With respect to cervical epidural steroids, one brief report claimed excellent to complete pain relief for over 4 months in 14 of 95 patients.[125] Subsequent reports have all been uncontrolled, retrospective reviews of experience.

In patients with cervical pain, greater than 75% relief of pain has been reported in "most" of 45 patients,[25] in 16 of 25 cases,[116] in 18% of 96 patients reviewed of an original sample of 155,[124] in 38% of 40 patients,[93] and in 42% of 33 patients.[111]

What is striking about these figures is the low percentage of patients obtaining substantial relief in the majority of studies, sometimes less than what one might expect as a placebo response. No controlled studies have been conducted on cervical epidural steroids, and in the absence of any greater, documented clinical experience, the value of this procedure remains unproven.

Overall, the literature on epidural steroids indicates that there has been widespread endorsement

---

*References 28, 35, 36, 43, 75, and 83.

Table 22-4

Results of Klenerman et al.[81] with the use of lumbar epidural injections

Response	Normal Saline	Depo-Medrol	Treatment Bupivacaine	Needling	Total	
Failed	5	4	5	2	16	25%
Not failed	11	15	11	10	47	75%

of the procedure over the past 30 years. More than 40 papers have described experience with over 4000 patients. Only four of these papers have been unfavorable to the procedure. However, most of the literature on caudal and lumbar, epidural steroids are uncontrolled trials. Few controlled studies have been conducted.

The literature on cervical epidural steroids is meager and is only anecdotal in quality. The greater part of the literature describes the use of caudal epidural and lumbar epidural steroids, which by and large have been used only for patients with radicular pain or pain referred to as "sciatica." There is no worthwhile data vindicating their use for other lumbar pain problems.

Such benefit as may occur as a result of lumbar epidural steroids is of limited duration. The apparent effect is evident for up to 3 months after treatment but attenuates thereafter.

The two controlled studies of caudal epidural steroids appeared to indicate a superiority of epidural steroids over control but, on closer analysis, failed to achieve convincing statistical significance because of small size. Of the five controlled trials of lumbar epidural steroids, one is methodologically flawed, two have been supportive, and two have been unfavorable.

Thus, despite the enthusiasm that has been shown for epidural steroids there are no data stemming from controlled trials, let alone double-blind controlled trials, that unreservedly vindicates their use.

Transforaminal Steroids

To date, transforaminal steroids have not been used and studied as a therapeutic technique. The literature refers only to their prognostic value. They have been used only to predict the outcome of surgical intervention. In this regard they have a proven value.

Surgical outcome correlates with the degree of pain relief at 1 week following nerve-root blocks with local anesthetic and steroids; the prolonged response is ascribed to the steroid and is referred to as the "steroid response."[37] The "steroid response" is of

limited value in patients with symptoms of less than 1 year's duration but had good negative predictive power in patients with longer durations of symptoms (Table 22-5). Patients who fail to obtain sustained relief of radicular pain are unlikely to benefit from surgery.

Controversies

Whereas epidural steroids have been an accepted part of medical practice in the rest of the world, they have attracted considerable criticism in Australia to the extent that manufacturers of certain steroid preparations have recommended against their intraspinal use.[68,69] The effects of this criticism may have repercussions in the rest of the world. The background to this problem and its details are outlined elsewhere.[12]

In essence, the problems surrounding epidural steroids concern their perceived efficacy, their morbidity, and the confusion between the morbidity from epidural steroids and the morbidity from intrathecal steroids.

As outlined above, it is clear that the popularity of epidural steroids is based on the results of uncontrolled trials. No controlled studies have properly vindicated their use. Meanwhile, the procedures are associated with known side effects and complications.

Table 22-5

Correlation between surgical outcome and steroid response in 51 patients with leg pain lasting longer than 1 year who underwent selective nerve-root blocks[37]

	Surgical Outcome		
	Positive	Negative	Total
Steroid Response			
Positive	11	2	13
Negative	2	36	38
Total	13	38	51

What has been most controversial is the ascription by an American physician[103-108] of serious neurologic complications to the use of epidural steroids, and the claims by large numbers of patients in Western Australia of having been seriously injured by epidural steroids. The public alarm raised by these claims led the National Health and Medical Research Council of Australia to commission a report on epidural steroids.[12]

That report found that in the context of *epidural* steroids the concern was unjustified.[12] None of the agents commonly injected into the epidural space, nor any of their constituents, were found to be hazardous if accurately injected into the epidural space. Nor were any of the side effects or complications of accurately performed epidural injections considered to be of a nature or prevalence as to justify banning the procedure. However, the report was mindful of the hazards of inadvertent, *intrathecal* injection of steroid preparations.

Consequently, the National Health and Medical Research Council of Australia recommended that in view of the lack of convincing evidence of the efficacy of epidural steroids, the procedure should be performed only with the fully informed, written consent of the patient, and in view of the potential hazards of the procedure being performed by unskilled physicians, the procedures should be performed only subject to approval by an ethics committee or a hospital accreditation committee.

These recommendations place a major restriction on the practice of epidural steroid injection in Australia. In essence, doctors wishing to perform the procedures must prove their technical skill and their awareness of the complications and putative benefits of the procedure, and the patients must provide fully informed consent.

Such restrictions have not been applied elsewhere in the world, but they do reflect legitimate concerns. There is an urgent need either to vindicate properly the use of epidural steroids or to abandon their use. Moreover, there is an imperative to ensure that if the procedures are performed they are performed with consummate skill.

Acknowledgements

Much of the text of this chapter was adapted from the Report of the Working Party on Epidural Steroids,[12] which was prepared by the senior author with advice from the other members of the Working Party. The descriptions of the techniques for transforaminal steroids were adapted from a contemporary publication by the authors—Bogduk N, Aprill S, Derby R: Selective nerve root blocks. In Wilson D, editor: Interventional radiology of the skeletal system, London, Edward Arnold (in press).

References

1. Abram SE: Perceived dangers from intraspinal steroid injections, *Arch Neurol* 46:719, 1989 (letter).
2. Abram SE, Cherwenka RW: Transient headache immediately following epidural steroid injection, *Anesthesiology* 50:461, 1979.
3. Abram SE, Hopwood MB: *What factors contribute to outcome with lumbar epidural steroids.* In Bond MR, Charlton JE, Woolf CJ, editors: *Proceedings of the VIth World Congress on Pain,* Amsterdam, 1991, Elsevier, p 495.
4. Andersen KH, Mosdal C: Epidural application of corticosteroids in low-back pain and sciatica, *Acta Neurochir* 87:52, 1987.
5. Barry PJC, Kendall PH: Corticosteroid infiltration of the extradural space, *Ann Phys Med* 6:267, 1962.
6. Beliveau P: A comparison between epidural anaesthesia with and without corticosteroids in the treatment of sciatica, *Rheum Phys Med* 11:40, 1971.
7. Benzon HT: Epidural steroid injections for low back pain and lumbosacral radiculopathy, *Pain* 24:277, 1986.
8. Berman AT, Garbarinbo JL, Fisher SM, Bosacco SJ: The effects of epidural injection of local anesthetics and corticosteroids on patients with lumbosciatic pain, *Clin Orthop* 188:144, 1984.
9. Beyer W: Das zervikale and lumbale Bandscheibensyndrom und seine Behandlung mit Novocain-Prednisolon-Injektionen an die Nervenwurzeln, *Munch Med Wochenschr* 102:1164, 1960.
10. Biella A, Cicognini P: L'acetato di idrocortisone nel trattamento della sindrome sciatalgica. *Min Med* 1:1863, 1954.
11. Bogduk B, Cherry D: Epidural corticosteroid agents for sciatica, *Med J Aust* 143:402, 1985.
12. Bogduk N, Christophidis N, Cherry D, et al.: *Epidural use of steroids in the management of back pain and sciatica of spinal origin.* Report of the Working Party on Epidural Use of Steroids in the Management of Back Pain, Canberra, Australia, 1993, National Health and Medical Research Council.
13. Breivik H, Hesla PE, Molnar I, Lind B: *Treatment of chronic low back pain and sciatica: comparison of caudal epidural injections of bupivacaine and methylprednisolone with bupivacaine followed by saline.* In Bonica JJ, Albe-Fessard D, editors: *Advances in pain research and therapy,* vol. 1, New York, 1976, Raven Press, p 927.
14. Bridenbaugh PO, Greene NM: *Spinal (subarachnoid) neural blockade.* In Cousins MJ, Bridenbaugh PO, editors: *Neural blockade in clinical anaesthesia and management of pain,* ed 2, Philadelphia, 1988, JB Lippincott, p 213.
15. Brown FW: Management of diskogenic pain using epidural and intrathecal steroids, *Clin Orthop* 190:72, 1977.
16. Brownridge P: The management of headache following accidental dural puncture in obstetric patients, *Anaesth Intensive Care* 11:4, 1983.

17. Bullard JR, Houghton FM: Epidural treatment of acute herniated nucleus pulposus, *Anesth Analg Curr Res* 56:862, 1977.

18. Burn JMB, Langdon L: Lumbar epidural injection for the treatment of chronic sciatica, *Rheum Phys Med* 10:368, 1970.

19. Burn JMB, Langdon L: Duration of action of epidural methyl prednisolone. A study in patients with the lumbosciatic syndrome, *Am J Phys Med* 53:90, 1974.

20. Bush K, Hillier S: A controlled study of caudal epidural injections of triamcinolone plus procaine for the management of intractable sciatica, *Spine* 16:572, 1991.

21. Canale L: II desametazone per via epidurale sacrale nelle lombosciatalgie, *Gaz Med Ital* 122:210, 1963.

22. Cappio M: II trattamento idrocortisonico per via epidurale sacrale delle lombosciatalgie, *Reumatismo* 9:60, 1957.

23. Cappio M, Fragasso V: Osservazioni sull'uso dell'idrocortisone per via epidurale ed endorachidea nelle lombosciatalgie, *Riforma Med* 22:605, 1955.

24. Cappio M, Fragasso V: II prednisolone per via epidurale sacrale nelle lomboschiatalgie. *Reumatismo* 5:905, 1957.

25. Catchlove RFH, Braha R: The use of cervical epidural nerve blocks in the management of chronic head and neck pain, *Can Anaesth Soc J* 31:188, 1984.

26. Chan ST, Leung S: Spinal epidural abscess following steroid injection for sciatica: case report, *Spine* 14:106, 1989.

27. Cicala RS, Westbrook L, Angel JJ: Side effects and complications of cervical epidural steroid injections, *J Pain Symptom Manage* 4:64, 1989.

28. Coomes EN: A comparison between epidural anaesthesia and bed rest in sciatica, *BMJ* 1:20, 1961.

29. Corrigan AB, Carr G, Tugwell S: Intraspinal corticosteroid injections, *Med J Aust* 1:224, 1982.

30. Cousins MJ, Bromage PR: *Epidural neural blockade*. In Cousins MJ, Bridenbaugh PO, editors: *Neural blockade in clinical anaesthesia and management of pain*, ed 2, Philadelphia, 1988, JB Lippincott, p 253.

31. Cronen MC, Waldman SD: Cervical steroid epidural nerve blocks in the palliation of pain secondary to intractable tension-type headaches, *J Pain Symptom Manage* 5:379, 1990.

32. Cuckler JM: Correspondence, *J Bone Joint Surg* 68A:789, 1986.

33. Cuckler JM, Berini PA, Wiesel SW, et al.: The use of epidural steroids in the treatment of radicular pain, *J Bone Joint Surg* 67A:53, 1985.

34. Czarski Z: Leczenie rwy kulszowej wstrzykiwaniem hydrokortyzonu i nowokainy do rozworu krzyowego, *Przeglad Lekarski* 21:511, 1965.

35. Daly P: Caudal epidural anesthesia in lumbosciatic pain, *Anaesthesia* 25:346, 1970.

36. Davidson JT, Robin GC: Epidural injection in lumbosciatic syndrome, *Br J Anaesth* 33:595, 1961.

37. Derby R, Kine G, Saal J, et al.: Response to steroid and duration of radicular pain as predictors of surgical outcome, *Spine* 17:S176, 1992.

38. D'Hoogue R, Compere A, Gribmont B, Vincent A: Peridural injection of corticosteroids in the treatment of the low back pain/sciatica syndrome, *Acta Orthop Belg* 42:157, 1976.

39. Dilke TFW, Burry HC, Grahame R: Extradural corticosteroid injection in management of lumbar nerve root compression, *BMJ* 2:635, 1973.

40. Dooley JF, McBroom RJ, Taguchi T, McNab I: Nerve root infiltration in the diagnosis of radicular pain, *Spine* 13:79, 1988.

41. Dougherty JH, Fraser RAR: Complications following intraspinal injections of steroids, *J Neurosurg* 48:1023, 1978.

42. El-Khoury G, Ehara S, Weinstein JW, et al.: Epidural steroid injection: a procedure ideally performed with fluoroscopic control, *Radiology* 168:554, 1988.

43. Evans W: Intrasacral epidural injection in the treatment of sciatica. *Lancet* 219:1225, 1930.

44. Fisher RH: Correspondence, *J Bone Joint Surg* 68A:789, 1986.

45. Forrest JB: The response to epidural steroid injection in chronic dorsal root pain, *Can Anaesth Soc J* 27:40, 1980.

46. Fragasso V: II prednisolone idrosolubile per via epidurale sacrale nelle lombosciatalgie, *Gaz Med Ital* 118:358, 1959.

47. Franson RC, Saal JS, Saal JF: Human disc phospholipase A2 is inflammatory, *Spine* 17:S190, 1992.

48. Gardner WJ, Goebert HW, Sehgal AD: Intraspinal corticosteroids in the treatment of sciatica, *Trans Am Neurol Assoc* 86:214, 1961.

49. Gerest MF: Le traitement de la nevralgie sciatique par les injections epidurales d'hydrocortisone, *J Med Lyon* 261, 1958.

50. Gertzbein SD: Degenerative disk disease of the lumbar spine: immunological implications, *Clin Orthop* 190:68, 1977.

51. Gertzbein SD, Tile M, Gross A, Falk R: Autoimmunity in degenerative disk disease of the lumbar spine, *Orthop Clin North Am* 6:67, 1975.

52. Gilly R: Essai de traitement de 50 cas de sciatiques et de radiculalgies lombaires par le Celestene chonodose en infiltrations pararadiculaire, *Marseille Med* 107:341, 1970.

53. Goebert HW, Jallo JS, Gardner WJ, Wasmuth CE: Painful radiculopathy treated with epidural injections of procaine and hydrocortisone acetate: results in 113 patients, *Anesth Analg* 140:130, 1961.

54. Gordon J: Caudal extradural injection for the treatment of low back pain, *Anaesthesia* 35:515, 1980.

55. Goucke CR, Graziotti P: Extradural abscess following local anaesthetic and steroid injection for chronic low back pain, *Br J Anesth* 65:427, 1990.

56. Green PWB, Burke AJ, Weiss CA, Langan P: The role of epidural cortisone injection in the treatment of diskogenic low back pain, *Clin Orthop* 153:121, 1980.

57. Harley C: Extradural corticosteroid infiltration, *Ann Phys Med* 9:22, 1967.

58. Hartman JT, Winnie AP, Ramaurthy S, Meyers HL: Intradural and extradural corticosteroids for sciatic pain, *Orthop Rev* 3:21, 1974.

59. Hasueisen DC, Smith BS, Myers SR, Pryce ML: The diagnostic accuracy of spinal nerve injection studies: their role in the evaluation of recurrent sciatica, *Clin Orthop* 198:179, 1985.

60. Hellens A: Lumbar nerve-root compression treated with epidural hydrocortisone, *Duodecim* 78:28, 1962.

61. Herron LD: Selective nerve root block in patient selection for lumbar surgery: surgical results, *J Spinal Dis* 2:75, 1989.

62. Heyse-Moore GH: A rational approach to the use of epidural medication in the treatment of sciatic pain, *Acta Orthop Scand* 49:366, 1978.

63. Hickey RF: Outpatient epidural steroid injections for low back pain and lumbosacral radiculopathy, *N Z Med J* 100:594, 1987.

64. Husemeyer RP, White DC: Topography of the lumbar epidural space, *Anaesthesia* 35:7, 1980.

65. Irsigler FJ: Mikroskopische Befunde in den Ruckenlarkswurzeln beim lumbalen und lumbosakralen (dorsolateral) Diskusprolaps. *Acta Neurochir* (Wien) 1:478, 1951.

66. Ito R: The treatment of low back pain and sciatica with epidural corticosteroids injection and its pathophysiological basis, *J Jpn Orthop Assoc* 45:769, 1971.

67. Jackson DW, Rettig A, Wiltse LL: Epidural cortisone injection in the young athletic adult, *Am J Sports Med* 8:239, 1980.

68. Jacobs D: Intrathecal and epidural/extradural injection of depo medrol, *Med J Aust* 2:301, 1981.

69. Jacobs D: Intraspinal injection of depot corticosteroids, *Med J Aust* 140:49, 1984.

70. Jacobs S, Pullan PT, Potter JM, Shenfield GM: Adrenal suppression following extradural steroids, *Anesthesia* 38:953, 1983.

71. Jamison RN, VadeBoncouer T, Ferrante FM: Low back pain patients unresponsive to an epidural steroid injection: identifying predictive factors, *Clin J Pain* 7:311, 1991.

72. Johansson A, Hao J, Sjolund B: Local corticosteroid application blocks transmission in normal nociceptive C-fibres, *Acta Anaesthesiol Scand* 34:335, 1990.

73. Jurmand SH: Corticotherapie peridurale des lombalgies et des sciatiques d'origine discale, *Concours Med* 94:5061, 1972.

74. Katz JA, Lukin R, Bridenbaugh PO, Gunzenhauser L: Subdural intracranial air: an unusual cause of headache after epidural steroid injection, *Anesthesiology* 74:615, 1991.

75. Kelman H: Epidural injection therapy for sciatica pain, *Am J Surg* 64:183, 1944.

76. Kepes ER, Duncalf D: Treatment of backache with spinal injections of local anesthetics, spinal and systemic steroids: a review, *Pain* 22:33, 1985.

77. Kikuchi S, Hasue M, Ito T: Anatomic and clinical studies of radicular symptoms, *Spine* 9:23, 1984.

78. Kikuchi S, Hasue M: Combined contrast studies in lumbar spine diseases: myelography (peridurography) and nerve root infiltration, *Spine* 13:1327, 1988.

79. Kirkaldy-Willis WH: The relationship of structural pathology to the nerve root, *Spine* 9:49, 1984.

80. Kirkpatrick AF: Correspondence, *J Bone Joint Surg* 72A:948, 1990.

81. Klenerman L, Greenwood R, Davenport HT, et al.: Lumbar epidural injections in the treatment of sciatica, *Br J Rheumatol* 23:35, 1984.

82. Knight CL, Burnell JC: Systemic side-effects of extradural steroids, *Anaesthesia* 35:593, 1980.

83. Knutsen O, Ygge H: Prolonged extradural anesthesia with bupivacaine at lumbago and sciatica, *Acta Orthop Scand* 42:338, 1971.

84. Korbon GA, Rowlingson JC, Carron H: Correspondence, *J Bone Joint Surg* 68A:788, 1986.

85. Krempen JF, Smith BS: Nerve root injection: a method for evaluating the etiology of sciatica, *J Bone Joint Surg* 56A:1435, 1974.

86. Krempen JF, Smith BS, de Freest LJ: Selective nerve root infiltration for the evaluation of sciatica, *Orthop Clin North Am* 6:311, 1975.

87. Lievre JA, Bloch-Michel H, Pean G, Uro J: L'hydrocortisone en injection locale, *Rev Rhum* 20:310, 1953.

88. Lindblom K, Rexed B: Spinal nerve injury in dorsolateral protrusions of lumbar disks, *J Neurosurg* 5:413, 1949.

89. Lindhal O, Rexed B: Histologic changes in spinal nerve roots of operated cases of sciatica. *Acta Orthop Scand* 20:215, 1951.

90. Lindholm R, Salenius P: Caudal, epidural administration of anaesthetics and corticoids in the treatment of low back pain, *Acta Orthop Scand* 1:114, 1964.

91. MacArthur C, Lewis M, Knox EG: Investigation of long term problems after obstetric epidural anaesthesia, *BMJ* 304:1279, 1992.

92. Mahner A: Die peridurale Injektion von Novocain und Kortikosteroiden in der Therapie des lumbalen radikularen Syndrom, *Zbl Chir* 85:625, 1960.

93. Mangar D, Thomas PB: Epidural steroid injections in the treatment of cervical and lumbar pain syndromes, *Regional Anesth* 16:246, 1991.

94. Marshall LL, Trethewie ER: Chemical irritation of nerve-root in disc prolapse, *Lancet* 2:320, 1973.

95. Marshall LL, Trethewie ER, Curtain CC: Chemical radiculitis: a clinical, physiological and immunological study, *Clin Orthop* 190:61, 1977.

96. Matthews JA, Mills SB, Jenkins VM, et al.: Back pain and sciatica: controlled trials of manipulation, traction, sclerosant and epidural injections, *Br J Rheumatol* 26:416, 1987.

97. McCarron RF, Wimpee MW, Hudkins PG, Laros GS: The inflammatory effect of nucleus pulposus: a possible element in the pathogenesis of low back pain, *Spine* 12:758, 1987.

98. McCulloch JA, Waddell G: Variation of the lumbosacral myotomes with bony segmental anomalies, *J Bone Joint Surg* 62B:475, 1980.

99. Mehta M, Salmon N: Extradural block. Confirmation of the injection site by x-ray monitoring. *Anaesthesia* 40:1009, 1985.

100. Mount HTR: Hydrocortisone in the treatment of intervertebral disc protrusion, *Can Med Assoc J* 105:1279, 1971.

101. Mount HTR: *Epidural injection of hydrocortisone for the management of the acute lumbar disc protrusion.* In Morley TP, editor: *Current controversies in neurosurgery,* Philadelphia, 1976, WB Saunders, p 67.

102. Murphy RW: Nerve roots and spinal nerves in degenerative disk disease, *Clin Orthop* 190:46, 1977.

103. Nelson D: Arachnoiditis from intrathecally given corticosteroids in the treatment of multiple sclerosis, *Arch Neurol* 33:373, 1976 (letter).

104. Nelson D: Methylprednisolone acetate, *Arch Neurol* 36:661, 1979 (letter).

105. Nelson D: Dangers from methylprednisolone acetate therapy by intraspinal injection, *Arch Neurol* 45:804, 1988.

106. Nelson DA: Safety of intrathecal steroids in multiple sclerosis. *Arch Neurol* 46:718, 1989 (letter).

107. Nelson DA: Dangers from methylprednisolone acetate therapy by intraspinal injection, *Arch Neurol* 46:721, 1989 (letter).

108. Nelson DA, Vates TS, Thomas RB: Complications from intrathecal steroid therapy in patients with multiple sclerosis, *Acta Neurol Scand* 49:176, 1973.

109. Norlen G: On the value of the neurological symptoms in sciatica for the localisation of a lumbar disc herniation, *Acta Chir Scand Suppl* 95:1, 1944.

110. Park WW, Watanabe RYO: The intrinsic vasculature of the lumbosacral spinal nerves, *Spine* 10:508, 1985.

111. Purkis IE: Cervical epidural steroids, *Pain Clin* 1:3, 1986.

112. Renier JC: L'infiltration epidurale par le premier trou sacre posterieur, *Rev Rhum Malad Osteoartic* 26:526, 1959.

113. Ridley MG, Kingsley GH, Gibson T, Grahame R: Outpatient lumbar epidural corticosteroid injection in the management of sciatica, *Br J Rheumatol* 27:905, 1988.

114. Robechhi A, Capra R: L'idrocortisone (composto F): prime esperienze cliniche in campo reumatologico, *Min Med* 98:1259, 1952.

115. Rosen CD, Kahanovitz N, Bernstein R, Viola K: A retrospective analysis of the efficacy of epidural steroid injections, *Clin Orthop* 228:270, 1988.

116. Rowlingson JC, Kirschenbaum LP: Epidural analgesic techniques in the management of cervical pain, *Anesth Analg* 65:938, 1986.

117. Ruggieri F, Capello A: L'idrocortisone nel trattamento della lumbosciatalgica, *Min Ortop* 7:388, 1956.

118. Ryan MD, Taylor TKF: Management of lumbar nerve-root pain, *Med J Aust* 2:532, 1981.

119. Rydevik B, Brown MD, Ludborg G: Pathoanatomy and pathophysiology of nerve root compression, *Spine* 9:7, 1984.

120. Saal JS, Franson RC, Dobrow R, et al.: High levels of inflammatory phospholipase A2 activity in lumbar disc herniation, *Spine* 15:674, 1990.

121. Sharma RK: Indications, technique and results of caudal epidural injection for lumbar disc retropulsion, *Postgrad Med J* 53:1, 1977.

122. Sharrock NE: Correspondence, *J Bone Joint Surg* 67A:981, 1985.

123. Shealy CN: Dangers of spinal injections without proper diagnosis, *JAMA* 197:1104, 1966.

124. Shulman M: Treatment of neck pain with cervical epidural steroid injection, *Regional Anesth* 11:92, 1986.

125. Shulman M, Nimmagadda U, Valenta A: Cervical epidural steroid injection for pain of cervical spine origin, *Anesthesiology* 61:A223, 1984.

126. Simon D, Carron H, Rowlingson J: Correspondence, *J Bone Joint Surg* 67A:981, 1985.

127. Simon DL, Kunz RD, German JD, Zivkovich V: Allergic or pseudoallergic reaction following epidural steroid deposition and skin testing, *Regional Anesth* 253, 1989.

128. Smyth MJ, Wright V: Sciatica and the intervertebral disc: an experimental study. *J Bone Joint Surg* 40A:1401, 1959.

129. Snoek W, Weber H, Jorgensen B: Double blind evaluation of extradural methyl prednisolone for herniated lumbar discs, *Acta Orthop Scand* 48:635, 1977.

130. Stambough JL, Booth RE, Rothman RH: Transient hypercorticism after epidural steroid injection, *J Bone Joint Surg* 66A:1115, 1984.

131. Stanley D, McLaren MI, Euinton HA, Getty CJM: A prospective study of nerve root infiltration in the diagnosis of sciatica: a comparison with radiculography, computed tomography, and operative findings, *Spine* 15:540, 1990.

132. Stanton-Hicks M: Therapeutic caudal or epidural block for lower back or sciatic pain, *JAMA* 243:369, 1980.

133. Swerdlow M, Sayle-Creer W: A study of extradural medication in the relief of the lumbosciatic syndrome, *Anaesthesia* 25:341, 1970.

134. Tajima T, Furukawa K, Kuramocji E: Selective lumbosacral radiculography and block, *Spine* 5:68, 1980.

135. Tuel SM, Meythaler JM, Cross LL: Cushing's syndrome from epidural methylprednisolone, *Pain* 40:81, 1990.

136. Warfield CA: Correspondence, *J Bone Joint Surg* 67A:980, 1985.

137. Warr AC, Wilkinson JA, Burn JMB, Langdon L: Chronic lumbosciatic syndrome treated by epidural injection and manipulation, *Practitioner* 209:53, 1977.

138. White AH: Injection techniques for the diagnosis and treatment of low back pain, *Orthop Clin North Am* 14:553, 1983.

139. White AH, Derby R, Wynne G: Epidural injections for diagnosis and treatment of low-back pain, *Spine* 5:78, 1980.

140. Williams KN, Jackowski A, Evans PJD: Epidural haematoma requiring surgical decompression following repeated cervical epidural steroid injections for chronic pain, *Pain* 42:197, 1990.

141. Wiltse LL: Therapeutic caudal or epidural block for lower back or sciatic pain, *JAMA* 243:369, 1980.

142. Winnie AP, Hartman JT, Meyers HL, et al.: Pain clinic II: intradural and extradural corticosteroids for sciatica, *Anesth Analg* 51:990, 1972.

143. Yamazaka N: Interspinal injection of hydrocortisone or prednisolone in the treatment of intervertebral disc herniation, *J Jpn Orthop Assoc* 33:689, 1959.

144. Yates DW: A comparison of the types of epidural injection commonly used in the treatment of low back pain and sciatica, *Rheum Rehab* 17:181, 1978.

145. Zappala G: Iniezione peridurale segmentaria di Hydrocortone nella sindrome dolorosa da ernia discale, *Policlinico Sez Prat* 62:1229, 1955.

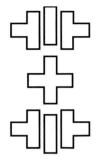

PART V

Conservative Treatment and Rehabilitation

Section I
The Patient with Structural Degenerative Disease

Chapter 23

Education: The Primary Treatment of Low-Back Pain

William Evans

Medical and Surgical Management of Spine Pathology

Health

Contemporary Educational Therapy

Barriers to Health Education

patient expectations
information overload
physician expectations
state and insurance carrier expectations
pharmaceuticals

Conclusion

Debates on medical care are being fueled by changing disease patterns, accelerating medical expenses, and mounting long-term disability costs. None of these changes are independent of psychosocial factors. In America, the doubling time for medical care expenditures is now less than 5 years.[66] To turn this condition toward better health at the least cost, we must educate and activate the latent resource of responsible patient behavior.

Early in their training, nearly all physicians have seen a patient in congestive heart failure decompensate as a result of not understanding or adhering to a prescribed no-salt diet. Virtually all physicians learned that the medical treatment of choice in this condition is not a pill or procedure, but education that results in appropriate behavior. Optimal medical management requires responsible patient compliance. When there is a lack of patient cooperation, or when a physician inappropriately takes over the patient's power and duties, there may be adverse consequences. Educational successes are being reported with better medical outcomes[38-40] and decreased costs in a wide range of problems[54,75,100] Previous attempts to decrease low-back pain by educational,[14] ergonomic, or treatment methods have generally failed.[79] However, the mounting epidemic demands that we re-examine education in light of successes in other medical fields. In spine care, education could be especially useful in rectifying the imbalances in the distribution of responsibilities between the patient and society and the patient and physician.

In spine care, teaching patients to take responsibility for their backs will not be enough. Education of the general public and the policy makers who influence the psychosocial factors that promote and encourage unnecessary illness behavior and disability will also be required. Although further improvement in our diagnostic and therapeutic skills is needed, it is obvious that something important is lacking. The growing burden of spine costs cannot continue to be borne by the employers and nations of Europe and North America.[13,28,80,94] The patient must participate in the management of his/her low-back pain. Treatment failures, prolonged recoveries, and increased costs associated with treating patients in the workers' compensation system are already known to physicians and surgeons.[29,41,93] In 1989 one insurance carrier paid "almost $4 million per working day for low back claims" with 65.8% of these costs consumed by worker lost time and 32.4% by medical expenses.[103] The distinctions between backaches, back injuries, and back disabilities have become blurred.[42] However, it is clear that no nation can afford to give everyone who complains of a backache a disability pension.

The prevalence of lumbar disc degeneration increases with advancing years to become a nearly universal phenomenon, but in most cases this is an aging change tolerated with little or no associated disability.[8,25,89,107] However, a treatment system that lacks goals, methods, and a purpose for managing chronic illness[58] will find itself increasingly uncertain and inept when confronted by the medical and psychosocial dilemma of low-back pain. The path from backache to disability has now become a highway,[13,34,80] and children can learn from the behavior of their parents.[90] Complex problems are easily oversimplified. However, it is equally true that complexities can obscure the fundamentals of a problem. New treatment guidelines[36,64,96] and suggestions in health care reform proposals[26,66,100] offer the opportunity to emphasize patient participation in shared decision-making and self-care responsibilities. Because adverse outcomes in spine management can result in failed back syndromes, we must balance our accelerating ability to diagnose and treat clinically irrelevant pathology[8,25,52,89,107] with an effort to educate patients, politicians, and employers about the benefits of low-back self-care and the prevention of disability. The pathology model can often fail to predict low back pain.[45,80]

Medical and Surgical Management of Spine Pathology

Medical care is most often an external service to the patient provided in a paternalistic relationship at the time of illness or injury. Both patients and physicians understand that medical care consists largely of the art and science of a practitioner's actions aiding the patient's own homeostatic mechanisms. Because nonsteroidal anti-inflammatory drugs (NSAIDs) are effective in treating acute low-back pain[19] it is understandable that patients feel that their solution must be in a pill or, if this does not effect a cure, in surgery. However, spine physicians and surgeons know the limitations as well as the benefits of medication and that even with sciatica due to lumbar disc injury surgical intervention is necessary in only a select few cases.[11]

Spine care is the distillation of knowledge and wisdom, stemming from the legacies of Hippocrates, Galen, Vesalius, Andry, Mixter, Barr, Hirsch, and many other teachers. Since the seventeenth century, medicine has been identifying the disease that underlies the patient's distress as the most effective way to treat symptoms. From pathologically based medical practice and research grew the specific and effective medical management and surgical treatment of many conditions. In 1934, Mixter and Barr realized the significance of a displaced nucleus pulposus and operated on the first patient with the preoperative diagnosis of a ruptured intervertebral disc.[76] "Surgeons throughout the world quickly rushed to adopt disc removal."[110] In selected cases not responding to conservative care, this is an effective treatment for a focal acute disc herniation. On the other hand, surgical failures can contribute to iatrogenically induced disability.[10,35,62]

Dubos referred to the tradition wherein understanding a disease meant understanding its cause as the "doctrine of specific etiology."[22] Despite the success of the disease-illness paradigm in some disorders, it has limitations that cannot be disregarded. Some features of illness, low-back pain included, may be independent of the physiologic derangement. Some diseases "do not necessarily produce illness, and the quality of the illness may not be predictable from knowledge of the disease,"[109] as is the case with the distinction between disc degeneration and disc disease. Adherence to the doctrine of specific etiology has obstructed our understanding that disease can also occur from adaptive failure[78] or be multifactorial.[33] Salk observed, "Until we see the sources of pathology as partly attributable to ignorance of what is required for maintaining health, we will continue to search for causes which can be eliminated or prevented, when, in fact, some of the pathology we seek to suppress is the result of our failure to do certain things that actively evoke and maintain a state of balance."[92] Historically, patients actively sought to cope and stay functional despite their low-back pain. Today the predominant focus in low-back pain is still on the physician-led search for spine pathology and intervention; it is not yet on maintaining activity and balance. The discovery of disease is rewarded. Disability is reinforced by a system that enables illness behavior.

Fortunately, Waddell has emphasized the natural history of low-back pain as a benign self-limited condition and has explained the relevance of the biopsychosocial medical model to understanding low-back disability. He calls attention to the success of low-back pain management by rehabilitation and restoration of function rather than rest.[101] The boundaries between a healthy spine and a diseased one are often unclear, and this is the daily problem faced by physicians treating patients with backaches and back injuries. A degenerative lumbar disc will occur in 30% to 60% of a normal asymptomatic population under

age 35,[8,25,89,107] and 20 percent of the normal population under 60 will have an asymptomatic herniated lumbar disc on imaging studies.[8,107] Twenty-four percent of an asymptomatic population between 18 and 76 years of age had an abnormal lumbar disc on myelography.[52] Jensen et al. found that only 36% of 98 asymptomatic subjects had normal lumbar discs.[59] In order to proceed with appropriate active medical intervention for back pain without risking an iatrogenic aggravation, the physician must distinguish whether a patient's lumbar spine pathology is significant. This is often a dilemma, but physicians and surgeons involved in spine care have recognized the dangers of ignoring psychosocial factors and are joining cognitive practitioners in adopting the biopsychosocial medical model.[101]

Nevertheless, Cats-Baril and Frymoyer report that U.S. Social Security low-back disability claims are increasing at 14 times the rate of population growth.[13] Nachemson has compiled an international comparison of disabling low-back pain that shows that the workers of Canada, Great Britain, West Germany, the Netherlands, and Sweden all annually have a greater number of back-related days absent from work than those in the United States.[80] An increase in spine disease does not seem a reasonable explanation for this international explosion of lumbar disability; rather, psychosocial factors are likely the most significant cause.[4,5] Sweden leads the world in low-back disability, not because of more injuries or increased pathology, but, says Nachemson, because it has the highest take-home pay of any nation in the world for those sick or injured.[81] Hadler, who has urged physicians to return to being "patient advocates in the service of clinical truth,"[44] points out that in many nations physicians have become involved in a complex "pivotal role" in disability programs when they are asked to judge whether an injury is consolidated (maximum medical improvement). While understanding pathology and its significance is fundamental to modern medicine and results in effective treatment of selected cases, today's collective medical intervention has not achieved control of the low-back disability epidemic with pharmacologic and surgical methods. Given the complexity of this dilemma it is useful to look at the responsibilities and expectations of patients and physicians.

With the progress of medicine over the past 100 years, it is understandable that the public has come to expect effective answers from the medical community. Although a cure is not available for all human ailments, with some authentic cures has come the hope and expectation that medical science will have a cure for every discomfort, disorder, and disease. This expectation is unrealistic and has led to an imbalance in patient-physician responsibilities. The infectious diseases early in this century—tuberculosis and pneumonia—are no longer the problem they were. Chronic diseases, including low-back pain and destructive living patterns, have become today's costly medical concerns.[61] The truth is that physicians are now often asked and tempted to intervene actively in problems and domains that are the patient's own health care responsibility. The power of medicine is not all-encompassing, and medical practitioners increasingly acknowledge the role the patient plays in maintaining his/her own health.[43,46,61,68]

In the past, the individual with back pain was challenged to be responsible for his/her health, strength, and coping strategies. Given what we know from history and current Third World experience, this approach works. Patients have abilities and resources that should not be ignored. Physicians' words are known to influence healthful behavior.[68] But as the Institute of Medicine[57] and others[87] have noted, this traditional trust is being questioned. Today, modern medicine and compensation systems can reward dependence and disability rather than promote independence and health. Many physicians have become so involved in mastering the technical aspects of disease management and are so hassled by the barriers to caring for people in modern practice they have little time for teaching about coping, independence, and healthful behavior. If the patient wants a "healthy back," he/she must become active and responsible, and the physician must understand and promote healthful action.[43]

Health

The pathologically based medical model views health as the absence of disease and may make it difficult to see many "normal" people as healthy. If we instead view health as the ability to work and love we can encourage patients to function despite their backaches and degenerative discs. Kass argues, "Health is a state of being, not something that can be given. . . . It no more makes sense to claim a right to health, than a right to wisdom or courage. . . . To make my health someone else's duty is not only unfair, it imposes a duty impossible to fulfill. . . . Doctors and public health officials have only limited powers to improve our health. Health is not a commodity that can be delivered. Medicine can only help those who help themselves."[60] Health resides in the power and action of the individual. In health care, the patient is the autonomous manager and the

physician is a resource, teacher, or partner. While general education programs can convey large amounts of information to large numbers of people, there has not yet been a substitute developed for conversing one-on-one with a physician. Often the moment of greatest potential for turning someone toward balance and health occurs when the patient seeks out a physician for the problem or condition that disturbs him/her. When the complaint is heard, the doctor determines whether the treatment of choice is education, medication, surgery, or a combination, for doctor in Latin means "teacher; one who gives instruction in some branch of knowledge."[85] A teacher of health is one who has the knowledge, experience, insight, and skill to communicate with compassion to the patient, recognize the essence of his/her problem, and lead that person toward the self-care skills necessary to achieve optimal recovery and independence. Talking with people is time-intensive. Will the physician have the time and necessary resources to do this, or will he/she only write a prescription to dull the symptoms, an action that alone could also regrettably dull the patient's sense of healing capacities and self-accountability? If we only operate or medicate, when in reality the treatment of choice also calls for education, we take away the patient's power—perhaps his/her health potential. However, skillful physicians have always aspired for their patients to move from medical care to health, and much of the current practice of health education results from the work of dedicated clinicians and researchers.

Contemporary Educational Therapy

The greatest successes today in health education can be seen in two great medical problems—heart disease[82] and cancer.[17] "During the past two decades, there have been substantial reductions in death rates from acute myocardial infarction in both men and women in the United States. These reductions, which have occurred in both whites and blacks, are attributable to efforts in primary prevention as well as improved therapies for myocardial infarction."[68] Hadler, however cautions we have accomplishd more in terms of medicalization than health promotion over the past 50 years. (Hadler N personal communication 1993). He argues that physicians perhaps out of self interest, fail to inform the layman about how to deal with the claims and counter claims offered as dogma by medicine. Nevertheless, as a result of education, "the prevalence of smoking has decreased substantially, from 40 percent in 1965 to 29 percent in 1987."[68]

Despite these successes, serious questions have been raised about whether education is a viable primary treatment approach to low-back pain. One published low-back educational trial found that physician training resulted in improved knowledge, confidence, and behavior with low-back pain patients. However, this program did not result in improved patient outcome satisfaction.[14]

The purpose and outcome measurement of education as the primary treatment of low-back pain cannot be based solely on patient satisfaction. The confounding effect of psychosocial factors in workers reporting low-back pain make it clear that the solution to their psychosocial problem(s) may not exist in spine therapy. In this paper, the rationale for education as the primary management of low-back pain is based on respect for that fundamental principle *primum non nocere* and the fact in the historical record and in the Third World there is no evidence of a large-scale low-back disability problem. Spine practitioners can learn from the methods and success of education in other medical fields, but we must recognize that this educational program cannot be measured only by patient reports of satisfaction. To apply these principles to spine care, physicians must balance how they legitimize and treat low-back pain with a strong and effective strategy of educating and informing not only patients, but also employers, community populations, insurance systems, political leaders, and policy makers. Education is needed to avoid expropriating patient power, inducing iatrogenic disability and misusing medical care to fix a psychosocial problem.

Despite Waddell's recommendation of a new clinical model,[101] most physicians treating low-back pain currently think first of intervention with medication, next of surgery, and last of education. Many insurance systems reinforce this thinking by refusing to compensate for patient education. The first priority ought to be education. An education-based low-back paradigm is inexpensive, beginning with providing reassuring information to the patient.[43] The seeds of the educational approach exist in back schools,* functional restorative programs,[49,70,71] and innovative prevention and rehabilitation strategies.[37,72] What does not yet exist is sufficient focus and emphasis on education in the primary management of low-back pain. In this case, the objective of

education is to help patients learn to help and trust themselves. This may be done by a variety of methods, but the attitude with which education is delivered is key. Adequate training and skills in teaching health education to a patient take time and commitment, as do all medical and surgical care. Information can best be received and integrated in a safe and trusting relationship.[86] The purpose of education is not to coddle or unduly protect; nor is it a license to substitute only education for necessary patient medical or surgical treatment or to deny legitimate disability. The physician must be guided by both his understanding of the patient's pathology and by a coherent concept of the biocultural basis of health[15,18]—both personal and social. Holding the tension between when to intervene in the pathology and how to activate the patient's self responsibility is the challenge. The ability to identify personality types and recognize learning styles helps a clinician to adjust his/her teaching and instruction methods[30,51,73,98,104] (see box below). There will be pathologic conditions which will take precedence and override this educational paradigm.

Even in acute management, patient education begins at the first visit to the clinician with an explanation and interpretation of the history and the physical examination findings. The overwhelming majority of patients at that time are in pain and frightened but can be reassured that they will not need surgery and

*References 7, 12, 31, 50, 71, and 111.

Candidates for Patient Education

Inclusion Criteria

Patients experiencing low-back pain with or without leg pain due to sprain, strain, degenerative disc disease, bulging or herniated discs, or stenosis.

Exclusion Criteria

Patients suspected of having a malignancy.

Patients with an infectious process of the spine.

Surgical emergencies—cauda equina syndrome or progressive neurologic deficit.

Patients with cognitive impairment or language barriers.

Adapted from Treatment Choices for Low Back Pain, Foundation for Informed Decision Making and Massachusetts General Hospital.

are appropriate candidates for conservative care. "You will get better. You will not be paralyzed." Improvement occurs within 6 to 12 weeks in 85% to 90% of low-back-injured patients.[1,95,99] Therefore, reassurance that low-back pain is most often benign and self-limited is calming and can reduce fear. LaCroix found that 94% of patients with a good understanding of their condition returned to work, whereas only 33% of patients with a poor understanding of their condition returned to employment.[63] Rest for low-back pain may be helpful for up to 2 to 3 days.[21] With a disc herniation, bed rest for no more than 1 to 2 weeks is highly effective.[102,108] Longer inactivity may be deleterious.[47,53,69,111] Reassurance that activity is helpful promotes return to function.* Pain is an inevitable part of being alive. Some pain treatment can heal and relieve, but there is much it cannot rectify. The myth that life should be pain-free may promote excessive use of medication and unnecessary avoidance of activity and problem solving. In the absence of severe sciatic pain or stenosis, walking is often the preferred initial activity, and performing daily activities and working restores confidence. Patients are told they must do two things—become active to regain their strength, and become informed about how their back is built in order to avoid creating unnecessary aggravations. In a randomized series, Weber followed 280 patients with sciatica due to a herniated lumbar disc and found that *both* the patients who had surgery and those who didn't adjusted to their strenuous Norwegian daily activities in spite of their back disease.[102]

Back school provides information on spine anatomy and function, and was found to be one of only three interventions identified by the Quebec Task Force on Spinal Disorders[96] as effective for patients in randomized, controlled trials. Back school is highly effective between 7 days and 6 weeks postinjury and has resulted in returning patients to work 1 week earlier. Acute patients are instructed to avoid lifting heavy objects, to stand close to the work site, to avoid bending the back, to avoid twisting, to change position frequently, to avoid sitting in low chairs, and to use a lumbar support and arm rest when sitting.[79] Back school uses simple words and illustrations to point out the importance for patients of moving around their center of gravity. They learn to locate their center of gravity, which is in front of their lumbar spine—where they experience pain. Patients are reminded of the importance of careful

*References 32, 55, 56, 77, 105, and 106.

Goals for Patient Education

1. Assign responsibility—90% of patients with low-back pain who leave the primary physician's office need to know they have a patient-managed condition.

2. Reassure—the natural history of most low-back pain is one of improvement.

3. Prescribe and direct patient behavior—rest rarely needs to exceed 3 days; encourage activation and return to function.

4. Instruct in spine function, injury prevention, strengthening, and stabilization.

body mechanics in preventing another injury or aggravation. When they see the lack of rotation in the low back resulting from the relationship of the facet joints, patients understand the dangers of twisting. They can practice the safe way to turn with proper footwork or in chairs or vehicle seats. Patients learn that back pain may recur and are warned to be prepared to handle aggravations, as well as guided to recognize the changes that do require a physician evaluation. Because many of us now live in a world defined by automobiles, machinery, computers, telephones, and television, it is useful to remind urban patients that they are living beings who must balance activity and rest (see box above).

Physical activity restores confidence as well as tissue and aerobic strength. Functional restoration is the key to the rehabilitation of chronic low-back pain.[49,69-71] Some patients need coaching to identify their safe zone of movement when they begin conditioning. Pacing and quality of movement are developed for the years ahead. In the recovery process, it is necessary to challenge patients not only physically but also mentally by establishing both short- and long-term goals. Specific goals for improvement on quantitative physical function tests guide the rehabilitation programs and include trunk strength and flexibility and cardiovascular (aerobic) fitness, with the ultimate goal of independence and return to work.[69] Patients are advised that there is a greater prevalence of disc degeneration in smokers as compared to nonsmokers.[6] For patients with permanent structural injury and impairment, the rehabilitation process provides "the handicapped person with the knowledge and skills to overcome barriers."[88] The educational components of this process are accepting the handicap, goal setting, understanding the barriers, pain management methods, and reinforcement through repetition (see box on next page).[88]

Physician Guidelines

1. See the patient as a powerful and useful person.

2. Education is the link to hold the tension between the patient's responsibilities and pathology.

3. Know when overriding the patient's power and responsibility with intervention can result in an improved outcome.

(from Mulley, AG *Clinician's Guide*)

In some cases the clinician will point out to patients that not only will their lives and work depend on their successful recovery, but that their children will learn from their coping skills.[90] Children will either learn illness behavior and dependency or that "I had a parent with a backache, but he got better and learned to live with it." For those whose injury results in a catastrophic disruption of their lives—family, work, recreation, and social support system—it is useful to explain the process of adapting and rebuilding lives. As Mitchell says, "It's not what happens to you. It's what you do about it" (Mitchell W: personal communication, 1991). Successful education is achieved through effective communication. Patients are counseled that the path of disability focuses on pathology and is accompanied by atrophy and depression. On the other hand, health focuses on the ability to work and love, which is possible even in the presence of aging changes and injury. Instruction in stabilization skills enables patients with symptomatic disc injuries to improve truncal strength and function[91] (see boxed material at the top of p 352).

Success with health education has also been demonstrated in patients who have undergone spinal surgery and patients with arthritis as well as victims of spinal cord injuries. Surgeons have incorporated preoperative patient educational programs into their practices,[72] and this model has been so successful it is being replicated in multiple locations (Selby D: personal communication, 1992). Lorig and Holman report that patients in the Arthritis Self-Management Program showed a 19% reduction in pain and a 43% reduction in physician visits even after 4 years. The project showed that if 1% of Americans suffering from rheumatoid arthritis and osteoarthritis achieved the same benefits as did the participants in its 4-year follow-up, the reduction in medical costs would be $2.9 million and $14.5 million dollars, respectively.[54] They identified self-efficacy (confidence) as a positive psychologic factor that correlated better with improved health outcomes than did behavioral changes.[37] In spinal cord rehabilitation, Menter describes the goals of health education philosophy: "In an acute spinal cord injury the rehabilitation team has a responsibility to undertake a course of paternalism in which decisions are made for, and in the best interest of, the individual. The process of acute rehabilitation is one of gradually returning responsibility and autonomy to the individual consistent with his or her medical stability and knowledge and the ability to make decisions. However, the interaction of an individual with chronic illness with health care professionals is different. This is now a partnership of mutual responsibility for *education, learning, and planning*."[74] (Emphasis added.) "Think First" is an innovative nationwide program developed by America's neurosurgeons to prevent spinal cord and head injuries in young people—the population at highest risk.[27] It is too early to have significant data yet, but the magnitude and quality of the program are impressive. From nonspecific low-back pain to spinal cord rehabilitation, the goal of patient independence is primary and achieved through education.

A national low-back educational program has been recommended by the author to the North American Spine Society. The Foundation for Informed Medical Decision-Making has developed generic interactive video programs and written materials[20] for patient education in nonspecific low-back pain, spinal stenosis, and herniated disc. In the latter, the patient is given a balanced presentation of the possible advantages and disadvantages of surgery. Risks of disc surgery, overall results, and outcomes at 4 and 10 years for surgical versus nonsurgical management are provided.

The vision of health education today is expanding. Recently, the U.S. Public Health Service published *Healthy People 2000,* a concept of the future of American health—332 objectives in 22 broad categories, using "three approaches of health promotion, health protection, and preventive (educational) services as organizing categories, but running through the priority areas and the objectives is a common theme of shared responsibility for carrying out this national agenda. Achievement of the agenda depends heavily on changes in individual behaviors. . . . It calls on medical and health professionals to prevent, not just to treat, the diseases and conditions that result in premature death and chronic disability." For the spine, specific goals are to increase by at least 50% the proportion of work sites with 50 or more employees that offer back injury prevention and rehabilitation programs and to reduce activity limitation due to chronic back conditions to no more than 19 per 1000 people (base line, average of 21.9 per 1000 during 1986-1988).[16]

Physicians can now educate employers that perceptions of work, job satisfaction, and other psychosocial factors have been found to play a greater role in industrial back pain complaints than did the physical measures studied.[4,5] These findings are consistent with those of other studies,[2,65] but some employers still view the worker as a throw-away component in the production process. The Juan de Fuca hospital system found instead that the most effective treatment for an injured employee was a telephone call from the immediate supervisor affirming his value by stating "you're so valuable, we can't afford to replace you. You are a vital part of the hospital team. Your work is important and your job is waiting for you."[112] The solution to the social-economic pathology that inappropriately rewards and promotes disability calls for physicians knowledgeable not only about spine management but also about social and political educational challenges. Physicians can educate politicians and insurance systems that the settlement of claims and decreased litigation speeds return to work. When disability payments for low-back pain increase, low-back disability increases. Nachemson has discussed the political problems of low-back disability and reported the proceedings of the U.S. Senate Hearings which, in 1976, documented that the threshold of increased disability claims lies at about 55% of net income. If the income received during sickness or injury exceeds this percentage, the number of claims increases drastically.[79]

Health education is growing in some medical and surgical practices and succeeds in blending technology with teaching. While this chapter is concerned primarily with physicians and patients, a successful low-back education paradigm will demand that insurance systems and political programs provide for those truly disabled but no longer encourage the able-bodied to lean on disability. To achieve control and balance with the low-back pain problem, all parties, including unions, employers, insurance policy makers, and politicians must promote patient stability and independence. However, even then significant obstacles will exist.

Barriers to Health Education

Scientific progress and validated studies do not necessarily result in healthful behavior. Patient reassurance takes time and is not always easily achieved, especially with workers' compensation patients. Modifying behavior is more easily said than done, and this is the case for physicians as well as patients. The ancient medical tradition of advocacy for healthful behavior and balanced living has been neglected. What was once the trunk of the tree of medicine—patient education—does not support and balance today's growth of specialized medical and surgical branches. Most of academic medicine and most physicians are now more oriented toward new pharmaceuticals and technical procedures than toward teaching. The skills and methods of health education and behavioral change are not in the core medical education curriculum. There are, thus, mixed signals on the horizon for health education and, in fact, the current expectations of patients, physicians, and insurance carriers pose significant barriers.

Patient Expectations

Over this century, many patients seem to have moved away from taking responsibility for their behavior and their medical care. The success of pharmaceuticals has led patients to expect a quick solution to pain. Another possible explanation may be that even before they fall victim to sickness or injury, some Americans suffer from a lack of confidence and belief in their own abilities and judgment. In overcrowded urban concentrations, they are increasingly subject to job layoffs and economic fluctuations beyond their control. It stands to reason that if sedentary urban dwellers lose power and a sense of meaning in their lives, they no longer retain ethics of self-sufficiency and responsibility. They will tend to assume a more passive attitude regarding their health. Physicians may want to consider when intervention should be balanced with education if they want to stop contributing to further deterioration of patient capacities and instead to promote patient empowerment.

Information Overload

Confusing or excessive information may promote dependence and exacerbate a patient's tendency to transfer responsibility to physicians. Never in history has there been more information and knowledge available to more people; never has wisdom been more needed or endangered. Much televised information is accompanied by advertising—which may be misinformation. The message is that technology can solve all problems, and foolish ways of living may be encouraged. The role of parents in the education of their children is decreasing; male parent teaching began to diminish years ago with the industrial revolution and now, female parent teaching is decreasing with the entry of more mothers into the working world. The ability to absorb wisdom may be impaired when the cognitive overload becomes excessive. Because of the potential for confusion during information overload, the need for meaningful, individualized patient-physician communication is increased.

Physician Expectations

More medical care does not always result in better health. It can have the opposite effect.[9,23,25,97] It will remain fragmented from the wholeness of health, despite the power of modern medicine today, until it can more effectively unite with patient health education. Teaching patients has become overshadowed by the powerful diagnostic and therapeutic armamentarium available to the contemporary physician.

But the astute clinician who knows when to say, "A pill or procedure is not the answer here," can be influential. On the other hand, a patient may be understandably stopped from action or reflection if he/she is told "there is nothing that can be done"; this is regrettable if in reality the patient's condition would benefit from education. Education has yet to find its full role in connecting medicine and surgery to health.

State and Insurance Carrier Expectations

The compensation system to a large degree determines what is performed in medical care and health care. American physicians do not expect to be paid for educational services. Current compensation regulations discourage physician teaching. For reasons they have never chosen to reveal, most medical insurance companies have taken a strong anti-health-education posture, although they have enthusiastically embraced the term *health care* for marketing purposes. "No serious national (American) educational effort will take place until the problem of reimbursement is solved. The present blanket exclusion of preventive (educational) services from federal health insurance programs is not responsive to the current state of knowledge.[57]

Pharmaceuticals

While nonsteroidal antiinflammatory medications are highly effective in the first 3 months of both non-specific low-back pain and lumbar disc herniation, dependence on these medications often exceeds 3 months. Long-term use of opiates or semisynthetic analgesics can contribute to a patient's increasing disability, and their use is basically incompatible with a functional restoration approach.[69] Drugs have always had the ability to seduce and addict. Their current potency is enhanced by new levels of refinement and specificity. Seldom are medications withheld when they are "indicated." Unfortunately, distinc-

tion is not always made between drugs that are curative or life essential, those that have a limited but specific therapeutic window, and the prescriptions that may be unnecessary. It is when drugs are used excessively or unnecessarily to do what the patient would better do for himself that problems occur. The unnecessary prescription written as a "ticket out the door" may actually be a stumbling block to a patient's recovery and health. Osler counseled, "One of the first duties of the physician is to educate the masses not to take (unnecessary) medicine."[3] Imperative drugging—the ordering of medicine in any and every malady is no longer regarded as the chief function of the doctor."[84] When to medicate and when to educate is a challenging question because a prescription can be written quickly, while talking and teaching require more time and care.

Conclusion

The health education paradigm for managing low-back pain is patient-centered rather than physician-centered. The power is given to the patient, who will do with it as he/she chooses. This orientation presumes the individual to be the key decision-maker with respect to his/her own back and health. Education provides information to aid decisions and is a low-cost, low-technology initial approach to back pain; it encourages and empowers patient participation in the process and outcome of treatment. It does not preclude effective medical and surgical intervention in carefully selected patients. Knowledgeable clinicians will be expected to override the educational paradigm when the pathology dictates. However, if this educational construct receives acceptance from the spine care and larger community, physicians and surgeons will need to tighten the criteria by which they intervene and expropriate from the patient control of back-pain management.

The goal of independent patient self-care contrasts with the current pathologically dominated view. Overutilizing pharmacologic and surgical methods to treat low-back pain too often promotes patient dependence, which in turn is supported by an enabling disability-compensation system. The question physicians face daily is whether a patient's condition is to be treated by medical care (intervention by the clinician on the patient's behalf) or rather by health education to induce action by the patient for his/her own benefit. The educational process not only involves patients but also employers, community populations, insurance systems, political leaders and policy makers. This view will need to earn acceptance from patients, physicians, academic medicine, insurance carriers, and governments.

In most cultures, the physician-patient relationship is a clearly stated and acknowledged equal partnership; doctors teach patients as well as intervene on their behalf. Western medicine has become so powerful that this balance now seldom exists. However, for the most effective medical care and virtually all of spine care, greater patient responsibility is needed. Both patients and physicians share responsibilities in health education. Payment reform for educational services is necessary. Forty years ago, in 1952, Macnab, speaking in London on "Structural Changes in the Lumbar Intervertebral Discs," chose "*to avoid confusion,*" (Emphasis added.) and not to use the term *disc degeneration* except when changes in the disc occurred prematurely or to an unusual degree.[48] Low-back education chooses to avoid confusing and frightening patients and is able to reassure nearly all of them that they will get better and most certainly can and need to continue with active lives and work. "The vital necessity to know as much about the patient who has the backache as about the backache the patient has,"[67] can only be achieved by talking with the person and in that conversation resides the opportunity to affirm and bless the patient's value and usefulness.

References

1. Abenhaim L, Suissa S: Importance and economic burden of occupational back pain: a study of 2500 cases representative of Quebec, *J Occup Med* 29:670, 1987.
2. Andersson GBJ: *The epidemiology of spinal disorders.* In Frymoyer J, editor: *The adult spine,* New York, 1991, Raven Press, p 129.
3. Auden W, Kronenberger L: *Aphorisms.* New York, 1966, Viking.
4. Battie M, Bigos S, Fisher L, et al.: A prospective study of the role of cardiovascular risk factors and fitness in industrial back pain complaints, *Spine* 14:141, 1989.
5. Bigos S, Spengler D, Martin N, Zeh J, et al.: Back injuries in industry: a retrospective study. III. Employee related factor, *Spine* 11:252, 1986.
6. Battie M, Videman T, Gill K, et al.: Smoking and lumbar intervertebral disc degeneration: an MRI study of identical twins, *Spine* 16:1015, 1991.
7. Blair SN, Oiserchia PV, Wilbur CS, Crowder JH: A public health intervention model for work-site health promotion: impact on exercise and physical fitness in a health promotion plan after 24 months, *JAMA* 255:921, 1986.
8. Boden S, Davis D, Dina T, et al.: Abnormal magnetic resonance scans of the lumbar spine in asymptomatic subjects, *J Bone Joint Surg* 72A:403, 1990.
9. Brennan T, Leape L, Laird N, et al.: Incidence of adverse events and negligence in hospitalized patients—results of the Harvard Medical Practice Study I, *N Engl J Med* 324:370, 1991.
10. Burton C, Kirkaldy-Willis W, Yong-Hing K, et al.: Causes of failure of surgery on the lumbar spine, *Clin Orthop* 157:191, 1981.
11. Bush K, Cowan N, Katy D, et al.: The natural history of sciatica associated with disc pathology, *Spine* 17:1205, 1992.
12. Cady LD, Thomas PC, Karwasky RJ: Program for increasing health and physical fitness of firefighters, *J Occup Med* 2:111, 1985.
13. Cats-Baril W, Frymoyer J: *The economics of spinal disorders.* In Frymoyer J, editor: *The adult spine,* New York, 1991, Raven Press.
14. Cherkin D, Deyo R, Berg A: Evaluation of a physician education intervention to improve primary care for low-back pain. II. Impact on patients, *Spine* 16:1173, 1991.
15. Conger J: Behavioral medicine and health psychology in a changing world, *Child Abuse Neglect* 11:443, 1987.
16. Department of Health and Human Services: Healthy People 2000, Washington, D.C., 1991, Office of the Asst Sec for Health (DHHS pub. no. (PHS) 91-50213).
17. Department of Health and Human Services: Reducing the health consequences of smoking. 25 years of progress: a report of the Surgeon General, Washington, D.C. 1989, Government Printing Office (DHHS pub. no. (CDC) 89-8411).
18. Dever G: Community health analysis. Gaithersburg, MD, 1991, *Aspen.*
19. Deyo R: Conservative therapy for low back pain: Distinguishing useful from useless therapy, *JAMA* 250:1057, 1983.
20. Deyo R: Patient treatment choices for low back problems, 1992, Foundation for Informed Medical Decision Making.
21. Deyo R, Diehl A, Rosenthal M: How many days of bed rest for acute low back pain, *N Engl J Med* 315:1064, 1986.
22. Dubos R: *Man adapting.* New Haven, CT, 1965, Yale University Press.
23. Dvorak J, Ganchat M, Valach L: The outcome of surgery for lumbar disc herniations, *Spine* 13:1418, 1987.
24. Dvorak J, Valach L, Euhrimann P: The outcome of surgery for lumbar disc herniation II, *Spine* 13:1423, 1988.
25. Evans W, Jobe W, Seibert C: A cross sectional prevalence study of lumbar disc degeneration in a working population, *Spine* 14:60, 1989.
26. Evans W: Where is the health in health care reform? Unpublished.
27. Evans W: Think first, *Colo Med* 88:98, 1991
28. Federspiel C, Guy D, Kane D, Spenger D: Expenditures for nonspecific back injuries in the workplace, *J Occup Med* 31:919, 1989.
29. Flynn J, Hogue M: Anterior fusion of the lumbar spine: end result study with long-term follow up, *J Bone Joint Surg* 61:1143, 1979.
30. Ford C: Illness as a life style: the role of somatization in medical practice, *Spine* 17:10S:338, 1992.
31. Fordyce WE, Brockway JA, Bergman JA, Spengler D: Acute back pain: a control-group comparison of behavioral vs. traditional management methods, *J Behav Med* 9:127, 1986.

32. Forrsselt M: The back school, *Spine* 6:104, 1981.
33. Frymoyer J: Back pain and sciatica, *N Engl J Med* 318:291, 1988.
34. Frymoyer J, Cats-Baril W: Predictors of low back pain disability, *Clin Orthop* 21:89, 1987.
35. Gill K, Frymoyer J: *The management of treatment failures after decompressure surgery.* In Frymoyer J, editor: *The adult spine,* New York, 1991, Raven Press, p 1849.
36. Goldman B, Evans W, Fitzgerald E, et al.: Low back pain guidelines. Denver, CO, 1992, Colorado State Department of Labor.
37. Gonzalez V, Goeppinger J, Lorig K: Four psychosocial theories and their application to patient education and clinical practice, *Arthritis Care Res* 3:133, 1990.
38. Greenfield S, Kaplan SH, Ware JE Jr: Expanding patient involvement in care: effects on patient outcomes, *Ann Intern Med* 104:520, 1985.
39. Greenfield S, Kaplan SH, Ware JE Jr, et al.: Patient participation in medical care: effects on blood sugar control and quality of life in diabetes, *J Gen Intern Med* 3:448, 1988.
40. Greenfield S, Kaplan S, Ware J, Martin E: Expanding patient involvement in care: effects on blood pressure control, Presented at the National Conference on High Blood pressure Control, April, 1985.
41. Greenough H, Fraser R: The effects of compensation on recovery from low back injury, *Spine* 14:947, 1989.
42. Hadler N: Regional backache, *N Engl J Med* 325:1090, 1986.
43. Hadler N: The predicament of the backache. *J Occup Med* 30:449, 1988.
44. Hadler N: Disabling backache in France, Switzerland and the Netherlands: contrasting sociopolitical constraints on clinical judgement, *J Occup Med* 32:823, 1989.
45. Haldeman S: Failure of the pathology model to predict back pain, *Spine* 15:718, 1990.
46. Hamburg D, Elliott G, Parron D: *Health and behavior: frontiers of research in the biobehavioral sciences,* Washington, D.C., 1982, National Academy Press.
47. Hansson T, Roos B, Nachemson A: Development of osteopenia in the fourth lumbar vertebra during prolonged bed rest after operation for scoliosis, *Acta Orthop Scand* 46:621, 1975.
48. Harris R, Macnab I: Structural changes in the lumber intervertebral discs, *J Bone Joint Surg* 36B:304, 1054.
49. Hazard R, Fenwick J, Kalisch S, et al.: Functional restoration with behavioral support and a one year prospective study of patients with chronic low back pain, *Spine* 14:157, 1989.
50. Hazard RG, Fenwick J, Kalish S, et al.: Functional restoration with behavioral support: a one year prospective study of chronic low back pain patients. Presented at the ISSLS Meeting, Miami, Florida. April 13-17, 1988.
51. Hendler N, Mollett A, Talo S, et al.: A comparison between the Minnesota Multiphasic Personality Inventory and Mensana Clinic Back Test for validating the complaint of chronic pain, *J Occup Med* 30:98, 1988.
52. Hitselberger W, Witten R: Abnormal myelograms in asymptomatic patients, *J Neurosurg* 18:1720, 1968.
53. Holm S, Nachemson A: Variations in the nutrition of the canine intervertebral disc induced by motion, *Spine* 8:866, 1983.
54. Holman H, Margonson P, Long K: Health education for self management has significant and sustained benefits in chronic arthritis, *Trans Assoc Am Physicians* 102(204):204, 1989.
55. Hurri H: The Swedish back school in chronic low back pain. Part I. Benefits, *Scand J Rehab Med* 21:33, 1989.
56. Hurri H: The Swedish back school in chronic low back pain. Part II. Factors predicting the outcome, *Scand J Rehab* Med 21:41, 1989.
57. Institute of Medicine. Medical education and societal needs: a planning report for the health professions, Washington, D.C., 1983, National Academy Press.
58. Jennings B, Callahan D, Caplan A: Ethical challenges of chronic illness, Hastings Cent Rep Suppl. Feb/Mar, 1988.
59. Jensen M, Brant-Zawadzki M, Obuchowski N, Modic M, et al.: Magnetic resonance imaging of the lumbar spine in people without back pain, *N Eng J Med* 331:69-73, 1994.
60. Kass L: *Toward a more natural science,* New York, 1985, The Free Press, p 157.
61. Knowles J, editor: *Doing better and feeling worse: health in the United States,* New York, 1977, WW Norton.
62. Kostuik J, Frymoyer J: *Failures after spine fusion.* In Frymoyer J, editor: *The adult spine,* New York, 1991, Raven Press, p 2027.
63. LaCroix J, Powell J, Lloyd G: Low back pain, factors of value in predicting outcome, *Spine* 15:495, 1990.
64. Lee C: Low back pain treatment guidelines, *Spine,* 1991.
65. Levine M: Depression, back pain, and disc protrusion: relationship and proposed psychophysiotopic mechanisms, *Dis Nerv Syst* 32:41, 1971.
66. Lundberg G: National health care reform: The aura of inevitability intensities, *JAMA* 267:2521, 1992.
67. Macnab I: *Backache,* Baltimore, 1977, Williams & Wilkins.
68. Manson J, Tosteson H, Ridker P, et al.: The primary prevention of myocardial infarction, *N Engl J Med* 326:1406, 1992.
69. Mayer T, Gatchel R: *Function restoration for spinal disorders: the sports medicine approach,* Lea and Febiger. 1988, Philadelphia.
70. Mayer T, Gatchel R, Kishino N, et al.: Objective assessment of spine function. Following industrial industry, *Spine* 10:489, 1985.
71. Mayer T, Gatchel R, Mayer H, et al.: A perspective two-year study of functional restoration in industrial low back injury: an objective assessment procedure, *JAMA* 258:1763, 1989.
72. McCoy S, Selby J, Henderson R: Patients avoiding surgery: pathology and one year life status follow up, *Spine* 16(Suppl 6):198, 1991.
73. Melzack R, Katz J, Jean M: The role of compensation in chronic pain: analysis using a new method

of scoring the McGill Pain Questionnaire, *Pain* 23:101, 1985.

74. Menter R: *Aging with spinal cord injury,* New York, 1992, Demos Publications, p 327.

75. Miller L, Goldstein J: More efficient care of diabetic patients in a county hospital setting, *N Engl J Med* 286:1388, 1972.

76. Mixter W, Barr J: Rupture of the intervertebral disc with involvement of the spinal cord, *N Engl J Med* 211:210, 1934.

77. Moffett J, Chase S, Portek I, et al.: A controlled, prospective study to evaluate the effectiveness of a back school in the relief of chronic low back pain, *Spine* 2:120, 1986.

78. Moore L, Arsdale PL, Glittenberg J, Aldrich R: *The biocultural basis of health,* Prospect Heights, IL, 1980, Waveland Press.

79. Nachemson A: Work for all, *Clin Orthop* 179:77, 1983.

80. Nachemson A: Newest knowledge of low back pain, *Clin Orthop Relat Res* 279:8, 1992.

81. Nachemson A: *The solution: challenge of the lumbar spine,* San Antonio, TX, 1988.

82. National Center for Health Statistics: Vital statistics of the United States, 1968-1988, Washington, DC, Government Printing Office, 1968-1988.

83. Neuwelt E, Coe M, Wilkinson A, et al.: Oregon head and spinal cord injury, prevention program and evaluation, *Neurosurgery* 24:453, 1989.

84. Osler W: *Counsels and ideals,* Birmingham, England, 1985, Classics of Medicine Library, p 191.

85. Oxford English Dictionary. 1961 reprint of 1933 edition.

86. Platt F, McMath J: Clinical hypocompetence: the interview, *Ann Intern Med* 91:898, 1979.

87. Plomp N: Workers attitude toward the occupational physician, *J Occup Med* 34:893, 1992.

88. Pope M, Frymoyer J, Andersson G: *Occupational low back pain,* New York, 1984, Praeger.

89. Powell M, Wilson M, Szzyprt P, et al.: Prevalence of lumbar disc degeneration observed by magnetic resonance in symptomless women, *Lancet* 2:1366, 1986.

90. Rickard K: The occurrence of maladaptive health-related behaviors and teacher-related conduct problems in children of chronic low back pain patients, *J Behav Med* 11:107, 1988.

91. Robison R, Saal J: *The new back school stabilization training, parts I and II.* In White L, editor: *Back School,* Philadelphia, 1991, Hanley & Belfus.

92. Salk J: *The survival of the wisest,* New York, 1973, Harper & Row.

93. Sander R, Meyers J: The relationship of disability to compensation status in railroad workers, *Spine* 2:141, 1986.

94. Snook S: *Cost.* In Pope M, Frymoyer J, Andersson G, editors: *Occupational low back pain,* New York, 1984, Praeger.

95. Spendler D, Bigos S, Martin N, et al.: Back injuries in industry: a retrospective study, *Spine* 11:241, 1986.

96. Spitzer W, LeBlanc F, Dupuis M: Scientific approach to the assessment and management of activity related spinal disorders: report of the Quebec Task Force on Spinal Disorders, *Spine* 12:51, 1987.

97. Steel K, Gertman P, Crescenzi C, Anderson J: Iatrogenic illness on a general medical service at a university hospital, *N Engl J Med* 304:638, 1981.

98. Talo S, Rytokoski U, Puukka P: Patient classification: a key to evaluate pain treatment, *Spine* 17:998, 1992.

99. Vallfors B: Acute, subacute and chronic low back pain: clinical symptoms, absenteeism and working environment, *Scand J Rehab Med* 11(suppl):1, 1985.

100. Vickery D, Iverson D: *Medical self-care and use of the medical care system.* In O'Connell MP, Harris JS, editors: *Health promotion in the work place,* ed 2, Albany, NY, Delmar (in press).

101. Waddell G: A new clinical model for the treatment of low back pain, *Spine* 12:632, 1987.

102. Weber H: Lumbar disc herniation: a controlled, prospective study with ten years of observation, *Spine* 8:131, 1983.

103. Webster B, Snook S: The cost of 1989 worker's compensation low back pain claims, *Spine* 19:1111-1116, 1994.

104. Weighill V: Compensation: neurosis, *J Psychosom Res* 27:97, 1983.

105. White A, Mattmiller A, White L: *Back school and other conservative approaches to low back pain,* St. Louis, 1983, Mosby.

106. White L: *Back school state of the art reviews.* Philadelphia, 1991, Hanley & Belfus.

107. Wiesel S, Tsourmas N, Feffer H, et al.: A study of computer-assisted tomography. I. The incidence of positive CAT scans in an asymptomatic group of patients, *Spine* 9:549, 1984.

108. Wiesel S, Cuckler J, Deluca F, et al.: Acute low back pain: An objective analysis of conservative therapy, *Spine* 5:324, 1980.

109. Williams M, Hadler N: The illness as the focus of geriatric medicine, *N Engl J Med* 308:1357, 1983.

110. Wiltse L: *The history of spinal disorders.* In Frymoyer J, editor: *The adult spine,* New York, 1991, Raven Press.

111. Woo SL-Y, Buckwalter JA, editors: *Injury and repair of the musculoskeletal soft tissues: American Academy of Orthopaedic Surgeons Symposium,* Savannah, GA, 1987, American Academy of Orthopaedic Surgeons.

112. Wood D: Design and evaluation of a back injury prevention program within a geriatric hospital, *Spine* 12:77, 1987.

Acknowledgement

The author gratefully acknowledges the teaching and writing of Alf Nachemson, John Frymoyer, and Arthur White. Charles Durnin encouraged the writing of this manuscript, and Nortin Hadler, Larry VanGenderen, and Bert Goldberg kindly offered criticism. The author thanks Claudia Putnam, Lee Tilton, Jodeen Sanders, and Connie Platt for their assistance.

Chapter 24
Evaluation of Outcome Studies
Jerome A. Schofferman

Great challenges face us in the field of spinal medicine and surgery. Clinicians must continue to search for the most cost-effective ways to treat patients with spinal disorders. In this new era of medical economics the drive to lower the costs of medical care is great. Increasingly payers in the private, government, and workers' compensation sectors are insisting that the treatments we render be proven effective before they will be reimbursed. Spinal care is under especially hard scrutiny because of the large costs incurred treating patients with spinal disorders.

Many of the treatments we recommend are being challenged in a subtle way. Payers are not saying that some treatments are ineffective. Instead they say that some treatments have not been *proven* effective. Proof in the minds of payers means randomized, controlled trials (RCT). In some ways the scientific spine community has been lax. We have depended too long on uncontrolled studies with poorly defined end points and outcome criteria.[15] We have failed to insist on RCT to prove our treatments effective.

The problem is compounded further because currently there is no consensus in spine medicine regarding the preferred means to evaluate or measure the outcome of treatment. It appears axiomatic that clinicians and researchers must have the means to evaluate response to treatment. Practitioners must be able to assess an individual patient's response to treatment. Researchers must have a means to compare different treatments and to compare outcomes from one center to another.

This issue is not just academic. Treatment of a patient with spine pain must be based on scientific research, not on unproven beliefs or anecdotes. An evaluation of a patient's response to treatment or a comparison of different treatments depend on an assessment of the outcome of each patient before and after treatment.

Outcome assessment in turn depends on having a reliable method to assess a patient's status. Consensus must emerge regarding what to measure, how to measure it, and how to interpret the measurements clinically. To date, no such consensus has emerged. Any assessment technique must be "patient- and physician-friendly." It must be easy to administer and easy to score.

In response to the need for a simple and reliable way to evaluate the outcome of both conservative and surgical treatment of the patient with low-back pain, the North American Spine Society (NASS) has developed an outcome questionnaire (refer to Chapter 6). The NASS Questionnaire will always be in evolution in response to feedback from patients, clinicians, and researchers. The NASS Questionnaire can readily be modified to be used in cervical spine problems (refer to Chapter 6).

Problem of Outcome Measurement

Howe and Frymoyer demonstrated the complexity and by inference, the importance of methodology when measuring outcome.[7] They evaluated 207 patients 10 or more years after a single lumbar spine surgery. A questionnaire, which was composed of 14 other questionnaires that had been used previously in published studies to assess outcome, was administered to each patient. The composite questionnaire was then broken down into its 14 separate questionnaires. Depending on which of the 14 questionnaires was used to measure surgical success, the percentage of patients with satisfactory outcome could be varied from 60% to 97%.

These authors came to several important conclusions. A researcher can greatly influence the reported success rate of any treatment by virtue of the choice of outcome parameters. An author's bias regarding what constitutes success or failure can affect the reported outcome as much as and perhaps more than the treatment itself. The best treatment results reported are obtained when questionnaires depended heavily on subjective criteria. In general, evaluations that depend more on objective criteria show less favorable results.

The way an author chooses to categorize patients also influences outcome. Many authors classify patients into broad categories such as excellent, good, fair, or poor and arbitrarily define each category based on personal biases about what is important. One author's "good" result may be another's "fair." The lack of agreement on the criteria to define success or failure makes comparing results from different centers extremely hazardous.

It is important to consider that there are different points of view about what constitutes successful outcome. Despite considerable overlap patients, physicians, and insurers have different concerns. An individual patient may be seen as a success from one perspective but as a failure from another.

A *patient* is primarily concerned with reduction of pain and think that if pain were eliminated or reduced other problems would also improve. However, *clinicians* realize that pain reduction may not be possible, and other aspects of life such as return to work or improvement in function must be considered when evaluating outcome.

Furthermore, pain is difficult to measure. The examiner is totally dependent on the report of the patient to evaluate pain. Despite the use of questionnaires, analog scales, or other techniques, there is no way to objectify pain, nor is there a way to compare one patient's pain to another's. Any measurement of pain or change in pain is at best merely a way to quantify a subjective experience. The difficulty with reliable assessment and quantification of change in pain is a reason that many outcome studies avoid such a "soft" criterion altogether. This is particularly ironic since pain is the issue considered most important by the patient and is usually the reason the patient seeks care.

A similar "soft" criterion is patient satisfaction with treatment outcome. Most authors choose to disregard patient satisfaction. Mayer and Gatchel call patient self-report, "unreliable . . . insufficient to help judge outcome."[11] Yet the clinician's goal is to satisfy the patient. Therefore, it is reasonable to include patient satisfaction as an outcome measure.

Researchers tend to look at parameters that can be identified quickly and reliably. These include return to work; improvement in strength, range of motion, or neurologic deficits; need for future medical visits; and reduction in the use of medication.[1,11,18,19] However, there are problems with using these indirect measures as outcome criteria.

The use of return to work as the major determinant of success has pitfalls. Return to work is an outcome parameter biased toward the population who are injured on the job and part of the workers' compensation system. However, most patients with spine problems are not injured workers and are not receiving disability benefits. In fact, many patients with spinal problems are working at the time they seek treatment and continue to work during treatment. If a patient is working when first seen, using the fact that they are working at final assessment as an outcome criterion significantly biases the outcome toward success whether there is actual improvement or not.[10]

There are other reasons patients do not work besides the spine problem. Some are retired. Others work in their homes. Some have other disabling medical problems.

Decreased use of medication as a determinant of success is also subject to bias. Medication use is dependent on the philosophy of both the patient and the treating physician. If a physician does not prescribe opioids for the treatment of spinal pain, then patients who "require" no opioids would be considered successful because of the prescribing patterns of the doctor rather than whether the patient is improved.[1,19]

Insurers are not concerned with pain reduction as a determinant of success. They consider return to work, future disability payments, future lost work days, reinjury rates, and future health care costs as the important criteria of success. However, many of these indices of outcome apply best to injured workers. They do not apply to large segments of the population—such as students, house spouses, or retired persons—who also are treated for spinal pain and therefore must be included in research studies.[2]

Another pitfall of outcome evaluation is to consider only the final status of a patient when determining success or failure rather than comparing the status of the patient before and after treatment. It is not reasonable to expect patients who have had multiple spine surgeries or who are extremely disabled and in severe pain to do as well as patients who have not had prior surgery or who are only mildly disabled. Groups of patients must be assessed before and after treatment to draw valid conclusions.

Review of Available Assessment Instruments

Overview

There are as many ways to evaluate outcome as there are ways to treat back pain. Assessment of outcome ranges from the use of the history and physical examination to the use of sophisticated questionnaires and/or expensive devices to quantify strength or range of motion.

Most investigators choose to look at so-called hard data, which are considered to be findings that are reproducible and reliable.[2,5] "Soft" data consist of information reported by the patient, which many investigators think is too subjective to be meaningful. However, results from questionnaires about symptoms have been found to be highly reproducible and reliable. In addition, interobserver agreement is much higher regarding the history than the physical examination, which has low interobserver agreement and may be influenced by motivation, effort, and psychologic state.[2,11,12]

Deyo has summarized many of the problems inherent in the assessment of the functional status of a patient and defines functional status as the ability to perform the usual tasks of living.[2] He suggests five criteria for the evaluation of questionnaires, indices, instruments, and techniques used to evaluate functional status.

A questionnaire or test must be *practical*. It must be easy for the patients to understand, preferably be self-administered after simple instructions, be able to be quickly administered in an office setting without the need for additional staff, and require only a short time to score.

A questionnaire should be *comprehensive*. It should measure functions of daily life and abilities. It may take more than one tool to obtain sufficient information.

The results of a test must be *reproducible*. It must be reliable and yield the same results with retesting if the patient's status has not changed. It must be internally consistent and there must be good correlation between different parts of the test that measure the same thing.

The test must be *valid*. It must measure that which it is designed to measure. This may be the most difficult goal, since there is no acknowledged gold standard. The variable and only modest correlation between structural pathology and symptoms further compounds this difficulty.

Lastly, any test must be *responsive to change*. It should be able to detect small but meaningful changes in the patient's condition.

In addition to the above requirements of the measurement instruments and techniques, study design plays a very important role in evaluating outcome.[15] As discussed previously the most useful studies are prospective and randomized. Retrospective studies are much less reliable. At least 90% of the patients entered into a study should be available for evaluation at the conclusion of the study. If not, analyses must consider these patients lost to follow-up, and adequate statistical adjustments must be made.

Functional Assessment Questionnaires

Functional assessment questionnaires are designed to quantify function and reflect change in function over time that usually reflects clinical response to treatment. Many questionnaires have been available for decades, but few have become accepted. The following section briefly reviews and evaluates some of the available questionnaires. Each is described in terms of practicality, comprehensive nature, reproducibility, validity, and responsiveness to change.

Oswestry Low Back Pain Disability Questionnaire (OSW)

The OSW was described in 1980 as a tool to quantify a patient's performance compared to a fit person.[4] It is easily self-administered by the patient in

3.5 to 5 minutes and takes less than 1 minute to score by hand. It is quite comprehensive. The OSW examines a person's ability to care for himself/herself in activities of daily living. It examines a patient's ability to lift, walk, sit, and stand. It evaluates sleep, sexual function, social life, ability to travel, and pain intensity. Higher scores reflect a greater degree of disability.

The OSW has been shown to be internally consistent and valid. It is sensitive to change over time and to treatment.[2,4] It is useful both when administered a single time to describe degree of disability and is even more useful when administered serially over time to assess changes in function.

The OSW was developed in England and its language is decidedly British in flavor. Therefore, the NASS Outcome Committee made minor revisions in the language of the OSW to reflect a North American population. In addition, the category addressing medications was removed. The Committee thinks these changes improve the instrument, but to date this has not been tested.

Sickness Impact Profile (SIP)

The SIP was designed to be a health status indicator for chronic diseases and was not designed specifically for evaluating low-back pain.[2] It is not practical. It takes 20 to 30 minutes to administer. Scoring is complex and cumbersome and is best done by computer. It is comprehensive, reproducible, and valid. The SIP examines both physical and psychosocial dimensions. Because of its length, time to administer, and complex scoring methods, it has not gained wide acceptance clinically but is useful for some research purposes.

Roland Adaptation of Sickness Impact Profile (ROL-SIP)

Roland and Morris won the 1982 Volvo award for their questionnaire designed to measure disability in low-back pain.[17] They selected 24 items from the SIP and added the phrase, "because of my back," to each. Each item is answered yes or no.

The ROL-SIP is practical, easy to use, and may be self-administered in 3 to 5 minutes. It is easily scored. It does not measure any psychosocial parameters. It has been found to be reproducible, valid, and sensitive to change.

However, despite these positive factors, the ROL-SIP also has not been widely accepted as an outcome measure. Patients have found it frustrating to use because of its dichotomous yes-or-no format with no opportunity for continuous variables. Some have complained to us that there is no opportunity to describe small or moderate changes in status that they feel are important.

Million Questionnaire (MIL)

Million et al. won the 1981 Volvo award for their attempt to evaluate the progress of the patient with back pain.[14] Again, their format has not become accepted by spine clinicians and researchers.

The MIL consists of 15 visual analog scales. It appears to me to be vague, unfocused, and unbalanced. There is attention to some specific areas of function, such as ability to sit in various types of chairs (2 of 15 items). There are 5 items that attempt to quantify pain or discern whether "anything that you do" makes pain worse. Mixed in are several global items such as "overall handicap in your complete lifestyle."

The MIL is reasonably simple to administer, but it has not been tested in a self-administered format. It is simple to score. It is reproducible. Validity is not clear, nor is it sensitive to change, except in a small study comparing rigid to soft corsets.

Waddell Disability Index (WADDELL)

The WADDELL consists of nine items, which are answered in a yes-or-no format.[21] Limits are proposed that separate a normal person from a disabled person in the areas of lifting, sitting, standing, travel by car, social life, sleep, sexual activity, and ability to put on one's own footwear. There is no opportunity to quantify each item.

The WADDELL is simple and quick to administer and score. It is not comprehensive. It appears to be reproducible and has fair to good correlation with OSW. It is not clear that it is sensitive to change, especially to small or moderate changes.

Functional Rating Scale (FRS)

Evans and Kagan described the FRS in 1986,[3] but it has not gained wide acceptance. The FRS is a rating system that depends on asking the patient specific questions. It is not in questionnaire form but is readily adapted. There are typographic errors in the essential table in the original publication that should be corrected before use.

The FRS is easy to administer. Scoring takes less than 1 minute by hand. It assigns points for various activities, including vocational status, independence with activities of daily living, down time, use of medications, and reliance on aids such as corsets, braces, or cane. It does not examine psychologic or social factors. The lower the FRS score, the greater the degree of disability.

The FRS appears most useful in patients who are significantly disabled at the beginning of treatment and does not appear responsive to small levels of improvement, especially in patients who are only minimally disabled at the beginning of treatment.

Evaluation of Change in Pain

Overview

The challenge of using pain reduction as an outcome measure is to find an easily administered, reliable, and reproducible way to objectify and quantify a subjective experience. Multiple instruments to measure pain are useful when used appropriately.[8-10] Some have been shown to be extremely practical, reproducible, and sensitive to change over time with treatment. It is essential to realize that these pain-measurement instruments or questionnaires are not meant to compare the pain of one person to the pain of another, nor to state whether pain is "appropriate for the structural findings," "real," or "psychogenic."

There are many assessment techniques available to show change in pain over time. Several of the better-studied ones are discussed below.

Assessment Instruments

McGill Pain Questionnaire (MPQ)

The MPQ has been used extensively to quantify pain. It is generally considered the gold standard against which other pain measurement instruments are compared.[13] There are 78 adjectives or pain descriptors arranged in 20 categories. Scoring is done by assigning a rank value to each word in each category. The word in each category signifying the least pain has a value of 1, the next word has a value of 2, etc. A total summary score, the Pain Rating Index (PRI) is the total point value of all words chosen.

The MPQ produces scores for three dimensions of pain, sensory (items 1 to 10), affective (items 11 to 15), evaluative (item 16), and there is a miscellaneous category (items 17 to 20). There is debate regarding whether it is more useful to report only the PRI or whether it is better to report a score for each dimension of pain. It has been shown that the affective subscore of the MPQ is a good measure of pain-related emotional distress independent of the intensity or quality of the pain.[6]

The MPQ is readily self-administered by the patient in 4 to 5 minutes and takes less than 1 minute to score by hand. It has proven practical, reliable, valid, and sensitive to change over time and with treatment. It is very comprehensive.

There may be language difficulties and difficulties following instructions, especially with patients choosing more than one word in each category or feeling the need to choose a word in every category. Patients who are recovering from surgery or anesthesia or who have some degree of cognitive impairment due to medications or illness may make errors.

Visual Analog Scale (VAS)

A VAS is a line, usually 10 cm in length, which represents a continuum of quantity of pain.[6,8,9] The patient is instructed to mark the VAS line at the point that best represents the severity of pain. The line is anchored by a phrase such as "no pain" at one end and "worst possible pain," at the other. The VAS can also be used to measure pain relief after a test, medication, or procedure. In this use it would be anchored with "complete relief" at one end and "no relief" at the other. A VAS can be used to measure mood; therefore, comprehensive assessment is possible, but it requires two or more scales.[6]

The VAS is simple to use and score. It appears to have a greater capacity to reflect change than simple verbal descriptors. it has been shown to be reproducible, valid, and responsive to change.

However, there are limitations. It can be used only in written form. A patient who rates pain at the end of the line, "worst possible pain," but then gets worse has no way to reflect this deterioration. There may be a 5% or higher incidence of failure to follow instructions, and this rate may be even higher in older patients.[9] Completing the VAS requires some degree of hand-to-eye coordination, which may lead to errors after anesthesia or by patients taking sedating amounts of opioids or other drugs. There are two steps to use—estimate of pain by the patient and scoring by the clinician. The VAS should be photocopied carefully, as this may lengthen the line.

Pain Drawing

The use of pain drawings to evaluate the patient with spinal pain has been popular since 1976, when it was proposed that drawings are useful to screen for psychologic disturbances in patients with low-back pain.[16] Subsequent studies have found that drawings have low sensitivity and low specificity for finding psychologic problems in patients with low-back pain.[20]

Drawings have uses, however. The anatomic distribution of pain in the drawing may offer an opportunity to make a differential diagnosis quite quickly. In addition, some studies have shown that the percentage of body-surface area covered by the drawing can be quantified.[10] Unfortunately, no studies have been performed to show the effect of treatment on the change in body-surface area.

Verbal Numerical Scale (VNS)

To use the VNS the examiner asks the patient, "On a scale of 0 to 10 (or 0 to 100) where 0 is no pain and 10 (or 100) is the worst pain you could imagine, what is the level of your pain?" This scale is obviously simple to administer and score. It is easy to understand. No hand-to-eye coordination is necessary. It has been shown to be reliable, valid, and responsive to change. It measures only pain intensity and therefore is not comprehensive.

The VNS, despite its simplicity, is very useful in the clinical setting and may be useful in a research setting as well.

Numerical Rating Scale (NRS) 11 or 101

To use the NRSS-11 or NRS-101 the patient is asked to write the number between 0 and 10 (or 0 and 100) that best describes the pain "where 0 is no pain and 10 (or 100) is the worst pain you could imagine."

The NRS has been well studied and may be preferred in patients with chronic nonmalignant pain.[8,9] It is practical and simple to administer and score, and there does not appear to be increased error with age. The NRS is reproducible and valid. It measures only pain intensity.

Verbal Descriptor Scale (Verbal Rating Scale) (VRS)

The VRS is actually a written instrument in which the patient is given a choice of phrases and asked to choose the one that best describes their degree of pain.[8,9] The VRS can be given as 4, 5, or 15 items, and the results are generally equally sensitive and discriminative. An example from the NASS questionnaire is shown. Each descriptor can be assigned a numerical score if quantification is desired.

The VRS is practical but there may be language problems. It has been shown to be reproducible,

Verbal Rating Scale

	None at all	Slightly bothersome	Bothersome	Very bothersome	Extremely bothersome
Back pain					
Leg pain					
Neck pain					
Arm pain					

valid, and responsive to change. It measures only pain intensity in the form most often used.

11-Point Box Scale (11-BS)

Another technique is the use of an 11-point scale where the patient rates the pain from 0 to 10 by choosing a box of 0 to 10.[9] The 11-BS has been shown to be practical, reproducible, valid, and responsive to change.[9] It is very simple to use and is a good choice for both clinical and research settings. An example follows.

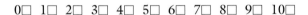

0☐ 1☐ 2☐ 3☐ 4☐ 5☐ 6☐ 7☐ 8☐ 9☐ 10☐

Evaluation of Patient Satisfaction

Ultimately, an appraisal of the results of treatment depend on whether the patient is satisfied with the outcome and whether the outcome met the patient's expectations. Different types of patients will have different outcomes; therefore, both patient and clinician must have appropriate expectations. The patient who has had multiple prior surgeries can rarely expect to have the same outcome as a patient with a large disc extrusion with radiculopathy.

Most studies do not consider patient satisfaction as a criteria for success. It is a "soft" outcome criterion totally dependent on subjective factors. Nonetheless, because patient satisfaction is a global phenomenon and embraces the whole person, it does not seem reasonable to omit it when considering treatment outcome.

My colleagues and I have used a simple 4-item choice:

1. The results of the treatment completely met my expectations.

2. The results of the treatment were not as good as I expected, but I would go through the same treatment for the same result.

3. I am improved but I would not undergo the same treatment for the same result.

4. I am the same or worse compared to before treatment

Conclusion

It has become apparent that evaluation of outcome is an essential part of clinical care and research. It is no longer acceptable to use vague outcome measures that are nonstandardized and unproven. The spine community will be held accountable to prove our treatments are effective in randomized, clinical trials.

This chapter presented an overview of the currently available outcome measurement tools. Each clinician must choose those that best fit the clinical and/or research needs of his or her practice.

References

1. Blumenthal S, Baker J, Dossett A, Selby D.: The role of anterior lumbar interbody fusion for internal disc disruption, *Spine* 13:566, 1988.

2. Deyo R: Measuring the functional status of patients with low-back pain, *Arch Phys Med Rehab* 69:1044, 1988.

3. Evans J, Kagan A: The development of a functional rating scale to measure the treatment outcome of chronic spinal patients, *Spine* 11:277, 1986.

4. Fairbank J, Couper J, Davies J, O'Brien J: The Oswestry low back pain disability questionnaire, *Physiotherapy* 66:271, 1980.

5. Feinstein A: Clinical biostatistics: hard science, soft data, and challenges of choosing clinical variables in research, *Clin Pharmacol Ther* 22:4854, 1977.

6. Fishman B, Pasternak S, Wallenstein S, et al.: The Memorial pain assessment card: a valid instrument for the evaluation of cancer pain, *Cancer* 60:1151, 1987.

7. Howe J, Frymoyer J: The effects of questionnaire design on the determination of end results in lumbar spine surgery, *Spine* 10:804, 1985.

8. Jensen MP, Karoly P, Braver S: The measurement of clinical pain intensity: a comparison of six methods, *Pain* 27:117, 1986.

9. Jensen MP, Karoly P, O'Riordan EF, et al: The subjective experience of actual pain: an assessment of the utility of 10 indices, *Clin J Pain* 5:153, 1989.

10. Margolis R, Tait R, Krause S: A rating system for use with patient pain drawings, *Pain* 24:57, 1986.

11. Mayer T, Gatchel R: Introduction and overview of the problem. In Mayer T, Gatchel R, editors: Functional restoration for spinal disorders: the sports medicine approach, Philadelphia, 1988, Lea & Febiger, 183.

12. McCombe P, Fairbank J, Cockersole B, Pynsent P: Reproducibility of physical signs in low back pain, *Spine* 14:908, 1989.

13. Melzack R: The McGill pain questionnaire, major properties and scoring methods, *Pain* 1:277, 1975.

14. Million R, Hall W, Nilsen K, et al.: Assessment of the progress of the back pain patient, *Spine* 7:204, 1982.

15. Nachemson AL, La Rocca H: *Spine*, 12:427, 1987 (editorial).

16. Ransford A, Cairns D, Mooney V: The pain drawing as an aid to the psychologic evaluation of patients with low back pain, *Spine* 1;127, 1976.

17. Roland M, Morris R: Study of natural history of back pain, part I: development of a reliable and sensitive measure of disability in low-back pain, *Spine* 8:141; 1983.

18. Saal J, Saal J: Nonoperative treatment of herniated lumbar intervertebral disc with radiculopathy, an outcome study, *Spine* 14:431, 1989.

19. Selby D, McCoy E, Henderson R: A study of post surgical narcotic use, Presented at the 4th Annual Meeting, North American Spine Society, Quebec City, Canada, June 29-July 2, 1989.

20. Von Baeyer C, Bergstrom K, Brodwin S, Brodwin M: Invalid use of pain drawings in psychological screening of back pain patients, *Pain,* 16:103, 1983.

21. Waddell G, Pilowsky I, Bond M: Clinical assessment and interpretation of abnormal illness behavior in low back pain, *Pain* 39:41, 1989.

Chapter 25
Conservative Care—Pulling It All Together

Arthur H. White

There are hundreds of nonoperative methods for treating spine pain. Which one should we choose for our patient? There is great confusion and billions of dollars being spent on disorganized, arbitrary selection of one failing method of conservative treatment after another.

It is easy to understand the development of such a vast array of conservative care methods when one considers the vague nature of back pain, its spontaneous resolution in most cases, and the poorly understood areas of placebo response, subjective pain experience, and psychologic and social factors affecting pain and suffering.* This has led to a chaotic array of treatment programs, none of which have strong scientific bases or deserve major space in this book.

Unfortunately, some patients progress from acute to chronic back pain. Chronic low-back pain, because of its great cost to society has stimulated the development of scientifically founded structured programs of conservative care that are broadly accepted in comparison to questionable short-term programs.[2,9,15,29] These pain and functional restoration programs of conservative care are described in detail in Chapters 32 and 38 of this book.

In order to help clarify the confusion, the preceding chapters of this book have pointed out that it is essential that we define the pain generator in any unresolved case of back pain. We can then select a treatment plan aimed at the pain generator and can monitor our progress in returning the patient to normal function. If success is not rapidly forthcoming we must question our diagnosis and/or switch to other measures. Conservative care incorporates most nonoperative care.

Selection of Treatment Plan

Conservative care should be considered a dynamic changing process. Unfortunately, conservative care in many medical communities is a static process that either works or does not. Conservative care as we use it in this book cannot be just one set of things given to the patient. It is a changing dynamic process that builds from the working diagnosis and is altered depending on the response to the previous treatments. There is a reasonable method of selection for the conservative measure that is most likely to work for a given working diagnosis. The least expensive, most effective, and safest conservative measures are used first. If they do not work adequately, the next most reasonable conservative care measure is added.

*References 2, 9, 16, 26, 40, and 43.

Conservative care is abandoned when reasonable measures have failed. Unfortunately, the decision for abandonment is frequently made by surgeons or other specialists who do not have full knowledge of conservative care. The most reasonable selection of treatment is based on

- Knowing the pain generator
- Understanding the variable effects of the pain on an individual patient
- Knowledge of the physical and emotional resources of the patient
- Familiarity with the treatment methods, actions, application, responses and time frames.

When we are not moving adequately toward normal function, one of five situations exists:

1. We are treating the wrong diagnosis.

2. We are using the wrong conservative care measures for the correct diagnosis.

3. We have a therapist inadequately administering the proper treatment for the correct diagnosis.

4. We have a patient who is unwilling to receive and use the proper treatment for the correct diagnosis.

5. The underlying pathologic condition is too severe to be successfully treated by conservative measures.

Time Frames

There are well accepted time frames for each conservative treatment measure.[3] For example, education can be given relatively quickly and should demonstrate some improvement in function as the patient learns which activities to avoid. With education, noticeable changes should occur within hours to a few days. Patients should quickly become conversant with terms and be able to demonstrate alternative body mechanics in the examining room.[31,49,56]

Stabilization training and learning new proprioceptive movements take considerably longer. An athlete devoting several hours a day to this type of training can progress from poor to excellent in a few weeks. Less coordinated and less motivated individuals can take months to improve performance.[46,49,51]

Strengthening also takes time. Gross strength and endurance can safely increase 10% per week with good training techniques. This rate decreases at the high end of human potential.[58]

The patient should show some noticeable improvement in pain and function after a few treatments of manual therapy and manipulation. In an average nonspecific low-back problem the patient should be well on the way to independent function after 10 such treatments. It is assumed that exercise and education will be quickly added to the manual therapy and soon become the maintenance program.

Modalities such as ice, heat, ultrasonography, acupuncture, electric stimulation, and traction should never be the mainstay of conservative care. They are used in addition to manual therapy early during the acute phase to bring pain or inflammation under control. Immediate benefit should be observed or the treatment should be discontinued within a few treatments. Later, during active training and exercise, if pain is an inhibiting factor, modalities can be used as long as they are reliably moving the patient forward in his/her program.

Nonoperative Conservative Care Programs

There are myriad nonoperative conservative care programs commonly used today. Many have developed into formalized practices that have been widely taught and written about. A few of the best known are McKenzie, Williams, Rolfing, and Feldenkreis.[4] Less well known are Reike, Heller, Aston and Alexander.[35,36,58] Each has well-defined techniques and applications, but few have rigid time frames. They can be used for selected patients to help move them toward normal function when more conventional measures are not working.

The alternative care subspecialties listed in the box have survived because patients find them valuable. There may be an underlying scientific basis for pain relief that we do not understand. Each of their proponents has a theory as to why they work. The public is unhappy with typical Western medicine, which tells them to take a pill and go to bed or go to "shake and bake" physical therapy. Patients look for alternative care to give them relief. It is well known that manipulation and acupuncture give relief to patients with back and neck pain. All the alternative care specialties mentioned have had success with patients for whom the more conventional approaches have failed. We will not attempt to describe any of these subspecialties. Each has volumes of teachings available.

It is important that the reader understand in general that all conservative treatments should have as their chief aim pain relief and/or improvement of function. Each school or method of care will include one or more of the following:

- Central pain relief—hypnosis, medication, meditation, endorphins
- Peripheral pain relief—needles, massages, ice, acupuncture
- Alteration of structural alignment—manipulation, traction, surgery
- Alteration of posture/strength/movement—Feldenkreis, Williams, stabilization, work hardening

Alternative Care Sub-Specialties

Acupressure	Macrobiotics
Acupuncture[40]	Manipulation[13,27]
Akido[15a]	Martial arts[15a]
Alexander technique[15a]	Massage[40,15a]
	McKenzie technique[50]
Aston patterning[15a]	Medication[40]
Back school[5,58]	Meditation[25,43]
Bioenergetics	Megavitamins[40]
Biofeedback[4]	Needling–dry/wet
Blocks	Orthomolecular
Body jackets	therapy
Braces	Pain clinics
Chiropractic[13]	Physical therapy[15a]
Cold packs	Pilates
Corsets	Pool therapy[15a]
Cortisone	Postural integration
Craniosacral manipulation[27,40]	Prolotherapy
	Proprioceptive neuro
Cryotherapy	facilitation (PNF)
Dance therapy[15a]	Psychocybernetics[15a]
Diathermy	Psychotherapy
Drugs[40]	Reflexology
Electrostimulation	Reike[15a]
Epidural blocks[27]	Relaxation therapy[15a]
Facet blocks[27]	Rolfing[3,15a]
Feldenkreis[40,15a]	Sclerotherapy
Functional	Self-hypnosis
restoration[44]	Stabilization[38]
Ginseng	Sympathetic blocks
Heller work[3]	Tai chi[15a]
Herbs[40]	Traction
Hypnosis[40]	Trigger points
Ice	Ultrasound
Imagery[43,15a]	Wedges
Injections[27]	Williams exercise
Inserts	Yoga[40]
Lifts	Zen[40,15a]

Because of the great expense created by the chaotic array of conservative care measures and the arbitrary selection of these measures by different subspecialists, several agencies and organizations have developed guidelines for acute conservative care. A few of these organizations are the Quebec Task Force,[27,45] the National Back Injury Network (1992), the Agency for Health Policy Reform (1993), and the San Francisco Spine Institute (1987–1993). The aim of these organizations is to provide the best scientifically validated conservative care in the most efficient and economical fashion.

In the box below are treatment outlines and plans for conservative care and treatment of patients with acute degenerative spinal pain. Treatment programs for patients with chronic pain, tumor, trauma, and infection follow a much different algorithm.

A Cookbook for Conservative Care

Acute Nonspecific Low-Back Pain

Days 1 through 7

Rest the back	Maximum 2 days bed rest
Pain control	Ice and aspirin
Educate	Books, tapes, back school
Exercise	Walk, swim, stabilization

Weeks 2 through 4

Return to work	As soon as possible
Alternative treatments	Manipulation, medication, injections, acupuncture
Accelerate education	
Exercise	

Weeks 4 through 6

Get accurate diagnosis	Scans, blocks, electromyography, psychosocial and functional testing
Develop long-range plan	Surgery, rehabilitation, job change

Acute Back and Leg Pain (Neurologic Involvement)

Days 1 through 7

Rest, ice, aspirin, cortisone, epidural block

Weeks 2 through 4

No progress	Early diagnostic tests
Some progress	Rehabilitation—physical and psychosocial

Phases of Care

The conservative care of degenerative spinal problems, as with most other diseases, falls into three phases of acute, subacute, and chronic conditions. The time frame for the acute phase is a matter of only days. The subacute phase generally lasts for weeks, and after 6 weeks most are considered chronic. These phases coincide with progression of the degenerative cascade. The treatment plan will vary with the severity of the pain and with the addition of leg pain, which indicates neurologic involvement.

Acute Phase

Nonspecific Low-Back Pain

Most acute injuries are early disc, muscle, or joint problems that spontaneously resolve within a few weeks. Inflammation in the first few days creates acute pain and may lead to reactive muscle spasm. Residual inflammation may remain for several weeks. The more severe conditions such as herniated discs or spinal stenosis may not completely subside or have recurrent acute episodes. The plan for such patients is delineated in the next section.

Days 1 to 7 As with most muscular skeletal injuries the injured area should be rested for a day or two using pain relief methods such as ice. Oral antiinflammatory medications such as aspirin can also be valuable. It is important to teach the patient how to rest his/her injured spine while going about normal activities. Bed rest is recommended for only a day or two, during which time the patient should be educated about his/her condition and how to not reinjure his/her spine by improper bending, sitting, and daily activities. Reading materials and video tapes are two means of education.[34] Exercise should start within a day or two to help realign the injured spinal area and strengthen the muscles required to maintain a pain-free balanced position.[1,54] Walking or swimming may be all that is necessary. More complex education and exercise is commonly called "Back School."* There are specific exercise programs such as the McKenzie program,[50] Williams exercises, and others that may provide rapid relief for specific spinal conditions. If the practitioner does not know how to select a specific exercise program, then a painless balanced range or neutral body mechanics program is usually quite adequate.[52,53] This amounts to finding the pain-free range and moving about painlessly by using the trunk and pelvic musculature to stabilize the spine while the lower extremities do the work of positioning the body for daily activities. Reassurance, education, and communication help prevent frustration and negative attitudes toward work and recurrences.

*References 17, 18, 21, 23, 24, and 57.

Abnormality   **Treatment**

Normal ——————————— None

Mild ——————————— Exercise and Education
                                              +
Moderate ——————————— Stabilization training, injections, work hardening, modalities, medication, manipulation
                                              +
Moderately Severe ——————— Train, surgery, disability rating, vocational training
                                              +
Severe ——————————— Disability rate and/or surgery, vocational training

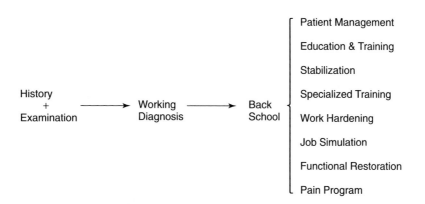

Weeks 2 to 4 Return to work as soon as possible (even part-time) and use the workplace for training in movement patterns, body mechanics, and stabilization training. If the patient cannot return to reasonably normal activities in 1 week, alternative treatments may be valuable. Manipulation, acupuncture, trigger-point injections, or other alternatives have little scientific basis but may be acceptable if they are clearly moving the patient rapidly toward normal function and are not expensive or dangerous.[37]

If the patient has not returned to work or had significant movement clearly indicating impending return to normal activities by 4 weeks, a diagnostic plan should be instituted so that an accurate diagnosis can be made. One can then make a realistic prognosis and help the patient, family, and employer make plans for the future. The pathoanatomy should be evaluated using scans, x-ray studies, or electrodiagnostics, and the motivation, psychopathology, and social ramifications of the case should be explored. The patient's physical resources such as strength, flexibility, endurance, and movement patterns should also be evaluated.

Weeks 4 to 6 When a patient has not returned to normal function by 6 weeks there is usually some residual pathology that is not going to "spontaneously heal." From a pathoanatomic standpoint this usually means some new unstable degree of disc degeneration, disc bulging or herniation, facet arthri-

tis, or stenosis.[10] If we hope to return the patient to normal function we will have to alter the patient's job, activities, or make some changes in his/her physical structure to compensate for the anatomical weaknesses.[8] This compensation may occur in the form of strength, endurance, flexibility, or movement patterns. It might even require some form of surgical intervention.

Continued use of pain treatment methods and medication, rest, or passive forms of treatment are not likely to change the underlying pathoanatomy.[7,11,12] We therefore must assess the patient's reserves, strength, flexibility, and movement patterns and decide how much change would be required to compensate for the underlying pathoanatomic weakness. Minor pathoanatomic abnormalities are easier to compensate for than severe conditions with neurologic deficits. A small bulging disc, for example, in a deconditioned patient is much more likely to improve with a work-hardening program than a major herniated disc in an already well-conditioned but very disabled patient. We therefore select the program most appropriate for the individual patient.[14] This might be a general exercise program in a gym, a specific work-hardening program with job simulation, or a high-level stabilization program as presented in the next chapters.[48,49]

Because of the great interest in cost containment it is important that we follow these patients closely and verify that our program is working. Gains in strength, flexibility, and endurance should be verified. Increases in functional activities should be commensurate with gains in training. We should be able to predict when maximum return in function will occur. All individuals affected by the patient's illness should be kept apprised of the current assessment and future predictions. When no further significant gains are occurring, the condition can be considered stable with minimal expected future improvement. If a disability rating is necessary at such a time, it should be formulated.[47]

If the patient has not returned to normal function by 6 weeks, we have a complete diagnosis and can develop a long-range plan for this patient with chronic back pain. If there is insurmountable pathoanatomy, the patient may need to change jobs, retire, or have surgery, if there is a reasonable likelihood of returning the patient to a significantly more acceptable level of function. If the physical pathology is not overwhelming, a long-range physical strengthening, flexibility and training program can begin.[28] This could be in the form of a work-hardening or high-level stabilization program.[30,32,38,39,46] If there is significant psychopathology or social pathology, it should be dealt with by counselors, occupational medicine physicians and nurses, functional restoration programs, or pain programs.[6,19,20,22,41]

If there is no movement toward more normal activities within a few weeks, there is clearly something wrong with the plan or diagnosis. Further help may be necessary in the form of a multidisciplinary program of diagnostics. A new plan should be forthcoming, which may include a disability rating or invasive diagnostics such as diagnostic blocks or discograms. In the most efficient and economical system the case would be finalized by 3 months at the earliest and 6 months at the latest.

Specific Back and Leg Pain

Although tumor, trauma, or infection can cause neurologic deficit, patients with degenerative cascade and neurologic deficit usually have a herniated disc or spinal stenosis. The patient may have only leg pain but frequently also has back pain. There is neurologic deficit in the form of reflex loss, sensory loss, and/or motor loss or deficit. Frequently, there have been previous episodes of back pain of a nonspecific nature. The patient is now more incapacitated than previously and needs more rapid diagnostic measures and should be more closely monitored and supervised during treatment. Although conservative care has a good likelihood of improving this patient with time, they do not typically resolve in the 1- to 6-week time frame, as do other patients with low-back pain. The diagnosis is made by thorough history and examination. The source of the pain and neurologic deficit can be determined by history, imaging studies, electrodiagnostics, and diagnostic blocks. Resolution of the patient's symptoms or decisions regarding surgery and recovery may take several months. It is therefore important to delineate the pathologic condition early in the disability so that the prognosis can be made.

Days 1 to 7 Bed rest may be necessary for a day or two. If the patient cannot progress from bed rest with education and training, he/she may need some oral or epidural steroids to relieve the inflammation. Ice and aspirin are still indicated. Alternative methods such as manipulation are of little value and may be dangerous if they give the patient a false sense of security or move the patient in an improper or dangerous position.

Weeks 2 to 4 If the patient has moved from bed to household activities, he/she should be placed in a formalized education and training program and will hopefully progress to light work activities by 4 weeks. If he/she is not progressing, diagnostic procedures can be started as early as the first week. If insurmountable pathoanatomy is identified, surgery may be necessary as early as the first month, but if there is some improvement with conservative measures, surgery should be postponed for a month or two until the patient reaches a plateau at an unacceptable level of maximum improvement.

Moderate pathology (bulging, discs, moderate stenosis) can respond to aggressive conservative care. This may include injection procedures such as epidural cortisone and may require months of slow but progressive education and training in strengthening, flexibility, body mechanics, and stabilization. Work hardening may be necessary. If there are extensive psychosocial factors, these should be treated appropriately with counseling, functional restoration, and work-hardening or pain programs.[41,44]

Weeks 4 to 12 A few patients have transient neurologic involvement that subsides within days and allows return to work within weeks. Some patients with neurologic involvement will reach a final plateau by 3 months and require surgery or a permanent disability rating with a change of job or retirement. Most cases with significant neurologic involvement, however, take 6 months or longer to resolve or to build enough strength and stabilization body mechanics to overcome the underlying pathoanatomic condition. If high-level psychosocial disability develops during such a long period of recuperation, there is great danger of multiple failed spine surgeries and tremendous personal and economic expense. These patients should be referred as soon as possible to multidisciplinary centers that are accustomed to handling such complex cases.[6,42]

Chronic Pain and Psychosocial/ Conservative Care

Definition and Diagnosis

Patients in this category represent the 10% of patients that cost 90% of the dollars. They are most likely to be misdiagnosed, receive unnecessary treatments and unnecessary or inappropriate surgery, and develop a cascade of complexities that are physical, psychosocial, and industrially related. There are warning signs along the path of diagnosis and treatment that should alert the clinician that the patient's case is in danger of becoming a complex multidisciplinary one.[55] As soon as warning signs develop, the patient should be transferred to the care of someone who understands the complexities of this type of case. The physical anatomic diagnostic categories can range from herniated disc and spinal stenosis to internal disc disruption, and the patients frequently have multiple failed spine surgeries. The psychosocial diagnoses include depression, somatoform disorders, addiction and social or psychologic premorbid conditions affecting the underlying structural disorder, and many others. (See the psychosocial chapters in this book.)

These diagnoses are made by delving into the historical relationship of the patient to his/her work environment, lifestyle, and relationships. Physical examination will demonstrate inconsistencies and measurable abnormalities known to be associated with psychosocial disease. Details of these can all be found in other chapters.

Conservative care for patients in the chronic pain and psychosocial disease categories should include education and exercise activities valuable in acute and subacute low-back-pain conditions. In addition, however, there are specific treatments that are absolutely essential if the psychosocial factors are to be treated successfully. Depression needs to be medically treated. Abnormal work situations need to be corrected; counseling may be important with regard to job satisfaction, aging, relationships, with employers and fellow workers. Drugs, alcohol and suppressed childhood experiences of desertion and abuse need to be identified and treated.

Chronic tertiary care patients require extreme coordination between multidisciplinary health providers who can resolve a patient's condition, in most cases without surgery. Even if surgery is necessary, intensive conservative care before and after surgery is essential to a successful outcome.

References

1. American College of Sports Medicine: *Guidelines for exercise testing and prescription,* ed 4, Philadelphia, 1991, Lea & Febiger.
2. American Medical Association Committee on Impairment: *Guides to the evaluation of impairment.* Chicago, 1989, AMA Press.
3. Anderson R: *Diagnosis and treatment of low back pain since 1850.* In White A, Anderson R, editors: *Conservative care of low back pain.* Baltimore, 1991, Williams & Wilkins, p 8.
4. Asfour SS, Khalil TM, Waly SM, et al.: Biofeedback in back: muscle strengthening, *Spine* 15:510, 1990.
5. Attix E, Tate M: Low back school: a conservative method: for treatment of low back pain, *J Miss State Med Assoc* 20:4, 1979.
6. Bartorelli D: Low back pain: a team approach, *J Neurosurg Nurs* 15:41, 1983.
7. Bigos S, Battie M: Acute care to prevent back disability: ten years of progress. *Clin Orthop* 221:121, 1987.
8. Caruso L, Chan D, Chan A: The management of work-related: back pain, *Am J Occup Ther* 41:11, 1987.
9. Department of Health and Human Services: *Report of the Commission on the evaluation of pain,* Washington, DC, 1987, Government Printing Office.
10. Deyo RA: Conservative therapy for low back pain, *JAMA* 250:1057, 1983.
11. Deyo RA, Mayer DG, Peidnoff S, et al.: The painful low back: keep it moving. *Patient Care* 21:47, 1987.
12. Donatelli R, Owens-Burkhart H: Effects of immobilization on the extensibility of periarticular connective tissue, *J Orthop Sports Phys Ther* 3:67, 1981.
13. Dutro C, Wheeler L: Back school and chiropractic practice, *J Manipulative Phys Ther* 9:209, 1986.
14. Fahrni W: *Backache and primal posture,* Vancouver, 1976, Musqueam Publishers, Ltd.
15. Fahrni W: *Backache assessment and treatment.* Vancouver, 1976, Musqueam Publishers, Ltd.
15a. Fields, R, et al: *Chop Wood, Carry Water,* New York, 1984, The Putnam Publishing Group.
16. Felten D: *The brain and the immune system.* In Moyers B, editor: *Healing and the mind,* New York, 1993, Doubleday, p 213.
17. Fisk J, DiMonte P, Courington S: Back schools: past, present and future, *Clin Orthop* 179:18, 1983.
18. Forsell M: The back school, *Spine* 6:104, 1981.
19. Fredrickson BE, Treif PM, VanBeveren P, et al.: Rehabilitation of the patient with chronic pain, *Spine* 13:351, 1988.
20. Hall H: *The back school.* In Tollison C, Kreigel M, editors: *Interdisciplinary rehabilitation of low back pain,* Baltimore, 1989, Williams & Wilkins, p 291.

21. Hayne C: Back schools and total back-care programmes—a review, *Physiotherapy* 70:14, 1984.

22. Holzman A, Turk D: *Pain management: a handbook of psychological treatment approaches,* New York, 1986, Pergamon Press.

23. Hurri H: The Swedish back school in chronic low back pain. Part I. Benefits, *Scand J Rehab Med* 21:33, 1989.

24. Hurri H: The Swedish back school in chronic low back pain. Part II. Factors predicting the outcome, *Scand J Rehab Med* 21:41, 1989.

25. Kabat-Zinn J: *Meditation.* In Moyers B, editor: *Healing and the mind,* New York, 1993, Doubleday, p 115.

26. Kirkaldy-Willis WH: *Managing low back pain,* ed 2, New York, 1988, Churchill-Livingstone.

27. LeBlanc F: Scientific approach to the assessment and management of activity-related spinal disorders: a monograph for clinicians. Report of the Quebec task on spinal disorders. *Spine* (European edition) 12:75, 1987.

28. Liang M, Daltroy L, Pallozi L: The patient's responsibility in therapy for low back pain. *J Musculoskel Med* 3:43, 1986.

29. Liang M, Komaraoff A: Roentgenograms in primary care: patients with acute low back pain: a cost-effectiveness analysis. *Arch Intern Med* 142:1108, 1982.

30. Lichtner R, Hewson J, Radke S, et al.: Treatment of chronic low back pain: a community-based comprehensive return-to-work physical rehabilitation program, *Clin Orthop* 190:115, 1984.

31. Martin L: Back basics: general information for back school participants, *Spine State Art Rev* 5(3):333, 1991.

32. Matheson L: *Capacity evaluation: systematic approach to industrial rehabilitation,* Anaheim, 1986, ERIC.

34. Mattmiller A: The California back school, *Physiotherapy* 66:118, 1980.

35. McKenzie R: *Treat your own back.* Lower Hutt, New Zealand, 1980, Spinal Publications.

36. McKenzie R: *The lumbar spine: mechanical diagnosis and therapy,* Waikanae, New Zealand, 1981, Spinal Publications.

37. Mooney V: Alternative approaches for the patient beyond the help of surgery. *Orthop Clin North Am* 6:331, 1975.

38. Morgan D: Concepts in functional training and postural stabilization for the low back injured, *Top Acute Care Trauma Rehab* 2:8, 1988.

39. Morgan D, McGoniga T, Moore M, et al.: *Education in manual therapy: training the patient with low back dysfunction,* Folsom CA, 1986, Folsom Physical Therapy.

40. Moyers B: *Healing and the mind,* New York, 1993, Doubleday.

41. Murphy T, Anderson S: *Multidisciplinary approach to managing pain.* In Benedetti C, Chappman R, Moricca G, editors: *Advance in pain research therapy,* New York, 1984, Raven Press, p 359.

42. Novak J: *The back loser: Liberty Mutual back pain symposium,* Boston, 1981, Liberty Mutual, p 52.

43. Olness K: *Self regulation and conditioning.* In Moyers B: *Healing and the mind,* New York, 1993, Doubleday, p 71.

44. Polatin P: The functional restoration approach to chronic low back pain, *J Musculoskel Med* 7:17, 1990.

45. Quebec Task Force on Spinal Disorders: Scientific approach to the assessment and management of activity-related spine disorders: a monograph for clinicians, *Spine* 12:7S, 1987.

46. Robison R: The new back school prescription: stabilization training, Part I, *Spine State Art Rev* 5:341, 1991.

47. Rosomoff H, Steel-Rosomoff R: Nonsurgical aggressive: treatment of lumbar spinal stenosis. *Spine State Art Rev* 1:383, 1987.

48. Saal JA, Saal JS: Nonoperative treatment of herniated lumbar intervertebral disc with radiculopathy: an outcome study, *Spine* 14:431, 1989.

49. Saal JA: The new back school prescription: stabilization, training, Part II, *Spine State Art Rev* 5:357, 1991.

50. Stankovic R, Johnell O: Conservative treatment of acute low back pain: a prospective randomized trial: McKenzie method versus patient education in "mini back school," *Spine* 15:120, 1984.

51. Steel-Rosomoff R: The pain patient, *Spine State Art Rev* 5:417, 1991.

52. Tollison C, Kreigel M: Physical exercise in the treatment of low back pain. Part I: A review, *Orthop Rev* 17:724, 1988.

53. Tollison C, Kreigel M: Physical exercise in the treatment of low back pain. Part II: A practical regimen of stretching exercises, *Orthop Rev* 17:913, 1988.

54. Tollison C, Kreigel M: Physical exercise in the treatment of low back pain. Part III: A practical regimen of stretching exercises, *Orthop Rev* 17:1002, 1988.

55. Waddell G, McCulloch J, Kummel E, et al.: Nonorganic physical signs in low-back pain, *Spine* 5:117, 1980.

56. White A, Mattmiller A, White L: *Back school and other conservative approaches to low back pain,* St. Louis, Mosby, 1983.

57. White A, et al.: *The back school: an audiovisual team approach to low back pain,* St. Louis, Mosby, 1984.

58. White Lynne A, editor: Back school, *Spine State Art Rev* 5:1, 1991.

Chapter 26
The Physiologic Basis of Therapeutic Exercise*

Jeffrey L. Young

Joel M. Press

*Modified from Young JL: *Physiologic basis of sports rehabilitation*. In Press JM, editor: *Rehabilitation clinics of North America*, 5 ed, pp 9-36, 1994, WB Saunders, Philadelphia.

Regardless of the decision to treat a patient surgically or nonsurgically, incorporation of a precisely prescribed exercise program is essential to a successful outcome. When physiologic principles are adhered to, and when exercise is performed in a systematically progressive manner, skeletal muscle adapts favorably, and higher levels of human performance or function are obtained. On the other hand, should the physician, physiologist, therapist, or trainer fail to develop a program that includes activity, specific exercise, and adequate rest, maladaptation occurs and performance is jeopardized. The purpose of this section is to provide the reader with an overview of the physiologic basis of exercise and the training response.

Skeletal Muscle

Skeletal muscle is the largest internal organ, comprising approximately 40% of the human body.[47] Each muscle is made of large numbers of fibers, which for the most part, run the entire length of the muscle. Each muscle fiber contains hundreds to thousands of myofibrils, and each myofibril is sequentially subdivided into functional units of contraction called "sarcomeres."[5,47,68,71]

The sarcomere itself contains the contractile proteins actin and myosin (thin and thick filaments, respectively), which lie in parallel to the long axis of the fiber. The actin filaments are structurally fixed to the outer margins of the sarcomere (Z disks), while the myosin filaments are located centrally, linked through their middle portions by the protein containing M line. There is considerable overlap of the filaments when the muscle is at its resting length (schematically shown in Fig. 26-1). The darker A band, which runs the length of the thick filament, has continuous overlap except at its center (H zone). The thin filament is bare only through the outermost portion of the sarcomere, within the light I band.[5,47,68,71] Electron microscopic examination of muscle cross sections reveals that the thin filaments actually form a hexagonal lattice about the thick filaments, with each thin filament equidistant from three thick filaments.[47,65,68,71] The thick and thin filaments are then linked to one another via cross bridges, which emerge from the myosin molecule. It is this cross-bridge system that forms the basis for increasing the amount of myofilament overlap and shortening of the whole muscle.

Myosin filaments are made up of approximately 200 myosin molecules.[47] Specific examination of the myosin molecule reveals that it has a "head" region and a "tail" region and is composed of one pair of heavy and two pairs of light chains.[47,68,71] The tail region is a coiled α-helical structure, derived from the greater portion of the heavy-chain pair.[47,71] The head region is actually a two-headed globular structure that projects out from the plane of the tail and is derived from the remainder of the heavy-chain pair and the two light-chain pairs.[47,71] Actin and ATP binding sites are on the head region.[47,71] The transition zone between the two regions (a heavy-chain "arm") serves as a flexible two-part hinge that allows the head portion to be extended out from or drawn close to the rest of the molecule. The arm and the heads together form the cross bridge. Simplified, the entire structure resembles two identical golf clubs lined up side by side, with the shafts twisted around each other (the tail) and the two club heads projecting off one end. Myosin subunits are then joined to one another, tail over tail, so that the filament as a whole has a thick body with hundreds of cross bridges projecting out on either side of a small area devoid of cross bridges in the middle.[47,63,71]

The thin actin filament is made from three different protein components—actin, troponin, and

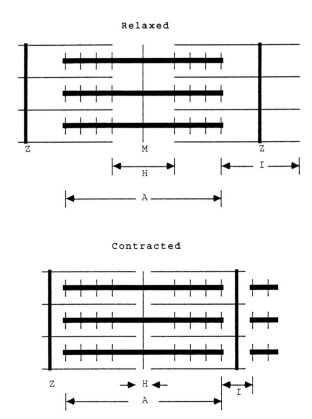

Fig. 26-1

Schematic representation of sarcomere under relaxed and contracted conditions. *(From Young JL: Physiologic Basis of Sports Rehabilitation. In JM ed, Rehabilitation Clinics of North America. 5:1., p 9-36, 1994, WB Saunders, Philadelphia.)*

tropomyosin.[5,48,68,71] G-actin globules are assembled into F-actin strands, which are wound into a double-stranded helix.[5,47,71] Each G-actin molecule has an active site with a molecule of ADP attached to it, and there are approximately 13 G-actin molecules per each helical revolution along each strand.[47] Tropomyosin is distributed along the grooves of the helix and blocks the active sites, preventing actin-myosin interaction at rest.[5,47,63,68,71] Troponin, another regulatory protein, is located near the tropomyosin. Troponin is a complex of three subunits, one with a high affinity for calcium (Tn-C), one with strong affinity for tropomyosin (Tn-T), and the third, (Tn-I), with affinity for actin.[47,63,71]

The final structural component to be considered before discussing the mechanism of contraction is the intracellular tubule system. The sarcoplasmic reticulum (containing longitudinal tubules), runs parallel to the myofibril. These tubules terminate in "terminal cisternae," vesicles capable of sequestering or releasing Ca^{2+}. Running perpendicular to the myofibril, is the transverse (T) tubule system. The T tubules communicate with the exterior of the cell membrane at one end, and meet up with cisternae, near the Z lines, on the inside. A "triad" is the junction between the two tubular systems and refers to a single T tubule accompanied by two terminal cisternae. The triad and T-tubule system serve as conduits for electrochemical information (i.e., waves of depolarization) from the outside of the cell to deep within the cell.

Once a wave of depolarization is propagated into the muscle cell, it rapidly reaches the level of the triad. Calcium ions are released from the cisternae, and come in contact with the troponin-tropomyosin complex. It is postulated that Tn-C, in particular, is affected by calcium, and undergoes a conformational change such that tropomyosin is drawn away from the active site on the actin molecule, leaving actin to interact freely with myosin.[47,63,71] Binding results in formation of an actomyosin complex, which is a highly active ATPase. This actomyosin ATPase can then split ATP into ADP plus a high-energy phosphate (P) and energy. The energy is used to produce movement of the cross bridge, with further overlap of the myofilaments, and tension is generated. Uncoupling of the complex occurs when myosin binds with the next available ATP molecule. As long as the sarcoplasmic level of calcium ions remains high, this process of coupling and uncoupling will continue and the filaments will continue to "slide" over one another ("sliding filament" theory).[54] Referring back to Fig. 26-1, the contraction process results in the Z lines moving toward one another, disappearance of the I band, and shrinking of the H zone.*

When stimulation of the muscle halts, calcium is resequestered by the tubule system, tropomyosin activity is no longer blocked by Tn-C, and the binding of actin to myosin is once again inhibited.[47,71] At this point, the sarcomere returns to its resting length.

The amount of tension produced by contracting muscle is highly influenced at a cellular level by the degree of actin-myosin overlap, and at a gross level by the length of the whole muscle. At the sarcomere level, the potential force generation is low under two conditions. The first is when sarcomere length is so great that there is little to no actin-myosin overlap and an adequate number of effective cross-bridge links cannot be made.[47,68,71] The second is when the sarcomere is already contracted to the point at which the Z disks approximate the outer margins of the thick filaments and the actin filaments from opposite sides are overlapping, which precludes any further shortening.[47,71] Potential force generation is maximal when the sarcomere is at a length of 2.0 to 2.2 μm, a range in which there is complete actin-myosin overlap, but no actin-actin overlap.[5,29,47,71] This corresponds roughly to the normal resting length of the sarcomere.[47,71] At a whole-muscle level, active force generation is also at a maximum when the sarcomere is at its resting length. However, if the muscle is stretched to slightly (10% to 20%) more than its resting length, the viscoelastic properties of surrounding connective tissue can be taken advantage of to generate even more force without loss of the potential force generation at the sarcomere level.[47,68,71] This is schematicized in Fig. 26-2. Note that the upper

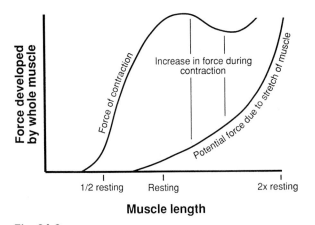

Fig. 26-2

Potential force generation by muscle relative to whole muscle length. *(From Young JL: Physiologic Basis of Sports Rehabilitation. In JM ed, Rehabilitation Clinics of North America. 5:1., p 9-36, 1994, WB Saunders, Philadelphia.)*

*References 5, 47, 54, 65, 68, and 71.

curve, which represents the potential force generation of whole muscle is maximized when the muscle is stretched to just beyond its resting length. This may have significant implications for athletic performance, as will be discussed later. Further stretching does confer greater tension in the connective tissue, but reduces the amount of tension that can be generated by the muscle at the sarcomere level for reasons described above.

Types of Muscular Contraction

Depending on the external resistance applied to the musculotendinous unit and the specific demands of the athletic activity, muscular contraction may be described in a number of ways as discussed below.

Concentric

During concentric contraction, the muscular force generated is able to overcome an applied external resistance, and the whole muscle length is reduced. As a result, at least one of the two limb segments spanned by the contracting muscle moves, with the assigned origin and insertion being brought closer to one another. For example, the combined concentric contractions of the middle deltoid and rotator cuff muscles produces elevation (abduction) of the humerus. Concentric contractions are also important because they are utilized to accelerate the more distal link segments in the kinetic chain. Combined concentric contractions of the pectoralis major and the latissimus dorsi enable a quarterback to accelerate rapidly, in sequence, the upper arm, the lower arm and wrist, and the football.

Eccentric

A contraction is considered to be eccentric when development of increased muscle tension is accompanied by muscle lengthening. Motion occurs, but the assigned origin and insertion move away from one another. The slow lowering of abducted humerus to the side of the body is an example of an eccentric contraction. Eccentric contractions are also essential for deceleration of kinetic link segments that have acquired large amounts of kinetic energy. Once the quarterback's arm has accelerated forward and the football is released, the eccentric firing of scapular stabilizer muscles and rotator cuff muscles are necessary to retain normal glenohumeral relationships and prevent the humerus from flying toward the receiver with the ball.

Isometric

Under isometric conditions, the length of the whole muscle is unchanged, and there is no net movement of the link segments spanned by the contracting muscles. While a gymnast holds himself in an L position on the parallel bars, the shoulder depressors, pectoralis major, latissimus dorsi, and triceps contract isometrically to stabilize the upper body, while the abdominal muscles, hip flexors, and knee extensors isometrically contract to maintain the 90-degree angle between the legs and the torso.

Isotonic versus Dynamic

When originally used, the term *isotonic* encompassed contractions of both the eccentric and concentric type.[65] This term implies that either the tension within the muscle or the torque generated by the muscle is constant throughout the arc of motion. This is an imprecise term, at best, since muscle tension changes constantly with alteration of joint angle, even when the speed of the contraction is kept constant.[30,65,68] Therefore, it is more appropriate to use the term *dynamic* when categorizing contractions as those associated with limb motion.

Isokinetic

Literally taken, isokinetic contractions are those that take place at a constant velocity. Computerized machines that can calculate external torque generation by a muscle group within a predetermined arc of motion and at a predetermined velocity are necessary to evaluate isokinetic strength. Although it is common for therapists, trainers, and researchers to utilize isokinetic data when evaluating strength and performance, it is important to recognize that isokinetic contractions do not occur in real life, making extrapolation from isokinetic data to clinical situations rather limited.

Plyometric

Plyometric exercise is designed to utilize the viscoelastic properties of the whole muscle to produce greater forces than by sarcomere shortening alone. A rapid overload (prestretch) is placed on the muscle immediately prior to a concentric contraction. This both stretches the connective tissue and places an eccentric load on the muscle, which facilitates subsequent concentric force generation.[63,68,88]

It is important to note the relative amount of force that can be generated under isometric and dynamic conditions. Muscles are capable of generating greater forces under eccentric conditions than either isometric or concentric conditions, and more isometrically than concentrically.[5,47,63,68] Thus, it is easier to hold a weighted barbell still than actually to lift it, and it is even easier to lower the barbell gradually than to hold it still. This relationship is further modified by the speed of muscle contraction. Rapid eccentric contractions generate more force than slow ones (slower eccentric work approximates isometric), and slower concentric contractions generate more force than rapid ones.[5,47,65] Eccentric contractions are also more efficient than concentric contractions (i.e., require less oxygen) at the same tension and contraction velocity.[36,62] The time to reach peak tension is also faster during eccentric contractions than during concentric contractions.[13,62]

Muscle-Fiber Types and Ultrastructural Considerations

Skeletal muscle is not an entirely homogeneous structure. When special staining techniques are used, it is evident that muscle is, instead, a "mosaic," with different fiber types. The two major groups of muscle fibers are referred to as either "slow twitch" or "fast twitch." Their categorization is primarily determined by their contractile and metabolic profiles, which will be discussed in this section.

Historically, it has generally been accepted that a muscle fiber's properties are conferred on it by its innervating neuron.[5,29,30,47] This concept has been challenged, as there is some evidence that early differentiation of muscle is somewhat independent of neuromuscular connection and that the role of innervation is, instead, to help organize the tissue functionally.[59] The majority of skeletal muscle differentiation occurs prenatally.[17,38] Distinction between fast- and slow-twitch subtypes may be made on the basis of the particular myosin isozyme expressed.[38] However, approximately 20% of fibers are still undifferentiated at birth, and it is not until about 6 years of age that the adult pattern is identified.[8,17] The stimulus for the assumption of the final adult pattern has not yet been identified.

Slow-twitch fibers, also referred to as "Type I" or "red" fibers, are the smaller-sized of the two fiber groups and contain the slow myosin isozyme.[4,38,40,41] They are innervated by smaller motor-nerve fibers and are the first fibers recruited during submaximal muscular contraction.[57] They are designed for repetitive, low-intensity work as evidenced by their highly oxidative capabilities. They have many mito-chondria and have high levels of stored myoglobin, both of which confer a reddish color on this fiber type.[5,19,20,68] There is a relatively high capillary density about these fibers, and they have high levels of oxidative enzymes such as succinic dehydrogenase.[5,20,47,68] These fibers are the ones typically trained by long, slow distance running, cross country skiing, and distance cycling.

Fast-twitch fibers, also referred to as "Type II" or "white" fibers, are the larger-sized fibers and contain fast myosin isozymes.[5,38,47,68,71] They are innervated by large-diameter motoneurons, are designed to develop large amounts of tension within a short time, and are recruited when the force-generating capacity of the smaller-caliber fibers is no longer adequate to meet the needs of the assigned task.[57] They are suited for short work periods, as evidenced by their relative paucity of oxidative machinery but high levels of ATPase and glycolytic enzymes, such as phospho-fructokinase.[5,68] They produce more lactic acid than Type I fibers.[5,98] The sarcoplasmic reticulum is extensive in these fibers so that there can be rapid release of calcium ions to initiate contraction.[5,47,71] These fibers are typically trained by sprinting, weight lifting, and high jumping.

It is also well recognized that fast-twitch fibers may be subdivided further into at least two subgroups—Type IIa and Type IIb. A smaller subpopulation, Type IIc, will also be discussed briefly. Type IIb are the "classic" fast-twitch fibers, with properties as described above. However, Type IIa fibers appear to be intermediate in their properties relative to the Type I and Type IIb fibers, and are sometimes called "FOG" (fast oxidative glycolytic) fibers. They are large, have large-diameter innervating motorneurons, and generous amounts of sarcoplasmic reticulum, but the also contain a relatively high number of mitochondria and oxidative enzymes.[29,41,69] During work of progressively increasing intensity, they are recruited after Type I fibers, but earlier than Type IIb.[29,57] It appears that this intermediate group has the capability of being trained for either endurance or short-burst activities.[4,5,18,19,40] This is significant because there still is controversy over whether athletic training can convert Type I fibers into Type IIb fibers or vice versa.[5,47,68]

Type IIc fibers are relatively rare, generally comprising less than 5% of the total fiber population in healthy humans.[55] They are undifferentiated and may represent fibers involved in motor unit transformation or when reinnvervation occurs following denervation.[55,56] It has been speculated that these fibers are actually derived from Type I fibers rather than IIa or IIb subtypes, and that transformation

Table 26-1

Major fiber types of human skeletal muscle

Characteristic	Type I	Type IIa	Type IIb
Contraction time	Slow	Fast	Fast
Oxidative capacity	High	Moderate	Low
Number of mitochondria	High	Moderate	Low
Myoglobin content	High	Moderate	Low
Fatigability	Low	Low	High
Glycolytic capacity	Low	Moderate	High
ATPase activity	Low	High	High
Stored phosphagens	Low	High	High

from Type I to Type IIc can be encouraged by intense anaerobic training.[56] Table 26-1 summarizes the key characteristics of the major fiber types in human skeletal muscle.

While there is little evidence to support that Type I and Type II fiber interconvertability takes place in humans, it is well known that there are considerable differences in fiber-type distribution between different types of athletes and between trained and untrained individuals.* Untrained individuals have about 50% of both Type I and Type II fibers. Elite endurance athletes, such as cross-country skiers, may have as high as 90% Type I fibers.[9,68] Strength athletes and sprinters may have as high as 65% to 75% Type II fibers.[5,9,20,68] Again, it is not entirely clear if these high percentages exist as a function of genetics or if the many years of intense training that most of these athletes undergo has induced fiber transformation. Furthermore, fiber type composition has not been shown to be a good independent predictor of performance.[20] On the other hand, there is little argument that under the influence of regular physical conditioning, there appears to be considerable plasticity within the Type II group.† Endurance-type training is associated with a relative increase in the proportion of Type IIa fibers, while anaerobic training (or inactivity) increases the relative proportion of Type IIb fibers.[4,19,55,56]

Energy Metabolism

In order for muscle to contract, energy is needed. Energy is stored in the body as adenosine triphos-

*References 47, 52, 55, 56, 60, 68, 98, and 99.
†References 3, 5, 18 to 20, 52, 55, 56, and 68.

phate (ATP), and is released when ATP is hydrolyzed into adenosine diphosphate (ADP) plus a free phosphate (Pi):

$$ATP + H_2O + ATPase \rightarrow ADP + Pi + energy \ (7.3 \ kcal/mol)$$

ADP may also be hydrolyzed yielding the monophosphate, AMP, a second Pi, and more energy.[3,5,47,68,71] The supply of ATP stored within cells is rather limited, and during intense exercise can be depleted within a few seconds. In order for muscular activity to continue, the ATP supply must be replenished through resynthesis of this molecule.

ATP regeneration may take place either in the absence or presence of oxygen. The first line of reserve is via the high-energy compound creatine phosphate (CP). CP is readily broken down into creatine (C) and Pi, with this Pi used to regenerate ADP from AMP or ATP from ADP[3,5,47,68,71]:

$$CP + AMP + creatine \ kinase \rightarrow ADP + C$$
$$CP + ADP + creatine \ kinase \rightarrow ATP + C$$

Splitting of CP yields 10.3 kcal/mol.[5,47,68] Intracellular CP is two to four times more plentiful than ATP, and it allows for an additional 5 to 6 seconds of exercise.[47,71] In all, the phosphagen system, which does not require oxygen, can provide maximal power for approximately 8 to 10 seconds.[5,47,71] This system is both nonaerobic and alactic.[5,47,68,78] Myoglobin, the iron-containing protein found in Type I fibers, serves as a limited reservoir of oxygen for energy release in the Type I fibers during this time.[5]

A second metabolic pathway, also not requiring oxygen, and taking place in the cytoplasm, is capable of ATP resynthesis. This pathway is often referred to as the "anaerobic" or "nonoxidative" pathway and revolves about the generation of ATP from the breakdown of glycogen or glucose.[12,47,67] In an all-out exercise task, the anaerobic pathway provides 85% of the needed energy output at 10 seconds, 65% to 70% at 1 minute, 50% at 2 minutes, and no more than 30% at 4 minutes.[5] This again reflects that ATP can be resynthesized much more rapidly by the pathways that do not require oxygen. The phosphagen system can form ATP 4 times as quickly and the glycolytic/glycogenolytic pathway 2.5 times as quickly as the oxidative pathway.[47]

The important biochemical reactions of glycogenolysis/glycolysis are summarized below:

$$glucose \ (6 \ carbons) + 2 \ ATP \leftrightarrow fructose\text{-}1,6\text{-}diphosphate \ (1)$$
$$2 \ phosphoglyceraldehyde + 2 \ NAD^+ \leftrightarrow 2 \ pyruvic \ acid +$$
$$4 \ ATP + 2[NADH + H^+] \qquad (2)$$
$$pyruvic \ acid + NADH + H^+ \leftrightarrow lactic \ acid + NAD^+ \ (3)$$

In reaction 1, key enzymes are phosphorylase, which regulates glycogenolysis, and phosphofructokinase (PFK), which is a rate-limiting enzyme for glycolysis.[5,47,68,71] Two ATP are expended. In reaction 2, a pair of three-carbon molecules, phosphoglyceraldehyde, and nicotinamide adenine dinucleotide (NAD) combine to yield pyruvic acid. Four ATP are generated for immediate use, thus yielding a "net" of 2 ATP.[3,5,12,47,71] The two NADH are eventually shuttled into the mitochondria, where they are oxidized, yielding four more ATP, and "freeing" NAD again.[3,5,88] As long as the rate of hydrogen ion production is relatively matched by hydrogen oxidation, pyruvic acid is the major end product of this scheme. On the other hand, if the ratio of NADH to NAD starts to rise (i.e., nonoxidative conditions), glycolysis will come to a stop, unless some molecule (in this case, pyruvate) acts as an oxidizing agent. Reaction 3 is catalyzed by lactic dehydrogenase and provides another mechanism for freeing NAD again.[5,12,47,68]

Once lactic acid is formed, it has a number of possible fates. It can undergo oxidation in muscle, the liver, and the heart.[11,91-93] It can be converted back into glucose in the liver or kidney.[11,12] It can combine with bicarbonate to form carbon dioxide and water.[3,5,68] Thus, it serves as a metabolic intermediate, between carbohydrate stores and metabolic end products.

Regulation of lactate accumulation during exercise is rather complicated. Appearance of lactate is a function of changes in muscle lactate concentration, blood flow, pH, and resistance to lactate efflux from muscle.[12,82,91,92] It is crucial to understand that a rise in blood lactate does not mean that muscle is working under "anaerobic" or hypoxemic conditions—it merely implies that the rate of lactic acid entry into the blood exceeds its rate of removal.[12,68,81] Under resting or low-intensity exercise conditions, lactic acid is produced, but usually does not accumulate because lactate clearance matches production.* During more intense exercise, significant accumulation may occur. This is particularly true at the onset of exercise when the limited supply of the phosphagen pathway has been exhausted and the more sluggish mitochondrial driven oxidative pathway is not yet ready to oxidize large volumes of lactate.[12,15,78,91,92] Under these conditions, glycolysis must proceed at a rapid rate to continue producing ATP, more lactate is formed, and more spills into the blood stream.† Lactate production is also greater when there is increased sympathetic nervous system (specifically β-adrenergic) drive.[91,92] Epinephrine is a powerful stimulator of phosphorylase, which increases glycogenolytic activity.[12,91,92]

*References 3, 5, 11, 12, 91, and 92.
†References 5, 11, 12, 68, 91, and 92.

The consequences of increased lactate accumulation are well documented. Muscular fatigue, muscular pain, and increased perceived effort are all observed.[5,10,14,68] Lowering of pH depresses myofibril contractility and interferes with key enzyme activity, thereby limiting exercise performance.[12,82] In addition, the drop in pH and the increase in CO_2 production (from buffering with bicarbonate), are associated with increased ventilatory drive.[3,5,68,101]

The final pathway to be considered is the oxidative energy system. This system has the lowest peak power but the greatest total capacity for ATP regeneration. As opposed to the phosphagen system, which relies on stores, and the glycolytic pathway, which is restricted to carbohydrates, the oxidative pathway has the distinct advantage of being able to utilize any of the major fuel sources. The entire pathway takes place in the mitochondria and in the presence of oxygen. It consists of two major parts—the Krebs cycle and the electron transport system (oxidative phosphorylation). In the Krebs cycle, the acetyl portion of acetyl coenzyme A (CoA) initially combines with oxaloacetic acid to form citric acid. CoA is released (so that it may be reused with another pyruvate molecule), and the remaining portion is gradually broken down to CO_2 and hydrogen atoms.[47] The overall reactions are as follows:

$$pyruvate + NAD^+ + CoA \rightarrow acetyl\ CoA + CO_2 + NADH + H^+ \quad (4)$$

$$2\ acetyl\ CoA + 6\ H_2O + 2\ ADP \rightarrow 4\ CO_2 + 16H + 2\ CoA + 2\ ATP \quad (5)$$

Thus, for every molecule of glucose, there is a net gain of only 4 ATP from all the reactions prior to the electron transport system (reactions 1, 2, and 5). Oxidative phosphorylation utilizes NAD and FAD (flavin adenine dinucleotide) to oxidize the hydrogens generated from glycolysis and Krebs cycle and via a cascade of reactions, generates another 32 ATP, for a total of 36 ATP.[5,47,68]

As noted above, the aerobic pathway demonstrates the slowest kinetics of the three energy systems. In an all-out exercise task, it provides 15% of the contribution to total energy output at 10 seconds, 30% to 35% at 1 minute, 50% at 2 minutes, and 70% by 4 minutes.[5] During events lasting upward of 1 hour, virtually all the energy needs are met by the oxidative system.[5] As the length of the task increases there is also a gradual shifting of substrate metabolism as well. Initially, aerobic metabolism shares in the use of carbohydrates as the primary fuel source, first from blood-borne glucose and then from muscle glycogen.[12,68,88] But, as the body begins to adjust to the task, there is lessening of the insulin:glucagon ratio, activation of lipases, and mobilization of free fatty acids (FFA) from adipose tissue.[5,47,68] This leads to assumption of fat as the primary fuel source. Fatty acids are transformed into the acetyl portion of acetyl CoA through β-oxidation, which involves breaking down long fatty acids into two carbon chains.[5,68] The advantage of utilizing fat as a fuel source is striking. While the total body stores of carbohydrate represent less than 2000 kcal, usable adipose reserves contain approximately 100,000 kcal.[68] Trained endurance athletes tend to be able to utilize fats more effectively during exercise and in doing so demonstrate a "glycogen-sparing" effect.[5,68] This is, in part, due to the fact that they accumulate less lactic acid than untrained individuals at the same work output.[5] Lactate interferes with FFA mobilization, thereby reducing its availability to the cell.[5] Furthermore, endurance training is associated with decreased body fat and increased insulin sensitivity, both of which lead to lower systemic levels of insulin and decreased reliance on carbohydrates as a fuel source during exercise.

The last fuel source to be considered is protein. Protein is never the major fuel source in eumetabolic individuals, but may be utilized during prolonged exercise. In order to enter the Krebs cycle, certain amino acids (aspartate, leucine, glutamate, valine), undergo deamination, and then usually enter the cycle as a smaller molecule, such as alanine or glycine.[3,5,68]

Fuel-source utilization during exercise may be estimated via collection and analysis of expired respiratory gas. Since glucose, protein, and fat all require different amounts of oxygen to be combusted into carbon dioxide and water, measuring the relative amounts of O_2 and CO_2 enables us to identify the predominant fuel source being utilized. The respiratory quotient (RQ) is calculated as follows:

RQ = VCO_2/VO_2 = volume of CO_2 expired divided by the volume of oxygen consumed

For carbohydrate, RQ is 1.0; for fat, 0.7; and for protein, 0.8. During submaximal exercise, RQ usually reflects mixed substrate utilization (i.e., RQ = 0.84). As exercise intensity increases and more carbohydrate is used, the RQ approaches 1.0. However, once exercise is of sufficient intensity to induce metabolic acidosis, CO_2 collected from the lungs is not only a product of fuel combustion, but a product of the body's bicarbonate buffering system as well.[3,5,90,101] Under these conditions, collection at the lung level no longer reflects cellular metabolism and the respiratory exchange ratio (R) no longer reflects RQ.

The Exercise Response

With the onset of dynamic exercise of large muscle groups, the body reacts in a way that is analogous to the "fight-or-flight" response seen under any condition of physiologic stress.[5,47] There is both vagal nerve inhibition and an increase in sympathetic nervous system activity with an outpouring of adrenocortical hormones.[5,47,68] Rapid central and local circulatory adjustments occur, yielding increases in cardiac output and muscle blood flow but restricted splanchnic flow.[5,68] Alveolar ventilation increases in anticipation of greater oxygen requirements.[5] There is increased gluconeogenesis and a rise in glucose uptake by the skeletal muscles.[5,68] This is a generalized response, which becomes more focused as exercise progresses. The two major factors controlling the extent of the cardiorespiratory and metabolic responses to exercise are the intensity and duration of the selected activity. The exercising individual's state of training, familiarity with the specific activity, nutritional status, the extent of recovery from any recent exercise, and the environmental conditions are all modifiers of this response. This section will address the major physiological events associated with dynamic exercise.

Cardiovascular

The heart and central cardiovascular system respond to the stress of exercise by increasing contractility and pumping frequency of the heart. Heart rate (HR) increases linearly with respect to work or VO_2.[3,5,68,88] Initially, the rise in HR is due primarily to vagal withdrawal, while rates in excess of 120 beats per minute are due to sympathetic stimulation.[5] Maximal HR in a young athlete is typically between 190 and 200 beats per minute. Maximal HR is often estimated as 220 − age.[3] Resting HR may be as low as 40 beats per minute in a well-trained endurance athlete.[5] Figure 26-3 illustrates the effect of endurance training on HR response to incremental work. Although the highest HR achieved is the same in the two individuals, the slope of the HR line is less in the trained subject, with the trained person able to do more work at a given heart rate (A), and exhibit a lower HR for a given intensity of work (B).

Stroke volume (SV) is influenced by numerous factors. These include central venous return (how much blood is available for filling and how much stretch myocardial fibers will undergo), afterload (the downstream pressure against which the heart must contract), the state of myocardial contractility,

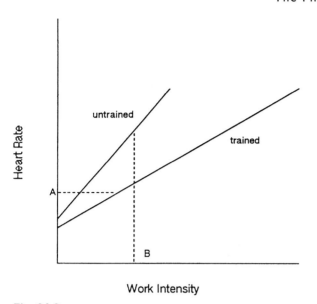

Fig. 26-3

Heart rate response to progressively increasing exercise intensity in untrained and trained states. In trained state, more work can be performed at any absolute heart rate (*A*), and heart rate is lower for given work intensity (*B*). *(From Young JL: Physiologic Basis of Sports Rehabilitation. In Press JM ed, Rehabilitation Clinics of North America. 5:1., p 9-36, 1994, WB Saunders, Philadelphia.)*

and the heart rate, which influences diastolic filling time.[3,5,47,68] SV will increase by approximately 40% simply by assuming a supine posture[5,68] due to the facilitation of venous return.[3,5] In the upright posture, the exercising athlete can achieve a maximal SV of 150 to 200 ml/beat, which typically occurs around 40% to 50% of VO_{2max}.[3,5,68] Highly trained individuals exhibit higher maximal SV than untrained subjects.[3,5,68]

Cardiac output (Q_{CO}), which is the product of HR and stroke volume, also increases linearly with respect to work and VO_2.[3,5,68] The relationship between Q_{CO} and VO_2 is that there is approximately a 6 liter/min increase in Q_{CO} for every 1 liter/min increase in VO_2.[3,68,78] Well-trained individuals have maximal cardiac outputs over 30 liters/min, and elite athletes up to 40.[5,88] The cardiac output is directly dependent on the venous return. If venous return is interfered with or there is a drop in central circulating blood volume, cardiac output will be acutely lowered.[3,5,47]

Peripheral Circulation

Muscle blood flow (MBF) increases dramatically with dynamic exercise. At rest, 10% to 15% of the total cardiac output is sent to muscle. During in-

tense exercise, 85% of the total cardiac output will go to muscle.[3,5] Peak MBF is a function of the amount of muscle used, how many muscles are active, and is usually expressed in milliliters per 100 mg of muscle tissue.[16,77] If a smaller muscle mass is utilized at a given level of cardiac output, then the MBF is higher. While central blood flow is clearly limited by the cardiac output, the upper limit of MBF, expressed in milliliters per 100 mg tissue, is a matter of debate.[83] In any event, a conservative estimate would be that MBF may increase sixtyfold to seventyfold, with peak values in excess of 150 ml/100 mg.[77,83] Ultimately, if exercise is carried out long enough, MBF will also be limited by the diversion of central blood flow to skin for thermoregulatory purposes.[5] Maximal MBF increases with endurance training.[5,77,83]

Respiratory

Minute ventilation (V_E) may approach 200 liters/min in a large, highly trained athlete.[5] During early stages of a progressive exercise test, V_E remains linear with respect to VO_2, or with respect to work.* The relationship frequently reported is 25 liters V_E to 1 liter VO_2.[3,5,68,88] However, as the intensity surpasses a critical threshold (generally 50% to 70% VO_{2max}), a disproportionate rise in V_E is observed, and from that work stage on, V_E rises curvilinearly

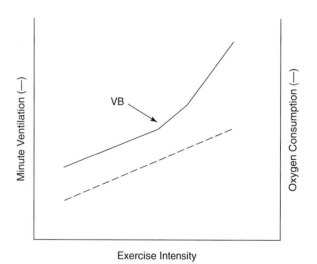

Fig. 26-4

Minute ventilation (V_E) and oxygen consumption (VO_2) during incremental exercise. The ventilatory breakpoint is indicated by V_B. *(From Young JL: Physiologic Basis of Sports Rehabilitation. In Press JM ed, Rehabilitation Clinics of North America. 5:1., p 9-36, 1994, WB Saunders, Philadelphia.)*

*References 3, 5, 12, 27, 68, and 88.

with respect to VO_2.* This inflection point, demonstrated in Fig. 26-4, may be referred to as V_B, or the ventilatory breakpoint. Two important stimuli for the rapid rise in V_E are the lowering of pH, and an increase in CO_2 production, both of which are associated with the increased presence of lactic acid in the blood.† In the past, attempts were made to use V_B as a noninvasive marker for the onset of lactic acid production or accumulation.[26,27,101] However, it is now thought that these two events, while related, do not represent the same physiologic phenomenon and should not be used interchangeably.[5,12,91,92] The exercise intensity at which V_B occurs, though, is valuable, because it is positively correlated with the pace that many endurance athletes will attempt to approximate during competitive events.[64,79,96] With training, the V_B occurs at a higher level of exercise; highly trained endurance athletes exhibit higher V_B, both in absolute terms and when expressed as a percentage of VO_{2max}.[1,5,22,67]

Oxygen Consumption

Oxygen consumption is reflective of the circulatory and pulmonary systems' ability to deliver oxygen to the working muscles and the ability of those muscles to utilize that O_2.[5,12,67] It can be calculated via the Fick formula, which takes the cardiac output and arteriovenous oxygen difference (av O_2D) into account:

$$VO_2 = HR \times SV \times av\ O_2D$$

*References 5, 26, 27, 68, 88, and 101.
†References 3, 5, 12, 26, 27, 64, and 101.

The arterial oxygen content of blood is 20 ml/100 ml blood and the av O_2D is approximately 5 ml/100 ml blood at rest. During maximal exercise it increases to approximately 16 ml/100 ml blood.[3,5,88]

The oxygen deficit refers to the delay in oxygen utilization at the muscle level with the onset of exercise.[3,5,68,88] In order to meet metabolic demands, anaerobic metabolism (i.e., lactic acid metabolism) must come into play to provide energy for work. At low levels of work this deficit is transient (less than a minute or so), but as work intensity increases, it takes a longer time for oxidative metabolism to fully "catch up" and achievement of a "steady state" or "steady rate" is delayed.[5,68,88] Figure 26-5 illustrates this relationship. Although not illustrated here, this phenomenon of achieving a steady rate does not occur ad infinitum—at very high intensities (i.e., over 90% VO_{2max}), a leveling off of VO_2 is not observed.[5,68]

Following cessation of exercise, oxygen consumption remains considerably above resting values for minutes to hours, depending on how long and intense the exercise bout was.[5,68] This VO_2 in excess of resting is referred to as the "oxygen debt."* It is important to note that the O_2 debt is not merely a 1:1 repayment of the deficit, and that as the intensity of exercise increases, the extra O_2 consumed in recovery greatly outweighs the deficit at the onset of exercise.[3,5,88] Trained muscles are characterized by a faster rise of the VO_2 during the "unsteady" portion of the oxygen uptake curve.[16]

*References 3, 5, 47, 68, 78, and 88.

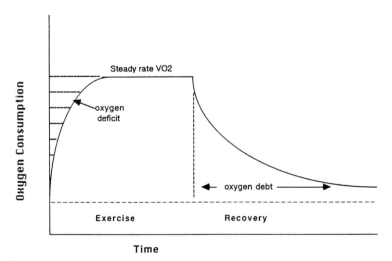

Fig. 26-5

Oxygen consumption (VO_2) at onset and during and after cessation of constant load exercise. *(From Young JL: Physiologic Basis of Sports Rehabilitation. In Press JM ed, Rehabilitation Clinics of North America. 5:1., p 9-36, 1994, WB Saunders, Philadelphia.)*

During a progressive exercise test, VO_2 increases in a fairly linear manner with respect to increased work rate.* Eventually a work rate is reached at which there are no further increases in VO_2. This is referred to as the "maximal oxygen consumption" (VO_{2max}) and is defined as the highest level of oxygen uptake possible during physical work at sea level[3,5,12,68]:

$$VO_{2max} = HR_{max} \times SV_{max} \times av\ O_2D_{max}$$

Obviously, there are many factors that influence the VO_{2max}, with a dynamic interplay between the availability and utilization of O_2 dictating the value in any given individual. Minute ventilation and the ventilation perfusion ratio directly affect the amount of oxygen delivered to the arterial system.[5,95] The blood volume and the total body hemoglobin influence the amount of O_2 that can be carried in the blood.[3,5,68,100] A 1-liter decrease in blood volume or a 6 g/dl decrease in hemoglobin will result in a 20% decrease in VO_{2max}.[100] The cardiac output directly influences the amount of oxygenated blood that can be delivered to the peripheral circulation.[3,87,95] The affinity of hemoglobin for O_2 will affect unloading at a tissue level.[3,44,95] Muscle blood flow, the size of the active muscle mass, capillary density, and diffusion gradients dictate how much O_2 is delivered to the muscle cell.[3,5,87,95] Finally, the number of mitochondria, the amounts of key rate-limiting enzymes, and sarcolemmal function (ability to sequester and release CA^{2+}, the ability to fire repetitively) control VO_{2max} at the cellular level.[44,95]

VO_{2max} is an important determinant of endurance performance.[5,22,79] However, it is much more valuable for events that take 3 to 8 minutes to complete than for longer events, such as marathons, which are dependent on factors such as running economy and fractional utilization of the VO_{2max}.[5,22,72,79,96] Thus, if one is interested in the 1500-m run, training to improve VO_{2max}, should improve performance in this event. Levels as high as 90 ml/kg/min have been recorded in athletes.[5] The highest values are generally found in cross-country skiers; among runners, milers tend to have the highest values.[5] VO_{2max} decreases by 9% per decade after age 25.[3] Values of near 40 ml/kg/min may still be observed in runners 80 years of age.[46] This is particularly impressive when one considers that an acceptable value for VO_{2max} in a healthy 25-year-old man is 50 ml/kg/min.[3]

*References 3, 5, 12, 47, 68, and 88.

Lactic Acid Metabolism

The essentials of lactic acid metabolism have been discussed in greater detail above. As noted, lactate is produced at rest and at all intensities of exercise.[5,11,12,68,88] During dynamic exercise of progressively increasing intensity, accumulation stays relatively close to that of resting levels until approximately 50% to 70% VO_{2max}.[3,5,88] Following the surpassing of this "lactate threshold" or onset of blood lactate (OBLA), it accumulates in substantial amounts, inducing the aforementioned increases in CO_2 production and ventilation.[3,5,68,88] The lactate threshold observed during a treadmill running test is highly correlated with running performance in events of various distances, but most highly with longer-duration activities.[22,35,64,96] This is important, because while VO_{2max} is a relatively good predictor of performance among a heterogeneous group of athletes (i.e., varied $VO_{2max}s$), the usefulness of VO_{2max} when runners have similar maximal aerobic capacities is rather limited.[5,22,72,79] The running speed, or percentage of VO_{2max} at which increased accumulation of lactate is observed, is a much more sensitive predictor of performance.[22,79,96] Regular endurance training promotes alterations in skeletal muscle that favor improvement in the lactate threshold. These include increased percentage of Type IIa fibers, increased capillary density, increased numbers of mitochondria, improved utilization of free fatty acids, and increased numbers of oxidative enzymes.* Faster O_2 kinetics at the onset of exercise are also associated with these favorable changes.[15] Figure 26-6 illustrates the pattern of lac-

*References 1, 3, 19, 20, 52, 53, 72, and 76.

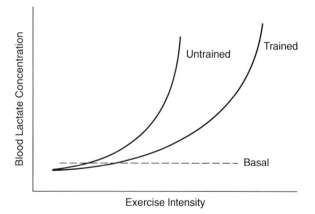

Fig. 26-6

Blood lactate accumulation during progressive exercise in untrained and trained states. *(From Young JL: Physiologic Basis of Sports Rehabilitation. In Press JM ed, Rehabilitation Clinics of North America. 5:1., p9-36 1994 WB Saunders, Philadelphia.)*

tate accumulation during exercise in the untrained and trained states.

Upper- versus Lower-Body Exercise

Although the phrase *large muscle group exercise* typically conjures the thought of leg exercise, many athletes utilize their arms to generate part (rowers, swimmers) or almost all (wheelchair athletes) of the forces needed for their preferred activity.[5,15,48,80,89] The differences between the physiologic responses to "arm" and "leg" exercise are outlined in this section.

Cardiovascular

In general, for any given work rate, heart rate is greater during arm work than during leg work.[3,5,68,70] The relationship between heart rate and oxygen consumption remains linear, but the heart rate during arm work is higher for any given VO_2 as well.[3,5,68,70,77] However, at least at low intensities, the time for adjustment to the steady-state heart rate (HR) is roughly the same under both conditions, with half time to steady state ($t_{1/2}ss$) heart rate being slightly under 20 seconds.[77] Cardiac output (Q_{CO}) increases linearly in both forms of exercise, but there is a more blunted increase in stroke volume during arm work.[5,70,77] Decreased venous return from the extremities results in a smaller end diastolic volume and decreased contraction efficiency.[3,5,77] Systolic and diastolic blood pressures are higher during arm work. The greater HR and systolic blood pressure (SBP) result in a higher rate pressure product (HR × SBP = RPP), which reflects a higher myocardial oxygen consumption.[3,5]

The vascular resistance of the entire systemic circulation, or total peripheral resistance (TPR), decreases during both upper- and lower-body work.[5,47,70,71] In both cases, the large drop in resistance within the active muscle circulatory bed plus the modest drops across skin and coronary vessel resistance overmatch the vasoconstriction within the inactive muscle and splanchnic beds.[5,47,70] However, the TPR is higher during arm work.[5,47,70] There have been a number of possible mechanisms cited, including the following:

1. Exercise with the arms that includes grasping (i.e., kayak) introduces an isometric component to the work, thereby increasing resistance within the active muscle bed.[15,70,77]

2. The sympathetic nervous system induces constriction within inactive muscles. Since the total level

of constriction is inversely proportional to the active muscle mass, and the mass of the arms is smaller than the legs, this reduces the patent total body vascular cross-sectional area.[70,77]

3. For a given power output, a smaller muscle mass must work at a greater percentage of its contraction maximum.[5,70,77,78] If this work requires contraction forces of more than 15% to 20% of the maximum voluntary contraction, the muscular activity itself may result in occlusion via mechanical compression of vessels.[70]

4. There is slightly greater plasma efflux during arm work resulting in a slightly greater blood viscosity.[70]

Respiratory

In untrained subjects, minute ventilation is greater relative to either work rate or oxygen consumption during arm exercise.[3,5,68,77] A higher breathing frequency rather than increased tidal volume is observed.[5] This may be due to greater proprioceptive (neural) drive, earlier accumulation of metabolic byproducts (see below), and greater changes in pH.[5] The ventilatory breakpoint (i.e., the exercise intensity above which minute ventilation rises disproportionately to further increases in VO_2), occurs at lower work loads during arm work as well.[3,5,68,77]

In addition, the half-time to a steady state of oxygen consumption, ($t_{1/2} VO_2ss$), during submaximal exercise tends to be slower during arm work.[15,77,78] This results in a larger relative oxygen debt with a concomitant greater accumulation of anaerobic metabolites.[5] Once a steady state for a given work load is achieved, VO_{2arms} tends to be higher than VO_{2legs}.[5,15,77] This is associated with poorer mechanical efficiency during arm work.[5,15,77,78]

At maximum effort, in untrained or non-arm-trained subjects, $VO_{2max_{arms}}$ is typically on the order of 40% to 70% $VO_{2max_{legs}}$.[5,68,77] However, elite kayakers are capable of achieving roughly the same VO_{2max} with either arms or legs, indicating that with specific training the arms are as adaptable as the legs.[78,89] Rowers have very high values of VO_{2max} (over 6 liters/min or above 65 ml/kg/min), but they, clearly, also involve their legs and back in the generation of power output.[48,80]

Muscle Blood Flow

Muscle blood flow increases markedly during arm exercise, and flow (ml/100 g of muscle tissue/min) rivals,[77] and may even exceed,[83] MBF_{legs} at the same relative percent maximum HR. The kinetics of MBF are rapid, and as with leg work, the steady state for MBF_{arms} is reached well before the steady state for VO_2 or cardiac output.[15,78] However, the total body VO_2 at a given MBF is usually higher during leg work, implying poorer extraction by the arms particularly in the untrained state.[78]

Lactic Acid Metabolism

In association with the observed slower O_2 kinetics and greater O_2 deficits, the onset of lactate accumulation is earlier during arm exercise.[5,68,77,78] There is also a greater accumulation of lactate during arm work than leg work at the same workload.[3,5,61,68,77] Again, as with VO_{2max}, arm-trained individuals demonstrate superior responses than untrained subjects, with lesser accumulation of lactate during submaximal work.[5,15,68,78]

Response to Resistance Exercise

Weight lifting and isometric activities promote a different exercise response than do the dynamic exercises referred to above. To begin with, these exercises tend to be of a higher intensity and are "anaerobic," and can only be carried out for limited periods.[3,5,31,88] Furthermore, because they generally require force generation in excess of 20% of a muscle's maximal voluntary contraction (MVC), the contraction itself often results in muscle blood vessel occlusion.[3,5,88]

Strength may be defined as the maximum force or tension that a muscle or a muscle group can generate with a single contraction.[5,7,30,68] The time that it takes to perform this contraction is not an issue, unless power (output over time) is being considered. Strength is classically assessed via a single maximal effort (the one repetition maximum or 1 RM), but may also be estimated from the knowledge that 70% to 80% of the 1 RM can usually be lifted 8 to 10 times.[5,30]

During maximal effort, skeletal muscle may develop 3 to 4 kg of force per square centimeter.[5,29,30] Thus, the maximum potential force that a muscle may develop is highly related to its size, or the number of sarcomeres in cross section of the muscle.[29,30,47] The major determinants of strength, in addition to muscle size, include fiber-type profile, muscle-tendon lever relationships, and neuromuscular issues such as firing patterns of motor units.[5,29,30,63] Weight lifters generally demonstrate greater percentages of their area occupied by Type II fibers and often have higher percentages of Type II fibers as well.[5,68,97] Lever relationships come into play because the amount of torque a muscle can generate is influenced by the point in its range of motion at which strength measurement is being made. When the perpendicular distance between the line of muscular pull and the joint axis is increased, the measured torque increases.[30,65] Increased force generation is also possible if the person lifting is able to activate motor units more fully within the prime movers for the specific movement.[85] This neural adaptation of motor units is reflected by an increased integrated electromyogram, which is commonly seen after strength training.[85]

The most impressive acute responses to resistance exercises are seen in the cardiovascular system. Blood pressures as high as 320/250 mm Hg and heart rates up to 170 beats/min have been recorded during maximal double leg presses.[5,34] The larger the muscle mass involved, the greater the magnitude of the response will be.[5,34] The explanation for this incredible rise in pressure has not been entirely clarified. Increased cardiac output, increased intraabdominal and intrathoracic pressures, increased intramuscular pressure and utilization of the Valsalva maneuver have all been suggested.[5,34] Trained body builders do exhibit slightly less of this pressor response.[34] Over time, resistance training is associated with increased left ventricular wall thickness and ventricular mass.[3,5,34,68] Left ventricular volume is unchanged.[5,34] Oxygen uptake is elevated to less than 50% maximum, unless the athlete is participating in a training circuit with greater numbers of repetitions at multiple lifting stations.[31,39] Long-term resistance training leads to only small increases in VO_{2max} at best.[5,31,32,67,68]

Short- and long-term metabolic responses, again, reflect the anaerobic nature of these exercises. ATP, CP, and glycogen all decrease during lifting sessions.[31] Mitochondrial density, creatine kinase, myofibrillar ATPase, PFK, and citrate synthetase levels decrease with long-term resistance training; LDH appears to be unaltered.[5,31,98] Lactic acid accumulation during submaximal leg work does appear to be lowered following leg training.[67] This may relate to increases in leg strength (i.e., the contractions are being performed at a lesser percentage of MVC).[67] Capillary density decreases with resistance training.[3,5,18,68] This is partially because of the larger size of the muscle fibers and partially because resistance exercises have not been shown to promote neocapillarization.[5,68,94,97]

The primary adaptation to long-term resistance training is hypertrophy, or increased cross-sectional area of the muscle. Hypertrophy is due to an increase in the number and size of myofibrils.[5,7,66,97] Synthesis of contractile proteins is accelerated, more so in Type II than in Type I fibers.[97] Other changes that consistently occur with resistance training include increased tendinous and ligamentous strength and mass and increased bone density.[5,94] Much more controversial is the suggestion that some of the increase in muscle size is due to splitting of and formation of "new" fibers, or *hyperplasia*.[42,43,63,68] This has been demonstrated in the flexor carpi radialis of cats following high-resistance training, but not conclusively in humans.[29,42,43,68]

Strength training regimens are quite variable, and there is no single approach that has been deemed the best. Success may be found with the DeLorme technique (utilizing progressively increasing percentages of the 10 RM through the workout), by using "pyramid" routines, in which each set consists of lifting weights which are closer and closer to the 1RM, or other routines.[28-30] Regardless of the approach, it is essential to alternate muscle groups to promote balance between muscle groups and to facilitate recovery of the exercised groups. It is extremely important for the novice lifter to be coached in appropriate technique to reduce risk of acute injury as well. A reasonable starting prescription for the aspiring weight lifter is to perform one to three sets of lifting a weight that can be lifted 8 to 12 times, three times per week. If the weight cannot be lifted at least 8 times during the final set, the weight is too great and needs to be reduced. If the lifter can lift the weight 12 times all three sets, it is reasonable to increase the resistance, but by no more than 10%. Competitive lifters may lift 5 to 6 days per week for hours at a time.[7] However, these lifters still rotate the groups exercised and also alternate between heavy- and light-lifting days. Lifting to improve power can entail lifting somewhat lighter weights so that more repetitions may be performed (i.e., 15 to 20 repetitions), or so that the movements involved in the left can be done more quickly. Utilization of the stretch-shortening cycle also increases power output during training sessions.[63]

Healthy, previously untrained college males may increase their strength by 20% to 40% over a 2- to 4-month period.[7] Measurable strength gains and muscular hypertrophy have also been documented in both postpubescent children and elderly individuals.[37,103] Prepubescent youths tend to demonstrate increased strength without appreciable increases in muscle mass.[103]

Prescription of Exercise

The prescription of exercise for development of strength, power, or endurance is based on a relatively simple principle. The SAID (specific adaptation to imposed demand) principle recognizes that the human body will respond to given demands with specific and predictable adaptation.[2] An important corollary of this is that although muscle is extremely adaptable and can "learn" to do many different things, it can probably do only one thing best. Although one can improve in more than one area of fitness at a time (i.e., "cross-training"), one cannot attain maximal gains in both strength and marathon-type endurance at the same time.[5,32,51,86] This implies that when designing conditioning programs, it becomes important to identify what the goals of that program are and then select exercises that maximize the likelihood that the desired training effect will be achieved. The basic components of the exercise prescription are described below.

Intensity

Essentially, this describes how difficult the exercise is. For aerobic training, the exercise should be carried out at 40% to 85% VO_{2max}, or 55% to 90% of maximal heart rate.[3] Lower intensities may promote a training effect, but they must be carried out for lengthy periods of time to do so.[3,5,88] For recreational exercisers, use of the rating of perceived exertion (RPE) scale may be a convenient method of ensuring that approximately the same intensity is selected on a day-to-day basis.[10,14] Exercising in the range between "somewhat hard" and "hard" will promote a cardiovascular training effect. For sprint or anaerobic training, the intensity will be "supramaximal" (i.e., the athlete will be exercising at work rates in excess of that necessary to elicit VO_{2max}).[3,5,69] Intensities that promote endurance training effects do not have an effect on anaerobic capacity.[69] However, if one employs Fartlek ("speed play")-type training, in which short fast bursts of running are interspersed within the running workout, there may be development of some anaerobic qualities as well.[25]

Duration

This indicates how long the session is. Exercise should be carried out for between 15 and 60 minutes to develop an aerobic training effect, and may be done continuously or discontinuously.[3] Continuous-type training can have different outcomes, depending on the exercise intensity selected. Specificity dictates that if the athlete trains at high intensities for shorter periods, a tolerance for lactate will be built up and VO_{2max} will likely improve.[5,68,69] If exercise is carried out near the intensity of the lactate threshold, then this is the parameter most influenced.[69,76] Exercise at lower intensities carried out for upward of 1 hour allows for large total energy expenditure without exposure to high levels of stress and promotes more efficient utilization of FFA stores.[67,69,88]

Interval training is a method of discontinuous training with alternating "work" and "relief" periods.[5] The work interval typically consists of exercise that is a very high percentage of maximum for a short period, followed by the relief period, which is of low intensity. The relief interval allows for resynthesis of phosphagens and decreases the need for glycolytic metabolism when the high-intensity work interval is started over.[5,68] When the cumulative exercise time is examined, it becomes apparent that this scheme potentially enables the individual to work for long periods at an intensity that would normally cause fatigue in a few minutes.[5,68] Daniels recommends that a 1:1 work:relief ratio be used with the work bouts kept less than 5 minutes.[25]

Frequency

The frequency of exercise is typically 3 to 5 days per week.[3] Exercise can be performed safely every day if different muscle groups are stressed on different days or if different energy systems are relied on. The ultimate example of this are competitive triathletes who must carefully balance exercise stress and recovery so that three events can be trained for with more than one training session per day.

Mode of Exercise

The key issue to remember for mode of exercise is that if improvement in fitness is of interest, the athlete should be tested in a manner that resembles the mode of training as much as possible. A bicycle-trained athlete should be tested on a bike, a runner on a treadmill, and a swimmer in a flume. Failure to do so will often result in underprediction of the training effect. For patients with spine problems, mode is also critical because while two exercises may have the same potential cardiovascular benefit, one may place less stress on the three-joint complex. For example, the person with a lateral L4-L5 disc extrusion may perform better on a stationary ski machine, where posture is upright and the spine is maintained in neutral or mild extension, than on a stationary bicycle, where there is increased loading due to the forward lean and seated posture.

Muscular Overwork

Exercise that is too intense, or that involves a significant amount of eccentric overload, may induce excessive postexercise muscular soreness, reflecting a condition of acute muscular overwork. In general, if exercise results in elevation of blood levels of creatine kinase, lactate dehydrogenase, or myoglobin some level of rhabdomyolysis has occurred.[33] This is apparent within 24 hours of exercise. Extremes of either intensity or duration are capable of producing these enzymatic changes, although intensity appears to be the more critical factor.[33,39]

Intense eccentric exercise is associated with numerous disturbances of muscle ultrastructure. Forced lengthening of contracted muscle produces damage that includes sarcolemmal rupturing, degeneration and disorganization of myofibrils, and increased numbers of inflammatory cells have all been reported.[21,36,84,102] Eccentric exercise that induces delayed-onset muscle soreness (24 to 72 hours post exercise) is also associated with decreased ability to resynthesize glycogen during this time frame.[21,74] If the athlete is not allowed adequate recovery following eccentric overload, microscopic breakdown will occur, increasing the likelihood that a maladaptive response to exercise will occur, with ultimate worsening of performance or injury.

Overtraining

The fitness boom of the past decade, along with an increased number of individuals participating in ultraendurance events has made "overtraining" a relatively common phenomenon. Put simply, overtraining is the product of an imbalance between overload (training) and recovery. The individual who overtrains exhibits symptoms and findings of muscular and systemic breakdown (maladaptation) that are, unfortunately, frequently overlooked until athletic performance begins to suffer.

From a subjective standpoint, the person who is overtraining may complain of feeling "stale," of not being as motivated as usual, or of being generally fatigued.[5] Sleep patterns may be disturbed, and the athlete may report that he or she is always tired on arising in the morning. The school-aged or college athlete may admit having a difficult time keeping up in classes or receiving poorer grades. Teammates or family members may note that the athlete is more irritable or more difficult to talk to. Loss of appetite is common.[90] Complaints of pain and soreness of muscles and joints, often in the absence of overt cause, is another clue that the person is overtraining and a "chronic athletic fatigue" syndrome is present.[90]

Objective findings include elevation of the morning resting heart rate by more than 5 beats per minute, immunosuppression with an increased frequency of respiratory illnesses, and weight loss.[5,58,90] Testosterone levels tend to drop, while cortisol levels tend to rise, suggesting hypothalamic dysfunction.[6,73] Glycogen depletion which can be caused by repeated heavy bouts of exercise accompanied by inadequate ingestion of carbohydrates may also contribute to muscular fatigue.[90] Certain muscle enzyme concentrations (creatine kinase, lactate dehydrogenase, transaminase) and myoglobin rise rather dramatically following single bouts of heavy exertion, signifying muscle damage, but in and of themselves are not reliable markers of chronic overtraining.[33,90,99] Recurrent stress fractures, at the very least, indicate some repetitive biomechanical overload. Although full discussion of this issue is beyond the scope of this chapter, when stress fractures are discovered in a lean female athlete, the athlete's dietary habits and menstrual history should be investigated. Consultation with a sports psychologist and formal endocrinologic evaluation may be required as well.

Ultimately, prevention of overtraining is more critical than its detection and treatment. Prudent recommendations include ensuring that the athlete matches energy expenditure with caloric intake, allowing the athlete to obtain adequate sleep every night, and increasing training frequency, duration, or intensity by small increments. "Periodization" of training (i.e., varying the volume and intensity of training sessions) at different times of the year, so that the athlete "peaks" near competitions but does not have to maintain peak form year-round is critical. Tapering the volume of training in the weeks prior to competition allows for reduction of muscular soreness, recovery from injury and restoration of metabolic stores.[88]

Consequences of Detraining

The consequences of deconditioning are well recognized by all professionals who work in rehabilitation medicine. Joint contractures, disuse atrophy of muscle, and disturbances of metabolism, cardiovascular, and respiratory systems function are all observed in patients subjected to prolonged bed rest.[49]

VO_{2max} decreases up to 25% after 3 weeks of bed rest.[3,45] Patients with chronic back pain are prone to deconditioning and muscle atrophy due to their restricted activity in order to avoid pain. Unfortunately, this only leads to further deconditioning, muscle atrophy, and diminished ability to withstand physical stress or recover from exertion. While it is unusual for an athlete to refrain from all physical activity, conditions may arise that necessitate tapering or discontinuation of training. The presence of an acute or chronic injury, a surgical procedure and the associated postoperative care, or simply the end of a competitive season all serve as examples. It is important to recognize that although athletes typically start at much higher levels of fitness than the general population, they are not immune to the effects of interrupted training regimens.

Detraining results in a relatively rapid decrease in VO_{2max}.* The beneficial effects of 7 weeks of endurance training disappears within 8 weeks of detraining, with approximately half of the endurance training effect lost within the first 2 weeks.[75] The decrease in maximal aerobic power is related to reduction of the maximal cardiac output, which in turn, is highly related to the drop in maximal stroke volume.[5,23,45,75,88] Reduction of stroke volume is primarily a result of reduced blood volume.[5,23,24] Neither depressed myocardial function nor change in ventricular wall dimensions is the cause.[5,23,24,88] Mitochondrial activity, which rises by approximately 30% following 2 to 4 months of endurance training, will drop to pretraining levels by only 1 to 2 months with detraining.[50,60] The number of capillaries within trained muscle may decrease by up to 25% within 3 weeks.[68,88] Mildly encouraging is the finding that the changes above are somewhat attenuated, (but not eliminated), in those who have trained for years.

The most logical approach to this potential problem is to remain fit all year round. This may be particularly difficult in athletes who are injured or feel that a break from sports will prevent mental staleness. The purpose of the "out of competition" training program is therefore just to maintain some type of "base" from which the athlete can springboard into the next competitive season. This may be accomplished with as few as two good workouts per week. It should be stressed to the athlete that it is better to decrease frequency rather than totally discontinue training, and that by continuing to maintain fitness, he or she will have an easier time getting into shape and will be able to spend more time on skill training at the start of the next season.

*References 5, 23, 24, 45, 75, and 88.

Conclusions

Exercise is the cornerstone of spine rehabilitation. Optimization of strength, flexibility, and endurance in conjunction with a program focused on restoration of normal spine mechanics requires the coordinated efforts of the entire spine treatment team. For the professional who intends to work with patients with spinal dysfunction, an understanding of the basic principles of exercise physiology and exercise prescription is essential. It is hoped that this chapter will serve as the foundation on which a greater breadth of spine rehabilitation knowledge may be built.

References

1. Acevedo EO, Goldfarb AH: Increased training intensity effects on plasma lactate, ventilatory threshold, and endurance, *Med Sci Sports Exerc* 21:563, 1989.
2. Allman FL: *Exercise in sports medicine*. In Basmajian JV, editor: *Therapeutic exercise*, ed 9, Baltimore, 1984, Williams & Wilkins.
3. American College of Sports Medicine: *Guidelines for exercise testing and prescription*, ed 4, Philadelphia, 1991, Lea & Febiger.
4. Andersen P, Henriksson F.: Training induced changes in the subgroups of human type II skeletal muscle fibres, *Acta Physiol Scand* 99: 123, 1977.
5. Astrand PO, Rodahl K: *Textbook of work physiology*, New York, 1986, McGraw-Hill, Inc.
6. Barron GL, Noakes TD, Levy W, et al.: Hypothalamic dysfunction in overtrained athletes, *J Clin Endocrinol Metab* 60:803, 1985.
7. Basford JR: Weightlifting, weight training and injuries, *Orthopedics* 8:1051, 1985.
8. Bell RD, MacDougall JD, Billeter R, et al.: Muscle fiber types and morphometric analysis of skeletal muscle in six year old children, *Med Sci Sports Exerc* 12:28, 1980.
9. Bergh U, Thorstensson A, Sjodin B, et al.: Maximal oxygen uptake and muscle fiber types in trained and untrained humans, *Med Sci Sports Exerc* 10:151, 1978.
10. Borg GAV, Linderholm H: Perceived exertion and pulse rate during graded exercise in various age groups, *Acta Med Scand Suppl* 472:194, 1967.
11. Brooks GA: Current concepts in lactate exchange, *Med Sci Sports Exerc* 23:895, 1991.
12. Brooks GA, Fahey TD: *Fundamentals of human performance*. New York, 1987, Macmillan Publishing Company.
13. Cavanagh PR, Komi PV: Electromechanical delay in human skeletal muscle under concentric and eccentric contractions, *Eur J Appl Physiol* 42:159, 1979.
14. Ceci R, Hassmen P: Self monitored exercise at three different RPE intensities in treadmill vs field running, *Med Sci Sports Exerc* 23:732, 1991.
15. Cerretelli P, Pendergast D, Paganelli, et al.: Effects of specific muscle training on VO_2 on-response and early blood lactate, *J Appl Physiol* 47:761, 1979.
16. Claussen J, Lassen N: Muscle blood flow during exercise in normal man studied by the ^{133}xenon clearance method, *Cardiovasc Res* 5:245, 1971.
17. Colling-Saltin A: Enzyme histochemistry of skeletal muscle of the human fetus, *J Neurol Sci* 39:169, 1978.
18. Costill DL, Coyle EF, Fink WF, et al.: Adaptations in skeletal muscle following strength training, *J Appl Physiol* 46:96, 1979.
19. Costill DL, Daniels J, Evans W, et al.: Skeletal muscle enzymes and fiber composition in male and female track athletes, *J Appl Physiol* 40:149, 1976.
20. Costill DL, Fink WJ, Pollock ML: Muscle fiber composition and enzyme activities of elite distance runners. *Med Sci Sports Exerc* 8:96, 1976.
21. Costill DL, Pascoe DD, Fink WJ, et al.: Impaired muscle glycogen resynthesis after eccentric exercise, *J Appl Physiol* 69:46, 1990.
22. Costill DL, Thomason H, Roberts E: Fractional utilization of the aerobic capacity during distance running, *Med Sci Sports Exerc* 5:248, 1971.
23. Coyle EF, Hemmert MK, Coggan C: Effects of detraining on cardiovascular responses to exercise: role of blood volume, *J Appl Physiol* 60:95, 1986.
24. Coyle EF, Martin WH, Bloomfield SA, et al.: Effects of detraining on responses to submaximal exercise, *J Appl Physiol* 59:853, 1985.
25. Daniels J: Training distance runners—a primer. *Sports Sci Exch Gatorade Sports Sci Inst* 1:11, 1989.
26. Davis JA: Anaerobic threshold: review of the concept and directions for future research, *Med Sci Sports Exerc* 17:6, 1985.
27. Davis JA, Vodak P, Wilmore JH, et al.: Anaerobic threshold and maximal aerobic power for three modes of exercise, *J Appl Physiol* 41:544, 1976.
28. DeLorme TL, Watkins AL: Techniques of progressive resistance exercise, *Arch Phys Med* 29:263, 1948.
29. Dillingham MF: Strength training, *Phys Med Rehab State Art Rev* 1:555, 1987.
30. DiNubile N: Strength training, *Clin Sports Med* 10:33, 1991.
31. Dudley GA: Metabolic consequences of resistive-type exercise, *Med Sci Sports Exerc* 20:S158, 1988.
32. Dudley GA, Djamil R: Incompatibility of endurance- and strength-training modes of exercise, *J Appl Physiol* 59:1446, 1985.
33. Evans WJ: Exercise-induced skeletal muscle damage, *Physician Sports Med* 15:89, 1987.
34. Fleck SJ: Cardiovascular adaptations to resistance training, *Med Sci Sports Exerc* 20:S146, 1988.
35. Foster C, Costill DL, Daniels JT, et al.: Skeletal muscle enzyme activity, fiber composition and VO_{2max} in relation to distance running performance, *Eur J Appl Physiol* 39:73, 1978.
36. Friden J, Sjostrom M, Ekblom B: Myofibrillar damage following intense eccentric exercise in man, *Int J Sports Med* 4:170, 1983.
37. Frontera WR, Meredith CN, O'Reilly F, et al.: Strength conditioning in older men: muscle hypertrophy and improved function, *J Appl Physiol* 64:1038, 1988.
38. Gauthier GF, Lowey S: Distribution of myosin isozymes among skeletal muscle fiber types, *J Cell Biol* 81:10, 1981.

39. Gettman LR, Ayres JJ, Pollock ML, et al.: The effect of circuit weight training on strength, cardiorespiratory function, and body composition of adult men, *Med Sci Sports Exerc* 10:171, 1978.

40. Gollnick PD, Armstrong RB, Saltin B, et al.: Effect of training on enzyme activity and fiber composition of human skeletal muscle, *J Appl Physiol* 34:107, 1973.

41. Gollnick PD, Armstrong RB, Saubert CW, et al.: Enzyme activity and fiber composition in skeletal muscle of untrained and trained men, *J Appl Physiol* 33:312, 1972.

42. Gonyea WJ: Role of exercise in inducing increases in skeletal muscle fiber number, *J Appl Physiol* 48:421, 1980.

43. Gonyea WJ, Sale DG, Gonyea FB, et al.: Exercise induced increases in muscle fiber number, *Eur J Appl Physiol* 55:137, 1986.

44. Green HJ, Patla AE: Maximal aerobic power: neuromuscular and metabolic considerations, *Med Sci Sports Exerc* 24:38, 1992.

45. Grimby G, Saltin B: Physiological effects of physical training, *Scand J Rehab Med* 3:6, 1971.

46. Gutin B, Zohman L, Young JL: Case report: an 80 year old marathoner, *J Cardiac Rehab* 1:344, 1981.

47. Guyton AC: *Textbook of medical physiology*, ed 8, Philadelphia, 1991, W.B. Saunders Co.

48. Hagerman FC: Applied physiology of rowing, *Sports Med* 1:303, 1984.

49. Halar EM, Bell K: *Contracture and other deleterious effects of immobility.* In DeLisa JA, editor: Rehabilitation medicine, Philadelphia, 1988, J.B. Lippincott.

50. Henriksson J, Reitman JS: Time course of changes in human skeletal muscle succinic dehydrogenase and cytochrome oxidase activities and maximal oxygen uptake with physical activity and inactivity, *Acta Physiol Scand* 99:91, 1977.

51. Hickson RC: Interference of strength development by simultaneously training for strength and endurance, *Eur J Appl Physiol Occup Physiol* 45:255, 1980.

52. Hickson RC, Heusner WW, Van Huss WD: Skeletal muscle enzyme alterations after sprint and endurance training, *J Appl Physiol* 40:868, 1975.

53. Hickson RC, Rennie MJ, Conlee RK, et al.: Effects of increased plasma fatty acids on glycogen utilization and endurance, *J Appl Physiol* 43:829, 1977.

54. Huxley HE: The mechanism of muscular contraction, *Sci Am* 213:18, 1965.

55. Jansson E, Kaijser L: Muscle adaptation to extreme endurance training in man, *Acta Physiol Scand* 100:315, 1977.

56. Jansson E, Sjodin B, Tesch P: Changes in muscle fibre type distribution in man after physical training, *Acta Physiol Scand* 104:235, 1978.

57. Johnson E, editor: *Practical electromyography,* ed 2, Baltimore, 1988, Williams & Wilkins.

58. Keast D, Cameron K, Morton AR: Exercise and the immune response, *Sports Med* 5:248, 1988.

59. Kelley AM, Rubenstein NA: Development of neuromuscular specialization, *Med Sci Sports Exerc* 18:292, 1986.

60. Klausen K, Andersen LB, Pelle I: Adaptive changes in work capacity, skeletal muscle capillarization and enzyme levels during training and detraining, *Acta Physiol Scand* 113:9, 1981.

61. Klausen K, Rasmussen B, Clausen JP, et al.: Blood lactate from exercising extremities before and after arm or leg training, *Am J Physiol* 227:67, 1974.

62. Knuttgen HG, Bonde Petersen F, Klausen K: Oxygen uptake and heart rate responses to exercise performed with concentric and eccentric contractions, *Med Sci Sports* 3:1, 1971.

63. Komi PV, editor: *Strength and power in sport,* London, 1992, Blackwell Scientific Publications.

64. Lafontaine TP, Londeree BR, Spath WK: The maximal steady state versus selected running events, *Med Sci Sports Exerc* 13:190, 1981.

65. Lehmkuhl LD, Smith LK: *Brunnstrom's clinical kinesiology,* ed 4, Philadelphia, 1985, F.A. Davis Company.

66. Luthi JM, Howald H, Classen H, et al.: Structural changes in skeletal muscle tissue with heavy resistance exercise, *Int J Sports Med* 7:123, 1986.

67. Marcinik EJ, Potts J, Schlabach G, et al.: Effects of strength training on lactate threshold and endurance performance, *Med Sci Sports Exerc* 23:739, 1991.

68. McArdle WD, Katch FI, Katch VL: *Exercise physiology: energy, nutrition and human performance,* ed 3, Philadelphia, 1991, Lea & Febiger.

69. Medbo JI, Burgers S: Effect of training on the anaerobic capacity, *Med Sci Sports Exerc* 22:501, 1990.

70. Miles DS, Cox MH, Bomze JP: Cardiovascular responses to upper body exercise in normals and cardiac patients, *Med Sci Sports Exerc* 21:S126, 1989.

71. Murphy RA: *Muscle.* In Berne RM, Levy MN, editors: *Physiology,* ed 3, St. Louis, 1993, Mosby.

72. Noakes TD: Implications of exercise testing for a prediction of athletic performance: a contemporary perspective, *Med Sci Sports Exerc* 20:319, 1988.

73. O'Connor PJ, Morgan WP, Raglin JS, et al.: Selected pseudoendocrine responses to overtraining, *Med Sci Sports Exerc* 21:S50, 1989.

74. O'Reilly KP, Warhol MJ, Fielding RA, et al.: Eccentric exercise-induced muscle damage impairs glycogen repletion, *J Appl Physiol* 63:252, 1987.

75. Orlander J, Keissling KH, Karlsson, et al.: Low intensity training, inactivity and resumed training in sedentary men, *Acta Physiol Scand* 101:351, 1977.

76. Pate RR, Branch JD: Training for endurance sport, *Med Sci Sports Exerc* 29:S340, 1992.

77. Pendergast DR: Cardiovascular, respiratory and metabolic responses to upper body exercise, *Med Sci Sports Exerc* 21:S121, 1989.

78. Pendergast D, Cerretelli P, Rennie DW: Aerobic and glycolytic metabolism in arm exercise, *J Appl Physiol* 47:754, 1979.

79. Peronnet F, Thibault G, Rhodes EC, et al.: Correlation between ventilatory threshold and endurance capability in marathon runners, *Med Sci Sports Exerc* 19:610, 1987.

80. Pyke FS, Minikin BR, Woodman LR, et al.: Isokinetic strength and maximal oxygen uptake of trained oarsmen, *Can J Appl Sports Sci* 4:277, 1979.

81. Reeves JT, Wolfel EE, Green HJ, et al.: *Oxygen transport during exercise at altitude and the lactate paradox: lessons from Operation Everest II and Pikes Peak*. In Holloszy JO, editor: *Exercise and sports sciences reviews,* vol 20, Baltimore, 1992, Williams & Wilkins.

82. Roth DA: The sarcolemmal lactate transporter: transmembrane determinants of lactate flux, *Med Sci Sports Exerc* 23:925, 1991.

83. Rowell LB: Muscle blood flow in humans: how high can it go? *Med Sci Sports Exerc* 20:S97, 1988.

84. Russell B, Dix DJ, Haller DL, et al.: Repair of injured skeletal muscle: a molecular approach, *Med Sci Sports Exerc* 24:189, 1992.

85. Sale DG: Neural adaptation to resistance training, *Med Sci Sports Exerc* 20:S135, 1988.

86. Sale DG, MacDougall JD, Jacobs I, et al.: Interaction between concurrent strength and endurance training, *J Appl Physiol* 68:260, 1990.

87. Saltin B, Strange S: Maximal oxygen uptake: "old" and "new" arguments for a cardiovascular limitation, *Med Sci Sports Exerc* 24:30, 1992.

88. Sharkey BJ: *Training for sport*. In Cantu RC, Michelli LJ, editors: *ACSM's guidelines for the team physician,* Philadelphia, 1991, Lea & Febiger, p 34.

89. Shepard RJ: Science and medicine of canoeing and kayaking, *Sports Med* 4:19, 1987.

90. Sherman WS, Maglischo EW: Minimizing chronic athletic fatigue among swimmers: special emphasis on nutrition, *Sports Sci Exch Gatorade Sports Sci Inst* 4:35, 1991.

91. Stainsby WN, Brooks GA: *Control of lactic acid metabolism in contracting muscles and during exercise*. In Pandolf KB, editor: *Exercise and sports sciences reviews,* vol 18, Baltimore, 1990, Williams & Wilkins.

92. Stainsby WN, Brechue WF, O'Drobinak DM: Regulation of muscle lactate production, *Med Sci Sports Exerc* 23:907, 1991.

93. Stanley WC: Myocardial lactate metabolism during exercise, *Med Sci Sports Exerc* 23:920, 1991.

94. Stone MH, Wilson GD: Resistance training and selective effects, *Med Clin North Am* 69:109, 1985.

95. Sutton JR: VO$_2$max—new concepts on an old theme, *Med Sci Sports Exerc* 24:26, 1992.

96. Tanaka K, Matsuura Y: Marathon performance, anaerobic threshold and the onset of blood lactate accumulation, *J Appl Physiol* 57:640, 1984.

97. Tesch PA: Skeletal muscle adaptations consequent of long-term heavy resistance exercise, *Med Sci Sports Exerc* 20:S132, 1988.

98. Tesch P, Sjodin B, Karlsson J: Relationship between lactate accumulation, LDH activity, LDH isozyme and fibre type distribution in human skeletal muscle, *Acta Physiol Scand* 103:40, 1978.

99. Tiidus PM, Ianuzzo CD: Effects of intensity and duration of muscular exercise on delayed soreness and serum enzyme activities, *Med Sci Sports Exerc* 15:461, 1983.

100. Warren GL, Cureton KJ: Modeling the effect of alterations in hemoglobin concentration on VO$_2$max, *Med Sci Sports Exerc* 21:526, 1989.

101. Wasserman K, Whipp BJ, Koyal SN, et al.: Anaerobic threshold and respiratory gas exchange during exercise, *J Appl Physiol* 35:236, 1973.

102. Waterman-Storer CM: The cytoskeleton of skeletal muscle: is it affected by exercise? A brief review. *Med Sci Sports Exerc* 23:1240, 1991.

103. Webb DR: Strength training in children and adolescents, *Pediatr Clin North Am* 37:1187, 1990.

Chapter 27

Low-Back School and Stabilization: Aggressive Conservative Care*

Robin Robison

* Modified from Robison R: The new back school prescription:
stabilization training, part I, *Spine State Art Rev* 5(3):341-356,
1991.

The SpineCare model of aggressive nonoperative care focuses on the importance of education and training in the complete rehabilitation of the patient with spinal disease and dysfunction. Although it technically falls under the heading of conservative care, the aggressive nature of the exercise and training would not be considered conservative by the program participants. The SpineCare program is based on the "Back School" and "Stabilization Training" model, which evolved as a multifaceted program of education, flexibility, strength, coordination, and endurance training to prevent the repetitive microtrauma to the spinal structures responsible for pain and degeneration.[52] It is an active patient participation program that gives patients the responsibility and the power to manage their low-back problems and prevent further injury.[40] Epidemiologic studies show a staggering frequency of low-back pain, between 60% and 80%, with 20% to 30% suffering at any one time.[36] Although most low-back pain is self-limiting, with a spontaneous recovery rate of 80% to 85% in 8 to 12 weeks, the 60% recurrence rate of back pain demonstrates that healing may not have taken place.[13,36] Additionally, it is reported that there has been a rapid increase of 168% from 1971 to 1981 in the number of individuals with more chronic disabling back symptoms.[25] These statistics reinforce the need for a program that addresses the components that fortify the spinal structures and educates the patient to avoid harmful maneuvers. Fortunately, there has been a recent trend in spine injury rehabilitation toward a more aggressive nonoperative approach in contrast to the previous treatment of analgesics and bed rest or surgery.[77] Unfortunately, there has been a great deal of controversy over which treatment philosophy provides the greatest reduction in pain and return to functional activities.[4,76] This has prompted the need for clarification of a sound education- and exercise-based approach that can be applied individually to various pathologic conditions.

History

The exercise-base approach, termed "stabilization training," is not a new entity, but a compilation of known theories and practices such as back school,[17,44] proprioceptive neuromuscular facilitation (PNF),[38] orthopedic sports medicine,[13,51,55] manual therapy,[8,9,13,16,22,59] and sound exercise principles as set forth by the American College of Sports Medicine.[1,3]

A clear understanding of the anatomy and physiology of the spine and how they relate to movement and function is imperative in accurate assessment and treatment of spinal dysfunction.[20,22,50,53] Recent advances in the understanding of the complex chemical and biomechanical aspects of the spinal structures have guided the development of the stabilization principles.* Kirkaldy-Willis's concept of the degenerative cascade clearly demonstrates the need for trunk muscle control, especially during the unstable phase. One of the earliest references to the concept of stabilization was made by Kendall and Jenkins in 1968 in a study comparing Williams' flexion and McKenzie's extension exercises. They found that the most successful programs avoided further strain to damaged structures while encouraging a posture of minimum stress to improve function and limit disability.[34]

Continuing-education programs have emerged in the past 5 years teaching the concepts of stabilization training.[26,30,48] Also, the techniques of stabilization training and neutral spine have been more clearly defined in the literature.[47,63,64,70] The term *stabilization* has drawn controversy because of the inference of rigidity. The term *neutral* is also felt to imply a fixed position. Other terms have been proposed to describe more accurately *neutral spine* as a position of function or functional range, and these terms are often used interchangeably. The most recent term for stabilization, *methods for limiting and controlling movement*, implies a more dynamic approach.[47] Since the term *stabilization* is more concise and clearly describes the goal of movement control, it would appear to be the best term available at this time.

Research on the efficacy of stabilization and neutral spine training is just beginning. Many articles reference the term *conservative care* with the use of exercise and education without specific mention to the type of training.† Other studies are searching for muscoloskeletal predictors of back injury or success in the rehabilitation process.[17,66] Many studies list exercises for all patients, independent of diagnosis.[33, 57,72,73,74] The P.R.I.D.E. program advocates a multidisciplinary approach called "functional restoration" to the patient with chronic pain.[55] The focus of this program is to restore the functional capacity by having the deconditioned patient work through the pain in a work-hardening and strengthening program. The success rate is 80% to 85% as measured by the ability of the patient to return to work. In a recent Swedish study, patients with nonspecific mechanical low-back pain were treated with a graded

---

* References 5, 14, 15, 20, 26, 30, 47, and 72.
† References 2, 7, 10, 17, 18, 28, 29, and 39.

activity program including trunk strengthening and mobility as well as cardiovascular training and work simulation. This program showed significant increases in mobility, strength, and fitness in addition to an earlier return to work.[41] Specific use of stabilization training in the nonoperative rehabilitation of herniated lumbar disc pain with radiculopathy was reported by Saal and Saal to have 90% good to excellent results, with a 92% return to work rate.[63] This study utilized the SpineCare model of stabilization training, along with a multidisciplinary management team for medical and psychologic intervention. The purpose of this chapter is to outline the specifics of this conservative yet aggressive model of spine rehabilitation.

Diagnosis and Evaluation

A stabilization and neutral spine program of training can be applied to a variety of conditions throughout the phases of degeneration including disc herniation, stenosis, facet syndrome, and spondylolisthesis. An accurate diagnosis is important to identify indications and contraindications.[8,9,32,64,77] Additionally, a thorough evaluation is necessary to obtain subjective and objective information such as limitations in strength, coordination, and range of motion as well as behavior of symptoms, habit patterns, and functional limitations. This information quantifies and qualifies the pain and dysfunction to identify the pain-generating lesion and contributing areas of dysfunction.[13,22] An evaluation will define the patient's current level of function and available pain-free range and identify certain sensitivities to position, load, pressure, or stasis.[47,70] With this information a treatment plan can be developed with definable goals. This base-line information is important not only in program development, but also to identify progress, therefore assisting in treatment evaluation and patient motivation.

Phases of Rehabilitation

Neutral spine and stabilization training begins in the initial phase of rehabilitation or the pain control phase[64] and is carried through to the patient's discharge and then throughout the rest of his or her life. Education in proper movement patterns prevents irritation and reinjury and allows initial healing to begin. Early reconditioning has been shown to assist healing by increasing circulation and promoting an increase in bone density and tissue remodeling.[56] Bed rest for more than 2 days has been shown to be detrimental.[11] Beyond the initial stages of rehabilitation, stabilization progresses into the restoration and strengthening phases. Specific exercise and training provide the patient with greater strength, coordination, and endurance to participate in work-related and home activities without pain and reinjury. Training includes not only task-specific strengthening, but also flexibility and general cardiovascular fitness. One study demonstrated the importance of endurance training for trunk musculature in prevention of injury to passive structures during prolonged activities.[54] Advanced training allows the patient to engage in heavier sport and recreational activities, promoting a more physically active and healthier lifestyle.

Stabilization and Neutral Spine Concepts

It is important to define the terms used in stabilization training to promote a uniform understanding of techniques. *Neutral spine* is a position or range of movement defined by the patient's symptoms, pathology, and current musculoskeletal restrictions. It is a position in which a vertical force exerted through the spine allows equal weight transference into the weight-bearing surfaces.[30] In sitting, these surfaces are the ischial tuberosities and in standing, the feet (Figs. 27-1 and 27-2). The *Functional position* or *range* is defined as the most stable and asymptomatic position for each individual task,[47] and is usually the midrange of the available degrees of pain-free motion. In the patient with acute pain, the neutral functional range may be quite narrow. In therapy, patients learn to identify and improve support within their functional range determined by existing pathology and sound biomechanical principles of spinal movement.* Stenotic and facet conditions may make a patient tend toward slight flexion, while an active disc lesion may dictate greater extension. Techniques such as mobilization or manipulation, stretching, and soft-tissue massage may be used to improve available range, followed by muscular stabilization to control the new motion. The goal is to achieve the maximum range of motion possible as dictated by pain and pathology to promote normal functional movement. Neuromuscular training must then progress through the full range of motion to allow strength and control toward the end of the range where injury occurs. This neuromuscular coordination and control is the goal of stabilization training. It has been shown that the spinal column

---

*References 12, 15, 17, 24, 27, 54, and 75.

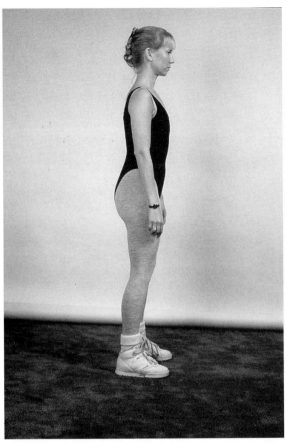

Fig. 27-1

Neutral spine positioning in standing position. *(From Robison R: The new back school prescription: stabilization training, part I,* Spine State Art Rev *5(3):344, 1991.)*

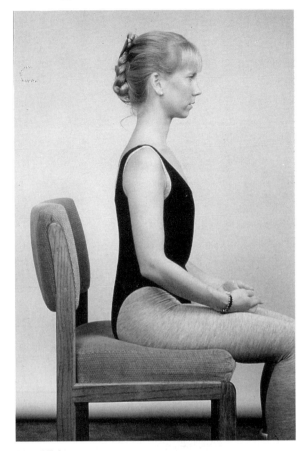

Fig. 27-2

Neutral spine positioning in sitting position.

alone, without muscular support is unable to carry normal physiological loads.[15] Hence, the purpose of stabilization training is to educate and strengthen the patient to maintain the functional range and to facilitate proper movement patterns that control, prevent, or eliminate low-back injury.[63,64] This response must become an automatic neuromuscular skill, counteracting the varied and unpredictable loads placed on the body.[26] Emphasis is placed on achieving quality and grace in movement with the kinesthetic awareness to control spinal posture automatically. The patient can develop this response only through exhaustive practice.

The key muscles responsible for trunk control are the abdominals, especially the oblique muscles, and the spinal extensors controlled obliquely by the multifidus. Much research has been conducted on the importance of these muscles to spinal stability.* Inadequate back extensor strength has been implicated as a predictor of low-back injury.[6,43,67,68] The

*References 15, 19, 31, 49, 54, 68, and 71.

YMCA study reported greater pain reduction with substantial improvement of trunk muscle strength.[36] Use of the oblique abdominal muscles, called "dynamic abdominal bracing," was thought to stabilize the spine through an increase in intraabdominal pressure.[19,35,49] Recent studies have not demonstrated this phenomena, but have found the stabilizing force to come through tensing of the thoracolumbar fascia. This, in combination with a tightening of the posterior ligamentous system, acts as a corset to fortify the spinal elements against torque and shear forces.[19] This tensing is produced by the oblique muscles through their attachment to the lumbodorsal fascia. In forward-bending activities, the internal oblique muscles are needed to counteract the shear forces of the extensor muscles.[19,64] Training of proper abdominal recruitment is difficult. Patients tend to use the rectus abdominus exclusively without oblique contribution. Education in abdominal bracing, emphasizing oblique recruitment is the key to stabilization training. This phase of the education process may be the most time consuming and frus-

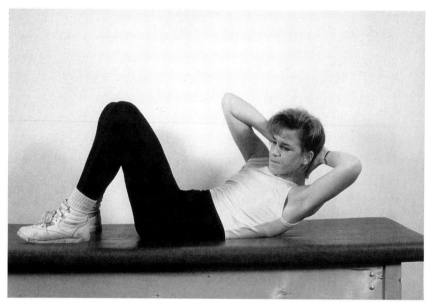

Fig. 27-3

Diagonal curls. Strengthening of oblique abdominal muscles can be more easily achieved on diagonal to minimize excessive recruitment of rectus abdominus. *(From Robison R: The new back school prescription: stabilization training, part I, Spine State Art Rev 5(3):347, 1991.)*

trating for both the patient and the clinician, but advancement cannot be made until this skill is obtained. The clinician must be able to demonstrate proper technique and then facilitate recruitment in the patient through verbal or tactile cuing. Electrical stimulation and electromyographic biofeedback have been shown to facilitate abdominal training.[26,31] Studies have also shown that greater abdominal muscle-fiber recruitment is obtained with concentric exercise (Fig. 27-3).[31] Electrical stimulation may also facilitate strength training in the spinal extensor musculature, but eccentric exercises have been shown to promote greater strength gains in extensor musculature.[31,68] This difference relates easily to function, as the flexors more commonly work in a concentric fashion while the extensors function more eccentrically.

Flexibility

A complete stabilization program addresses not only strength but all factors that may influence stability of the spine. This includes specific spinal segmental mobility for equal movement contribution and extremity flexibility.[42,46,65] Each part of the body must contribute its fair share of movement, or another area will have to compensate to allow adequate movement for daily and work activities. A study from the University of Miami demonstrated that aggressive stretching of spinal and extremity musculature

Table 27-1

Muscle requiring optimal flexibility for postural alignment and spine safe maneuvers

Upper Extremity	Lower Extremity
Pectoralis major/minor	Hamstrings
Subscapularis	Quadriceps
Teres major	Psoas major/minor
Latissimus dorsi	Iliacus
Levator Scapula	Quadratus lumborum
Trapezius	Gluteus maximus, medius, minimus
	Piriformis
	Iliotibial band
	Gastrocnemius
	Soleus

From Robison R: The new back school prescription: stabilization training, part I, *Spine State Art Rev* 5(3):345, 1991.

significantly improved the patient's functional abilities while decreasing pain.[37] Muscles attaching to the pelvis or vertebrae such as the hamstrings, iliacus, psoas, quadriceps, quadratus lumborum, hip rotators, gluteals, hip abductors and abductors, and the

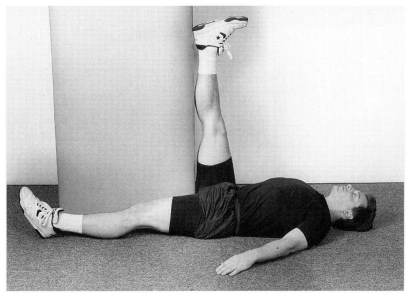

Fig. 27-4

Hamstring stretch. Wall is used to allow relaxation during stretching. Floor support gives spinal stability with ability to overcorrect in flexion (opposite knee bent) or extension (opposite knee extended or towel roll under lumbar curve).

iliotibial band, directly influence spinal and pelvic symmetry (Table 27-1) (Fig. 27-4). Restriction or weakness of other peripheral joints and their surrounding musculature can cause undue compensation in movement through the spinal elements. Muscle tightness in the upper trunk and extremities such as the pectorals, rotator cuff, and latissimus can change the postural alignment and resultant movement patterns (Fig. 27-5). For example, a tennis player with weakness in the rotator cuff with resultant tendonitis may use excessive lumbar extension for overhead shots. Tightness of the triceps surea complex can modify lifting techniques by decreasing balance and base of support (Fig. 27-6). Thoracic mobility must also be addressed, as loss of extension and rotation in this area will have to be absorbed by the lumbar spine.

Stabilization Continuum

Stabilization training progresses from the simplest non-weight-bearing supported positions to complex high-speed functional activities. Each program is individualized for the patient's current pathology, goals, and needs. Each exercise is designed to improve either flexibility, strength, cardiovascular endurance, or coordination while reinforcing safe spine movement. All exercises must be performed with an emphasis on proper technique, and progression is undertaken only after a new skill has been completely

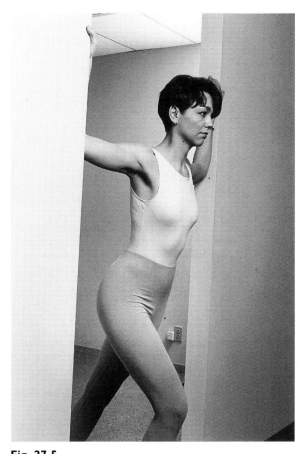

Fig. 27-5

Chest stretch. Doorway or corner can be used to stretch both extremities simultaneously. Attention must be paid to lumbar spine position as tendency is to lean through doorway, causing lumbar extension.

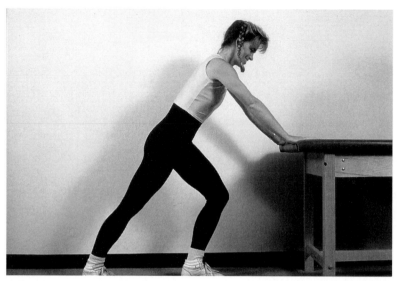

Fig. 27-6

Gastrocnemius stretch. Flexibility of gastocnemius and soleus muscle is important for proper balance in deep lifting activities.

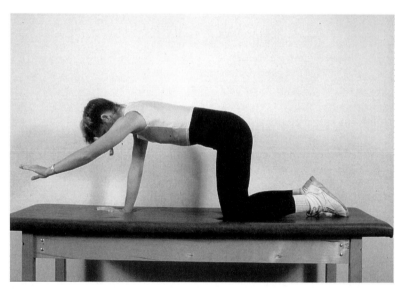

Fig. 27-7

Quadruped single arm lift. Although this exercise appears easy, it challenges both abdominals and extensors to maintain balanced posture while moving arm. This exercise correlates well to household functions such as cleaning the floor or bathtub or to outside activities such as gardening.

mastered. The entry point for each individual patient, based on this continuum of training, is determined through the evaluation process. Symptoms, signs, and sensitivities will determine the need for initial load reduction or position-specific exercise and training. Initial strength, endurance, flexibility, coordination, and body awareness will not only establish a starting point but direct the speed of progression. Constant reassessment is vital to the success of a stabilization program.

Phases of Progression

In the acute or painful state, training can begin with passive prepositioning of the patient in his or her position of comfort.[30,47,48] For example, this may be accomplished in the supine position with the legs and hips supported at 90 degrees of hip and knee flexion. This position greatly reduces the load and biases the lumbar spine in slight flexion, preventing movement into a potentially painful part of the range

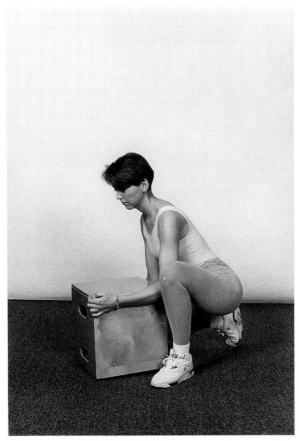 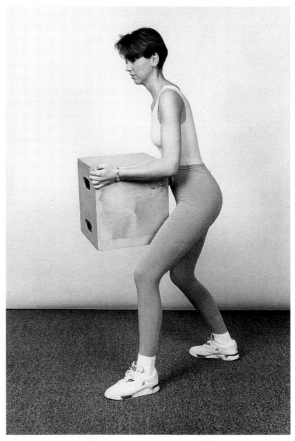

Fig. 27-8

Training proper body mechanics during complex pivoting and lifting movements is critical to complete understanding and application of biomechanical principles to daily work and household activities.

of motion. From this position, the patient can begin to isolate abdominal and extensor muscle contraction and then explore control over lumbopelvic movement. Since muscle contraction does apply a compressive load, traction can be used in this position to further decrease the load, especially in load-sensitive individuals. Removing the external support to provide positional overcorrection is the next progression, called "active prepositioning."[47,48] The patient's own muscular control is used to position the pelvis. In this phase the patient can be taught varying degrees of abdominal control to accommodate to increasing loads and more demanding positions. Dynamic stabilization begins to address more functional activities as limb and body movement is introduced. The patient is taught to control spinal movement through activation of several trunk muscle groups while superimposing extremity movement (Fig. 27-7). Accommodating to changes in stress and load by altering muscle tension is difficult to learn but, once mastered, is less fatiguing and more natural than the overcorrected position.[47]

Learning to control the movement of the lumbar spine while performing normal functional activities is the goal of the final transitional phase.[47,48] Progress is made by increasing from simple to complex transitional movements needed for home, job, or sport activities. This training phase begins with simple sagittal plane movement but must progress to oblique and torsional movements. Whole body movement such as sitting to standing progresses to complex multiangle activities such as lifting (Fig. 27-8). Stabilization exercises should closely resemble functional activities to reinforce proper technique in daily tasks. Exercises are advanced as strength is gained and technique is mastered. Practice in various positions and situations allows the patient to develop problem-solving skills for future activities and demands on the spine. The overriding principle in stabilization training is that exercise will improve function without increasing pain. Progression must therefore be made within the constraints of the patient's pathology and ability. An increase in pain may be caused by poor technique or lack of trunk strength

Table 27-2

Stabilization progression levels: trunk exercises

Level I

Supine	Sidelying	Quadruped	Prone
Abdominal bracing	Hip abduction	Four-point rock	Gluteal sets
Pelvic clock	Four-point arm/leg lift		Short arc upper/lower half extensions
Opposite hand-knee push			
Supported dying bug (alternate arm and leg lift)			
Short arc bridging			
Isolated free-weight training			
Theraband exercise			

Level II

Supine	Sidelying	Quadruped	Prone
Partial/diagonal curls	Hip adduction	Four-point reciprocal arm/leg	Upper/lower half extensions
Unsupported dying bug	Bilateral leg lift	Fire hydrant	
Single straight leg lowering	Fire hydrant		
Air bike			
One-legged bridge			
Bridging with leg lift			

Standing
Free-weight training/isolated weight equipment
Theraband resistance training

Level III

Supine	Prone	Weight Training (increase endurance or weight)
Unsupported dying bug (add wrist and ankle weights)	Full range of movement back extensions over ball (combined with sets of alternate arm lifts)	Free weights
Partial and diagonal curls (on incline or with chest weight)	Bilateral leg extensions over ball (combined with sets of alternate leg flutter)	Weight machines
Bilateral straight-leg lowering	Prone dying bug (alternate arm/leg lift)	
Ball walk/tremble point		
Ball bridging		

Level IV

Ball exercises (increase lever arm/balance difficulty)	Equipment
Bridge	Standing chair (hip flexion with knee extension)
Push-up	Roman chair (back extension)
Partial/diagonal curls with medicine ball	Combine pulley (advanced job-/sport-specific)

From Robison R: The new back school prescription: stabilization training, part I, *Spine State Art Rev* 5(3):349, 1991.

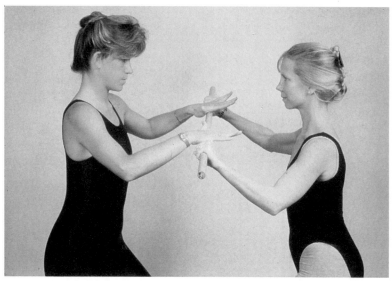

Fig. 27-9

Rhythmic stabilization and slow reversals. PNF techniques can be applied easily using a stick. Pushing and pulling activities can be reproduced slowly or quickly for unanticipated training reactions.

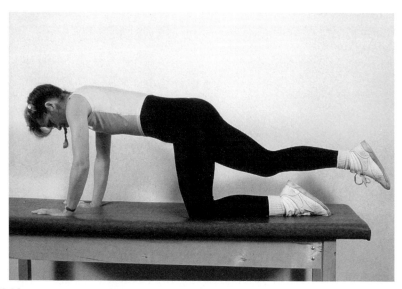

Fig. 27-10

Quadruped alternate leg lift requires cocontraction of oblique abdominals, gluteals, and spinal extensors for spinal stability in neutral. Advancement is achieved by adding reciprocal arm and leg movement or wrist and ankle weights. *(From Robison R: The new back school prescription: stabilization training, part I, Spine State Art Rev 5(3):350, 1991.)*

and control for the specific exercise.[69] The use of manual PNF techniques such as approximation, rhythmic stabilization, slow reversal, and graded resistance can be used to facilitate postural responses and correct body positioning to promote training advancement (Fig. 27-9).[30,35]

Specific Stabilization Exercises

Exercises are divided into four categories of difficulty—level I, beginning; level II, intermediate; level III, advanced; and level IV, sport- and job-specific training, i.e., work hardening (Table 27-2). Most supine exercises challenge and strengthen the flexor musculature while prone activities use the extensor

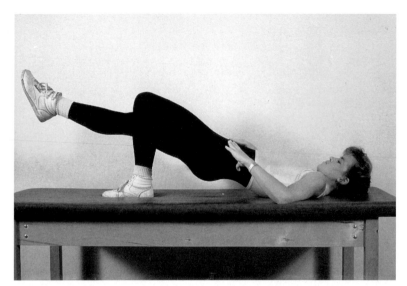

Fig. 27-11

Bridging with alternate leg lift. Gluteal contraction is balanced by oblique abdominal recruitment while superimposing long-lever extremity movement. Maintenance of neutral positioning is monitored for flexion and extension as well as rotation. *(From Robison R: The new back school prescription: stabilization training, part I,* Spine State Art Rev *5(3):351, 1991.)*

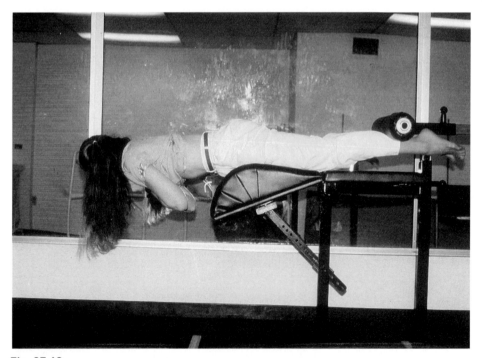

Fig. 27-12

Roman chair back extensions. Back extensors can be strengthened throughout full range of motion by using back extension bench. Saba bench shown allows multiple angle settings for individual patient progression.

musculature.[45] Bridging, sidelying, and quadruped exercises activate cocontraction of multiple muscle groups for control of movement. Standing exercises give whole-body strengthening for proper execution of functional activities.[21] Patients progress in each category as skill and strength levels advance. Each stabilization level increases in complexity and demand on the strength and postural reflexes as external support and stability is removed (Figs. 27-10, 27-11, and 27-12). Exercises are progressed in dif-

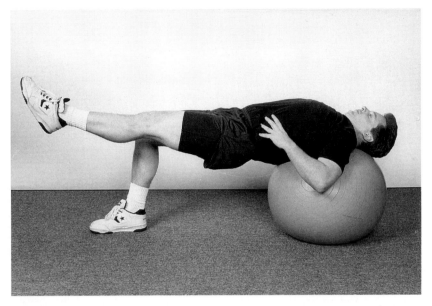

Fig. 27-13

Ball bridging adds a component of balance to strengthening. Use of the gymnastic ball promotes proprioceptive control for automatic postural response.

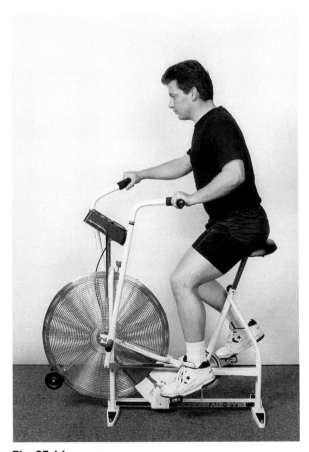

Fig. 27-14

Proper positioning on exercise equipment is critical especially in long aerobic activities.

ficulty by increasing vertical load, resistance, balance requirements, time or repetitions, complexity, and spontaneity. Advanced exercises involve unanticipated stabilization using the gymnastic ball, medicine ball, or external manual resistance (Fig. 27-13). These exercises train the musculature to accommodate rapidly and synergistically to sudden changes in loads and stresses without advance notice.[26]

Aerobic exercise is an integral part of the program from the beginning stages.[28,29] A frequently cited study on firefighters listed optimal cardiovascular fitness as one of the important parameters for prevention of back injuries.[7] Supine or reclined cycling may be substituted for greater weight-bearing exercises in early rehabilitation. Progression to an aerobic exercise that the patient enjoys will promote greater compliance. Proper posture during aerobic exercise is critical, as prolonged positioning is often required (Fig. 27-14).

Use of weight training to facilitate specific strength gains can be used in all levels as adequate stabilization skills and trunk strength are achieved.[23] Specific muscle groups such as the latissimus and rhomboids are addressed for additional spinal and postural stabilization (Table 27-3). Attachment of the latissimus dorsi muscle to the lumbodorsal fascia provides additional lumbar stability (Fig. 27-15). Dynamic muscles such as the biceps, gluteus maximus, and quadriceps require strengthening to ensure adequate extremity strength for execution of

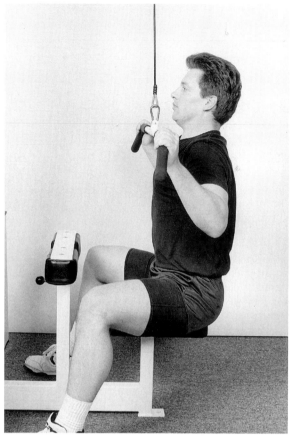 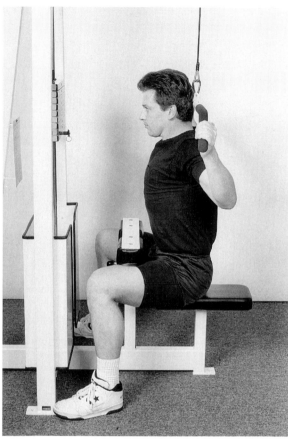

Fig. 27-15

Latissimus pull exercise can be performed behind or in front of neck for complete muscle fiber recruitment. Care should be taken to maintain full neutral spine positioning (cervical, thoracic, and lumbar).

Table 27-3

Muscles requiring strengthening for optimal lifting and postural support

Upper Extremity	Lower Extremity
Biceps	Gluteals
Triceps	Quadriceps
Deltods	Gastrocnemius/soleus
Latissimus dorsi	Hamstrings
Rhomboids	
Pectorals	
Serratus	

From Robison R: The new back school prescription: stabilization training, part I, *Spine State Art Rev* 5(3):352, 1991.

proper body mechanics (Fig. 27-16). Care should be taken in execution of each technique, not only in the actual lift, but the racking of the weight and positioning on weight equipment. Exercises should be advanced according to the needs and lifestyle de-

mands of each individual patient.[60] For example, a young mother may need considerable upper and lower extremity strength in addition to trunk control to lift her growing child.

Realistic goals should be set to avoid injury or discouragement. Although certain pathologic conditions may dictate an initial bias toward flexor (e.g., stenosis) or extensor (e.g., herniated disc) strength training, as the neutral range improves and sensitivities decrease, the program should be revised to include a greater balance of muscular training. Current research tends to support the need for symmetry in abdominal and extensor strength to balance the shear and stress forces.[15] The final home exercise program should include aerobic exercise, trunk strengthening, and isolated extremity exercises as dictated by job, sport, and lifestyle demands.

Stabilization Evaluation

Frequent testing of strength and skills in movement patterns and body mechanics is important for patient

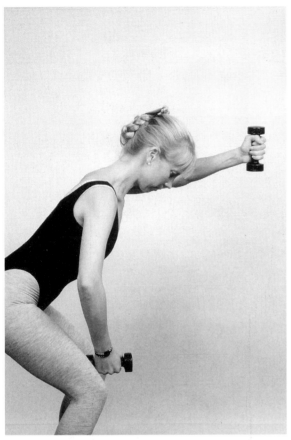

Fig. 27-16

Sumo shoulder flies. Use of sumo position for free-weight training demands synergistic extensor and abdominal control during lifting. *(From Robison R: The new back school prescription: stabilization training, part I, Spine State Art Rev 5(3):353, 1991.)*

motivation and treatment planning but also serves as a valuable measure of patient progress for reporting to physicians, employers, and third-party payers. Areas of difficulty can be isolated and emphasized in the treatment program. Testing enables the practitioner to have a clear picture of patient compliance and depth of understanding of stabilization and neutral spine principles and their application to daily activities. A "Functional Gym Stabilization Evaluation" (Table 27-4) has been developed to quantify strength levels of major muscle groups influencing spinal control and proper body mechanics. Strict adherence to the protocol for conducting the stabilization evaluation ensures consistency among those administering the test. A "Functional Activities Assessment" (Table 27-5) quantifies understanding and ability to control lumbopelvic movement in activities of daily living. A point system is used in both assessments to establish a grading of strength and skill. Research is currently

underway to determine the reliability of these measures and to establish normal values for optimal health and function as well as determining individual needs for varying pathologies and physical demands.

Functional Gym Stabilization Evaluation: Protocol

The stabilization evaluation was designed to test the functional strength of a patient undergoing spine rehabilitation without the use of elaborate or expensive machinery that may not be available in all clinics. With this in mind, the hope was to find a universal way to measure the strength of certain muscles that have been shown to either control spinal mobility or provide movement and strength for activities of daily living. Three categories or levels of testing of strength and control coordinate with the three levels of exercise progression. A point system was devised to allow categorization per level independently of one area of deficit (i. e., inability to do advanced extension-based exercises because of pain or weakness but able to do advanced abdominal exercises). Simply add the scores listed for each successfully completed exercise to determine the patient's stabilization level. Determining which level of exercise to test should be based on the current level of exercise in the patient's home or clinic exercise program. If the patient feels underchallenged or overstressed, you can repeat the test on another day at a different level. In reporting your results, areas of pain or weakness should be outlined along with a plan for treatment and exercise to correct each deficit. Additional testing for specific extremity strength, aerobic capacity, position tolerance, or job-related activities Work Capacity Assessment (WCA) are also recommended.

This test can be performed in approximately 30 to 45 minutes. Although it is listed by muscle groups tested, it is advisable to alternate between abdominal-based exercise and extensor-based exercises to avoid excessive fatigue and promote active resting of one muscle group. The following is a detailed description of each exercise in each level of the test to promote consistency of testing between clinicians.

The partial sit up (PSU) tests primarily abdominal strength and is begun in the hooklying position (supine with knees bent and feet flat on the floor). The patient's hands are placed behind the head to determine level of difficulty not to lift through pulling on the head. Through contraction of the abdominal muscles (especially the internal and exter-

Table 27-4

Functional gym stabilization evaluation

	Level I	Level II	Level III
Partial sit-ups	3 × 10 forward	3 × 10 forward	3 × 10 forward
	3 × 10 right	3 × 10 right	3 × 10 right
	3 × 10 left	3 × 10 left	3 × 10 left
	Hands behind head	Hands behind head	Hands behind head
		Hips 90/knees 90	Hips 60-70/knees extended
	1 pt.	2 pts.	3 pts.
Dying bug	Supported	Unsupported	Unsupported
			UE/LE with 3 lb/5 lb
	2 minutes	2 minutes	2 minutes
	1 pt.	3 pts.	5 pts.
Bridging	Slow reps	Alternate LE extension continuously	Alternate LE extension with 5 lb continuously
	3 minutes	3 minutes	3 minutes
	1 pt.	3 pts.	5 pts.
Prone	Alternating BUE/BLE Slow reps	Alternating BUE/BLE over chair 15-sec holds	Superman over chair
	1 minute	2 minutes	3 minutes
	1 pt.	2 pts.	3 pts.
Quadruped	Reciprocal	Reciprocal	Reciprocal
	UE/LE	UE/LE	UE/LE with 3 lb/5 lb
	Slow reps	15-sec holds	Slow reps
	5 sec holds		5-sec holds
	2 minutes	2 minutes	3 minutes
	1 pt.	2 pts.	3 pts.
Functional squat	75 reps	150 reps	250 reps
	1 pt.	2 pts.	3 pts.

Point Scale

Stabilization I:	0-9 pts.
Stabilization II:	10-16 pts.
Stabilization III:	17-22 pts.

Stabilization Total:

Patient		Date
Therapist	Person administering test	

From Saal J: The new back school prescription: stabilization training, part II, *Spine State Art Rev* 5(3):364, 1991.
BLE = bilateral lower extremity; BUE = bilateral upper extremity; LE = lower extremity; UE = upper extremity.

nal obliques which cause a flattening of the abdominal wall with contraction), the patient lifts his/her upper torso until the scapulas lift off the floor. Each repetition is done slowly with minimal to no time at rest on the floor between repetitions. The abdominal contraction must be maintained throughout the entire repetition both concentrically and eccentrically. Additionally, the patient must not hold his/her breath during the exercise, but inspiration and expiration can occur with either the concentric or eccentric portion of the exercise. In level I, the patient performs one set of 10 repetitions forward, right, and left and then repeats the circuit three times. The left and right partial sit-ups (D.S.U., or diagonal sit-ups) are done on a very narrow diagonal. Both scapulas still must clear the floor with the left or right

Table 27-5
Functional activities assessment

Activity	Date: Score	Date: Score	Date: Score
Sit to stand and return			
Sit to supine and return			
Roll supine to sidelying and return			
Overhead reach			
Stand to squat and squat to floor			
Total score			
Initials of tester:			

Patient Name   Chart #

Physical Therapist

Key to scoring:

0 = cannot perform with verbal cuing

1 = can perform correctly with verbal cuing

2 = can perform correctly without verbal cuing

From Saal J: The new back school prescription: stabilization training, part II, *Spine State Art Rev* 5(3):364, 1991.

being slightly higher depending on direction. In level II the starting position is modified from a feet flat position to a feet elevated position so that the knee and hip angles are 90 degrees. This increases the level of difficulty. The rest of the exercise progression is the same. Level III increases the level of difficulty by extending the knees relatively straight while lowering the angle of the hip to the floor to 60 to 70 degrees. Again, the rest of the exercise is exactly the same, with three sets of 10 repetitions in all three directions. In all positions, the patient must not only be able to complete the repetitions but to do so while maintaining neutral spine posture.

The dying or dead bug exercise, as it is called interchangeably, also primarily test abdominal strength but requires more movement and transitional control due to the extremity movement. Level I begins in the hooklying position. This is called the "supported position," as there will be two extremities in contact with the floor at all times. The exercise involves lifting of one arm and the opposite leg and

extending them until the arm is flexed to 160 to 180 degrees, and the knee is straight with the hip angle to the floor being 60 to 70 degrees. The exercise continues with a constant alternating of the arms and legs (i.e., right arm + left leg then left arm + right leg) for 2 minutes without the loss of neutral spine position. Failure would be determined if the patient was unable to complete the time or was unable to control and limit lumbar movement into extension caused by the forces of the arm and leg movement. Level II increases the level of difficulty of the exercise by removing the leg support. In this level, the starting position is exactly like level II in the PSU exercise, known as a 90/90 position. Again, the patient must be able to alternate the arm and leg movement nonstop for 2 minutes without loss of neutral spine position. Level III introduces wrist (3 lb) and ankle (5 lb) weights to increase the level of difficulty. Otherwise the exercise is the same.

The bridging exercise tests primarily gluteal, quadriceps, and hamstring strength. Additionally, the abdominals and spinal extensors must co-contract to control spinal movement and assist in lifting the middle torso. The starting position is the hooklying position and the patient lifts his/her buttocks off the floor, hinging at the hip joint, until they make a straight line from shoulders to knees. The patient should not hyperextend or hyperflex the spine beyond neutral position throughout the exercise.

No time should be spent resting on the floor between repetitions. In level I, repetitions should be performed continuously for 3 minutes. The level II exercise increases the level of difficulty by adding additional leg movement to challenge rotational control. The legs are alternately extended to a knee straight and hip angle at a 60- to 70-degree position. This leg activity is done continuously for 3 minutes without the buttocks ever being lowered back to the floor. Completion of the exercise is determined not only by time but the ability of the subject to avoid lumbar flexion, extension, and rotation during the entire 3 minutes. The level III exercise is identical except for the addition of 5-lb weights to the ankles to increase the level of difficulty.

Prone exercises primarily challenge and test the strength of the extensor mechanism but require additional spinal control through the abdominals to avoid hyperextension of the spine. The level I exercise begins with the patient in prone position over two to three pillows situated under their abdomen centered at their navel. The exercise involves lifting of both arms and then lowering them and lifting both legs. This exercise should be done slowly and fluidly with little to no rest between the arm and leg switches for a total of 1 minute. The start position for level II and III is prone over a well padded armless chair placed at the same level as the pillows. This increases the range of motion through which the exercise can be performed. The level II exercise increases in difficulty by requiring an isometric hold of the arm and then the leg lifts for 15 seconds and adds an additional 1 minute to the overall exercise, for a total of 2 minutes. The level III exercise requires a continuous isometric hold of both arms and legs at the same time for a total of 3 minutes.

The quadruped exercise tests the rotatory control of the extensors and abdominals especially testing the multifidus and the oblique abdominals. The starting position is the same in all levels, with the patient on hands and knees with the shoulder, hip and knee angle at 90 degrees. The level I exercise requires lifting of the right arm and left leg and then slowly switching to the opposite arm and leg lift. This should be done continuously for 2 minutes with 5-second holds in each position. Again there should

be no rest time, with all four extremities on the floor. The tester is looking for smooth transitional movement control during the switching of extremities lifted with no evidence of rotation, flexion, or extension in the spine. The level II exercise increases the level of difficulty by challenging endurance and balance with 15-second holds in each position. The level III exercise further challenges strength, balance and endurance by adding 3-lb weights to each wrist and 5 lb to each ankle. The holds are only 5 seconds, but the total exercise time is 3 minutes.

The functional squat exercise tests primarily lower extremity strength, especially the quadriceps, gluteals, hamstrings, and gastrocnemius/soleus muscle groups but requires abdominal and extensor stabilization control throughout a transitional movement. Starting position is a staggered stance (right or left leg slightly forward) with the legs abducted 45 degrees and the hips and knees relatively straight. The patient then performs a squat until the hips and knees are flexed at 100 degrees. This would place the patient's hands at their knees with their torso angled forward and their buttocks shifted backward. They must maintain a balanced center of gravity over their base of support. In level I, this exercise is repeated for 75 repetitions. Level II increases the difficulty to 150 repetitions, and level III requires 250 repetitions. Again, form is as important as number, and the patient must be able to maintain neutral position throughout the entire number of repetitions.

Summary

Stabilization training in neutral spine is an integrated approach of education in proper posture and body mechanics along with exercise to improve strength, flexibility, muscular and cardiovascular endurance, and coordination of movement. It is a self-help and self-management program relying heavily on individual responsibility. The goal is to reduce stress on the spinal structures while promoting optimal function. This program is not reserved only for patients with existing back pathology, but should be applied prophylactically in all individuals to prevent spinal injury and disability. Furthermore, it is not a standalone method for the treatment of low-back dysfunction. Other physical therapy interventions such as manual therapy may be needed to correct mechanical dysfunction and diminish pain. Use of selective injections or medications can decrease the pain inhibition to exercise and training. An accurate diagnosis is imperative to allow proper planning of an individualized treatment program. Additionally, treatment of spine dysfunction does not end at patient discharge. The changes in body mechanics and the exercise routines must become permanent lifestyle changes. It is helpful to have the patient return for follow-up testing and program revisions at 1-, 3-, 6-, and 12-month intervals. This not only helps in patient motivation for program compliance but allows modification of the exercise routine toward a more balanced program as continued healing occurs. The use of exercise and proper movement patterns for the treatment of spine dysfunctions is just beginning to show sophistication and specific individual design and application. Future study should uncover even greater technical advances, which may help streamline programs and play a greater part in prevention as well as treatment of low-back pain.

References

1. American College of Sports Medicine: *Guidelines for exercise testing and prescription,* ed 4, Philadelphia, 1991, Lea & Febiger.
2. Asfour S, Ayoub M, Mital A: Effects of an endurance and strength training programme on lifting capability of males, *Ergonomics* 27:435, 1984.
3. Berger RA: *Applied exercise physiology,* Philadelphia, 1982, Lea & Febiger.
4. Bigos S, Battie M: Acute care to prevent back disability, *Clin Orthop Relat Res* 221:121, 1987.
5. Bogduk N, Twomey T: *Clinical anatomy of the lumbar spine,* Melbourne, Australia, 1987, Churchill-Livingstone.
6. Brady T, Cahill B, Bodnar L: Weight training-related injuries in the high school athlete, *J Sports Med* 10:1, 1982.
7. Cady L, Bischoff D, O'Connell E, et al.: Strength and fitness and subsequent back injuries in firefighters, *J Occup Med* 21:269, 1979.
8. Cyriax J: *Textbook of orthopedic medicine,* vol 2, ed 11, New York, 1984, Baillière-Tindall.
9. Cyriax J: *Textbook of orthopedic medicine,* vol 1, ed 8, New York, 1982, Baillière-Tindall.
10. Delauche-Cavallier M-C, Budet C, Laredo J-D, et al.: Lumbar disc herniation: computed tomography scan changes after conservative treatment of nerve root compression. *Spine* 17:927, 1992.
11. Deyo R, Leoser J, Bigos S: Herniated lumbar intervertebral disc, *Ann Intern Med* 112:598, 1990.
12. Dolan P: Commonly adopted postures and their effects on the lumbar spine, *Spine* 13:197, 1988.
13. Donatelli R, Wooden M: *Orthopedic physical therapy,* New York, 1989, Churchill-Livingstone.
14. Donatelli R, Owens-Burkhart H: Effects of immobilization on the extensibility of periarticular connective tissue, *J Orthop Sports Phys Ther* 3(2):67, 1981.
15. Farfan H: Muscular mechanism of the lumbar spine and the position of power and efficiency, *Orthop Clin North Am* 6:135, 1975.
16. Farrell J, Twomey L: Acute low back pain: comparison of two conservative treatment approaches, *Med J Aust* 1:160, 1982.
17. Forssell M: The Swedish back school, *Physiotherapy* 66(4):112, 1980.
18. Fredrickson B, Trief P, Van Beveren P, et al.: Rehabilitation of the patient with chronic back pain, *Spine* 13:351, 1988.
19. Gracovetsky S, Farfan H, Helleur C: The abdominal mechanism, *Spine* 10:317, 1985.
20. Gracovetsky S: The optimum spine, *Spine* 11:543, 1986.
21. Gunnari H, Evjenth O: *Sequence exercise,* Oslo, 1983, Dreyer.
22. Grieve, G: *Common vertebral joint problems,* ed 2, Edinburgh, 1988, Churchill-Livingstone.
23. Gustavsen R: *Training therapy,* New York, 1985, Thieme Inc.
24. Hart D, Stobbe T, Jaraiedi M: Effect of lumbar posture on lifting, *Spine* 12:138, 1987.
25. Hazard R, Fenwick J, Kalisch S, et al.: Functional restoration with behavioral support: a one year prospective study of patients with chronic low back pain, *Spine* 14:157, 1989.
26. Headley BJ: *The "play-ball" exercise program,* St. Paul, MN, 1990, Pain Resources, Ltd.
27. Hedtmann A, Steffen R, Methfessel J, et al.: Measurement of human lumbar spine ligament during loaded and unloaded motion, *Spine* 14:175, 1989.
28. Jackson C, Brown M: Analysis of current approaches and a practical guide to exercise prescription, *Clin Orthop Relat Res* 179:46, 1983.
29. Jackson C, Brown M: Is there a role for exercise in the treatment of patients with low back pain? *Clin Orthop Relat Res* 179:38, 1983.
30. Johnson G, Saliba V: *Post-graduate courses in orthopedic and neurological manual therapy and exercise training,* Institute of Physical Art.
31. Kahanovitz N, Nordin M, Verderame R, et al.: Normal trunk muscle strength and endurance in women and the effect of exercise and electrical stimulation, *Spine* 12:105, 1987.
32. Kapandji I: *The physiology of the joints,* vol. 3, The trunk and vertebral column, New York, 1974, Churchill-Livingstone.
33. Kellett K, Kellett D, Nordholm L: Effects of an exercise program on sick leave due to back pain, *Phys Ther,* 71:283, 1991.
34. Kendall P, Jenkins J: Exercises for backache: a double blind controlled trial, *Physiotherapy* 54:154, 1968.
35. Kennedy B: An Australian programme for management of back problems, *Physiotherapy* 66(4):108, 1980.
36. Kirkaldy-Willis WH: *Managing low back pain,* ed 2, New York, 1988, Churchill-Livingstone.
37. Kjalil T, Asfour S, Martinez L, et al. Stretching in the rehabilitation of low-back pain patients, *Spine* 17:311, 1992.
38. Knott M, Voss D: *Proprioceptive neuromuscular facilitation,* ed 2, New York, 1968, Harper & Row.
39. Kraus H, Nagler W: Evaluation of an exercise program for back pain, *Am Fam Physician* 28:153, 1983.

40. Liang M, Daltroy L, Pallozzi L: The patient's responsibility in therapy for LBP, *J Musculoskel Med* 3:43, 1986.

41. Lindstrom I, Ohlund C, Eek C, et al.: Mobility, strength, and fitness after a graded activity program for patients with subacute low back pain, *Spine* 17:641, 1992.

42. Locke J: Stretching away from back pain and injury, *Occup Health Saf* 52:8, 1983.

43. Manniche C, Hesseloe G, Bentzen L, et al.: Clinical trial of intensive muscle training for chronic low back pain, *Lancet* 1473, 1988.

44. Mattmiller A: The California back school, *Physiotherapy*, 66(4):118, 1980.

45. McKenzie R: *Treat your own back*, New Zealand, 1983, Spinal Publications.

46. Mellin G: Correlations of hip mobility with degree of back pain and lumbar spine mobility in chronic low-back pain patients, *Spine* 13:668, 1988.

47. Morgan D: Concepts in functional training and postural stabilization for the low back injured, *Top Acute Care Trauma Rehab* 2(4):8, 1988.

48. Morgan D, McGonigal T, Moore M, et al.: *Education in manual therapy: training the patient with low back dysfunction*, Folsom Physical Therapy.

49. Morris J, Lucas D, Bresler B: Role of the trunk in stability of the spine, *J Bone Joint Surg* 43A:327, 1961.

50. Nachemson A: The lumbar spine: an orthopedic challenge, *Spine* 1:59, 1976.

51. Nicholas, JA, Hershman EB: *The lower extremity and spine in sports medicine*, St Louis, Mosby, 1986.

52. Oakley R: *History of stabilization in California, master's thesis*, pp 8-12, 1990, University of California.

53. Paris S: Anatomy as related to function and pain, *Orthop Clin North Am* 14:475, 1983.

54. Parnianpour M, Nordin M, Kahanovitz N, Frankel V: The triaxial coupling of torque generation of trunk muscles during isometric exertions and the effect of fatiguing isoinertional movements on the motor output and movement patterns, *Spine* 13:982, 1988.

55. Polatin P: The functional restoration approach to chronic low back pain, *J Musculoskel Med*, 7:17, 1990.

56. Porter R, Adams M, Hutton W: Physical activity and the strength of the lumbar spine, *Spine* 14:201, 1989.

57. Plum P, Rehfield J: Muscular training for acute and chronic back pain, *Lancet* 1:453, 1985.

58. Robison R: The new back school prescription: stabilization training, part I, *Spine State Art Rev* 5(3):341-356, 1991.

59. Roy S, Irvin R: *Sport medicine—prevention, evaluation, management, and rehabilitation*, Englewood Cliffs, New Jersey, 1983, Prentice-Hall, Inc.

60. Rutherford O, Jones D: The role of learning and coordination in strength training, *Eur J Appl Physiol* 55:100, 1986.

61. Saal J: The new back school prescription: stabilization training, part II, *Spine State Art Rev* 5(3):357-366, 1991.

62. Saal J: General principles and guidelines for rehabilitation of the injured athlete, *Phys Med Rehab State Art Rev* 1:523, 1987.

63. Saal J, Saal J: Nonoperative treatment of herniated lumbar intervertebral disc with radiculopathy: an outcome study, *Spine* 14:431, 1989.

64. Saal J: Rehabilitation of sports-related lumber spine injuries, *Phys Med Rehab State Art Rev* 1:613, 1987.

65. Saal J: Flexibility training, *Phys Med Rehab State Art Rev* 1:537, 1987.

66. Selby D: Conservative care of the industrial back, *AAOS Instruct Lect*, p 177, 1982.

67. Sorensen F: Physical measurements as risk indicators for low-back trouble over a one-year period, *Spine* 9:106, 1984.

68. Smidt G, Blanpied P, White R: Exploration of mechanical and electromyographic responses of trunk muscles to high-intensity resistive exercise, *Spine* 14:815, 1989.

69. Sweeney T, Prentice C, Saal J, Saal J: Cervicothoracic muscular stabilization, *Phys Med Rehab State Art Rev* 4:335, 1990.

70. Syms J: Stabilization training can help your back patients gain control, *Back Pain Monitor* 8(7):101, 1990.

71. Tesh KM, Dunn JS, Evan JH: The abdominal muscles and vertebral stability, *Spine* 12:501, 1987.

72. Tollison C, Kriegel M: Physical exercise in the treatment of low back pain, part I: A review, *Orthop Rev* 17:724, 1988.

73. Tollison C, Kriegel M: Physical exercise in the treatment of low back pain, part II: a practical regimen of stretching exercises, *Orthop Rev* 17:913, 1988.

74. Tollison C, Kriegel M: Physical exercise in the treatment of low back pain, part III: a practical regimen of strengthening exercises, *Orthop Rev* 17:1002, 1988.

75. Troup J: Biomechanics of the vertebral column, *Physiotherapy* 65:238, 1979.

76. Waddell G: A new clinical model for the treatment of low-back pain, *Spine* 12:632, 1987.

77. Waddell G, McCulloch J, Kummel E, Venner R: Nonorganic physical signs in low-back pain, *Spine* 5:117, 1980.

Chapter 28

Cervicothoracic Muscular Stabilization Techniques[*]

Tara Sweeney P.T.
Carol Prentice

[*]From Sweeney T, Prentice C, Saal JS, Saal J: Cervicothoracic muscular stabilization techniques, *Phys Med Rehab State Art Rev* 4:335, 1990.

This chapter introduces the concept and basis of cervicothoracic stabilization training (CTST). Traditionally, the patient with cervicothoracic pain has been treated with cervical collars, cervical traction, ultrasound, electric stimulation, soft-tissue massage, and joint mobilization.[1,8] Although these techniques may form an integral part of the early treatment process, they also rely more heavily on the practitioner rather than on active patient participation.

Rehabilitation of the patient with cervicothoracic spine pain requires a comprehensive approach. To be successful, a program must include active patient participation. The program should teach the patient to assume control of his/her cervicothoracic condition. The primary goals of the CTST program should be to maximize return of function, to limit progression of degenerative changes, and to prevent further injury. Additionally, functional improvement gives the patient realistic goals and expectations as well as an objective outcome. The overall rehabilitation program should be designed with the individual's needs, lifestyle, available training time, and occupation taken into consideration.

Cervicothoracic stabilization training emphasizes balanced postural alignment, segmental control of mobility, and appropriate use of stabilization skills. The program is divided into multiple phases: the musculoskeletal evaluation, the patient education phase, the postural reeducation phase, and the stabilization training phase.

Assessment of Physical and Functional Capacity

Prior to the commencement of the training program, accurate assessments of the patient's physical and functional capacity are required. A thorough musculoskeletal evaluation, complete functional examination, and an accurate diagnosis provide rational and effective rehabilitation goals.

Location and character of symptoms will assist in the education phase of the treatment plan, while identification of bony and soft-tissue restrictions will guide the manual part of the treatment. Evaluation of muscular weakness, postural imbalance, and compensation of movement patterns will direct the progression of muscular stabilization training. Specific exercises, postures, and stretches can be prescribed for pain relief. Stretching exercises and segmental mobility training may be used to increase the available range of motion. Resistance exercises are individualized for functional requirements, current strength levels, and patient's stabilization skills. Careful cor-

relation of the patient's history, mechanism of injury, and physical and functional examinations determines the balance between mobility training and stability training in a treatment regiment.

The cervical spine must provide support of the head while allowing great degrees of movement to optimize function of the sensory organs housed within the cranium. Cervical spine mobility should allow an individual to look quickly behind him/her over his/her shoulders, up at the stars, and down at a newspaper. The cervical spine moves in flexion, extension, lateral flexion, and rotation. Lateral flexion and rotation are considered combined movements.[2,4,6]

Total movement of the cervical spine is the composite of segmental motion of all the cervical vertebrae. The major portion of rotational movement occurs in the upper cervical portion between the occiput, the atlas, and the axis.[2] The remaining motion occurs at the lower cervical segments C4 to C7.[2]

Poor posture and irregular movement patterns alter the normal segmental use of cervical vertebrae. Postures considered "poor" or undesirable are those that aggravate dorsal thoracic kyphosis, resulting in a rounding of the shoulders. The faulty posture thrusts the head forward from the lower cervical spine and increases the upper cervical lordosis with compensatory occipital-atlas extension[3,8] (Fig. 28-1). Poor posture during lifting, carrying, pushing, and pulling activities may contribute to additional forward translation and compression stresses on cervical structures.

Movement patterns on a poor postural base contribute to repetitive microtrauma of cervical structures including facets, discs, ligaments, articular capsules, and muscles. These patterns of movement contribute to habitual overuse of isolated motion segments while minimizing normal movement at others. Habitual dysfunction of isolated segments may generate bony hypertrophy, ligamentous laxity, and breakdown of disc and facet articulations.[11] The underlying combination can perpetuate itself in pain, spasm, and the dysfunction cycle.[9,11]

Correct dispersal of segmental movement depends on the balance postural alignment between the head (occiput), the cervical spine and the thoracic cage. This balanced postural alignment is termed the "position of optimal function (POF) (Fig. 28-2). POF is a position that optimizes the biomechanical balance between the thoracic "base" and the "motion" segments of the cervical spine. POF does not mean eliminating all lordosis by forcing a dorsal glide into a military posture. Rather POF is a balanced alignment combining slight occipital-atlas

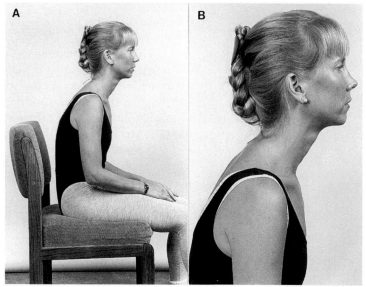

Fig. 28-1

A, Note increase in thoracic kyphosis associated with scapular protraction and reversion of lumbar lordosis. **B,** Note leading chin position and exaggeration of cervical lordosis. *(From Sweeney T, Prentice C, Saal JS, Saal J: Cervicothoracic muscular stabilization techniques, Phys Med Rehab State Art Rev 4:336, 1990.)*

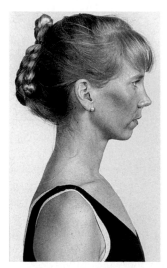

Fig. 28-2

Note chin-down position coupled with scapular retraction. *(From Sweeney T, Prentice C, Saal JS, Saal J: Cervicothoracic muscular stabilization techniques, Phys Med Rehab State Art Rev 4:337, 1990.)*

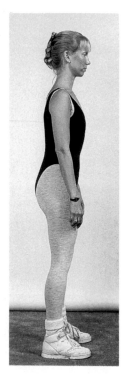

Fig. 28-3

Note balanced lumbar posture itself to balanced cervicothoracic curve. *(From Sweeney T, Prentice C, Saal JS, Saal J: Cervicothoracic muscular stabilization techniques, Phys Med Rehab State Art Rev 4:338, 1990.)*

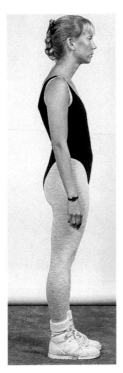

Fig. 28-4

Note increase in lumbar lordosis that will necessitate second counterbalancing of increase of thoracic kyphosis, finally leading to cervical lordosis in chin and stooped-shoulders posture. *(From Sweeney T, Prentice C, Saal JS, Saal J: Cervicothoracic muscular stabilization techniques, Phys Med Rehab State Art Rev 4:338, 1990.)*

flexion with a mild degree of cervical lordosis available to each individual.

Alteration of this cervical alignment may not be attempted without consideration of the entire spine. All spinal curves transect a plumb line to remain in balance with gravity[2] (Fig. 28-3). An increase in any one curve must be compensated by a proportionate increase or decrease in the other curves (Fig. 28-4). For example, lumbar flexion associated with slump sitting contributes to collapsing of the thoracic cage or increased thoracic kyphosis (see Fig. 28-1). The increased thoracic kyphosis and rounded shoulders provide a poor base of support for the cervical spine. This poor base thrusts the head forward at the cervicothoracic junction. A forward head position results in a flattened lower cervical spine with a compensatory occipital-atlas extension position.

Stabilization of the Total Spine

Training the balanced cervical spine must, therefore, include postural stabilization retraining of the entire spine. Lumbar spine stabilization offers a properly aligned base of support for the thoracic cage. If the thoracic cage is conceptualized as the platform on which the cervical spine rests, the thoracic cage position is the key to postural control of the balanced cervical spine.

The critical components of a balanced spine are muscular strength and symmetry. The anterior and posterior muscles of the thoracic cage may be thought of as cables that effectively influence the articular interaction of the thoracic spine, scapulothoracic articulation, and glenohumeral joints.

A shortening of the anterior musculature including pectoralis major, pectoralis minor, and anterior deltoid contributes to a shortened, narrow, and collapsed thoracic cage. Pectoralis minor muscle fibers run inferiorly, obliquely, and medially from the tip of the coracoid process to the anterior third through fifth rib. The fibers pull the anteroscapulae laterally and anteriorly, resulting in a rounded-shoulder postural position.

A lengthened, widened, and opened thoracic cage requires equivalent soft-tissue extensibility between these muscle groups. Additionally, the posterior interscapular musculature including the middle and lower fibers of the trapezius, rhomboids, and serratus anterior must be both flexible and strong enough to support the "shoulders back, chest out" posture and an aligned cervical spine.

The muscles with force vectors that lay anteriorly and posteriorly to the cervical spine also act as cables that influence the joint alignment and symmetry of the head and cervical spine in relation to the thoracic cage. A shortening of the suboccipital, sternocleidomastoid, upper trapezius, levator scapulae, splenius capitis, longissimus capitis, spinalis capitis, and semispinalis capitis musculature contribute to a flattened lower cervical spine with a compensatory occiputatlas extension position. Lengthening of these muscles in balance with the anterior flexors frees up the motion segments to attain a balanced position of the occiput resting on the atlas. The balance cervicothoracic spine offers an appropriate base for training segmental mobility and stabilization exercises.

The stability of the cervical column depends on ligaments and dynamic muscular control. The musculature must be strong and symmetrical for position maintenance during cervicothoracic training. This will reduce compression forces, chronic soft-tissue strain, and excessive forces on the cervical intervertebral discs.

Cervicothoracic Stabilization Training

Cervicothoracic stabilization training (CTST) requires specialized training and coordination using body mechanics, posture, movement principles, and active exercise. The principles of stabilization training include retraining the musculature to control and use cervical mobility and stability of the diseased (painful) spinal segment. CTST promotes the necessary strength, coordination, and endurance to maintain the cervical spine in a stable and safe position during loading, mobility, and weight-bearing activities. Stabilization training optimizes the cervicothoracic spine's capacity to absorb loads in all directions while minimizing direct stress and strain in relation to individual cervical tissues. It eliminates repetitive microtrauma to the cervical segments and limits progression of injury, thereby, allowing healing to take place.[11]

Cervicothoracic stabilization training focuses on the balance of neutral spine or POF, restoration of segmental mobility, dynamic muscular control, and the appropriate use of stabilization principles. The components of training must, therefore, encompass mobility as well as stability within a functional range.

Mobility

The emphasis of the mobility phase is restoration of segmental movement within a functional range from a balanced position. Proper movement sequencing establishes segmental control of newly acquired movement. It is important to develop dynamic stability while avoiding cervical joint fixation and soft-tissue rigidity. Additionally, restoration of motion may be limited by pain and pathologic changes.[10] A fine line exists between a tolerable range of movement and its end range that will exacerbate the patient's symptoms. Proper flexibility and mobility exercise applied to area of restriction gives the patient a valuable tool for controlling pain and improving function.[10] Flexibility training geared at restoring lost movement is discussed later in this chapter.

Stability

While mobility provides an important function in daily living, stabilization in the balanced position is essential when lifting, carrying, pushing, and pulling objects. Isometric control of the head and neck maintains the balanced position during tasks that require use of upper and lower extremities independent of the trunk/spine. Spinal stabilization training focuses cocontraction of axial musculature while allowing isolated movement at the peripheral joints.

Dynamic stabilization encounters a large range of muscular activity, depending on the task. For example, an activity such as backing a car out of a driveway requires mobility in conjunction with contraction of muscles to place the head in a position to increase the visual field. An activity such as lifting an object requires muscular stabilization of the cervical spine in a safe position while transmitting the forces away from the spine to the upper and lower extremities. For this reason, strength and endurance exercises are established for segmental control of mobility and for maintaining correct posture during use of the extremities. Mobility and stability are challenged by altering the type of exercise, the position of exercise, the resistance of exercise, and related functional activities.

Initial Patient Education

During an acute phase of pain, rest to the injured areas and use of cervical supports may be indicated. The cervical supports should hold the neck in a comfortable, balanced position. Initial patient education entails neck first aid, positions of comfort, time-contingent activity and rest, application of ice, and body mechanics. The patient learns independent techniques to control symptoms while performing activities of daily living. This control is a vital tool in eliminating fear of movement and promoting active participation in the healing process.

The training phase begins with the patient's education in "neck and back schools." The purpose of "back school" is to instruct an individual who has either a low-back or cervicothoracic injury about the basic concepts of spine care, spinal anatomy, POF, and stabilization. Work ergonomics are addressed to promote correct head and neck posture during work.

Postural Reeducation

Following back and neck school principles, postural reeducation begins. A balanced posture is the "state of muscular and skeletal balance that protects supporting structures of the body against injury or progressive deformity regardless of the attitude."[2]

The cervical spine is a very flexible structure that can be tilted, rotated, and lowered by contracting the muscles attached to it. Balanced on top of the cervical spine is the head, with its center of gravity anterior to its base, the atlas.[2] It is the ligaments and muscles of the neck with their insertion points at the base of the skull that play a key role in maintaining a balanced position of the head in relation to the cervical and thoracic spine[2] (see Figs. 28-2 and 28-3).

The therapist begins by having the patient sit with front and side mirror views. This positioning enables the patient to see any postural deviations of the spine. It is important for the patient to see his/her habitual posture in order to facilitate change (see Fig. 28-1).

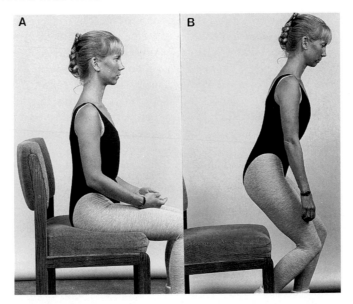

Fig. 28-5

A, Note reduction of thoracic kyphosis and associated flattening of cervical spine. **B,** Transition position: note lack of cervical extension that should correctly accompany position transition, as opposed to extension synergy pattern. *(From Sweeney T, Prentice C, Saal JS, Saal J: Cervicothoracic muscular stabilization techniques, Phys Med Rehab State Art Rev 4:341, 1990.)*

Next, the therapist helps the patient find a neutral balanced position of the lumbar and cervicothoracic spine. Instruction includes both verbal and very subtle hands-on cueing. With the patient's feet on the floor in front of him/her, he/she sits balanced on the ischial tuberosites in a stabilized lumbar spine position. The therapist then demonstrates to the patient where the thoracic cage and cervical spine neutral position are in relationship to the lumbar spine. Generally, this involves lengthening the anterior and posterior soft tissues, with special attention to releasing the posterior neck muscles, thereby, allowing the head to assume a slightly forward and balanced position on the cervical spine. If the patient is in a more acute stage, this training may need to begin in the supine position.

The next phase of postural reeducation is to use the balanced neutral position in a basic movement sequence such as a transition from sitting to standing. In this sequence the patient has a tendency to extend the head back and down, as well as to tighten the posterior and posterolateral muscles of the neck. The therapist instructs and directs the patient to move forward from the hips while maintaining a neutral spine and allowing the chin to drop slightly as the patient leaves the chair (Fig. 28-5). Most patients will not realize that they are pulling their heads back and tightening their neck muscles in this ha-

TABLE 28-1
Soft-tissue flexibility training: major areas of concern

Anterior Muscles	Posterior Muscles
Sternocleidomastoid	Rectuc capitis posterior major
Scaleni	Rectus capitis posterior minor
Pectoralis major	Obliquus capitis inferior
Pectoralis minor	Obliquus capitis superior
Biceps (long head)	Levator scapulae
	Superior trapezius
	Latissimus doris
	Teres major
	Subscapularis
	Rhomboids
	Middle trapezius
	Lower trapezius
	Serratus anterior

(From Sweeney T, Prentice C, Saal JS, Saal J: Cervicothoracic muscular stabilization techniques, *Phys Med Rehab State Art Rev* 4: 1990.)

bitual movement pattern. A hand on the back of the neck helps demonstrate this pattern and provides kinesthetic feedback.

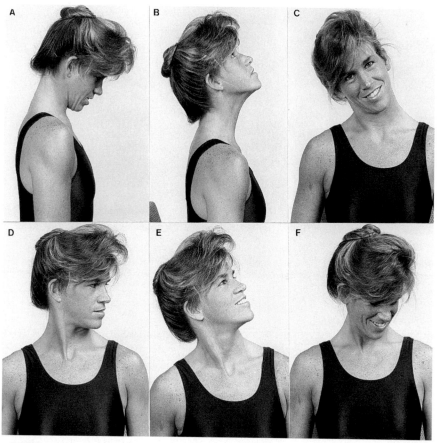

Fig. 28-6

A, Forward flexion stretching posterior soft tissues. **B,** Extension stretching anterior soft tissues. **C,** Lateral flexion principally stretching contralateral upper trapezius. **D,** Cervical rotation stretching combination of posterior lateral and anterior tissues. **E,** Combined extension: rotation principally stretching contralateral, deep anterior soft tissues. **F,** Combined flexion: rotation principally stretching contralateral, upper lateral soft tissues. *(From Sweeney T, Prentice C, Saal JS, Saal J: Cervicothoracic muscular stabilization techniques, Phys Med Rehab State Art Rev 4: 1990.)*

Flexibility

If the patient is unable to attain the POF because of soft-tissue or joint restrictions, the next step involves flexibility training before proceeding. Flexibility is an integral component of cervicothoracic stabilization training. Adequate flexibility of the anterior chest wall, interscapular region, and cervical musculature restores a cervicothoracic balanced posture.

Isolation of upper extremity movement without compensatory cervicothoracic motion requires adequate flexibility of the shoulder girdle musculature, especially the internal rotators. Additionally, restoration of normal scapulothoracic movement must be accomplished.[8,9]

The two components of cervical flexibility are joint mobility and soft-tissue extensibility. Joint mobility is accomplished through mobilization techniques. Mobilization describes the application of a force along the rotational or translational planes of motion of a joint.[12] Specific joint mobilization may be accomplished through a gentle active range of motion as demonstrated in Fig. 28-6. Clearly defined beginning and ending positions with careful attention to movement of the segment in question are essential to correct execution of the exercise. An appropriate exercise applied improperly does not achieve the desired effect.[10] Proper movement sequencing establishes segmental control of newly acquired movement.

Stretching techniques provide increased soft-tissue extensibility. Stretching defines an activity that applies a deforming force along a linear plane of motion.[12] The shortened musculature in the cervical, scapulothoracic, and shoulder girdle areas are the chief targets for stretching (Table 28-1). The specific muscle groups can be divided into anterior and posterior groups. The anterior muscle groups include

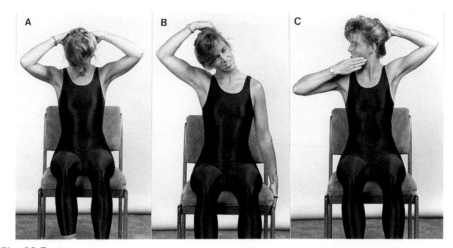

Fig. 28-7

A, Position neck stretch. **B,** Cervical lateral flexion stretch. **C,** Cervical rotational stretch. *(From Sweeney T, Prentice C, Saal JS, Saal J: Cervicothoracic muscular stabilization techniques,* Phys Med Rehab State Art Rev 4: 343, 1990.)

the sternocleidomastoid, scaleni, pectoralis major, pectoralis minor, and the long head of the bicep. The posterior muscle groups contain the deep occipital muscles—rectus capitis posterior major and minor, obliques capitis inferior and superior, levator scapulae, superior trapezius, latissimus dorsi, teres major, subscapularis, tricep, and posterior deltoid.

Techniques proven effective in promoting musculotendinous flexibility include ballistic stretching, passive stretching, static stretching, and neuromusculature facilitation. Ballistic stretching is not recommended, as repeated bouncing stretches contracting muscle and may lead to further injury. Early passive stretching by the treating practitioner should be performed with caution. A sustained stretch beyond the patient's safe and available range may contribute to prolonged duration of symptoms or additional injury. It is advisable to instruct the patient to initiate static stretching between or near the end of the tolerable range of motion. Static stretching requires spine safe techniques. The stretch is initiated from the POF. Prevention of collapsed thoracic cage and forward head positioning minimizes abnormal stretching patterns. A position that applies a gradual stretch to the cervical musculature (Fig. 28-7) and upper-extremity musculature (Fig. 28-8) are achieved and maintained for a 15- to 60-second period.

An improved range of shortened soft-tissue musculature restores capacity for normal movement patterns. Full range is desired for tissue health and function. It minimizes and/or prevents abnormal excursion, which contributes to adaptive shortening and functional disability. Finally, it establishes adequate extensibility of tissues for dynamic stability versus protective rigid stability.

It is important to stabilize the shoulder girdle prior to stretching the cervical musculature. This stabilization may be accomplished by grabbing the base of a chair to depress and stabilize the shoulder girdle from moving (see Fig. 28-7, *B*). Once the shoulder girdle is stabilized, the head is directed away from the shoulder in rotation, lateral flexion, or combined patterns. As the available excursion improves, a steady application of additional force may be added by the use of proper hand placement. If deficits in range of motion remain after patient instruction, then passive stretching and neuromuscular facilitation techniques are appropriate. These methods require a skilled practitioner to perform hold-relax and contract-relax methods to the appropriate shortened musculature. As normal range of both joint and soft-tissue is achieved, muscle strength, endurance, and coordination can be addressed through stabilization routines.

Exercise Program

A good cervicothoracic program begins with a lumbar stabilization program. Lumbar stabilization programs include exercises such as partial sit-ups, diagonal sit-ups, prone reciprocal arm and leg, and lifts. Necessary precautions in monitoring and supporting the spine during this initial phase are important so as not to exacerbate cervical symptoms. The lumbar stabilization exercise program strengthens and aligns the lumbopelvic base of support for a neutral cervicothoracic posture.

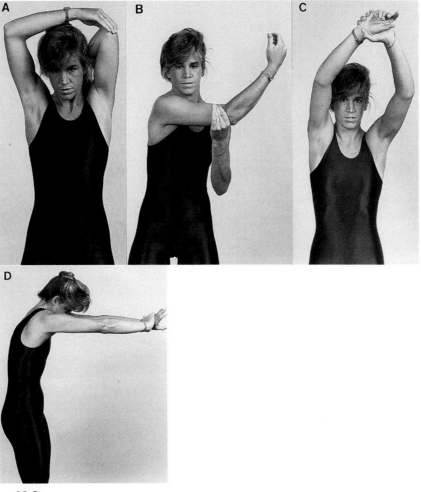

Figure 28-8

A, Triceps and interior shoulder capsule stretch. **B,** Posterior deltoid and posterior shoulder capsule stretch.
C, Latissimus dorsi and teres major stretch. **D,** Interscapular/rhomboid stretch. *(From Sweeney T, Prentice
C, Saal JS, Saal J: Cervicothoracic muscular stabilization techniques, Phys Med Rehab State Art Rev 4:344, 1990.)*

Treatment Phases

A. Stabilization Program
  1. Finding neutral position
    a. Supine
    b. Prone
    c. Sitting
    d. Standing
    e. Sumo squat position (flexed hip-hinge position)
    f. Jumping
  2. Supine pelvic bracing
    a. Abdominal program
      1. Curl-ups
      2. Dying bug
        a. Supported
        b. Unsupported
      3. Diagonal curl-ups

      4. Diagonal curl-ups on incline board
      5. Straight leg lowering
  3. Prone gluteal squeezes
    a. With arm raises
    b. With alternate arm raises
    c. With leg raises
    d. With alternate leg raises
    e. With arm and leg raises
    f. With alternate arm and leg raises
  4. Bridging progression
    a. Basic position
    b. One leg raised
    c. With ankle weights stepping
    d. With ankle weights balanced on gym ball
  5. Quadruped
    a. With alternating arm and leg movements
    b. With ankle and wrist weights

6. Kneeling stabilization
    a. Double knee
    b. Single knee
    c. Lunges
        1. Without weight
        2. With weight
7. Wall-slide quadriceps strengthening
8. Position transition with postural control
    a. Gym program
        1. Latissimus pull-downs
        2. Angled leg press
        3. Lunges
        4. Hyperextension bench
        5. General upper-extremity weight exercises
        6. Pulley exercises to stress postural control

Regional Exercises

Cervicothoracic stabilization training may be divided into regional exercises for the cervical, interscapular, chest, and upper-extremity musculature. The patient must learn to use the muscle groups in an isolated fashion as well as in cocontraction patterns, performing increasingly difficult tasks and demands applied to the body.

The cervical spine regional musculature includes cervical spinal extensors and anterior musculature—rectus capitis anterior, rectus capitis lateralis, longissimus, cervicis, and longus capitis. The anterior musculature stabilizes the cervical spine in the neutral position during muscular contraction of the sternocleidomastoid as when raising a patient's head off the table while in the supine position (see Fig. 28-10, C). Additionally, emphasis is placed on the cervical extensors to balance shear stress on the intervertebral segments (see Fig. 28-10, B).

The primary thoracic stabilizers are the abdominal, spinal extensor, and latissimus dorsi muscles. In the scapulothoracic area, the major muscles of concern include the middle and lower trapezius, serratus anterior, and rhomboids. Latissimus dorsi and scapulothracic muscles are developed for scapular depression. The chest wall musculature on which to concentrate includes the clavicular head of the pectoralis major and pectoralis minor. The upper extremity musculature also requires training using the supraspinatous, bicep, tricep, and deltoid.

Exercise Progression

As the exercise program advances, the patient is instructed in cocontraction techniques, which consist of isometric control of the trunk stabilizing muscles to balance the spine during tasks that require use of upper and lower extremities independent of the trunk/spine. Advancing the type, position, and resistance of the exercise provides a progression of cervicothoracic stabilization training (Table 28-2). Cervicothoracic exercises presented here are arranged according to these principles of program progression (Table 28-3). The types of exercise selected challenges the individual's stabilization skills by altering the activity from static positioning to dynamic balancing. Each exercise incorporates varying degrees of upper-extremity movement, progressing from unilateral arm raises to reciprocal arm raises to bilateral arm raises. The patient's stabilization skills may continue to be challenged with transitional movements. Transitional movements include a change of position such as sitting to standing or entire body movement in space such as pivoting and turning. The movement from the supine position to the sitting position may be a difficult stabilization skill for the patient to achieve. Once stabilization skills are mastered in the transitional movement phase of the program, predictable loading and unexpected loading may be added. The patient's balance may be challenged with the use of the Swiss gymnastic ball. Power drills involving speed, strength, falls, and contact require the highest level of stabilization skills.

Exercise Position

Varying exercise position determines the required amount of trunk stabilization. Initially, exercises can be performed in the supine position with the head supported in the balanced position. Exercises progress to the sitting, kneeling, and standing positions. Finally, the prone and the flexed hip-hinge stance positions may be introduced into the program. The flexed hip-hinge stance is a standing position with varying degrees of knee and hip flexion (see Fig. 28-17).

Resistance Exercises

The type of resistance advances from isometric to isotonic contractions. During isometric contractions, the muscle remains at a constant length. Isometrics vary the patient's positioning and direction relative to gravity, resulting in direct stabilization of the cervical spine. Initially, the patient may begin isometrics in the supine position with the head supported. He/she then progresses to isometrics in the seated position (Fig. 28-9). or off the edge of a table against gravity (Fig. 28-10). Exercises are performed with

TABLE 28-2
Variables for cervicothoracic stabilization progression

Training Level	Trunk Position	Exercise Pattern	Resistance Type
I	Supine	Reciprocal arm	Theraband
	Sit	movement	(elastic resistance)
Basic	Kneel	Unilateral arm	
	Stand	movement	
	Flexed hip-hinge		
	position (0-30°)*		
	Prone		
II	Supine	Reciprocal arm	Weight machine
	Sit	movement	Pulleys
Intermediate	Kneel	Unilateral arm	Free weights
	Stand	movement	
	Flexed hip-hinge		
	position (30-60°)*		
	Transition positions:		
	Sit-stand		
	Supine-sit		
III	Supine	Reciprocal arm	Weight machine
	Sit	movement	Pulleys
Advanced	Kneel	Unilateral arm	Free weights
	Stand	movement	Free form objects
	Flexed hip-hinge	Bilateral arm	
	position (60-90°)*	movement	
	Prone	Predictable	
	Balanced challenge:	loading†	
	Swiss ball		
	Transition positions:		
	Sit-stand		
	Supine-sit		
IV	Free form	Specialized sports	Live sports activity
		drills†	
Advanced		Unexpected loading‡	
Athlete		Falls	
		Contact (football	
		tackling and blocking)	
		Power Drills§	

(From Sweeney T, Prentice C, Saal JS, Saal J: Cervicothoracic muscular stabilization techniques, *Phys Med Rehab State Art Rev* 4:347, 1990.)
*See Fig. 28-17.
†Tasks that involve cervicothoracic load placement accomplished in definable postural positions, e.g., lifting a box from a high shelf.
‡Loads placed on the cervicothoracic spine that occur without warning and in various postural positions, e.g., catching a falling object or bracing for a sudden fall.
§High-speed movement patterns using near-maximal loads.

TABLE 28-3

Progression of cervicothoracic stabilization exercises

	Cervicothoracic Stabilization Levels		
	I Basic	II Intermediate	III Advanced
Direct Cervical stabilization	Cervical active range of motion	Cervical gravity	Cervical active
Exercises	Cervical isometrics	Resisted isometrics	Range gravity resisted
Indirect Cervical stabilization Exercises			
Supine, head supported	Theraband chest press Bilateral arm raise Supported dying bug	Unsupported dying bug	Chest flies Bench press Incline dumbbell press
Sit	Reciprocal arm raise Unilateral arm raise Bilateral arm raise Seated row Latissimus pulldown	Swiss ball reciprocal Arm raises Chest press	Swiss ball bilateral Shoulder shrugs Supraspinatus raises

Stand	Theraband reciprocal
	Chest press
	Theraband straight
	Arm latissimus
	Pulldown
	Theraband:
	   Chest press
	   Latissimus pulldown
	Standing rowing
	Crossovers
	Tricep press
		Standing rowing
		Bicep pulldown
			Upright row
			Shoulder shrugs
			Supraspinatus raises

Flexed hip-hinge position	0-30° Reciprocal arm raise Unilateral arm raise Bilateral arm raise Interscapular flies	30-60° Incline prone flies Reciprocal deltoid raise Cable crossovers	60-90° Bilateral anterior Deltoid raises Interscapular flies
Prone	Reciprocal arm raise Unilateral arm raise Bilateral arm raise	Quadruped Head unsupported Swiss ball bilateral Anterior deltoid raises Swiss ball prone Rowing Swiss ball prone flies	Head supported Prone flies Latissimus flies
Supine, head unsupported	Not advised for Level I	Partial sit-ups Arm raises	Swiss ball chest flies Swiss ball reciprocal

(From Sweeney T, Prentice C, Saal JS, Saal J: Cervicothoracic muscular stabilization techniques, *Phys Med Rehab State Art Rev* 4:345, 1990.)

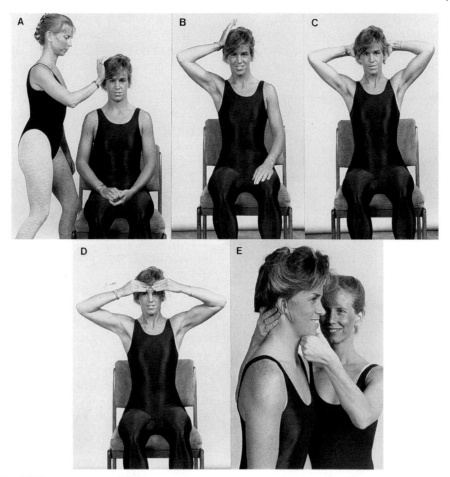

Fig. 28-9

A, Isometric lateral flexion. **B,** Isometric lateral flexion. **C,** Isometric extension. **D,** Isometric forward flexion. **E,** Isometric upper cervical flexion. *(From Sweeney T, Prentice C, Saal JS, Saal J: Cervicothoracic muscular stabilization techniques, Phys Med Rehab State Art Rev 4:348, 1990.)*

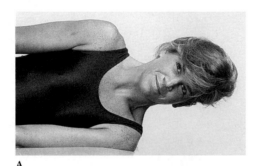

A

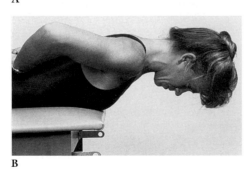

B

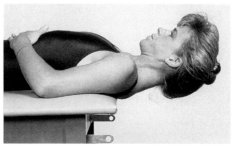

C

Fig. 28-10

A, Gravity resisted: isometric lateral flexion. **B,** Gravity resisted: isometric extension. **C,** Gravity resisted: isometric forward flexion. *(From Sweeney T, Prentice C, Saal JS, Saal J: Cervicothoracic muscular stabilization techniques, Phys Med Rehab State Art Rev 4:349, 1990.)*

the cervical spine in the POF. An active range of resistance results in dynamic stabilization of the cervical spine (Figs. 28-11 and 28-12). The dynamic cervical stabilization requires great segmental control from the POF. It is restricted to the tolerable range available to each patient. Avoidance of end-range movement can minimize the exacerbation of symptoms.

Training the interscapular, shoulder, and upper-extremity musculature provides indirect stabilization support for the cervical muscles. The training must couple cocontraction of cervicothoracic stabilizers with isotonic contractions of interscapular, shoulder, and upper-extremity musculature and against resistance. Methods of resistance during isotonic contractions progress from rubber tubing or theraband (Figs. 28-13 and 28-14) to pulley systems (Fig. 28-15) and free weights (Figs. 28-16, 28-17, 28-18, 28-19, and 28-20) and finally, free-body weights such as boxes. Rubber tubing, theraband, a Swiss gym ball, and 3-to 6-lb dumbbells can provide the diversity necessary for a successful home program.

Prior to gym training, the patient must demonstrate consistent postural control and stabilization skill. Gym training challenges the stabilization ability of the patient; therefore, skill level assessment is necessary prior to advancement. The training goals include increasing muscular strength and endurance of trunk stabilizing and extremity musculature in a spine-safe technique. The targeted exercises for the shoulder girdle are listed in Table 28-4 and targeted exercises for the upper trunk or interscapular region are listed in Table 28-5. Table 28-6 provides the targeted groups for the upper extremities.

Resistance exercises also train strength, power, and endurance. The type of resistance, number of sets, and repetitions determine whether strength, power, or endurance will be trained. Specificity of training with sets and repetitions must match with the individual's activities of daily living, occupation, and sports.

Exercises must be constantly matched with the patient's strength, endurance, and stabilization ability. Pain is one guide for exercise progression. An increase in axial or radicular pain requires a reevaluation of the exercise program. The pain increase may be due either to poor technique or to inadequate coordination of available strength and endurance. Additionally, the degree of pathology may present a limitation to progression in the exercise program.

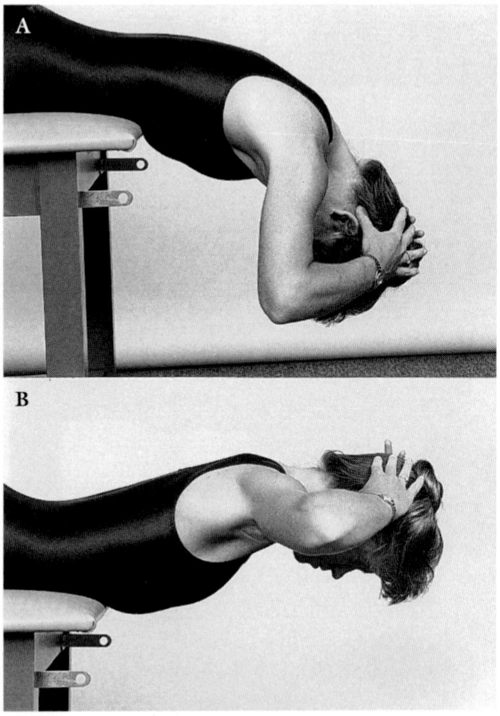

Fig. 28-11

A, Initial position: active gravity resisted cervicothoracic extension position. **B,** Final position: active gravity resisted cervicothoracic extension. *(From Sweeney T, Prentice C, Saal JS, Saal J: Cervicothoracic muscular stabilization techniques, Phys Med Rehab State Art Rev 4: 1990.)*

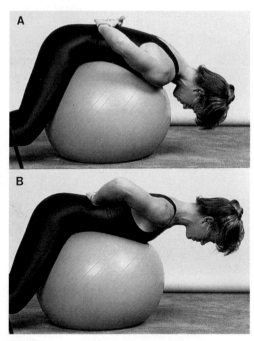

Fig. 28-12

A, Initial position: Swiss ball active, gravity-resisted cervicothoracic extension start position. **B,** Final position: Swiss ball active, gravity-resisted cervicothoracic extension. *(From Sweeney T, Prentice C, Saal JS, Saal J: Cervicothoracic muscular stabilization techniques, Phys Med Rehab State Art Rev 4:350, 1990.)*

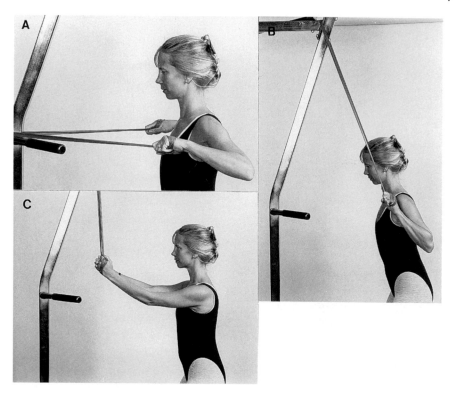

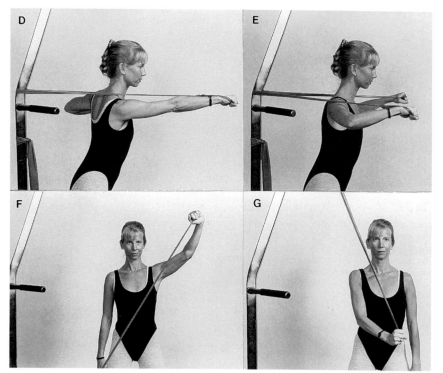

Fig. 28-13

A, Theraband-resisted rowing while standing. **B,** Theraband-resisted rowing during pull-down. **C,** Theraband-resisted pull-down. **D,** Theraband-resisted reciprocal chest press. **E,** Theraband-resisted chest press while standing. **F,** Theraband-resisted diagonal external rotation. **G,** Theraband-resisted diagonal internal rotation. *(From Sweeney T, Prentice C, Saal JS, Saal J: Cervicothoracic muscular stabilization techniques, Phys Med Rehab State Art Rev 4: 1990.)*

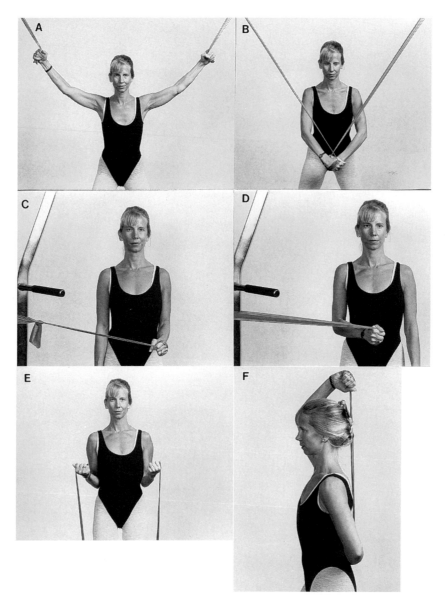

Fig. 28-14

A, Initial position: theraband-resisted diagonally symmetrical internal rotation. **B,** Final position: theraband-resisted diagonally symmetrical internal rotation. **C,** Theraband-resisted external rotation pulls. **D,** Theraband-resisted internal rotation pulls. **E,** Theraband-resisted biceps curl in standing position. **F,** Theraband-resisted triceps curl in standing position. *(From Sweeney T, Prentice C, Saal JS, Saal J: Cervicothoracic muscular stabilization techniques,* Phys Med Rehab State Art Rev 4:352, 1990.)

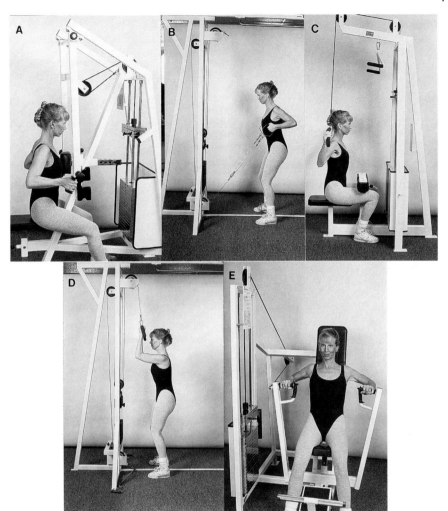

Fig. 28-15

A, Seated rowing. **B,** Rowing from low pulley while standing. **C,** Closed hand pull-down. **D,** Open-hand pull-down. **E,** Chest press. *(From Sweeney T, Prentice C, Saal JS, Saal J: Cervicothoracic muscular stabilization techniques, Phys Med Rehab State Art Rev 4:353, 1990.)*

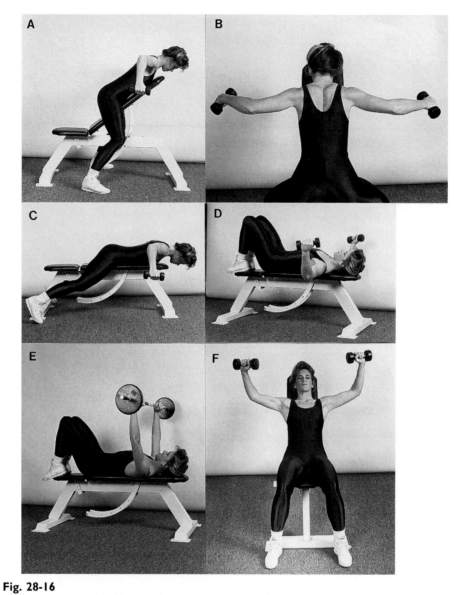

Fig. 28-16

A, Incline prone flies, final position. **B,** Incline prone flies, posterior view. **C,** Prone flies. **D,** Chest flies.
E, Bench press. **F,** Incline dumbbell press. *(From Sweeney T, Prentice C, Saal JS, Saal J: Cervicothoracic muscular stabilization techniques, Phys Med Rehab State Art Rev 4:354, 1990.)*

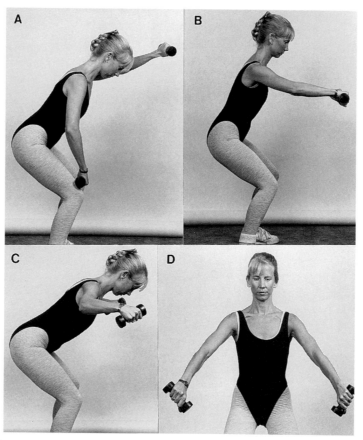

Fig. 28-17

A, Flexed hinge-hip position: reciprocal arm raise. **B,** Flexed hinge-hip position: anterior deltoid raises. **C,** Flexed hinge-hip position: reverse flies (interscapular flies). **D,** Supraspinatous raises in standing position. *(From Sweeney T, Prentice C, Saal JS, Saal J: Cervicothoracic muscular stabilization techniques,* Phys Med Rehab State Art Rev *4:355, 1990.)*

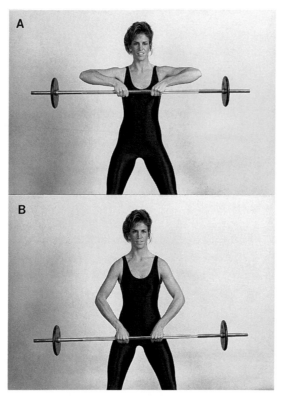

Fig. 28-18

A, Initial position: upright rowing. **B,** Final position: upright rowing. *(From Sweeney T, Prentice C, Saal JS, Saal J: Cervicothoracic muscular stabilization techniques, Phys Med Rehab State Art Rev 4:356, 1990.)*

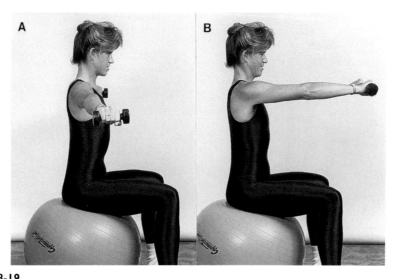

Fig. 28-19

A, Lateral deltoid raises while seated on Swiss gym ball. **B,** Anterior deltoid raises while seated on Swiss gym ball. *(From Sweeney T, Prentice C, Saal JS, Saal J: Cervicothoracic muscular stabilization techniques, Phys Med Rehab State Art Rev 4:356, 1990.)*

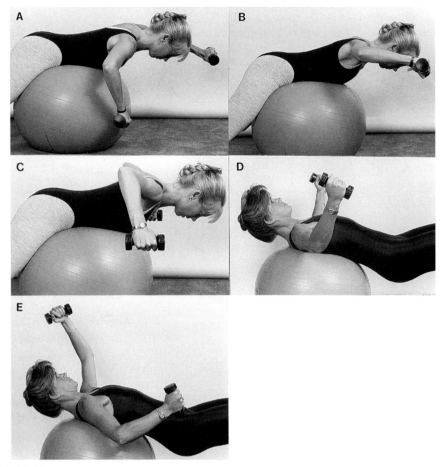

Fig. 28-20

A, Prone reciprocal arm raise while on Swiss gym ball. **B,** Bilateral arm raises while on Swiss gym ball. **C,** Prone flies while on Swiss gym ball. **D,** Chest flies while on Swiss gym ball. **E,** Supine reciprocal arm raises while on Swiss gym ball. *(From Sweeney T, Prentice C, Saal JS, Saal J: Cervicothoracic muscular stabilization techniques, Phys Med Rehab State Art Rev 4:357, 1990.)*

TABLE 28-4

Shoulder girdle muscle strengthening exercises useful in cervicothoracic stabilization training[*]

Exercise Routines	Figures	Primary Muscle Groups
Theraband-resisted reciprocal chest press	28-13, D	
Therband-resisted chest press while standing	28-13, E	Pectoralis major
Initial and final positions: Theraband-resisted diagonally Symmetric internal rotation	28-14, A & B	
Chest press	28-15, E	Pectoralis major and minor, anterior deltoid
Bench press	28-16, E	Pectoralis major and minor, anterior deltoid
Incline dumbbell press	28-16, F	Anterior deltoids, pectoralis major and minor, serratus anterior
Chest flies and chest flies while on Swiss gym ball	28-16, D & 28-20, D	Pectoralis major and minor
Supine reciprocal arm raises while on Swiss gym ball	28-20, E	Anterior deltoids, pectoralis major and minor, serratus anterior
Initial and final positions: upright rowing	28-18, A & B	Deltoid, pectoralis major and minor
Reciprocal arm and anterior deltoid arm raises	28-17, A & B and 28-19, B	Anterior deltoids
Lateral deltoid raises	28-19, A	Middle deltoids
Prone reciprocal arm raise	28-20, A	Posterior deltoid
Supraspinatus raises in standing position	28-17, D	Supraspinatus
Theraband-resisted diagonal internal rotations	28-13, G & 28-14, D	pectoralis major, subscrapularis
Theraband-resisted diagonal external rotations	28-13, F & 28-14, C	Infraspinatus

[*]Cocontraction of direct cervical and thoracolumbar stabilizers must accompany these exercise routines. (*From Sweeney T, Prentice C, Saal J: Cervicothoracic Muscular Stabilization techniques,* Phys Med Rehab State Art Rev *4: 1990.*)

TABLE 28-5

Interscapular muscle strengthening exercises useful in cervicothoracic stabilization training*

Interscapular Muscle Strengthening Exercises	Figures	Primary Muscle Groups
Seated rowing	28-15, A	Latissimus dorsi, rhomboids, middle trapezius, posterior deltoid
Theraband-resisted rowing while standing and rowing from a low pulley while standing	28-13, A & 28-15, B	Trapezius
Theraband-resisted pulldown and closed hand pulldown	28-13, B & 28-15, C	Serratus anterior, latissimus dorsi
Theraband-resisted pulldown	28-13, C	Serratus anterior, latissimus dorsi
Open hand pulldown	28-15, D	Latissimus dorsi, rhomboids, middle trapezius, posterior deltoid
Incline prone flies: final position	28-16, A & B	Rhomboids, middle trapezius, thoracic lumbar paraspinals
Prone flies, bilateral arm raises while on Swiss gym ball and prone flies while on Swiss gym ball	28-16, C and 28-20, A & B	Rhomboids, middle trapezius, thoracic lumbar paraspinals
Prone reciprocal arm raise while on Swiss gym ball	28-20, A	Rhomboids, middle trapezius, thoracic lumbar paraspinals
Reverse flies while standing in a flexed hip-hinge position	28-17, C	Rhomboids, middle trapezius, thoracic lumbar paraspinals

*Cocontraction of direct cervical and thoracolumbar stabilizers must accompany these exercise routines. (From Sweeney T, Prentice C, Saal JS, Saal J: Cervicothoracic muscular stabilization techniques, Phys Med Rehab State Art Rev 4:358, 1990.)

TABLE 28-6

Upper-extremity muscle-strengthening exercises useful for cervicothoracic stabilization training*

Upper-Extremity Muscle-Strengthening Exercises	Primary Muscle Groups
Biceps pulldown	Biceps brachii
Standing biceps curl	Biceps
Standing triceps press	Triceps brachii

*Cocontraction of direct cervical and thoracolumbar stabilizers must accompany these exercise routines. (From Sweeney T, Prentice C, Saal JS, Saal J: Cervicothoracic muscular stabilization techniques, Phys Med Rehab State Art Rev 4:359, 1990.)

Summary

Cervicothoracic stabilization training is a specialized program requiring coordination of body mechanics, posture, movement principles, and exercise to optimize spine function. It requires the balance of neutral spine, restoration of segmental mobility, and the appropriate use of stabilization principles. Stabilization training optimizes the cervicothoracic spine's capacity to absorb loads in all directions while minimizing direct stress-strain relations to individual cervical tissues.

When the patient becomes an active integral part of the rehabilitation process, carryover and consistency of the stabilization training occurs. The patient learns independence through self-management of symptoms and progress in the home program. The patient's heightened awareness of aggravating factors and the newly acquired ability to manage them with relieving positions, proper body mechanics, problem solving, and favorable ergonomic design improves the patient's overall function. Training, thereby, can control cost expenditure by reducing treatment time and limiting recidivism.

References

1. Basmajian JV, *Therapeutic exercise*, Baltimore, 1984, Williams & Wilkins.
2. Bland JH: *Disorders of the cervical spine*, Philadelphia, 1987, W.B. Saunders Co.
3. Caplan D: *Back trouble: a new approach to prevention and recovery*, Gainesville, FL, 1987, Triad Publishing Co.
4. Foreman SM, Croft AC: *Whiplash Injuries: the cervical spine acceleration deceleration syndrome*, Baltimore, 1988, William & Wilkins.
5. Gorman D: *The body moveable*. Vol. 1: The trunk and head.
6. Gracovetsky S: *The spinal engine*, New York, 1988, Springer-Verlag Wien.
7. Gracovetsky S, Farfan H: The optimum spine, *Spine* 10:543, 1986.
8. Gustavsen R: *Training therapy: prophylaxis and rehabilitation*, New York, 1985, Thieme, Inc.
9. Knott M, Voss D: *Proprioceptive neuromuscular facilitation: patterns & techniques*, New York, 1956, McGraw-Hill.
10. Saal JS: Non-operative treatment of lumbar pain syndromes, *Spine* 14 (4): 1989, p 431.
11. Saal JS, Flexibility training, *Phys Med Rehab State Art Rev* 1: 1987.
12. Sweeney T, Prentice C, Saal JS, Saal J: Cervicothoracic muscular stabilization techniques. *Phys Med Rehab State Art Rev* 4:335, 1990.

Chapter 29

Validity and Basis of Manipulation

John J. Triano
Dennis Skogsbergh
Marion McGregor

Historical Review

An integral relationship between the spine and health was first suspected by the early Greeks. Hippocrates (470 to 357 BC) is reported to have written "look to the spine for disease," and to have given methods of repositioning vertebrae considered displaced.[46,58] Since then, the significance of the role of the spine in disease has held varied acceptance. Manipulative therapy for spine-related disorders has been received similarly. A continued controversy over the use of manipulation has focused on the chiropractic profession. This is probably due to the fact that chiropractors now administer 94% of all manipulative therapy in the United States[69] as a health delivery system parallel to the orthodox medical community. That chiropractic has maintained a separate and distinct professional culture probably stems from two primary factors.[88] The first is the significant historical influence on the profession by the fervent personalities of its early leaders. Their convictions were fueled by political and sociologic climates that surrounded them, leaving a heritage that still may be felt in chiropractic today. Second, barriers promoted by organized medicine opposed broader sanction of chiropractic. As a result, the profession persisted as an isolated and relatively ostracized participant in health care. Oddly, that isolation, from both intrinsic and extrinsic factors may have facilitated the advancement of its parallel education and delivery system.

Recently, however, medical sociologist Wardwell[88] has reported findings of a "currently entrenched legal status, its solid acceptance by the public and its developing collegial relations with MDs." More importantly, research over the past decade has presented good evidence of the therapeutic merits of manipulation[3,23,54,69] [also known as spinal manipulative therapy (SMT), spinal adjustment] for musculoskeletal complaints related to the spine, providing support for the vast majority of chiropractors who use it as their intervention of choice.

Today, the controversy has narrowed more to the scope of practice and the selection of appropriate patients to receive SMT. An objective assessment of chiropractic was given first by the New Zealand Report in 1979.[17] Their findings support conclusions that training and skills place the chiropractor "in a strong position to diagnose and treat musculoskeletal (Type M) spinal complaints . . . that will respond to manual therapy or associated musculoskeletal components of Type O (organic or visceral) disorders." This report, by noting the need for effectiveness research, coincided with an unprecedented scrutiny of health care delivery beginning in the 1980s. Emphasis on treatment outcomes represents the next era in public health policy making. The paradigm has shifted from apprenticeship-based to evidence-based clinical care.[28] Unfortunately, insufficient evidence exists for much of what is done to or for patients today, regardless of the provider's discipline. In this respect chiropractic is no different. Further research is needed to define more clearly the boundaries and benefits of treatment. In the interim, the provider is faced with the practical problem of trying to abate human suffering with the best knowledge available.

Early in 1992, the chiropractic profession formally responded to this challenge by developing a set of guidelines based on research and expert consensus to recommend appropriate practice parameters.[41] This development was sponsored by the broadest coalition of professional groups yet assembled. This chapter will focus on the modern application of chiropractic manipulation reflected in the current guideline recommendations. Specifically, it will present an overview of what is understood technically regarding how SMT works, the procedures that are available, and the approaches used to manage complaints associated with mechanical disorders of the spine.

Technical Data

The Manipulable Lesion

The manipulable lesion may arise *de novo* or as a coexisting problem with more widely recognized disorders, including discopathy, stenosis, instability, entrapment, and myofascial pain syndromes.[13] There are three main hypotheses (see box below) on the pathomechanics of spine dysfunction. Associated changes include inflammation, soft-tissue injury, intermittent nerve irritation, and dysfunction arising from local peak tissue stresses or focal hypomobility or both.* It is unknown, in scientific terms, whether SMT interacts with the primary pathology directly or with coincident factors that contribute to symptom expression and impairment. In view of the multiple diagnoses for which there is evidence of benefit from SMT, the latter perspective seems logical. Consequently, most clinical and experimental investigations of SMT and the manipulable lesion rely on descriptive characteristics. Kirkaldy-Willis[53] first attempted to reconcile clinical observations from pa-

---

*References 11, 34, 39, 78, 81, and 84.

tients with spine pain by articulating a unified theory relating a progression from joint dysfunction through pathologic degeneration, instability, and restabilization.

Theoretical Pathomechanics of Manipulable Lesions

- Blocked vertebral motion
    Connective-tissue shortening
    Intracapsular adhesions
    Synovial tags/inclusions
    Degenerative joint proliferation
- Dysponesis of intrinsic spinal muscles
- Motion segment buckling

Limitation of intersegmental motion is a common clinical observation considered as one indication for use of manipulation and may represent a passive blocking of movement of the joint.[68,84] Sedentary life styles, trauma, and postinjury deconditioning provide opportunities for ligament shortening, adhesions, and cartilage degeneration. Manipulative treatment is designed to achieve local effects, including connective-tissue lengthening, disruption of adhesions, and restoration of motion and normal tissue stresses.[26,34,74] Advanced degenerative joint disease may bring about a permanent limitation of motion that is unaffected by SMT. Other authors have proposed that intracapsular meniscoids or fibrotic synovial tag "inclusions" (Fig. 29-1) can become incarcerated, leading to anomalous motion, tissue irritation, and symptoms.[7,57,84] Treatment is intended to release the inclusion and relieve secondary hypertonic muscle reactions.

High internal forces acting on the motion segment can be generated by inappropriate or dysponetic muscle recruitment patterns.[10,34,48] Muscular tension with mechanical shortening or inhibition and weakness in response to external loading can result in high stresses on the motion segment. It is uncertain whether altered muscle tension arises from a manipulable lesion, is reinforced by it, or stems from a habitual movement pattern. Unilateral low-back pain associated with hypertonic paraspinal muscle has been confirmed using cerebral evoked responses from magnetic stimulation.[92] Cerebral evoked potentials were restored to normal amplitude and paraspinal spasm was resolved following SMT.

Buckling responses of motion segments have been observed in biomechanical tests[90] that may resemble the clinical events associated with patient reports of "giving way" during exertion. Data on flexion and lateral-bending buckling is extended to axial rotation in Fig. 29-2, *A* for comparisons with computer model simulation of the effects of SMT. Simply described, buckling occurs under specific load conditions when small increases in load result in large, nonlinear rotations or translations. Triano[77] has reviewed the hypothetical relationship to manipulable

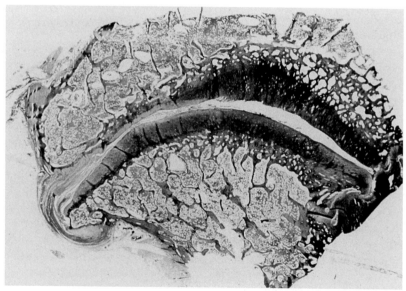

Fig. 29-1
Horizontal section through left lumbar zygapophyseal joint with intracapsular meniscoid (synovial tag) *(From Cassidy JD, Potter GE: Motion examination of the lumbar spine,* J Manipulative Physiol Ther 2:151, 1979.)

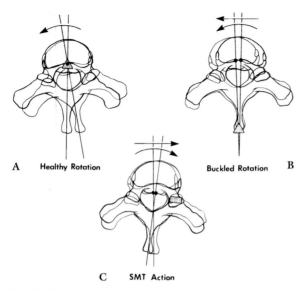

Fig. 29-2

Schematic drawings portray concepts of rotation and buckling as it may effect rotation. **A,** Healthy rotation has anatomically constrained centers of rotation *(dot, stippled triangle).* **B,** Buckled rotation incorporating high translation and rotations around abnormal center *(stippled triangle).* **C,** SMT action results initially in rotation until facets come into contact forming pivot point and fulcrum for unbuckling action *(stippled rectangle).*

lesions in greater detail. Buckling occurs more readily after exposure to vibration, a feature in common with the risk of low-back pain. Following deformation, the motion segment assumes a new stable orientation from which it operates (Fig. 29-2, *B*). Other than changes in compliance, no morphologic damage has been reported in biomechanical tests of motion segments. The buckling analogy carries into the effect of treatment by manipulation. That is, buckled structures remain deformed until external corrective forces are applied. Triano and Gudavalli[79] have used computer models to study motion segment biomechanics and shown a pivoting action on the facets that may explain how SMT could produce an unbuckling action (Fig. 29-2, *C*).

Procedures

Successful case management with SMT proceeds with three principal elements in sequence—(1) patient selection, (2) treatment procedure-patient matching, and (3) outcome monitoring. Depending on the nature of the lesion and its severity, the treatment plan may have to be modulated in terms of the specific methods, dosage, duration, and any cointerventions used.

In the traditional pathoanatomic model of disease, the indications for treatment are directly related to the diagnosis. For spine pain, this model is of limited value.[40] Instead, descriptive models that classify patients by the pattern of clinical findings, for example the presence of radiating leg pain and coincident pathology, is more useful.[56,75] For instance, patients with a herniated nucleus pulposus at L5-S1 may or may not be disqualified for treatment with SMT.[15,79] The determining factors will rest on the balance of clinical findings suggesting neurologic deficit and the types of treatment procedures available for this purpose.

Patient Selection

The immediate purpose of manual procedures is to reduce abnormal intersegmental kinematics and any functional or pathophysiological sequelae. As a result, the examiner must seek findings related to local joint dysfunction in addition to the traditional pathoanatomic findings. The box below lists the common elements of the examinations that are used.*

Local Findings Associated with Joint Dysfunction

- Joint pain with motion
- Altered passive flexibilities
    Midrange
    End-range
- Altered paths of motion
- Soft-tissue tenderness around affected joint
- Decreased muscle compliance to manual pressure
- Variations in skin temperature and texture

Fig. 29-3 illustrates palpatory procedures that may be used to search for local spinal joint dysfunction. Reproduction of the patient's pain or symptoms often is possible by imitating particular positions or movements related to symptoms evoked during activities of daily living. Sensitive tissues may be isolated in this way and the mechanism of pain production made obvious. Joint compression, local point tenderness, pain response to active or assisted range of motion, and passive flexibility testing (end-

*References 13, 26, 31, 32, 51, 57, and 85.

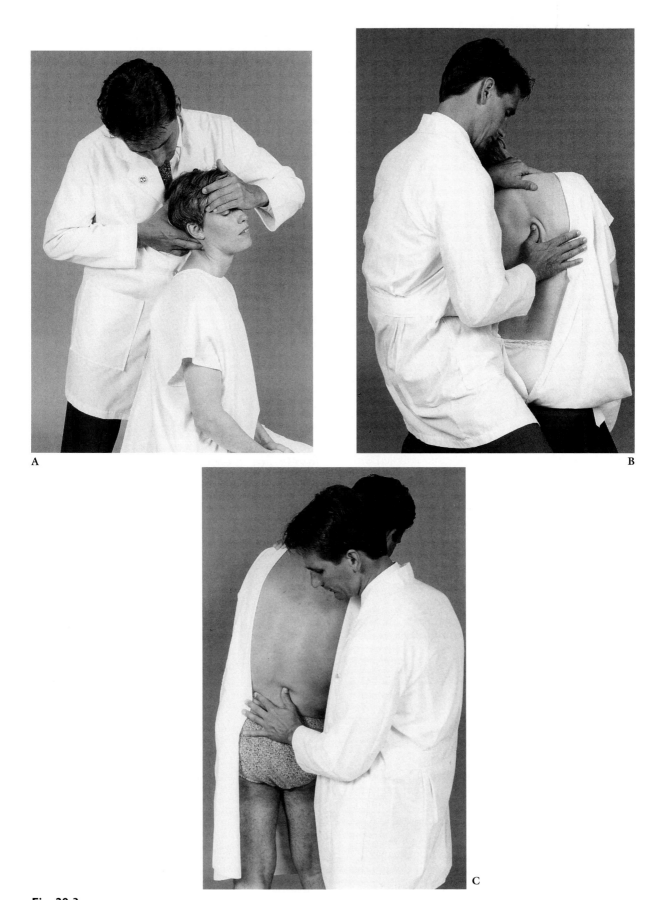

Fig. 29-3

Reproduction of the patient's pain, and localization of joint dysfunction and pain-sensitive tissues by physical procedures. **A,** Motion augmented palpation of posterior cervical facet joints. **B,** Estimating joint play in thoracic region. **C,** Assessing end-feel characteristics in lumbar spine.

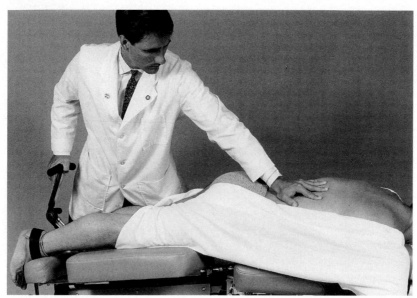

Fig. 29-4

Graded loading of lumbar spine with flexion-distraction technique.

feel characteristics, joint play estimates, and over-pressure testing) are used to assess articular kinematics. An absence of contraindications coupled with significant alteration in pain-free flexibility justifies a therapeutic trial of SMT.

The main conditions that would contradict the use of SMT are represented by the typical red-flag disorders reviewed in Table 29-1. Diagnostic efforts to confirm the presence of any of these conditions include the standard laboratory tests, specialty tests, or imaging appropriate to the provider's suspicion.

Procedure-Patient Matching

A number of procedures are available to treat each level of the spine. The selection of the appropriate method is guided by considerations of the severity of coexisting pathology, response to provocative joint preloading, history of previous treatment, provider skill, and preference. Parameters of the procedures that may be modified to accommodate underlying complications include the location of SMT loading, speed and amplitude of movements, and magnitude of the preload and impulse loads applied. In the presence of pathology (e.g., compressive neuropathy), more restrained procedures using graded loads as in flexion-distraction techniques[18] may be used initially (Fig. 29-4). Following regression of the signs of inflammation and nerve irritation, more aggressive strategies may be introduced if needed. Fig. 29-5 shows prone (drop), lateral recumbent and

Table 29-1

Contraindications to SMT at affected levels and associated key diagnostic factors

Condition	Key Factors
Severe neuro-logic deficit	Urinary retention/incontinence
	Decreased sphincter tone
	Fecal incontinence
	Rapidly progressive weakness
	Saddle anesthesia
Infection and malignancy	History of cancer
	Unexpected weight loss
	Urinary infection
	Intravenous drug use
	Corticosteroid use
	High ESR (erythrocyte sedimentation rate) > 50 years of age
	Abnormal complete blood count, serum protein
Fracture	History of serious trauma > 70 years of age
	Prolonged steroid use
Acute arthro-pathies	History and physical findings
	Conventional radiography
Joint instability	History of serious trauma
	Physical findings
	Stress radiography

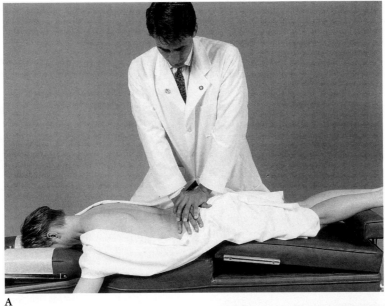

A

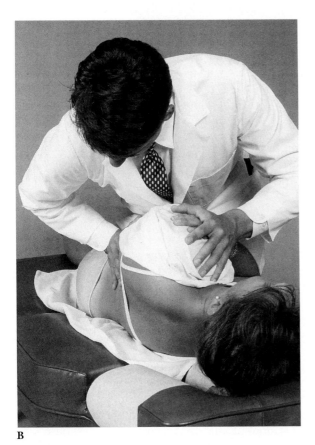

B

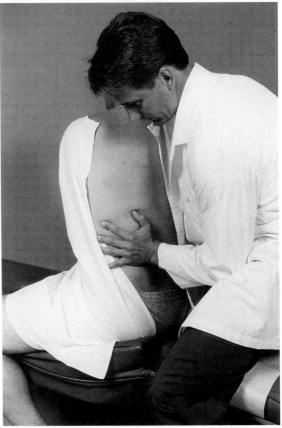

C

Fig. 29-5

Illustrative lumbar SMT procedures and location of intended loading. **A,** Prone "drop" position. At initiation of SMT, pelvic support suddenly releases to fall about 0.25 in., giving an added impulse load to joint. **B,** Lateral recumbent posture. **C,** Seated position. Not illustrated is torso rotation action produced by tractioning patient's left arm.

seated positioning for manipulation techniques applied to the lumbar region. Similar options are available for the other spinal and paraspinal joint regions.

Provocative joint preloading is accomplished by positioning the patient for the candidate procedure and using graded, subthreshold forces in the direction of the intended thrust. Patients who respond with sharp pain, reproduction of symptoms, or rigid muscular guarding to preloading are poorly matched with the treatment method. Procedures may be modified and provocatively tested again. If still unsuccessful, a different type of procedure should be attempted or the condition determined as being unfit for SMT. Successful manipulation usually can be carried out without the patient experiencing undue distress or apprehension.

Outcome Monitoring

Evaluation of patient response to treatment of spine pain is a function of the prognosis from the natural and treatment histories for uncomplicated cases.[41,75,82] Expectations for therapeutic outcomes based on the documented patterns can be effectively modified to account for extenuating circumstances unique to each case. The more important modifiers of treatment prognosis are listed in the box below.

Factors Effecting Treatment Prognosis[41,71,73]

- Pain severity at presentation
- Duration of pretreatment symptoms
- Number of prior episodes
- Exertional demands from activities of daily living
- Psychosocial components
- Job satisfaction

For the uncomplicated episode, short-range treatment objectives usually involve pain control and improvement of flexibility. Significant improvement in clinical status toward these aims should be anticipated within 2 weeks from the onset of treatment intervention. This pattern has been observed for patients with acute or chronic spine pain.[80,82,83] Presence of modifiers can result in a prolonged recovery period, generally about 1.5 to 2 times the expected rate. Available evidence[12,49,91] suggests that a more

aggressive initial treatment frequency may be the best approach. Depending on the patient's status, care administered five times per week for 2 weeks followed by up to three times per week for 3 months, may be warranted.[61] Cassidy et al.[15] advocate similar treatment protocols for management of lumbar intervertebral disc herniations as a safe and effective method to resolve symptoms, without the use of surgery in many cases. A very low incidence of complications has been reported,[42] but the potential benefits for properly selected candidates may be strong enough to initiate a therapeutic trial before operative interventions are contemplated.

In patients with symptoms beyond 16 weeks, passive manual care is probably appropriate for acute episodic exacerbation only. The treatment emphasis should shift to a supervised rehabilitation program and an alteration of life style. When the patient does not return to preepisode status, a declaration of maximum therapeutic benefit for the existing treatment plan should be considered. Whenever several efforts to withdraw treatment continue to result in significant deterioration of the clinical status, ongoing supportive care may be appropriate. However, such therapeutic effort may be improper when it interferes with other appropriate care or whenever the risk of physician dependence outweighs the benefits of supportive care.

Relationship To Other Subspecialties

Medical management through the use of nonsteroidal antiinflammatory drugs (NSAIDs) and epidural injection to manage severe pain with coexisting pathologies occasionally may prove useful over the short term, especially in chronic pain patients experiencing acute exacerbation.[2,24,65,67] As always, the balance of benefit versus the potential complications should be weighed on a case-by-case basis.

Sufficient information on the recovery of patients with musculoskeletal complaints of the spine exists to warrant a sense of urgency when the rate of recovery begins to lag. Pending chronicity is signaled by several factors. One of the more obvious is a set of symptoms that is stationary or unresponsive to passive treatment. Persistent symptom severity for 2 to 3 weeks should result in reevaluation of diagnosis and psychosocial and ergonomic influences affecting the patient. In these cases, modifying the treatment plan to deemphasize passive care methods, and to move into patient activation and rehabilitation is warranted. Patient assessment and the development of quantitative, quota-based, supervised rehabilitation may be carried out effectively by centers dedicated to management of these cases.[43,76] Such plans cut across health discipline boundaries to the advantage of the patient. Programs may involve the assistance of physical and occupational therapists, psychologists, and exercise physiologists.

Patients who are already expressing chronic spine disorders have been shown to benefit from a short course of manipulation to control symptoms, followed by implementation of back education programs designed to teach avoidance of mechanically stressful circumstances.[83]

Clinical Relevance

Treatment Effectiveness

The concept of treatment effectiveness is perhaps one of the most important in health care today. The relative term *effectiveness* speaks to the ability to discern patient improvement when a treatment is used under "real-world" experience.[16,30] That is, conditions that include the variety of ways in which patient compliance and additional confounders (such as natural history, socioeconomic status, general health, and sometimes education) seen in actual practice settings affect the treatment outcome. Typically, the investigation of treatment effects begins at the scientifically rigorous level of therapeutic "efficacy." In other words, under rigid experimental circumstances, does the treatment work?[16,30] Conditions under these study methods typically translate to the creation of a randomized clinical trial, during which comparison is made between a treatment intervention and a placebo. This may be difficult to accomplish, since for example, it may be unethical in certain instances to use a placebo, or those that are available may not be realistic. In addition, rigid controlled trials are expensive and often require large research teams that must work effectively and consistently over months or years when patient compliance can be even more unpredictable.

The assumptions for chiropractic practice in the past are like those that have guided the paradigm of all health care. That is, in the absence of high-quality studies, unsystematic and empirical observations have directed decisions in diagnosis, treatment efficacy, and prognosis. In essence, traditional clinical training and common sense have been used as substitutes for sufficient clinical and technical expertise to evaluate new tests and treatments.[28] The

social trends toward accountability and evidence-based practice is changing that premise. More objective information is expected to be used, when available, for decision making in patient care. Chiropractors have long been known to treat spine complaints of many kinds, including those resulting in referred or radiating pain. There is now a rather small but scientifically more rigorous pool of evidence that supports the empirical experience. Reviews and meta-analyses specifying distinct criteria for study inclusion and some form of research quality assessment can be used to summarize the current state of the art for SMT. Review topics have included biomechanical studies involving SMT, types of procedures, and both treatment and cost effectiveness.*

Lumbar Spine

Since 1990, five reviews on the effectiveness of SMT for treatment of low-back pain have been published with systematic and consistent techniques of analysis.[1,3,23,54,69] Due to the diversity of research study methods, patient diagnoses, and types of manual treatments used, interpreting and contrasting the results from different studies has required the determination of a quality score for each. Koes et al.,[54] Shekelle et al.,[69] and Anderson et al.[3] all have conducted analyses of as many as 34 articles appearing since 1965. Two scoring methods were used. Both were designed to consider such factors as subject randomization and investigator blinding. Table 29-2 presents the 16 articles common to all three analyses and the quality rating scores for each based on a maximum value of 100. To give practical meaning to the ratings, a reference value can be created by considering the results from analysis of unrelated research that has had a broad impact on changing medical practice patterns. The study by Veronesi et al.[86] on lumpectomy as a technique for treating mammary carcinoma was ranked by Shekelle et al.,[69] producing a quality score of 64.

While some diversity can be expected in literature assessment, rigorous reviews of SMT have common conclusions. Most randomized clinical studies dealing with acute episodes of mechanical low-back pain have found that SMT provides pain relief with functional improvement at a faster rate contrasted either with the natural history or other physical methods. Shekelle et al.[69] compiled a preliminary profile of the patient most likely to have a favorable response to SMT, which is given in the following box.

*References 1, 3, 5, 9, 21 to 23, 37, 44, 50, 54, 56, 59, 63, and 69.

Profile of the Optimum Case for Response to SMT

- Nonradicular low back pain
- Less than 1 month duration
- No previous manipulation
- No complications
- No secondary gain

Only six true clinical trials have focused on patients with chronic low-back pain.* In five of them, significant benefit in favor of SMT was found on at least one parameter. The most strict randomized study of effectiveness in cases of chronic back pain[83] found substantial benefits of a 2-week program of daily SMT over use of a mechanical sham treatment or a back education program. Patients had history of low-back and/or leg pain lasting over 50 days. During treatment, improvement in pain control and activities of daily living were noted. While this in-

*References 4, 27, 33, 62, 83, and 87.

Table 29-2

Sixteen trials reviewed by three recent analyses (maximum score, 100)

First Author	Anderson	Koes	Shekelle
Arkuszewski[4]	13	31	22
Berquist-Ullman[6]	71	49	49
Coxhead[19]	44	38	41
Doran[25]	36	42	42
Farrell[29]	56	32	36
Gibson[33]	40	46	47
Glover[35]	56	39	44
Godfrey[36]	40	22	36
Hadler[38]	51	53	56
Hoehler[45]	62	35	43
Mathews[60]	49	41	45
Rasmussen[66]	24	33	33
Sims-Williams[70]	42	35	40
Waagen[87]	73	37	49
Waterworth[89]	38	31	48
Zylbergol[93]	42	33	34

formation is promising, data demonstrating the relative efficacy requires further study. Current application of a trial of SMT is warranted when there are no contraindications present.

Cervical Spine

There are few well-conceived clinical trials of the benefits from manipulation given to patients with neck pain. Cassidy et al.[14] reported results from a randomized clinical trial contrasting the immediate effects from SMT versus mobilization. Pain severity and neck flexibility were quantified in patients with unilateral neck symptoms and referred pain into the area of the trapezius muscle. A single procedure was administered to the cervical spine. SMT was used on 52 cases, while the remaining 48 were treated with mobilization. The range of motion was increased for both types of intervention, but those that received SMT more frequently reported reduced severity of pain. Howe and associates reported the benefits from manipulation for combined neck and upper limb pain in a controlled study.[47] Significant improvement in pain and stiffness of the neck with increased range of motion in rotation was maintained for the duration of a 3-week follow-up period. An immediate improvement seen in lateral flexion was not sustained. Improvement also was noted in the associated peripheral pain but to a lesser degree than the neck pain itself. A third small trial used intravenous diazepam as a cointervention across study groups to enhance patient naivete with respect to study methods. No statistically significant differences were reported, although there was an apparent trend in differences in pain and activity ratings. Both parameters favored the SMT group. Unfortunately, the total sample size of 38 patients had too low power to show statistically the clinically relevant results that may have been present.[72] Finally, a European study of chronic spine complaints included neck disorders as a part of the patient sample. Koes and his colleagues[55] randomized patients to receive either manual therapy (manipulation, mobilization), treatment by the general practitioner (medication, exercise, bed rest, etc.), physiotherapy (heat, electrotherapy, ultrasound, short-wave diathermy), and a placebo (detuned ultrasound and detuned short-wave diathermy). Manual therapy again was reported to produce a higher rate and greater improvement in physical functioning. Clearly, however, more information is necessary. The data thus far accumulated shows a promising outlook for SMT in neck-related complaints.

Thoracic Spine

Published scientific evidence for the effectiveness of SMT in dealing with thoracic spine and costovertebral complaints is minimal. Clinical wisdom derived empirically and from extrapolation of the evidence from the cervical and lumbar regions serves as the basis for decision making. Only one prospective observational study has been reported that has included cases with thoracic complaints.[82] Resolution of symptoms, on average, required 50% of the care observed for treatment in the lordotic spinal regions and probably reflects the structural buttressing offered by the multiple attachments from the rib cage.

Other Spine-Related Complaints

Several quasiexperimental and clinical studies of varying quality, have reported promising results in cases treated with SMT in which the problems were not typically considered mechanical in nature or to have involved disorders of extremity joints.[20] Chiropractic has a history of attempting to aid patient discomfort due to a variety of disorders, by providing manipulation.[17] The relative degree of success provided by such measures requires substantially more research. These conditions account for a small proportion of cases in most chiropractic practices.[20]

Perhaps the conditions most relevant to a discussion spinal SMT are the various categories of headache. Results from treatment of most types of headache are unavailable. Parker et al.[64] conducted a study comparing chiropractic manipulation, medical manipulation, and a mobilization control in the treatment of migraine. No statistical difference was found between groups for either mean disability or mean pain intensity.[23] Their conclusions are not compelling, however, since the sample size was relatively small and the clinical course for this condition is quite variable. Further, the mean duration in hours of attack reported for the chiropractic manipulation group at the beginning of the study was substantially higher than for the other two groups. Despite this fact, treatment was associated with a notably larger change in duration for the SMT group. Sample variations were not provided in the report and it is impossible to tell if this difference was statistically significant, but the clinical difference appears striking. Boline et al.,[8] on the other hand, have reported significant differences in response of headache severity, frequency, and duration from SMT to the neck and thoracic spine regions in contrast to an alternative therapy of medication.

Accumulated evidence from a series of studies over the past several years strongly supports the use of manipulation for spine-related disorders. The best evidence is available for the treatment of low-back pain. Similarities between spinal regions apparent clinically[52] and in prospective observational study[82] suggests that distinction in response to SMT need not be expected by region. There is also evidence that manual procedures are not all equally effective. The trial by Hadler et al.[38] established the clear superiority of SMT over mobilization in patients with back pain. The work of Cassidy et al.[14] speaks similarly for neck pain. For treatment of episodes of spine-related complaints in which there are no clear contraindications, one of the first treatment alternatives that should be considered is manipulation. The literature has established that patients receiving this type of care, on average, can expect more rapid control of their pain and improvement in functional performance.

Future

Like the art and skill of the surgeon, it is doubtful that the experience and practice of manipulation can be offset strictly by advances in scientific understanding. However, many questions remain to be settled on the use of manipulation in patients with spine complaints. Their resolution is likely to help improve on the clinical outcomes from utilization of these treatment methods. Research involving clinical and basic scientists and engineers will be required to determine the optimal utilization. Fundamental issues include the scientific description and effects of biomechanical treatment characteristics and refinement of patient triage into manipulation. The large selection of manipulation methods also must be studied to determine appropriate applications for those that have clinical utility and to reject the use of those that do not. Finally, the mechanisms of action and physiologic benefits from SMT need to be studied.

References

1. Abenhaim L, Bergeron AM: Twenty years of randomized clinical trials of manipulation for back pain—a review, *Clin Invest Med* 15:527, 1992.
2. Amlie E, Weber H, Holme I: Treatment of acute low-back pain with piroxicam: results of a double blind placebo-controlled trial, *Spine* 12:473, 1987.
3. Anderson R, et al.: A meta-analysis of clinical trials of spinal manipulation, *J Manipulative Physiol Ther* 15:181, 1992.
4. Arkuszewski Z: The efficacy of manual treatment in low back pain: a clinical trial, *Man Med* 2:68, 1986.

5. Bergmann TF: Short lever, specific contact articular chiropractic technique, *J Manipulative Physiol Ther* 15:591, 1992.

6. Berquist-Ullman M, Larsson U: Acute low back pain—a controlled prospective study with special reference to therapy and confounding factors, *Acta Orthop Scand* 170:1, 1977.

7. Bogduk N, Engel R: The menisci of the lumbar zygapophyseal joints: a review of their anatomy and clinical significance, *Spine* 9:454, 1984.

8. Boline R, Boline PD: *General health status of patients with muscle contraction headaches.* Presented at the 1992 International Conference on Spinal Manipulation, Chicago, May 1992.

9. Brunarski DJ: Clinical trials of spinal manipulation: a critical appraisal and review of the literature, *J Manipulative Physiol Ther* 7:243, 1984.

10. Bullock-Saxton JE, Janda V, Bullock MI: Reflex activation of gluteal muscles in walking, *Spine* 18:704, 1993.

11. Butler DS: *Mobilisation of the nervous system,* Melbourne, 1991, Churchill-Livingstone, p 55.

12. Capasso C: Occupational low back pain: prevention of chronic disability, *Wis Med J* 90:581, 1992.

13. Cassidy JD, Kirkaldy-Willis WH, Thiel HW: *Manipulation.* In Kirkaldy-Willis WH, Burton CV, editors: *Managing low back pain,* ed 3, New York, 1992, Churchill-Livingstone.

14. Cassidy JD, Lopes AA, Yong-Hing K: The immediate effect of manipulation versus mobilization on pain and range of motion in the cervical spine: a randomized controlled trial, *J Manipulative Physiol Ther* 15:570, 1992.

15. Cassidy JD, Thiel HW, Kirkaldy-Willis WH: Side-posture manipulation for lumbar intervertebral disk herniation, *J Manipulative Physiol Ther* 16:96, 1993.

16. Cochrane AL: *Effectiveness and efficiency: random reflections on health services,* London, 1972, Nuffield Provincial Hospitals Trust.

17. Commission of inquiry into chiropractic: *Chiropractic in New Zealand: Report,* Wellington, New Zealand, 1979, PD Hasselberg, Government Printer, p 56.

18. Cox JM: *Low back pain: mechanisms, diagnosis and treatment,* ed 5, Baltimore, 1990, Williams & Wilkins.

19. Coxhead CE, et al.: Multicentre trial of physiotherapy in the management of sciatic symptoms, *Lancet* 1:1065, 1981.

20. Cramer GD, et al.: Generalizability of patient profiles from a feasibility study, *J Can Chiro Assoc* 36:84, 1992.

21. Deyo RA: Conservative therapy for low back pain: distinguishing useful from useless therapy, *JAMA* 250:1057, 1983.

22. Difabio RP: Clinical assessment of manipulation and mobilization of the lumbar spine: a critical review of the literature, *Phys Ther* 66:51, 1986.

23. Difabio RP: Efficacy of manual therapy, *Phys Ther* 72:853, 1992.

24. Dilke TF, Burry HC, Grahame R: Extradural corticosteroid injection in management of lumbar nerve root compression, *BMJ* 16:635, 1973.

25. Doran DM, Newell DJ: Manipulation in treatment of low back pain: a multicentre study, *BMJ* 2:161, 1975.

26. Dvorak J, Dvorak V: *Manual medicine: diagnostics,* New York, 1990, Thieme Medical Publishers, p 72.

27. Evans DP, et al.: Lumbar spinal manipulation on trial. Part 1—clinical assessment, *Rheumatol Rehabil* 17:46, 1978.

28. Evidence-based medicine working group: Evidence-based medicine—a new approach to teaching the practice of medicine, *JAMA* 266:2420, 1992.

29. Farrell JP, Twomey LT: Acute low back pain: comparison of two conservative treatment approaches, *Med J Aust* 1:160, 1982.

30. Feinstein AR: *Clinical epidemiology: the architecture of clinical research,* Philadelphia, 1985, WB Saunders Co, p 219.

31. Fisher AA: Pressure threshold meter: its use for quantification of tender spots, *Arch Phys Med* 67:836, 1986.

32. Fisher AA: Pressure algometry over normal muscles—standard values, validity and reproducibility of pressure threshold, *Pain* 1:115, 1989.

33. Gibson T, et al.: Controlled comparison of short-wave diathermy treatment with osteopathic treatment in non-specific low back pain, *Lancet* 1:1258, 1985.

34. Gitelman R: *The treatment of pain by spinal manipulation.* In Goldstein M, editor: *The research status of spinal manipulative therapy,* Bethesda, MD, 1975, Government Printing Office (US DHEW publ. no. 76998), p 277.

35. Glover JR, Morris JG, Khosla T: Back pain—a randomized clinical trial of rotational manipulation of the trunk, *Br J Ind Med* 31:59, 1974.

36. Godfrey CM, Morgan PP, Schatzker J: A randomized trial of manipulation for low-back pain in a medical setting, *Spine* 9:301, 1984.

37. Greenland S, et al.: Controlled trials of manipulation: a review and a proposal, *J Occup Med* 22:670, 1980.

38. Hadler NM, et al.: A benefit of spinal manipulation as adjunctive therapy for acute low-back pain—a stratified controlled trial, *Spine* 12:702, 1987.

39. Haldeman S: Pain physiology as a neurological model for manipulation, *Man Med* 19:5, 1981.

40. Haldeman S: Presidential address, North American Spine Society: failure of the pathology model to predict back pain, *Spine* 15:718, 1990.

41. Haldeman S, Chapman-Smith D, Petersen DM: *Guidelines for chiropractic quality assurance and practice parameters,* Proceedings of the Mercy Center Consensus Conference, Burlingame, California, January 25-30, 1992, Gaithersburg, 1993, Aspen Publishers Inc.

42. Haldeman S, Rubenstein SM: Cauda equina syndrome in patients undergoing manipulation of the lumbar spine, *Spine* 17:1469, 1992.

43. Hazard RG, et al.: Functional restoration with behavioral support—a one-year prospective study of patients with chronic low-back pain, *Spine* 14:157, 1989.

44. Herzog W: Biomechanical studies of spinal manipulative therapy, *J Can Chiro Assoc* 35:156, 1991.

45. Hoehler FK, Tobis JS, Buerger AA: Spinal manipulation for low back pain, *JAMA* 245:1835, 1981.

46. Homola S: *Bonesetting, chiropractic and cultism.* Panama City, 1963, Critique Books, p 8.

47. Howe DH, Newcombe RG, Wade MT: Manipulation of the cervical spine—a pilot study, *J R Coll Gen Pract* 33:57, 1983.

48. Janda V: *Muscle weakness and inhibition (pseudoparesis) in back pain syndromes.* In Grieve G, editor: *Modern manual therapy of the vertebral column,* New York, 1987, Churchill-Livingstone, p 197.

49. Jarvis KB, Phillips RB, Morris EK: Cost per case comparison of back injury claims of chiropractic versus medical management for conditions with identical diagnostic codes, *J Occup Med* 33:847, 1991.

50. Johnson MR, Ferguson AC, Swank LL: Treatment and cost of back or neck injury—a literature review, *Res Forum* 1:68, 1985.

51. Juhl G, Bogduk N, Marsland A: The accuracy of manual diagnosis for cervical zygapophyseal joint pain syndromes, *Med J Aust* 148:233, 1988.

52. King PM: Outcome analysis of work-hardening programs, *Am J Occup Ther* 47:595, 1993.

53. Kirkaldy-Willis WH: *Managing low back pain.* New York, 1983, Churchill-Livingstone.

54. Koes BW, et al.: Spinal manipulation and mobilisation for back and neck pain—a blinded review, *BMJ* 303:1298, 1991.

55. Koes BW, et al.: A blinded randomized clinical trial of manual therapy and physiotherapy for chronic back and neck complaints—physical outcome measures, *J Manipulative Physiol Ther* 15:16, 1992.

56. Leblanc FE, et al.: Quebec Task Force on Spinal disorders: scientific approach to the assessment and management of activity-related spinal disorders, *Spine* 12:S1, 1987.

57. Lewit K: *Manipulative therapy in rehabilitation of the locomotor system,* ed 2, Boston, 1991, Oxford.

58. Ligeros K: *How ancient healing governs modern therapeutics,* New York, 1937, Putnam, pp 52, 65, 421.

59. Mannello DM: Leg length inequality, *J Manipulative Physiol Ther* 15:576, 1992.

60. Mathews JA, et al.: Back pain and sciatica—controlled trials of manipulation, traction, sclerosant and epidural injections, *Br J Rheumatol* 26:416, 1987.

61. North American Spine Society: Ad Hoc Committee on Diagnostic and Therapeutic Procedures, Common diagnostic and therapeutic procedures of the lumbosacral spine, *Spine* 10:1161, 1991.

62. Ongley MJ, et al.: A new approach to the treatment of chronic low back pain, *Lancet* 2:143, 1987.

63. Ottenbacher K, Difabio RP: Efficacy of spinal manipulation/mobilization therapy—a meta-analysis, *Spine* 10:833, 1985.

64. Parker GB, Tupling H, Pryor DS: A controlled trial of cervical manipulation for migraine, *Aust N Z J Med* 8:589, 1978.

65. Postacchini F, Facchini M, Palieri P: Efficacy of various forms of conservative treatment in low back pain—a comparative study, *Neuroorthopedics* 6:28, 1988.

66. Rasmussen GG: Manipulation in the treatment of low back pain—a randomized clinical trial, *Man Med* 17:8, 1979.

67. Ridley MG, et al.: Outpatient lumbar epidural corticosteroid injection in the management of sciatica, *Br J Rheumatol* 27:295, 1988.

68. Schneider W, et al.: *Manual medicine: therapy,* New York, 1988, Thieme Medical Publishers, p 14.

69. Shekelle PG, et al.: Spinal manipulation for low-back pain: review, *Ann Intern Med* 117:590, 1992.

70. Sims-Williams H, et al.: Controlled trial of mobilisation and manipulation for patients with low back pain in general practice, *BMJ* 2:1338, 1978.

71. Singer J, et al.: Predicting outcomes in acute low back pain, *Can Fam Phys* 33:655, 1987.

72. Sloop PR, et al.: Manipulation for chronic neck pain—a double-blind controlled study, *Spine* 7:532, 1982.

73. Tate DG: Worker's disability and return to work, *Am J Phys Med Rehabil* 71:92, 1992.

74. Threlkeld A: The effects of manual therapy on connective tissue, *Phys Ther* 72:893, 1992.

75. Triano J: *Standards of care: manipulative procedures.* In White A, Anderson R, editors: *Conservative care of low-back pain,* Baltimore, 1991, Williams & Wilkins, p 159.

76. Triano JJ: *Chiropractic rehabilitation practice.* In Hochschuler S, et al., editors: *Rehabilitation of the spine: science and practice,* New York, 1992, Springer-Verlag.

77. Triano JJ: *Interaction of spinal biomechanics and physiology.* In Haldeman S, editor: *Principles and practice of chiropractic,* Norwalk, CT, 1992, Appleton & Lange.

78. Triano J, Cramer G: *Patient information—anatomy and biomechanics.* In White A, Anderson R, editors: *Conservative care of low-back pain,* Baltimore, 1991, Williams & Wilkins, p 45.

79. Triano JJ, Gudavalli R: *Torque-rotation response of sagittally symmetric, facetectomized lumbar motion segments in flexion,* Presented at the International Conference on Spinal Manipulation, Montreal, April 1993.

80. Triano JJ, Hyde TE: *Nonsurgical treatment of sports-related spine injuries II. Manipulation.* In Hochschuler SH, editor: *The spine in sports,* Philadelphia, 1990, Hanley & Belfus Inc, pp 246-53.

81. Triano J, Luttges M: Nerve irritation: a possible model of sciatic neuritis, *Spine* 7:129, 1982.

82. Triano JJ, Hondras MA, McGregor M: Differences in treatment history with manipulation for acute, subacute, chronic and recurrent spine pain, *J Manipulative Physiol Ther* 15:24, 1992.

83. Triano JJ, et al.: *A randomized controlled clinical trial of manipulation for chronic low-back pain patients,* Presented at the World Federation of Chiropractic Congress, May, 1993, London.

84. Twomey L: A rationale for the treatment of back pain and joint pain by manual therapy, *Phys Ther* 72:885, 1992.

85. Vernon HT, et al.: Pressure pain threshold evaluation of the effect of a spinal manipulation in the treatment of chronic neck pain, *J Manipulative Physiol Ther* 13:13, 1990.

86. Veronesi U, et al.: Comparing radical mastectomy with quadrantectomy, axillary dissection, and radiotherapy in patients with small cancers of the breast, *N Engl J Med* 305:6, 1981.

87. Waagen GN, et al.: Short term trial of chiropractic adjustments for the relief of chronic low back pain, *Man Med* 2:63, 1986.

88. Wardwell W: *Why has chiropractic survived?* In Wardwell W, editor: *Chiropractic: history and evolution of a new profession,* St. Louis, 1992, Mosby.

89. Waterworth RF, Hunter IA: An open study of diflunisal, conservative and manipulative therapy in the management of acute mechanical low back pain, *N Z Med J* 98:372, 1985.

90. Wilder D, Pope M, Frymoyer J: The biomechanics of lumbar disc herniation and the effect of overload and instability, *J Spinal Disord* 1:16, 1988.

91. Wolk S: *An analysis of Florida workers' compensation medical claims for back-related injuries,* Boston, 1988, American Public Health Association.

92. Zhu Y, et al.: *Paraspinal muscle evoked cerebral potentials in muscle spasm,* Presented at the International Society for the Study of the Lumbar Spine, 7th Annual Meeting, Boston, May 1992.

93. Zylbergold RS, Piper MC: Lumbar disc disease—comparative analysis of physical therapy treatments, *Arch Phys Med Rehabil* 62:176, 1981.

Chapter 30

The Role of Manual Therapy in Spinal Rehabilitation*

Joseph P. Farrell

Janet Y. Soto

Carol Jo Tichenor

*Taken in part from Farrell JP: Cervical passive mobilization techniques: the Australian approach, *Phys Med Rehab State Art Rev* 4(2):309, 1990.

Manual therapy is an important aspect of the total management scheme for patients experiencing spinal symptoms of musculoskeletal origin. Manual therapy techniques include massage of the soft tissues, manually sustained or rhythmically applied muscle stretching, traction applied in the longitudinal axis of the spine, specific or general high-velocity manipulation, passive joint mobilization, and adverse neural tissue mobilization.[5,33,49,57] Grieve defines joint mobilization as passive, repetitive, oscillatory movements that can be controlled by the patient.[33] Joint mobilization techniques are applied to regions of the spine or to specific vertebral motion segments by the hands, fingers, or thumbs of the physical therapist. Maitland describes manipulation as a high-velocity small-amplitude movement applied generally to a region of the spine or specifically to one vertebral motion segment in a manner such that the patient cannot prevent the maneuver from taking place.[57]

In the United States, chiropractors, osteopaths, and physical therapists are the professionals most often associated with manual therapy (MT) or manipulative therapy. Manual therapy is not exclusive to any profession, and each group uses a variety of manual techniques. The practitioner, based on his or her education and clinical experiences and the patient's clinical profile, decides the force, amplitude, direction, duration, and frequency of MT treatment movements.[66] The role of the orthopedic manual physical therapist (OMPT) in spinal rehabilitation is to *methodically* assess pain and function, test tissue structures, and detect movement abnormalities of the musculoskeletal system, and subsequently design a treatment program that is *reassessed continually* and altered to optimize recovery of function.[36,57]

Patients with spinal musculoskeletal pathology who seek treatment are usually limited by pain. They generally complain of symptoms such as pain, numbness, tingling, burning sensations, and heaviness and coldness of the extremities. Manual therapy is a suitable treatment choice when these symptoms are aggravated by activity and selected postures and relieved by rest and other antalgic postures. In addition, patients who exhibit altered range of spinal motion, asymmetry of position, and tissue texture abnormalities may also benefit from MT.[36] For MT to be an effective treatment method, the practitioner must be skilled in evaluating spinal dysfunction, applying appropriate treatment techniques relating to treatment goals, and assessing changes in symptoms and function. The treatment goal is to eliminate or minimize symptoms so that the patient can resume a functionally normal lifestyle. Therefore, to achieve

optimal treatment outcomes, manual therapists must also utilize numerous physical therapy procedures (ergonomic analysis, modalities, education, and therapeutic exercise to improve endurance, strength, coordination, flexibility, and stabilization) in addition to passive movement techniques.[21]

The data that must be considered in the management of patients with spinal disorders is complex, requiring decisions based on current diagnosis, etiology, pathogenesis, prognosis, and treatment. The spinal joints, soft tissues, and related nervous, vascular and autonomic systems are anatomically complicated. Through careful examination of these systems the OMPT provides vital data related to the patient's overall functional abilities and musculoskeletal impairments that can assist the physician in clarifying a musculoskeletal diagnosis and in planning effective treatment. This sharing of expertise contributes to clinical decisions that will benefit the patient and lead, ultimately, to cost-effective health care.

This chapter will focus on the orthopedic manual physical therapy evaluation process, which leads to the successful application of MT techniques as a component of the spinal rehabilitation program. A brief review of clinical trials relating to MT techniques will be presented, followed by a discussion of the examination process, assessment/clinical decision-making process, and treatment planning aspects of spinal rehabilitation.

Clinical Trials Relating to Manual Therapy

Research investigating the efficacy of MT for treatment of pain and/or dysfunction of spinal origin is difficult to design and implement and has been limited in scope.[9,51,62] Despite the "pitfalls" that plague these clinical trials, the following findings in recent research should be recognized. The first is that MT hastens recovery in the short term in patients suffering from acute back pain. Studies comparing various manual therapies to passive modalities such as detuned diathermy, heat, medication, back school, or nonintervention report quicker relief from pain and increased spinal motion.[22,39,48,72] Other studies have examined the effect of MT on increasing sacroiliac joint innominate tilts bilaterally,[6] increasing straight-leg raise limitations in a controlled study of patients with low-back pain (LBP),[24] increasing serum β endorphins, which are associated with pain reduction,[78] and decreasing electromyographically measured skin resistance.[15]

Controlled clinical trials proving the efficacy of MT for the treatment of cervical dysfunction are few in number.[68,73] To our knowledge, no studies have been performed regarding the thoracic region of the spine. Studies of "back pain," though greater in number, are challenged for lack of standardization, researching isolated techniques with limited clinical relevance, and rigid adherence to grouping patients according to diagnosis.[9,10,51] In a study conducted in England, private out-patient chiropractic treatment was purported to be more effective than hospital out-patient physical therapy.[60] The study was biased to favor the outcomes. There was no control group, treatment methodology was poorly defined, and treatment settings were unequal.

The presence of true control groups, randomization, strict inclusion/exclusion criteria, concise description of experimental and control group treatment intervention, and blind assessment of outcome variables are critical factors when considering the validity of clinical trials. Lack of standardization is often levied as a criticism of studies of MT. Korr,[46] in *Neurobiologic Mechanisms in Manipulative Therapy*, stated " . . . manipulative procedures, even in the hands of the same practitioner, vary according to the findings and their changes in each visit; they vary from patient to patient and from visit to visit. Manipulative therapy is no more a uniform therapeutic entity than is surgery, psychiatry, or pharmaco-therapeutics."

However, attempts to control relevant experimental variable have led to clinical research that does not study how MT would be applied in a normal clinical setting. For example, rotatory manipulation for back pain is the most commonly studied MT technique.* Utilization of this isolated technique has not produced significant measurable functional changes in patients with acute or chronic back pain. The results did suggest that manipulation produced more favorable results in subjective pain relief than did modalities or patient education. To judge the value of spinal MT based on research of isolated techniques is dubious. An approach more consistent with clinical practice and therefore value would be an investigation of a system of MT examination and treatment techniques, since in the clinical setting, most patients will not respond to one technique or one application of a technique. This suggestion is supported by Ottenbacher and DiFabio,[67] who performed a meta-analysis of mobilization/manipulation studies. Their findings suggest that the effects of mobilization/manipulation were greater when MT was used in conjunction with other forms of treatment.

Another shortcoming of spinal research involves rigid adherence to the practice of grouping patients according to diagnosis. Most spinal studies center around the diagnosis of the patient's problem, despite the claim that 80% to 90% of patients with disabling back pain fail to receive a precise diagnosis.[11,75] Most experienced clinicians practicing MT have seen patients with the diagnosis of "herniated nucleus pulposus at L4-L5" who are able to bend forward and touch their toes in a painless manner, yet are functionally unable to sit, or drive for greater than 5 minutes, because of back pain. Another patient with the same diagnosis may be able to sit for an unlimited period of time, but has significant back pain that limits forward bending to the 50% range. Medical practitioners and other critics of MT should seriously look at refining the term *diagnosis* and consider the nature of research design faults within various clinical studies prior to disregarding its use in treating spinal dysfunction.

The Examination Process

The Subjective Data

The interview process during which the patient describes his or her symptoms is vital in determining the source(s) of the patient's complaint(s). By obtaining the location and behavior of the problem(s), the history, and any precautions to applying manual techniques, the clinician can formulate a "working hypothesis" of the disorder. The working hypothesis identifies the potential musculoskeletal structure(s) involved in the presenting pathology. The clinician uses this subjective information to rank the importance of each component of the working hypothesis according to its severity, irritability, and stage of pathology.[29,40,57]

The goals of the subjective examination are presented in the box on page 454 so the reader can acquire an appreciation of the detailed interview process required to understand the patient's major complaint. If the major complaint is not fully understood, the clinician risks applying manual techniques inappropriately or to the wrong body region, which may endanger the patient.

The subjective examination consists of four components[57]: the area of symptoms; the behavior of symptoms; necessary precautions to examination and treatment; and the history.

*References 8, 19, 24, 28, 35, and 65.

Goals of the Subjective Examination

- Understand the patient's lifestyle and the specifics of his or her working environment.

- Identify functional problems.

- Obtain a description of the patient's symptoms.

- Assess which body area(s) to emphasize during the interview physical examination.

- Understand how the problem affects the patient's lifestyle throughout the 24-hour day.

- Formulate a clinical working hypothesis related to the presenting pathology and progression of the pathology.

- Determine any contraindications to treatment or use of specific techniques.

- Assess the patient's perception of his or her problem and understand the patient's goals(s).

Area of Symptoms

The experienced clinician can quickly diagram the location of each symptom on a body chart and establish its relationship to the others. By studying the body chart (Fig. 30-1), and knowing the referral patterns of musculoskeletal problems, and observing the patient, the orthopedic manual physical therapist can begin to formulate the working hypothesis, which will continually be refined during the examination and treatment process.

Behavior of Symptoms

The next step is to find out how the symptoms vary with movements and positions: how severe the pain is, and how easily the pain is exacerbated. The clinician will use this information to be cautious in the vigor and extent of examination and treatment.

Precautions to Examination and Treatment

The third component of the subjective examination consists of questions to rule out serious medical conditions that may limit or preclude treatment with manual therapy. These conditions include malignancy involving the spinal column, signs and symptoms of spinal-cord compression, active inflamma-tory and infective arthritic conditions, advanced stages of rheumatoid arthritis affecting the ligaments of the cervical spine, bone diseases such as spondy-lolisthesis or osteoporosis, vertebrobasilar artery disease, cauda equina syndrome, and tethered cord syndrome.[32]

Several situations necessitate caution in the application of passive manipulation/mobilization techniques. In the presence of neurologic signs, techniques that compromise the intervertebral foramen on the side of the painful extremity should be avoided. Osteoporosis necessitates gentle application of mobilization techniques and precludes manipulation since loss of up to 40% of bone salts occurs prior to observable radiologic evidence.[52] Previous metastatic disease in tissues other than the spine does not necessarily contraindicate passive movement treatment. Similarly, passive mobilization of the cervical or lumbar spine may be performed if particular attention is paid to the history and behavior of the symptoms. Additional diagnostic testing to rule out spinal metastases is necessary if the cause of the patient's complaint is not related to movement or selected postures.

Dizziness is a common symptom associated with vertebrobasilar arterial disease. Regardless of the origin, every patient who presents with upper quarter dysfunction should be questioned in detail concerning the presence of dizziness, prior to cervical examination and treatment. Although the incidence of injury from manipulation of the cervical spine is small,[31,71] the potential danger for injury that may lead to permanent neurologic damage or death cannot be overlooked when examining the patient. The incidence of injury from passive cervical mobilization techniques has not been adequately explored in the literature. Details of the subjective and objective examination of the patient who presents with symptoms of dizziness have recently been reported.[1,29]

The History

Lastly, the manual therapist traces the present and past history of each area of symptoms. A sequential history provides important data pertaining to the nature of the problem (diagnosis) and the progression of symptoms. By understanding the progression of symptoms, the skilled clinician will be able to further rank, rerank, or reject the working hypothesis. In addition, the patient whose symptoms are worsening (e.g., progressive radiation of extremity symptoms plus numbness) will be examined quite differently from the patient who is progressively improving.

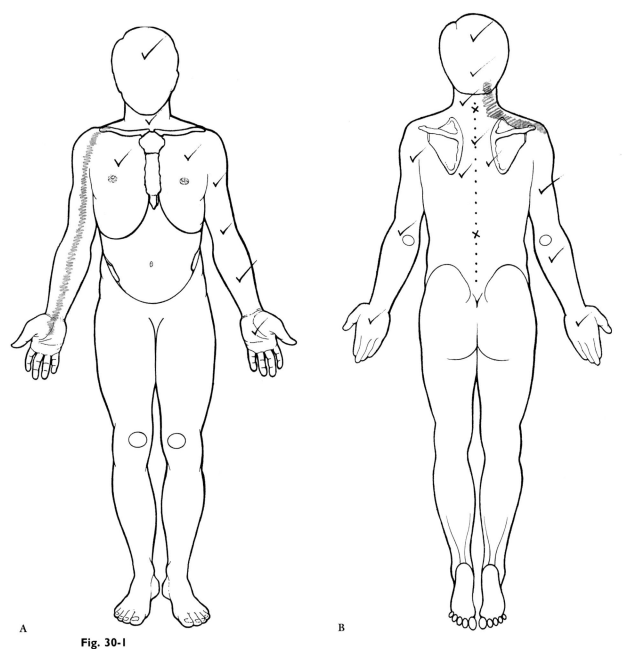

Fig. 30-1

Pain diagram: Areas and relationships of symptoms. When the constant deep neck ache (**A**) increases or is exacerbated, the intermittent deep arm ache (**B**) is exacerbated. In other words, the patient does not experience right arm symptoms without experiencing an increase in neck ache.

Often, past history of trauma, even from a decade prior to current presenting problems, is important in determining the diagnosis and prognosis. A thorough understanding of the etiology of each trauma consolidates the working hypothesis and priority of each problem in relation to the current complaint. Once the clinician assesses the subjective data, he or she is able to prioritize the physical examination and continue the process of refining the working hypothesis.

The Physical Examination

Critical analysis of the information gathered from the subjective examination enables the clinician to plan the physical examination. The analysis of subjective data aids the clinician in identifying a plan (first box) for examining the patient.[57] The points listed in the box enable the astute clinician to set individualized goals of the physical examination. These goals are described in general terms in the second box.

Analysis of Subjective Data/Plan of the Examination

- Identify structures that may be responsible for the symptoms.
- Differentiate structures or functional movements to prove or disprove a working clinical hypothesis.
- Note the irritability, nature, and stage of the pathology, which will dictate the vigor of the examination and treatment.
- Identify factors that might contraindicate any portion of the physical examination.
- Arrive at a possible rationale for symptoms (e.g., lifestyle, repetitive nature of the patient's work, any other predisposing factor) so that the examination and treatment lead to total patient management.

Aims and Goals of the Physical Examination

- Identify movement patterns and restriction of movement that relate to pain-provoking and pain-easing factors reported by the patient.
- Reproduce the patient's complaint via movement testing and palpation of all structures that can potentially cause the problem.
- Differentiate which structures are causing various components of the complaint.
- Confirm the irritability of the condition.
- Confirm the cause(s) of the patient's complaint based upon the subjective data collected.
- Determine the patient's neurologic status.

The emphasis of the physical examination will vary according to the assessment of subjective data synthesized during the plan of the physical examination.

For example, if the major complaint is right low cervical aching radiating down the central aspect of the arm to the palm of the hand, the clinician must examine the cervical spine, shoulder complex, elbow complex, and wrist region and must perform a neurologic examination to determine the cause of the problem. Further tests of adverse neural tissue tension are in order[4,5,18] because of the presenting pain pattern. The detail necessary in examining the peripheral joint and soft tissue structures depends on the working hypothesis. If the clinician determines the problem to mainly arise from the cervical spine, slightly from the shoulder, and moderately from adverse neural tissue tension, the cervical spine will be examined in far greater detail than the shoulder. However, if the problem appears to have a larger shoulder component, the shoulder portion of the examination will be more detailed and precise than in the first scenario.

Observing the Patient

Skillful observation of the patient performing functional activities such as undressing or opening the door, or of the posture with which the patient holds the head or upper extremity, can supply considerable information about the severity of the disorder and the way the patient reacts to the complaint. These functional aggravating activities can be used to differentiate and incriminate which structure or region of the body is the source of the patient's dysfunction.[77] They also yield information as to the ergonomic advice required for the long-term management of the patient's condition.

The clinician analyzes the functional activity to determine which component of the activity or which aggravating position is causing the symptoms. The clinician uses the sequential method of adding or eliminating components to test the working hypothesis. The first step is to reproduce the symptoms by asking the patient to reach backwards as if she is reaching for her purse in the back seat of the car (Fig. 30-2). The next step is to return the cervical spine to a neutral position (Fig. 30-3). If the neck and arm symptoms disappear when eliminating the cervical rotation/side-flexion/extension component, the cervical spine is implicated as a region of the body that is contributing to the neck and arm complaint. If the symptoms are still present when the cervical spine is held in neutral, then the symptoms may be arising from the shoulder, elbow, or any soft-tissue structure in the upper limb or cervical muscles, or from adverse neutral tissues tension.

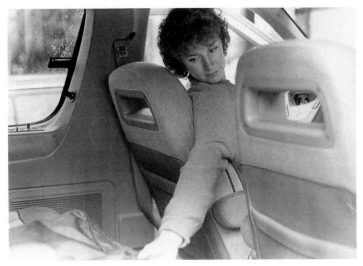

Fig. 30-2
Patient reaching backward as if reaching for purse in back seat of car. Cervical spine: right rotation, right side-flexion, extended.

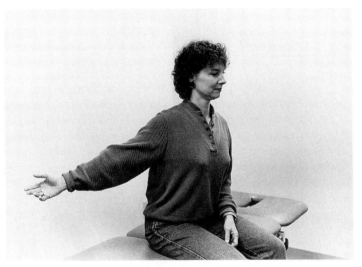

Fig. 30-3
Return cervical spine position to neutral for differentiation purposes.

This ongoing assessment process aids the clinician in prioritizing the remainder of the physical examination. Further testing will confirm or dispute the hypothesis that the neck region is a major contributor to the symptoms in this patient example. The authors will refer to this brief case study example to illustrate the clinical decisions required for the OMPT to examine a patient successfully.

Movement Testing

Referring back to the body chart in Fig. 30-1, we use knowledge of pain referral patterns, aggravating factors, and the description of the functional differentiation tests to prioritize our movement testing. Let's assume that our assessment of subjective data suggests that the symptoms are not stopping the patient from performing his or her daily work and lifestyle activities. When the symptoms are aggravated, they settle within a minute, suggesting a nonirritable condition. The history suggests a stable state of the pathology and no progression of symptoms distally for over 6 months. Cervical traction, postural instruction, and heat had failed over a period of 6 weeks to change functionally the patient before this evaluation.

Based upon the data presented, the clinician needs to examine all potential structures that may cause the patient's complaint. Most OMPTs embark quickly onto a screening process to test and confirm the working clinical hypothesis (see box). Testing is best performed bilaterally for comparison of the normal extremity with the abnormal extremity.

Working Clinical Hypothesis: Case Study Example

1. Cervical dysfunction
2. Shoulder dysfunction
3. Elbow dysfunction
4. Adverse neutral tissue tension
5. Muscle length/strength
   a. Scalenes
   b. Upper trapezius
   c. Rotator cuff
   d. Biceps
   e. Pectoralis major/minor
6. Postural dysfunction

Information Needed to Obtain Reproducible Baseline Data During Movement Testing

- Resting symptoms.
- Location and behavior of symptoms during movement testing.
- Quality and duration of symptoms reproduced.
- Effect of movement upon each related and unrelated symptom.
- Quality of intersegmental movement through range.
- Presence and relevance of protective deformity.
- Effect of pressure at the end range of normal or pathologic anatomic limit.
- Whether any spinal movements ease a particular symptom, thus allowing their use as a treatment technique.

Traditional cervical active anatomic plane movements (flexion, extension, lateral flexion, and rotation) should be examined. Shoulder movements should include flexion, abduction, reaching the hand behind the back, external and internal rotation, and functional aggravating factors. Elbow flexion, extension, pronation, and supination are tested to confirm the role of the elbow complex. Specific muscle strength and length tests will yield information as to the muscular component of the hypothesis.

Adverse neural tissue tension testing[5,18] is indicated owing to the position of the shoulder and arm when reaching backward (shoulder abduction, horizontal extension, external rotation, coupled with forearm extension/supination). Elvey has shown the importance of this test for determining the contribution of neural tissue dysfunction in patients with neck/shoulder/arm symptoms.[16] (See the section below on adverse neural tissue tension.)

During the screening process the clinician acquires the following information to obtain reproducible baseline data (see box). These data are used to reassess change in movement and pain patterns as a result of a particular evaluation or treatment technique.[53]

Subjective data collection assists in dictating which movement tests will best confirm which region or structures are the source of functional limi-

tation. Therefore, if standard active movement tests do not reproduce the patient's complaint, the clinician should consider sustaining movements, performing repeated movements, compressing or distracting the cervical spine, performing movements under compression or distraction, altering the speed of the movement test, or performing combined movement testing.[13,14] In this case example, one may consider sustaining right side-flexion if symptoms are not reproduced with standard cervical movements. This movement is the logical choice, since holding the phone in a right cervical side-flexion causes the patient's symptoms. Another reasonable test is combining the cervical movements of right rotation, right side-flexion, and extension to reproduce the neck complaint, since this mimics the cervical spine position when reaching backward for an object in the rear seat of a car.

Adverse Neural Tissue Tension

Manual therapists are routinely confronted with the difficulties of differentiating the cause of shoulder and arm pain. Pain may be referred from the cervical spine or from a multitude of structures. Experimental studies on human beings have produced pain in the shoulder region and upper extremity by stim-

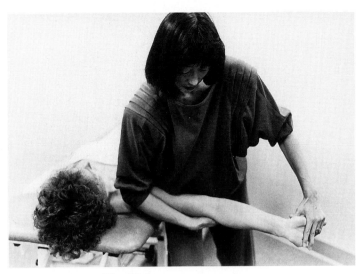

Fig. 30-4

ULTT base test: median nerve bias.

ulating interspinous ligaments,[23,43] cervical intervertebral discs,[7] paraspinal and scapular musculature,[42] and the cervical nerve roots via mechanical distortion.[25] Pathologic and degenerative changes that occur in the cervical spine may be accompanied by fibrosis and adhesion formation in and around nerve roots. Nerve roots are susceptible to irritation from tensile stresses arising from mechanical interfaces such as disc bulges and osteophytes or uncovertebral and zygoapophyseal joints, which may inhibit mobility or extensibility. Formation of fibrous tissue can develop within the nerve root sheath and nerve root as a result of the inflammatory process following trauma or disease.[63] Clinical examples of this presentation are evident when patients present with a stiff and painful shoulder or tennis elbow, which is often caused by proximal pathology such as cervical radiculopathy.[2,34] Orthopedic manual therapists originated the method of differentiating the contribution of adverse neural tissue tension[3] to various musculoskeletal presentations. Maitland first described the slump test, which combines trunk flexion, neck flexion, knee extension, dorsiflexion, and hip flexion, as a test for mobility of neural structures within the intervertebral canal, intervertebral forearm, and the peripheral extensions of the nerves into the lower extremity.[54] Others documented use of the slump test in differentiation of posterior thigh pain thought to be of hamstring muscle origin from immobility of neural tissue.[45]

Elvey first documented in 1979 the brachial plexus tension test to differentiate which anatomic structures are responsible for upper quarter symp-

toms.[17] He found that despite sophisticated diagnostic tests such as MRI, the specific pathology was often not determined. This is especially evident when patients present with shoulder and cervical signs that singularly or together contribute to the musculoskeletal symptoms. Through dissection studies and clinical experience, Elvey devised the brachial plexus tension test (BPTT), which is analogous to the straight-leg raising test of the lower extremity.[17] The BPTT or upper limb tension test (ULTT) places tension on the neural tissues of the upper quarter throughout its length, from the cervical spine to the periphery of the arm and hand. This test procedure combines shoulder depression, shoulder abduction, horizontal extension, lateral rotation, forearm supination, elbow extension, and wrist/finger extension (Fig. 30-4). The major cervical nerve roots affected are C5-C6, and the median nerve peripherally is most stretched. Other "tension tests" for the ulnar nerve (Fig. 30-5) and radial nerve (Fig. 30-6) are performed when signs and symptoms are thought to be arising from these nerves (e.g., radial bias test for tennis elbow, or ulnar bias test for medial forearm aching). Many clinicians in Australia have studied Elvey's maneuver and have offered modifications to the test[4,5] and conducted studies documenting normative responses.[44]

In our hypothetical patient (page 456), the rationale should now be obvious for testing for adverse neural tissue tension as a component of the working hypothesis. Elvey's ULTT should be tested since it stresses the C5-C6 nerve roots and the median nerve, which may be causing symptoms in our pa-

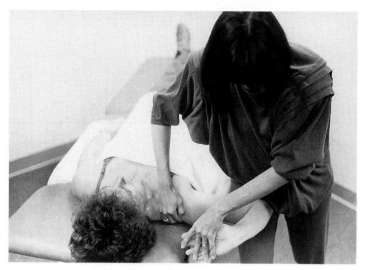

Fig. 30-5

ULTT: ulnar nerve bias.

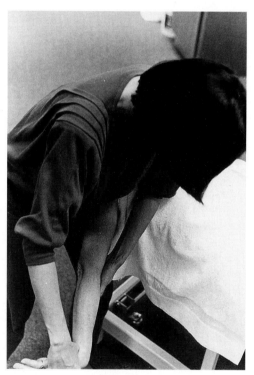

Fig. 30-6

ULTT: radial nerve bias.

tient example. The presence of adverse neural tissue tension is confirmed when the symptoms are reproduced by the ULTT and either decreased when tension is decreased on neural tissues or increased by movement of the cervical spine away from the tested side (Fig. 30-7).

Palpation of the Spine and Associated Regions

Skillful palpation is becoming a lost art in the field of medicine. Most OMPTs believe that palpation of the spine and all associated areas that contribute to the presenting symptoms may be the most informative aspect of the physical examination.[55] The clinician assesses the findings to confirm further which structures contribute to the dysfunction and to formulate the rationale for treatment of appropriate structures. The findings also verify how each structure relates to the working hypothesis.

As a general rule, OMPTs palpate all regions of the spine that may contribute to the dysfunction. For example, if a patient presents with upper cervical pain and stiffness extending to T8-T9 and sits as pictured in Fig. 30-8, the OMPT would palpate all muscles and soft tissues from the occiput to T10-T-11 and evaluate the vertebral and rib mobility as a routine portion of the examination. Particular attention would be paid to the occipito-atlantal (O/A) and atlanto-axial (A/A) motion segments, owing to the head-on-neck posture, and to the C7-T1 (C/T) junction, owing to the positioning of the neck on the trunk. Both of these regions are transitional zones, where the function of the spinal column changes.[50] The O/A segment is the site where tonic neck reflexes influence muscle tone throughout the trunk musculature. If there is dysfunction at this vertebral motion segment the posterior postural muscles exhibit hypertonus, which can be palpated at times along the corresponding dermatome. Korr[47] calls this "a facilitated segment."

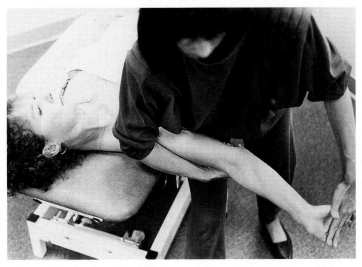

Fig. 30-7

ULTT base test: median nerve bias, sensitized by cervical side flexion away from tested limb to confirm ANTT.

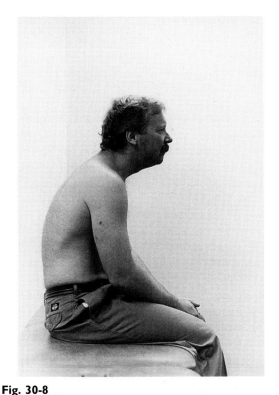

Fig. 30-8

Patient seated in slump position to illustrate upper extension and truncal flexion.

The A/A segment is very important for rotation of the cervical spine. If dysfunction is evident at this motion segment, the remainder of the cervical spine is forced to take over this rotation. The C/T junction is the region of the spine where the most mobile section of the spine is joined to the most rigid,

the thoracic spine and rib cage. Muscles of the upper extremity and shoulder girdle attach at this zone and should therefore be carefully examined for length and strength as contributors to any dysfunction.

A study by Jull and associates[41] in Australia evaluated an orthopedic manual physical therapist's ability to identify cervical zygoapophyseal joint syndromes in 20 patients, all of whom had complained of chronic neck pain or headaches for at least a year. Two research questions were proposed:

1. Can OMPTs actually sense abnormalities in the joint by palpating movements between specific vertebra?

2. Are the allegedly palpated abnormalities diagnostic or are they nonspecific signs?

The study used a crossover design. In one group of 11 patients, the presence or absence of a symptomatic joint was established by radiologically controlled diagnostic nerve blocks. The OMPT examined the patients 1 to 4 weeks after the nerve block. The OMPT was unaware of the medical diagnosis. In the second group, consisting of 9 patients, the order of events was reversed.

The OMPT first examined the patients, gave an opinion as to whether there were symptoms present and, if present, at what vertebral motion segment. Neither the OMPT nor the medical team had any knowledge of the cause of the patient's symptoms. Of the 20 patients in both groups, the OMPT correctly identified all 15 with proven symptomatic zygoapophyseal joints and correctly concluded that the other five patients were free of symptoms. The authors of this study[41] concluded that for the diagno-

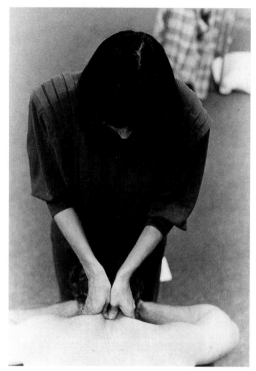

Fig. 30-9

Cervical posterior-anterior (P-A) pressure.

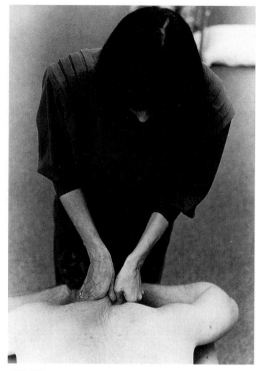

Fig. 30-10

Unilateral P-A pressure over cervical zygoapophyseal joint.

sis of symptomatic cervical zygoapophyseal joints, the manual examination by a trained OMPT is as accurate as expensive radiologically controlled diagnostic blocks. In addition, the OMPT could not possibly have made accurate clinical diagnoses so consistently had one not in fact been able to palpate and assess the specific vertebral motion segments.

The palpation techniques used in the Jull study have been described in detail in Maitland[57] and are also performed as treatment techniques. These movements cannot be voluntarily performed by the patient. Mennell[61] calls these movements "joint play," and all joints must have normal joint play to function. For example, it is impossible for an individual to move actively one vertebral motion segment in an anterior-posterior direction, yet these movements are required of a motion segment to flex the spine. These passive accessory movements include the following:

- Posterior-anterior (P-A) pressures on the spinous processes of the vertebral motion segment (Fig. 30-9).
- Unilateral P-A pressures applied along the laminae and adjacent to the spinous processes moving lateral to the zygoapophyseal joints (Fig. 30-10).
- Transverse pressures performed against the lateral aspect of the spinous process (Fig. 30-11).

The variations of these movements are endless. The position of the palpating thumbs or the direction of the movement (medial, lateral, cephad, caudad) may be altered so that the pressure placed upon the zygoapophyseal joint and intervertebral discs are different. The OMPT angulates the passive accessory intervertebral movement (PAIVM) in an effort to reproduce the patient's complaint in a manner that the patient experiences. The aim of the palpation assessment by the OMPT is to reproduce the most comparable symptoms and signs. This is essential in determining the correct treatment technique and the appropriate region of the spine at fault, and in determining the directions, patient position, and vigor of the technique.

Of equal importance is the evaluation of passive physiologic intervertebral movements (PPIVMs) (Fig. 30-12), which are described in numerous texts.[57,76] The region of the spine is systematically tested at each vertebral motion segment (flexion, extension, lateral flexion, rotation) to detect range of motion, quality of movement, and end feel. The extremities or spine are moved in a passive manner while the fingers are used to palpate the facet joint or interspinous space in an effort to detect motion. In a joint with restricted mobility (hypomobility), the "springing" or "giving" of the joint is lost and

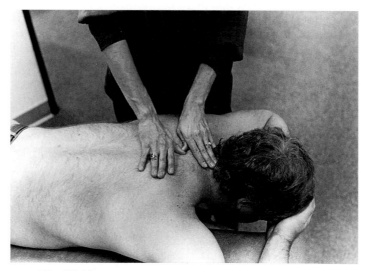

Fig. 30-11
Transverse pressure performed at lower cervical motion segment.

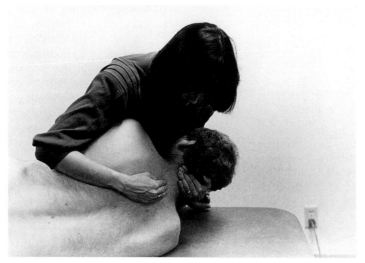

Fig. 30-12
Passive physiologic intervertebral motion testing (upper thoracic flexion).

the clinician may abruptly feel blockage to movement. The restriction in vertebral movement is often accompanied by muscular tension or spasm which, with experience, is detected easily and is an indication that the mobility of the vertebral motion segment is altered. Passive physiologic intervertebral movement testing in skilled hands also may give information relating to excessive movement of a vertebral motion segment (hypermobility), which necessitates musculature stabilization rather than mobilization. Often, the movement restrictions detected by PAIVM and PPIVM correlate to yield significant evidence that a particular vertebral motion segment is contributing to the patient's dysfunction.

Muscle Length and Strength

The evaluation of muscle length and strength is a routine component of the evaluation process. The mobility of spinal musculature is important, as shortened muscles lead to joint limitations, which may facilitate a pain cycle that is difficult to break.[37,70] Numerous texts[20,38] outline the specific methods of testing for muscle length and specific stretching techniques.

When testing for muscle strength it is commonplace to test myotonally to detect neurologic deficits coupled with sensation and reflex testing. Functional muscle testing is also of significance. Often, traditional muscle tests yield normal muscle grades. The patient may still be limited in his or her ability to lift repetitively, for example, and may tire at work secondary to weakness of the quadriceps and gluteals and back pain. A simple functional test is to have the patient bring a tire into the clinic so that he or she can actually lift and carry the object that is required of his or her work. From this test the OMPT may ascertain the strength and endurance of the quadriceps and gluteals by documenting the number of lifts and carries prior to fatigue. Body mechanics and coordination may be concurrently assessed. In this example, the OMPT should pay particular attention to the patient's ability to control the lumbopelvic region during the lifting, carrying, or pivoting activities. This portion of the evaluation assists in formulating a total treatment program that is functional in nature. Concrete data collection of this sort is reproducible and may be reassessed as the treatment program progresses.

Assessment: Its Role in Clinical Decision Making

Assessment is an appraisal or evaluation of information collected. Data are routinely assessed at the conclusion of the subjective examination, during and at the conclusion of the physical examination, prior to administration of a particular treatment technique, during the application of the treatment technique, and at the conclusion of the initial treatment.[57] From this assessment, realistic goals are established. Between treatments, it is important to assess the effect of treatment on the patient's functional limitations as they relate to lifestyle and work environment as well as the movement signs and symptoms that relate to the clinical working hypothesis.

The clinician must continually reassess the effect of each modality, exercise, or treatment technique on the presenting history and nature of the problem in order to appreciate the changing nature of the patient's problem. Continual reassessment aids the clinician in determining the validity of the treatment technique(s) of choice and yields information as to which structures are most likely contributing to the patient's complaint. If a patient's signs, symptoms, and functional limitations are not changing at an appropriate rate, the clinician needs to reassess the working hypothesis and alter the treatment accordingly.

The OMPT assessment is of great benefit to the patient. By quickly terminating ineffective treatment and instituting more appropriate measures, the patient's potential for recovery to a functional lifestyle is enhanced. The cost savings to the "health care system" should be obvious, since prolonged treatment

is avoided. To further illustrate the concept of assessment as used by the OMPT, a case study is presented to demonstrate the clinical reasoning and decision-making skills required to employ successfully manual therapy techniques.

Case Study to Illustrate Assessment

Subjective Data

Profile

34-year-old male working in real estate. Drives 300 miles/week. Hobby: Snow skiing.

Major Complaint

See pain diagram: constant left buttock ache, intermittent "pulling" posterior thigh (Fig. 30-13).

Aggravating Factors

Sitting or driving for more than 1 hour reproduces the left buttock ache. Maximum time: 1.5 hours secondary to posterior thigh aching and pulling. Symptoms settle in 5 minutes to normal resting level. Walking more than 1 mile or getting into his car (neck flexion component) causes the left pulling sensation in the thigh. At the end of a work day he generally feels that the left buttock ache is worse.

Current History

Three months prior to evaluation the patient noticed left low back/buttock pain when attempting to open a heavy fence gate that was not releasing. While driving away from the work site, he noticed left posterior thigh ache/pull that did not extend past the knee. Next morning the patient noticed a right lumbar shift and walking was limited to 0.5 mile. He sought medical evaluation. He received a Demoral injection, which helped for about 4 hours. MRI was performed revealing an L4-L5 and L5-S1 herniated nucleus pulposus. No OMPT treatment was administered. Within the week, the patient drove from Texas to California. All symptoms were exacerbated. Patient then received an epidural injection and was referred for physical therapy (PT) to consist of exercise and instruction in body mechanics. The epidural and PT assisted in decreasing the intensity of symptoms and he felt he was able to walk up to 1 mile before increasing left posterior thigh symptoms. The patient had not missed any work due to this episode nor was there any past history of back or leg symptoms. He believed that over the past 2 months his sitting and driving tolerance had improved to about 1 hour.

(Continues on page 466)

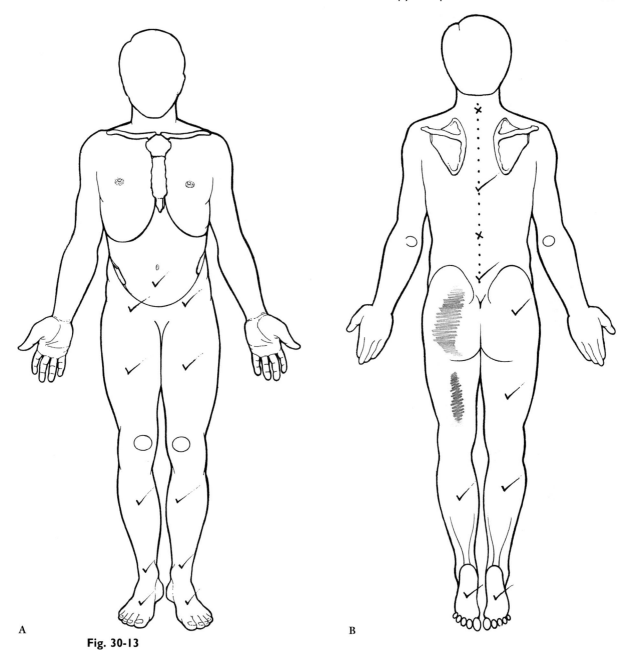

Fig. 30-13

Lumbar case study: the patient had no complaints of numbness or tingling or signs or symptoms of cauda equina syndrome.

Case Study to Illustrate Assessment (Continued)

Observation

Sits slumped in flexion. Slight lumbar list to the right. No change with correction to the list. Moderate left calf atrophy, minimal gluteal and hamstring atrophy. Symmetric pelvis.

Neurologic Signs

Absent left ankle jerk; sensation intact to pin-prick; left gastrocsoleus (unable to toe raise); left extensor hallucis longus, extensor digitorum longus, and peroneals (4−/5); left gluteals and hamstrings (4+/5).

Trunk and lower-extremity muscle strength: Abdominals 4+/5, erector spinae 5−/5, functionally able to squat repetitively 25× before tiring.

Active Lumbar Movement Testing

Flexion: 50% range, left buttock and thigh ache, worse with neck flexion.

Extension: 10% range, reproduces left low-back pain.

Repeated extension in standing: increased buttock and thigh ache.

Left-side flexion: 40% range, increased left buttock ache.

Right-side flexion: 55%, painless, eased left buttock ache.

Adverse Neural Tissue Tension

Passive neck flexion: 80% range, reproduced left buttock pain.

Right SLR: 70 degrees.

Left SLR: 40 degrees, left buttock and thigh pulling, worse when dorsiflexion was added.

Slump test to first increase in symptoms (P1): Trunk flexion (painless), neck flexion (reproduces back pain), left-knee extension −40 degrees (left buttock and thigh pulling), neck extension eased symptoms while left knee was able to extend to −10 degrees, right knee extension in slump −5 degrees.

Palpation

P-A pressures over the spinous process of L4-L5 reveal a 60% limitation of intervertebral mobility with reproduction of buttock pain upon pressuring L5. Left unilateral P-A pressures over the facet joints reveal increased muscle tone and local back pin. Passive physiologic movements showed limited mobility in left rotation and flexion at L4-L5 and L5-S1.

Assessment of Subjective Data

The following discussion is a form of clinical reasoning that is routine to OMPT.[30,40] This is the first stage of formulating a working hypothesis.

The patient presents with a nonsevere problem in that he is able to limit his lifestyle (e.g., driving and sitting) and still work. Aggravating factors such as driving and sitting longer than 1 hour (1.5 hours maximum) reproduce distal symptoms; however, they settle quickly, suggesting a nonirritable problem. The patient reports that he has a documented diagnosis of L4-L5, L5-S1 herniated nucleus pulposus (HNP). The buttock pain when sitting could arise from the intervertebral disc.[64] Adverse neural tissue tension (ANTT) probably exists because the HNP, acting as mechanical interfaces, may inhibit nerve root mobility.[5] The neck flexion component when getting into a car also suggests ANTT in that neck flexion pulls the spinal cord, meninges, and nerve root proximally when the trunk is flexed.[3,56,69] The proximal movement of neural structures may contribute to the aggravation of left posterior thigh pulling when walking or getting into the car. The neck extension component of the slump test eased the thigh "pulling," therefore, evidence for ANTT is stronger.

The history suggests that the pathology is stable and slightly improving over a 2-month period. But looking at the total picture, it appears that this patient's pathology is worsening in that he had never experienced back or leg symptoms in the past.

Assessment After the Physical Examination

The physical examination confirms that several positive movement signs are contributing to the patient's problem. The working hypothesis would include: (1) L4-L5, L5-S1 HNP with chronic nerve root irritation (S1 > L5); (2) adverse neural tissue tension; (3) truncal/left lower extremity weakness; and (4) poor body mechanics. The discogenic component of the hypothesis is supported by the limited lumbar flexion and left SLR.[64,74] The S1 > L5 nerve root irritation is based on the greater number of S1 myotomal muscles revealing weakness as compared with L5 myotomal muscles, the limited left SLR, and the dermatomal pain pattern. Because repeated extension increases the posterior thigh symptoms, it can be hypothesized that the extension movement is compressing a nerve root or the disc itself. The ANTT is strongly represented by the positive passive neck flexion test,[69] the left SLR of 40 degrees that worsens with dorsiflexion,[26] and the very positive

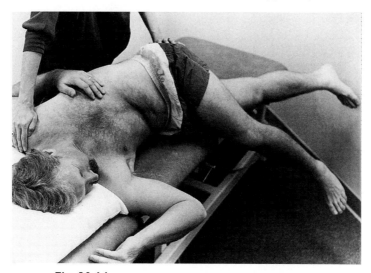

Fig. 30-14

Lumbar rotation IV+ performed as a treatment technique.

slump test,[5,57] which differentiates ANTT from hamstring tightness or strain. Truncal and lower extremity weakness are documented via basic manual muscle tests and the poor body mechanics observed while the patient is sitting.

Treatment

Trial Treatment

The initial treatment session must affect some or all components of the working hypothesis so that the clinician can further refine or rank which structures are contributing most to the total clinical picture. The general principle of technique selection is based on whether one is treating pain, stiffness, spasm, or weakness. The nature of the pathology is also important: which movements increase or decrease the symptoms and the irritability of the problem. This patient's problem appears to be stiffness more than pain, and it is affecting the disc. The clinician will have to perform some end-range technique to affect the discogenic component.[57] Extension as a treatment technique is commonly used when the disc is involved[59]; however, in this case, extension is contraindicated since it increases distal symptoms. Clinical experience[57] and clinical studies[58] have proven that lumbar rotation does affect discogenic disorders. Fisk[24] also showed that lumbar rotation positively improved SLR in patients with limited unilateral SLR. The movement testing revealed that right side flexion relieved the buttock and thigh aching. Biomechanically, right side flexion couples with left rotation.[76] Therefore, clinical reasoning points to the choice of left lumbar rotation (painful side up), as this technique affects the intervertebral disc and SLR, is pain easing, and opens the intervertebral canal, which is desirable when neurologic signs are present.[57] This technique can be performed (Fig. 30-14) in a painless manner as an end-range Grade IV or IV+.[57]

The process of assessment after an application of a particular treatment technique is routine in orthopedic manual physical therapy to prove its value and effectiveness on each component of the working clinical hypothesis. In this patient example, the following signs that relate to the working hypothesis should be tested:

1. lumbar flexion;
2. left SLR plus dorsiflexion;
3. left ankle jerk;
4. muscle strength: left gastrosoleus, extensor hallucis longus, peroneals; and
5. palpation signs: P-A and unilateral P-A at L4-S1 motion segments to test for pain reproduction, mobility, and muscle tone.

Satisfactory change for the first visit would be lumbar flexion increasing to 65%, left SLR to 60 degrees (a 20% improvement), and no change in the neurologic signs, especially since an examination was performed prior to treatment. If treatment is too vigorous on Day 1, and the patient returns worse, it would be difficult to determine what made the patient worse: the examination or the treatment. Instruction in basic body mechanics (getting out of bed, dressing, and sitting) should also be done at the first visit to begin the education process for long-term management.

Subsequent Treatments

Decisions made in subsequent treatments depend on the change in subjective reports and key physical examination signs. For example, if the patient has maintained the 20% improvement from Day 1, it is reasonable to continue with rotation as a treatment technique. If the patient has regressed, the clinician must determine the cause. Is it secondary to the treatment, to something the patient has done, or to the natural progression of the disorder? With careful questioning, appropriate decisions to alter or supplement treatment can be made.

In the initial phase of spinal rehabilitation, the clinician works to control pain and the inflammatory process. By applying gentle passive mobilization techniques to the appropriate vertebral motion segment(s), segmental mobility and functional range of motion may improve and pain may lessen. The mobilization technique is progressed further into the available range of motion for that segment. The clinician continues the technique until movement is painless or no functional change is detected.

If both joint and soft tissue limitations exist, the OMPT should assess the effect of the joint mobilization technique on the soft tissue component. If little or no change is seen in the soft tissue component, specific muscle stretching or soft tissue massage techniques should be applied to improve the condition of the soft tissues. Likewise, if ANTT is present, the effects of joint mobilization and/or soft tissue techniques on the tension signs must be assessed. If no change is noted, specific techniques that treat ANTT should be used.

As the irritability of the condition decreases and functional range of motion improves, specific exercises to strengthen and stretch the spinal region and extremity muscles should be taught to assist in maintaining spinal mobility. Furthermore, instruction in body mechanics and self-treatment techniques reduces dependence on the clinician and aids patients in assuming some responsibility for their care.

When the patients perform repetitive tasks at work and during recreational activities, they require specific training in their rehabilitation program. Endurance and coordination should be addressed and should be sport or job specific. The clinic should be equipped with exercise apparatus such as pulley systems, free weights, aerobic machines, gymnastic balls, and assorted household items to train the patient functionally. Such equipment is also easily adaptable and inexpensive for patients to use for long term management through home exercise programs.

Modalities such as ice, electric stimulation, or ultrasound may be used in conjunction with MT techniques as long as the value of the modality is assessed. Any medications prescribed by the physician as an adjunct to treatment during the inflammatory phase of the condition should also be assessed.

Conclusion

Manual therapy in spinal rehabilitation requires much skill on the part of the practitioner. Meticulous examination and assessment determine the propriety of its role in the total treatment scheme. Some patients may not have responded to treatment with modalities and specific stabilization exercises aimed at strengthening and stretching the spine and associated structures. These patients may require a thorough MT evaluation. Specific joint limitation, soft tissue immobility, and ANTT may be present and hinder the rehabilitation process. If the structures at fault are not initially identified, they may not be addressed with the exercise program.

The OMPT must, therefore, be able to thoroughly evaluate pain and its relationship to the patient's lifestyle, functional activities, and movement abnormalities as they relate to the neuromusculoskeletal system. Using the clinical reasoning outlined in this chapter, the OMPT formulates a working hypothesis based on clinical experience, in-depth knowledge of the anatomy and biomechanics of the neuromusculoskeletal system, and the patient's clinical presentation. Treatment is designed and implemented to improve movement abnormalities, decrease pain, and improve the quality of the patient's functional abilities.

With further clinical reasoning, the OMPT proves or disproves the initial working hypotheses and ranks and reranks them according to the evolving clinical picture and functional responses to treatment. Techniques are appropriately altered or added to address all aspects of the patient's dysfunction. When the patient is ready, exercises and functional training should be incorporated into the total treatment program. Logical decision making skills and continual reassessment aids the therapist in appropriate selection of technique and contributes to a successful outcome for the patient.

With increasingly complex technology, rapid changes in the delivery of health care, and increasing regulations affecting accountability in medical settings, the demands on health professionals to make prudent, cost-effective clinical decisions are tremendous. Never before have health professionals had so many treatment options for their patients. Never before have there been so many medical specialties that can contribute to the care of the patient. With these increasing options come obligations and opportunities for health professionals to share expertise to make possible the best treatment outcome for the patient. The OMPT can provide subjective and objective data to assist the physician in clarifying his or her diagnosis and in establishing an effective plan for the patient. Rapid identification of musculoskeletal pathology and logical decision-making skills do lead to efficient patient management, and, ultimately, cost-effective, prudent, and accountable medical care.

References

1. Aspinall W: Clinical testing for cervical mechanical disorders which produce ischemic vertigo, *Ortho Sports Phys Ther* 11:176, 1989.
2. Bogduk N: *Neurology of the neck/shoulder complex.* Proceedings of the M.T.A.A. Symposium, Brisbane, 19-29, 1983.
3. Breig A: *Adverse mechanical tension in the nervous system.* New York, 1978, John Wiley & Sons.
4. Butler DS: Adverse mechanical tension in the nervous system: a mode for assessment and treatment, *Aust J Physiother* 35:227, 1989.
5. Butler DS: *Mobilization of the nervous system,* Edinburgh, 1991, Churchill-Livingstone.
6. Cibulka MT, Delitto A, Koldehof RM: Changes in innominate tilt after manipulation of the sacroiliac joint in patients with low back pain: an experimental study. *Phys Ther* 68(9):1359, 1988.
7. Cloward R: Cervical diskography, *Ann Surg* 150:1052, 1959.
8. Coyer AB, Curwen IHM: Low back pain treated by manipulation: a controlled series, *BMJ* 1:705, 1955.
9. DiFabio RP: Clinical assessment of manipulation and mobilization of the lumbar spine: a critical review of the literature. *Phys Ther* 66:1:51, 1986.
10. DeFabio RP: Efficacy of manual therapy, *Phys Ther* 72(12):853, 1992.
11. Dillane JB, Fry J, Kalton J: Acute back syndrome: study from general practice, *BMJ* 2:82, 1966.
12. Doran MI, Newel DJ: Manipulation in the treatment of low back pain: a multicentre study. *BMJ* 2:161, 1975.
13. Edwards BC: Combined movements in the cervical spine (C2-7): their value in examination and treatment choice, *Aust J Physiother* 26:165, 1980.
14. Edwards BC: *Combined movements of the cervical spine in examination and treatment.* In Grant R, editor: *Physical therapy of the cervical and thoracic spine,* Edinburgh, 1988, Churchill-Livingstone, p 125.
15. Ellestadt SM et al.: Electromyographic and skin resistance responses to osteopathic manipulative treatment for low back pain, *J Am Osteopath Assoc* 88(8):991, 1988.
16. Elvey R: The treatment of pain associated with abnormal brachial plexus tension, *Aust J Physiother* 32:225, 1986.
17. Elvey RL: *Brachial plexus tension tests and the pathoanatomical origin of arm pain.* In Glasgow EF, Twomey LT, editors: *Aspects of manipulative therapy.* Melbourne, 1979, Lincoln Institute of Health Sciences. p 105.
18. Elvey RL: *Brachial plexus tension tests and the pathoanatomical origin of arm pain.* In Idczak RM, editor: *Aspects of manipulative therapy,* Carlton, Australia, 1981, Lincoln Institute of Health Sciences, p 116.
19. Evans DP, et al.: Lumbar spinal manipulation on trial. Part I. Clinical assessment, *Rheumatol Rehab* 17:46, 1978.
20. Evjenth O, Hamberg J: *Muscle stretching in manual therapy: a clinical manual, vol 2,* Sweden, 1984, Alfta Rehab.
21. Farrell JP, Jensen GM: Manual therapy: a critical assessment of role in the profession of physical therapy, *Phys Ther* 72(12):843, 1992.
22. Farrell JP, Twomey LT: Acute low back pain, comparison of two conservative treatment approaches, *Med J Aust* 1:160, 1982.
23. Feinstein B, et al.: Experiments on pain referred from deep somatic tissues, *J Bone Joint Surg* 36A:981, 1954.
24. Fisk JW: A controlled trial of manipulation in a selected group of patients with low back pain favouring one side, *N Z Med J* 89:346, 1979.
25. Frykholm R: Cervical root compression resulting from disc degeneration and root sleeve fibrosis, *Acta Chir Scand Suppl* 1960, 1951.
26. Gajdosik R, LeVeau B, Bohannon R: Effects of ankle dorsiflexion on active and passive unilateral straight leg raising, *Phys Ther* 65:1478, 1985.
27. Glover JR, Morris JG, Khosla T: Back pain: a randomised clinical trial of rotational manipulation of the trunk, *Br J Ind Med* 31:59, 1974.
28. Godfrey CM, Morgan PP, Schatzker J: A randomized trial of manipulation for low back pain in a medical setting, *Spine* 9(3):301, 1984.
29. Grant R: *Dizziness testing and manipulation of the cervical spine.* In Grant R, editor: *Physical therapy of the cervical and thoracic spine,* Edinburgh, 1988, Churchill-Livingstone, p 111.
30. Grant R, Jones M, Maitland GD: *Clinical decision making in upper quadrant dysfunction.* In Grant R, editor: *Physical therapy of the cervical and thoracic spine,* Edinburgh, 1988, Churchill-Livingstone, p 51.
31. Green D, Joynt R: Vascular accidents associated with neck manipulation, *JAMA* 170:522, 1959.
32. Grieve G: *Common vertebral joint problems,* Edinburgh, 1981, Churchill-Livingstone.
33. Grieve GP: *Mobilization of the spine: notes on examination, assessment and clinical method,* ed 4, Edinburgh, 1984, Churchill-Livingstone.
34. Gunn CC, Milbrant WE: Tennis elbow and the cervical spine, *CMA* 114:803, 1976.
35. Hadler NM, et al.: A benefit of spinal manipulation as adjunctive therapy for acute low back pain: a stratified controlled trial, *Spine* 12(7):703, 1987.

36. Haldeman S: Spinal manipulative therapy: a status report. *Clin Orthop* 179:62, 1983.

37. Janda V: *Muscle and joint correlations.* In Lewit K, Gutman G, editors: *Functional pathology of the motor system*, Rehabilitacia, Bratislava, Obzov Suppl 10–10, 154, 1975.

38. Janda V: *Muscle function testing,* London, 1983, Butterworths.

39. Jayson MIV, et al.: Mobilization and manipulation for low back pain, *Spine* 6(4):409, 1981.

40. Jones MA: Clinical reasoning in manual therapy, *Phys Ther* 72(12):875, 1992.

41. Jull G, Bodguk N, Marsland A: The accuracy of manual diagnosis for cervical zygoapophyseal joint pain syndromes, *Med J Aust* 148:233, 1988.

42. Kellegren J: Observations on referred pain arising from muscle, *Clin Sci* 3:175, 1938.

43. Kellegren J: On the distribution of pain arising from deep somatic structures with charts of segmental pain areas, *Clin Sci* 4:35, 1939.

44. Kenneally M, Rubenach H, Elvey R: *The upper limb tension test: the SLR test of the arm.* In Grant R, editor: *Physical therapy of the cervical and thoracic spine*, Edinburgh, 1988, Churchill-Livingstone, p 1967.

45. Kornberg C, Lew P: The effect of stretching neural structures on grade one hamstrings injuries, *J Orthop Phys Ther* 10:481, 1989.

46. Korr IM: *Neurobiologic mechanisms in manipulative therapy.* Preface. New York, 1978, Plenum Press, p xvi.

47. Korr IM: Proprioceptors and somatic dysfunction, *J Am Osteopath Assoc* 74:638, 1975.

48. Kuo PP, Loh A: Treatment of lumbar intervertebral disc protrusions by manipulation, *Clin Orthop Rel Res* 215:47, 1987.

49. Lamb D: *A review of manual therapy for spinal pain: with reference to the lumbar spine.* In Grieve GP, editor: *Modern manual therapy.* New York, 1986, Churchill-Livingstone, p 605.

50. Lewit K: *Manipulative therapy in rehabilitation of the locomotor system,* London, 1985, Butterworths.

51. Lindahl O: Methods for evaluating the therapeutic effect of nonmedical treatment, *Scand J Rehab Med* 11:151, 1979.

52. Mackinnon J: Osteoporosis: a review, *Phys Ther* 68:1533, 1988.

53. Magarey ME: *Examination and assessment of spinal joint dysfunction.* In Grieve GP, editor: *Modern manual therapy of the vertebral column*, Edinburgh, 1986, Churchill-Livingstone, p 401.

54. Maitland G: Negative disc exploration: positive canal signs, *Aust J Physiother* 25:129, 1979.

55. Maitland GD: Palpation examination of the posterior cervical spine: ideal, average, and normal, *Aust J Physiother* 28:3, 1982.

56. Maitland GD: The slump test: examination and treatment. *Aust J Physiother* 31:215, 1985.

57. Maitland GD: *Vertebral manipulation,* ed. 5, London, 1986, Butterworths.

58. Mathews JA, Yates DAH: Reduction in lumbar disc prolapse by manipulation, *BMJ* 2:696, 1969.

59. Mckenzie RA: *The lumbar spine: mechanical diagnosis and therapy,* Waikanae, New Zealand, 1981, Spinal Publications.

60. Meade TW, et al.: Low back pain of mechanical origin: randomized comparison of chiropractic and hospital outpatient treatment, *BMJ* 300:1431-1437, 1990.

61. Mennell J: *Back pain,* Boston, 1960, Little Brown.

62. Moritz U: Evaluation of manipulation and other manual therapy: criteria for measuring the effect of treatment, *Scand J Rehab Med* 11:173, 1979.

63. Murphy RW: Nerve roots and spinal nerves in degenerative disc disease, *Clin Orthop* 129:46, 1977.

64. Nachemson A, Morris JM: In vivo measurements of intra discal pressure. *J Bone Joint Surg* 46:1077, 1964.

65. Nwuga VCB: Relative therapeutic efficacy of vertebral manipulation and conventional treatment in back pain management, *Am J Phys Med* 61:6:273, 1982.

66. *Orthopaedic physical therapy terminology.* Orthopaedic section, American Physical Therapy Association, LaCrosse, WI, 1991, Orthopaedic Section.

67. Ottenbacher K, DeFabio RP: Efficacy of spinal manipulation/mobilization therapy: a meta-analysis, *Spine* 10(9):833, 1985.

68. Parker G, Tupling H, Pryor D: A controlled trial of cervical manipulation for migraine, *Aust N Z J Med* 8:589, 1978.

69. Reid J: Effects of flexion-extension movements of the head and spine upon the spinal cord and nerve roots, *J Neurol Neurosurg Psychiatry* 23:214, 1960.

70. Reynolds M: Myofascial trigger point syndromes in the practice of rheumatology, *Arch Phys Med Rehab* 62:111, 1981.

71. Schellhas K, et al.: Vertebrobasilar injuries following cervical manipulation, *JAMA* 244:145, 1980.

72. Sims-Williams H, et al.: Controlled trial of mobilization and manipulation for low back pain: hospital patients, *BMJ* 24:1318, 1979.

73. Sloop P, et al.: Manipulation for chronic neck pain: a double blind study, *Spine* 7:532, 1982.

74. Smyth MJ, Wright V: Sciatica and the intervertebral disc: an experimental study, *J Bone Joint Surg* 40A:1401, 1418, 1959.

75. Spratt KF, et al.: A new approach to the low back physical examination: behavioral assessment of mechanical signs, *Spine* 15(2):96, 1990.

76. Stoddard A: *Manual of Osteopathic technique,* London, 1961, Hutchinson.

77. Trott P: *Differential mechanical diagnosis of shoulder pain.* In Proceedings of the Manipulative Therapists Association of Australia, 4th Biennial Conference, Brisbane, 1985.

78. Vernon HT, et al.: Spinal manipulation and beta endorphin: a controlled study of the effect of a spinal manipulation on plasma beta-endorphin levels in normal males, *J Manip Physiol Therapeutics* 9(2):115, 1986.

Section 2
The Patient within the Socioeconomic Cascade

Chapter 31
Ergonomic Intervention for the Prevention and Treatment of Spinal Disorders[*]

Chris C. Shulenberger

[*]Modified from Shulenberger CC: Ergonomics in the workplace: evaluating and modifying jobs. In White LA, editor: Back School, *Spine State Art Rev* 5:429–436, 1991.

Manifold is the harvest of diseases reaped by certain workers from the crafts and trades that they pursue. All the profit they get is injury to their health that stems mostly, I think, from two causes. The first and most potent is the harmful character of the materials that they handle, noxious vapors and very fine particles, inimical to human beings, inducing specific diseases. As a second cause I assign certain violent and irregular motions and unnatural postures of the body, by reason of which the natural structure of the living machine is so impaired that serious diseases gradually develop therefrom.

Bernardino Ramazzini
De Morbis Artificum
(About Diseases of Workers), 1700

As stated above, the first cause (noxious vapors and very fine particles) falls into the realm of the contemporary industrial hygienists. The second cause (violent and irregular motions and unnatural postures) constitutes the area in which the ergonomists most often function. Low back injuries, repetitive motion problems of the upper extremity, cervical strains and sprains—these are all examples of gradually developing problems referred to by Ramazzini. In one way or another, all these problems as well as stress-related disorders involve a mismatch between the worker's capabilities (physical, emotional, intellectual) and the workplace demands.

Historically, and at present, there are many examples of ergonomic interventions. During World Wars I and II, much of industry was modified to meet the lifting, carrying, and reaching abilities of women, who became much more predominant in the workforce. Recently public bathrooms, sidewalks, and buildings, have been modified to meet the functional needs of wheelchair riders and others with special mobility needs. Unfortunately, most of U.S. industry has just begun to understand the importance of ergonomics from the standpoints of both safety and productivity. Pushing this movement are several pieces of federal and state legislation that have or will require ergonomic evaluations and modifications to workplaces.

Various federal and state Occupational Safety and Health (OSHA) offices are writing citations regard-

ing ergonomics based on the general-duty clause, which requires an employer to maintain a safe working environment. OSHA has begun to enforce ergonomic guidelines regarding manual material handling and cumulative trauma disorders (e.g., National Institute of Occupational Safety and Health [NIOSH] Lifting Guidelines and Meat Packing Industry Guidelines, respectively). By 1995, it is anticipated that there will be specific OSHA guidelines covering cumulative trauma disorders.

The recently passed Americans With Disabilities Act will require all employers to accommodate individuals with disabilities unless it creates undue financial hardship or a significant safety risk. This applies to newly hired workers, on-the-job injuries, and injuries that occur off-the-job.

States have passed legislation such as California's Senate Bill 198, which requires employers to identify problems and hazards, to develop systems to correct them, to maintain comprehensive safety and health programs, and to develop methods to ensure compliance.

Employers who have embraced ergonomics as a way of doing business have already begun to reap benefits. Some of the major benefits to good ergonomic design are improved safety leading to fewer injuries, fewer accidents, and less risk taking; improved efficiency, leading to increased productivity and fewer errors; improved well-being, leading to less fatigue, less discomfort, less occupational disability, and improved worker health; and improved job satisfaction, leading to less absenteeism, less labor turnover, better cooperation, and better attitude toward work.

These benefits translate directly to dollars earned or dollars saved by an employer. However, injuries to the spine are still the number one workers' compensation claim. They result in the most lost work days and the highest costs to employers. So, where do we start, given the importance and the requirement to improve the ergonomics of the industrial work environment? The most logical place to begin is with a better understanding of the job.

Job Analysis

The job analysis is the foundation on which other decisions are based. Without a complete working knowledge of the job, proposed problem solutions are at best an educated guess. At worst they are misdirected, expensive, and ineffective. But what is a job analysis? One functional definition is as follows: A job analysis is an objective and systematic evaluation of the work environment that documents job demands and task requirements. These demands can include the basic physical demands (e.g., lifting, carrying, pushing, pulling, etc.) and the environmental conditions (exposures to heat, cold, vibrations, mechanical hazards, etc.). However, more complex situations may require a working knowledge of population-based standards of performance such as for lifting and energy expenditure and/or of anthropometric (human factors) data. These data can relate to the general worker population or specific subgroups such as gender, ethnic variations, and special needs of the aged or disabled. Clearly, the job analysis requires much more than just a working knowledge of human anatomy, physiology, and good body mechanics.

The word *objective* is a key part to the definition of job analysis. All too often a job analysis is prepared based on the perceptions of the workers, supervisors, and managers. The importance of subjective input should not be discounted; however, a comprehensive job analysis also validates the subjective perceptions with data that is measurable, reliable, and reproducible (i.e., objective). Therefore, a complete job analysis gathers data from several sources:

1. Review of records
   a. OSHA 200 logs
   b. Workers' compensation claims
   c. Health benefits utilization
2. Review of programs and practices
   a. Hiring procedures
   b. Safety training
   c. Injury investigations
   d. Return to work, including restricted/modified duty
3. Interviews with
   a. Upper management
   b. Supervisors
   c. Line and staff workers
4. On-site observations documented with photos and/or videotapes
   a. Methods of execution
   b. Site variances
   c. Changes due to environmental conditions (snow, rain, darkness, etc.)
   d. Shift variances
5. Physical measurement
   a. Forces
   b. Distances
   c. Frequencies
   d. Postures
   e. Duration

The Americans with Disabilities Act adds another aspect to the job analysis process. It requires that employers make personnel decisions based on an individual's ability to perform the "essential functions" of the job with or without accommodation. This means that employers need to understand the overall purpose of the job and to consider the performance standards or objectives of the functions. Employers can no longer just focus on the "usual and customary methods" currently being used to complete job tasks. For example, lifting and carrying are really methods of transporting materials between locations and can be accommodated in several ways (mechanical lifts, carts, etc.).

This change in the required process clearly has an impact on the hiring, promotion, and return to work of individuals with spinal injuries. At present, nearly 20% of all claims filed with the Equal Employment Opportunity Commission (EEOC) are related to back disabilities. In addition, approximately 80% of claims are related to current employees, not newly hired workers. Therefore, the job analysis process used by employers needs to address the purposes of the essential functions, not just the tasks and methods. Once the essential functions are determined, then the accommodation process can evaluate whether those functions can be accomplished by different methods.

Essential Function Analysis

Determining the "essential functions" of the job is the responsibility of the employer. However, the EEOC encourages employers to solicit incumbent input during the development of job descriptions and other human resource and risk management documents. This information can then be used for a variety of purposes, such as hiring decisions, preplacement medical evaluations, accommodation options, and return-to-work determinations after on- or off-the-job injuries. The job analyst must be skilled at developing the essential function information from the review of documents, incumbent and supervisor interviews, onsite observations, and management review. However, job analysis references and "expert system" software have been developed to guide employers through this legal labyrinth.[17,22] In general, such an analysis should consider the following information when developing the essential functions of a job.

1. What is the overall purpose of the job? (e.g., custodian-to maintain a clean, sanitary and secure work environment)
2. For each of the worker actions:
   a. What action is being performed? (e.g., washes)
   b. To whom or what is the action directed? (e.g., windows, sinks, toilets, and floors)
   c. For what purpose is the action occurring? (e.g., to maintain a clean appearance and sanitary condition)
   d. What are the usual and customary methods used? (e.g., manual methods using bucket, wringer, detergents, mop, disinfectants, brushes, and squeegee)
   e. What is the performance standard for this action? (e.g., no missed areas and completed within specified time limits)

For more completeness and legal defensibility, it is helpful to consider areas such as the justification for calling a function essential versus marginal, and the physical/sensory/mental/environmental requirements and exposures of the job.

Job Analysis Tools and Equipment List

The tools used in most job analyses to document the physical demands of the job are not overly expensive, nor are they overly complex and technical. Knowing what to measure and how to measure it are skills. In some cases, it is better to call in an expert in a specific field than to "estimate" based on your limited working knowledge. The following list of tools can be used to complete most physical demands analyses, along with a brief description of what they are used to measure.

Recommended

1. A 35-mm camera, usually not an instant-type, and/or video camera in order to record and document critical information. Care should be taken not to distract workers with a flash and/or bright lights.
2. Tape measure to determine reach distances, heights, and widths, generally not exceeding 15 or 20 ft (Fig. 31-1).
3. Force gauge to measure weights as well as push/pull forces (Figs. 31-2 and 31-3).
4. Torque wrench to determine turning forces on rotating parts such as steering wheels, bolts, and screws (Fig. 31-4).
5. Pedometer to measure longer distances normally associated with pushing, walking, and carrying tasks.
6. Level used to measure angles and slopes particularly of walking surfaces and controls (e.g., ramps, steering wheels).
7. Goniometer to measure joint angles of workers and working angles of equipment.
8. Stopwatch to measure precise intervals of time for calculation of task duration and cycle frequency.
9. Event counter to count accurately the number of repetitions of a specific event or cycles within a specified period.

Optional

1. Heart-rate monitor, particularly useful for indirect measurement of endurance.
2. Thermometer to measure the temperature in usually hot or cold environments.

Special Equipment

1. Oxygen uptake measurement devices ($VO_{2\,max.}$) for use when endurance appears to be a critical issue.
2. Noise-measuring devices.
3. Air-quality–measuring devices.
4. Muscle-activity–measuring devices (electromyograph).

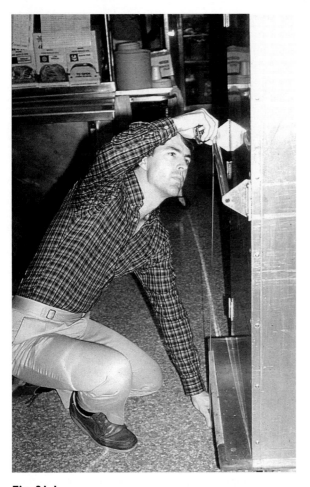

Fig. 31-1

Use of tape measure to determine height of handle on food delivery cart.

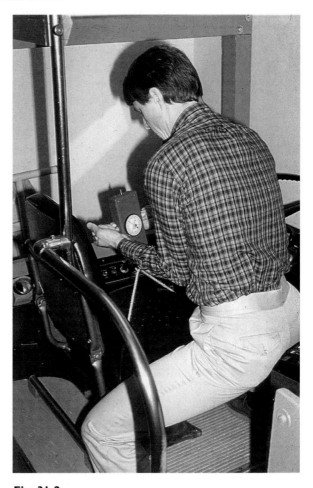

Fig. 31-2

Use of force gauge to determine lifting force necessary to adjust bus-driver seat manually.

Applications

Assuming a comprehensive job analysis has been obtained, how can it be used in the industrial environment to reduce worker injury/reinjury and to improve the rehabilitation process? The following list describes 15 ways that a job analysis can be used in the industrial environment. This should not be considered all-inclusive, because there are probably at least several others if the subtle uses of job analysis information are considered.

Preplacement Medical Standards

Job-related medical standards for preplacement enable a physician to compare a diagnosed medical condition to the job demands in an objective and systematic way. This is a nondiscriminating method of accurately placing individuals who may put themselves or others at imminent and substantial risk of injury without unduly discriminating against individuals with disabilities.

Physical Abilities Testing for Preplacement and Maintenance

Not all people can do all aspects of a specific job. The job analysis is used to identify the strength, endurance, range of motion, and other physical factors required by the job and to help identify tests that are appropriate for evaluating applicants for those positions. These tests can also be used to promote fitness of the incumbent population and as the basis for accommodation.

Safety Hazard Evaluations

This identifies the sources of the injuries that are the result of a worker/workplace mismatch. By doing a complete ergonomic evaluation of the worker(s) and

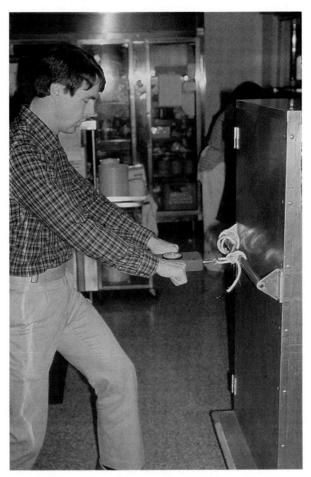

Fig. 31-3
Use of force gauge to determine push/pull force necessary to move loaded food delivery cart.

workplace, injury-producing mechanisms can be reduced or eliminated. These mechanisms can be caused either internally (person; e.g., posture, movement patterns, work techniques, and physical condition [strength, endurance, and range of motion]) or externally (workplace; e.g., environment, workstation design, work flow/processes, tool and equipment design, and psychologic stressors).

Injury Prevention Training Programs

Back schools and other training programs that are not job-specific have not been shown to be statistically effective. Only programs that integrate the job requirements into the training program show statistically significant results.

Workstation Design

Workstation designs and modifications require knowledge of the job as well as the worker group. This is particularly important when considering seated versus standing tasks and single-person versus multiple-user workstations such as computer workstations and manufacturing/assembly lines.

Tool Design

Many different kinds of tools, including manual material handling equipment, hand and power tools, and seating systems, are dependent on the task be-

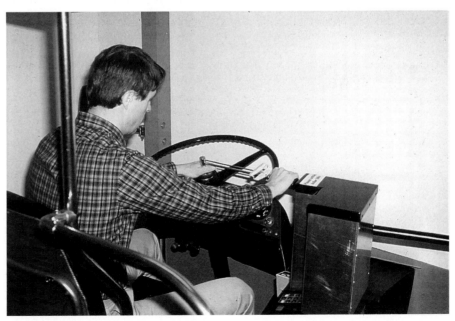

Fig. 31-4
Use of torque wrench to determine push/pull force necessary to turn manual steering bus.

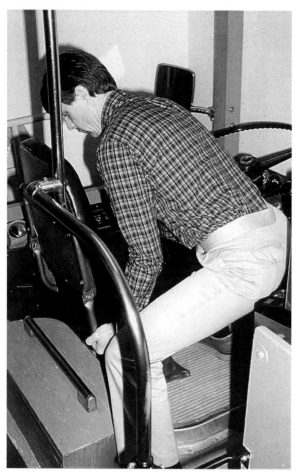

Fig. 31-5

Demonstration of body mechanics training for application to bus-seat adjustment task.

ing performed. Limited knowledge of the job often leads to poor decisions about design and/or selection of tools and equipment. For example, a chair may be perfectly suitable for computer work but not functional for desk work or laboratory microscope use. If a change in task frequency occurs, power equipment may be preferable to manual tools.

Work Procedures and Protocols

In some cases, decisions are made that increase short-term productivity but create a mismatch between the worker and the work tasks, resulting in a long-term inefficiency and/or injury. Examples include cardiovascular and muscular fatigue with increased repetitions of specific tasks such as lifting, positioning of parts or products, and static postures with computer use.

Reasonable Accommodation for the Disabled Individual

When dealing with the disabled individual, his/her physical capacity is often different from that of general population norms. Therefore, the essential parts of the job, as well as the specific mismatches between the job requirements and the abilities of the disabled individual (e.g., reaching distances, lifting capacity) need to be identified. Without this job knowledge, reasonable accommodation becomes difficult to implement effectively.

Basis for Physical Rehabilitation Programs

Job knowledge enables the treatment team to set specific goals and directions. This approach emphasizes function as the rehabilitation objective rather than just reduction of symptoms (Fig. 31-5).

Functional Capacity and Work Tolerance Testing Parameters

The job analysis is the base line for comparison when determining someone's ability to return to his/her usual and customary occupation, alternate duty, or modified position (Fig. 31-6).

Work-Hardening Program Guidelines

The job analysis sets the performance level that should be attained prior to returning an individual to his/her usual and customary occupation. This often occurs after more traditional physical rehabilitation programs are completed.

Qualified Injured-Worker Determinations

Accurate determination of a person's eligibility for vocational rehabilitation requires a comparison of job task demands to worker function. Without an accurate assessment of both components, the vocational rehabilitation system is too subjective and therefore very expensive and less effective than is otherwise possible.

Development of Work Samples at Vocational Evaluation Centers

Specific job knowledge is essential to the development of a test that accurately predicts successful job performance.

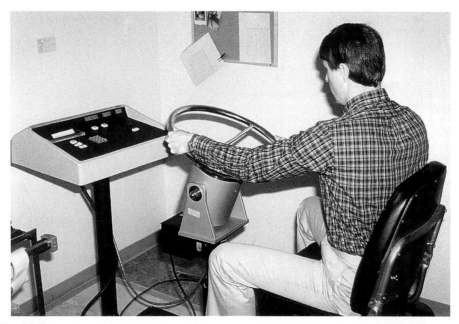

Fig. 31-6
Use of BTE to evaluate worker ability to performing manual steering of buses safely. Also useful in work-hardening program.

Job Modification for Return to Work or Reasonable Accommodation

Job modifications either reduce task demands or increase worker function. The job analysis identifies the specific part of the job that may exceed the individual's work capacity. This then allows for the task demand to be reduced or the worker's function to be increased through tool selection, workplace reorganization, selected assistive devices, training, job task rotation/elimination, or other job-modification strategies.

Evaluation and Selection of Appropriate Rehabilitation Plans

A preplacement job analysis helps to ensure a fit between the physical capacities of workers and new job task demands. Failure to analyze prospective jobs leads to higher failure rates, extended training programs, and higher costs.

Americans with Disabilities Act— Case Study

Physicians, chiropractors and other health care providers are often called on to assist employers with preplacement, fitness-for-duty, and return-to-work employment decisions. As a result, it can be argued that they are functioning as an agent of the employer. If so, then this decision may well be covered under the Americans with Disabilities Act. To avoid claims of discrimination and to assist with the safe employment of all individuals, disabled or not, medically related decisions should consider the "essential functions" of the job as well as the "usual and customary methods" of performance.

For example, the following communication was sent to the treating doctor in order to clarify his position related to a specific individual with a disability.*

*Client has a diagnosis of ankylosing spondylitis, an inflammation of the vertebrae resulting in a progressive stiffening of the spine and resulting in loss of movement and flexibility.

Re: Client
        Senior Building Inspector—Structural
        The Employer

Dear Dr. ,

I am writing to you at the request of The Employer. The Employer is attempting to determine what, if any, accommodations are needed or possible in order to return Client to his usual and customary occupation as a Senior Building Inspector. In order to accomplish this task, it is critical that we have very specific information related to his function ability to perform safely the essential functions of his job.

Your report of May 7, 1992, stated the following:
1. No repetitive bending
2. No repetitive twisting
3. No repetitive lifting
4. No heavy lifting

Your report also stated, "that he should no longer take part in his previous job description with duties of climbing ladders, crawling under houses and through small spaces." These medical restrictions indicate the function of on-site building inspection (Worker Action #3) is problematic in some cases. A summary is included for your review.

Once you have reviewed your records and this information, please complete the attached form, which asks for specific job-related abilities/limitations. If you need additional information prior to completing this form, please feel free to contact me directly.

Thank you for your prompt attention to this matter. Without your medical input, the process of accommodation cannot proceed appropriately.

Respectfully,

Chris C. Shulenberger, M.S. Engr.
Rehabilitation Engineer/Ergonomist
cc: Representative, The Employer
     Client's Attorney

WORKER ACTION SUMMARY #3

DESCRIPTION OF ESSENTIAL FUNCTION: Inspect commercial and residential facilities for the purpose of checking structural work in progress; reviewing compliance with work permits and plans; completing intermittent and final structural inspections.

PERFORMANCE STANDARD/S DESCRIPTION: Accurate, complete, and timely.

CURRENT OR CUSTOMARY METHOD OF PERFORMING FUNCTION: On-site visual inspection, visual review of plans, discussions with contractors, reference to code books as required, written documentation of activities. Requires walking over uneven and/or slippery surfaces, climbing ladders (6 to 25 ft), accessing flat and sloped roofs (generally not more than 10 in. rise:12 in. run). See physical demands/environmental conditions for more details.

THE MANNER IN WHICH THE JOB IS CURRENTLY PERFORMED
INVOLVES USING: (MTEWA [MACHINE/S, TOOL/S, EQUIPMENT, WORK AID/S]): ladders (supplied by contractor), work plans/permits (supplied by contractor), code books as required, and note-taking materials.*

*Photographs are usually sent to the doctor to show a series of typical tasks performed and situations encountered related to the essential function. This allows the doctor to visualize the actual work activity more clearly and accurately than possible by written and verbal description alone.

Physical Abilities Performance Sheet

Patient/Injured Worker: Client
Employer: The City

This form is designed for the treating doctor to indicate which job related task(s) the injured worker can perform safely. Space is available after each section for comments regarding the need for accommodations or other information related to the return-to-work process.

☑ Indicates the ability to perform the task safely.

Bending/Stooping and/or Crouching/Kneeling: The movements are required in order to perform on-site inspections (Essential Function #3) as shown in the photos. The frequency of these activities varies from intermittent throughout the day to highly repetitive and nearly continuous on a large commercial construction project.

- ☐ Foundation and/or pier work under houses.
- ☐ Passing through or leaning out from windows or other spaces to inspect a roof and/or shear walls.
- ☐ Working at/near ground level to measure joist and rebar spacing.

Comments:

Twisting: The body movement occurs intermittently throughout the day while performing the following tasks:

- ☐ Moving to/from ladder and roof.
- ☐ Looking out a window at a shear wall nailing pattern.
- ☐ Accessing confined spaces in and under construction.

Comments:

Climbing: A variety of different climbing situations occur on various building sites. These include but may not be limited to:

- ☐ Step ladders from 6 to 12 ft high.
- ☐ Vertical ladders, routinely up to 20 ft, inside or outside commercial buildings for roof access and on scaffolds.
- ☐ Sloped earth surfaces that may be muddy and have construction debris present.
- ☐ Over retaining walls and roof beams with 30–36 inch heights not unusual.
- ☐ Roofs with slopes of 7 to 10 in. (rise):12 in. (run) being common, with 17:12 occurring on rare occasions (footing boards used as shown in figures).

Comments:

Movement in Confined Spaces: These tasks can occur on any job, particularly residential remodeling. The duration of the task is variable but could well be 15 to 30 minutes when inspecting footings, foundation changes, or attic/roof changes.

☐ Working under homes in basements or crawl spaces.

☐ Working in attics or roof crawl spaces.

Comments:

Exposure to Slips/Trips/Falls: This exposure is nearly continuous on all job duties.

☐ Uneven surfaces.

☐ Construction debris.

☐ Walking across open floor joist and rebar patterns.

Comments:

Additional Comments:

Please return the completed form in the enclosed addressed envelope.

Thank you.

Completed by: The Doctor

Signature: Date Completed:

Problem Solving

With a better match between the worker and the workplace, we can affect many areas important to industry. For example:

1. Improve efficiency
   a. Reduce errors
   b. Improve productivity
2. Improve well-being
   a. Reduce discomfort
   b. Improve health
   c. Reduce occupational disability
3. Improve safety
   a. Reduce risk-taking behavior
   b. Reduce accidents
   c. Reduce workers' compensation injuries

4. Facilitate return to work
   a. Original job
   b. Restricted duty
   c. Modified job
   d. Alternate job
5. Improve job satisfaction
   a. Reduce absenteeism
   b. Reduce labor turnover rates
   c. Promote positive work attitudes
   d. Reduce personal complaints about the work environment
6. Improve cooperation with labor
   a. Reduce sabotage
   b. Decrease grievances
   c. Improve teamwork among workers and between workers and management.

In order to accomplish the goal of improved worker/workplace interface, an ergonomic problem-solving process needs to be used. This is not a difficult process, and follows a general problem-solving method. Many of the "failures" in industrial ergonomics result from skipping one or more of the essential steps.

1. Problem as stated or given. Each client will normally present a problem to the consultant. Some problem statements will be more fully developed and/or specific than others. It is important to recognize that the problem as it is initially stated may reflect only one aspect or impression of the entire problem.

2. Fact finding. Often there is a lot more to the problem than is originally presented by the employer or the worker(s). Several activities are often valuable when "getting to know the problem." These include, but may not be limited to, the review of OSHA and medical records, review of programs and practices, interviews with various levels of employees, on-site observations, and direct measurements that were previously discussed. It is the job analysis portion of the process that serves as the foundation for a more complete understanding of the real problem.

3. Problem as understood. Once you have a more complete understanding of the problem and what is needed, it is often valuable to restate the problem in a concise form. This allows the ergonomic consultant and the employer or client to reaffirm that both parties are focused on the same appropriate goal.

4. Ideation (Brainstorming). There are often many solutions to a problem. Therefore, it is helpful to generate a large number of possible solutions before deciding on the one(s) to be recommended or implemented. Evaluating ideas as you go often stifles the creative process. The brainstorming step allows the creative side to be active before the analytic side evaluates the possible solutions.

5. Solution evaluation and selection. Once several possible solutions are generated, one or more will be selected for implementation. The basis for selection varies from client to client. Several factors may come into play, depending on the nature of the problem. Some of these will include, but not necessarily be limited to, cost, feasibility, ease of implementation, impact on others (e.g., co-workers, unions, etc.) and safety.

6. Implementation. Once the overall approach is selected, a plan for implementation must be developed. This may involve the activities of people from one or more departments (e.g., Safety, Medical, Risk Management, Human Resources). Therefore, it is important to develop a plan of action for implementation, which may include, but not be limited to, budgeting, purchase versus internal fabrication of tools and equipment, installation and maintenance of equipment, evaluation criteria, and time lines.

7. Follow-up plan. Even the best solutions may have components that do not work out precisely. Therefore, there should be a follow-up plan to check on the results and to respond as appropriate. Therefore, your plan should consider the following questions: (a) How will I know if the changes are working? What are the criteria for success? (b) Whom should I contact and how often? (c) What else can I do to help ensure success? (d) What are my options if things are not going according to plan?

Case Study Results

In the case study previously presented, the accommodations were not overly complex. They included:

- Assignment to inspection of commercial versus residential buildings to reduce twisting, climbing and exposure to confined spaces and slips/trips/falls.
- Use of a mechanical lift normally available on commercial job sites to further reduce climbing.
- Use of a long-handled mirror to reduce bending/stooping/crouching/kneeling when inspecting rebar.
- Use of a lightweight, portable surface to eliminate walking over exposed areas (e.g., partial section of plastic carpet protector).

Summary

The process outlined above works. The more comfortable ergonomists become with problem-solving methodology, the more efficient and effective they become. By applying good problem-solving analysis and synthesis techniques to ergonomic problems, engineers, physicians, and therapists can all contribute significantly to the solutions. Decisionmakers within factories, office buildings, and corporate headquarters are beginning to look for help to trained ergonomists and health-care professionals with ergonomic experience.

Research currently being conducted in ergonomics around the country and the world serves as the basis for the evaluation of the data collected. However, good job analysis and problem solving are the primary cornerstones of ergonomics and are ones that require not only education but also experience in order to be most effective. In a field as complex and multidisciplinary as ergonomics, it is important to recognize the benefits of other disciplines. Problem-solving is often most effective when approached in a cooperative fashion. The industrial client and the field of ergonomics are often best served by a multidisciplinary team.

Additional Readings

1. Alexander D, Pulat BM: *Industrial ergonomics—a practitioner's guide*. Norcross, GA, 1985, Industrial Engineering and Management Press.
2. Chaffin D, Andersson G: *Occupational biomechanics*, New York, 1984, John Wiley & Sons.
3. Eastman Kodak: *Ergonomic design for people* at work, Belmont, CA, 1983 (vol 1), 1986 (vol 2), Lifetime Learning Publications.
4. Grandjean E: *Fitting the task to the man*, ed 4, New York, 1988, Taylor & Francis, Ltd.
5. Huchingson RD: *New horizons for human factors in design*, New York, 1981, McGraw-Hill Book Co.
6. Kantowitz BH, Sorkin RO: *Human factors*. New York, 1983, John Wiley & Sons.
7. Konz S: *Work design: industrial ergonomics*. Columbus, OH, 1983, Grid Publishing Co.
8. McCormick E, Sanders M: *Human factors in engineering and design*, ed 6, New York, 1989, McGraw-Hill Book Co.
9. National Institute for Occupational Safety and Health: *Work practices guide for manual lifting*, Washington, DC, 1981, Government Printing Office.
10. National Institute for Occupational Safety and Health Technical report: *Work practices guide for manual lifting*, Washington, DC, 1981, Government Printing Office, publ. no. 81-122.
11. National Safety Council: *Ergonomics guidebook*, Chicago, 1983, National Safety Council.
12. National Safety Council: *Making the job easier—an ergonomics idea book*, Chicago, 1988, National Safety Council.
13. Putz-Anderson V, editor: *Cumulative trauma disorders: a manual for musculoskeletal diseases of the upper limbs*, London, 1988, Taylor & Francis.
14. Rodgers SH: *Working with backache*, New York, 1985, Perinton Press.
15. Silverstein BA, Fine LJ: *Evaluation of upper extremity and low back cumulative trauma disorders: a screening manual*, Ann Arbor, MI, 1983, School of Public Health, Occupational Health Program.
16. Tichauer ER: *The biomechanical basis of ergonomics: anatomy applied to the design of work situations*, New York, 1978, John Wiley & Sons.
17. Thrush RA, *ADA essential function identification*, El Cajon, CA, 1993, Access Ability Press.
18. United Auto Workers International Union: *Strains and sprains*, Detroit, MI, 1986, United Auto Workers.
19. U.S. Department of Justice and Equal Employment Opportunity Commission: *Americans with Disabilities Act handbook*. Washington, DC, 1991, Government Printing Office, publ. no. EEC-BC-19.
20. U.S. Department of Labor, Bureau of Labor Statistics: *Recordkeeping guidelines for occupational injuries and illnesses*, Washington, DC, 1986 (and on), Government Printing Office, publ. no. OMB 1220-0029.
21. U.S. Department of Labor, Occupational Safety and Health Administration: *Ergonomics program management guidelines for meatpacking plants*, Washington, DC, 1990, Occupational Safety and Health Administration.
22. Watters GM: *TaskMaster expert system*, Pleasant Hill, CA, 1992, Occupational Management Systems.

Chapter 32
Work Simulation, Work Hardening, and Functional Restoration
Peter B. Polatin

While the probability for full recovery after a back injury is good, the longer an individual remains disabled, the poorer the prognosis becomes. From the onset of symptoms, 50% of patients recover within 2 weeks, 70% within 1 month, and 90% within 4 months.[2] However, of those patients still symptomatic at 4 months, most will go on to chronic, long-term disability, costing the majority of health expenditure for this category.[14,25] It is therefore in the interest of both good patient care and health-cost containment to provide timely conservative and rehabilitation care to prevent chronic low-back disability.

Tissue Healing

The duration of tissue healing after low back injury is somewhat variable,[1] but 2 to 4 months should be sufficient for even severe derangements to achieve primary healing.[18] However, facilitation of tissue healing by early motion and exercise has been noted for tendon, ligament, cartilage, and bone,[1] and argues strongly for early mobilization of the injured patient, as do studies noting the deleterious effects of prolonged bed rest on outcome.[6]

Complicating Factors with Chronicity

With persistence of low back pain (LBP), secondary behavioral and physical effects develop that contribute to prolonged disability and therapeutic failure. Patients become *pain avoidant* to even momentary pain exacerbations, with reactive fearfulness, hypervigilance, and avoidance of any physical activity that might precipitate pain.[27] The result is enforced restriction of activity and development within a relatively short time of the deconditioning syndrome,[17] characterized by joint stiffness, ligament elasticity, muscle atrophy, decreased cardiovascular endurance, and impaired neuromuscular coordination.[24,26] At the same time other psychosocial barriers may be developing, such as depression, substance abuse, and secondary gain issues,[3,13,28] which compound the original problem and make treatment more difficult.

Conservative Care: Primary, Secondary, and Tertiary

Since this progression of symptoms is so commonly observed, therapeutic efforts must incorporate an awareness of these complicating factors. The treatment of a recently injured patient is far less complex than the treatment of a patient with chronic LBP.

Primary care is delivered to acute cases of very limited severity, within the first 4 to 6 weeks after the onset of symptoms, when the primary goals of therapy are pain relief and mobilization. During this time passive modalities, that is, treatments done *to* a patient to palliate pain during a normal early healing period, are indicated. Such things as traction, heat, ice, manipulation, and medications to relieve pain and muscle spasm are included in this category. An acute McKenzie protocol to centralize radicular pain would also be appropriate. Since the majority of patients recover during the initial few weeks, expensive treatment protocols are rarely justified, but a timely return to even modified function, both at home and in the workplace, should be encouraged. To this purpose, "activation" of a symptomatic patient, that is, supervised stretching, aerobics, and even initial progressive resistance exercises, may begin almost immediately and even in conjunction with initial passive modalities.

Secondary care represents "reactivation," and is actually the initial phase of rehabilitation for individuals who have been unable to return to productivity through the normal healing process of the first few weeks. The focus here should be on facilitating the return to productivity before chronic disability supervenes. It is individualized, but limited in intensity and time, and is designed to prevent chronic disability, advanced deconditioning, and the development of psychologic barriers to work return. *Work hardening* and *work conditioning* approaches fall into this category, and are designed to be used near the end of a normal soft-tissue healing period.

Tertiary care is interdisciplinary, individualized, intensive treatment designed for patients demonstrating changes consistent with chronic disability (after 4 to 6 months of back pain and lack of productivity). As opposed to secondary care, which is therapist-driven, tertiary care is doctor-driven; incorporates psychologic and disability (or pain) management resources, in addition to the physical and occupational therapies comprising secondary care; and requires more specific physical and psychologic assessments. Additionally, in contrast to secondary care, tertiary care, which is "end of the line" conservative care, should lead to a therapeutic end point (maximum medical recovery or permanent and stationary) in every case. Function restoration and pain management are the available tertiary care resources for chronic LBP.

Functional Capacity and Physical Capacity: To Quantify or Not

The issue of quantification of functional or work capacity in the treatment of LBP is somewhat controversial. Some clinicians believe that since lifting in the workplace corresponds closely to psychophysical capacity,[22] real lifting tasks and actual material handling should be used for assessing ability to work.[15] Others have found isometric[5,7] and isokinetic[19] testing equipment important in assessing patients' functional capacity and rehabilitation progress.

This conflict may be at least partially resolved by clearly defining some terms. *Physical capacity* refers to assessment of specific aspects of the performance of a particular joint or region of the body. In the spine this would refer to range of motion or strength of trunk extensors and flexors. *Functional capacity,* on the other hand, focuses on whole-body tasks that incorporate the impaired region. In the lumbar spine this would include such things as lifting capacity, bending, reaching, twisting, pulling, and sitting tolerance.

Functional and work capacity tests may include a variety of different human performance measures, but the whole-body task performances will be most relevant to matching the patient to physical job requirements.

Measures of Work Capacity: To Determine Work Readiness

Essential to analyzing work capacity is an accurate job description. Also helpful is a work site evaluation. With the aid of this information, accurate testing of the patient may be accomplished without the use of isometric, isokinetic, or isodynamic equipment, to answer specific questions.[9]

1. Is the patient able to do this specific set of physical activities?
2. Are safety precautions necessary to prevent reinjury?
3. Do residual physical limitations prevent long-term job performance?

Such a series of tests, *specific to the demands of the job for which the patient is being tested,* assess the patient's general fitness, agility, strength, and ability to perform job-related tasks. Depending on the job, certain general measurements might be included such as cardiovascular fitness, grip strength, or psy-chophysical lifting ability.[10] Additional tests of job-specific capacity include such measurement devices as the Functional Measurement Laboratory[12]; the BTE (Baltimore Therapeutic Equipment, Inc., Baltimore, MD), which measures hand and arm strength in tool use; the Multiple Tasks Obstacle Course[11]; and the Employment and Rehabilitation Institute of California (ERIC) Work Tolerance Screening Battery.[16]

Measures of Work and Physical Capacities to Guide Rehabilitation: Different Uses in Secondary and Tertiary Care

In secondary care, work capacity measures to help to identify an end point to therapy and to document ongoing improvement. Physical capacity measures (i.e., range of motion and trunk extensor strength), while not useful for job matching, nevertheless offer additional feedback on the efficacy of the physical training. One assumption inherent in secondary care programs is that psychosocial barriers are not prominent and therefore a primarily physically focused program will be effective. Assessment of effort, while desirable, is not of paramount importance.

In functional restoration, a tertiary rehabilitation program, measures of functional and physical capacity must also be used to monitor compliance and effort throughout the rehabilitation program. Therefore both tester observation and intratest consistency are essential. Patients who verbalize full effort but clearly demonstrate less than this on testing must be confronted, and the data must be irrefutable to maximize success.

Measuring the Medical Measurement

To be meaningful, a measure of functional or physical capacity must fulfill certain criteria.[4] It must be relevant in that it validly measures what it claims to measure. For example, whole-body lifting tests do not measure trunk extensor or flexor strength. It must be accurate and reproducible, with good correlation of intertest and interrater reliability. The measurement system should not alter the function being tested, should be safe to use, and should be user friendly. The measurements should distinguish between normal and abnormal and therefore a normative data base is essential. Finally, an effort assessment is essential, so that test results may be clearly defined as representing true capacity.

Quantification of Physical Capacity

Range Of Motion Measures

A number of tests have been used to assess spinal mobility, including goniometric measures, fingertip to floor distance, the Schober technique, utilization of flexicurves, and roentgenographic assessment. The dual inclinometer technique, well described in the literature,[11] successfully discriminates between hip and lumbar intersegmental motion, fulfills validity criteria, and also assesses effort. Inclinometer measures are taken at T12-L1 (for gross motion) and over the sacrum (for hip motion). True lumbar motion may then be derived by subtracting hip from gross motion. Supine straight leg raise is also measured by inclinometer and should correlate within $10°$ to $15°$ with total hip mobility (flexion plus extension). If the most limited straight leg raise exceeds hip motion by $15°$, poor effort is suggested.

Trunk Strength Measures

Devices to measure accurately the strength of abdominal flexor and trunk extensor musculature require isolation of the lumbopelvic unit. Methods of measurement include (1) keeping distance and velocity at 0 while measuring the maximal force of the muscular contraction (isometric technology); (2) keeping velocity at a constant and restricting distance while measuring the torque (isokinetic technology); and (3) allowing acceleration and velocity to increase in proportion to the degree to which torque exceeds a preset minimum (isodynamic technology). A number of testing devices are available commercially that provide some of these capabilities. Cybex (Ronkonkoma, NY) offers two separate units—the TEF (trunk extension-flexion unit) and the TR (torso rotation unit)—that can measure isometrically and isokinetically, with well-established protocols, a large normative data base, and an objective measure of effort, by comparing computer generated curves for "average points variance." Lido Back System (Loredan; Davis, CA) also offers a device that measures both isometrically and isokinetically in the sagittal plane. Kin-Com (Chatteck Corp.; Chattanooga, TN) and Biodex (Biodex Inc.; Shirley, NY) offer a back-testing attachment to their extremity systems, also utilizing both isometric and isokinetic capability. Med-X

(Med-X; Ocala, FL) has an isometric lumbar extension testing device that also has a training capability. Isotechnologies B-200 (Isotechnologies; Hillsboro, NC) provides a unique isodynamic approach, with no isometric or isokinetic capability. It has been found to be a good training tool, but is probably not the best choice for testing.

Quantification of Functional Capacity

Lift Testing

Lifting is the most essential whole-body functional task to involve the lumbar spine, and may be assessed isometrically, isokinetically, and psychophysically. The Cybex Liftask (Cybex; Ronkonkoma, NY) and the Lido Lift (Loredan; Davis, CA) are two commercial devices that offer both isometric and isokinetic protocols, with the same advantages as previously described for trunk strength testing; that is, analysis of acceleration, torque, power, and effort.

Psychophysical testing of lifting capacity, while not providing the "high tech" capability to analyze isolated variables, nevertheless allows accurate quantification of whole-body lifting performance in a "real life" setting, without the need to purchase costly quantification testing devices. The Progressive Isoinertial Lifting Evaluation (PILE) is a simple protocol involving the repetitive lifting of weights in a plastic box, from floor to waist and waist to shoulder height. The two test distances are evaluated separately, with men beginning with a 10-lb load and women with a 5-lb load. Four lifting movements (two round trips) are carried out in a 20-second period, at which time additional weight equal to the initial load is added, up to an end point determined by either subject fatigue (psychophysical end point), aerobic goal of 85% of maximum heart rate (aerobic end point), or "safe limit" of approximately 50% of body weight (safety end point). Maximum weight lifted, work, and power consumption may be derived, with an effort assessment provided by test observation and comparison of the heart rate achieved to target heart rate.

The West 2 (Work Evaluation Systems Technology; Huntington Beach, CA) is a simple device to test lifting isoinertially. The subject raises and lowers a bar with weights by holding it along a frame with projecting bolts, through a preselected range. The test requires sufficient neuromuscular coordination to hook the bar repetitively up and down the frame.

Task Performance Testing

Other devices exist, with normative data bases, for the assessment of workplace tasks. The BTE (Baltimore Therapeutic Equipment, Inc.; Baltimore, MD) provides a computerized system to measure hand and arm strength in the use of different tools. The Functional Measurement Laboratory assesses with computer assistance a large number of musculoskeletal and neurologic parameters, including balance, postural stability, reaction time, and coordination.[12] The Multiple Task Obstacle Course assesses the subject's ability to perform a number of work tasks, including pushing, pulling, twisting, crawling, and climbing.[11]

Aerobic Capacity Testing

Cardiovascular endurance is relevant to any repetitive task performance and therefore should be measured in any physical capacity assessment battery. A submaximal protocol using bicycle ergometry has been found to be useful. Standardized nomograms based on work rate and heart rate allow conversion of predicted oxygen consumption to a Vo_2 max and fitness level. An upper-body ergometer is useful for determining endurance of the upper extremities, utilizing increasing work rate at regular intervals to a fatigue or aerobic end point.

"Bare Bones" Quantification

To perform secondary or tertiary spinal rehabilitation, the clinician benefits by using *some* quantification measures. While the isokinetic, isometric, and isodynamic devices are useful, they are not essential except in treating the most refractory chronic patients with several barriers to recovery. A "low-tech" battery might consist of (1) dual inclinometer ROM assessment; (2) the one-repetition maximal back extension and abdominal flexion capacity on a progressive resistance exercise device; (3) bicycle ergometry assessment; and (4) a psychophysical lifting protocol.

Work Hardening

Work hardening is defined by the American Occupational Therapy Association (AOTA) as a "structured, productivity oriented program using real or simulated activities as its principle means of treatment," with the goal of returning an injured patient to the workplace. Therapy occurs in a setting similar to a workplace milieu and focuses on improving an individual's work tolerance, work rate, and basic workplace behaviors, including punctuality, attendance, and hygiene. Work hardening attempts to replicate the workplace. While it may begin as a 2-hours-a-day program, in its full form it should progress to 6 to 8 hours a day, 5 days a week, and usually lasts from 4 to 6 weeks, as defined by the Commission on Accreditation of Rehabilitation Facilities (C.A.R.F.). While work hardening may integrate a number of disciplines, there is a certain range of variability in different programs.[10] *Physical therapy* in work hardening addresses the physical deconditioning through a structured program of mobilization and progressive resistance exercises. For the motivated, uncomplicated patient, this may be all that is required to facilitate a return to work. *Occupationally therapy*–driven programs are more activity oriented, focusing on work simulation and behavioral skills, and more closely monitored job performance. These two disciplines may be integrated into a work-hardening program that provides both reconditioning and work performance refinement. *Vocational rehabilitation* focuses on work adjustment and the acquisition of alternative job skills or the provision of an altered work environment for an individual previously handicapped by disease or injury. This usually requires some period of assessment independent of physical activities and includes counseling the patient on job-seeking skills, exploration of job options, and possibly actual job placement. These services may be provided on an independent, consultative basis, or may be integrated into a more interdisciplinary program of work hardening.

There are, therefore, a number of different interlocking components of work hardening after initial evaluation has taken place. The patient enters the therapeutic milieu having had a work-capacity evaluation that has defined his or her physical capabilities as currently inadequate for the workplace. *Reconditioning* prepares the body to do work activities by correcting loss of muscle strength and endurance, decreased aerobic capacity, stiffness, and coordination dysfunction. If, for example, trunk extensor weakness exists such that a patient must use substitution patterns or poor body mechanics to perform a task, work simulation will be premature. Initially, the patient requires exercises to improve the strength and endurance of weak muscles, after which further work-specific activity may proceed safely. *Aerobic conditioning* is essential for the deconditioned patient, who may be able to perform brief tasks, but does not have the stamina to perform repetitive tasks over an 8-hour day. Therefore, aerobic training is an essential component of the reconditioning process.

Work Simulation

Work simulation consists of job-specific activities developed for an individual patient from a job description, to restore lost work ability. The focus is on improving body mechanics and progression of physical activities with improved tolerance until the full range of the actual job activities is being replicated in the milieu. This requires innovation and flexibility, as well as a large work space so that individual pieces of equipment used on a particular job may be incorporated into the individual's therapeutic activities.

Patient education should address such essential work-related topics as safe body mechanics, vocational skills (interviewing, communication, goal setting, attendance, hygiene), stress reduction, and disability issues where applicable.

Integrated work hardening, as defined by Matheson,[16] represents an extended, interdisciplinary approach, in which the patient initially goes through a detailed evaluation phase of "work tolerance screening" and "specific vocational exploration." This information is then integrated into a second phase of career development, during which the patient is encouraged to pick a vocational goal. A third phase consists of reconditioning and work simulation tasks to get the patient to the desired vocational level. The "core team" consists of a physical therapist, occupational therapist, psychologist, and vocational specialist, as well as technicians, who work in a coordinated fashion, with regular staff meetings, to facilitate progress in the work-hardening program.

Functional Restoration

As opposed to work hardening, functional restoration is applicable to the chronically disabled patient with LBP who has multiple barriers to recovery, including deconditioning, lack of motivation, psychologic dysfunction, and secondary gain issues.[23] Inherent in this treatment approach are the assumptions that the patient may not participate willingly in therapy and that symptom magnification and therefore invalid self reporting may be present. An interdisciplinary approach is essential, integrating physical therapy, occupational therapy, vocational therapy, psychology, nursing, and the physician. Functional and physical capacity testing are used not only to initially define pretreatment deconditioning and dysfunction, but also to drive the treatment program. The interdisciplinary team must be completely comfortable with the objective meaning of the functional capacity measures, which will be utilized to confront patients who fail to progress or are otherwise noncompliant. Pain is acknowledged and treated sympathetically, but function drives the program and sets the therapeutic goals.

As opposed to work hardening, to which patients may be referred by their physicians, functional restoration is a physician-driven program. The medical director is the first team member to see the patient. At the initial medical evaluation a detailed history and physical examination takes place, as well as screening for symptoms of psychologic distress. A deconditioning syndrome is defined for the patient and the rationale for functional restoration is explained. The patient then undergoes a full functional capacity evaluation, including a psychologic interview and vocational counseling intake. All members of the interdisciplinary team are involved with the patient from the very beginning of therapy. Once the entire initial evaluation has been completed, the patient then returns to the medical director who reviews with him or her the results of the functional capacity testing and psychologic interview and initiates the functional restoration treatment program. When applicable, psychotropic medication may be started at this time.

The patient has regular appointments with the medical director throughout rehabilitation, during which progress is reviewed, medications adjusted, and compliance issues addressed. After the second appointment with the physician, the patient begins the initial phase of rehabilitation, which consists of supervised stretching, aerobics, and light work-simulation exercises for 2 hours twice a week. Initial focus is on improving mobility, overcoming neuromuscular inhibition and pain sensitivity, and increasing cardiovascular endurance. After a maximum of 12 appointments, over a 4- to 6-week period, rehabilitation is intensified to the "comprehensive phase," during which the patient is present at the rehabilitation facility for 10 hours a day, 5 days a week, for a total of 3 weeks. There the patient in engages vigorous stretching and aerobics classes, and performs progressive resistance exercises twice a day under the supervision of a physical therapist. In the occupational therapy component, the patient undergoes daily work-simulation tasks, lifting drills, and position tolerance training exercises similar to work hardening. Several times a week he or she is trained on testing equipment, and at the end of each week undergoes a functional capacity evaluation by which progress is assessed. In both exercise and work simulation, the physical demand on the patient is increased regularly and aggressively, and is monitored carefully by serial quantifications.

Concurrently, the patient also participates in classes on goal setting, work issues, stress management, and interpersonal skills development, under the supervision of the psychologist. Active planning for return to work is initiated and monitored by the vocational therapist. The patient will not be permitted to complete this phase of functional restoration without a work plan, and will be terminated if he or she refuses to make such a plan.

At the completion of the comprehensive phase, the patient enters a less intensive follow-up phase, during which reconditioning and work hardening continue and the vocational therapist is particularly active in assisting the patient to finalize return-to-work plans. At the end of follow-up, the patient receives a work release from the medical director, with functional limitations as indicated, and the, it is hoped, returns to work. The patient continues to be seen at less frequent intervals, for periodic functional capacity reevaluations and assessments by the physician and interdisciplinary team to ensure good progress in the workplace and maintenance of adequate conditioning in a prescribed home program. One- and two-year outcome studies have delineated an 80% to 85% success rate, as defined by return to work, with this approach.[8,20]

Clinical Dilemmas in Delivering Secondary and Tertiary Care to Patients with Spinal Pain

Quantification In Secondary And Tertiary Care

Not all patients with spinal pain will require physical or functional quantification or rehabilitation. Most will recover within the first few weeks, with minimal periods of disability and a rapid progression to full duty. However, when a patient fails to progress to full work capacity within 6 weeks in spite of appropriate early activation (mobilization, progressive resistance exercise, aerobic training), secondary care should be considered. At this time some initial quantification to identify insufficient work capacity is helpful. Periodic work capacity assessments thereafter will identify readiness for work. Assuming good effort and motivation and the absence of psychosocial barriers, testing with built-in effort assessments

and normative data bases are less essential, since the critical issue is matching the work capacity with a particular job's demands.

In a patient who has failed to recover at 4 months in spite of good secondary care, with emerging psychosocial barriers evident, quantification becomes more essential to driving the tertiary rehabilitation, and documentation of effort becomes critical. It is at this juncture that a more complete battery of physical and functional capacity tests is important.

When Is A Patient At Maximum Medical Improvement?

Maximal medical improvement (MMI) refers to the point at which a patient is "as good as he is going to get," and is therefore at the end point for further medical treatment. This does not necessarily mean that the patient is "cured" and symptom-free, nor that further improvement may not occur over time. A patient who has progressed through secondary or tertiary care such that he or she is able to return to full duty may be at maximum medical improvement, even though some symptoms are still present. Conversely, a patient who has failed to progress to full duty release, but has nevertheless received full and optimal medical and surgical treatment, may be at MMI, even with residual disability. Therefore, the major determining issues are (1) functional recovery or (2) complete medical/surgical care beyond which nothing further can be accomplished.

Functional Capacity Versus Workplace Demands

The therapeutic goal in treating patients with spinal pain is to get them back to work, preferably at the level of previous job demands. However, if a patient reaches MMI but is not at full job capacity, the options become (1) vocational placement with or without retraining or (2) permanent disability. Hopefully, with the impact of the Americans with Disabilities Act (ADA) on society, fewer sufferers of spinal pain will have to take the choice of disability.

Are Patients Receiving Workers' Compensation Different Than Unsubsidized Injured Workers?

Patients who injure their backs and are then disabled from work face the same issues for recovery. It is a common clinical assumption that patients receiving disability payments may be less motivated to progress in therapy and return to work than those patients not receiving such payments. However, regardless of the context of the injury, with increasing chronicity, pain avoidance, deconditioning, and psychosocial barriers become more prominent, requiring a progression from secondary to tertiary care.

Summary

The nonsurgical treatment of LBP becomes progressively more complicated and intensive with increasing chronicity. Very little is required in the first few weeks after injury, when most patients recover. With time, however, more and more of an interdisciplinary approach is required. Work hardening incorporates not only progressive work simulation activities, but also reconditioning and vocational counseling, depending on the individual patient's needs. Functional restoration integrates elements of work hardening, but is always an interdisciplinary, medically driven rehabilitation approach encompassing physical, occupational, and vocational therapies, as well as psychologic management for the more complicated chronically disabled patient with LBP. While work hardening may use some quantification to define the beginning and end points of therapy, functional restoration depends on quantification to drive therapy, giving the treatment team and the patient feedback of ongoing progress or lack thereof.

It is essential that medical practitioners involved in the assessment and treatment of LBP be aware of the continuum of care available for the prevention of longstanding disability in this group of patients. Work hardening and functional restoration are two important interdisciplinary treatment techniques in this armamentarium.

References

1. Akeson W and others: *Concepts of soft tissue hemostasis and healing.* In Mayer T, Mooney V, Gatchel R, editors: *Contemporary conservative care for painful spinal disorders,* Lea & Febiger, Philadelphia, 1991, p 84.
2. Andersson G: Epidemiological aspects of low back pain in industry, *Spine* 6:53, 1981.
3. Capra P, Mayer T, Gatchel R: Adding psychological scales to your back pain assessment, *J Musculoskel Med* 2(7):41, 1985.
4. Chaffin D, Andersson G: *Occupational biomechanics,* 1984, John Wiley.
5. Chaffin D, Herrin G, Keyserling W: Pre-employment strength testing: an updated position, *J Occup Med* 20:403, 1978.
6. Deyo R, Diehl A, Rosenthal M: How many days of bed rest for acute low back pain?: a randomized clinical trial, *N Engl J Med* 315:1067, 1986.
7. Harber P, Soohoo K: Static ergonomic strength testing in evaluating occupational back pain, *J Occup Med* 26:77, 1984.
8. Hazard R and others: Functional restoration with behavioral support: a one year prospective study of patients with chronic low back pain, *Spine* 14(2):157, 1989.
9. Isernhagen S: *Functional capacity evaluation and work hardening perspectives.* In Mayer T, Mooney V, Gatchel R, editors: *Contemporary conservative care for painful spinal disorders,* Philadelphia, 1991, Lea & Febiger, p 328.
10. Isernhagen S: *Work injury management and prevention,* 1988, Aspen Publication.
11. Keeley J: *Quantification of function.* In Mayer T, Mooney V, Gatchel R, editors: *Contemporary conservative care for spinal disorders,* Philadelphia, 1991, Lea & Febiger, p 290.
12. Kondraske G and others: A computer based system for automated quantification of neurological function, *IEEE Trans Biomed Eng* 31:401, 1984.
13. Leavitt F and others: Organic status, psychological disturbance, and pain report characteristics in low back pain patients on compensation, *Spine* 7(4):398, 1982.
14. Leavitt S, Johnson T, Byers R: The process of recovery: patterns in industrial back injur, *In Med Surg* 40:7, 1971.
15. Lichter R: *"Work hardening"—using work for rehabilitation.* In White A, Anderson R, editors: *Conservative care of low back pain,* Baltimore, 1991, Williams & Wilkins, p 371.
16. Matheson L: *Integrated work hardening.* In Mayer T, Mooney V, Gatchel R, editors: *contemporary conservative care for painful spinal disorders,* Philadelphia, 1991, Lea & Febiger, p 346.
17. Mayer T: Rehabilitation of the patient with spinal pain, *Ortho Clin North Am,* 3(14):623, 1983.
18. Mayer t: *The shift from passive modalities to reactivation.* In Mayer T, Mooney V, Gatchel R, editors: *Contemporary conservative care for painful spinal disorders,* Philadelphia, 1991, Lea & Febiger, p 270.
19. Mayer T, Gatchel R: *Functional restoration for spinal disorders: the sports medicine approach,* Philadelphia, 1988, Lea & Febiger.
20. Mayer T and others: A prospective two year study of functional restoration in industrial low back injury: an objective assessment procedure, *JAMA* 258(13):1763, 1987.
21. Mayer T and others: Use of noninvasive techniques for quantification of spinal range of motion in normal subjects and chronic low back dysfunction patients, *Spine* 9(6):588, 1984.
22. Nordin M, Ortengren R, Andersson G: Measurements of trunk movements during work, *Spine* 9:465, 1984.
23. Polatin P: The functional restoration approach to chronic low back pain, *J Musculoskel Med* 7(1):17, 1990.

24. Smidt G and others: Assessment of Abdominal and back extensor function: a quantitative approach and results for chronic low back pain patients, *Spine* 8:211, 1983.

25. Spengler D and others: Back injuries in industry: a retrospective study. I. Overview and cost analysis, *Spine* 11:241, 1986.

26. Tipton C, Vailas A, Matthas F: Experimental studies on the influences of physical activity on ligaments, tendons, and joints: a brief review, *Acta Med Scand Suppl* 711:157, 1985.

27. Troup J, Slade P: Fear avoidance and chronic muscular skeletal pain, *Stress Med* 1:217, 1985.

28. Waddell G and others: Chronic low back pain, psychological distress and illness behavior, *Spine* 9(2):209, 1984.

Section 3

The Chronic Pain Patient within the Psychologic Cascade

Chapter 33
Pain and Its Meaning:
A Biocultural Model
David B. Morris

> *"Nature has placed mankind under the governance of two sovereign masters, pain and pleasure. It is for them alone to point out what we ought to do, as well as to determine what we shall do."*
>
> Jeremy Bentham, *Principles of Morals and Legislation* (1789)

Pain is such a familiar event within medicine—the most common symptom bringing doctor and patient together—that (paradoxically) it often tends to go unnoticed, like the air we breathe. Its role in diagnosis is frequently crucial, but once pain has served as a diagnostic aid, doctors often find it of little importance. Even 20 years after the appearance of a ground-breaking study indicating widespread medical undertreatment for pain, a 1993 survey in *The American Journal of Public Health* reports that 8 of 10 health-care professionals believe that undertreatment is a serious problem in their facilities.[1] Fears that patients might become addicted to opiates and opioid narcotics are simply unfounded. A well-known report shows that the rate of addiction among a hospital population is far less than 1%.[2] The undertreatment of pain in medical settings must have sources that run far deeper than statistics.

Our culture, as expressed in the assumptions we take to be common sense, helps to explain much about the dismissive attitudes that most people—not just health-care professionals—hold toward pain. We learn very quickly that time and drugs will usually bring relief. Life in modern Western industrial societies teaches almost everyone that drugstores contain a pharmacopoeia of well-advertised medications that effectively, if temporarily, cancel pain. When pain plays by the ordinary rules, then, when it disappears after a reasonable time and proves responsive to various drugs, it doesn't merit a second thought, and we seem entirely justified (if not entirely accurate) in describing it as merely transient and meaningless. But the same terms might be used to describe dynamite.

There is good reason for questioning the dismissive attitude we have learned to adopt toward pain and for seeking to recover the perspective common

to eras before the invention of aspirin and modern anesthetics. The metaphors that utilitarian philosopher Jeremy Bentham employed in the opening sentence of his *Principles of Morals and Legislation* (1789)—quoted in the epigraph—suggest that pain holds the same role in the life of an individual as the king or sovereign power holds in the state. Its normal function is to provide an ultimate underlying stability. When something goes seriously wrong in our normal relation to pain, the change can prove as threatening and incomprehensible as if terrorists blew up the White House or fire-bombed Buckingham Palace.

Two Pictures of Pain

The future may look a little clearer if we contrast two very different but representative pictures of pain.[3] The first is the well-known kneeling figure that Descartes in the seventeenth century included as an illustration in his *Treatise of Man* (Fig. 33-1). Cartesian physiology still used the old idea that the body moves with the assistance of small organisms called "animal spirits" produced and stored in the brain. These minute rarefied particles travel through nerves supposed to resemble hollow tubes containing tiny filaments that terminate in the brain.[4] The bodily response to pain, as Descartes described it, works like a simple mechanism. The fast-moving particles of fire disturb the filaments in the nerve. The disturbance passes along the length of the nerve until it reaches the brain, where it activates the animal spirits, which in turn travel down through the nerves to the muscles, producing the movement that removes, say, foot from flame. The nerve impulse traveling from the site of injury to the brain, Descartes explains, produces pain "just as, pulling on one end

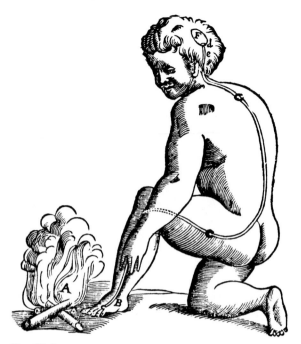

Fig. 33-1
Kneeling Figure: From Descartes: De l'homme (1664).

of a cord, one simultaneously rings a bell which hangs at the opposite end."[5]

Descartes's mechanistic, rope-pull model of pain is a direct precursor of the standard medical model developed (from Cartesian principles) in the mid-nineteenth century and still going strong. Doctors and researchers adhering to the medical model now talk about nociceptive impulses and endorphins rather than about filaments and animal spirits, but the basic idea is the same. They view pain as the result of an internal mechanism sending a signal from the site of tissue damage to the brain.

Some implications of this mechanistic view will be evident if we consider what is absent from the Cartesian picture. Notice how Descartes suspends his human figure in a limbo outside of time or space. There is literally almost no ground to stand on. The diagram cannot tell us whether the kneeling figure is male or female, aristocrat or commoner, French or English, Christian or Jew. The blankness of the diagram probably reflects a desire to situate scientific truth in an abstract or universal realm beyond the irrelevant historical accidents of a specific time and place. But the emptiness of the drawing is exactly the point. Descartes, in this early version of the medical model, gives us what amounts to a picture of pain in a vacuum.

The model of pain depicted by Descartes is not just a quaint, antiquarian diagram but reflects a de-

liberate assault on earlier ways of understanding pain that Cartesian science judged wholly inadequate. The extensive discourses on pain in theology, literature, philosophy, art, and folklore, for example, are implicitly commanded to fall silent. As a way of imagining what has been lost in the shift to a Cartesian view of pain, consider a second illustration that suggests how far Descartes and his successors have succeeded in stripping away the complex fabric of personal and cultural experience that once enfolded pain.

The enigmatic painting "The Flagellation" by Piero della Francesca, created some 200 years before Descartes—about 1450—ranks among the most famous artifacts of the early Renaissance (Fig. 33-2) and depicts a somewhat confusing drama played out in historical space and time. In fact, the painting depicts two specific and vastly different spaces and times. The trio of figures standing to the right clearly inhabits the contemporary world of quattrocento Italy. Within the interior, however, we see another trio who lived some 1400 years earlier: the two torturers who stand on either side of Jesus with their whips upraised, as Pontius Pilate and a mysterious turbaned figure look on.

The painting, like pain itself, is full of questions. Who are the three well-dressed contemporary figures? What are they doing at this biblical scene of flagellation? Why does the flagellation (whose theologic importance is paramount) proceed in the background? Such questions have sparked a variety of ingenious and often conflicting explanations, but none of the commentators directly addresses the question we need to ask here. How does the painting invite us to think about pain? The answer turns out to be closely entwined with an account of Piero's strange mixture of disparate historical places and times.

The best explanation of the painting has been proposed by Marilyn Aronberg Lavin.[6] She identifies the contemporary group on the right as portraying two powerful Renaissance figures: Ludovico Gonzaga, a nobleman, and Ottaviana Ubaldini della Carda, a famous astrologer. (As befits his occult profession, Ottaviana wears an exotic, eastern-style hat.) Both men, she shows, had each recently lost a son, one to death, the other to crippling disease. The barefoot youth standing between the two bereaved fathers thus represents an idealized, angelic "son" figure—whose loss brings them together. Their loss, meanwhile, is also what helps explain why Piero should represent them as if standing alongside the biblical scene of flagellation. The subject of the painting, we might say, is pain ancient and modern, visible and invisible. It is pain that draws the two disparate historical scenes into a single field of thought. Jesus in effect

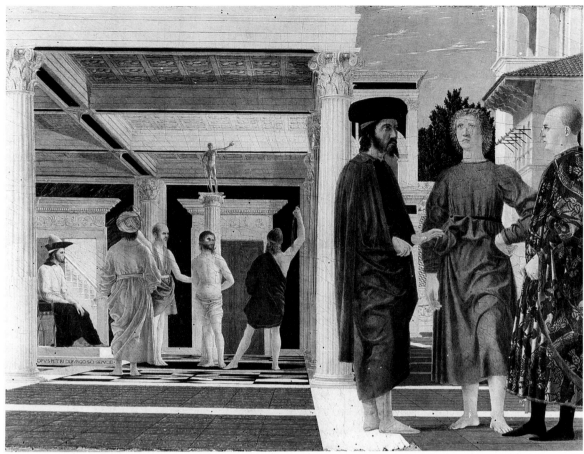

Fig. 33-2

Piero della Francesca (c. 1420–1492). *The Flagellation* (c. 1450). Galleria Nazionale delle Marche, Plazzo Ducale, Urbino, Italy. Courtesy Alinari/Art Resource, N.Y.

accepts the blows of the two torturers with a calm that offers guidance for the bereaved fathers. The painting may have served both as a memorial and as a meditative consolation. Lavin shows that its dimensions exactly fit a space in front of the altar in Ludovico's private chapel.

Piero and Descartes, then, offer very different perspectives on pain. Piero seeks to make pain comprehensible by placing it within a complexly layered historical world of religious meaning, social values, and personal loss. Equally important, he assumes that the pain of emotional loss finds a precise parallel in the pain of flagellation: there is no break between (what the legacy of Cartesian dualism has mistaught us to call) physical pain and mental pain. Descartes, two centuries later, not only divides mind from body but also strips away the social, theologic, and psychologic meanings of pain to expose almost an x-ray picture of a universal human nervous system. Pain is now everywhere and completely equivalent to tissue damage.

It is probably high time that the automatic flagellation of Descartes should stop, because he distinguishes himself from his later mechanistic followers by insisting that we do not feel pain until the physical motion of the nerve fibers and animal spirits is perceived by the mind or soul. (This insistence explains his otherwise bizarre claim that animals do not feel pain; animals, he believed, do not possess minds or souls.) Whatever his ultimate responsibility for developing the medical model of pain, however, the modern world has very successfully outdescarted Descartes. In rejecting the earlier view represented by Piero, it has perfected a picture of pain so stripped down that it contains almost no meaning and no social value at all. The problem is not only that this Cartesian picture is so bleak that it may help to explain the despair felt by many patients with pain whom medicine cannot as yet relieve. The medical model of pain, I want to argue, the model built on Cartesian principles during the nineteenth century, is fundamentally incorrect.

The Dimensions of Crisis

We need to respect the destructive, panic-inducing power of pain because many patients today find themselves in a situation in which time and drugs fail to bring relief. Such pain, even while doctors and patients alike continue to regard it as transient and meaningless, may expand to fill the patient's entire world and to create permanent disability.[7] A life filled with intractable pain is not just arduous and fundamentally disordered. Pain in laboratory animals has been shown to depress the immune system and to destroy cancer-fighting cells.[8] It can certainly lead to suicide. Moreover, the social costs are immense. Pain in the United States alone results, each year, in more than 900 million lost workdays at a total cost to the GNP of $120 billion.[9] Patrick Wall—coauthor with Ronald Melzack of the well-known "gate-control" theory—calls pain "the greatest health problem of our age."[10] Something, clearly, is amiss.

The dimensions of the problem have begun to approach crisis. Some 20 million Americans suffer from arthritis and another 7 million from low-back pain. Three percent of the population experiences daily headaches, and ten percent suffers weekly headaches. A trio of representative modern illnesses—AIDS, cancer, and depression—add an immeasurable weight of pain and misery. Meanwhile, in 1989 Americans spent $1 billion for prescription analgesics, another $2.2 billion for over-the-counter painkillers, while the annual world output of aspirin rose to 30,000 tons. As the grim statistics mount, there seems good reason to ponder Norman Cousins's claim that no form of illiteracy in the United States is more widespread or costly as ignorance about pain: "what it is, what causes it, how to deal with it without panic."[11]

If the public is ignorant about pain, the medical profession has certainly not provided a sound alternative education. A 1988 study of 28 British medical schools revealed that four had no teaching about intractable pain and that the others averaged just over 3 hours in 5 years.[12] In a 1992 survey, the distinguished anesthesiologist and pain-specialist John J. Bonica reviewed 17 top textbooks in medicine, surgery, and oncology, finding just 1/2 of one percent of the space devoted to "a detailed description of the symptomatic treatment of acute postoperative, post-traumatic, visceral and cancer pain."[13] In a 1989 interview Bonica described the general situation bluntly: "No medical school has a pain curriculum."[14]

We are left, then, with a large-scale crisis of pain that our systems of public and professional education are so far unable to address effectively. They are ineffective, I believe, largely because, whether through silence or misinformation, they simply perpetuate the errors of the standard medical model, which has of course been absorbed into our general cultural thinking about pain over the past 150 years. A model that defines pain as solely a matter of nerves and neurotransmitters, while it incorporates important scientific discoveries, falls far short of providing a full understanding. Its shortcomings merely reinforce current myths and errors, including the error of medical undertreatment. The result is widespread suffering and a health-care system nearly overwhelmed by an epidemic of chronic pain.

A Conflict of Models

My proposal is that the best features of the medical model of pain be absorbed into a more comprehensive model that I would call biocultural. The supporting argument that I developed at length in *The Culture of Pain* (1991) can be summarized in four main points:

1. Pain is more than a medical issue and more than a matter of nerves and neurotransmitters.

2. Pain is historical, psychologic, and cultural.

3. Meaning is fundamental to the experience of pain.

4. Minds and cultures (as makers of meaning) have a powerful influence on pain, for better or worse.

Unfortunately, this approach, given the strength of current social and medical assumptions based on the medical model, seems instantly counterintuitive. British gerontologist Ray Tallis articulates what I take to be the prevailing opinion when he asserts: "I have a prejudice against pain, believing that, once it has done its job of warning us of danger, it is meaningless. . . ."[15]

The meaninglessness of pain seems evident if we consider pain to be merely an electrochemical signal transmitted over nerve pathways from the site of tissue damage to the brain. Pain, on this standard view, is chiefly a problem in biochemistry, a problem that medicine understands reasonably well, allowing for a few unlucky gaps in our knowledge of pain mechanisms. Doctors committed to the medical model thus have no need to consider meanings because the medical model assumes from the start that meaning is irrelevant. Pain from this point of view has no more meaning than an alarm bell or a neurotransmitter.

The alternative, biocultural model of pain that I propose, while it greatly values medical knowledge about nociception, holds that the problem of pain is far from solved and that pain is never entirely a matter of nerves and neurotransmitters. Pain, according to a biocultural model, taps into our emotional, psychologic, and cultural experience in ways so entangled with the meanings we make that pills and surgery often not only fail to bring relief but sometimes constitute a serious component of the problem. As the biocultural model recognizes, pain serves as far more than a warning of danger, a service that in any case it performs quite inconsistently. "The truth is," writes Patrick Wall, "that pain is a very poor reporting system."[16]

A biocultural model, among its other advantages, corrects the error of the medical model in treating all pain as if it were acute pain. The crucial distinction between acute pain and chronic pain is one of the chief facts that Descartes's illustration and the medical model ignore. Indeed, the medical model breaks down notoriously when confronted with the ambiguities of chronic pain. Rajan Roy, in *The Social Context of the Chronic Pain Sufferer* (1992), offers a scrupulous review of current research indicating how chronic pain eludes the clinician who seeks to understand it through tissue damage alone.[17] Chronic pain, moreover, is not an anomaly or marginal case. It is so widespread and so resistant to traditional treatment as to highlight the need for a better, more inclusive model of pain that I am calling biocultural.

A new model of pain, whatever it comes to be called, seems an inevitable result of the new knowledge we are receiving almost daily. Small wonder that a model built in the nineteenth century has trouble accommodating recent research. Pain-specialist Tony Yaksh, quoted in a 1992 *JAMA* article, helpfully articulates both the extent of recent changes and the still-unfinished state of current understanding:

> At this moment, we're becoming just barely sufficiently sophisticated to say that all pain is not the same, and therefore to know why some analgesics may be very effective in some pain states and less effective in others. We need to learn the precise nature and mechanism of all the pain producers.[18]

In fact, the medical literature on conditions from arthritis and diabetes to irritable bowel syndrome and panic disorder suggests that there are almost as many varieties of pain as of roses. We may assume, I trust, that pain is always accompanied by (measurable) biochemical changes and physiologic processes. Anyone concerned with "all" the pain producers, however, cannot stop short just at the point where cortical activation begins to open the Pandora's box of human consciousness. An adequate model will need to tell us how human pain is created not in the nervous system alone but at the complex point where biology and culture intersect.

Toward a Biocultural Model

What kinds of thinking and research support the shift to a biocultural model of pain? I would like to look briefly at five areas that offer evidence of major change: redefinition, cross-cultural studies, inter-ethnic studies, psychologic research, and studies of pain beliefs. My aim is to be selective and suggestive rather than exhaustive. No single study can provide all the evidence or arguments needed to justify a change in models of pain. Together, however, they add up to a persuasive case against thinking about pain in the old ways. They imply that it will take nothing short of a new model to explain, for example, why the two strongest predictors of on-the-job back injury should turn out to be job satisfaction and social relations in the workplace.[19]

Scientific redefinitions of pain provide a basic index of change. At its founding, the International Association for the Study of Pain (IASP) set up a Subcommittee on Taxonomy, and the definition it published in 1979 is fascinating for the steps it takes to loosen up the medical model. "Pain," the IASP authors write, "is an unpleasant sensory and emotional experience associated with actual or potential tissue damage, or described in terms of such damage."[20] Notice that Cartesian mind–body dualism comes under implicit rebuke in the phrase "sensory and emotional experience." Notice that the strategic "or"s eliminate a direct one-to-one link between tissue damage and pain. Henry K. Beecher, in his classic work on Second World War battlefield injuries, demonstrated persuasively that tissue damage is not directly correlated with reports of pain.[21] No longer is pain regarded simply as the response to a stimulus.

The most illuminating changes in the IASP definition occur in the annotations. There the authors openly insist that pain must be understood as an "emotional experience" and as "always subjective." Further, they distinguish sharply between pain and nociception. "Activity induced in the nociceptor and nociceptive pathways by a noxious stimulus," they insist, "is not pain, which is always a psychological state. . . ."[22] We should not be surprised that the revolutionary impact of these ideas gets somewhat muted in the one-sentence definition. It is common practice in the history of science to announce revolutionary findings in a way that makes them appear no more than afterthoughts.[23]

The revolutionary distinction between nociception and pain runs parallel to another key distinction between pain as sensation and pain as perception. The medical model treats pain as a sensation: the response to a stimulus. This way of thinking, of course, proves especially inadequate in dealing with chronic pain, in which tissue damage is often not evident and where the persistence of pain over many months enlists the modifying influence of mind, emotion, and social context. All pain, however, is perception, even the most commonplace acute pain. The frequent failures of medical treatment in cases of chronic pain simply create a more obvious role for the perceiving mind. Neurosurgeon John D. Loeser reminds us that the brain is the organ responsible for all pain. "All sensory phenomenon, including nociception," he comments, "can be altered by conscious or unconscious mental processes."[24]

Many of the insights contained in recent biomedical thinking are captured by the noted pain specialist Allan I. Basbaum, Professor of Anatomy and Physiology at the University of California (San Francisco). As he writes:

> Pain is not just a stimulus that is transmitted over specific pathways but rather a complex perception, the nature of which depends not only on the intensity of the stimulus but on the situation in which it is experienced and, most importantly, on the affective or emotional state of the individual. Pain is to somatic stimulation as beauty is to a visual stimulus. It is a very subjective experience.[25]

If pain is always subjective and always a psychologic experience, the implications seem clear. Animal models, however useful in exploring anatomic and physiologic mechanisms, can achieve only limited power in explaining human pain, because they cannot tell us enough about human mental processes. Human subjectivity cannot somehow be washed out as an impure and undesirable variant in the analysis of pain. Further, subjectivity is never merely a private or individual state, because individual humans exist only within the intersubjective framework of specific cultures. Cultures, as they help to shape and to constrain human mental processes, thus necessarily play a role in pain.

If culture plays a role in pain, then it follows that pain should differ across cultures. The evidence supporting a new biocultural model of pain gains strength as we turn to the growing literature on cross-cultural studies. Carron, DeGood, and Tait (1985) studied patients with low-back pain (LBP) in the U.S. and New Zealand, concluding that American patients not only used more medication and were more likely to receive pretreatment compensation but also experienced greater "emotional and behavioral disruption."[26] A similar comparison of Japanese and American patients with LBP found that Japanese patients were significantly less impaired in "psychological, social, vocational, and avocational

functioning."[27] A more extensive study—comparing patients with LBP in America, Japan, Mexico, Colombia, Italy, and New Zealand—again found that American patients were "clearly most dysfunctional."[28] Dysfunction and impairment are not simply reactions *to* pain, linked but forever separate and distinct, as if pain were stimulus A and impairment were response B. Rather, pain as a perception comes to *include* (as a constituent of the pain) the culturally reinforced meaning that an individual is dysfunctional and impaired.

The range of cross-cultural meanings and experience that pain can encompass has been explored recently by participants in the Harvard Program in Medical Anthropology. The volume that describes their findings—*Pain as Human Experience: An Anthropological Perspective* (1992)—offers abundant illustrations showing how a purely biologic approach misses an essential component of pain. Even the taxonomy of pain changes significantly across cultures. The Sakhalin Ainu people of Japan, for example, distinguish among at least three different kinds of headaches: "bear headaches" (like the heavy steps of a bear), "deer headaches" (like the light steps of running deer), and "woodpecker headaches" (like a woodpecker pounding on a tree trunk).[29] These headaches among the Sakhalin Ainu are described primarily through *sound*. Is it relevant that the sounds are all drawn from birds and animals (rather than from, say, jackhammers or chain saws)? Medical anthropology would suggest that we cannot fully understand a person's pain without taking into account the values, beliefs, and social context of whatever culture helps shape our individual experience.

Cross-cultural approaches to pain find support in the parallel exploration of interethnic experience. The pioneering interethnic study is unquestionably Mark Zborowski's *People in Pain* (1969).[30] Zborowski studied hospitalized U.S. veterans in the aftermath of World War II, and his findings indicate that members of specific ethnic groups—in this case, Italians, Jews, Irishmen, and Old Americans (slang: WASPS)—experience pain quite differently. Two cautions are important. First, Zborowski's veterans are males, and a full-scale interethnic study must pay equal attention to the experience of women, whose physiology and social context may present significant differences. (Migraine headaches, for example, occur three times more often in women than in men, suggesting an estrogen connection.) Second, Zborowski does more than discover how specific ethnic groups *respond* to pain. The responses should be regarded, more accurately, as integral to an experience that (the IASP insists) is both sensory *and* emotional. What Zborowski with striking clarity describes is how the experience of pain changes across lines of culture and ethnicity.

Zborowski's stoic Irishmen and hyperverbal Jews may look today like cardboard stereotypes. Yet, if Zborowski's 1950s Jews and Irishmen hardly resemble their assimilated grandchildren, the differences help illustrate how our own experience of pain is no less mediated by the cultural forces of our own time and place. The *Nuprin Pain Report* (1985), for example, indicates that second- or third-generation Americans are more likely than their first-generation counterparts to report suffering from headaches, backaches, muscle pains, and stomach pains.[31] Howard P. Greenwald's "Interethnic Differences in Pain Perception" (1991) finds significant variance among ethnic groups in the "affective" dimension of pain, even when measures of pain sensation remain similar.[32] Other researchers, extending their analysis to Poles, French Canadians, and Hispanics, conclude that variations in pain intensity may be affected by differences in "attitudes, beliefs and emotional and psychological states associated with the different ethnic groups."[33] Such studies usually indicate their distance from rock-solid certainty, yet they too lend credence to a new biocultural model of pain.

The degree of credence increases when we look at research that might be broadly described as psychologic. Such research has proliferated massively since the 1978 publication of *The Psychology of Pain*, edited by Richard A. Sternbach, now in its second edition.[34] Today it is routine to associate chronic pain with psychologic states such as fear, loss, and anger, while the strong but elusive link between pain and major clinical depression has recently generated a small library of studies.[35] The impetus for much psychologic research on pain no doubt comes from George L. Engel's classic study "'Psychogenic' Pain and the Pain Prone Patient" (1959). In his clinically based analysis, Engel found that so-called "pain prone" patients tended to be individuals for whom psychologic conditions during childhood create a template for adult experiences of pain and suffering. As students of abnormal psychology have long recognized, some individuals need to inflict pain or to suffer it, often in the form of punishment.[36] The English word *pain*, of course, derives from the Latin word for punishment (*poena*), and we should not be surprised if people who feel a need for punishment eventually find their way to pain.

The concept of psychogenic pain—pain generated in the absence of an organic lesion—remains controversial, but a recent study from the Baylor College of Medicine strongly suggests that for some people the mind plays a crucial role in pain. One hundred paid volunteers were told that the experiment in which they would participate involved an electric current that might produce a headache. The volunteers were not informed, however, that the electric stimulator was set at a level that could not produce a painful charge. The result? Fifty percent of the volunteers reported pain.[37] We see a similar phenomenon in the condition known as "couvade syndrome," in which the male partners of expectant mothers undergo various symptoms of pregnancy, including abdominal pain.[38] The power of the mind to generate pain seems matched by a mysterious power to eliminate it. The placebo effect is normally dismissed as an irritating variable in drug trials, and pain specialist Patrick D. Wall has good reason to call it an "unpopular" topic. In demystifying common ideas about placebos, Wall argues against the widespread belief that a fixed fraction of the population (one third) responds to placebos. The figure, he argues, ranges all the way from almost zero to near 100 percent, depending on the circumstances of the trial.[39] What can't be demystified is the plain fact that placebos somehow prove effective in eliminating pain. Although the mechanism still remains obscure, the placebo effect (by definition) requires patients to believe that they are receiving effective treatment. Placebos thus offer another instance in which mind and belief and culture (centering here on beliefs about medical treatment) are deeply relevant to pain.

Studies in the personal and social psychology of pain radiate in so many directions that it is easy to lose sight of the central concern they share with the role of mind and meaning. In *Somatization Disorder in the Medical Setting* (1991), G. Richard Smith, Jr., describes a condition in which pain establishes itself in the absence of tissue damage. Pain in fact is the single most common symptom of somatization disorder. Its routes may be very circuitous: Smith cites research showing that a large percentage of women with pelvic or abdominal pain report childhood incidents of sexual abuse.[40] Moreover, social conflict, whether in the home or on the job, often influences pain, so that fear about the future or family stress regularly complicates treatment. Even the diagnosis may aggravate pain. One study showed that patients with arthritis reported significantly less pain than patients with the more ambiguous diagnosis of myofascial disorders.[41] Other research offers compelling evidence that even pain with demonstrable organic origins can be exacerbated by events that are largely mental and emotional. Jay D. Summers and colleagues emphasize the importance of anger and "negative cognitions"—especially punishing responses from family members—in the patient's experience of pain from chronic spinal-cord injury.[42]

The need for replacing the medical model of pain with a biocultural model is further supported by research in the area of pain beliefs. Psychologists, whether leaning toward cognitive or behaviorist principles, usually agree on one fundamental point: pain involves learning.[43] They disagree over whether what is learned should best be understood as behaviors or as beliefs. Some influential pain specialists are willing to say that the learning concerns *both* behaviors and beliefs.[44] The disagreement, however, has implications that extend beyond the normal turf wars to treatment. If clinicians treat behaviors only, without attending to beliefs that the behaviors embody, then there seems a serious risk of relapse. Moreover, an understanding of individual pain beliefs can assist in the development of personalized coping strategies.[45] Many pain treatment programs, of course, incorporate behaviorist techniques that have proven effective. Donald S. Ciccone and Roy C. Gresiak argue that the operant conditioning of traditional behaviorist treatment proves effective, however, precisely because (even if unknowingly) patients develop "new thinking skills."[46]

The work on assessing beliefs about pain began in the 1980s with the use of an educational videotape to present specific statements about pain, with which patients registered their agreement or dissent.[47] Several sophisticated instruments have since been developed to measure pain beliefs, including the Pain and Impairment Relationship Scale (PAIRS) and the Pain Beliefs Questionnaire.[48] These instruments are not trouble-free. (The Pain Beliefs Questionnaire perpetuates the myth that pain comes in two flavors: organic or psychologic.) Nonetheless, the study of pain beliefs shows interesting results. David A. Williams examines what he calls "core beliefs" about pain, which involve issues of self-blame, causation, and duration. Core beliefs, he argues, are predictive of pain intensity, and their identification can lead to effective cognitive–behavioral coping strategies.[49] Mark P. Jensen and colleagues suggest that patients function better when they believe that they have some control over their pain, when they do not catastrophize, when they believe in the value of medical services, when they believe that family members care for them, and when they believe that they are not severely disabled.[50] Shutty, DeGood, and Tuttle, studying 100 patients, show that pain beliefs correlate directly with treatment outcomes.[51]

Disability is the area in which beliefs and pain seem today most clearly tied to culture. As specialists insist, disability is not equivalent with impairment. Left-handed pitcher Jim Abbott plays baseball at the major league level despite having been born without a right hand. He is impaired but not disabled. Disability is in effect a malleable category reinvented by Western industrial social welfare systems to provide compensation for individuals deemed unable to perform normal work. It also has special relevance for back pain. In Sweden between 1952 and 1982, permanent disability status for patients with rheumatoid arthritis showed no increase, whereas awards for back injury increased almost 4,000 percent.[52] Either a vast number of Swedes injured their backs during a freakish 30-year period or the creation of disability status has encouraged people with back pain to regard themselves as disabled.

Culture, embodied in government, now regulates pain in ways that may well increase, prolong, or even create it. Doctors are called on by the state not only to treat pain but also to judge whether it merits compensation. Such a dual role for the physician creates a potential conflict—between medical and bureaucratic demands—that for the patient can turn countertherapeutic.[53] The promise of compensation undoubtedly can influence the patient's experience of pain. Although George Mendelson rejects the notion that patients suffering with pain who have claims pending often exhibit something called "compensation neurosis," he confirms that claims for compensation both complicate and impede effective treatment.[54]

Pain in our culture, then, includes the meaning that, under certain circumstances, it can be certified as disabling and thus exchanged for cash. We must be very careful, as Nortin M. Hadler argues, to know whether we are talking about a person in pain, a patient with pain, or a claimant.[55] Not everyone with pain seeks medical help, and not everyone who seeks medical help has a claim pending. Each will likely have different stories to tell about their pain, or, rather, their pain will express quite different meanings, some of which remain completely unsuspected. Effective therapies may need to address not only the pain but also the invisible meaning it conveys.

The Multiple Voices of Pain

Cultures, of course, often attribute multiple meanings to pain, which we can find almost anywhere we look. The engineer at a radio station told me how pain had begun to wreck the marriage of her elderly parents. Her mother insisted that pain was a symptom of serious illness, whereas her father dismissed pain as merely a sign of ageing. The husband regarded his wife as a hypochondriac, while the wife regarded her husband as a fool, and their different beliefs about pain had put them at each other's throats. Other meanings remain almost invisible. The pain of the elderly, like the pain of children, is a topic about which we know very little.[56] A full exploration will explode the medical myths that deny infants and geriatric patients adequate pain relief, and it will also help us understand how the meanings of pain may differ at different stages in the process of human growth.

Indeed, when we look beyond the boundaries of medicine, we find an immense proliferation of cultural meanings that accrue to pain. Although many Western physicians may not share the religious beliefs of the patients whom they treat, religion has for centuries offered numerous explanations for pain, from the Old Testament view of pain as divine punishment to the New Testament view of pain as a sacrificial act of love. A mother may understand the pain of childbirth as a test or as an obligation; a weight lifter may regard pain as a kind of growth tonic; a ballet dancer may look at her bloody toes as a sign of luck. Teenagers today understand pain through sexualized rock songs or rap lyrics, with their aura of body-piercing, masochism, and self-mutilation. The hottest fashion model in Paris, as of March 1993, is 21-year-old Eve Salvail, who at the back of her closely shaved head sports a serpentine dragon tattoo. Why the tattoo? "It symbolizes pain," she told *Women's Wear Daily*.[57] Pain, it seems, can even make a fashion statement.

One reason we don't recognize the multiple meanings of pain all around us is because we have so fully accepted the medical model. We assume that pain is meaningless and see only what we assume. We also assume that pain comes in two kinds: physical and mental. These assumptions have real effects. Thus, as pain came to be understood solely as the transmission of nerve impulses from the site of tissue damage to the brain, nineteenth-century women who could not produce evidence of lesions found themselves regarded by doctors as hysterics whose pain was bogus or imaginary: all in the head. Today many patients reach pain specialists only after a disheartening experience with health-care professionals who indicate a belief, in words or action, that the patient's pain is not "real." Real pain means physical pain: pain anchored in tissue damage; pain understood in the old nineteenth-century medical model as a meaningless shuttle of electrochemical impulses.

Modern culture, then, has trapped us in a contradiction that, for many people, makes the experience of pain especially difficult. The prestige of medical science encourages us to believe that pain has no meaning whatsoever. (Put a little differently: the one allowable meaning of pain is that it has no meaning.) On the other hand, while accepting this belief, we continue to endow pain with a variety of invisible or subterranean meanings, such as the belief that pain on some occasions translates directly into a cash payment or that it signifies old age or that it makes a powerful fashion statement. So we continue to create meanings out of pain while believing, incorrectly, incoherently, that pain is meaningless.

The point is not simply that, like the innovative Wisconsin Cancer Pain Initiative, we need to educate doctors and patients about the means to treat pain effectively. We need to understand that pain is meaningless only when we *believe* it is meaningless, in which case we have provided simply one more example of how pain always wraps itself in meaning. Medicine ignores at great cost both the meanings of pain and its own role in promulgating the myth of meaninglessness. The pertinent question—in the clinic and elsewhere—is not whether pain is meaningless but whether the personal and cultural beliefs we bring to pain are accurate, positive, and helpful or inaccurate, negative, and detrimental.

Culture and Pain

My general argument about the intrinsic relationship between pain and meaning is not something I can prove here, where I offer it as a hypothesis that lends itself, more or less convincingly, to support and illustration. The support comes not just from recent biomedical literature, however, but from places rarely visited by textbooks of medicine. A community health center in Australia, for example, published a small booklet of writings by patients with chronic pain entitled *People With Pain Speak Out* (1990). Janet Boyd provided one of the contributions:

A Snowball
Pain is like a snowball engulfing all in its path.
My path.
A snowball of pain careering out of control,
Boring down, planing off my sanity.
The swirling whiteness of pain blotting out
My attempts to live normally.
The crushing weight of the unfettered snowball
Leaves me fighting for survival.[58]

A biocultural model of pain would assume that even a nonmedical document like a poem can contain useful medical information.

Janet Boyd's poem illustrates how medicine could benefit from examining the beliefs that enfold pain in meaning. It tells us the following things. She believes, first, that her pain is so all-consuming as to force out of her life anything that is not pain. She believes that it threatens her sanity. In this sense, the foundation of her world—her ability to reason—is under direct assault. She believes that her pain not only eliminates normalcy but also plunges her into a living nightmare, as if a crushing, inexorable outside force were bearing down on her. She believes, finally, in what is surely pertinent medical information, that her survival is at stake. A doctor who failed to learn what Janet Boyd believed about her pain would lack relevant, perhaps crucial, facts for helping her to deal with it.

Beliefs are not always recognized or understood by those who hold them. Patients who have learned to assume that pain is meaningless will find it difficult or impossible to discuss what their pain means. Meanings will often emerge only gradually and indirectly. The work of understanding must thus fall to others. Fortunately, multidisciplinary pain clinics today usually include psychologists skilled in reading the roundabout signs of human communication. Very few clinics will include staff from cultural anthropology, women's studies, philosophy, history, or literature. Such scholars, however, may be especially well trained to help interpret the meanings with which patients or cultures have endowed the experience of pain. A biocultural model will challenge multidisciplinary pain clinics to stretch even further the borders of medical knowledge and practice.

Imagine what a cultural historian might add to our education about pain. Many of the finest nineteenth-century physicians believed that black slaves did not feel pain, unlike white slave-owners. Pain was also divided across class as well as race: for years medicine lent its prestige to beliefs that aristocratic classes possessed finely tuned and sensitive nervous systems that left them more vulnerable to pain than the coarse laboring masses. Women, ever since Plato described the womb as an animal roaming freely within the body, have had their pain reinterpreted within patriarchal cultures devoted to myths about male power and female weakness. Explorations in the cultural history of pain offer a challenge and a paradigm for examining the ways in which our own experience of pain is framed within the social institutions of our time and place—institutions such as sport, entertainment, welfare, and higher education.

The future, even without the help of cultural historians, is likely to see the old one-dimensional medical model replaced with a new multidimensional model that encompasses the intersecting physiologic,

emotional, cognitive, and social aspects of pain. The new model will insist that pain is not a static, universal code of nerve impulses but rather a complex perceptual experience that continues to change as it passes through culture, history, and individual consciousness. The challenge of a biocultural model is to supersede the two contrary pictures of pain we see illustrated in Piero della Francesca and in Descartes. Each picture contains a portion of the truth. Pain is, of course, an event of the nervous system. But the human nervous system also interacts in complicated ways with the environment, especially with the immensely complex environment we call human culture. We need a new picture.

Putting together a new model of pain will not be easy. Ronald Melzack, after his ground-breaking work in the 1960s on the gate-control theory, now works with quadriplegics who have suffered complete verified sections of the spinal cord such that no nociceptive impulses from the periphery can reach the brain. Yet the patients still feel pain. For Melzack, the problem of pain has shifted its main focus directly to the brain. It does not surprise him that researchers shy away from this region. As he writes: "It is difficult to deal with such problems as consciousness, awareness of one's own body, and the brain's capacity to create perceptions, memories, and every other aspect of cognitive activity.[59] As the brain and consciousness open out finally onto the multifarious field of human culture, we can expect the difficulties to mount exponentially.

Difficulties, however, are preferable to errors or illusions. In 1896 the internationally famous neurologist (and popular American novelist) S. Weir Mitchell delivered a poem he had composed for the fiftieth anniversary of Ether Day. This annual celebration commemorated the first successful demonstration (by John Collins Warren at Massachusetts General Hospital) of the surgical use of ether: a truly epoch-making event that initiated the era of modern anesthesia. Mitchell, invited to Mass General, read to the assembled medical audience a poem he entitled "The Birth and Death of Pain." It included these bold lines:

> Whatever triumphs still shall hold the mind,
>   Whatever gift shall yet enrich mankind,
>   Ah! here no hour shall strike through all the years,
> No hour so sweet as when hope, doubt, and fears,
>   'Mid deepening stillness, watched one eager brain,
>   With Godlike will, decree the Death of Pain.[60]

Pain has not died with the advent of effective surgical anesthesia, as Mitchell expected. If anything, it has multiplied alarmingly. Another new wonder drug to kill pain may be less important today than a new model that allows us to understand why pain, with its roots in human consciousness and culture, is so very hard to kill.

References

1. M. Z. Solomon et al., "Decisions Near the End of Life: Professional Views on Life-Sustaining Treatments," *The American Journal of Public Health* 83 (1993): 14-23. See the pioneering study by Richard M. Marks and Edward J. Sachar, "Undertreatment of Medical Inpatients with Narcotic Analgesics," *Annals of Internal Medicine* 78 (1973): 173-181; and also John P. Morgan, "American Opiophobia: Customary Underutilization of Opioid Analgesics," *Advances in Pain Research and Therapy*, vol. 2, eds. C. Stratton Hill, Jr. and William S. Fields (New York: Raven Press, 1989), 181-189.

2. Jane Porter and Hershel Jick, "Addiction Rare in Patients Treated with Narcotics," *New England Journal of Medicine* 302 (1980): 123. See also Barry Stimmel, *Pain, Analgesia, and Addiction: The Pharmacologic Treatment of Pain* (New York: Raven Press, 1983).

3. The following section, with its comparison of Descartes and Piero della Francesca, draws upon my book *The Culture of Pain* (Berkeley: University of California Press, 1991).

4. See Edwin Clarke, "The Doctrine of the Hollow Nerve in the Seventeenth and Eighteenth Centuries," in *Medicine, Science, and Culture: Historical Essays in Honor of Owsei Temkin*, eds. Lloyd G. Stevenson and Robert P. Multhauf (Baltimore, Md.: Johns Hopkins University Press, 1968), 123-141. On the origin and development of the term "animal spirits," see Walther Riese, *A History of Neurology* (New York: MD Publications, 1959), 50-52.

5. René Descartes, *Treatise of Man*, trans. Thomas Steele Hall (Cambridge, Mass.: Harvard University Press, 1972), 34. The *Traité du l'homme* was published posthumously—and imperfectly—in 1662.

6. Marilyn Aronberg Lavin, *Piero della Francesca: The Flagellation* (London: Allen Lane The Penguin Press, 1972). The strongest competing interpretation is by John Pope Hennessy ("Whose Flagellation?", *Apollo* 124 [September 1986]: 162-165).

7. See Elaine Scarry, *The Body in Pain: The Making and Unmaking of the World* (New York: Oxford University Press, 1985); and *Pain and Disability: Clinical, Behavioral, and Public Policy Perspectives*, eds. Marian Osterweis, Arthur Kleinman, and David Mechanic (Washington, DC: National Academy Press, 1987).

8. John Liebeskind, "Pain *Can* Kill," *Pain* 44 (1991): 3-4.

9. John J. Bonica, "Pain Research and Therapy: History, Current Status, and Future Goals," in *Animal Pain*, eds. Charles E. Short and Alan Van Poznak (New York: Churchill Livingstone, 1992), 2.

10. Patrick D. Wall and Mervyn Jones, *Defeating Pain: The War Against a Silent Epidemic* (New York: Plenum Press, 1991), 15.

11. Norman Cousins, *Anatomy of an Illness as Perceived by the Patient: Reflections on Healing and Regeneration* (New York: W. W. Norton, 1979), 37, 89.

12. D. Marcer and S. Deighton, "Intractable Pain: A Neglected Area of Medical Education in the UK," *Journal of the Royal Society of Medicine* 81 (1988): 698-700.

13. John J. Bonica, "Pain Research and Therapy," in *Animal Pain*, eds. Short and Van Posnak, 7.

14. In Richard S. Weiner, "An Interview with John J. Bonica, M.D.," *Pain Practitioner* 1 (Spring 1989): 2.

15. Ray Tallis, "Terrors of the Body," *Times Literary Supplement* (London), 1 May 1992, 1.

16. Patrick D. Wall and Mervyn Jones, *Defeating Pain: The War Against a Silent Epidemic* (New York: Plenum Press, 1991), 44. They add: "The doctrine that pain is a useful signal needs heavy qualification."

17. Ranjan Roy, *The Social Context of the Chronic Pain Sufferer* (Toronto: University of Toronto Press, 1992).

18. Quoted in *JAMA* 267 (1992): 1579.

19. Stanley J. Bigos et al., "A Prospective Study of Work Perceptions and Psychosocial Factors Affecting Report of Back Injury," *Spine* 16 (1991): 1-6; and T. Dwyer and A.E. Raftery, "Industrial Accidents Are Produced by Social Relations at Work: A Sociological Theory of Industrial Accidents," *Applied Ergonomics* 21 (1991): 167-178.

20. "Pain Terms: A List with Definitions and Notes on Usage," *Pain* 6 (1979): 249-252.

21. Henry K. Beecher, "Pain in Men Wounded in Battle," *The Bulletin of the U.S. Army Medical Department* 5 (April 1946): 445-454.

22. "Pain Terms: A List with Definitions and Notes on Usage," *Pain* 6 (1979): 249-252.

23. Paul Feyerabend, *Against Method: Outline of an Anarchistic Theory of Knowledge* (1975; rpt. London: Verso Edition, 1978), 81-90.

24. John D. Loeser, "What Is Chronic Pain?", *Theoretical Medicine* 12 (1991): 215-216.

25. Allan I. Basbaum, "Unlocking the Secrets of Pain: The Science," *1988 Medical and Health Annual*, ed. Ellen Bernstein (Chicago: Encyclopedia Britannica, 1987), 84-103.

26. Harold Carron, Douglas DeGood, and Raymond Tait, "A Comparison of Low Back Patients in the United States and New Zealand: Psychosocial and Economic Factors Affecting Severity of Disability," *Pain* 21 (1985): 77-89.

27. Steven F. Brena, Steven H. Sanders, and Hiroshi Motoyama, "American and Japanese Low Back Pain Patients: Cross-Cultural Similarities and Differences," *The Clinical Journal of Pain* 6 (1990): 113-124.

28. Steven H. Sanders et al., "Chronic Low Back Pain Patients Around the World: Cross-Cultural Similarities and Differences," *The Clinical Journal of Pain* 8 (1992): 317-323.

29. *Pain as Human Experience: An Anthropological Perspective,* eds. Mary-Jo DelVecchio Good et al. (Berkeley: University of California Press, 1992), 1. The authors here draw upon the work of Ohnuki-Tierney.

30. Mark Zborowski, *People in Pain* (San Francisco: Jossey-Bass, 1969).

31. *The Nuprin Pain Report* (New York: Louis Harris and Associates, 1985), 7.

32. Howard P. Greenwald, "Interethnic Differences in Pain Perception," *Pain* 44 (1991): 157-163.

33. Maryann S. Bates, W. Thomas Edwards, and Karen O. Anderson, "Ethnocultural influences on variation in chronic pain perception," *Pain* 52 (1993): 101-112. See also B. Berthold Wolff, "Ethnocultural Factors Influencing Pain and Illness Behavior," *The Clinical Journal of Pain* 1 (1985): 23-30.

34. *The Psychology of Pain,* ed. Richard A. Sternbach, 2nd ed. (New York: Raven Press, 1986).

35. See Jennifer A. Haythornthwaite, William J. Sieber, and Robert D. Kerns, "Depression and the Chronic Pain Experience," *Pain* 46 (1991): 177-184. For a biocultural approach to depression, see *Culture and Depression: Studies in the Anthropology and Cross-Cultural Psychiatry of Affect and Disorder* ed. Arthur Kleinman and Byron Good (Berkeley: University of California Press, 1985).

36. George L. Engel, "'Psychogenic' Pain and the Pain-Prone Patient," *American Journal of Medicine* 26 (1959): 899-918.

37. Timothy Bayer, Paul E. Baer, and Charles Early, "Situational and Psychophysiological Factors in Psychologically Induced Pain," *Pain* 44 (1991): 45-50.

38. Jesse O. Cavenar, Jr. and William W. Weddington, Jr., "Abdominal Pain in Expectant Fathers," *Psychosomatics* 19 (1978): 761-768.

39. Patrick D. Wall, "The Placebo Effect: An Unpopular Topic," *Pain* 51 (1992): 1-3.

40. G. Richard Smith, Jr., *Somatization Disorder in the Medical Setting* (Washington, DC: American Psychiatric Press, 1991), 22, 58.

41. Julia A. Faucett and Jon D. Levine, "The Contributions of Interpersonal Conflict to Chronic Pain in the Presence or Absence of Organic Pathology," *Pain* 44 (1991): 35-43.

42. Jay D. Summers et al., "Psychosocial Factors in Chronic Spinal Cord Injury," *Pain* 47 (1991): 183-189.

43. Wilbert E. Fordyce, "Pain Viewed as Learned Behavior," *Advances in Neurology,* vol. 4, ed. John J. Bonica (New York: Raven Press, 1974), 415-422; also Fordyce's influential book *Behavioral Methods for Chronic Pain and Illness* (St. Louis: C.V. Mosby, 1976).

44. See, for example, Dennis C. Turk, Donald Meichenbaum, and Myles Genest, *Pain and Behavioral Medicine: A Cognitive-Behavioral Perspective* (New York: Guilford, 1983).

45. See Gerhard Schüssler, "Coping Strategies and Individual Meanings of Illness," *Social Science and Medicine* 34, no. 4 (1992): 427-432.

46. Donald S. Ciccone and Roy C. Gresiak, "Cognitive Dimensions of Chronic Pain," *Social Science and Medicine* 19 (1984): 1339-1345.

47. David P. Schwartz, Douglas E. DeGood, and Michael S. Shutty, "Direct Assessment of Beliefs and Attitudes of Chronic Pain Patients," *Archives of Physical Medicine and Rehabilitation* 66 (1985): 806-809.

48. See John F. Riley et al., "Chronic Pain and Functional Impairment: Assessing Beliefs about their Relationship," *Archives of Physical Medicine and Rehabilitation* 69 (1988): 579 ff.; and Lindsey C. Edwards et al., "The Pain Beliefs Questionnaire: An Investigation of Beliefs in the Causes and Consequences of Pain," *Pain* 51 (1992): 267-272.

49. See David A. Williams and Beverly Thorn, "An Empirical Assessment of Pain Beliefs," *Pain* 36 (1989): 351-358; and David A. Williams and Francis J. Keefe, "Pain Beliefs and the Use of Cognitive-Behavioral Coping Strategies," *Pain* 46 (1991): 185-190.

50. See Mark P. Jensen et al., "Coping with Chronic Pain: A Critical Review of the Literature," *Pain* 47 (1991): 249-283; and Mark P. Jensen and Paul Karoly, "Pain-Specific Beliefs, Perceived Symptom Severity, and Adjustment to Chronic Pain," *The Clinical Journal of Pain* 8 (1992): 123-130.

51. Michael S. Shutty, Jr., Douglas E. DeGood, and Diane H. Tuttle, "Chronic Pain Patients' Beliefs About their Pain and Treatment Outcomes," *Archives of Physical Medicine and Rehabilitation* 71 (1990): 128-132. See also Douglas E. DeGood and Michael S. Shutty, "Assessment of Pain Beliefs, Coping, and Self Efficacy," *Handbook of Pain Assessment,* eds. Dennis C. Turk and Ronald Melzack (New York: Guilford, 1992), 214-234.

52. E. Nettelbladt, "Subjects on Permanent Disability in Sweden," *Opuscula Medica* (Sweden) 30, no. 2 (1985): 54-56.

53. Mark D. Sullivan and John D. Loeser, "The Diagnosis of Disability: Treating and Rating Disability in a Pain Clinic," *Archives of Internal Medicine* 152 (1992): 1829-1835.

54. George Mendelson, "Compensation and Pain," *Pain* 48 (1992): 121-123.

55. Norton M. Hadler, "Backache and Humanism," *The Adult Spine: Principles and Practice,* ed. John W. Frymoyer, 2 vols. (New York: Raven Press, 1991), 2: 55-60.

56. See Pamela S. Melding, "Is There Such a Thing as Geriatric Pain?", *Pain* 46 (1991): 119-121. As Melding writes: "Each year over 4000 papers (Medline data) are published on pain, but less than 1% of these focus on pain experience or syndromes in the elderly person."

57. Elizabeth Snead, "Tattooed scalp signals a model of rebellion," *USA Today,* 23 March 1993, D1.

58. *People With Pain Speak Out,* eds. Christine Nyhane and Brian Sardeson (Ballarat, Australia: The Writing Project Group, 1990).

59. Ronald Melzack, "Central Pain Syndromes and Theories of Pain," *Pain and Central Nervous System Disease: The Central Pain Syndromes,* ed. Kenneth L. Casey (New York: Raven Press, 1991), 59-64.

60. S. Weir Mitchell, "The Birth and Death of Pain," *The Wager and Other Poems* (New York: The Century Company, 1900), 18.

Chapter 34
Use of Medication for Pain of Spinal Origin
Jerome A. Schofferman

Medications have a significant role in the treatment of patients with acute and chronic pain of spinal origin. All physicians who treat spinal pain will prescribe medications at some time in the course of treatment.[1,52,58] In some patients medications are very important, while in others, medications do not help and may even prove detrimental. It is imperative that physicians understand the many medication options available, the complexities of drug use, and how to optimize the risk–benefit ratio to best help their patients.

Medications, like surgery, are just one part of an overall treatment program. For most patients medications are adjunctive treatment to help control symptoms and perhaps create a therapeutic window during which patients may participate in other treatments, such as physical therapy, that previously had been difficult because of excess pain. Although it is true that for certain patients at certain times, medications may be the most important part of the treatment, medications alone rarely prove sufficient in the long term.

However, some medications may address an underlying process. Medications such as corticosteroids or nonsteroidal antiinflammatory drugs (NSAIDs) may decrease inflammation and pain may improve. Other medications address the neurophysiology of pain, such as the use of antidepressants for neuropathic pain.

Medications are not without cost. Any medication can have side effects. Side effects can be subtle and lead to gradual worsening, such as depression secondary to long-term use of opioids or benzodiazepines. Others can be devastating, such as gastrointestinal hemorrhage due to NSAIDs.

Many classes of medications are used in the management of pain of spinal origin. These are shown in the box opposite. The spine physician should have a working knowledge of a few drugs from each class.

Acute Pain Versus Chronic Pain

When managing spinal pain with medications, the clinician must consider the differences between acute and chronic pain, because medication use differs greatly between them. If one treats a patient with chronic pain with an acute pain model, the treatment is often doomed to failure.

Acute pain has well known characteristics. The onset is clear and usually well defined. Often there is a precipitating event or injury. The pain is usually well localized and is described in clear and unambiguous terms. There may be signs of sympathetic hyperactivity such as dilated pupils, tachycardia, increased blood pressure, and sweating.

Categories of Medications Used for Pain of Spinal Origin

- Analgesics
    - Peripherally acting
    - Centrally acting
- Sedative-hypnotics
- Muscle relaxants
- Antidepressants
- Antihistamines
- Stimulants
- Glucocorticosteroids
- Anticonvulsants
- Miscellaneous
    - α-Adrenergic blocking agents
    - Antiarrhythmic drugs
    - Capsaicin
    - Colchicine

Acute pain appears to serve a useful purpose such as keeping a person from overusing the injured body part while healing occurs.[62] The "endorphin system" and other pain-modulation systems become activated. Because both patient and physician have experience with acute pain, they expect it to resolve completely in a short time based on the natural history of the particular injury.

Chronic pain is very different.[62] Some experts define chronic pain as pain that has been present for 6 or more months. However, it seems more useful to define chronic pain as pain that persists well beyond the expected resolution based on the natural history of the problem.

The onset may or may not have had a specific precipitant. Pain topography may remain clear and distinct, but often there is a diffuse and less specific location and referral pattern. The descriptors of the pain also may be less clear, and the terms used to describe the pain sound less physiologic. Chronic pain no longer serves any useful purpose. Behaviors that may be appropriate for acute pain, such as rest and inactivity, may be deleterious in chronic pain and lead to deconditioning with even more pain due to disuse. Sympathetic overactivity has dissipated and is replaced by vegetative symptoms of low energy, sleep disturbance, and change in appetite and weight.

Medications used for acute pain are often different than in chronic pain and, when the same drugs are used, they may be used differently. For example, opioids are effective for acute pain but are often ineffective and may be deleterious in chronic pain.[12,57]

Nonsteroidal antiinflammatory drugs and acetaminophen (APAP) are also effective in acute pain but appear less effective for chronic pain.

Selection Of Medications

Many factors must be considered when choosing medications to treat pain. Some of these are listed in the boxes below.

Patient Factors

* Type of pain
* Severity of pain
* Duration of pain
* Expected time course of resolution
* Coexisting medical problems
* Coexisting psychologic problems
* History of current or past chemical dependence or addiction
* Other medications being taken
* Experience with similar medications

The natural history of the problem determines how medications are used. Acute anulus tears of a cervical or lumbar disc can be expected to resolve in weeks in most patients. Pain is usually worst initially and decreases over time. Therefore, the first choice of medication may be an NSAID and if necessary a low potency opioid for 1 to 2 weeks. Nonsteroidal antiinflammatory drugs may be continued, but opioids are rarely indicated for longer. If the patient has not improved, alternative treatments might be considered.

The severity of pain will determine whether or not opioids are necessary and the potency of the opioid chosen.[36,37,44,64] Mild or moderate pain that is not responsive to peripherally acting analgesics will usually respond to codeine or a codeine equivalent such as hydrocodone.[1,47]

Some patients with low-back pain (LBP) or neck pain (NP) have other medical problems. Hepatic or renal disease may alter drug metabolism, which may necessitate adjustment of dose or dosing intervals. The elderly often experience fewer cumulative side effects when shorter-acting drugs are used. Aspirin and other NSAIDs may be relatively contraindicated if there is a history of ulcer, especially if there has been gastrointestinal (GI) bleeding. Depressed patients may worsen with the use of sedative-hypnotics or opioids

Drug interactions must be considered. Nonsteroidal antiinflammatory drugs may adversely affect the action of some antihypertensives, especially diuretics. Obviously, patients on anticoagulants cannot be given aspirin or other NSAID.

Patients who have a history of alcoholism, prior addiction to opioids or sedative-hypnotics, or other chemical dependencies are at increased risk for relapse when given opioids or benzodiazepines.[54] This is true even if there has been a long interval during which the patient has remained drug free. It has been suggested that many patients with chronic pain who develop addiction had problems with drug abuse or addiction prior to the pain problem.[46]

It is useful to know about a patient's prior experience with medications. Patients who have had a previous favorable response to an antidepressant or NSAID often do well when treated with the same medication.

It is important to know that a drug that is being considered has been proven to be effective and appropriate for the clinical situation. The medication must be safe and the risk–benefit ratio must weigh in favor of using it. The drug must be affordable. Dosing schedules must fit the patient's lifestyle, which may mean choosing a drug that can be given once or twice per day rather than every 6 hours.

Drug Factors

* Effective
* Safe
* Affordable
* Convenient
* Appropriate

Dosing Intervals

Analgesics can be prescribed in either a pain contingent or time contingent dosing regimen. *Pain contingent* means taking the analgesic when pain occurs ("prn"). *Time contingent* means taking it on a regular schedule based on the analgesic half-life of the drug (e.g., every 6 hours around the clock). There is usually better analgesia and fewer side effects with time contingent dosing, although pain contingent dosing is prescribed more frequently.

Choice Of Medications

Based on the principles outlined above, medication management can be approached logically. It is useful to explain to each patient that there are no miracle drugs and that medication management often requires serial trials until the best regimen is found. Avoid the use of terms such as "trial and error."

Analgesics

Analgesics may be divided into peripherally acting analgesics, which are useful for mild to moderate pain, and centrally acting analgesics, which are used for severe pain.* When choosing an analgesic, it is best to start with a peripherally acting agent. If analgesia is not adequate, a centrally acting analgesic may be added to, not substituted for, the peripherally acting drug.[7,47]

Many analgesics have a ceiling effect—the maximum analgesia that can be obtained from that drug. Increasing the dose does not provide increased analgesia. With some drugs the ceiling is created by significant side effects that do not permit dose escalation. With others the ceiling is neurophysiologic. Peripherally acting drugs all have a ceiling effect. The weak opioids such as codeine or hydrocodone have a ceiling effect, but the potent opioids such as morphine do not.

Peripherally Acting Analgesics

The prototype peripherally acting analgesics are acetaminophen (APAP) and aspirin (ASA). Despite the introduction of many other analgesics, ASA remains the standard for comparison.[64]

Acetaminophen is effective for mild to moderate pain. It is primarily an analgesic although it may have minimal antiinflammatory action. There is a linear dose response curve, with higher doses producing greater analgesia, until a ceiling at 600 to 1000 mg. Analgesia from 300 to 600 mg lasts about 4 hours, but at 1000 mg, analgesia lasts up to 6 hours.

Acetaminophen is extremely safe, without significant hepatic or renal toxicity in doses below 4 g per day except in patients who drink large amounts of alcohol. Of course, a single massive ingestion can cause severe and fatal hepatic necrosis.

Aspirin (ASA) is effective for mild to moderate pain. There is progressive analgesia with increasing dose until a ceiling at 650 to 1000 mg. Analgesia at

doses of 325 mg to 650 mg lasts about 4 hours. At 1000 mg, analgesia lasts 6 hours.

Aspirin has the potential for many more side effects than APAP. Gastrointestinal side effects are the most common, and are discussed in detail below. Tinnitus occurs at high serum levels.

Nonaspirin nonsteroidal antiinflammatory drugs have become the mainstay of treatment of mild to moderate acute and subacute pain.[7,36,47,64] There are little or no data to document their efficacy in chronic pain.

The explanation of the mechanisms of action of ASA and other NSAIDs is still evolving.[71] Nonsteroidal antiinflammatory drugs appear to produce analgesia via a peripheral mechanism of action.[36,37,64] It has been established that NSAIDs inhibit synthesis of prostaglandins by blocking the enzyme cyclooxygenase.[37,64,71] Prostaglandins sensitize and/or activate peripheral nociceptors. Therefore, blockade of prostaglandin synthesis reduces inflammation and results in analgesia. However, it has been established that the antiinflammatory action and the analgesic effect of NSAIDs is disproportionate.[34] Analgesia produced by NSAIDs occurs quickly, long before antiinflammatory activity occurs; in addition, analgesia is observed in painful conditions in which inflammation does not have a significant role. Therefore, other mechanisms of analgesia must be at work.[37]

All NSAIDs have much in common and therefore can be discussed as a group. It is interesting to note, however, that while the NSAIDs share a common mechanism of action, their effectiveness and side effects vary greatly from patient to patient, a finding that is neither explainable nor predictable by the chemical class of the NSAID.[36] Therefore, the selection of an NSAID is somewhat empiric. It appears clinically useful to use speed of onset and duration of analgesia as well as prior response to determine the choice of drug and dosing schedule. Despite the value of time contingent dosing, there are circumstances in which pain contingent dosing is preferred. In this case a drug with a more rapid onset of analgesia is preferred. In general, these drugs have a shorter duration of analgesia and need to be taken more frequently, usually three or four times daily. When time contingent dosing is used it may be preferable to choose an NSAID with longer half-life. It is presumed that compliance will be better because the drug will have to be taken only once or twice per day.

It is important to offer an adequate trial of any NSAID before it is considered a failure, discontinued, and another tried. An adequate trial should last about 2 weeks.

*References 1, 7, 36, 37, 47, and 64.

Table 34-1

Nonsteroidal antiinflammatory drugs: dosing suggestions

Generic Name	Brand Name	Starting Dose	Maximum Dose
Short Half-Life			
Aspirin		650 mg q6h	4000-6000 mg
Flurbiprofen	Ansaid	50 mg q6h	300 mg
Ibuprofen	Motrin	400 mg q6h	4200 mg
Ketoprofen	Orudis	50 mg q6-8h	300 mg
Intermediate Half-Life			
Choline salicylate	Trilisate	1500 mg once, then 1000 mg b.i.d.	4000 mg
Diflunisal	Dolobid	1000 mg once, then 500 mg b.i.d.	1500 mg
Diclofenac	Voltaren	50 mg q6-8h	225 mg
Etodolac	Lodine	400 mg once, then 200 mg q8h to 300 mg q12h	1200 mg
Nabumetone	Relafen	500 to 750 mg b.i.d.	2000 mg
Naproxen	Naprosyn, others	375 mg q8-12h	1250 mg
Sulindac	Clinoril	100 mg q12h	400 mg
Long Half-Life			
Piroxicam	Feldene	20 mg q24 h	40 mg

Table 34-1 shows the dose recommendations for several commonly used NSAIDs. They are arbitrarily separated into short, intermediate, and long half-lives based on the duration of analgesia. Some of the distinctions are blurred, and patient response may vary. It is preferable to start at lower doses and work up to the maximum dose.[47,64]

It is instructive to compare the relative analgesic efficacies of different NSAIDs. The data are incomplete for final conclusions to be reached and there are few direct analgesic comparisons of one nonaspirin NSAID to another. However, it has been shown repeatedly that ibuprofen 400 mg is more effective than aspirin 650 mg and about equally effective to the combination of aspirin 650 mg plus codeine 65 mg.

Ketoprofen 25 mg is equianalgesic to aspirin 650 mg, and 50 mg is superior to aspirin.[64] Diclofenac and indomethacin are roughly equivalent to aspirin. Diflunisal 500 mg is superior to aspirin. Flurbiprofen is superior to aspirin. Piroxicam 20 mg is equivalent to aspirin but has a longer duration of analgesia.

Naproxen 500 mg provides greater analgesia than aspirin 650 mg and usually provides about 8 hours of analgesia. Therefore, when using naproxen as an analgesic, administer a loading dose of 500 mg and follow it with 250 to 375 mg every 8 to 12 hours to a total daily maximum dose of 1250 mg.[7,64]

It is also instructive to examine the relative effectiveness of NSAIDs versus the "weak" opioids—propoxyphene, codeine, hydrocodone, dihydrocodeine, and pentazocine. Most studies compare these analgesics in acute pain such as tooth extraction or post-operative pain. Data are also available for patients with cancer pain. None of the weak opioids when used alone (not in combination products) has been shown to be more effective than 650 mg of aspirin![8] Codeine 60 mg or pentazocine 50 mg are each consistently as effective as 650 mg of either aspirin or APAP. Propoxyphene 65 mg has been shown to be less effective than 650 mg of aspirin.

Most often, codeine or its equivalent is prescribed as combination products with APAP or aspirin. These combinations have additive analgesic effects and also offer the advantage of fewer side effects for similar degrees of analgesia, since less opioid is needed.[8] In most studies the combination of codeine 65 mg plus aspirin or APAP 650 mg is much more effective than either drug alone.

***Side Effects* Gastrointestinal** The gastrointestinal (GI) tract bears the brunt of most of the adverse effects of NSAIDs. Problems include dyspepsia, superficial mucosal damage, gastric ulcer, duodenal ulcer, reflux esophagitis, and colitis.[5,14,42] Much less common are ulcerations of the distal small bowel and large intestine. Up to 60% of patients who take NSAIDs chronically have silent mucosal damage of the stomach or duodenum. The issue of adverse GI effects due to NSAIDs is best examined by considering prevalence, primary prevention, treatment of side effects, and secondary prevention.

Dyspepsia occurs in 30% of patients who take NSAIDs.[14] However, the correlation between dyspepsia and the presence of active ulcers or erosions is only modest.[61] In patients *with* dyspepsia 50% have erosions or petechiae, 30% have gastric ulcers, but 20% have normal mucosa on endoscopy.[14,39] Conversely, in the 70% of patients *without* dyspepsia, 45% have erosions or petechiae, 5% have gastric ulcers, and only 50% have normal mucosa.[14]

Based on summary data, the approximate relative risk of gastric ulcer in patients taking NSAIDs compared with those not taking them is about 4.8, and the relative risk of bleeding from gastric ulcer is between 2.8 and 9 to 1. The relative risk of duodenal ulcer is only about 1.1 but the relative risk of bleeding from duodenal ulcer is between 2.7 and 6.5 to 1. The relative risk of perforation from either gastric or duodenal ulcer is between 1.6 and 7.3 to 1.[39] Unfortunately, many NSAID-associated ulcers that bleed or perforate had been silent clinically.

Risk factors have been identified that may predispose to GI side effects. These include age greater than 60, history of peptic ulcer disease, high dose of NSAID, use of more than one NSAID, prolonged NSAID use (equivocal), cigarette use, alcohol use, and serious concomitant medical disease.[14]

No good data document any regimen as being effective in the prevention of dyspepsia. In a randomized controlled study designed to compare misoprostol to sucralfate in the prevention of gastric ulceration in patients taking NSAIDs, neither drug was effective in preventing dyspepsia.[2] Dyspepsia occurred in 31% of patients taking misoprostol and in 24% of those taking sucralfate.

Neither cimetidine nor ranitidine has been demonstrated to be effective in preventing gastric mucosal lesions in patients taking NSAIDs.[39,42] However, both drugs have been shown to be effective in preventing duodenal ulcers.[39,42] There are no data to help in choosing one drug over the other. In one study, misoprostol was more effective than sucralfate in the prevention of gastric ulcer.[2]

In summary, no data document the efficacy of any drug regimen in the prevention of dyspepsia. Both cimetidine and ranitidine are effective in preventing duodenal ulcer. Misoprostol has been shown to be effective in preventing gastric ulcer.[2] In patients at high risk, it may be prudent to use an H_2 blocking agent or omeprazole, although their efficacy has not been established.

The data regarding recommendations for treatment of established symptoms also is not definitive. Treatment for dyspepsia is empiric and is based on the importance of continuing the NSAID therapy and the individual risks of the patient. In most patients dyspepsia will dissipate quickly simply by stopping the NSAID, and no further action is necessary.

If symptoms continue or there is pressing need to continue an NSAID several options are available, although none is proven effective. Anecdotally, some patients will have dyspepsia with some NSAIDs but not with others. It is therefore reasonable to try a different NSAID when dyspepsia has resolved after stopping the first NSAID. Choline magnesium salicylate and salsalate have less potential for causing ulcer than other NSAIDs.[47] Either might be tried to see if analgesia can be obtained without dyspepsia.

If a more potent NSAID is necessary and/or symptoms recur, secondary prophylaxis may be considered. The available drugs for prophylaxis include H_2 blockers, synthetic prostaglandins (misoprostol), or omeprazole (ATPase inhibitor). Anecdotally, all have been effective in some patients. I usually start with an H_2 blocker because they are much less expensive, and switch to omeprazole only if the H_2 blocker is not effective.

The treatment of small gastric ulcers and duodenal ulcers is quite satisfactory and either usually heals with H_2 blockade or treatment with omeprazole despite continued use of NSAID. The healing of larger gastric ulcers is probably impaired if NSAIDs are continued.

The large intestine can be affected by NSAIDs. Colitis has been seen occasionally in patients treated with NSAIDs.[5] It may be more common in the elderly and occurs after months to years of use. Patients present with abdominal pain, blood in the stool, and weight loss. They are anemic and have markedly elevated sedimentation rates. It is difficult to distinguish NSAID-induced colitis from true ulcerative colitis. However, in most patients the disease resolves after withdrawal of the NSAID. Reactivation of quiescent ulcerative colitis has also been seen after NSAID use.[61]

Side Effects **Hepatic** Risk factors for NSAID hepatic effects include age greater than 60, renal insufficiency, high dose, prolonged therapy, and alcohol

Recommendations Regarding Gastrointestinal Side Effects of NSAIDs

- Use the lowest dose of NSAID that is effective for the patient.

- Document that the NSAID is effective before continuing therapy.

- It is not appropriate to place all patients on prophylactic therapy.

- In patients who are at high risk, consider prophylaxis with H$_2$ blocker.

- If symptoms occur, stop the NSAID if possible.

- Treat uncomplicated dyspepsia by discontinuing the NSAID. If continued NSAID therapy is necessary, try H$_2$ blockade or omeprazole (probably superior but more expensive).

- If symptoms persist, endoscopy may be necessary

use.[5] In large-scale studies of 7000 patients taking NSAIDs, 3% developed persistent elevation of more than one liver function test (LFT). Clinical hepatitis, cholestasis, and severe hepatic necrosis are rare. Abnormalities of liver function almost always revert to normal after the drug is discontinued.[14]

Salicylates appear to be direct hepatotoxins. The effects are dose and time related. The abnormal LFTs seen with other NSAIDs may be hypersensitivity reactions and usually occur within the first 4 to 6 weeks of therapy.[14] The earliest LFT abnormality is elevation of the alanine aminotransferase (ALT, previously called SGPT). Other hepatic problems manifest within 3 months.

Based on the known time course of NSAID-induced liver changes, patients at low risk should undergo LFTs within the first 3 months of therapy and repeated every 6 to 12 months thereafter. In patients at high risk, LFTs should be tested after 1 month of therapy and repeated every 3 to 6 months. A threefold elevation of ALT should prompt discontinuation of NSAID.

Side Effects **Hematologic** Aspirin and other NSAIDs alter platelet function. Aspirin irreversibly binds platelet cyclooxygenase for the life of the platelet, while the NSAIDs block the enzyme reversibly and platelet inhibition lasts only as long as the drug is

present. The clinical importance of this platelet inhibition varies and will lead to an increased risk of bleeding in some patients but not others. Choline magnesium salicylate and salsalate have less potential for causing ulcer than other NSAIDs and do not impair platelet function.[47]

Because of the potential risk of increased bleeding with surgery or invasive procedures, discontinuing NSAIDs before such procedures is often considered.[19] In fact, in one study, patients who were taking NSAIDs at the time of total hip arthroplasty had a higher incidence of bleeding complications than patients who were not taking NSAIDs.[19] Perioperative complications in the NSAID group increased by 5.8. No significant differences occurred in intraoperative transfusion requirements, wound drainage, fall in hematocrit, or length of hospital stay. The NSAID group had a higher estimated intraoperative blood loss, but this was not clinically significant. The NSAID group also had a higher incidence of GI hemorrhage and postoperative hypotension.

Side Effects **Renal** NSAID have various adverse renal effects.[32,63] The most common are renal insufficiency, edema, interstitial nephritis (renal insufficiency and proteinuria), and ischemic necrosis. Less common are hyponatremia and hyperkalemia. Exacerbation of controlled hypertension may occur. Most of the complications can be attributed to blockade of renal prostaglandin synthesis.

The deterioration of renal function is usually reversible after the NSAID is discontinued. Occasionally, severe cases have required dialysis. In mild cases renal function usually returns to baseline within 3 to 5 days of stopping the NSAID.

Risk factors include age greater than 60, atherosclerotic cardiovascular disease, concomitant diuretic use, preexisting renal insufficiency, hypovolemia, and diseases such as cirrhosis, nephrotic syndrome, or congestive heart failure.[63] Problems are more likely to occur at higher, antiinflammatory doses, rather than lower, analgesic, doses.

Side Effects **Central Nervous System** There are several types of central nervous system (CNS) side effects seen with NSAIDs. The most common are tinnitus, headache, and hearing loss. However, rarely, cognitive dysfunction, psychosis, and aseptic meningitis[33] have been seen.

A retrospective study based on subjective recall reported that cognitive function deteriorated in 15% to 20% of elderly patients given naproxen or ibuprofen.[32] Problems cleared within 2 weeks of stopping NSAIDs. A prospective study to test this hypothesis was of borderline significance in a small number of patients. Most experts believe that some elderly patients may be susceptible to cognitive impairment and that patients should be warned about and observed for mental status changes. Depression may also occur in a small number of patients.

Indomethacin is well known, however, for causing significant CNS effects including headache, psychosis, and hallucinations.[33] This is particularly true in the elderly.

***Side Effects* Respiratory** Asthma, particularly in patients with nasal polyps and hypersensitivity to aspirin, has been documented. Nonsteroidal antiinflammatory drugs may exacerbate asthma, particularly in patients with airway sensitivity to aspirin.

***Side Effects* Dermatologic** Rash develops in about 3% of patients who take NSAIDs. Urticaria is common. Also, photosensitivity with vesiculobullous eruptions occurring in sun-exposed areas has been reported, most often with piroxicam but also with sulindac and indomethacin. Fixed-drug eruption has been reported with naproxen and ibuprofen.

The Use of NSAIDs

- Usually drug of choice for mild to moderate acute pain

- Generally more effective if used in time-contingent manner

- No good data to help select one NSAID over another

- No proven effectiveness for *chronic* spine pain but definitely worth serial trials of 4 or 5 different NSAIDs

- Two-week trial before changing to another NSAID

- Screen for side effects by periodic clinical and laboratory surveillance

- Prophylaxis for dyspepsia or ulcer indicated only in high-risk patients

Centrally Acting Analgesics

Opioids Opioids have an extremely important role in the management of acute pain and pain secondary to cancer.[1,47] Opioids have an important role in the treatment of acute pain.[1] Pain after initial injury, painful procedures, occasional flares, or postoperative pain are clear indications for short term opioid use. There is controversy regarding the role of long term opioid use in chronic pain of nonmalignant origin (CNMP)[48,49,57]

The opioids share a common mechanism of action. They produce analgesia by binding with opiate receptors in the CNS. They may have some peripheral analgesic action as well.

Opioids may be arbitrarily classified into weak or potent, although there is overlap. Weak opioids include propoxyphene, codeine, dihydrocodeine, pentazocine, oxycodone, and hydrocodone. Each of these drugs appears to have a ceiling effect that limits analgesic efficacy. Potent opioids include morphine, meperidine, methadone, levorphanol, hydromorphone, fentanyl, and others. Potent opioids do not have a ceiling effect and there is increasing analgesia with increasing dose. Although one opioid may be more potent than another on a milligram-for-milligram basis, equivalent analgesia can be obtained from each with proper dosing. Patient responsiveness is individualized, however.[28]

The choice of medication is based on the clinical circumstances. If the pain is mild or moderate and not controlled with a peripherally acting analgesic, a weak opioid is added. If pain is moderate or severe or uncontrolled by a weak opioid, a more potent opioid is then used.

Opioids can be administered by oral, sublingual, rectal, transdermal, intramuscular, subcutaneous, intravenous, or intraspinal routes. Choice of route depends on the clinical circumstances.

Dosing intervals must be based on the analgesic half-life of the particular drug. Meperidine produces 2 to 3 hours of reliable analgesia and therefore must be given quite frequently. Morphine reliably produces 4 hours of analgesia. For most patients who have pain severe enough to warrant opioids, time contingent dosing is usually indicated.

Side effects are common to all opioids, but some patients are more sensitive than others. Nausea with or without vomiting may occur with all opioids and with any route of administration. Nausea is due to stimulation of the chemoreceptor trigger zone, and prophylaxis or therapy should be directed toward this site.[43] Most commonly, prochlorperazine 10 mg orally or 25 mg rectally every 6 to 8 hours is used. If not effective, transdermal scopolamine can be added. If nausea persists, haloperidol in doses of 0.5 to 1.0 mg is very effective when substituted for prochlorperazine.

Constipation occurs in most patients. In any patient on long term opioids, prophylaxis is important. Dioctyl sodium sulfate 100 to 200 mg twice daily plus senokot 1 to 2 tablets nightly is usually effective.

Sedation is common, particularly at initiation of treatment or when doses are adjusted upward. Subtle alterations of mental status may occur. Postoperative confusion may be seen in the elderly, especially after several days of use.

Most patients who undergo surgery of the spine require opioid analgesics in the early postoperative period.[1] There is wide variability in dose and dosing interval from patient to patient. Factors such as prior opioid exposure, magnitude and type of surgery, pain tolerance, patient personality, and patient expectations all play a part in determining the amount of opioid necessary. Because there is such variability, many clinicians now administer postoperative opioids by patient controlled analgesia (PCA).

Patient controlled analgesia offers several advantages.[1] Patients receiving PCA generally are more comfortable than patients who are treated with traditional intramuscular doses in a pain contingent manner. Overall opioid use is less in the PCA group. Patient controlled analgesia is probably cost effective after considering the amount of nursing time necessary to answer the patient's call, determine the analgesic requirement, prepare medication for injection, and then administer the drug.

The Use of Opioids in Chronic Pain of Non-malignant Origin The use of long term opioids (LTOs) to treat chronic pain of nonmalignant origin is controversial.[48,57] Until recently most physicians believed LTOs had almost no role in this setting. Clinical experience led most physicians to believe that opioids were not efficacious in chronic pain and in fact made patients worse.

However, in 1986 Portenoy and Foley reported their experience treating a small group of patients with CNMP using LTOs.[49] Many of their patients had favorable outcomes, and their article reawakened the controversy. More recently, Portenoy summarized his position in a thought provoking paper that fanned the flames of the controversy.[48] The Portenoy experience is very instructive and shows that in expert hands, patients with CNMP of nociceptive origin may do well with LTOs. He did not state or imply that all patients with chronic spine pain or other pain problems should be treated with LTOs. His patients all had well defined pain stimuli or neuropathic pain and treatment was in expert hands.

Many of the issues involved with LTO use can be reviewed briefly.[48,57] In my opinion the only true controversy regarding LTO use in CNMP is efficacy. Does LTO therapy improve pain and increase level of function with an acceptable risk of side effects? Other issues are far less important.

Tolerance does not seem to be a limiting factor. The use of LTOs in patients with cancer who survive for years has provided a model to show that tolerance is not a true clinical problem. However, no good prospective studies address the potential problem of tolerance in CMNP.

Toxicity is not an issue.[48] There is no evidence to suggest that LTO therapy causes renal, hepatic, or other organ toxicity or damage. Side effects such as sedation, constipation, and nausea or vomiting are common but are readily managed. Respiratory depression in ambulatory persons without significant comorbid conditions is not generally seen.

Fear of disciplinary action should not be a reason to withhold opioids.[18,67] Physicians who carefully evaluate their patients and prescribe opioids for appropriate clinical indications are acting well within the scope of good medical practice.[18,67] Periodic reevaluation is necessary. Patients should be given good informed consent, including a discussion of the controversy; also, monitoring of medication use and good record keeping are important.[18]

The illicit use of prescription opioids is always a concern. However, in patients who are treated for pain, this rarely occurs but bears careful monitoring. Strong suspicion of drug diversion or other illicit use should mandate termination of the LTO program.

The area of addiction is well covered elsewhere.[54] Addiction is greatly misunderstood. Addiction implies both physical dependence and psychologic dependence. Obviously, any patient treated with LTOs will become physically dependent with a withdrawal syndrome upon abrupt termination. It is rare to see psychologic dependence in a patient with pain who has no preexisting drug problems or psychologic problems.

A better definition of addiction is the continued use of a psychoactive substance despite biologic, psychologic, or social harm.[54] There is compulsive use, loss of control, and continued use despite harm (biologic, psychologic, or social). The incidence of true addiction in patients treated with LTOs for CNMP is quite low. However, there may be other more subtle problems, such as depression, cognitive impairment, and increased dysfunction and disability.[57]

Once again, the major controversy is efficacy. It would be extremely useful to determine in what clinical circumstances LTO therapy is useful. The widespread bias against LTO use is experientially based. Most experienced clinicians have seen patients treated with LTOs do poorly. Patients may respond initially but over time the improvement wanes. Patients return with more pain and decreased function. There may be increased depression, mild cognitive impairment, and a medication-centered lifestyle. On the other hand, a small group of patients do well. It is a challenge to carefully select appropriate patients for LTO therapy.

It is useful to hypothesize the process of deterioration that occurs when inappropriately chosen patients are treated with LTOs.[57] Many people who suffer acute injuries are treated appropriately with opioid analgesics for acute pain. However, in some people the acute injury does not resolve as expected and pain continues. These patients seek further medical care and because they still have pain, opioids are renewed. The cycle of continued pain and opioid renewals may repeat itself several times. Patients try to minimize the opioid use and often extend the period between doses and begin to experience a subtle withdrawal syndrome between doses.[12] This subtle withdrawal may manifest as increased pain with or without irritability and sleep disturbance. The patient is unable to distinguish between nociceptive pain and opioid withdrawal and takes more opioids. Some relief ensues. The patient attributes this to the analgesic effect of the opioid but in fact much of it is treating an opioid abstinence syndrome.

However, there is a group of patients with chronic pain of spinal origin who appear to do better with LTOs.[49,72] In general, these are patients with well-defined nociceptive stimuli or neuropathic pain that is not treatable by more definitive means. Patients with chronic pain syndrome who have pain and disability far out of proportion to the peripheral stimulus, patients with nonspecific low back or neck pain, or patients with premorbid psychologic abnormalities are generally not candidates for LTO therapy. In a study by Polatin and colleagues,[46] most patients with chemical dependence and chronic LBP had a history of chemical dependence at some time prior to their current pain. Therefore, a history of prior addictive disease is at least a relative contraindication to LTO use. Before committing to LTO use patients should undergo a clinical trial with decreased pain and increased function documented. Detailed reviews of this subject appear elsewhere.[48,57]

For me it has been useful to divide patients with chronic pain into three categories. Category I comprises patients with ongoing nociception that is not amenable to other treatments either because there is no good treatment available or because there are medical or other contraindications to definitive therapy. Examples of such problems might include arachnoiditis, neuropathic radiculopathy, osteomyelitis of the spine, or severe spinal stenosis with instability in the presence of severe coronary artery disease.

Category II comprises patients with ongoing nociception of a mild to moderate nature that is refractory to treatment by other means. These patients can be maintained on low doses of opioids such as the equivalent to 120 to 180 mg of codeine per day. They have increased function and no manifest side effects. Examples might be advanced osteoarthritis or multilevel degenerative disc disease.

Category III is the typical chronic pain patient. These patients have pain and disability far greater than expected for the structural peripheral stimulus. They may be depressed. Typically these patients have seen multiple physicians and tried many treatments without success. Often they are already taking low to moderate doses of opioids when first seen.[46] Psychologic factors are often playing a role in perpetuating the pain and disability cycle. They are usually not working. Many have been injured on the job. Many are seeking the cure for the problem and are not able to accept the pain as a chronic problem that requires learning coping skills, reconditioning, and functional restoration despite ongoing pain.

Category III appears to me to be the largest group and it is my impression that it is in this group of patients that opioids are often used inappropriately and appear to do more harm than good. In my opinion the controversy about the use of opioids in chronic pain is based on the experience physicians have had with Category III patients, not patients in Categories I or II.

Intraspinal Opioids An increasing number of patients with chronic LBP are being treated with intraspinal opioids. There are little data to demonstrate the efficacy of this treatment for CNMP. Before a patient is considered for intraspinal opioids, that patient must be a candidate for LTOs in general. That patient should have serial trials of at least three or four oral or transdermal opioids that fail because of poor analgesia or persistent side effects. Only then should the intraspinal route be considered.

Sedative-Hypnotics

The role of sedative-hypnotics in acute or chronic spinal pain is extremely limited.[45] When necessary, however, the benzodiazepines are the preferred drugs. There is essentially no role for barbiturates or drugs such as Placidyl, chloral hydrate, or others. Benzodiazepines do have some muscle-relaxant qualities through an effect on the CNS. If a patient is going to be at bedrest for 2 to 3 days, these medications may occasionally be used. If the patient with acute pain is unable to sleep, a benzodiazepine of intermediate half-life might be used for just a few days. The sedative-hypnotic drugs are generally not indicated in other situations.

The Use of LTOs

- The use of opioids for chronic nonmalignant pain is controversial.
- There is no role for use of LTO in nonspecific LBP or NP.
- There is a role for LTO for patients with documented nociceptive or neuropathic pain that is not amenable to definitive treatment.
- Careful informed consent is necessary.
- LTO treatment should be administered by experienced clinicians.
- It is good medical practice to do a therapeutic trial to document effectiveness in terms of pain reduction and improved function before making a long-term commitment.
- The patient must be seen regularly and the benefits of opioids must be evident to justify continued use.
- Surveillance is necessary to detect drug related problems.

It is certainly true that many patients with spinal pain have difficulties with sleep. However, because of the many detrimental effects of long term sedative-hypnotic use, sedating antidepressants are usually preferable.

The Use of Sedative-Hypnotics

- Sedative-hypnotics are greatly overused.
- Sedative-hypnotics are rarely indicated in acute pain and then only for a very short time.
- They are almost never indicated in chronic pain.
- There is a high incidence of physical dependence with significant withdrawal syndrome upon termination.
- Rebound insomnia may be severe after termination.
- Cognitive impairment may be subtle.
- Consider antidepressant use instead in chronic conditions when sleep is impaired.

The long-term use of sedative-hypnotics is fraught with problems. Long acting drugs such as diazepam or fluazepam may produce daytime sedation. In the elderly, there is a high risk for drug accumulation and the production of cognitive deficits. If used for many days or weeks, rebound insomnia may occur.

These drugs have the potential to produce physical dependence and can precipitate addictive behavior.

Muscle Relaxants

Muscle relaxants are frequently prescribed to patients with nonspecific LBP or NP under the theory that muscle strain or sprain is the cause of pain. These drugs do not selectively relax tight muscles. Their effect is generalized and is due to a CNS effect. Muscle relaxants are sedating. The muscle relaxants most commonly used and their usual doses are shown in Table 34-2.

No satisfactory studies have been performed to differentiate which muscle relaxant is best in any clinical situation.[25] Most of the studies that have been performed have looked at only the short term use of these drugs. There are no studies on the long term use.[52]

Many patients with LBP or NP complain of "muscle spasm."[6] Patients are more likely experiencing referred pain from a disc or facet joint, especially in the chronic situation. Usually, muscle pain is a secondary phenomenon due to overuse of muscles that are not sufficiently strong to provide support for the torso or head. There may well be visible or palpable muscle spasm in this circumstance. However, because patient and clinician believe that the source of pain is in the muscle itself, muscle relaxants are often prescribed. In fact, it is rare to see a patient with neck or back pain for more than a few weeks who has not had muscle relaxants prescribed.

It is my experience that muscle relaxants have significant detrimental effects. They are sedating and there appears to be physical dependence with a withdrawal syndrome upon abrupt discontinuation.

Table 34-2
Commonly used muscle relaxants

Generic Name	Brand Name	Common Doses
Carisoprodol	Soma	350 mg t.i.d. and h.s.
Baclofen	Lioresal	10 mg to 20 mg q6h
Chlorzoxazone	Parafon forte	250 mg to 500 mg t.i.d.
Cyclobenzaprine	Flexeril	10 mg h.s. to 10 mg t.i.d.
Methocarbamol	Robaxin	500 mg to 750 mg t.i.d.
Orphenadrine	Norflex	100 mg b.i.d.

There may be rebound insomnia in patients who take muscle relaxants at night. Therefore, before choosing to use muscle relaxants, it is important to examine the available data.

In a prospective study comparing cyclobenzaprine, 5 mg twice daily; diflunisal, 500 mg twice daily; combined therapy; and placebo in patients with LBP of 2 or fewer days' duration, there was no difference between the four groups at days 2, 7, or 10, although at day 4 combined therapy was better.[6] The cyclobenzaprine dose was quite low, and no loading dose of diflunisal was given. Data could not be analyzed in 31 of the 206 patients.

Dapas and colleagues conducted a randomized prospective study of 200 patients given baclofen versus placebo for the treatment of acute LBP of less than 2 weeks' duration who had evidence of paravertebral muscle spasm on examination.[20] The author was Associate Medical Director of the manufacturer. Patients were kept at bedrest for 4 days and longer "if necessary," and local heat was used three times per day. Patients were initially classified into one of two groups: those with moderate LBP or those with both moderately severe or severe LBP. Baclofen was prescribed at an initial dose of 80 mg per day and tapered to 0 by day 13.

At days 4 and 10 the patients in the second group had a statistically significant improvement. There was no difference in the group with moderate LBP. There is no mention of change in function or long-term benefits. Baclofen was tolerated by 76.5% of patients, but only 41% were able to tolerate the full 80 mg per day dose.

The author's conclusion that baclofen is a safe and effective drug is not well supported by the data. The drug was effective only in those patients who were able to tolerate high doses and who had moderately severe or severe pain, not in patients with moderate pain. There was no improvement in function. There were frequent side effects, which required dose reduction in many patients. There is no report of any long term benefit.

In an evaluation of meperidine alone versus a combination of meperidine plus baclofen plus diazepam in patients who underwent lumbar or cervical spine surgery, there was no difference between groups in terms of frequency or amount of opioid use or of pain severity.[10] There was a difference in complaint of muscle spasm, but this was not believed to be important by the author since there was no difference in overall pain between groups.

In 1980, Elenbaas reviewed the available literature on the muscle relaxants.[25] She believed that the effects of these drugs had been measured by subjective response and the evidence of efficacy was difficult to document. However, all these drugs, except diazepam, appear better than placebo. Studies were not available to compare muscle relaxants to sedatives or analgesics nor to show any one muscle relaxant to be superior to another.

In fibrositis, a controversial condition manifested by widespread nonspecific muscular pain associated with multiple tender trigger points, cyclobenzaprine has been compared with placebo.[9] The cyclobenzaprine group showed a significant reduction of pain and improvement in quality of sleep and in the number of tender trigger points. The authors point out that cyclobenzaprine is a tricyclic compound similar in structure to amitriptyline. It is possible that the efficacy is due to the improved sleep or analgesic effects similar to amitriptyline.[68,69]

Based on the available literature and the large clinical experience with these medications, empiric guidelines can be established. Muscle relaxants may be useful for 2 to 3 days after injury in patients with acute LBP or acute NP who have visible and/or palpable muscle spasm.[21] Muscle relaxants should probably be combined with an NSAID, which can then be continued if necessary after the muscle relaxant is stopped. Patients should be encouraged to use ice and stretching for muscle pain. There are no data to suggest long term efficacy of muscle relaxants.

The Use Of Muscle Relaxants

- Efficacy is not well documented.
- They are sedating.
- There are no data to help choose one drug over the other.
- They may be useful for short term use after an acute injury, especially if muscle spasm is documented on examination and NSAIDs have failed.
- They probably produce dependence and are rarely appropriate for long term use. A withdrawal syndrome may be seen upon abrupt termination, with rebound insomnia occurring frequently; seizures may occur after rapid withdrawal from baclofen.

Table 34-3

Biochemical activity of commonly used antidepressants

	Norepinephrine	Serotonin	α-Adrenergic
Amitriptyline	I	2	3
Desipramine	3	0	I
Doxepin	2	I	2
Fluoxetine	0	3	2
Nortriptyline	2	< I	I
Trazodone	0	I	2

Scale: 0 = no effect; 1 = slight effect; 2 = moderate effect; 3 = large effect (Modified from Potter WZ, Rudorfer MV, Husseini M: The pharmacologic treatment of depression, *N Engl J Med* 325:633, 1991.)

Antidepressants

The use of antidepressants for adjunctive treatment of patients with chronic LBP or NP has become commonplace.* They have been shown to be effective for pain relief, for the treatment of depression secondary to chronic pain, and for treatment of endogenous depression.† Sedating antidepressants are useful to promote sleep.

Antidepressants presumably act by blocking the presynaptic reuptake of monoamine neurotransmitters such as serotonin or norepinephrine, thereby increasing their action at the postsynaptic receptor sites (Table 34-3). However, they are also potent blockers of several different receptors, which may account for some of the benefits and some of the side effects. Improvement in pain is thought to be secondary to an effect on the descending modulating system, although some antidepressants may possess inherent analgesic action as well. The view that antidepressants improve pain through the treatment of a "masked" depression is no longer held.

It is not fully established which bioamine—serotonin or norepinephrine—is more important in pain modulation. Recent studies suggest norepinephrine is more important.[41] Virtually all studies showing effectiveness of antidepressants in neuropathic pain have used drugs that block norepinephrine, and recent data suggest no effectiveness with fluoxetine, a pure serotonergic reuptake blocker.[41]

Side effects are common with all antidepressants and may interfere with compliance if the medication is not titrated carefully. Side effects vary in frequency and intensity according to the specific drug. There

*References 37, 44, 45, 46, and 51.
†References 45, 46, 50, 66, 68, and 69.

is significant patient variability (Table 34-4). Excess daytime sedation, dry mouth, difficulty with visual accommodation, urinary retention, constipation, weight gain, and/or orthostatic hypotension may be seen with most heterocyclic antidepressants. Usually, side effects are mild and can be readily managed, but occasionally the drug must be changed.[66] Therefore, it is necessary for the clinician to be familiar with several different antidepressants. Finding the best regimen for each patient often requires a program of trial and retrial.

Side effects are related to the degree of blockade of reuptake of specific monoamine neurotransmitters or blockade of α_1- and α_2-receptors, histamine receptors, muscarinic cholinergic receptors, and dopamine receptors. Knowing the relative potency for neurotransmitter or receptor blockade of each antidepressant allows the clinician to predict the side effect profile (see Tables 34-3 and 34-4).

Side effects may be used to the patient's advantage. If the patient has a sleep disturbance, sedating antidepressants may be preferred. Conversely, if the patient sleeps excessively, a nonsedating drug that tends to produce insomnia might be tried first. If the patient has diarrhea, a drug with more anticholinergic activity might be used.

Many studies have looked at the effectiveness of antidepressants in chronic pain. Ward and associates compared doxepin with desipramine in a randomized fashion in patients who suffered from both LBP and depression.[69] They found the drugs to be equally effective. Both provided significant pain relief in 60% of patients. Patients with significant structural pathology were excluded from study. It was not made clear whether depression predated the LBP or occurred as a result of the pain. There was no placebo group, although there was a trial period before the actual study in which placebo responders were eliminated. Only 30 patients completed the study; there is no indication of how many dropped out owing to side effects. Alcoff and colleagues also were able to show a beneficial effect on pain relief in a group of patients with LBP in a controlled trial of imipramine versus placebo.[3]

Pilowsky and associates were not able to demonstrate significant improvement in pain in a double-blind crossover study comparing amitriptyline with placebo in patients with chronic pain.[44] While there was improvement in the active treatment group at 2 and 4 weeks, no difference could be demonstrated at 6 weeks. A large number of patients withdrew from the study, which may have affected the results. Patients in this study reflected a chronic pain popu-

Table 34-4

Relative side effects of commonly used antidepressants

	Sedation	Insomnia	Orthostasis	Anticholinergic[*]
Amitriptyline	3	0	3	3
Desipramine	1	1	1	1
Doxepin	3	0	3	2
Fluoxetine	0	2	0	0
Nortriptyline	2	0	1	1
Trazodone	3	0	2	0

Scale: 0 is no effect, 1 is mild, 2 is moderate, 3 is major.
[*]Anticholinergic side effects include blurred vision, dry mouth, sinus tachycardia, constipation, urine retention, and memory dysfunction.

lation and were not selected for the presence or absence of depression or LBP. Jenkins and colleagues also were not able to show a beneficial effect of imipramine in patients with chronic LBP.[35]

Most studies that have examined specific pain syndromes such as diabetic peripheral neuropathy or postherpetic neuralgia have consistently shown a beneficial effect of antidepressants. In a recent study both amitriptyline and desipramine were shown to be significantly better than placebo in improving the pain of diabetic neuropathy.[41] Fluoxetine was no better than placebo. There were slightly more side effects in the amitriptyline group. Doses of 75 to 150 mg of either drug were most effective, but there was no correlation between dose or serum concentration and beneficial effect.

Zitman and associates compared amitriptyline with placebo in 39 patients with chronic pain of various origins.[74] They reported a small but definite improvement in pain and sleep but no benefit with respect to analgesia or improvement in performing daily activities. They believed that because chronic pain is often so refractory to treatment, even modest gains are worthwhile.

Based on the available studies and clinical experience, it is clear that antidepressants have a useful and important role in the treatment of patients with chronic spine pain. They are probably most effective in patients with both pain and depression. However, results are not predictable. Patience and a good deal of trial and retrial is essential when using antidepressants as adjunctive treatment.

To use antidepressants effectively, dosing guidelines may prove useful. If patients have a significant sleep disturbance, it may be best to begin with a sedating antidepressant such as doxepin or amitriptyline. I start with an initial dose of 10 mg of either

and titrate the dose upward in 10 mg increments every 3 to 4 days to a dose of 50 mg. After that I titrate upward in 25 mg increments. Endpoints include a good night's restorative sleep, significant reduction in pain, or lingering side effects. If possible the dose should be increased to at least 75 or 100 mg and maintained 3 to 4 weeks before a trial is considered unsuccessful.

The Use Of Antidepressants

- Definitely useful when pain and depression coexist.
- For axial skeletal pain alone, results are mixed.
- Definitely useful for some patients with neuropathic pain.
- Heterocyclic antidepressants appear most useful.
- Start at very low doses and titrate up slowly.
- No therapeutic serum range established for treatment of pain.

If a large component of the pain appears neuropathic, drugs of choice are amitriptyline, nortriptyline, desipramine, or doxepin. If there is a significant sleep disturbance, amitriptyline or doxepin are more sedating and may be tried first. If no significant sleep problem exists or it is anticipated that a particular patient will have problems tolerating side effects, nortriptyline or desipramine may be better choices. The dosing guidelines are essentially the same for each of these drugs and are discussed above. With desipramine, nortriptyline, and doxepin, serum levels can be measured. Therapeutic range has been established for the treatment of depression but not for the treatment of pain. However, serum levels in the therapeutic range assure compliance and absorption.

In patients who are not able to tolerate the heterocyclic antidepressants, it is worthwhile to try fluoxetine or other new serotonergic antidepressants, although there are no data to evaluate their efficacy in LBP or NP. Diamond and Freitag have shown fluoxetine to be an effective prophylactic medication for the treatment of migraine headaches.[22] We have had some empiric success in patients with LBP but have not looked at our results critically.

Antihistamines

Antihistamines have been used for many years to enhance the analgesic efficacy of opioids, to allow reduction of opioid dose, to relieve or prevent opioid-induced nausea or vomiting, to relieve opioid-induced itching, and as a sedative-hypnotic.*

Hydroxyzine at intramuscular doses of 75 to 100 mg has been shown to be equianalgesic to 8 mg of injected morphine.[4,8,47] There is no evidence to support an analgesic effect of hydroxyzine at the usual oral doses of 25 to 50 mg or at the doses of 25 to 50 mg often used parenterally in conjunction with injectable opioids. Hydroxyzine does have anxiolytic effects and sedative properties and is a useful low-potency antiemetic.

Diphenhydramine is often used to relieve opioid-induced itching, which is not a true allergy but is due to opioid-induced histamine release. Diphenhydramine is often used as a sedative but it may cause deterioration in mental performance[29] or confusion, particularly in the elderly, presumably owing to its anticholinergic effect. In a study of healthy men 50 mg of diphenhydramine produced significant drowsiness for 6 hours after a single oral dose. Significant mental impairment measured by automobile driving–simulator and digit symbol substitution was noted for 2 hours after a single dose.

The Use of Antihistamines

- At commonly used doses, there is no meaningful enhancement of analgesia or opioid-sparing effect.
- Antihistamines may cause sedation and deterioration of mental performance.

*References 12, 24, 43, 53, and 60.

Caffeine and Other Stimulants

There have been many attempts to enhance the analgesic efficacy of peripherally acting analgesics. Caffeine has been added to different over-the-counter (OTC) analgesics to enhance analgesia. In a review of 30 clinical studies published before 1984, Laska and associates concluded that 65 mg of caffeine enhanced the analgesic effect of OTC preparations by a meaningful degree.[38] They concluded that to derive the equivalent analgesia without caffeine, a dose of analgesic 40% higher would be necessary.

Schachter and associates compared the analgesic efficacy of caffeine plus ASA versus ASA alone versus placebo for sore throat pain.[55] Aspirin plus 64 mg of caffeine resulted in a 23% to 44% improvement in analgesia when compared with ASA alone. Superior analgesia was noted within 15 minutes and was sustained throughout the evaluation period of 2 hours.

Ward and associates compared caffeine, 130 mg alone, with placebo, APAP, and APAP plus caffeine for nonmigraine headache.[70] They found that caffeine had a direct analgesic effect. In addition, caffeine produced some improvement in depression, fatigue, and vigor of the patients.

The mechanism of action of caffeine has not been established. It has a direct analgesic effect.[70] Caffeine is well known for creating a sense of "well being." This mild mood alteration may contribute to the enhanced analgesia. Caffeine may enhance the absorption of ASA.[55]

We have observed headaches in postoperative patients that appear to be due to caffeine withdrawal. When the patient is able to take liquids by mouth, they are given coffee or tea and the headaches resolve quickly.

Both methylphenidate and dextroamphetamine have been shown to enhance the analgesia of opioids and to reduce the sedative effect of the opioids in chronic cancer pain and postoperative pain.[13,27]

Glucocorticosteroids

Glucocorticosteroids can be given orally, intravenously, intramuscularly, or by intra- or perispinal routes. In pain of spinal origin short courses of oral or epidural corticosteroids are used frequently for acute LBP or NP or severe exacerbation of chronic spinal pain that has failed to respond to NSAIDs.

There is controversy regarding the efficacy of both intraspinal steroids and facet joint injections. A part of the controversy is due to a misunderstanding of the goal of epidural or facet injection. Neither is meant to cure the structural pathology nor to produce very long term pain relief. These techniques are meant for short term symptom control so the patient can participate in physical therapy or other treatments that have long term efficacy. They are quite effective when used in this manner.

The decision whether to use intraspinal versus oral steroids is clinical and economic. Obviously, it is much more expensive to employ the intraspinal route. In addition, the technical expertise must be available. It seems to us that side effects are less frequent and less severe with this route than with the oral-systemic route. The oral route is very inexpensive and universally available. In addition, it has been my experience that patients with painful degenerative disc disease without intraspinal pathology do better with oral than epidural steroids.

Prednisone, 10 mg, may be given initially as 2 tablets three times daily for 3 days and then tapered by 10 mg each day to 0. This is a safe technique that is used frequently in asthma or other inflammatory illnesses. Obviously, the patient should not take NSAIDs at the same time. Good data to demonstrate efficacy of oral steroids is lacking, although empirically they seem to be helpful. Many patients wish to minimize the systemic effects of steroids and therefore the intraspinal route is used.

Anticonvulsants

The use of anticonvulsants for pain of spinal origin is primarily reserved for patients with neuropathic pain. Swerdlow and Cundill suggest the drugs should be used in the following order: carbamazepine, clonazepam, phenytoin, and then valproate.[65] It appears that anticonvulsants are most effective for lancinating pains or shooting pains.[26,65]

Carbamazepine is started at 100 mg orally twice daily and increased by 100 to 200 mg each day until there is pain relief or symptoms or signs of toxicity. Plasma level should be measured because of individual variation in absorption and metabolism. We usually measure the level after the patient is at a steady dose for 5 days. Pain relief, when it occurs, is seen at plasma levels of between 5 and 10 μg/ml, but toxicity may be seen at levels above 8 μg/ml so there may be a narrow window for clinical efficacy. Side effects include sedation, nausea, vertigo, and blurred vision.[26] Mild leukopenia can be seen and very rarely irreversible aplastic anemia occurs. Therefore monitoring of the hematologic profile is necessary and the drug should not be continued unless there is documented pain reduction.

Clonazepam, a benzodiazepine, is also useful for lancinating pain of neuropathic origin.[26] It is a safe drug but does cause sedation. It is initiated at low doses of 0.5 mg three times daily and increased by 0.5 mg per dose every 2 to 3 days until pain relief occurs or side effects become significant.

Phenytoin may also prove effective. It can be given once daily with a starting dose of 200 mg and titrated upward according to the plasma level. The therapeutic range is 10 to 15 μg/ml.

Valproic acid has been used successfully for a variety of painful conditions including trigeminal neuralgia, cluster headache, and migraine. There appear to be a few patients with lancinating neuropathic pain who also respond. Dose is started at 600 mg twice daily and increased gradually. Plasma levels are monitored and the dose is adjusted to maintain a level of 100 μg/ml measured before the morning dose. Drowsiness may limit its usefulness.

Phenothiazines and Other Neuroleptics

Some clinicians have advocated the use of combining neuroleptic drugs such as haloperidol or flupentixol with antidepressants to enhance their effectiveness. Zitman and associates compared amitriptyline alone with amitriptyline plus flupentixol to treat patients with somatoform pain disorder.[73] Both treatments resulted in significant pain reduction; there was no difference between the two groups. There is the potential for significant side effects with the use of neuroleptic drugs for pain. Tardive dyskinesia has been reported and at times it may not abate after the neuroleptic is discontinued.[17]

There is scant evidence that any neuroleptic has a role in the treatment of acute or chronic pain of spinal origin. However, many clinicians use promethazine in an attempt to augment opioid analgesia although in fact no such benefit has been demonstrated.[4,60] In fact promethazine has been shown to increase pain over baseline and to diminish meperidine-induced analgesia.[4,24,60]

Miscellaneous Drugs

Some patients suffer painful nerve injuries after spinal disorders.[40] Nerves may be damaged from the initial injury; longstanding nerve compression may lead to permanent damage, which can be painful; and nerve damage can occur at the time of surgery. In some instances of neuropathic pain, the pain is sympathetically maintained, while in others it is not. The diagnosis of sympathetically maintained pain can be made when the pain is eliminated or markedly reduced by sympathetic block or intravenous phentolamine testing.[15]

Drugs that interfere with α-adrenergic function may be useful in sympathetically maintained pain.[15,30] Prazosin has been useful in some patients.[15] Phenoxybenzamine has been useful in causalgia but we have not had similar dramatic and prolonged relief.[30] It is started at 10 mg every 8 hours and gradually increased to a maximum of 40 mg every 8 hours. Orthostatic hypotension and palpitations are common and may limit the drug's usefulness. Guanethidine has also provided pain relief but it is not often used because of the high incidence of side effects.

Capsaicin is a topical analgesic cream that causes the depletion of substance P in small unmyelinated nociceptors. It has been used to treat painful peripheral neuropathy and recently it has been noted to be effective in osteoarthritis and rheumatoid arthritis. Capsaicin has been shown to be effective in some patients with reflex sympathetic dystrophy as well.[16] There are no data regarding its effectiveness in spinal disorders.

Colchicine has been popularized as a treatment for all types of lumbar spine pains.[51] It is initially administered intravenously and then continued orally. We were unable to demonstrate any efficacy of intravenous colchicine in a 10 patient pilot study.[59] Schnebel and Simmons were unable to show efficacy for oral colchicine.[56]

The antiarrhythmic medications mexilitine and tocainamide have a limited role in some patients with neuropathic pain.[47] In most instances these medications are best used by pain management specialists.

Summary

Medications have an important adjunctive role in the treatment of patients with pain of spinal origin. Clinicians should be familiar with the various medication options available and the scientific foundations that guide their use. No medication is a cure for spinal pain and every medication has the potential for side effects. Careful thought regarding the risks versus benefits of each medication, and the ability to be patient while trying and retrying medication regimens, will result in meaningful benefit to many patients.

References

1. Acute Pain Management Guideline Panel: *Acute pain management: operative or medical procedures and trauma: clinical practice guideline.* AHCPHR Pub. No. 92-00332. Rockville, MD: Agency for Health Care Policy and Human Research, Public Health Service, U.S. Dept. of Health and Human Services. February 1992.
2. Agrawal NM and others: Misoprostol compared with sucralfate in the prevention of nonsteroidal anti-inflammatory drug induced gastric ulcer, *Ann Intern Med* 115:195, 1991.
3. Alcoff J and others: Controlled trial of imipramine for chronic low back pain, *J Fam Pract* 14:841, 1982.
4. Atkinson JH: *Psychopharmacologic agents in the treatment of pain syndromes.* In Tollison CD, editor: *Handbook of chronic pain management,* Baltimore, 1989, Williams and Wilkins, p 69.
5. Babb RR: Gastrointestinal complications of nonsteroidal anti-inflammatory drugs, *West J Med* 157:444, 1992.
6. Basmajian JV: Acute back pain and spasm: a controlled multicenter trial of combined analgesic and antispasm agents, *Spine* 14:438, 1989.
7. Beaver WT: Maximizing the benefits of weaker analgesics, IASP Refresher Course Syllabus, 1987, p 1.
8. Beaver WT, Feise G: *A comparison of the analgesic effects of morphine, hydroxyzine and their combination in patients with post-operative pain.* In Bonica JJ, editor: *Advances in pain research and therapy,* New York, 1976, Raven Press, p 553.
9. Bennett RM and others: A comparison of cyclobenzaprine and placebo in the management of fibrositis, *Arthritis Rheum* 31:1535, 1988.
10. Blumenkopf B: Combination analgesic-antispasmodic therapy in postoperative pain, *Spine* 12:384, 1987.
11. Bouckoms AJ: Analgesic aduvants: the role of psychotropics, anticonvulsants, and prostaglandin inhibitors, *Drug Ther* November 1981, p 41.
12. Brodner RA, Taub FA: Chronic pain exacerbated by long-term narcotic use in patients with nonmalignant disease: clinical syndrome and treatment, *Mt Sinai J Med* 45:233, 1978.
13. Bruera E and others: Methylphenidate associated with narcotics for the treatment of cancer pain, *Cancer Treat Rep* 71:67, 1987.
14. Bush TM, Shlotzhauer TL, Imai K: Nonsteroidal anti-inflammatory drugs: proposed guidelines for monitoring toxicity, *West J Med* 155:39, 1991.
15. Campbell JN, Devor M: *Basic and clinical aspects of neuropathic pain,* IASP Refresher Course, Syllabus. 1990, p 69.
16. Cheshire WP, Synder CR: Treatment of reflex sympathetic dystrophy with topical capsaicin: case report, *Pain* 42:307, 1990.
17. Clarke IMC: Tardive dyskinesia and chronic pain, *Pain* 45:167, 1991.
18. CMA-BMQA: *Guidelines for prescribing controlled substances for chronic conditions: a joint statement by the BMQA and the CMA,* Action Report, BMQA, November 5-6, 1985.

19. Connelly CS, Panush RS: Should nonsteroidal anti-inflammatory drugs be stopped before elective surgery?, *Arch Intern Med* 151:1963, 1991.

20. Dapas F and others: Baclofen for the treatment of acute low-back syndrome: a double-blind comparison with placebo, *Spine* 10:345, 1985.

21. Deyo RA, Diehl AK, Rosenthal M: How many days of bed rest for acute low back pain?, *N Engl J Med* 315:1064, 1986.

22. Diamond S, Freitag FG: The use of fluoxetine in the treatment of headache (letter), *Clin J Pain* 5:200, 1989.

23. Dillin W, Uppal G: Analysis of medications used in the treatment of cervical disk degeneration, *Orthop Clin North Am* 23:421, 1992.

24. Dundee JW, Love WJ, Moore J: Alterations in response to somatic pain associated with anesthesia, further studies with phenothiazines derivatives and similar drugs, *Br J Anaesth* 35:597, 1963.

25. Elenbass JK: Centrally acting oral skeletal muscle relaxants, *Am J Hosp Pharm* 37:1313, 1980.

26. Fields H: Anticonvulsants, psychotropics, and antihistaminergic drugs in pain management. In Fields J, editor: *Pain*, New York, 1987, McGraw-Hill, p 285.

27. Forest WH and others: Dextroamphetamine with morphine for the treatment of post-operative pain, *N Engl J Med* 296:712, 1977.

28. Galer BS et al: Individual variability in the response to different opioids: report of five cases, *Pain* 49:87, 1992.

29. Gengof, Gabos C, Miller JK: The pharmacodynamics of diphenhydramine-induced drowsiness and changes in mental performance, *Clin Pharmacol Ther* 45:15, 1989.

30. Ghostine SY and others: Phenoxybenzamine in the treatment of causalgia, *J Neurosurg* 60:1263, 1984.

31. Goodwin JS, Regan M: Cognitive dysfunction associated with naproxen and ibuprofen in the elderly, *Arthritis Rheum* 25:1013, 1982.

32. Heinrich WL: Analgesic nephropathy, *Am J Med Sci* 295:561, 1988.

33. Hoppmann RA, Peden JG, Ober SK: Central nervous system side effects of nonsteroidal anti-inflammatory drugs, *Arch Intern Med* 151:1309, 1991.

34. Hunskaar S, Berge O, Hole K: Dissociation between antinociceptive and anti-inflammatory effects of acetylsalicylic acid and indomethacin in the formalin test, *Pain* 25:125, 1986.

35. Jenkins DG, Ebbutt AF, Evans CD: Tofranil in the treatment of low back pain, *J Intern Med Res* 4:28, 1976.

36. Kantor TG: Control of pain by nonsteroidal anti-inflammatory drugs, *Med Clin North Am* 66:1053, 1982.

37. Kantor TG: The management of pain by pharmacological agents, *Clin J Pain* 5:121, 1989.

38. Laska EM and others: Caffeine as an analgesic adjuvant, *JAMA* 251:1711, 1984.

39. Loeb DS, Ahlquist DA, Talley NJ: Management of gastroduodenopathy associated with use of nonsteroidal anti-inflammatory drugs, *Mayo Clin Proc* 67:354, 1992.

40. Loeser JD: Pain due to nerve injury, *Spine* 10:232, 1985.

41. Max MB and others: Effects of desipramine, amitriptyline, and fluoxetine on pain in diabetic neuropathy, *N Engl J Med* 326:1250, 1992.

42. McCarthy D: Treatment and prevention of nonsteroidal anti-inflammatory drug-associated ulceration. In Soll AH, moderator: Nonsteroidal anti-inflammatory drugs and peptic ulcer disease, *Ann Intern Med* 114:307, 1991.

43. Peroutka SJ, Snyder SH: Antiemetics: neurotransmitter receptor binding predicts therapeutic actions. *Lancet* 1:658, 1982.

44. Pilowsky I and others: A controlled study of amitriptyline in the treatment of chronic pain, *Pain* 14:169, 1982.

45. Polatin PB: Psychoactive medications as adjuncts in functional restoration. In Mayer TG, Mooney V, Gatchel RJ, editors: *Contemporary conservative care for painful spinal disorders*, Philadelphia, 1991, Lea and Febiger, p 465.

46. Polatin PB and others: Psychiatric illness and chronic low back pain, *Spine* 18:66, 1993.

47. Portenoy R: *Pharmacotherapy of cancer pain.* In IASP Committee on Refresher Courses, editors: *IASP Refresher Courses on Pain Management*, Adelaide, Australia, April 1, 1990, p 101.

48. Portenoy RK: Chronic opioid therapy in nonmaligant pain, *J Pain Symptom Manage* 5:46, 1990.

49. Portenoy RK, Foley KM: Chronic use of opioid analgesics in nonmalignant pain: report of 38 cases, *Pain* 25:171, 1986.

50. Potter WZ, Rudorfer MV, Husseini M: The pharmacologic treatment of depression, *N Engl J Med* 325:633, 1991.

51. Rask MR: Colchicine use in five hundred patients with disk disease, *J Neurolog Orthop Surg* 1:351, 1980.

52. Robinson JP, Brown PB: Medications in low back pain, *Phys Med Rehab Clin North Am* 2:97, 1991.

53. Rumore MM, Schlichting DA: Clinical efficacy of antihistaminics as analgesics, *Pain* 25:7, 1986.

54. Savage SR: Addiction in the treatment of pain: significance, recognition, and management, *J Pain Symptom Manage* 8:265, 1993.

55. Schachtel BP and others: Caffeine as an analgesic adjuvant: a double-blind study comparing aspirin with caffeine to aspirin and placebo in patients with sore throat, *Arch Intern Med* 151:733, 1991.

56. Schnebel BE, Simmons JW: The use or oral colchicine for low-back pain, *Spine* 13:354, 1988.

57. Schofferman J: Long term use of opioids for the treatment of chronic pain of nonmalignant origin, *J Pain Symptom Manage* 8:279, 1993.

58. Schofferman J: The use of medications in failed back surgery, *Spine: State Art Reviews* 1:129, 1986.

59. Schofferman J, Schofferman L, Zucherman J: *Failure of intravenous plus oral colchicine to relieve low back pain.* Monterey, CA, August, 1990, North American Spine Society (abstract).

60. Siker ES and others: The earlobe algesimeter: the effect of pain threshold of certain phenothiazine derivatives alone or combined with meperidine, *Anesthesiology* 2:497, 1966.

61. Soll A: Nonsteroidal anti-inflammatory drugs and ulcers, *West J Med* 57:465, 1992.

62. Sternbach JRA: *Clinical aspects of pain.* In Fordyce

WE, editor: *Behavioral methods for chronic pain and illness*, St. Louis, 1976, Mosby, p 223.

63. Stillman MT, Schlesinger A: Nonsteroidal anti-inflammatory drug nephrotoxicity, *Arch Intern Med* 150:268, 1990.

64. Sunshine A, Olson NZ: *Non-narcotic analgesics*. In Wall PD, Melzack, R, editors: *Textbook of pain*, New York, 1989, Churchill Livingstone, p 670.

65. Swerdlow M, Cundill JG: Anticonvulsant drugs used in the treatment of lancinating pain: comparison. *Anaesthesiology* 36:1129, 1981.

66. Tollefson GD: Antidepressant treatment and side effect considerations, *J Clin Psychiatry* 52:4, 1991.

67. Verhaag DA, Ikeda R: *Prescribing for chronic pain*. Action Report, BMQA, June 3 and 14, 1991.

68. Ward NG: Tricyclic antidepressants for chronic low-back pain: mechanism of action and predictors of response, *Spine* 11:661, 1986.

69. Ward NG, Bloom VL, Friedel RO: The effectiveness of tricyclic antidepressants in the treatment of coexisting pain and depression, *Pain* 7:331, 1979.

70. Ward N and others: The analgesic effects of caffeine in headache, *Pain* 44:151, 1991.

71. Weissmann G: Aspirin, *Sci Am* January, 1991, p 84.

72. Zenz M, Strumpf M, Tryba M: Long-term oral opioid therapy in patients with chronic nonmalignant pain, *J Pain Symptom Manage* 7:69, 1992.

73. Zitman FG and others: Does addition of low-dose flupentixol enhance the analgesic effects of low-dose amitriptyline in somatoform pain disorder?, *Pain* 47:25, 1991.

74. Zitman FG and others: Low-dose amitriptyline in chronic pain: the gain is modest, *Pain* 42:35, 1990.

Chapter 35
Physical Correlates of the Deconditioning and Dehabilitation Cascade*
Tom G. Mayer

*Much of the author's research reported in this chapter was supported by grants to him from the National Institutes of Mental Health (MH46452 and MH01107).

The focus of medical clinicians is all too often exclusively directed at symptoms. Pain is the symptom which produces the majority of all initial medical contacts, and represents the highest proportion of disorders related to the musculoskeletal system. We use the terms *low-back pain* and *neck pain* to describe complex disorders of the musculoskeletal system, in which our attention to *symptoms* often obscures anatomic, physiologic, somatoform, and socioeconomic factors associated with these symptoms. While the clinician's attention is focused on pain and its alleviation, payors, in an increasingly cost-conscious reimbursement system, have their attentions riveted on direct and indirect expenses associated with dealing with the symptoms.

While most episodes of spinal dysfunction are relatively trivial occurrences, and respond to spontaneous soft tissue healing in short periods of time, the larger problems of *disability* are often overlooked by the busy clinician, intent on producing short-term symptom relief. Yet, disability probably represents the central problem from which all other problems arise. Lower productivity of individual workers certainly produces major losses to society. Disability itself may lead to mental and physical dysfunction, which perpetrates itself and produces a general decline in human performance, with greater dependence on the medical system. Yet, many treatments devoted solely to the alleviation of pain fail to assure a simultaneous goal of amelioration of disability. As clinicians, we may become personally frustrated, blaming the patient for therapeutic failures claiming "secondary gain" concomitants for the patient's failure to respond.

The Role Of Injury

The rising rate of low-back disability has been accelerating dramatically over the past 20 years,[21] with a staggering 14 times increase in disability in the United States in the 1970s.[8] This increase can no longer be ignored, particularly in view of the aging work force. Recognizing disability as the central problem related to lumbar dysfunction characterizes the functional restoration approach. The primary goal of functional restoration is the elimination of disability; once this has been accomplished, pain relief and cost control can be anticipated as secondary phenomena. Another published book describes the functional restoration approach in detail.[21]

Debilitation and/or *deconditioning* may be a response mediated *physically* by the injury, as well as *psychosocially* by a variety of secondary factors. Some of these may include injury-imposed inactivity, neurologically mediated spinal reflexes, iatrogenic medication dependence, and psychologically mediated responses to prior psychiatric distress, vocational adjustment problems and/or limited social coping resources. Over time, such factors may potentiate each other, particularly in view of a compensation system that encourages dependence while symptom complaints persist.[10] These secondary factors may lead to the creation of the "disease" of work disability or incapacity by reinforcing a variety of factors within the affected individual. Additional factors at play in the compensation system may include the adversary employee/employer relationship, limited occupational alternative, compensation factors,[1, 32] and family stressors. Thus, potentiation of debilitation may have both an endogenous and exogenous initiation.

When a spinal injury occurs, the pathology may be diffuse and difficult to clearly identify. Notwithstanding the problems of identifying specific pathology, certain mechanical and biochemical disruptions of homeostasis may be anticipated. While it is beyond the scope of this chapter to identify these pathologic changes, a brief review of mechanical problems leading to rapid spinal degenerative changes and predictable symptoms, can be useful. The disc, representing the largest structure in the body without a blood supply, appears to be the anatomic structure at greatest risk. Injury to this structure will result in extremely slow repair and likely accumulation of inflammatory chemicals. Inhibition of normal motion will impair both the normal healing process and removal of chemicals associated with noxious stimuli, leading to an extremely prolonged period of regional symptoms. During this period of splinting, secondary contracture of apophyseal joint structures and muscle-tendon units can be expected to occur, gradually worsening with the passage of time. Sudden resumption of strenuous activities can be expected to increase symptoms by sudden overuse of these disused musculoskeletal structures.

Following soft-tissue healing (that will routinely occur within a maximum of a few months if no systemic disease is present), scar tissue in any of the involved mesenchymal structures may continue to wreak mechanical havoc. Partial intrinsic contractures of the anulus, joint capsule, or musculotendinous units may lead to retearing of these structures when uncontrolled motions and loads are applied without sufficient preparation of the tissues. Disc narrowing, associated with dispersion and desiccation of the nucleus pulposus, creates further mechanical problems. Disc narrowing in the axial plant produces malalignment of apophyseal joints creating minor subluxations that contribute to more rapid apophyseal joint degeneration and greater symptom report. Disc narrowing, particularly when combined with postsurgical scarring in the spinal canal, leads to *dynamic* foraminal narrowing. Foraminal narrowing may be only symptomatic when local tissue swelling or muscular tightness (and spasm) produces sufficient foraminal narrowing to temporarily compress neural structures. In contrast to true stenosis, dynamic foraminal narrowing may be only intermittently symptomatic, and thus much more difficult to diagnose and treat.

The undesirable byproducts of surgical intervention may contribute to mechanical difficulties. The commonly performed discectomy may relieve severe mechanical or chemical irritation of a specific nerve root, but results in narrowing and dysfunction of the surgically treated disc. Handling of neural elements within the spinal canal, and/or post-traumatic bleeding, leads to localized scarring that binds nerve roots and may contribute ultimately to localized stenosis. Segmental arthrodesis, or fusion, produces an even greater impact on normal anatomy and physiology, often leading to local structural stenosis affecting neural elements. The long-term effects of spinal fusion on degeneration of contiguous segments has been well-documented.

It is also clear that the degenerative process in the spine is commonly associated with aging, and not necessarily associated with prolonged symptoms. The same, or greater, degree of degenerative change, which can be imaged, may be associated with lesser, or even nonexistent, degrees of symptoms. As such, a different mechanism of symptom production, unrelated to age, must be postulated to account for continued presence of pain following spinal injury. It is believed that the debilitation/deconditioning cascade, when combined with the mechanical and biochemical effects of injury cited above, can account for these symptoms physiologically. The arachidonic acid inflammatory cascade and inactivity-induced decrease in endorphin production may be important biochemical processes. Subsequent potentiation by psychosocioeconomic factors associated with the "pain-stress-tension cycle" may then account for prolonged disability.

The Deconditioning Cascade

Loss of capacity to perform physical tasks may be associated both with structural lesions and decrements in physical capacity. An example of the first factor would be a tibial fracture, while an example of the second is joint stiffness and muscle atrophy secondary to prolonged cast immobilization and pain-induced neural inhibiting influences while primary healing occurs. This example delineates general principles of response of the human organism following musculoskeletal injury. Soon after injury, effects of the trauma on structural factors predominate. Inflammation leads to repair of the tissue with the original mesothelial elements, or (in the case of large defects) replacement with collagenous scar equivalents.

The period of immobilization/inactivity may be prolonged, in more significant trauma, leading to dysfunctional behaviors, abetted by a variety of psychosocial and cultural factors. These dysfunctional behaviors may be followed by loss of physical capacity as measured by deterioration of a variety of basic elements of performance (BEPs) such as motion, strength, endurance, and agility.[17, 18] The longer the period of inactivity, the greater the opportunity for disuse to create physical capacity deficits leading to decreased human performance, and ultimately to a variety of psychosocial and affective concomitants such as depression, medication abuse, and disability habituation. Pain may be a parallel factor, but its direct relationship to changes in muscles or other mesothelial structures remains unsubstantiated.

Physical capacity deficits are rarely a factor in human performance in the early post-traumatic stages, but become a gradually increasing factor accompanying inactivity and disuse. As time progresses, functional deficits become the dominant physical impairment disabling the more chronic patient. Strength testing during the early post-traumatic time period will be hampered by invalid measurements due to pain-induced neuromuscular inhibition. Also, there is some limited concern that over-aggressive attempts to achieve performance might actually exacerbate the injury during acute phases of low-back pain (LBP). Given usual soft-tissue healing periods, such concerns should no longer be necessary one to two months post-trauma. While testing may be feasible from that point forward, deconditioning produced by inactivity is likely to make its appearance only after that acute time period. Epidemiologically, we would anticipate that about 75% of acute LBP cases will have resolved spontaneously by then.

Extremity deficits are easily noted because they are amenable to simple visual observation of atrophy by muscle circumference measurement and comparison with the contralateral side. For this reason, sports medicine programs have focused considerable effort on restoring strength/endurance in the paraarticular musculature as a natural part of any rehabilitation process. Generally, due to lack of visual feedback and a comparison side in the spine, these above clinical connections have not been made. Subtle forms of loss of trunk strength are not generally perceived, and therefore not taken into consideration as a cause of symptoms.

Do atrophy or contracture represent the whole problem? The term "deconditioning syndrome" has been applied to the cumulative disuse changes produced in the chronically disabled patient suffering from spinal dysfunction. It is initially produced by the immobilization and inactivity associated with injury, supplemented by disruption of spinal soft tissues, scarring resulting from degenerative change, surgical approaches, or repetitive microtrauma. As pain perception is enhanced, learned protective mechanisms lead to a vicious cycle of inactivity and disuse. As physical capacity decreases, the likelihood of fresh sprains/strains to unprotected joints, muscles, ligaments, and discs increases. The disruption of soft-tissue homeostasis accelerates pain and dysfunction, typically perceived by the patient as a "recurrence" or "reinjury," but is actually secondary to a cycle of healing contracture and deconditioning. The concept of joint and muscle *inhibition* must be introduced to account for much of the measured loss of human performance.

Measurement Of Human Performance

Consciously and unconsciously, measurement is a part of all of our activities of daily living (ADLs). We regularly utilize our senses to determine temperature, distance, size, or texture of objects. In many cases, a fairly qualitative evaluation will suffice, usually because there is no visual or tactile limitation on frequent repeated assessment of the object we are interested in, such as observing a moving vehicle in traffic or placing food in our mouths. In most situations we witness, one observation confirms another. In some cases, however, greater precision is necessary, usually occurring when the object at hand is *not* amenable to regular visual inspection or when contradictory observations occur. In these cases, a quantitative assessment in the axial skeleton must be accompanied by knowledge of a range of normal values (obtained by testing many "normal" subjects). Variation from a mean normative score in a patient is then used as a mechanism for evaluating the presence of disease, dysfunction, or the return to an improved state from an abnormal one. The spinal anatomy does not lend itself easily to visual or tac-

tile examination, and thus demands indirect, quantitative measurement to describe its performance.

Musculoskeletal clinicians have the privilege of direct measurement by visual observation. We have not had to develop the discipline of our hematologist and cardiologist brethren who must rely on indirect measurements (such as blood component, heart rate, and blood pressure) to diagnose abnormalities. While the quantitative measurement of joint motion or muscle strength have been available for many years, all too often a hasty qualitative assessment is substituted for the quantitative one. The novice physician or therapist soon learns that quantitative measurements are time-consuming and generally unnecessary for routine clinical practice. We "eyeball" the comparison between the motion of both knees and the size of a quadriceps (often without using a tape measure), reserving the use of a goniometer or isokinetic testing device for special occasions when an evaluation specifies quantification.

In the spinal anatomy, the small, inaccessible, three-joint complexes stacked upon each other do not lend themselves to easy inspection. Intersegmental spine movement is difficult to measure even with biplanar x-ray devices. Multiple small muscles interdigitate over a variable number of segments, and ligamentous structures may share surprising amounts of load and certain joint positions. Moreover, bilateral comparisons are difficult. Until recently, there were no valid indirect measurement methods available to assess spine function, producing ignorance of pathological processes in the vast majority of spine dysfunction cases not resolving spontaneously. Currently, however, though absence of direct visualization methodology persists, novel technology for assessing spine function has become part of the clinical routine. Yet, many clinicians persist in ignoring or refusing to use such technology. In so doing, therapeutic errors are encouraged, outcomes remain unevaluated, and fringe/fad treatments are perpetuated.

We must recognize our weaker clinical areas before we can expect to move forward. Lack of recognizing the deconditioning syndrome in the diagnosis of spinal disorders has adversely affected our therapeutic modalities. Many individuals currently embracing "work-hardening" (often as fervently as they favored "pain-management" previously) do so using eclectic therapies applied uniformly to all patients, rather than individualizing treatment on the basis of functional testing. Surgical treatment is performed on only 2 to 3% of patients with spinal disorders. Nevertheless, surgeons will search diligently for that small percentage of cases with a wide variety of sophisticated but expensive diagnostic tools (CT or MRI scanning, electromyography, myelography, etc.). A structural diagnosis, when made, may lead to the ability to correct an anatomic aberration, such as a prolapsed disc. For the remaining 97% of the back-injured population, spontaneous recovery may account for many successful outcomes. However, a substantial percentage of patients, perhaps as high as 30 to 40%, will show some evidence of disuse and deconditioning, making them candidates for physical retraining once the functional deficits are identified. Without quantification, the deficits are simply not recognizable, leading to inevitable over- or underutilization of therapeutic services secondary to the absence of quantification. This observation is not merely true for spinal disorders, nor has it escaped the attention of health care planners. Medicare requires periodic testing to document progress in other areas of rehabilitation. It is likely that similar rules will ultimately apply to the treatment of spinal problems, once their necessity becomes more generally perceived.

Specific Physical Human Performance Quantification

Methods are now available to objectively quantify the degree of deconditioning in spinal disorders. They fall into two general areas corresponding to the measurement of the injured joint or region (physical capacity testing) as opposed to *whole body performance measures incorporating the injured region* (functional capacity measures). The injured joint in the extremities is usually well-isolated by easily manipulated long bones, allowing assessment of the BEPs of localized motion and strength of support musculature. In the spine, one must make practical compromises, generally including measurement of combined motions of multiple segments in a given spinal region, as well as cumulative strength across that region. Functional measurements, on the other hand, do not need to be modified for spinal anatomy since they are whole-body measurements. For these, the primary issue is *relevance* to those functional activities specifically dependent on the injured spinal region. For a variety of reasons, *lifting capacity* often becomes the classic functional measurement technique believed relevant for spinal disorders, and is also one for which measurement devices and protocols are readily available. Other relevant functional ADLs may include reaching, bending, pushing, pulling, and twisting.

Spinal Motion

Spinal motion is a *compound* movement combining intersegmental regional motion components with movements below the region of interest. Inclinometers are used to measure the superior and inferior inclinations of the region involved in an inclination in each of the major planes to derive the *true* regional motion from the *neutral 0-degree position*.[15, 29] In the cervical region, six movements in three planes are of interest (sagittal flexion/extension, right/left lateral flexion, right/left rotation). Recent active/passive normative data bases have been described using either two inclinometers or careful shoulder stabilization with a single inclinometer or three-dimensional digitizer.[7, 25] In the thoracic area, the ribs make coronal plane motion negligible, so the movements of interest are sagittal flexion/extension and right/left rotation. Since extension is usually limited in the thoracic area, the convention of an *angle of minimum kyphosis* (full voluntary extension) is used, with flexion measured from this position between T1 and T12. Similarly, lumbar facets permit minimal rotation, so that the relevant movements are sagittal flexion/extension and right/left lateral flexion.[15] Particularly in sagittal flexion, the hip (sacral) motion component from the standing, erect posture represents a large aspect of the movement, making it vital to pay close attention to both components when assessing limitations of lumbar spine flexion inhibiting important forward bending functional activities. The relationship between sagittal hip flexion and the passive supine straight leg raise (SLR) can be used as an *accessory effort factor* for patient cooperation in sagittal lumbar active range of motion (AROM) activities. This complements reproducibility characteristics of repeated measures for AROM, and use of passive range of motion (PROM), for assessing patient effort.[6,7,25,29]

Because ROM is the only partially visible performance measurement of the spine, it has been accepted as the only functional capacity assessment tool to be used in impairment evaluation. As such, the demand for improved science in this vital process has led to incorporation of inclinometry into the *American Medical Association Guides to the Evaluation of Permanent Impairment*, bringing a recognition of compound spinal movement, repeatable measurement, and normative data base to this process.[6, 37] Both mechanical and computerized inclinometers are currently commercially available from multiple manufacturers, with more expensive three-dimensional digitizers also available for obtaining accurate

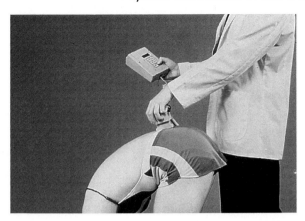

Fig. 35-1

The Cybex EDI-320 computerized inclinometer performs simple angular measurements on *continuous mode,* but also contains a microprocessor for utilizing the single optical scanner to be used for *compound mode* measurements.

regional spinal AROM and PROM measurements (Fig. 35-1).

Isolated Spinal Strength Tests

Literature on isolated spinal strength testing continues to grow dramatically.* Most work on spinal strength measurements have been performed on "trunk strength" measurement devices for assessing torque-production capability through a number of planes and a variety of static positions or dynamic movements. Torque is assessed around an axis usually placed at, or near, the lumbosacral junction with forces applied to the mid- to lower-thoracic spinal region. The anatomic justification for this choice appears to be the occurrence of true bilateral anatomy below the waist and above the lower border of the scapulae. However, it is also worth noting that strength performance in the cervical spine, necessary for stabilizing the head on the trunk, may also be worthy of measurement for patients having cervical and cervicothoracic deconditioning. While tools available for this purpose are less available and reliable than those used for the lumbar spine, a variety of hand-held dynamometers, and at least one computerized device, can be used for static *isometric* cervical strength measurements.[26] It is important to note here, however, that most patients with cervicothoracic injuries producing prolonged disability generally have their debilitation-deconditioning caused more by upper extremity and shoulder girdle dysfunctions than by cervical vertebral dysfunc-

tion, even though performance of both regions may be closely interrelated.

Irrespective of the region and measurement method chosen, two key points appear to be established:

1. Spinal muscle strength is one important physical performance measurement differentiating normals in patients.[2,26] Extensor deficits generally are greater than flexor deficits in the lumbar spine; axial deficits are least significant. Dynamic strength deficits are generally accompanied by even more dramatic endurance and agility deficits;

2. Because of the lack of visual feedback, mechanical devices to indirectly measure trunk strength objectively are increasingly recognized as essential for rehabilitation and work-capacity evaluations.

This brief chapter does not allow detailed discussion of the various devices currently available commercially for research or clinical use in testing isolated spinal strength or lifting capacity. We have reviewed these devices including effort factors and normative data in detail elsewhere.[21] However, it is important to point out that the back presents an area where the tools of measurement themselves have raised controversy over perceived commercial exploitation. It is clear that the various devices for measuring trunk strength will be ultimately recognized simply as measurement tools, as useful to the spine-muscle clinician/researcher as a treadmill/EKG is to the cardiologist.[9,30] An example of one of the newest such devices is shown, demonstrating a "modular unit" for back testing that can be attached to a dynamometer (Fig. 35-2). The Cybex dynamometer in turn, can also be connected to modules for extremity testing.

For the purposes of this chapter, the reader should recognize the difference between strength (and ROM) of an injured region, *physical capacity* of a particular region of the body versus *functional capacity* associated with whole body ADLs involving the injured area. As an analogy, injury to the knee generally produces vital losses of mobility and support muscle strength (quadriceps/hamstrings) relevant to the injured joint. In contrast, the most critical functional ADLs associated with the rehabilitated knee are activities such as walking, running, climbing, and "cutting." While one strives to rehabilitate for the ultimate performance of these functional ADLs, primary attention is focused on regaining the BEPs of the injured area. In this regard, serial measurements of knee motion and strength (isometric, isokinetic, or isoin-

*References: 5, 11, 20, 28, 33, 34, and 36.

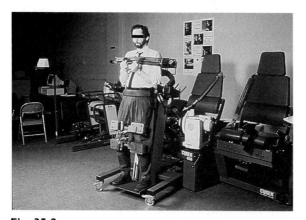

Fig. 35-2

The Cybex modular sagittal trunk extension/flexion (TEF) frame can be attached to the Cybex 6000 dynamometer, permitting both concentric and eccentric thoracolumbar sagittal strength measurements.

be very useful, aided by comparison to the presumed "normal" contralateral side providing intraindividual control. While spinal-strength measurements do not permit use of intraindividual control, large normative data bases tied to the specific spinal-strength measurement device have been derived and published by numerous research groups.

Lifting Tests

The previously discussed tests of mobility and strength focus primarily on the alterations in the localized spinal region induced by injury or disuse. Measurement of whole-body task performance represents the interaction of multiple functional unit "links in the biomechanical chain." Generic *functional capacity* tests involve all the major body functions which comprise components of more complex ADLs, including bending, climbing, reaching, lifting, pushing/pulling, running, sitting, etc. The clinician has two vital tasks in choosing *functional capacity tests* corresponding to a given injured joint or region: (1) choose the most *relevant* task(s); (2) choose tasks for which measurement devices and protocols permit *accurate* measurement, including some *effort assessment*.[12] *Lifting tests,* in this regard, appear to be among the most relevant and measurable functional tasks associated with spinal deconditioning, since they represent the transmission of forces from handling manual materials to foot-floor contact. The lumbar region is most involved in forces moved from floor to waist, while the cervicothoracic and shoulder-girdle region is most involved in movement from waist to overhead. While the body may utilize *substitution* of better performance by one body link for deficits in another (as in the case of

encouraging squatting rather than bending after a back injury), this acute choice is not necessarily the optimal biomechanical response to prolonged disability. Substitution may require frequent conscious compromises of function that predispose to recurrent injury. Optimal physical capacity involves the highest possible performance of *each* functional unit involved in a task and a relearning of coordination/agility dimensions linking the functional units to provide maximum safety and efficiency.

One approach taken at the Productive Rehabilitation Institute of Dallas for Ergonomics (PRIDE) is to perform multiple tests of varying complexity to examine a single task. A case in point is the examination of lifting, which has been implicated as a key risk factor in 60 to 70% of back injuries. Three separate tests of lifting are used, all performed along standardized protocols in the sagittal plane. An *isometric* test sequence is performed according to the NIOSH guidelines produced by Chaffin and colleagues.[4, 13] *Isokinetic* tests are performed using the Cybex Liftask, until very recently the only available isokinetic lifting device.[16, 21] Finally, a progressive *isoinertial* lifting evaluation (PILE) is performed to simulate "real world" lifting while using a standardized protocol controlling vertical distance, weight, and duration of lift to produce comparable data (Fig. 35-3).[22-24] Tests are normalized to age, gender, and body weight variables.

Other Tests

Aerobic capacity is an important factor in disability.[3] Inactivity leads to loss of cardiovascular performance also, particularly in older individuals spending unusual amounts of time reclining in order to protect painful spinal segments. Aerobic capacity tests can be performed using a variety of protocols with treadmill or bicycle ergometers. Oxygen consumption and fitness levels may be derived from standardized tables.

Position and activity tolerance is another area of interest in functional task measurement directed towards return to productivity. Following spine surgery, patients often cannot tolerate prolonged static positioning (sitting/standing) and often complain of an inability to perform various generic functional tasks such as squatting, pushing/pulling, carrying, or climbing. The PRIDE group has devised an obstacle course requiring the use of multiple positions in an attempt to assess the patient's tolerance of a variety of positions and daily living activities.

Measurement of *endurance* or *fatigue resistance* remains an elusive, but desirable goal. Ever sine the work of Ortengren, the use of electromyogram

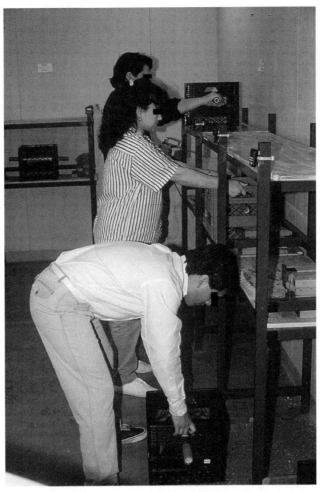

Fig. 35-3
Individual performing the PILE test using inexpensive equipment and a standardized protocol.

(EMG) spectral analysis has been touted as a potentially viable direct measurement of muscular endurance.[31, 35] However, controversy exists about the enthusiastic claims of earlier researchers, as direct comparison of sustained isometric maximum voluntary contractions with myoelectric spectral analysis has indicated that power spectrum change is much better correlated with *load* than with *fatigue*.[19,27] While sophisticated analyses of EMG signals offer exciting research potential for assessing muscle function, the many *sources of error* inherent in these measurements currently preclude any short-term promise of clinical implementation.

Summary

Quantification of physical function represents a new and important tool in assessing patients with chronic disabling low-back pain. Although measurements are in a relatively early stage of development and standardization, experience with extremity rehabilitation suggests that these tests will, become in time, an important supplement to our sophisticated but expensive imaging devices. Quantification of physical and functional capacity requires patient motivation, but since an "effort factor" can be identified with each functional capacity test, suboptimal effort can be recognized and used to validate actual test scores.[12,14]

Injury to soft-tissue spinal structures leads to debilitation and deconditioning through a combination of physically and psychosocially mediated mechanisms. These mechanisms produce a "weak link" in the *physical capacity* of the injured spinal (and/or extremity) region(s) which may lead to decreases in relevant *functional capacities*. Even if functional capacity can be maintained in short bursts, lowered *efficiency* of ADL performance can be anticipated in the long run. Recognition of the problem, through the appropriate measurement of physical and functional capacity, permits appropriate *prevention* and *functional restoration* modalities to combat this process. The ultimate goal is the elimination of disability associated with spinal disorders.

References

1. Beals R: Compensation and recovery from injury, *West J Med* 104:223, 1984.

2. Brady S, Mayer T, Gatchel R: Physical progress and residual impairment quantification after functional restoration, part II: isokinetic trunk strength, *Spine* 19:365, 1994.

3. Cady L and others: Strength and fitness and subsequent back injuries in firefighters, *J Occup Med* 21:269, 1979.

4. Chaffin D: Pre-employment strength testing: updated position, *J Occup Med* 10:105, 1978.

5. Davies G, Gould J: Trunk testing using a prototype cybex II isokinetic stabilization system, *J Orthop Sports Phys Ther* 3:164, 1982.

6. Doege T, editor: *American Medical Association Guides to the Evaluation of Permanent Impairment,* ed 3 rev, Chicago, AMA Press, 1990.

7. Dvorak J and others: Age and gender related normal motion of the cervical spine, *Spine* 17:S393, 1992.

8. Fordyce W, Roberts A, Sternbach R: The behavioral management of chronic pain: a response to critics, *Pain* 22:113, 1985.

9. Frymoyer J, Gordon S: *New perspectives on low back pain,* Chicago, 1988, AAOS Publication.

10. Hadler N: *Occupational Musculoskeletal Disorders,* New York, 1993, Raven Press.

11. Hasue M, Fujiwara M, Kikuchi S: A new method of quantitative measurement of abdominal back muscle strength, *Spine* 5:143, 1980.

12. Hazard R, Reeves V, Fenwick J: Lifting capacity indices of subject effort, *Spine* 17:1065, 1992.

13. Hazard R and others: *Functional restoration with behavioral support: a one-year perspective study of chronic low back pain patients.* Presented at the National Society for the Study of the Lumbar Spine, Miami, April, 1988.

14. Hazard R and others: Isokinetic trunk and lifting strength measurements: variability as an indicator of effort, *Spine* 13:54, 1988.

15. Keeley J and others: Quantification of lumbar function part five: reliability of range of motion measures in the sagittal plane and an *in vivo* torso rotation measurement technique, *Spine* 11:31, 1986.

16. Kishino N and others: Quantification of lumbar function part four: isometric and isokinetic lifting simulation in normal subjects and low back dysfunction patients, *Spine* 10:921, 1985.

17. Kondraske G: Human performance: measurement, science, concepts and computerized methodology, *Neurology* (in press).

18. Kondraske G: *Towards a standard clinical measure of postural stability.* In Kondraske G, Robison C, editors: *Proceedings of the Eighth Annual Conference of the IEEE Engineering in Medicine and Biology Society.* 3:1579, 1986.

19. Kondraske G and others: Myoelectric spectral analysis for human lumbar muscle fatigue assessment, *Arch Phys Med Rehabil* 68:103, 1987.

20. Lagrana N, Lee C: Isokinetic evaluation of trunk muscles, *Spine* 9:143, 1980.

21. Mayer T, Gatchel R: *Functional restoration for spinal disorders: the sports medicine approach to low back pain,* Philadelphia, 1988, Lea & Febiger.

22. Mayer T and others: Progressive isoinertial lifting evaluation, part I: a standardized protocol and normative database, *Spine* 13:993, 1988.

23. Mayer T and others: Progressive isoinertial lifting evaluation, part two: a comparison with isokinetic lifting in a disabled chronic low back pain industrial population, *Spine* 13:998, 1988.

24. Mayer T and others: Progressive isoinertial lifting evaluation: an erratum, *Spine* 15:5, 1990.

25. Mayer T and others: Noninvasive measurement of cervical tri-planar motion in normal subjects, *Spine* 18(15):2191, 1993.

26. Mayer T and others: A male incumbent worker industrial database, part II: cervical spinal physical capacity, *Spine* 19(7):765, 1994.

27. Mayer T and others: Lumbar myoelectric spectral analysis for endurance assessment: a comparison of normals to deconditioned patients, *Spine* 14:986, 1989.

28. Mayer T and others: Quantification of lumbar function part two: sagittal plant trunk strength in chronic low back pain patients, *Spine* 9:588, 1984.

29. Mayer T and others: Use of noninvasive techniques for quantification of spinal range-of-motion in normal subjects and chronic low-back patients, *Spine* 9:588, 1984.

30. Mayer T and others: Comparison of CT scan muscle measurements and isokinetic trunk strength in postoperative patients, *Spine* 14:33, 1989.

31. Ortengren R, Andersson B: Electromyographic studies of trunk muscles with special reference to functional anatomy of lumbar spine, *Spine* 2:44, 1977.

32. Polatin P: *Affective disorders in back pain.* In Mayer T, Mooney V, Gatchel R, editors: *Contemporary conservative care for painful spinal disorders,* Philadelphia, 1991, Lea & Febiger, p149.

33. Smidt G and others: Assessment of abdominal and back extensor function: a quantitative approach and results for chronic low-back patients, *Spine* 8:211, 1983.

34. Smith S and others: Quantification of lumbar function part I: isometric and multi-speed isokinetic trunk strength measures in sagittal and axial planes in normal subject patients, *Spine* 10:757, 1985.

35. Stulen F, DeLuca C: Muscle fatigue monitor: noninvasive device for observing localized muscular fatigue, *IEEE Trans Biomed Eng* BME-29:760, 1982.

36. Thorstensson A, Arvidson A: Trunk muscle strength and low-back pain, *Scand J Rehab Med* 14:69, 1982.

37. Waddell G and others: Objective clinical evaluation of physical impairment in chronic low back pain, *Spine* 17:617, 1992.

Chapter 36

Psychosocial Correlates of the Deconditioning Syndrome in Patients with Chronic Low-Back Pain

Robert J. Gatchel

As has been noted elsewhere, more than 90% of the time, back pain is a brief, time-limited condition for which the treatment chosen often appears irrelevant to the outcome.[6,10] From the onset of symptoms, about half the patients with acute low-back pain (LBP) are no longer disabled within 2 weeks, 70% have recovered in 1 month, and about 90% within 3 to 4 months. Yet, of those whose symptoms persist for more than 3 to 4 months, about 50% to 60% continue to be disabled at the end of the year, and the majority of these continue to be disabled after 2 years. For these individuals, extensive medical treatment, compensation costs, and settlement awards follow that make their contribution to the problem disproportionate to that of the entire group suffering acute LBP. Indeed, 10% of the cases cost about 80% of the compensation money in a variety of industries.[6,10] It is also these patients who demonstrate a "psychologic cascade" of problems that make them quite difficult and challenging to treat effectively.

Elsewhere in this text, Mayer has discussed the deconditioning syndrome that often develops in these patients, leading to their chronic disability. The longer the period of initial immobilization and inactivity, the greater the likelihood of developing dysfunctional behaviors. These dysfunctional behaviors may then be succeeded by further loss of physical capacity indices such as motion, strength, endurance, and agility. The longer the period of such inactivity, the greater the opportunity for disuse to create physical capacity deficits leading to decreased performance. This physical deconditioning is a progressive process related to disuse, with "mental" or psychologic deconditioning following as a natural consequence, and concurrently contributing to the development of dysfunctional behaviors and chronic disability. This chapter will discuss the psychosocial correlates of this deconditioning syndrome.

Mental Deconditioning

In addition to the physical deconditioning that can develop as a consequence of chronicity and disuse in patients with LBP, a collateral form of mental deconditioning also occurs.[6] This refers to the development of a "layer" of behavioral and psychologic problems that occur in response to the chronic pain and the patient's attempts to cope with it. These problems prevent the individual from maintaining a productive lifestyle. They prompt cessation or disuse of normal functioning, with all psychologic resources being expended in an attempt to deal with the prolonged pain and disability. In a sense, an "atrophy" of normal psychosocial functioning is present.

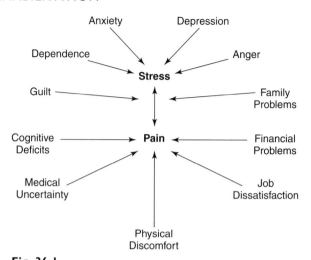

Fig. 36-1

Psychosocioeconomic factors magnifying the stress– chronic pain cycle.

Fordyce and Steger initially noted an important variable that differentiated acute pain from chronic pain—the type of anxiety experienced by the patient.[5] In acute pain experiences, anxiety increases as pain intensity increases, which is then followed by a reduction in anxiety after treatment begins. A reduction in anxiety generally results in a decrease in pain sensation. Thus, a cycle of pain reduction, followed by anxiety reduction, resulting in still more pain reduction, and so on is manifest. This cycle, however, is different for patients with chronic pain. For these patients, the initial anxiety associated with the pain persists, and eventually may result in feelings of greater anxiety, despair, and helplessness because of the health-care system's failure to alleviate the pain. This may stimulate a cascade of additional psychosocial problems that greatly complicate effective treatment of these patients. These may include a complex array of psychosocioeconomic problems that "feed into" this pain–stress relationship (Fig. 36-1).

Evidence that distinguishes patients with chronic pain from those with acute pain suggests that the former develop specific psychologic problems secondary to failed attempts to alleviate their pain. For example, Sternach and colleagues compared the Minnesota Multiphsic Personality Inventory (MMPI) profiles of a group of patients with acute LBP (pain present for less than 6 months) with those of a group of patients with chronic LBP (more than 6 months).[15] Results indicated significant differences between the two groups on the first three clinical scales (hypochondriasis, depression, and hysteria). The combined elevation of these three scales is often referred to as the "neurotic triad" because it is com-

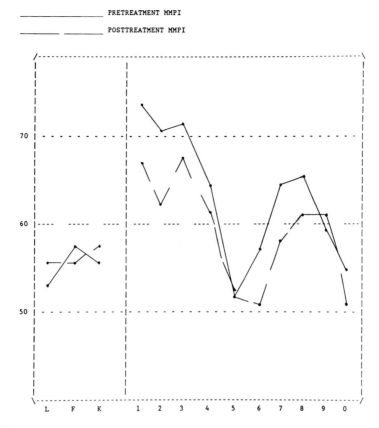

PRETREATMENT MMPI

POSTTREATMENT MMPI

Fig. 36-2

MMPI profile scores of patients before and after successful functional restoration treatment. *(From Barnes D and others: Changes in MMPI profile levels of chronic low back pain patients following successful treatment; J. Spine Dis, 3:353, 1990.)*

monly found in neurotic individuals who are experiencing a great deal of anxiety. These results indicate that during the early stages of pain, no major psychologic problems are manifest. However, as the pain becomes chronic in nature, psychologic changes begin to occur. These changes are most likely caused by the constant discomfort, despair, and preoccupation with the pain that comes to dominate the lives of these patients.

We found similar results from research conducted on patients with chronic LBP who participated in a functional restoration program at the Productive Rehabilitation Institute of Dallas for Ergonomics (PRIDE).[1] In this study, the first three clinical scales of the MMPI were significantly elevated before the start of the treatment program. However, a followup evaluation at 6 months after successful completion of this program showed these scales to be significantly *decreased* to normal levels (Fig. 36-2). Thus, these findings again suggest that the elevations of MMPI scores are most likely caused by the trauma and stress associated with the chronic pain

condition and not by some stable psychologic traits. When these patients with chronic pain are successfully treated, their MMPI scale elevations disappear.

The above results, therefore, suggest that one of the consequences of dealing with chronic pain is the development of emotional reactions such as anxiety and dysphoria produced by the long-term "wearing down" effects and drain of psychologic resources. This may produce a layer of behavioral and psychologic problems over the original nociception or pain experience itself. It is now generally accepted that chronic LBP is a complex phenomenon that does not merely result from some specific structural cause.

Biopsychosocial Conceptualizations of Pain

Indeed, Loeser originally formulated a model outlining four dimensions associated with the concept of pain: nociception, pain, suffering, and pain behavior.[9] *Nociception* refers to the actual physical units (chemical, mechanical, or thermal) that impact specialized nerve fibers and signal the central nervous system (CNS) that an aversive event has occurred. *Pain* is viewed by Loeser as the sensation arising as the result of perceived nociception. However, Loeser's definition of pain can be viewed as overly simplistic and less than certain because sometimes pain is perceived in the absence of nociception (e.g., phantom limb pain), or conversely, when nociception occurs without being perceived (an individual being severely wounded without immediately becoming aware of significant pain). Thus, pain is a much more complex phenomenon.

Nociception is meant to act as a signal to the CNS and represents a complex interaction within the CNS. In contrast, suffering and pain behavior are reactions to these phenomena that can be affected by past experiences as well as anticipation of future events. Specifically, according to Loeser, *suffering* refers to the emotional responses that are triggered by nociception or some other aversive event associated with it such as fear, threat, or loss. Because of a specific painful episode, the individual may lose his or her job and, as a consequence, develop anxiety and depression. *Pain behavior* refers to those things that people do or avoid doing when they are suffering or are in pain. For example, they may avoid exercise or any extended activity for fear of reinjury.

This biopsychosocial conceptual model of pain, which includes physical, psychologic, and social elements, moves away from an overly simplistic physical disease model of pain, and replaces it with an alternative multidimensional model. It draws upon the biopsychosocial concept of illness originally proposed by Engel.[3] A similar model has been presented by Waddell in discussing the treatment of chronic LBP.[16] Figure 36-3 presents these models.

A Physical and Mental Deconditioning Model of Low-Back Pain Disability

To date, little empirical research has been conducted to evaluate the above models or to assess the progression or development of the mental deconditioning process. Figure 36-4 represents my conceptual model, proposing a number of stages that may be involved.[6] The model is yet untested, but does present a number of directly testable hypotheses and important treatment implications. As can be seen, Stage 1 consists of emotional reactions such as fear, anxiety, and worry, that result as a consequence of the perception of pain. Pain or hurt is usually associated with

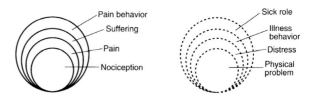

Fig. 36-3

The biopsychosocial conceptual models of pain and illness. *(From Waddell G: A new clinical model for the treatment of low-back pain,* Spine 12:63, 1987.)*

harm, and a very natural emotional reaction to the potential for the physical harm exists. Pain that persists past a reasonable acute period of time leads to progression into Stage 2. This stage is associated with a wider array of behavioral and psychologic reactions and problems, such as learned helplessness and depression, anger and distrust, and somatization, which are the result of suffering with the now chronic nature of the pain. It should be noted that a major assertion of this model is that the form these problems take primarily depends upon the *premorbid* or pre-existing personality and psychologic characteristics of the individual, as well as current socioeconomic and environmental conditions. Thus, an individual with a premorbid depressive personality who is seriously affected economically by loss of a job because of pain and disability, experiences depressive symptoms that are greatly exacerbated during this stage. Similarly, an individual who had premorbid hypochondriac characteristics, and who receives a great deal of secondary gain remaining disabled, will most likely display a great deal of somatization and symptom magnification. Environmental factors also may be quite important. For example, one of the major environmental factors that may play an important role is the presence or absence of social support, because social support has been shown to significantly buffer individuals from the impact of stress.[7] Other such environmental factors might be the secondary gain involved in being excused from normal responsibilities and obligations.

Obviously, this model does *not* propose that there is a preexisting "pain personality"; it is congruous with a great deal of research that has not found any such consistent personality syndrome. Rather, patients bring with them certain predisposing personality and psychologic characteristics (i.e., they have a *diathesis*) that is exacerbated by the stress of attempting to cope with the chronic pain. Basically, then, this is a *diathesis–stress* model of chronic pain. Indeed, the relationship between stress and exacerbation of mental-health problems has been documented in the scientific literature.[7] This is not to say

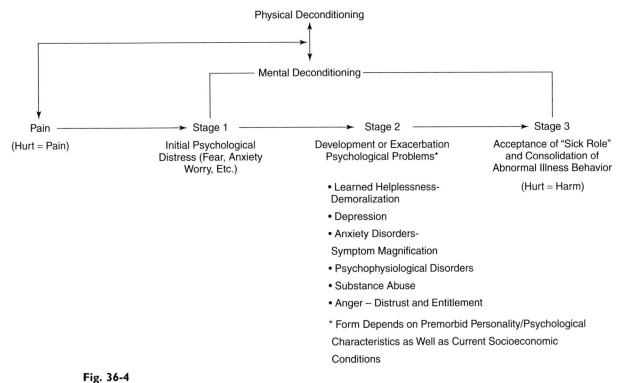

Fig. 36-4

Gatchel's conceptual model of the progression of the mental deconditioning process, and its interaction with physical deconditioning. *(From Gatchel RJ: Early development of physical and mental deconditioning in painful spinal disorders. In Mayer TG, Mooney V, Gatchel RJ, editors:* Contemporary conservative care for painful spinal disorders, *Philadelphia, 1991, Lea & Febiger.)*

that predisposing factors make chronic LBP a functional disorder and that it is "all in the patient's head." The chronic problem represents a complex interaction between physical factors and psychosocioeconomic variables.

Returning to our discussion of Fig. 36-4, as this "layer" of behavioral and psychologic problems persists, progression into Stage 3 manifests. This stage can be viewed as the acceptance or adoption of a sick role during which time the patient is excused from normal responsibilities and social obligations. This may become a potent reinforcer for not becoming healthy. The medical and psychologic disabilities (abnormal illness behaviors) are consolidated during this phase. Moreover, if compensation issues are still present, these behaviors can also serve as a disincentive for not becoming well again because compensation may be a critical factor in the persistence of disability.[2]

Superimposed on these stages is the physical deconditioning syndrome, which has been discussed in another chapter of this volume. Usually, a two-way pathway exists between the physical deconditioning and mental deconditioning processes. For example,

research has demonstrated clearly that physical deconditioning can feed back, negatively affecting the emotional well-being and self-esteem of individuals.[7] This can lead to further mental deconditioning. Conversely, negative emotional reactions such as depression can significantly feed back to physical functioning by, for example, decreasing the motivation to get involved in work or recreational activities and thereby further contributing to physical deconditioning.

Finally, these physical and mental deconditioning effects can also feed back to the initial pain perception process. For example, if the individual suddenly engages in an activity that produces acute soreness or tenderness, the activity may be erroneously interpreted as harmful. This can then retrigger or reinforce the emotions and psychologic problems associated with the other stages. Indeed, clinical researchers such as Fordyce suggest that patients with chronic pain must learn that hurt and harm are not the same thing.[4] They must be reeducated not to accept the traditional dogma that pain is always a warning signal. Pain often accompanies the early stages of physical reconditioning and does not necessarily mean that some physical harm is being produced.

Psychiatric Illness and Chronic Low-Back Pain Disability

The above conceptual model highlights the important role that psychosocial variables can play in the LBP disability process, especially as chronicity develops. With this model in mind, we have begun to evaluate systematically the relationship between psychopathology and chronic LBP disability because of its important treatment implications. In a recent study, Polatin and colleagues evaluated *DSM-III-R* disorders in a group of 200 with chronic LBP.[14] The American Psychiatric Association currently advocates the use of the *DSM-III-R* to express psychiatric diagnoses. Results of this study were quite striking in that high rates of psychopathology were found in these patients. For example, Table 36-1 presents the current and lifetime prevalence rates of major forms of psychopathology in these patients. As can be seen, even when the somewhat controversial category of somatoform pain disorder was excluded, 77% of the patients met lifetime diagnostic criteria and 59% demonstrated current symptoms for at least one psychiatric diagnosis. The most common of these diagnoses were major depression, substance abuse, and anxiety disorders. Additionally, 51% met criteria for at least one personality disorder. All these prevalence rates were significantly above base rates found for the general population.

Another extremely interesting finding in this study, besides the high rate of psychopathology, was that some of the patients with a positive lifetime history of psychiatric syndromes appeared to manifest these syndromes *prior* to the onset of back pain (54% of those with depression, 94% of those with substance abuse, and 95% of those with anxiety disorders). Such results are consistent with the earlier presented conceptual model of pre-existing psychologic disorders exacerbated by the stress of chronic pain. Of course, this was not a prospective study, and, therefore, these results cannot directly answer the question of whether psychopathologic disorders in patients with chronic pain is a consequence of experiencing the chronic pain, or whether preexisting disorders act as a "predisposition" to developing chronicity. We are currently conducting a prospective study that more directly addresses this issue.

Assessment and Treatment Implications

Just as one must address the important physical deconditioning issues in order to treat patients with chronic LBP effectively, one must be aware simultaneously of the significant mental deconditioning issues that are contributing to the chronicity. As reviewed above, one must be prepared to expect the presence of psychopathology in many patients with chronic LBP. Indeed, as illustrated in Fig. 36-4, a patient may progress through a number of stages as the pain and disability becomes more chronic. These stages may create formidable barriers to recovery if they are not effectively dealt with. The box below summarizes these barriers to recovery.

Barriers to Recovery: Important Psychosocial Concomitants of Chronic Low-Back Pain Disability

- General psychologic issues
- Compliance or resistance issues
- Financial disincentives
- Somatization or symptom magnification
- General emotional reactions
- Depression
- Anxiety and fear
- Anger
- Entitlement

Table 36-1
Lifetime and current prevalence rates of major psychiatric disorders in patients with chronic low-back pain

	Lifetime	Current
Somatoform disorders	99%	100%
Effective disorders	68%	49%
Substance abuse disorders	36%	19%
Anxiety disorders	19%	17%
Psychotic disorders	3%	3%

General Psychologic Issues

One can safely assume that the majority of patients in a chronic pain population (and who are not working or receiving compensation) are depressed and demoralized by their present physical, psychologic, and socioeconomic status. Only a small percentage of patients are consciously malingering or "faking" for personal gains. Indeed, most researchers agree that true malingering as a voluntary attempt to falsify symptoms and as a means of achieving some specific goal such as a case settlement is a rare phenomenon.[12,13]

By the time most patients reach a rehabilitation program, their lack of progress has left them with low self-esteem, feeling frustrated and discouraged, and almost always with significant and severe financial hardship. Most patients have been to several physicians, often receiving conflicting information in the process, resulting in frustration and distrust of medical systems. In addition, adversarial interactions in the workplace or with insurance companies may have left many patients feeling betrayed and cheated. Furthermore, longstanding work, family, and self-esteem issues come into play when the patient is injured and not fulfilling his or her usual social roles. All these experiences can lead to psychologic barriers to recovery. Once assessed, these barriers must be dealt with directly through a variety of interventions.

Compliance and Resistance Issues

Unlike athletes, who usually have to be restrained from doing too much too quickly, patients with chronic back disability tend to be reluctant to "work through" their pain. Often, this is related to fears of reinjury, depression, or other psychosocial barriers to recovery. In the early stages of treatment, when fear and trust are usually major issues for the patient, noncompliance or failure to progress is dealt with in a supportive and educational manner. A great deal of time and effort is spent explaining the treatment rationale to the patients, and working with them in a collaborative manner. At the same time, however, staff members must establish their roles as trained and experienced professionals who are experts so they can encourage patients to increase physical activity.

Financial Disincentives

A major set of barriers to recovery revolves around financial disincentives. Indeed, there can be no doubt that financial compensation may be a critical factor in the persistence of disability. Such disincentives serve as secondary gains for not getting better. Many patients entering a treatment program or evaluation procedure are receiving some type of financial supplement that will cease once the patient is no longer medically restricted from working. When the amount of the supplement approaches the patient's usual earnings, or is sufficient to support the patient's lifestyle, the economic incentive for returning to work is often removed. Patients may be involved in some type of injury-related litigation, which may or may not be affected by appearing "disabled" and in pain.

An anticipated monetary settlement may alter the patient's customary behavior patterns, slowing recovery, and increasing pain complaints. In many cases, such behaviors, if not arrested early, may lead to "illness behaviors" that are difficult to reverse.

Other financial disincentives or secondary gains for not getting better include hoping for early retirement, having loans paid by disability insurance, and hoping for a new or better job based on the patient being too "disabled" to perform the old job. The specifics of these financial issues vary, depending on state laws and whether the patient is involved in state, federal, Social Security, long-term disability, or FELA compensation systems. The treatment staff must be aware of financial disincentives for each patient because these issues have a major influence on motivation, pain reports, and adherence to treatment.

Somatization and Symptom Magnification Versus Malingering

As a result of multiple barriers to recovery, progressing the patient toward full physical functioning may be difficult at times. Moreover, psychosocial influences may lead the patient to be irritable, dependent, passive, or noncompliant, all of which may significantly tax the patience of health-care professionals. At these times the temptation exists to view these patients as malingerers and fakes. To maintain the sense of respect for the patient that is vital in any form of intensive treatment, it is important to understand that these individuals use their physical symptoms as a way of dealing with, and communicating about, their emotional lives (*somatization*). That is to say, in this type of symptom magnification, physical symptoms may be easier to accept as causing current unhappiness and discontent than admitting that some psychologic reason is contributing to it. Only rarely is a patient consciously "faking" disability, although many times symptoms may be exaggerated consciously or unconsciously. Symptoms may also be magnified as a way of "saving face" and justifying continued disability after a long period of dysfunction. This may, therefore, reflect conscious or unconscious illness-affirming aspects of the abnormal illness behavior. These processes are most apparent in the realm of self-report pain measures. It is essential for treatment personnel (e.g., the psychologist) to delineate carefully such issues and develop an appropriate strategy to deal with them effectively. It should also be noted that the issue of symptom magnification is so important in the area of chronic pain and disability that it is generating a great deal of research interest.

General Emotional Reactions

Certain emotional reactions can be expected in most patients with chronic LBP. The intensity of these reactions must be adequately assessed for all patients because it can greatly affect the treatment process. Assessment is essential for developing a comprehensive clinical picture of the patient. Indeed, adequately assessing and dealing with the emotional fallout of the patient's upheaval in lifestyle is important in every treatment approach. These important emotional reactions are described below.

Depression

Almost all patients with chronic back pain will be depressed to some degree (whether they acknowledge these feelings or not) because of the multiple losses they have sustained. Besides material and financial losses, these patients have lost jobs, family roles, important sources of their self-image and self-esteem, and, in some cases, their belief in "the system" (medical and otherwise). A severe, debilitating level of depression may have to be temporarily treated with antidepressant medication. This will have to be carefully evaluated and monitored by the medical and psychological staff.

Anxiety and Fear

Along with depression, almost all patients experience some degree of anxiety and fear. Often, a great fear of reinjury may significantly affect any effort in the physical reconditioning component of the program. Also, general anxiety is hardly surprising given the level of disruption that patients experience in their lives. Furthermore, lack of closure regarding the long-term effects of the injury on finances, careers, relationships, and physical capacity adds to patients' concerns.

Anger

Anger is perhaps the most obvious reaction among this population. There is usually a great deal of anger at the workplace, which may be longstanding, or may result from real or perceived mistreatment since the injury. By the time most of these patients reach a comprehensive rehabilitation program, they have also developed an adversarial relationship with their insurance company that leads to an intensification and generalization of anger. Frustration with the lack of physical progress and lack of consistency in medical treatment can produce dissatisfaction with medical systems in general. This same lack of progress leads to anger at family and friends, who may imply, because of the invisible nature of the physical handicap, that they are faking the injury. It is important for treatment staff to be sensitive to this anger and to defuse it whenever possible.

Entitlement

Along with a sense of anger, patients often have a sense of entitlement. This comes not only from the longstanding psychologic issues mentioned earlier, but also from a sense of feeling misunderstood, cheated, and betrayed. The financial and material losses they have sustained add to the belief that someone (or everyone) involved in the compensation process "owes me." Again, this emotional reaction must be adequately assessed because it can seriously jeopardize progression through a rehabilitation program.

The above barriers to recovery and emotional reactions obviously need to be dealt with for rehabilitation to progress smoothly. Often, when a suboptimal effort is manifest in physical rehabilitation, or when compliance is a problem, the barriers to recovery and emotional issues need to be addressed. Various psychologic treatment techniques have been developed and proved to be successful in dealing with these issues.

Multimodal Disability Management

I have described a Multimodal Disability Management Program (MDMP) elsewhere.[8,10] It is based on a cognitive–behavioral approach to crisis intervention, and focuses on overcoming physical and psychosocial difficulties that interfere with returning to a functional, productive lifestyle. Treatment issues deal with events in the present or the recent past, and patients are helped to understand how thoughts contribute to feelings and behaviors. Within this framework, therapists also maintain an awareness of early learning experiences and longstanding psychologic issues that can affect reactions to recent life experiences. For example, many patients come from family backgrounds in which there was some significant emotional deprivation. As a result, many experience chronic feelings of anger, depression, and low self-esteem. Relatedly, they also have a sense of entitlement stemming from a frustrated search for an idealized caretaker. These issues, along with the cognitions and emotions accompanying them, are rekindled quickly when the patients find themselves involved in a medical/compensation/disability system that fosters dependency.

The MDMP approach focuses on the disability associated with the pain behavior, and not merely the experience of pain. Basically, there are four major areas in this approach:

1. Individual and group counseling emphasizing a crisis intervention model (e.g., coping with family problems and unemployment).

2. Family counseling, during which family members are encouraged to take an active part in the rehabilitation process and are provided with information about the philosophy and specific details of MDMP.

3. Behavioral stress-management training that involves initial training in muscle relaxation, followed by exercises in guided imagery in which patients practice relaxing while imagining themselves in various stressful situations. Patients also receive EMG/temperature biofeedback sessions during which they refine their relaxation skills, with the understanding that these skills will help them cope more effectively with residual pain and discomfort.

4. Cognitive–behavioral skills training that includes instruction in assertiveness, rational versus irrational thinking, and stress and time management.

The above cognitive–behavioral treatment methods have been found to be effective when used in the overall context of functional restoration treatment approach.[10,11] In administering such treatment, however, it should be clearly kept in mind that each patient is unique and must be evaluated individually so the treatment program can be carefully tailored. Blindly administering the same disability management program to all patients, regardless of unique individual needs, will guarantee failure.

Summary

As we have discussed, the longer the period of initial immobilization and inactivity, the greater the likelihood that a patient with LBP will develop various dysfunctional behaviors associated with physical capacity indices such as motion, strength, endurance, and agility. Moreover, the development of mental deconditioning, and its interaction with physical deconditioning, in the progression from an acute-pain episode to a chronic stage can occur. The greater the opportunity for disuse to create physical capacity deficits leading to decreased performance, the greater the likelihood of a variety of psychosocial concomitants such as depression, medication abuse, and disability habituation. A comprehensive treatment approach must be used for the patient who has progressed to this stage of chronic disability.

References

1. Barnes D and others: Changes in MMPI profile levels of chronic low back pain patients following successful treatment, *J Spine Dis* 3:3, 1990.
2. Beals R: Compensation and recovery from injury, *West J Med* 140:233, 1984.
3. Engel GL: The need for a new medical model: a challenge for biomedicine, *Science* 196:129, 1977.
4. Fordyce WE: Pain and suffering: a reappraisal, *Am Psychol* 43:276, 1988.
5. Fordyce WE, Steger JC: Chronic pain. In Pomerleau OF, Brady JP, editors: *Behavioral medicine: theory and practice,* Baltimore, 1979, Williams & Wilkins.
6. Gatchel RJ: *Early development of physical and mental deconditioning in painful spinal disorders.* In Mayer TG, Mooney V, Gatchel RJ, editors: *Contemporary conservative care for painful spinal disorders,* Philadelphia, 1991, Lea & Febiger.
7. Gatchel RJ, Baum A, Krantz D: *Introduction to health psychology,* ed 2, New York, 1988, Random House.
8. Gatchel RJ, Mayer TG: Functional restoration for chronic low back pain. Part II: Multimodal disability management, *Pain Manage,* 2:136, 1989.
9. Loeser JD: Concepts of pain. In Stanton-Hicks J, Boaz R, editors: *Chronic low back pain,* New York, 1982, Raven Press.
10. Mayer TG, Gatchel RJ: *Functional restoration for spinal disorders: the sports medicine approach,* Philadelphia, 1988, Lea & Febiger.
11. Mayer T and other: A prospective randomized two year study of functional restoration in industrial low back injury utilizing objective assessment, *JAMA* 258:1762, 1987.
12. Mechanic D: The concept of illness behavior, *J Chronic Dis* 15:189, 1962.
13. Mooney V, Cairns D, Robertson J: A system for evaluating and treating chronic back disability, *West J Med* 124:370, 1976.
14. Polatin PB and others: Psychiatric illness and chronic low back pain: the mind and the spine—which goes first?, *Spine* 18:239, 1993.
15. Sternbach RA, Wolf SR, Murphy RW: Traits of pain patients: the low-back "loser," *Psychosomatics* 14:226, 1973.
16. Waddell G: A new clinical model for the treatment of low-back pain, *Spine* 12:632, 1987.

Chapter 37

Cognitive-Behavioral Treatment of the Patient with Chronic Pain

Thomas E. Rudy
Dennis C. Turk

Pain is one of the most complex of human experiences. It has been the focus of philosophical speculation and scientific attention for centuries, yet it remains one of the most challenging problems for the sufferer, health-care providers, and society. Individuals experiencing chronic pain frequently engage in a continual pursuit for relief, which often is elusive; this pursuit may lead to feelings of anger, helplessness, and demoralization and an incalculable amount of emotional suffering. Health-care providers frequently share similar feelings of frustration, as patients continue to report pain despite the health-care provider's best efforts. At a societal level, pain is a major health problem that affects millions of people in the United States and costs society billions of dollars in health care and lost productivity. Additionally, third-party insurance payers are confronted with escalating medical costs, disability payments, and frustration when pain patients remain disabled despite extensive treatment and rehabilitation efforts.

In this chapter we will (1) provide a description of conceptualizations of pain; (2) highlight some inadequacies of unidimensional models of pain, particularly of persistent pain; (3) discuss several multidimensional models of pain, with special emphasis on the cognitive-behavioral perspective; (4) review some of the supporting evidence for the cognitive-behavioral model; (5) outline some of the cognitive-behavioral treatment assumptions and strategies; and (6) suggest future directions of study that may clarify the role of psychologic factors in the evaluation and treatment of pain. Due to space limitations we will only be able to highlight these very complex topics and related issues.

Before beginning our discussion of psychologic factors relevant to understanding chronic pain, it is important to emphasize that understanding psychologic and psychosocial aspects of the pain experience is *essential* to the diagnosis and treatment of *all* pain patients. All too frequently, a highly artificial and erroneous distinction is made between structural or physical influences related to patients' pain conditions, and factors that are labeled as "psychologic." It is important for the reader to recognize that "psychologic factors" are far broader than "psychopathology." That is, understanding patients' attributions or beliefs about their condition (e.g., what the patient thinks causes their pain and how to treat it), the role of the spouse or other family members as allies or barriers to rehabilitation efforts, and so forth, are crucial to successful diagnosis and treatment, regardless of patients' degree of physical pathology. Thus, the cognitive-behavioral model or perspective of chronic pain described below should not be confused with "psy-

chogenic" or psychopathologic conceptualizations, which we believe create an overly simplistic and unhelpful mind-body dualism.

Psychologic Conceptualizations of Pain

Historically, pain has been viewed by medical investigators and practitioners as primarily a sensory-physiologic phenomenon. From this perspective, patients' reports of pain are believed to be associated directly with the extent of tissue damage or organ pathology. Advanced diagnostic imaging and laboratory procedures have been developed to evaluate the extent of tissue damage in the hope that locating the area and extent of the damage will explain the patient's reports of pain and thereby suggest the appropriate therapeutic intervention. Therapeutic interventions for patients with persistent pain derived from variations of the sensory-physiologic model have led to the development of surgical procedures to ablate the pain pathways from the periphery to the central nervous system and the synthesis of potent analgesic agents to block the transmission of signals along these pathways.

Over the past two decades, there has been increasing dissatisfaction with the purely sensory view of pain. Medical practitioners frequently noted that patients with ostensibly the same degree of tissue damage react very differently to identical therapeutic methods and that patients with similar diagnoses and organic findings respond quite differently to their conditions.[33] Moreover, despite rapid advances in neuroanatomy, physiology, and pharmacology, there continues to be a large number of patients and many pain syndromes for which no physical intervention consistently and permanently eliminates pain. Conversely, there are many individuals with extensive physical pathology who are asymptomatic and report no pain.

Psychogenic Model

The inability to identify specific organic pathology in many patients with chronic pain, continued reports of pain following correction of pathologic conditions, and continued complaints of pain following the expected period of resolution of an injury has led to two very different psychologically oriented approaches to conceptualizing chronic pain patients—a psychogenic model and a behavioral model. The psychogenic model of persistent pain suggests that pain reports in the absence of objective medical data can be explained by personality characteristics of the patient or the presence of a psychiatric disorder.

Empirical attempts to identify patient subgroups based on personality characteristics or psychiatric diagnoses have evolved from the psychogenic perspective.[3] Findings from these research efforts along with the results of sensory-based assessment approaches have led to a frequently used and often abused dichotomy, the cause of patients' pain complaints is classified as either "organic" or if not, ipso facto, "psychogenic." That is, if a physical basis can be found for patients' subjective pain reports, the pain is considered "real." However, if organic findings are absent or the patient's pain complaints are "disproportionate" to the amounts of tissue damage, the patient's pain is categorized as "functional" or "psychogenic." In the latter case, the basis for the patient's reports of pain is believed to be emotionally or motivationally rather than physically determined.

The organic-psychogenic distinction makes several unwarranted assumptions. First, it assumes that there are adequate means for reliably measuring the amount of pain experienced and that normative data are available for various pain syndromes against which to compare an individual's reports of pain to determine whether they are "excessive." However, as noted, it is recognized by many clinicians that people with very similar objective medical findings show quite diverse responses.

Additionally, this dichotomy assumes that current medical and diagnostic procedures can identify all sources of pathology likely to cause the pain reported by the patient. However, the predictive power of medical examinations and diagnostic tests (their sensitivity and specificity) are generally low for patients with persistent pain.[8,14] For example, physical examination, laboratory tests, and imaging procedures can be expected to lead to a definitive diagnosis in only 5% to 10% of patients with chronic low back pain.[48] Does this mean that 85% to 90% of patients with back pain have psychogenic pain? This dichotomy further assumes that there are no individual differences other than psychopathologic ones that influence pain perceptions (e.g., differences in sensory sensitivity). Finally, the organic-psychogenic dichotomy makes the implicit assumption that a psychiatric problem and a pain disorder cannot occur simultaneously in the same individual or that a psychiatric problem, when present, cannot result from a chronic physical disorder.

Operant Behavioral Model

Behavioral psychologists have emphasized that pain is a subjective phenomenon and, consequently, all that can be observed are behaviors emitted in response to the subjective experience of pain. Thus, behavioral manifestations are viewed as the means by which patients communicate pain and suffering and, especially in the case of chronic pain, it is these behaviors that should be assessed and treated, rather than pain per se. In other words, behavioral models of pain distinguish nociception, pain, suffering, and pain behavior. The first three are viewed as the "private" experience of pain; whereas, the latter is directly observable, quantifiable, and capable of eliciting responses that serve to perpetuate them, even in the absence of nociception.

According to Fordyce[13] behavioral operationalizations of pain—"pain behaviors"—include verbal complaints of pain and suffering, nonlanguage sounds (e.g., moans, sighs), body posturing and gesturing (e.g., limping, rubbing a painful body part or area), and displays of functional limitations or disability (e.g., reclining for excessive periods of time). It has been suggested that pain behaviors may provide a more "objective" means of assessing responses inferred to be pain-related than patients' self-reports, which may be biased or purposely distorted. Thus, subjective self-reports are suspect. Also, from an operant theory of behavior, if "pain" is considered to be comprised of observable behaviors, then we can consider the production and maintenance of those behaviors as being under environmental control through selective contingencies of reinforcement.

To illustrate the effect of environmental factors on reports of pain, it can be noted that significant others in the patient's environment, whether family, friends, or health care providers, respond to the patient's overt behavior. Significant others may reinforce these behavioral manifestations by providing attention or permitting the patient to avoid the performance of undesirable activities (e.g., physical activities), and thereby unwittingly contribute to the maintenance of these behaviors. Additionally, the insurance system may positively reinforce the expression of pain behaviors by providing financial incentives contingent on the emission of pain behaviors, positively reinforcing symptom magnification. Thus, although secondary gain factors may be involved in some patients, it is important for the reader to recognize that behavioral conceptualizations of pain are far more comprehensive than simply understanding behaviors that may be reflective of secondary gain.

The operant behavioral approach to pain becomes particularly relevant for persistent pain that extends over long periods. At an acute level, behavioral responses to injury and nociceptive stimulation may be appropriate in that they serve protective functions. However, when pain behaviors persist over extended periods they can become detrimental and problems in their own right. The behavioral responses of inactivity as well as limping, guarding, bracing, and so forth, for a patient with low-back pain leads to altered body mechanics and generalized deconditioning (e.g., reduction in muscle strength, mass, and flexibility; easy fatigability). Additionally, continuation of pain behaviors can lead to the reduction of previously enjoyed activities and the increase of psychologic distress (e.g., depressed mood). In essence, a vicious cycle may be initiated and perpetuated by the unwitting reinforcement of pain behaviors.

Although pain behaviors are important to consider, it is equally important to acknowledge that pain behaviors, like physical pathology, are unidimensional.[42] Pain behaviors should be viewed within the broader context that also includes cognitive, affective, psychosocial, and other behavioral factors (e.g., activities of daily living), as well as physiologic factors, all of which contribute to the experience of pain.

Gate Control Model

A dramatic shift from pain as a purely sensory phenomenon to pain as a perceptual event was given its greatest impetus in the mid-1960s by Melzack and his colleagues.[26,27] They proposed a new conceptual model of pain—the gate control model—designed to deal with the inconsistencies manifest by different sensory models of pain and to incorporate clinical experience.

According to this model, pain is not solely an automatic sensory phenomenon, but a highly personal, variable experience influenced by cultural learning, the meaning of the situation, attention, and other cognitive activities. The gate control model proposed that besides the traditionally recognized dimension of nociception (the sensory-discriminative component of the gate control model), there also existed motivational-affective and cognitive-evaluative components. In other words, Melzack and colleagues postulated that the perception of pain was the result of the simultaneous integration of motivational-affective, cognitive-evaluative, and sensory-discriminative factors.

This view of pain differed greatly from traditional sensory views that, when they considered psychologic factors at all, relegated them to reactions to

"pain" and, consequently, nuisance variables or at best epiphenomena. The gate control model did not give priority to sensory input, nor did it treat the sensory input as isomorphic with pain. Rather, pain was postulated to be the result of the integration and interpretation of sensory and psychologic processes, and, therefore, qualified as a perceptual process.

The gate control model also postulated that there were important physiologic pathways that are capable of augmenting or diminishing the subjective experience of pain. In addition to afferent pathways, some of the proposed pathways involved "top-down" processing, that is, the neurophysiologic influence of emotions and cognitive phenomena presumably travel down the spinal cord from the brain and can modulate sensory information traveling up the spinal cord toward the brain. Thus, the notion of a "gating" type action in the dorsal horn was proposed.

Although the gate control model has not been without its critics, particularly regarding the physical basis of the proposed gating mechanism,[30] it has been hailed as a resilient theory of pain with reasonable explanatory and heuristic value. Because it attributes the perception of pain to more than simply sensory stimulation, the gate control model provides some explanations as to why the surgical, electrical, or neurolytic ablation of pain pathways have not always been effective in eliminating pain. A natural consequence of the gate control model is that successful treatment of patients with chronic pain will require attention to all three components of the pain experience.

Cognitive-Behavioral Model

Although both the operant behavioral and gate control models departed significantly from sensory models of pain, each has a somewhat limited view and is inadequate to explain chronic pain by itself. The operant behavioral model fails to consider the contribution of cognitive appraisals of the patients as they influence patients' perceptions and responses to their physical problems. As pain persists, the gate control model does not consider the interaction of environmental influences, physical factors, and pain perceptions as they extend over prolonged periods.

An alternative model that emphasizes both the importance of environmental factors underscored by the operant approach and the psychologic contributions inherent in the gate control model has been formulated by Turk and his colleagues[43,45] and labeled a "cognitive-behavioral" perspective on pain. A comprehensive intervention model based on the cognitive-behavioral conceptualization has been developed and used with a diversity of pain syndromes (e.g., headaches,[17] temporomandibular pain disorders,[32] arthritis,[23] back pain,[15] cancer-related pain,[10] and heterogeneous pain syndromes[31]). Moreover, this approach has been applied to children,[36] adolescents,[24] and geriatric[34] pain populations.

Like the gate control model, the cognitive-behavioral perspective of pain is multidimensional in that it makes an important distinction between nociception, that is, activation of sensory transduction in the nerves that convey information about tissue damage capable of being experienced as pain, from *pain* per se. The cognitive-behavioral perspective places strong emphasis on the longitudinal impact of cognitive factors as they affect perception and behavioral responses to nociception.[43,45] It is hypothesized that people who experience chronic or recurrent nociception develop negative expectations about their ability to perform physical activities without pain,[38] adopt a negative mind-set about pain and how pain will affect their lives, and appraise their situation as one in which there is little they can do to cope with the nociception experienced.

Another central tenet of the cognitive-behavioral perspective is that patients' interpretations of nociception, their coping resources, and in general their situation and condition can have both direct and indirect effects on both physiologic and psychologic processes that may maintain and exacerbate pain. It is important to recognize that people not only respond to available stimuli and observe the consequences of their behavior, but also actively select from the information present and transform and categorize stimuli in idiosyncratic fashions, thereby partially determining some of the stimuli that impinge on them. Additionally, patients may have belief systems, some of which may be irrational, that determine or guide their responses to their condition. For example, patients may believe that they "should" be able to do tasks at preinjury levels or that they "must" try to engage in a strenuous task either out of bravado, guilt, or desperation or because they believe that they are "cured." In these cases, the patient will engage in a cycle of overactivity and flare-up, followed by pain and inactivity. Finally, cognitive processes may have a direct effect on physiologic parameters associated with pain perception, such as autonomic nervous system activation[11] and facilitation of the production of enkephalins.[2]

The cognitive-behavioral perspective also recognizes that cognitive processes reciprocally determine and redefine perception and patients' reports of unremitting pain. Because the experience of pain and subsequently the fear of pain is aversive, patients' expectations of the occurrence of pain in and of themselves become strong motivators for avoidance of situations or behaviors that are expected to produce nociception. Moreover, the belief that pain signals harm further serves to reinforce avoidance of activities believed to cause pain and increase physical damage. The persistence of avoidance will reduce physical activity and, consequently, the opportunities for experiencing disconfirmations. Moreover, avoidance of activity will contribute to further physical deconditioning, including reduction of muscle strength and flexibility.

To summarize, the cognitive-behavioral model adopts a broad perspective on pain, one that focuses on the patient and not just the symptom. That is, persistent pain, like any chronic disease, extends over time and affects all domains of the patient's life, vocational, familial, marital, social, psychologic, as well as physical. Rather than focusing on cognitive and affective contributions to the perception of pain in a static fashion, as in the gate control model, or exclusively on behavioral responses and environmental reinforcement contingencies and physical pathology, the cognitive-behavioral model entails a transactional view that emphasizes the ongoing reciprocal relationships among physical, cognitive, affective, and behavioral factors.

Research Support for the Cognitive-Behavioral Perspective of Chronic Pain

An increasing body of literature has emerged that supports many of the assumptions of the cognitive-behavioral formulation of the pain experience. Space limitations do not permit a comprehensive review of this literature; however, we will present illustrative research that demonstrates the important contribution of cognitive-behavioral factors in the maintenance and exacerbation of recurrent and persistent pain problems, and in the facilitation of disability.

A number of studies have been conducted to examine the contribution of the cognitive components of the pain experience.[44] These studies have focused on acute and laboratory pain research models, as well as the role of maladaptive cognitions in clinical pain. For example, Flor and Turk[12] examined the association between general and situation-specific pain-related thoughts, convictions of personal control, pain severity, and disability levels in patients with chronic low-back pain and patients with rheumatoid arthritis. The general and situation-specific cognitive variables were more highly related to reports of pain and disability than were disease-related variables for both samples. Moreover, these cognitive variables explained a significantly greater proportion of the variance in treatment outcome than did demographic or medical status variables.

How people cope with nociception may have both an indirect effect on pain through the influence on mood and behavior as well as a direct effect on nociception through the influence on the autonomic nervous system and the production and inhibition of select neurotransmitters. In a comprehensive meta-analysis of 46 laboratory studies, Fernandez and Turk[9] concluded that cognitive strategies do appear to have a major influence on pain perception or subjects' response to noxious stimulation. They further concluded that the effects of cognitive coping strategies are significantly greater than those effects displayed by placebo and expectancy control groups. In fact, subjects trained to use one or more cognitive strategies were found to be "better off" (i.e., were able to tolerate higher levels of noxious stimulation) than 80% of subjects not provided with specific coping strategies. Several studies with clinical samples have demonstrated the important role of coping strategies in the maintenance of pain disability and response to treatment.[21,35]

A central construct in the cognitive-behavioral model of chronic pain is self-efficacy.[1] A self-efficacy expectation is defined as a personal conviction that one can successfully perform certain behaviors in a given situation. It has been suggested that given sufficient motivation to engage in a behavior, it is an individual's self-efficacy beliefs that determine whether a given behavior will be initiated, how much effort will be expended, and how long effort will be sustained in the face of obstacles and aversive experiences. Support for the importance of self-efficacy as specifically related to pain has been demonstrated in laboratory studies,[7] with headache patients,[18] temporomandibular pain disorders,[16] back pain,[4] arthritis,[25] and heterogeneous clinical populations.[5,21]

Research by Dolce and his colleagues has focused on the significant associations that exist between exercise and self-efficacy. Dolce et al.[5] evaluated the role of setting exercise quotas on performance of exercise, concerns about engaging in exercise, and self-efficacy expectancies. Exercise quotas were shown to increase levels of previously avoided exercises. Additionally, when quotas were implemented, self-efficacy ratings were observed to increase, while patients' ratings of concern decreased. Self-efficacy expectancies were found to closely parallel increases in actual exercise levels during treatment ($r = 0.69$, $p < 0.001$). In another study, Dolce et al.[6] observed that patients with post-treatment self-efficacy ratings

of chronic pain were significantly correlated with exercise levels, medication use, and work status at follow-up periods ranging from 6 to 12 months.

The interrelationship between fear avoidance and self-efficacy has been illustrated in a study by Council et al.[4] They found that actual physical performances of patients with back pain were best predicted by self-efficacy ratings, which appeared to be determined by pain response expectancies. The authors interpreted these results as suggesting that daily pain experiences determine pain response expectancies for specific movements. Pain response expectancies appear to influence performance and associated pain behavior through their effects on efficacy expectancies. These findings also indicate that pain response expectancies associated with specific movements are based on generalized expectancies drawn from daily experiences, which suggest that patients with chronic pain have well-established ideas of how much pain they will experience in different situations. These beliefs about the results of activity may cause patients to avoid certain activities for fear of the consequences, including the belief that they may become more functionally impaired.

Evidence for the importance of the direct effect of cognitive factors on physical parameters in persistent pain is apparent in several psychophysiologic experiments.[12] For example, Flor, Turk, and Birbaumer[11] examined the association of paraspinal lumbar electromyographic reactivity of chronic-back-pain patients, non-back-pain patients, and healthy controls. All subjects participated in a psychophysiologic assessment that included four counterbalanced trials (discussion of personal stress, discussion of pain, performance of mental arithmetic, and a control condition [reciting of the alphabet]). Bilateral paraspinal and frontalis EMG, heart rate, and skin conductance levels were recorded continuously. The results indicated that back-pain patients displayed elevations and delayed recovery *only* in their paravertebral musculature and *only* when discussing personally relevant stress (the pain and stress trials). Neither of the other two groups displayed paravertebral hyperreactivity or delayed recovery. The extent of abnormal muscular reactivity was best predicted by depression and cognitive coping style rather than pain demographic variables (e.g., number of surgeries, duration of pain). Studies of patients with temporomandibular disorder[37] and musicians with upper-limb pain associated with occupational overuse[29] have replicated these findings. These tentative findings must be viewed with caution, but they are suggestive of the potential influence of cognitive factors on physiologic functioning in patients with chronic pain and warrant further investigation.

In sum, the results of these illustrative studies of self-efficacy, cognitive coping strategies, and psychophysiology underscore the important role of cognitive factors in disability maintenance of chronic pain and response to treatment. Moreover, these studies demonstrate that these cognitive factors may affect patients' reports of pain and use of the health care system as well as directly affect physiologic parameters believed to be associated with nociception.

Cognitive-Behavioral Treatment for Chronic Pain

Overview

To understand the cognitive-behavioral approach to the treatment of patients with chronic pain, it is important to understand that the techniques actually used are viewed as significantly less important than the more general philosophy and orientation, described above. By the time patients come to a treatment program for chronic pain they have received multiple evaluations and a range of treatments. A common feature across all patients regardless of diagnosis is that an array of interventions have failed to alleviate their suffering adequately. Thus, it is not surprising that by the time these patients are seen at a pain center they are quite demoralized, feel frustrated, feel their situation is hopeless, and yet still are seeking *the* cure for their suffering.

The general goal of a cognitive-behavioral pain treatment program is to assist patients to reconceptualize their view of their situation and their pain. Patients frequently come to pain clinics with a view of pain as a totally medical problem that is all-encompassing and over which they have little or no control. The cognitive-behavioral approach emphasizes both the effectiveness of the rehabilitation approach and the patient's ability to alleviate much of his or her pain and suffering if he or she is willing to work with the treatment team. In other words, the cognitive-behavioral treatment approach relies heavily on active patient participation and emphasizes a mutual problem-solving approach among the treatment team, the patient, and the significant others in the patient's environment.

Evaluation

Before embarking on specific cognitive-behavioral intervention techniques, it is critical for the therapist(s) who will be implementing these techniques to conduct a detailed evaluation. Regardless of

whether an organic basis for the pain can be documented or whether psychosocial problems preceded or resulted from the pain, the evaluation process can be helpful in identifying how biomedical, psychologic, and social factors interact to influence the nature, severity, and persistence of pain and disability. From a cognitive-behavioral perspective, factors such as emotional distress, depression, beliefs about the etiology of the pain, and social reinforcement of pain behaviors all need to be addressed. These and other factors to target during the assessment process are outlined in the box below.

Content Areas Covered in Cognitive-Behavioral Evaluation Interviews

- Secondary problems that have arisen because of persistent pain (e.g., vocational, familial, financial)
- Situational fluctuation of pain intensity, duration, and/or frequency
- How the patient expresses pain
- How others respond to the patient's complaints of pain and disability
- Behavioral manifestations of pain—pain behaviors (e.g., moaning, distorted ambulation or posture)
- What effect the patient believes the pain is having on others
- Whether the patient derives any benefits or secondary gains from having pain
- How the patient thinks about the pain and associated problems
- Pattern of medication use and substance abuse (current and previous)
- Current mood, evidence of affective distress, sleep and appetite disturbances
- What the patient has tried to do to alleviate pain
- Patient's work history (frequency of changes, satisfaction, whether the patient has a job to which he or she can/plans to return)
- Patient's expectancies from the physician and treatment
- Patient's views of previous physicians and treatments
- Prior history of pain problems of patient or family members
- Prior and current stressful life events
- Family (marital) relations (current and past)

To summarize, the primary purposes of the cognitive-behaviorally oriented evaluation are to (1) determine specific psychologic and behavioral contributors to pain behaviors, impairment in functioning, and suffering; (2) determine appropriate treatment targets and intervention strategies; and (3) provide pertinent information about aspects of a patient's psychosocial history and current situation that may have a bearing on responses to persistent pain.[40]

Interdisciplinary Team

We believe the most effective approach to treating patients with chronic pain is in the context of an interdisciplinary team. The core of the team is comprised of representatives from a variety of health care disciplines, including medicine, nursing, psychology, physical therapy, and occupational therapy. The specialty of the physician member of the team is less important than his or her commitment and dedication to working with pain patients. Additionally, we believe that it is essential for the treatment team to share a common philosophy so that patients are treated consistently regardless of the disciplines or techniques used by the various team members.[47]

Although the therapeutic team is often conceptualized as being comprised of professional members, we also believe that the team definition needs to be extended to include the patient and significant others as well.[45] Patients and their significant others need to be alerted to their important collaborative roles as part of the treatment team.

Too often the treatment team forgets about the importance of the family.[28,41] However, chronic pain, by virtue of extending over long periods, has an impact on all aspects of the patient's life, including his or her family life. Failure to include family members is likely to contribute to the problems of maintenance and generalization of treatment gains. At a minimum, families need to be aware of the nature and logic for the treatment goals and methods used. Some families may require additional involvement or family counseling if there is to be any hope for treatment success.

Essential Components of Cognitive-Behavioral Treatment

Following assessment, which should be considered an ongoing process throughout treatment, we believe that treatment should be comprised of at least four interrelated components: (1) education, (2) skills acquisition, (3) cognitive and behavioral rehearsal, and (4) generalization and maintenance.

Due to space limitations, we will provide only a brief overview of each of these components (see Turk and Rudy[45] for more complete descriptions).

Education

Presentation of the cognitive-behavioral perspective on pain and the control of pain (e.g., the role of thoughts, feelings, behavior, environmental, and physical factors) should begin at the outset of treatment and continue throughout. The presentation of cognitive-behavioral concepts needs to be provided in a simple, direct way with numerous examples that are customized to the specific patient and in a vocabulary that he or she can understand. We believe that when exploring with patients the cognitive-behavioral factors that may be associated with their pain condition, a collaborative rather than a didactic approach is more effective. That is, we believe that it is important to avoid the more traditional directive medical approach used in many settings, and to begin to communicate with patients in a manner that encourages them to begin to assume equal responsibility for their treatment. The approach is designed to be authoritative without being authoritarian.

The educational component of treatment also needs to address the unspoken fears that many patients have about their condition (e.g., fear of reinjury if they engage in certain exercises, fear that their condition is progressive, fear that health-care providers do not believe their pain is "real," etc.). It is necessary that this effort be interdisciplinary in nature, and include a review and lay-oriented discussion of the evaluation findings of the treatment team that incorporates biomedical, psychosocial, and behavioral results. During this process, it is important for the team, professional as well as patient, to identify patients' idiosyncratic beliefs and inaccurate understanding of the information presented. This information then can be used to begin the process of reconceptualization.

Skills Acquisition

Cognitive and behavioral treatment techniques consist of a range of methods and procedures that are designed to bring alterations in patients' perceptions of their situation and thus their ability to control their condition. A number of articles and textbooks have described these techniques in detail and the interested reader should consult these.[20,22,43] To reiterate, we believe that the mastery of the technical aspects of these techniques is less important than the manner in which they are presented and taught to patients. Specifically, we believe that these techniques need to be individualized to the specific patient, and described and taught to patients in a way that increases their perceptions of self-control and intrinsic motivation. Toward this goal, we prefer inclusion of techniques or skills that can be broadly categorized as self-management (e.g., stress-management, coping skills training, problem solving).

Cognitive and Behavioral Rehearsal

Teaching patients strategies and techniques to manage their pain and increase their level of functioning is of little value if they do not learn to apply them regularly in their home environments. The rehearsal component of cognitive-behavioral treatment emphasizes the importance of patients' practicing and consolidating the skills that they learn during the skills-acquisition phase. Rehearsal techniques can include mental practice, role-playing, and role-reversal. We find role-reversal particularly effective in evaluating specifically what the patient has learned. This technique simply involves the patient and therapist switching roles and the patient "teaches" skills to the therapist, who assumes the role of a new patient. Specific details of these rehearsal are described by Holzman et al.[19]

Homework

A closely related component of rehearsal is the assignment of specific homework tasks to patients so that they can practice skills learned during treatment sessions and report their results at the next session. We believe that the inclusion of significant others, whenever possible, can help to increase the effectiveness and the information obtained from homework assignments.

Homework assignments should be geared toward observable and manageable tasks—that is, tasks that are readily achievable—and then progressing to more difficult ones. Additionally, the goals and homework assignments should be customized to the particular condition, lifestyle, and unique assessment findings of each patient. Turk et al.[43] have described the general purposes of homework tasks between treatment sessions, and these are outlined in the box at right.

Generalization and Maintenance

Despite our best efforts and strategies, relapse remains a significant problem in the treatment of chronic pain.[46] To maximize the likelihood of main-

tenance and generalization of treatment gains, cognitive-behavioral therapists focus on the cognitive activity of patients as they are confronted with problems throughout treatment (e.g., failure to achieve specified goals, plateaus in progress on physical exercises, recurrent stresses). These events are employed as opportunities to assist patients in learning how to handle such setbacks and lapses since they are probably inevitable and will occur once treatment is terminated. Rehabilitation is not a cure.

In the final stage of treatment, discussion focuses on possible ways of predicting and avoiding or dealing with pain and pain-related problems following treatment termination. We have found it helpful to assist patients to anticipate future problems, stress, and pain-exacerbating events and to plan coping and response techniques before these problems occur.

It is important to note that all possible problematic circumstances cannot be anticipated. Rather, the goal during this phase, as for the entire treatment strategy, is to enable patients to develop a problem-

Purposes of Homework Assignments

- To assess various areas of the patient's and significant others' lives and how these influence and are affected by the pain problem

- To assess the typical responses of significant others and the patient to pain and pain behaviors

- To make the patient and significant others more aware of the factors that exacerbate and alleviate suffering

- To help the patient and significant others identify maladaptive responses to pain and pain behaviors

- To consolidate the use of coping procedures and physical exercises discussed during therapy sessions

- To increase physical activity levels

- To illustrate to the patient and significant others that progress can be made in living with pain but with less suffering

- To serve as reinforcers and as enhancers of self-efficacy as the patient achieves his or her goals

- To assist the therapeutic team, including the patient and significant others, in evaluating progress and in modifying goals and treatment strategies

solving perspective, in which they believe that they have the skills and competencies within their repertoires to respond in an appropriate way to problems as they arise. In this manner, attempts are made to help the patient learn to anticipate future difficulties, develop plans for adaptive responding, and adjust his or her behavior accordingly.

The generalization and maintenance phases serve at least two purposes: (1) it encourages the patient to anticipate and plan for the posttreatment period, when symptoms are greatly improved but not totally removed; and (2) it focuses on the necessary conditions for long-term success. More specifically, this phase gives the patient the understanding that minor setbacks are to be expected, but that they do not signal total failure. Rather, these setback should be viewed as cues to use the coping skills at which they are already proficient. It is important for the patient not to think of his or her responsibility as ending at the termination of treatment, but as entering a different phase of maintenance. Emphasis is placed on the importance of adherence to recommendations on an ongoing basis.

Future Directions

Most chronic pain syndromes represent a combination of contributing components in which both physical and psychologic influences are present. Throughout this chapter we have emphasized how psychologic factors can contribute to and augment pain problems. This is not to imply, however, that the presence of psychologic findings precludes the existence of physical pathology or that physical findings necessarily imply the absence of significant psychologic or behavioral contributors to pain and disability.

Although psychologists have made major contributions to theoretical conceptualizations of pain[13,26] and have developed innovative treatments for chronic pain problems,[39,43] challenges remain. We will underscore a major challenge that relates to treatment relapse and noncompliance. More specifically, psychologically oriented investigators need to give increased attention to cognitive and behavioral factors that may be predictive of relapse and patients' lack of adherence to treatment programs. Although the number of published treatment outcome studies for chronic pain has grown rapidly in recent years, relatively little attention has been given to the everpresent problem of relapse. Follow-up treatment data suggest that relapse rates, that is, regression back to pretreatment levels, for chronic pain patients range from 30% to 70%.[46] Long-term treatment success for many patients with chronic pain may depend on regular adherence to recommended self-care regimens. Yet high adherence rates for patients with chronic pain, as for other chronic diseases (e.g., diabetes, hypertension), are difficult to achieve. Research is needed to determine what psychologic factors and treatment strategies are associated with increased treatment adherence and what types of self-care behaviors are necessary and sufficient for patients with chronic pain to maintain therapeutic benefits.

Another challenge for the future is related to treatment matching. All too often patients with the same specific medical diagnosis or general label are treated as a homogeneous group and are provided with a standard treatment package. Although many patients benefit from this approach, others do not. A more efficient strategy would be one that evaluates patients and then selectively prescribes treatments customized to relevant patient characteristics. The important question to explore for the future is not what treatment is most effective for all patients with a common diagnosis, but rather what treatment components are most effective for patients with what set of characteristics. This approach may be especially appropriate for patients who do not respond to the usual treatment protocols.

Finally, given the complex, multidimensional nature of the pain experience, increased interdisciplinary research and treatment collaboration is needed, particularly among physicians and psychologists specializing in chronic pain.[47] The development of a common, comprehensive conceptualization of patients with chronic pain, the synthesis of the diverse sets of information from the evaluations by different pain specialists, the need to formulate more reliable differential diagnosis and treatment plans for each patient, and the willingness to share a common philosophy of pain treatment and disability management remain key issues that need further attention if chronic pain treatment is to advance.

References

1. Bandura A: Self efficacy: toward a unifying theory of behavioral change, *Psychol Rev* 84:191, 1977.
2. Bandura A, O'Leary A, Taylor CB, et al.: Perceived self-efficacy and pain control-opioid and nonopioid mechanisms, *J Personal Soc Psychol* 53:563, 1987.
3. Blumer D, Heilbronn M: Chronic pain as a variant of depressive disease: the pain-prone disorder, *J Nerv Ment Dis* 170:381, 1982.
4. Council JR, Ahern DK, Follick MJ, Kline CL: Expectancies and functional impairment in chronic low back pain, *Pain* 33:323, 1988.

5. Dolce JJ, Crocker MF, Moletteire C, Doleys DM: Exercise quotas, anticipatory concern and self-efficacy expectancies in chronic pain: a preliminary report, *Pain* 24:365, 1986.

6. Dolce JJ, Crocker MF, Doleys DM: Prediction of outcome among chronic pain patients, *Behav Res Ther* 24:313, 1986.

7. Dolce JJ, Doleys DM, Raczynski JM, et al.: The role of self-efficacy expectancies in prediction of pain tolerance, *Pain* 27:261, 1986.

8. Eisenberg RL, Hedgcock MW, Gooding GA, et al.: Compensation examination of the cervical and lumbar spine: critical disagreement in radiographic interpretation, *Am J Radoil* 134:519, 1980.

9. Fernandez E, Turk DC: The utility of cognitive coping strategies for altering pain perception: a meta-analysis, *Pain* 38:123, 1989.

10. Fishman B: *The cognitive-behavioral perspective on pain management in terminal illness.* In Turk DC, Feldman CS, editors: *Noninvasive approaches to pain management in the terminally ill,* New York, 1992, Haworth Press, p 73.

11. Flor H, Turk DC, Birbaumer N: Assessment of stress-related psychophysiological reactions in chronic back pain patients, *J Consult Clin Psychol* 53:354, 1985.

12. Flor H, Turk DC: The psychophysiology of chronic pain: do chronic pain patients exhibit symptom-specific psychophysiological response? *Psychol Bull* 105:215, A89.

13. Fordyce WE: *Behavioral methods for chronic pain and illness,* St. Louis, 1976, Mosby.

14. Haldeman S, Shouka M, Robboy S: Computed tomography, electrodiagnostic and clinical findings in chronic workers' compensation patients with back and leg pain, *Spine* 13:345, 1988.

15. Hazard RG, Benedix A, Genwich JW: Disability exaggeration as a predictor of functional restoration outcomes for patients with chronic low-back pain, *Spine* 16:1062, 1991.

16. Hijzen TH, Slangen JL, van Houweligen HC: Subjective, clinical and EMG effects of biofeedback and splint treatment, *J Oral Rehab* 13:529, 1986.

17. Holroyd KA, Nash JM, Pingel JD, et al.: A comparison of pharmacological (amitriptline HCI) and nonpharmacological (cognitive-behavioral) therapies for chronic tension headaches, *J Consult Clin Psychol* 59:121, 1991.

18. Holroyd KA, Penzien DB, Hursey KG, et al.: Change mechanisms in EMG biofeedback training: cognitive changes underlying improvements in tension headache, *J Consult Clin Psychol* 52:1039, 1984.

19. Holzman AD, Turk DC, Kerns RD: *The cognitive-behavioral approach to the management of chronic pain.* In Holzman AD, Turk DC, editors: *Pain management: a handbook of psychological treatment approaches,* Elmsford, NY, 1986, Pergamon Press, p 31.

20. Holzman AD, Turk DC: *Pain management: a handbook of psychological treatment approaches,* Elmsford, NY, 1986, Pergamon Press.

21. Jensen MA, Turner JA, Romano JM: Self-efficacy and outcome expectancies: relationship to chronic pain coping strategies and adjustments, *Pain* 44:263, 1991.

22. Kanfer FH, Goldstein AP: *Helping people change: a textbook of methods,* Elmsford, NY, 1986, Pergamon Press.

23. Keefe, FJ, Caldwell DS, Williams DA, et al.: Pain coping skills training in the behavioral management of osteoarthritic knee pain: a comparative study, *Behav Ther* 21:49, 1990.

24. Lascelles MA, Cunningham SJ, McGrath P, Sullivan MJL: Teaching coping strategies to adolescents with migraine, *J Pain Symptom Manage* 4:135, 1989.

25. Lorig K, Chastain RL, Ung E, et al.: Development and evaluation of a scale to measure perceived self-efficacy in people with arthritis, *Arthritis Rheum* 32:37, 1989.

26. Melzack R, Casey KL: *Sensory, motivational and central control determinants of pain: a new conceptual model.* In Kenshalo D, editor: *The skin senses,* Springfield, IL, 1986, Charles C Thomas, p 137.

27. Melzack R, Wall PD: Pain mechanisms: a new theory, *Science* 150:971, 1965.

28. Moore JE, Chaney EF: Outpatient group treatment of chronic pain: effects of spouse involvement, *J Consult Clin Psychol* 53:326, 1985.

29. Moulton B, Spence SH: Site specific muscle hyperreactivity in musicians with occupational upper limb pain, *Behav Res Ther* 30:375, 1992.

30. Nathan PW: The gate control theory of pain: a critical review, *Brain* 99:123, 1976.

31. Nicholas MK: *Relapse rates following treatment in pain management programs.* In Wilson PH, editor: *Principles and practice of relapse prevention,* New York, 1992, Guilford Press, p 259.

32. Olson RE, Malow RM: Effects of biofeedback and psychotherapy on patients with myofascial pain dysfunction who are nonresponsive to conventional treatments, *Rehabil Psychol* 32:195, 1987.

33. Osterweis M, Kleinman A, Mechanic D: *Institute of Medicine's Committee on Pain, Disability, and Chronic Illness Behavior, Pain and Disability: clinical, behavioral, and public policy perspectives,* Washington, DC, 1987, National Academy Press.

34. Puder RS: Age analysis of cognitive-behavioral group therapy for chronic pain outpatients, *Psychol Aging* 3:204, 1988.

35. Ressor KA, Craig KD: Medically incongruent chronic back pain: physical limitations, suffering, and ineffective coping, *Pain* 32:35, 1988.

36. Richter IL, McGrath PJ, Humphreys PJ, et al.: Cognitive and relaxation treatment of paediatric migraine, *Pain* 25:195, 1986.

37. Rudy TE: Psychophysiological assessment in chronic orofacial pain, *Anesth Prog* 37:1, 1990.

38. Schmidt AJM: Cognitive factors in the performance level of chronic low back pain patients, *J Psychosom Res* 29:183, 1985.

39. Sternback RA: *Pain patients: traits and treatments,* New York, 1974, Academic Press.

40. Turk DC: Psychological assessment of patients with persistent pain. II. Alternative views, *Pain Manage* 3:227, 1990.

41. Turk DC, Flor H, Rudy TE: Pain and families: I. Etiology, maintenance, and psychosocial impact, *Pain* 30:3, 1987.

42. Turk DC, Flor H: Pain > pain behavior: utility and limitations of the pain behavior construct, *Pain* 31:277, 1987.

43. Turk DC, Meichenbaum D, Genest M: *Pain and behavioral medicine: a cognitive-behavioral perspective,* New York, 1983, Guilford Press.

44. Turk DC, Rudy TE: Cognitive factors and persistent pain: a glimpse into pandora's box, *Cognitive Ther Res* 16:99, 1992.

45. Turk DC, Rudy TE: *An integrated approach to the treatment of chronic pain: beyond the scalpel and syringe.* In Tollison CD, editor: *Handbook of chronic pain management,* Baltimore, 1989, Williams & Wilkins, p 222.

46. Turk DC, Rudy TE: Neglected factors in chronic pain treatment—relapse, noncompliance, and adherence enhancement, *Pain* 44:5, 1991.

47. Turk DC, Stieg RL: Chronic pain: the necessity of interdisciplinary communication, *Clin J Pain* 3:163, 1987.

48. White AA, Gordon SL: Synopsis: workshop on idiopathic low-back pain, *Pain* 7:141, 1982.

Chapter 38

Understanding the Chronic Spine Pain Patient: The Attachment Theory

David J. Anderson
Robert H. Hines

Pain is an amazingly complex and mysterious phenomenon. It is not merely a sensation but an experience that provokes the imagination, memory, and emotions of the afflicted and challenges the patient and physician to comprehend it. The person with pain seeks the help of the caregiver (often a physician) to bring this noxious experience to an end. It is in and through the relationship with the caregiver that the pain experience may resolve. Most physicians relate to their patients through the prescriptions of medication, exercise, and procedures (diagnostic and therapeutic). The manner with which the patient consciously and unconsciously interprets these interventions is critical in determining the outcome of the pain experience.

All pain has psychologic components. Since most pain resolves, there is usually no need to consider these components. For patients in whom pain does not resolve, this chapter is relevant and offers another view. Psychologic factors are known to play a major role in the recovery from disabling spine injuries. Attempts have been made to define the factors that might portend a poor prognosis by using various psychologic tests, questionnaires, pain drawings, and/or interviews. The model presented in this chapter is rooted in the observations of researchers from different fields made over 30 years ago. George Engel, M.D., in his paper "Psychogenic Pain and the Pain-Prone Patient,"[5] hypothesized that various constellations of childhood psychologic neglect and abuse often led to the development of more pain than would be expected for the known peripheral stimulus. He based his hypothesis on the similar histories of his patients with chronic pain. His explanations were limited to psychoanalytic hypotheses that did not lend themselves to practical intervention. As a result, his observations did not receive much corroborative attention.

While Engel was working with patients with chronic pain, Mary Ainsworth[1] and other researchers in child development were empirically studying the natural development of early human relationships, known as "attachment," between children and their significant caregivers. What she and others discovered provides a very sound theoretical framework to help explain Engel's clinical observations.

Attachment Factors

Attachment research focuses on a readily observable basic system of behavior that is biologically rooted and unique. Attachment behavior (defined as any behavior designed to keep the primary caregiver in close proximity) is widespread and fundamental in the animal kingdom. For humans, an attachment figure is someone whom the individual perceives as stronger and wiser, whom the individual seeks out in times of danger, whose presence is comforting, whose unavailability is met with protest, and whose loss causes distress. The attachment figure provides the sense of comfort and security necessary for the child to venture out and explore the world.

Ainsworth studied systematically the quality of an infant's attachment to the significant caregivers (usually the mother). The quality of the attachment reflects the degree of security of this emotional bond and is measured by the ability of the infant to find comfort in his/her mother and to use that comfort to explore the environment.

A secure attachment allows an individual to have dynamic relationships that permit optimal autonomy in the context of emotional support. An insecure attachment will cause the individual to eschew emotional support or to require continuous reassurance to maintain autonomy. Research has demonstrated that these early behavioral patterns of attachment follow an individual throughout his/her life.[7] Other attachment studies demonstrate that the capacity of a distressed child to be consoled from either physical or emotional pain is directly linked to the security of his/her relationship to early caregivers.[9]

The following vignette is illustrative of the impact of caregiver sensitivity on attachment and subsequent response to physical and/or emotional trauma. A young child falls from a play structure and begins to cry. In one instance the caregiver may be physically or emotionally absent and may neglect the child. In another the caregiver may respond to the child in a variety of ways, including soothing reassurance, shattering humiliation, anxious smothering, or irritable impatience. If effective, the caregiver's intervention helps to restore order and well-being for the child. Interactions between child and caregiver occur hundreds of times in various contexts throughout childhood. As a result of these repeated interactions, a unique template of expectations, autonomic nervous system responses, and behaviors develop. This template becomes activated throughout life when physical and/or emotional stress is experienced. This activated template will also have pronounced effects on the nature and effectiveness of any caregiver's response to the distressed individual's request for help. The more insecure the early relationships, the less likely the adult will have the capacity to be consoled in a human relationship. This has obvious clinical implications for the health care provider who is accustomed to and expects the patient to receive consolation from his/her interventions. Indeed, the failure of the patient to respond favorably often leads to the clinician's frustration and often a reenactment of the patient's earlier untoward experiences with his/her primary caregivers.

Our early experiences working with patients with refractory spine pain led us to observe that patients who had not developed the capacity for healthy, secure attachments were much more likely to fail to improve after technically successful surgery. The spine injury and subsequent pain led to a marked loss or threatened loss of functioning. The patient is unable to recover from this loss with his/her own resources, including current attachment figures. The spine pain patient turns to the physician to provide the sense of security and comfort to reestablish a safe world in which to function. When this patient carries a history of insecurity of attachment, he or she will, in our experience, repeatedly look for the physician to provide comfort while expecting at a powerful and often unconscious level that the caregiver will fail.

Research

No objective scale of attachment security has yet been developed. Indirect measures must be used that either reflect the quality of attachment or the quantity of factors known to disrupt attachment. Initially, we designed a 100-item questionnaire to evaluate the extent of disturbing factors in the patient's attachment history. When this questionnaire proved to be cumbersome, we consolidated the factors potentially damaging to the development of a secure attachment to five types of experiences. These factors are by no means complete, and patients with none of these risk factors may have insecure attachments and may be missed. Nevertheless, these factors provide a gross indirect predictor of quality of attachment. Each factor is assessed during the course of a semistructured clinical interview based on the Adult Attachment Interview for Adults.[6]

Although we have designated factors that might be particularly damaging, it is vital to emphasize that it is not necessarily the presence of abuse or neglect that blocks development of a secure attachment, but the effect such events have had on the capacity of the individual to form consoling relationships. For example, some patients have a significant history of neglect or abuse but have found sanctuary through their relationship with a nurturing adult such as a high school coach or a favorite teacher or relative. In these relationships they have found a secure attachment figure that can compensate for the other damaging relationships. Other individuals have found refuge not in human relationships but in phys-

ical activities such as athletics or physical work. Such activities are severely disrupted by spine pain, leaving the individual without his/her familiar consoling activity.

These childhood experiences are considered factors that, if present, could endanger the establishment of a secure attachment and lead to increased vulnerability to pain. For the model we describe *childhood* is defined as age under 21 years, and *primary caregiver* as a parent or other significant adult who is entrusted with day-to-day of the child.

While very early experiences are perhaps most relevant to the security of attachment, attachment patterns tend to persist and be repeated throughout life. The factors are: (1) Physical abuse, which is considered present if the patient suffered a physical injury inflicted by the primary caregiver that was not accidental. The effects of physical abuse on attachment have been well established. Studies with abused and neglected children using the "strange situation"[6] confirm the grave consequences of violence in the family on security of attachment. These conclusions have been affirmed by Bowlby.[3] (2) Sexual abuse, which is considered present if a primary caregiver or other adult abused or exploited the child for the caregiver's sexual stimulation. The role of sexual abuse in the development of insecure attachments has been reviewed by Alexander.[2] (3) Alcohol or drug abuse in one or both primary caregivers, which is considered present if the patient states that the caregiver had problems with the use of alcohol or drugs. Substance-abusing mothers score negatively on variables of attachment more frequently than non-substance-using mothers.[14] (4) Abandonment, which is considered present if the patient suffered the loss of a primary caregiver that the patient perceived as abandonment. The adverse effects of repeated threats to abandon, let alone abandonment itself, on security of attachment is discussed by Bowlby in his 1988 book *A Secure Base*.[3] (5) Emotional neglect/abuse, which is considered present if the patient relates that the primary caregiver(s) were not available for emotional support or were actively and persistently critical, demanding, or rejecting of the child's emotional needs. Some of the most compelling evidence for the untoward effect of emotional unavailability on security attachment comes from studies of children with depressed caregivers.[9]

We have demonstrated in a retrospective study [10] a clear and significant correlation between the number of childhood risk factors and the success rate of lumbar spine surgery. We hypothesize that the number of risk factors is roughly equivalent to the severity of damage to attachment security. Patients who have had three or more risk factors had an 85% failure rate, whereas those with no risk factors had only a 5% failure rate. Conversely, in patients with a poor surgical outcome, the prevalence of three or more risk factors was 75%. The correlation was seen in single-level, multilevel, primary, and repeat surgeries. The correlation increased significantly with each additional risk factor. Factor analysis was not done to determine the relative strength of each risk factor or to determine which combination of risk factors might be more damaging.

Central to our understanding of vulnerability to pain is the adverse effect childhood traumas play on security of attachment. It is from the secure base that attachment can provide that one not only explores the world, but also weathers the inevitable traumas of life. Several authors[4,15,16] have found a high prevalence of early adverse childhood experiences in adults with painful medical illnesses. The focus in these studies was on the experiences alone, and not on the effects that the experiences had on attachment. We believe that it is not simply the presence of abuse or neglect in the history of the patient, but the effects such events may have had on the capacity of the individual to form consoling relationships (i.e., secure attachments). To understand better how these early childhood experiences damage attachment, some basic understanding of the psychology, neuropsychology, and neurophysiology of trauma must be understood.

Neuropsychology

Van der Kolk, a prominent researcher in psychologic trauma, states that "traumatization occurs when both internal and external resources are inadequate to cope with an external threat to one's existence. Trauma leads to hyperarousal states for which the victim's memory of the event can be state dependent or entirely dissociated. This hyperarousal state persists as chronic to the extent that the trauma is not adequately resolved and integrated."[12] Thus, a trauma only threatens to disturb the underlying attachment, but if the caregiver's interventions are inadequate, the consequences of the trauma persist. That is, lack of adequate consolation by the caregiver or lack of receptivity to such consolation by the patient serves to perpetuate the sequelae of the trauma.

A physiologic hyperarousal response left over from the earlier trauma is activated by stimuli reminiscent of it. These stresses or stimuli tend to be experienced as nonspecific somatic states (e.g., tics, tremors, wheezing, pain, panic attacks) rather than

as new specific events that require specific means of coping. Van der Kolk states that trauma victims "may respond to contemporary stimuli as if a return of the trauma has occurred without the conscious awareness that it is a *past* injury [e.g., physical or sexual abuse, abandonment] and *not* the current conscious stress that is identified by them that is responsible for the emergency hyperarousal state"[12] (emphasis and examples added by authors).

Trauma also induces long-term potentiation of memory tracts (flashbacks) that are also reactivated at times of subsequent arousal. Cognitively, this hyperarousal interferes with the victim's ability to make rational assessment about his/her experience and prevents resolution and integration of the previous trauma with current stresses. In addition, disturbances in the brain's catecholamines, serotonin, and endorphins participate in this confusing hyperaroused state. Further understanding of these biochemical disturbances is important if pharmacologic interventions are to become effective in facilitating resolution of the trauma. This is certainly true in the patient with mild to moderate low-back pain that seems to have activated a hyperarousal state based on past traumas.

Clinical Implications

During early development, when attachment patterns are being established, unmitigated trauma disrupts secure attachment. Traumas themselves only threaten the underlying attachment. The response of the caregiver to such traumas is critical. If the caregiver's interventions are inadequate, absent, or additionally traumatic, the trauma becomes enduring. Insecure attachment also leads to a hyperarousal pattern that can be incited by various stresses or stimuli without any conscious link to earlier trauma. This hyperarousal pattern becomes a part of the insecure attachment template. Van der Kolk's work on the effects of trauma supports this interdependent relationship between security of attachment, psychologic vulnerability, and trauma.[13] He concludes that "childhood trauma contributes to the initiation of self-destructive behavior, but lack of secure attachment helps to maintain it." He suggests that "vulnerability to posttraumatic stress disorder can be predicted on the *security of attachment* and that uncontrollable disruptions or distortions of attachment bonds precede the development of posttraumatic stress syndromes."[12] The latent hyperarousal, biochemical, and cognitive states of the earlier causative trauma await reactivation by any stress that threatens links to current attachment figures. The stresses of a spine injury, whether it be precipitous or of insidious onset, will evoke markedly different responses depending on the patient's earlier attachment and trauma history. When the clinician is confronted with pain and/or disability that does not appear to correlate with sufficient structural findings, consideration must be made as to what earlier unresolved traumata the stressors are stimulating in the patient.

Grossman and Grossman[7] suggest factors that may influence changes toward a more secure attachment in adults, including psychotherapy, supportive spouses, and emotionally significant others. Valliant,[11] in the prospective study of 100 male Harvard graduates, similarly found that the presence of long-term sustaining relationships in adults was not only positively correlated with emotional and physical health, but was a means of overcoming the untoward effects of unhappy childhoods. Certainly, these observations are consonant with our clinical experience: Where evidence for insecure attachment exists, strategic interventions are often effective. For patients not responding as expected to conservative care or for those who are being evaluated for possible surgery, psychiatric treatment planning begins with identification of factors from a developmental history that may make overcoming the rigors of a major surgery or rehabilitation problematic. When psychologic factors are identified, surgical intervention should be considered cautiously and only with adequate strategic psychologic intervention. Such intervention is necessary not only to enhance surgical and conservative care outcome but also to avoid evoking and not treating previously unresolved traumas and adding further to the patient's inconsolability.

Summary

Kolb has proposed an attachment-theory–based model of managing chronic pain patients.[8] Though his model does not include the vulnerability aspects of the model we propose, he does agree "that establishment of a trusting, expectant, and secure attachment base forms the fulcrum on which rests application of any indicated technical intervention to relieve painful distress."[8] It is our experience that the ability of the treating physician or team to form a consoling relationship with the patient is necessary to a successful outcome. This relationship sometimes entails a psychotherapeutic relationship in the more traditional sense, in which the "pain" of an upbringing in which caregivers abrogated their responsibility can be safely explored. Other times it involves the patient's successfully finding solace in the group environment, such as the variety of 12-step survivor groups or chronic pain groups. At still other times it may involve helping to find the appropriate (e.g., gender, character style, etc.) physical therapist or clinician with whom the patient can relate and form a consoling relationship. A patient with an insecure attachment often evokes significant negative responses in other caregivers, which can easily serve to perpetuate the patient's internal expectation of traumatizing relationships. The mental health professional in these situations must often serve as the consultant for the other involved professionals. In the model that we propose, chronic spine pain often represents a nonspecific plea for help in overcoming earlier unresolved traumas, traumas that have disrupted the most basic of human need — a secure attachment.

References

1. Ainsworth MDS, Bell SMV, Slayton D: *Individual differences in strange situation behavior in one-year olds.* In Schaffer HR: *The origins of human social relations,* London, 1971, Academic Press.
2. Alexander PC: Application of attachment theory to the study of sexual abuse, *J Consult Clin Psychol* 60:185, 1992.
3. Bowlby J: *A secure base,* New York, 1988, Basic Books, p 77.
4. Domino J, Haber J: Prior physical and sexual abuse in women with chronic headache: clinical correlates, *Headache* 27:310, 1987.
5. Engel GL: Psychogenic pain and the pain-prone patient, *Am J Med* 26:899, 1959.
6. George C, Kaplan N, Main M: *Attachment interview for adults,* Unpublished manuscript, 1984.
7. Grossman K, Grossman KE: *Attachment quality as an organizer of emotional and behavioral responses in a longitudinal perspective.* In Parks CM, Stevenson-Hinde J, Marris P, editors: *Attachment across the life cycle,* London, 1991, Tavistock/Routledge p 93.
8. Kolb L: Attachment behaviors and pain complaints, *Psychosomatics* 23:413, 1982.
9. Radke-Yarrow M: *Attachment patterns in children of depressed mothers.* In Parks CM, Stevenson-Hinde J, Marris P, editors: *Attachment across the life cycle,* London, 1991, Tavistock/Routledge, p 115.
10. Schofferman J, Anderson D, Hines R, et al.: Childhood psychological trauma correlates with unsuccessful lumbar spine surgery, *Spine* 17(Suppl): S138, 1992.
11. Valliant G: *Adaption to life: how the best and the brightest came of age,* Boston, 1977, Little Brown & Co.
12. van der Kolk BA: The compulsion to repeat the trauma: enactment, revictimization, and masochism, *Psychol Clin North Am* 12:389, 1989.
13. van der Kolk BA, Perry JC, Herman JL: Childhood origins of self-destructive behavior, *Am J Psychiatry* 148:1665, 1991.

14. Wachsman L, Schuetz S, Chan LS, Wingert WA: What happens to babies exposed to phencyclidine (PCP) in utero? *Am J Drug Alcohol Abuse,* 15:31, 1989.

15. Walker EA, Katon WJ, Harrop-Griffiths J, et al.: Relationship of chronic pelvis pain to psychiatric diagnoses and childhood sexual abuse, *Am J Psychiatry* 145:75, 1988.

16. Wurtele SK, Kaplan GM, Keairnes M: Childhood sexual abuse among chronic pain patients, *Clin J Pain* 6(2):110-113, 1990.

Chapter 39
Transcutaneous Electrical Nerve Stimulation, Acupuncture, Biofeedback, Hypnotherapy, and Spine Pain

Michael H. Moskowitz

The treatment methods of transcutaneous electrical nerve stimulation (TENS), acupuncture, biofeedback, and hypnotherapy are often called on by traditional practitioners when other methods of treating spine pain have failed to yield satisfactory results. Each of these approaches has its adherents and detractors. Often patients themselves, desperate for some measure of relief from their chronic pain, request one or more of these approaches. Much of the literature supporting these treatments is methodologically flawed, and this makes it difficult to evaluate them from an objective, scientific standpoint.[1,5,6,16,18] Often case studies or inadequate sample sizes or inadequate controls prevent proper conclusions from being drawn.[5,6] Many studies have been done to review the methods used to evaluate efficacy of these approaches, and as could be expected in such controversial situations, these studies also are split in most of their conclusions.[6] There is also a subjective quality to pain and its relief that cannot be evaluated properly in a rigorous scientific study, but contributes greatly to patient response. It is important to note than in examining these treatments, hypnotherapy and biofeedback are similar to each other, and TENS and acupuncture have much in common. There is little similarity in either of these two groups between each other. The author's clinical experience is weighted toward hypnotherapy; therefore, this will dictate the focus of this chapter.

Transcutaneous Electrical Nerve Stimulation

Transcutaneous electrical nerve stimulation (TENS) uses the principle of stimulating superficial nerves down to about 4 cm below the skin's surface by using externally mounted electrodes attached to the skin. A battery operated unit is attached to the electrodes and sends electrical pulses to the electrodes. These vary in amplitude and are controlled within a preset range, by the patient. In some chronic pain treatment, TENS may actually increase pain, although this seems more related to placement of the electrode than to the treatment itself. Its effectiveness had been studied in many different chronic and acute pain states, and its proponents tout it as effective, helpful in decreasing the use of analgesics, relatively long-acting, and particularly helpful in syndromes with some component of skin hypersensitivity and/or causalgia.[10,15,17] Its opponents say that most of the studies for chronic low-back pain are

flawed and that it is no more effective than placebo.[1] Theoretically, TENS is conceptualized by Wall and Gutnick as causing spinal cord inhibition of nerve cells through increased stimulation of inhibitory cells.[24] There is also speculation that inhibition of peripheral nerve cells occurs in a similar fashion.[13,17] Several papers discuss the various types of TENS for treating chronic back pain. Most authors agree that strong stimulation and continuous stimulation offer the best results.[10,13,16,17]

Acupuncture

Acupuncture is an ancient Chinese procedure developed four thousand years ago as part of the overall teachings of traditional Chinese medicine. As such, its traditional explanations make absolutely no sense to the Western medical model. This has led to a great deal of skepticism and attempts to delineate more clearly whether the treatment is truly effective and what might be the neurophysiologic process behind it. Ulett describes acupuncture as a means of stimulating the central nervous system through peripheral nerves.[23] He relates its effectiveness in controlling pain to its ability to stimulate serotonergic neurotransmission. He also states that there is a great body of evidence to support acupuncture stimulating increased central nervous system endorphin, dynorphin, and enkephalin release.[13,17] Other authors find that acupuncture does not stimulate endorphins.[19] Melzac and Wall state that acupuncture pain relief cannot be attributed solely to placebo effect.[17] They think that traditional acupuncture sites and needles are overly specific and that any strong sensory stimulation of a broad area surrounding the traditional acupuncture site is effective. Fox and Melzac did a study comparing the effectiveness of TENS and acupuncture, showing them both to be effective treatments for low-back pain and neither to be statistically more effective than the other.[8] Melzac and Wall postulate that the midbrain reticular formation cells receive strong signals from TENS and acupuncture stimulation and "close the gate to inputs from selected body areas.[17] Acupuncture for the treatment of chronic spine pain does have its detractors, as well. The National Council Against Health Fraud (NCAHF) conducted an extensive review of the literature on acupuncture and concludes that reports of its efficacy in any form of treatment is groundless. NCAHF feels that no good physiologic rationale has been advanced other than placebo response, distraction, or suggestibility.

Biofeedback

Biofeedback is actually quite similar to hypnotherapy. Basically, biofeedback uses hypnotic trance induction to alter a measurable physiologic function such as striated muscle tension, skin temperature, or blood pressure, while feeding back the changes via sound and/or light impulses to the patient and the therapist. Almost all the patients who suffer with chronic pain have difficulty handling life stresses. Many have initial difficulty with the idea of hypnotherapy, feeling that it represents a loss of control and a submission to someone else. This opinion is also held by many of the physicians referring patients for psychiatric care. Although this is not the case, it is often more palatable for patients and their primary physicians to enter into this type of work via the more technologically driven route of biofeedback. For patients it gives some objective evidence of the mind-body connection and in particular the mind's ability to influence physiologic processes. In treating spine-injured patients for pain, it is important for biofeedback to be aimed at weaning the patients off the biofeedback machines and tapes into a routine of self-hypnosis. Some patients do better with the initial biofeedback approach, and others do better with self-hypnosis. Biofeedback is a particularly useful method in the somatically preoccupied patient with a purely mechanistic view of spine disease. One of the main functions using this method is to educate the patient about the undeniable connection between mind and body.[4] By using biofeedback with this group, much unnecessary time dealing with resistances can be eliminated. A complete program of stress and pain reduction treatment should include a time-limited number of biofeedback or hypnotic sessions combined with self-hypnosis practice. These treatments are usually pleasant and relaxing, and it is easy for patient and therapist to continue them in an open-ended manner, thus unwittingly encouraging dependency on the part of the patient. Since the entire treatment approach is to emphasize independence my strong recommendation is to keep them time-limited with occasional reinforcement as clinically indicated.

Hypnosis and Hypnotherapy

Hypnosis is a state of consciousness that is part of the everyday experience of all people. It is one of the usual states of consciousness seen in people and animals. The famous Florida tourist attraction of watching a Seminole Indian wrestle an alligator is actually a demonstration of inducing the hypnotic state in the reptile by rolling it over on its back and rubbing its belly. An example of a more domesticated version of this practice is the purring and nursing behavior of a cat when being stroked on its head or neck. People are in and out of self-induced trance states on a daily basis. It is the state of consciousness entered prior to sleep, while reading a good novel, when daydreaming, during sexual activity, and in any other set of behaviors requiring focused attention. The key to attaining the hypnotic state is repetitive behavior and task focus.

Hypnotherapy is the clinical process of purposefully inducing the trance state in order to obtain some diagnostic or treatment result.[11,12] Merely inducing the state of hypnosis is not therapeutic. This is where many mistakes in using this technique are made by practitioners and patients alike. Often the technique used for pain control is done by the hypnotherapist to the patient, using posthypnotic suggestions to establish long-term pain relief. This approach is adequate in dealing with acute, time-limited pain, but is of little value with chronic pain. Additionally, it is often observed that in patients who are taught how to self-induce the trance state, there is no progression beyond attaining this pleasantly relaxed state of consciousness. Usually, this is because the patient erroneously believes that relaxing and relaxation therapy is the way to deal with pain. While this relaxation approach can be helpful in problems with sleep and anxiety, it is not particularly useful with chronic pain.

Hypnotherapy is a treatment method that is misunderstood and often maligned as "hocus-pocus." The reality is that there have been a multitude of studies that show the efficacy of this treatment.[13] Detractors exist here as well. They claim that the effect is placebo or based on the suggestibility of the patient. Perhaps a great deal of the problem with accepting this treatment comes from the stage hypnotist's dramatic and often embarrassing use of the hypnotic state to entertain an audience. Even the roots of the clinical application of this phenomenon rest with a controversial progenitor—Franz Mesmer, who established his theory of animal magnetism. Mesmer himself was quite a showman, treating his patients while he was dressed in a bejeweled robe, as they rested in a bathtub filled with iron filings. He would run a magnet over the patient, moving the iron filings, while inducing a trance state. Although the theory of magnetic forces being at play was a false one, Mesmer is credited with having discovered the clinical application of hypnosis.[14] This was a dubious distinction at best, having been rejected by the majority of medical and psychiatric practitioners until its period of resurgence following World War II. Mesmer himself was run out of town on numerous occasions and was labeled a fraud, dying a broken man. The method lay dormant as a treatment method until Freud discovered its usefulness in the late nineteenth century, while working as a neurologist under Charcot in France. Charcot used hypnotic-trance induction as a means of distinguishing organic epileptics from functional epileptics, relegating the latter group to the realm of hysteria. Freud found all this fascinating and incorporated trance technique into his early psychiatric treatment methods.[9] He had developed the "trauma theory" of psychology and used trance-induced recovery of memory to uncover early childhood trauma. It has been widely reported that Freud, an iconoclast, but still a product of Victorian morality, gave up the practice of hypnosis when one of his female patients threw her arms around him during a trance state and professed a strong sexual attraction to him. Whether this story is apocryphal or not, Freud not only gave up the use of hypnosis and abandoned the trauma theory of psychology, but he also admonished his students and followers against using this technique. Once again, hypnotherapy fell into disrepute.

It was not until Milton Erickson, the modern father of hypnotherapy came on the scene that hypnosis was again brought back into the legitimate clinical arena.[11,12] Dr. Erickson had suffered from polio as an adolescent and during his home convalescence in an iron lung, he accidentally discovered the use and value of self-hypnosis in his own recovery. When he attended his residency training in psychiatry, this treatment was considered inappropriate. He had to sneak it into his treatment regimen and research projects. He did so with a gift for ingenuity, and when he finished training, he established this approach as his major focus of clinical practice. Word of his success spread, and through papers and lectures hypnosis became established once again as a reasonable treatment approach. Currently, it is considered an effective treatment method for dissociative psychiatric conditions, recovery of repressed memory, habit control, sleep disturbance, stress reduction, and pain control.[2,3,14,20,21] The latter three clinical applications are particularly important to patients with back pain. It is important to add to these three the development in the patient of a sense of mastery over symptoms.

Patients with spine pain often present with symptoms of profound sleep disturbance, extremely high levels of stress, anxious and depressed emotional states, decreased frustration tolerance, social isolation and withdrawal, helplessness, loss of self-esteem, and severe pain. Most feel that the predictability and control in their lives has been dramatically curtailed. As with most patients, they enter into the medical care system with a certain sense of passivity and a need to be "fixed." There is frequently a sense of shock when they are told that they will have to learn to live with the condition that plagues them and causes such severe alterations in their lives and self-images. Unfortunately, they are often either given the message that this problem is all in their heads or they interpret the information to mean that they will have to learn to live with their spine pain problems as meaning nothing can be done to help them. This tends to increase despair, anger, anxiety, and frustration.

The patient with spine pain must be helped by the treating physician to understand that there are many approaches to treating the pain. Some of these are physical, some social, and some psychologic in nature. The problem they face is often one of understanding that they cannot be passively repaired, but that successful treatment will require their active participation in a course of treatment that will incorporate many methods, require trial and error approaches, and involve a cumulative effect of the various treatments to achieve success.

Hypnotherapy is one of these clinical approaches. When effectively taught and properly learned it can be a very useful part of the armamentarium against the ravages of spine-based pain. It requires active patient participation, diligent practice, and a creative approach to the individuals' experience of their own pain. There is a correct approach to this treatment, which should be used as a guideline, but needs to be customized by the practitioner and the patient.

The purpose of the rest of this chapter is to help all practitioners working with patients with spine-based pain to understand the uses and potential problems of hypnotherapy in helping these patients. Additionally, with some continuing medical education in clinical hypnotherapy, physicians should be able to incorporate it into their treatment plans for their patients. If the individual practitioner does not have time to add this to an already busy schedule, appropriate referral sources may be used.

Many articles have been written about the usefulness of hypnotherapy in treating acute and chronic pain, but few actually outline the actual treatment. I will review the clinical criteria for patients who should be considered for hypnotherapy, proper evaluation techniques, potential problem areas, specific treatment approaches and strategies, and reasonable treatment outcome expectations. I incorporate into this my own treatment approaches, which are geared toward short-term treatment, active patient participation, and a direct approach to the patient's pain.

I will describe several detailed trance inductions, techniques, and a typical overall treatment plan. This chapter reflects my own approaches and biases, and it should be interpreted as a guide and not the only hypnotherapeutic approach to the patient with spine-based pain.

The technique of hypnosis I use for patients with spine pain is that of teaching them self-hypnosis to control their pain. Hilgard cites several studies done at Stanford that show pain control and the hypnotic state to be directly related to the hypnotizability of the patient.[14] While this parallels my own clinical experience, I have found that hypnotizability is something that can be taught. People have an innate skill level at self-hypnosis, but almost all can be taught to improve this level. Exceptions may be people with attention-deficit disorders and severe depressive or anxiety states. It is my impression that even many of these patients may be worked with to improve their ability to achieve deeper hypnotic trances. Part of the logic to be applied here is the fact that the hypnotic state is not the exclusive purview of the skilled clinician. By teaching the patient how to use trance in a stepwise manner of increasingly rapid, self-directed inductions, a tool for pain control is combined with a sense of increased mastery over previously demoralizing symptoms. I approach this by teaching self-directed induction techniques, followed by trance-deepening techniques, pain-reduction metaphors, dissociative visualizations, age-regression techniques, and posthypnotic suggestion. This approach is then supplemented with several weeks of practice at home by the patient. it is followed up with reinforcement of techniques that work for the patient and rapid (less than 1 minute) trance-induction techniques. The patient is instructed to use the longer techniques at the end of the day and the more rapid stress-reducing techniques throughout the day. Additionally, I integrate hypnotherapy into the rest of the patient's treatment plan, with distinct approaches developed for the surgical patient, chronic pain patient, and functional restoration patient. Tapes should be used with caution. It is important for all hypnotherapeutic work to stress practice of the honing self-hypnotic techniques. It is all too easy for the patient to develop a passive attitude regarding hypnotherapy, and in my experience this is anathema to successful use of this technique. While tapes can be helpful reinforcers of technique, they should not be used as a substitute for the patient's own trance-induction and pain-reduction exercises and practice.

Patient Selection

Selection of patients for hypnotherapy for the treatment of spine-based pain is in many ways easier than choosing between other treatment methods. Successful hypnotherapy does not require a particularly psychologically minded patient, as does insight-oriented psychotherapy. Most patients with chronic pain are highly motivated to try almost anything to relieve their pain. They will often put themselves through costly and painful treatments in the hope of gaining relief. In contrast to this, hypnotherapy is relatively inexpensive, time-limited, and quite pleasant for most patients. The specific patients who may be poor candidates for hypnotherapy for pain control are those who have a concurrent psychotic disorder, severe anxiety disorder, profound depression, attention-deficit disorder, or some cultural or religious belief barring its use. Additionally, there are many patients who believe that this treatment is a form of mind control, and they may object based on this false belief. Finally there are a group of patients who feel that a referral for hypnotherapy means that their doctors believe the pain is psychologic. These are often people who have switched physicians frequently and are searching for the definitive physical answer to their problem and who remain unwilling to consider any psychologic contribution. Patients with any of these issues may still receive help with hypnotherapy, but proper preparation for a referral may be critical in obtaining the desired positive result.

For the patient with concurrent psychiatric problems the best approach is a general psychiatric evaluation and treatment before hypnotherapy is considered. In developing a therapeutic relationship and beginning treatment of the psychiatric disorder, basic trust is developed and the patient's ability to focus attention is enhanced. Often this evaluation may indicate the need for antidepressant or anxiolytic medications. These are not contraindicated for hypnotherapy when properly used.

Patients who are about to embark on spinal surgery may receive a good deal of help by learning self-hypnotic techniques to deal more effectively with postoperative pain. It can be of special benefit when anxiety levels are higher than usual regarding the impending surgery. If the patient expresses worries about dying from the surgery, fear of blood, fear of anesthesia, or fear of the specific surgical approach that are out of proportion, hypnosis may be quite helpful in allaying these concerns.

Patients with nonneuropathic chronic pain problems, multiple procedures and surgeries, generalized pain disorders such as fibromyalgia, and stress-increased pain problems will often have excellent results with hypnotherapy. Again, this should be presented as part of an overall treatment program that may include TENS or acupuncture, as well as physical therapy, blocks, nonsteroidal antiinflammatory drugs, antidepressants, etc., and not as the solution to the problem. The presentation of hypnotherapy is best broached with the patient as part of an overall treatment plan that does not ignore the physical aspects of the patient's pain and its treatment. The advantage of hypnotherapy is that it does not involve the use of medication, is painless, and is self-directed and self-controlled. Additionally, it is a generally relaxing therapy and is the basis for relaxation techniques. It should also be emphasized that hypnotherapy uses the mind's ability to change the patient's pain intensity positively.

Evaluation

Evaluations for hypnotherapy will share many of the elements of a psychiatric evaluation. The evaluator should look for any ongoing acute, reactive, or chronic intercurrent psychiatric disorder that might interfere with effective treatment. These include the above-mentioned psychosis, major depression, or severe anxiety, as well as current posttraumatic stress disorders. Patients with dissociative disorders are of special concern. Of significant importance is any past history of abuse or severe psychologic trauma. One should be aware of this or of unusual areas of memory dysfunction that often represent profound levels of repressive psychologic defense. The dissociative or highly repressed patient may experience an abreaction in hypnotherapeutic trance that can be quite frightening. These types of problems do not rule out the use of hypnotherapy, but patients should be forewarned of their possibility. Additionally, the specific types of trauma may play a role in the patient's current complex of psychologic symptoms and may point in the direction of hypnotherapeutic treatment. An example would be a patient who was severely abused and abandoned by parents and is now approaching a surgery. Once again that patient is in a situation of impending physical pain and potential abandonment by caretakers. Hypnotherapy should be aimed not only at helping the patient to reduce postoperative pain, but also to reassure the patient of continued support and help through the frightening postoperative recovery period.

Assessment of the patient's experience with hypnosis, biofeedback, meditation, visualization techniques, and relaxation techniques should be directed at understanding what has and has not worked in the past. Often this experience will not be related to pain, but the patient will be expert at achieving a trance. This expertise usually is a real advantage when starting hypnotherapy for pain control. Prior clinical success is an excellent predictor of good outcome of treatment.

Part of the initial evaluation should take into account the patient's preconceived concepts of hypnosis and hypnotherapy. This should involve a discussion with the patient of hypnosis and its application to the control of chronic pain. It should stress the concepts of self-hypnosis, active practice, self-control, and the use of the power of the unconscious mind to control pain.

When evaluation is complete, a treatment plan using specific approaches within the context of the patient's overall treatment plan should be delineated. These approaches should be spelled out and geared towards a time-limited approach directed at clear goals and focused on teaching mastery through self-hypnotic techniques. Most patients can be taught these techniques in three to five sessions with 2 or 3 weeks between sessions to practice. I discourage use of tapes in the beginning of treatment, in order to encourage the patient's own sense of mastery and creativity in using the techniques.

Specific Treatment Approaches

Most of my patients are treated in three sessions, following an initial evaluation session. The first session is started by asking if there are any further questions or concerns about the use of hypnotherapy. Once this is explored, actual treatment is begun. I always begin by asking the patient the locations, quality, and intensity of the pain. I ask them to quantify the pain in its various regions on a scale of 1 to 10. During this session I generally teach a simple light-trance induction technique, followed by a trance-deepening technique. I purposefully keep these simple and try to tie the previous technique into the subsequent one. Once in a deeper hypnotic trance I will give an explanation of hypnotherapy as using this normal state of focused attention to tap into the vast power of the unconscious mind to alter the perception of pain by the brain. I will give two or three pain-control techniques, followed by a visualization imbedded with an age-regression and posthypnotic suggestion. As with most of medicine, the words sound impressive and technical, but the underlying principles are really quite easy to understand. I end the session by bringing the trance work to an end and having a brief discussion with the patient about current pain levels, questions about what we did, and the necessity of practice on a twice daily basis. I also encourage the patient to use the trance inductions alone to help with sleep problems, but to make sure to use the rest of the techniques to help with pain control. Below is an example of the trancework done in the first session.

Trance Work in First Session

Close your eyes and relax. Let your attention drift to the feeling of the muscles in the soles of your feet. Take a nice deep breath all the way in and all the way out, and as you breathe out I want you to let go of all the tension in the muscles in the soles of your feet. Now let your attention drift up to your calf muscles, and let them relax as well, letting that sense of relaxation spread up to both the front and the back part of your thighs. Very, very relaxed. You can continue to let that sense of relaxation spread up to your buttocks, your pelvis, your abdomen, your low back. Very, very relaxed. You can relax that long set of muscles that runs up each side of your backbone from the base of your spine to the tip of your skull, letting that sense of relaxation spread out to the muscles of respiration between your ribs from your upper back to your chest and deep down into your diaphragm, the main muscle of respiration that separates your chest from your abdomen. Now let your attention drift to your hands and the feeling of the muscles in the palms of your hands. Let them relax, as well. Very, very relaxed, allowing that sense of relaxation to spread up to your forearms and your upper arms, into the muscles in your shoulders and your neck. These are muscles that can take on a great deal of tension with the stress of the day, so just let them relax, as well. Very, very relaxed. You can let that sense of relaxation spread up to your jaw muscle, which often clenches down when there is pain in your body. Relaxing that muscle and the muscles of facial expression around your mouth and nose and eyes, and out into your temples and forehead. Completely relax your scalp; you can feel the last bit of tension leaving your body, almost like the feeling of gooseflesh as it leaves.

Now I want you to count down from 10 to 0 with me, and with each number I want you to picture yourself on a safe, well-lit, carpeted flight of stairs 10 steps high. If you cannot picture this then you can picture the numbers or just listen to the sound of my voice. As you go down, each number will take you deeper and deeper into your own unconscious mind. Now before we do this it is important to understand that your mind and your brain are not the same organ. Your brain is a 3-lb organ that sits in the base of your skull. All nerves feed into it and it receives pain signals as part of its function. Your mind, however, has as much to do with your big toe as it does with your brain. It is a vast organ that we cannot see, we cannot x-ray, we cannot draw blood from, and we cannot operate on. It is the sum total of everything that has happened to you throughout your entire life. Your conscious mind is only a small part of the whole picture, with most of the information of your life stored in unconsciousness. Your unconscious mind forgets nothing. It even remembers what it is like to not hurt in your body. We are going to tap into the power of your unconscious mind to replace the feeling of conscious pain with the remembered unconscious experience of physical comfort. For this is the usual way things are supposed to be, with pain resting in unconsciousness and comfort in consciousness. Since this gets reversed in chronic pain, we are going to use the power of your unconscious mind to place things back in their proper or-

der. Turnabout is fair play. Now I am going to count down. Ten, deeper and deeper into your own unconscious mind. Nine, eight, seven, deeper and deeper. Six, five, four, three, two, one, zero, a profound state of trance.

Now, what I want you to do is picture a dial with the numbers 0 through 10 on it and wires running from the dial to your [pain locations]. The pointer on that dial is pointing to the number [whatever number the patient gave on the 1 to 10 scale for their pain prior to starting the trance induction]. We're going to turn that dial down, like lowering the volume on a stereo or a TV. As that dial lowers the volume so will the volume of your pain lower, like turning down the volume on a TV (then slowly count down the dial from the initial pain level).

Now, whatever pain is left I would like you to see as a sink full of water, a sink with a drain in the middle of it. I'm going to tell you to pull the drain plug and as you watch the water wash down the drain, I want you to feel the remaining pain drain out of your body. Now pull the plug and feel the remaining pain drain out of your body as the water swirls down the drain out of the sink.

While we're talking about water, I would like you to picture yourself standing on a beautiful white sand beach, on the part of the beach where the water tamps down the sand, with the waves washing in over the tops of your feet. I don't want you to just picture this beach, I want you to feel yourself there. Feel the contrast of the coolness of the water washing over your feet with the heat of the sun on your skin. You can feel the sand eroding under your feet as the waves roll in and out. Smell the sea air. Listen to the sound of the waves crashing in that wonderful one-note melody, rhythm, and harmony of the ocean playing against the beach. If you look out beyond the breakers all the way to the horizon, you can realize that the ocean goes on for thousands and thousands of miles. It not only possesses great distance, but great depth as well. The ocean represents the vastness of your unconscious mind and the beach represents consciousness. And just as when you walk away from the beach the ocean continues to wash against it so when you come out of this trance state your conscious mind will continue to be bathed by your unconscious mind and the pain control you have achieved in this state of trance will last for many hours after you return to regular consciousness.

The last thing I would like you to do before we bring you out of the trance state is to feel yourself walking down the beach, not now the way your body has been but several years ago, before you were ever hurt. I want you to feel the way your body moved and felt. Enjoy that sense of well being and comfort, and when you come up out of the trance allow that feeling to remain with you.

Now, when you are ready, open your eyes refreshed and relaxed, with your pain greatly reduced, knowing that this sense of comfort can last for hours after you have returned to normal activity.

The patient is sent home with instructions to practice this approach twice daily. An admonishment is given to not just go into the trance state to relax, but to practice the pain-control techniques. These are reviewed briefly. The patient is also encouraged to get creative with the approach and to make up personally more meaningful suggestions. At least 2 weeks are allowed to pass before the next scheduled session. The patient is told that we will review progress and build on what has worked during the practice period.

Second Session

During the next session the patient's progress is reviewed. Most often the complaint is heard that great depth of trance and pain relief were achieved in the office, but not in self-hypnosis practice. Most frequently, when this is explored it is determined that the patient did not set up routine practice times, used the technique only sporadically, only used the trance-induction phase, and did not try any self-directed creative approaches. Once again, the practitioner is faced with the learned approach of patient passivity in receiving medical care. The hypnotherapist must take on the role of coach, and it is usually in this second session that the use of a tape to substitute for the therapist must be resisted. This is best accomplished by agreeing to make a tape for the patient once success at self-induction and pain control has been achieved, with the tape to be seen only as a guideline to reinforce the proper approach.

During this session I often have patients demonstrate their own self-induction. I add to this a reinforcement of what worked well for them and may add a few new pain-control and visualization techniques. If the patient is having difficulty with trance induction, I will teach a more mechanical approach before repeating the simple countdown trance-deepening approach. This can take the form of a breathing technique or a repetitive phrase, such as the following:

Repeat three times "my feet are feeling comfortable and relaxed [wait 15 seconds between each suggestion]. My legs are feeling comfortable and relaxed. My thighs are feeling comfortable and relaxed. My buttocks are feeling comfortable and relaxed. My pelvis is feeling comfortable and relaxed. My abdomen is feeling comfortable and relaxed. My low back is feeling comfortable and relaxed. My upper back is feeling comfortable and relaxed. My chest is feeling comfortable and relaxed. My hands are feeling comfortable and relaxed. My forearms are feeling comfortable and relaxed. My upper arms are feeling comfortable and relaxed. My shoulders are feeling comfortable and relaxed. My neck is feeling comfortable and relaxed. My head is feeling comfortable and relaxed." Finish with the somewhat discordant final phrase of "My breathing is regular, my mind is clear, and I am relaxed."

At the end of this session the patient is instructed to practice all techniques and to be creative in approaching them all. Additionally, the boredom factor with hypnosis is acknowledged. It is a boring approach by nature and it is explained to the patient that this is part of how trance is induced. Time must be set aside for success. Once again a 2-week minimum period is set aside for practice.

Final Session

The final session is used to explore further success and failure. Rapid-eye-fixation 20- to 30-second trance inductions are taught by having patients focus their eyes on objects on the distant wall while remembering themselves into the trance state. In patients who have mastered the techniques this is quite a simple task. The following is an example:

I want you to stare at that light switch on the far wall. While you are staring at it you may notice it come in and out of focus or partially blur. You may even see it shift shape into something else. This is all part of going into rapid trance. While you are doing this I am going to time you after I say "Go." I want to see how fast you can drop into a trance state by staring at the switch and remembering the shift in consciousness that represents trance, while dropping into that state. I will try this several different times. You signal with your left pointer finger when you have achieved this state. "Go."

This is repeated several times. Most patients can achieve trance within 15 seconds. They are instructed to practice this technique to reduce stress 10 to 20 times daily. Conspiratorially, they are told that this will not be detected by anyone and they should practice this when in conversations with others, on walks, and during physical therapy. They are instructed to use these techniques with the longer trance-induction and pain-reduction techniques to be reserved for specific times during the day when they can set aside 15 to 20 minutes to do so. Practice is again emphasized, and it is at this time that a tape should be given if the patient still feels a need for it. Most often this is an issue of transference for the therapist and not one of actually requiring a tape.

Treatment Outcome

Reasonable treatment outcome expectation is that a patient will be able to reduce usual daily pain by 50%. Unusual flare-up pain is more difficult, but diligent application of the method should help to reduce down time and promote more rapid return to function. A well-trained patient in an acute flare-up may require one or two reinforcement sessions. Surgical patients should experience improved postoperative recovery with decreased use of pain medication if proper presurgical training was accomplished. It does no harm to use a tape during surgery, but the efficacy of this approach has yet to be demonstrated adequately. In my experience neuropathic pain does not yield well to hypnosis, and other approaches should be used in these types of patients. It must be stressed with all patients that no approach guarantees success all the time. There will be times when in even the best-trained patient, pain will break through. Sometimes this is because the pain is necessary because of new injuries or extensions of old injuries. Unlike pain medication, hypnotherapy will not mask this type of pain. Although a few truly outstanding hypnotic patients may be able to use the technique to mask serious new pain, this will not be a lasting effect, and the pain will break through the hypnotherapeutic control.

Summary

TENS, acupuncture, biofeedback, and hypnotherapy are effective tools in the struggle to control spine-based pain. Although all these approaches have their detractors, most of the criticism is directed at the quality of studies done for examining these techniques and the treatment of chronic low-back pain. There is certainly room for more rigorous controlled studies. To condemn treatments that have given relief to many patients in chronic pain, however, misses the point. Increased theoretical sophistication is being applied to each of these treatment approaches, and common ground clearly exists between acupuncture and TENS, as well as between biofeedback and hypnosis. More controlled studies are needed to determine long-term versus short-term relief, the benefit of one treatment with certain patient populations over another, and a standardization of treatment approaches within each of these treatment methods.

Because of the author's clinical experience, this chapter has focused on hypnotherapy. In the hands of the proper clinician it is clinically efficacious, time-limited, cost effective, and empowering to the patient. Proper patient screening, evaluation, and motivation are essential to its success. Emphasis on the active role of the patient and the benefit of self-directed creativity must be constantly reinforced. As part of an overall physical, psychologic, and social plan of treatment, hypnotherapy can help to block the pain cascade and help restore the patient with spine pain to comfort and function.

References

1. Acupuncture: The position paper of the National Council Against Health Fraud, *Clin J Pain*, 7:162, 1991.
2. American Society of Clinical Hypnosis: A syllabus on hypnosis and a handbook of therapeutic suggestions, 1973, *American Society of Clinical Hypnosis*, 1973.
3. Barber TX: The effects of hypnosis on pain: a critical review of experimental and clinical findings, *Psychosom Med*, 65:411, 1978.
4. Brener J, Clemens W: *The clinical application of biofeedback techniques,* Francis Xavier University

Council For Research and NRC grant no. A9938, Unpublished manuscript.
5. Deyo R: Conservative therapy for low back pain: distinguishing useful from useless therapy, *JAMA*, 250:1057, 1983.
6. Ernst E: Is acupuncture effective for pain control? *Pain Sympt Manage*, 9:72, 1994.
7. Fordyce WW: *Behavioral Methods for chronic pain and illness.* St. Louis, 1976, Mosby.
8. Fox EJ, Melzac R: Transcutaneous electrical stimulation and acupuncture: comparison of treatment for low back pain, *Pain*, 2:141, 1976.
9. Freud S: A case of successful treatment by hypnotism (1892–93), standard ed 1, 1:117-120, 1966, p 117.
10. Graff-Radford SB, et al.: Effects of transcutaneous electrical nerve stimulation on myofascial pain and trigger point sensitivity, *Pain*, 37:1, 1989.
11. Grinder J, et al.: *Patterns of the hypnotic techniques of Milton H. Erickson, M.D.*, vol 1 and 2, 1977, Meta Publications.
12. Haley J: *Uncommon therapy*, New York, 1975, W.W. Norton.
13. Han JS: Effect of low and high frequency TENS on Met-enkephalin-Arg-Phe and dynorphin A immunoreactivity in human lumbar CSF, *Pain*, 47:295, 1991.
14. Hilgard ER: A quantitative study of pain and its reduction through hypnotic suggestion, *Proc Natl Acad Sci U S A*, 57:1581, 1967.
15. Johnson MI, et al.: An in-depth study of long-term users of transcutaneous electrical nerve stimulation (TENS): implications for clinical use of TENS, *Pain*, 44:221, 1991.
16. Marchand S, et al.: Is TENS purely a placebo effect? A controlled study on chronic low back pain, *Pain*, 54:99, 1993.
17. Melzac R, Wall P: Acupuncture and transcutaneous electrical nerve stimulation, *Postgrad Med J*, 60:693, 1984.
18. Mendelson G, et al.: Acupuncture treatment of chronic back pain: a double-blind trial, *Am J Med*, 74:49, 1983.
19. Morel V, et al.: Mechanism of analgesia induced by hypnosis and acupuncture: is there a difference? *Pain*, 45:135, 1991.
20. Orne MT: Hypnotic control of pain: toward a clarification of the different psychological processes involved, *Research Publications Association in Nervous and Mental Disease* 58:155-172, 1980.
21. Sternbach RA, editor: *The psychology of pain*, New York, 1986, Raven Press.
22. Stroebel CR: Biofeedback and behavioral medicine: a paradigm shift for psychiatry? *Psychiatr Ann*, 11:11, 1981.
23. Ulett G: Scientific acupuncture: peripheral electrical stimulation for the relief of pain: Part 1. Basics, *Pain Manage*, May/June: 128, 1989.
24. Wall PD, Gutnick M: Ongoing activity in peripheral nerves. II. The physiology and pharmacology of impulses originating in a neuroma, *Exp Neurol*, 43:580, 1974.

Chapter 40
Pain Management by Electrical Implant

Charles S. Szabo

Historical Review

Spinal cord stimulation (SCS) is a reversible, non-destructive neuroaugmentative technique employed for the treatment of chronic intractable pain. Electrodes are positioned in the epidural space to create paresthesias over painful dermatomes and thus block the central transmission of unpleasant sensations. SCS has been proven to relieve pain in patients with failed back surgery syndrome (FBSS).[34] High success rates are evident when the technique is applied in the context of a comprehensive pain management program with extensive psychologic and technical support. Recent technical developments combined with a greater understanding of patient selection have made spinal cord stimulation an integral component in the treatment of chronic pain of spinal origin in properly selected patients.

The use of electrical stimulation for treatment of pain originated in ancient Rome, when electric eels were employed to provide relief to painful extremities.[45] Availability of electrical generators during the seventeenth and eighteenth centuries allowed more-controlled application of electricity. In the late nineteenth century, development of battery-powered transcutaneous electrical nerve stimulators (TENS) resulted in the use of commercially produced units. Development of solid-state electronics accounts for the products currently used.

Advances in cardiac pacemaker technology in the 1960s hastened neurologic applications. The "gate theory of pain" advanced by Melzac and Wall[27] provided a theoretical basis for pain control by electrical implant. It was hypothesized that the balance of activity in the large and small diameter fibers influenced the central transmission of pain. Electrical stimulation of the rapidly conducting large diameter fibers with a lower depolarization threshold would, theoretically, close the gate on the small C and A delta fiber activity that conveys the sensation of pain. Reynolds[42] supported the theory experimentally by performing laparotomies on rats with periaqueductal gray stimulation as the only analgesic. Mayer et al.[26] showed that electrical stimulation had an antinociceptive effect and termed the process "stimulation-produced analgesia" (SPA).

Clinical application of SCS was first described by Shealy et al.[48] Electrodes were placed via laminotomy over the posterior aspect of the spinal cord in an attempt to stimulate the dorsal columns, the small fiber termination site, and thus inhibit peripheral pain. The technique became known as dorsal column stimulation (DCS), but the actual sites and mechanisms of action are more complex and involve descending modulating pathways.[13,29] *Spinal cord stimulation* encompasses this broader understanding and is the term commonly used today for epidural neuroaugmentative analgesia.

Commercially manufactured units became available in 1970,[24] and with the initial reports of successful application, widespread interest followed. The first symposium on pain control by electrical stimulation was held in 1973.[40]

The theoretical basis for the use of SCS, the absence of serious side effects, the nonaddicting nature of the treatment, and the total reversibility of the implant combined to make SCS a very attractive method for control of chronic pain. Enthusiasm, however, waned when high complication rates developed secondary to technical malfunctions and when it became evident that the success of the technique was highly dependent on proper patient selection and appropriate electrode placement. Long-term follow-up studies showed a significant decrease in effectiveness several months after implantation.[11,19,30,37]

Initially, implants consisted of plate-type electrodes placed in a subdural or endodural position via laminotomy; eventually, however, the epidural placement became standard.[24] The power supply consisted of radiofrequency systems coupled with a receiver implanted in an accessible location on the torso.

It soon became obvious that screening techniques were needed to eliminate invasive procedures in patients who would not benefit from SCS. Hoppenstein[15] reported the percutaneous placement of stimulating electrodes that allowed for a trial period in which to determine effectiveness in each patient. This innovation greatly improved the overall long-term success rate of SCS.

The ease of placement and the decreased morbidity of the percutaneous trial electrodes led to the development of permanent percutaneously placed leads.[33,53] Initially, both unipolar and bipolar percutaneously placed leads were prone to migration and breakage. Improvements in electrode design and insulation have resulted in a lower rate of hardware failure and in the development of devices with multiple-channel capabilities. Over time these capabilities have reduced the negative effect of changes in electrode position.[35] However, problems with lead movement and malfunction of the implanted hardware continue to be major impediments to the overall success of SCS. Despite problems encountered with the percutaneously placed electrodes, most clinicians have discontinued the routine use of the laminotomy-placed electrodes.[32]

In 1982 a totally implanted and programmable SCS system was developed.[46] Today, both multi-channel percutaneously and laminotomy-implanted leads may be interfaced with either an implanted pulse generator or a radiofrequency-coupled receiver.

Since its inception, SCS has been the domain of neurosurgeons. However, with the advent of multi-disciplinary clinics devoted to pain management, anesthesiologists have begun to play a major role. It is estimated that nearly 50% of the spinal cord stimulating systems in the United States are implanted by anesthesiologists, usually with the aid of a surgeon for generator placement.[23]

Indications

What is the place of SCS in the treatment of spinal disorders? The technique does relieve pain in patients for whom all other therapies have failed. However, the application of SCS is time-consuming and may involve multiple reoperations. It is expensive, with an estimated cost of $20,000 to $30,000 per implant, but in many cases it can be cost effective. A dedicated team of health professionals is required for obtaining the maximum benefit from the technique. The general spinal practitioner should be aware of the technique and refer appropriate patients to a pain management specialist for evaluation.

Proper patient selection is the most critical factor in the ultimate success of SCS. Initially, the technique was attempted in a multitude of painful conditions, but long-term success rates were very disappointing. As a result, many clinicians abandoned the technique.[11,25,51,52] A dedicated group of practitioners continued to use SCS because many patients with intractable pain enjoyed some relief. With greater clinical experience a clearer picture of the indications for SCS has emerged. Several general guidelines must first be considered before this technique can be applied to treat specific pathologic conditions.

General Considerations

The patient must have the appropriate personality to use an implanted device. Psychiatric clearance should be obtained through an interview with a psychologist or a psychiatrist. Most centers use a variety of standard personality tests and other psychologic tools, including the Minnesota Multiphasic Personality Inventory, the Beck Depression Inventory and the McGill Pain Questionnaire. MMPI depression scale elevations are associated with SCS treatment failures. Other high-risk factors include mood and stress disorders, a history of being abused as children and pending litigation. The patient needs to understand the long-term commitment necessary for treatment. Narcotic medication should be eliminated or tapered to the maximum extent prior to trial stimulation. It has been suggested that patients older than 70 to 75 years may be unable to operate the unit properly. Our personal experience, however, has shown that this is not the case.

The patient's pain should be severe, chronic, and intractable. If possible, the cause of the pain should be determined and all other forms of therapy should be tried and found to be ineffective or unacceptable.

The painful areas should be distributed in a pattern amenable to treatment with SCS. Unilateral radicular pain is the ideal pattern; bilateral and axial pain patterns, on the other hand, are much more difficult to treat.

A trial of SCS should successfully decrease the level of pain and permit an increased activity level.

Efficacy studies over the past 20 years have yielded well-established principles for application of SCS. Neuropathic pain caused by injury to the central or peripheral nervous system has been responsive to treatment with electrical stimulation. In contrast, chronic nociceptive pain resulting from injury to other types of tissue is relatively resistant to SCS. Specific clinical conditions that have been successfully treated with SCS are listed below.

Specific Indications

Failed Back Surgery Syndrome

Failed back surgery syndrome (FBSS) is the most common indication for implantation in the United States. Arachnoid adhesions and/or epidural fibrosis are generally thought to be the causes of extremity pain associated with this syndrome.[32,34,39]

Sympathetically Maintained Pain

Reflex sympathetic dystrophy (RSD) and causalgia are two examples of this condition, with very high rates of success when treated with SCS.[2,6,43,44] Some post-spinal-surgery pain is sympathetically maintained and is amenable to treatment with SCS.

Peripheral Nerve Injury

Peripheral nerve injury includes surgical injury such as a cluneal neuropathy at bone graft harvesting sites.[47]

Peripheral Deafferentation Conditions

Peripheral deafferentation conditions include a wide variety of pathologic processes in which there is a loss of afferent nerve fibers, including postamputation stump and phantom pain, radiculitis, postherpetic neuralgia, and plexus injury.[12,19,28]

Spinal Cord Lesions

Spinal cord lesions include paraplegia secondary to trauma with pain at the level of the lesion, multiple sclerosis, and postcordotomy dysesthesias.[28,31,50]

Pain from Ischemic Peripheral Vascular Disease

The most common indication for SCS in Europe is pain from ischemic peripheral vascular disease. Improved healing of chronic lower extremity ulcers by the use of SCS has been well documented.[5,10,16]

Efficacy

The long-term efficacy of SCS has been a matter of debate. The difficulty of determining the overall clinical success of SCS may be explained by the absence of controlled double-blind studies. The technique relies on patient cooperation for determining optimal electrode placement in the epidural space. A true patient-blinded study is thus impossible to perform. Other evaluation problems include the lack of a consistent evaluation system, the small numbers of patients in each series, the combining of many diagnostic groups in a given report, and the questionable practice of implanters reviewing their own data. The literature indicates that the long-term success rate is in the range of 50% for the indicated conditions.[3,34,50] The percentage of pain relief, the decrease in narcotic intake, the increase in activity level, the return to employment or the ability to resume normal housework, and, finally, overall patient satisfaction have all been used as criteria of success. The average length of follow-up has varied widely from months to years. The inclusion of patients from multiple diagnostic groups in nearly all published studies makes it difficult to evaluate the treatment for individual pathologic conditions. The continued improvement in implantable hardware also requires that results of older studies be carefully compared with those reported in more recent studies. In general, patients with chronic pain and no other therapeutic alternatives may deem treatment successful even if the pain is only slightly alleviated. A relatively small increase in the activity level can be quite important to the patient's overall sense of well-being.

Continued low-back and lower extremity pain after lumbar surgery occurs in approximately 25% of cases.[7] Treatment of FBSS with SCS has yielded success rates from 23%[28] to 88%.[17] Other studies have reported success rates in the 50% range.[1,8,9,18,21,34,50] The success rates do not appear to depend on the length of trial stimulation. Racz et al.,[39] who implanted the permanent system immediately on determining the appropriate paresthesias, had an overall success rate of 65%. Meglio et al.,[28] on the other hand, reported that trial periods averaging 20 days yielded a long-term success rate of only 23% for FBSS patients. Of the original 18 patients with FBSS, Spiegelmann and Friedman[50] eliminated six after trial stimulation, and with the remaining 12 patients they achieved a long-term success rate of 63%, with an average follow-up of 13 months. Even with very strict criteria for permanent implantation, long-term success rates were no better than average in a published series by De la Porte and Van de Kelft.[8]

Many clinicians report an early failure rate of approximately 20% immediately after permanent system implantation.[5,34,50] It is unclear whether this failure rate is due to a placebo effect, technical problems, or unrealistic expectations on the part of the patients regarding the efficacy of the permanent implant.

Other clinical conditions indicated for SCS have success rates similar to that found for FBSS. Literature reviews have been published.[35,50] One indication meriting special mention is the sympathetically maintained pain syndrome. Robaina et al.[43] reported a long-term (27 months) success rate of 90% in patients with upper extremity RSD and Raynaud disease. In treating upper and lower extremity RDS, Sanchez-Ledesma[44] and Barolat[2] and their colleagues reported success rates of nearly 80%.

Complications

The safety of SCS is well documented. Major complications are exceedingly rare. Pain at the site of implanted hardware occurs in approximately 5% of patients. Gait disturbances in a small number of patients have been reported, and some patients complain of stimulation-induced headaches while using the device. Infection rates from 3% to 12% have been reported at the site of permanently implanted hardware. Treatment consists of removal of the hardware followed by reimplantation.*

*References 8, 9, 21, 28, 38, 39, and 50.

Electrode breakage has been a chronic problem, with reported incidences up to 14%[34] but more routinely in the 5%[8,9,20,34,38] range. Depletion of the implanted battery is expected in all cases if the system is successful in treating the patient and is used over the long term. However, early generator and receiver failures have been noted.

In a series of 53 patients with FBSS, 48% required a secondary procedure after implantation of a permanent spinal cord stimulator.[34] Probst[38] reported that 28% of FBSS patients with permanent epidural electrodes required reoperation; De la Porte and Van de Kelft[8] indicated a 55% complication rate in a similar group of patients. Devulder et al.[9] reported 174 revisions, including 69 battery changes, in 67 patients drawn from multiple diagnostic groups.

A major problem encountered after initial placement of the system is electrode migration, a condition resulting in paresthesias that no longer overlap the patient's symptomatic areas. The diagnosis of a malpositioned electrode is usually made on clinical grounds. X-ray films of the unit are usually nondiagnostic because the change in electrode position is frequently too small to be visualized. The advent of programmable multipolar systems has made it possible through the electronic reshaping of the stimulation pattern to avoid surgical electrode revision in many instances of minor electrode displacement. Unfortunately, surgical revision of multipolar electrodes has been required in 28% to 70%[35,49] of patients with percutaneous implants. Spiegelmann and Friedman[50] have reported a 3% incidence of migration with plate-type electrode (Medtronic Resume) placed by laminotomy under general anesthesia. This finding has prompted the observation that a return to this type of procedure should be considered routinely. The complication rate was 13%, but the overall success rate was no better than the average percutaneous implant series, with 42% of patients obtaining good to excellent relief after an average follow-up of 13 months.

Patient Evaluation

A multidisciplinary approach is used for patients referred for pain management. An orthopedic surgeon usually makes the referral to a pain management specialist. The source of the problem is identified, and any additional tests and scans are ordered. Therapy is initiated if the pain can be treated medically. If a correctable lesion is identified, surgery is indicated. If surgery is deemed inappropriate or is rejected by the patient, and medical treatment has been ineffective in reducing the patient's pain to a tolerable level, SCS treatment is discussed with the patient. Patients are then seen by a psychiatrist or psychologist who can identify other major psychologic issues that may interfere with treatment. Attempts are made to eliminate or at least reduce the use of narcotic medications.

Patients who are candidates for a trial of SCS are again seen by the pain management specialist. The procedure is then discussed in detail. The patient must understand that his or her subjective response to the electrical stimulus is required for proper placement of the electrode and for determining whether the permanent system is to be implanted. The possibility of reoperation is mentioned because, as noted in some publications, nearly 50% of patients required further surgical intervention. Preoperative teaching is initiated concerning the patient's operation and control of the implanted unit.

Trial Testing

A temporary percutaneous trial electrode may be placed in the operating room or in a fluoroscopy suite. Some practitioners believe placement of a simple monopolar or bipolar electrode removed after the trial stimulation provides enough coverage to determine whether a permanent system is appropriate and decreases the overall infection rate.[23,32] If the trial is successful, the electrode and generator are placed in a single surgical procedure in the operating room. Problems with this approach include movement of an electrode held in place by a dressing taped to the skin and the possibility that a difficult trial lead placement may not be reproduced successfully in the subsequent permanent lead placement.

At our institution the overwhelming majority of patients have a quadripolar trial lead placed and subcutaneously tunneled in the operating room. After a successful trial, the system is then internalized in a second operative procedure, with the trial lead left in place. In over 110 systems placed in this manner there have been no infections requiring system removal. Advantages include placement of a quadripolar lead that allows maximum flexibility of trial stimulation patterns and the secure attachment of the lead to the dorsal fascia, thereby decreasing the likelihood of lead movement during the trial. The major disadvantage of this approach is the added cost of two operating room procedures. Even if the trial is unsuccessful, the subcutaneously implanted lead must be removed surgically. In our practice, approximately 70% of patients who have undergone the trial period have had permanent systems placed.

Lead and Generator Placement

The patient, placed prone on an operating table that permits biplanar x-ray examination, is comfortably sedated by the anesthesiologist. Although sedated, the patient must be alert enough to guide the placement of the stimulating electrode.

Under local anesthesia, the dorsal fascia is exposed at the appropriate level. To obtain paresthesias in the lower extremities, the active electrodes are usually placed at the T9 or T10 vertebral levels, with entry made into the epidural space at the T12-L1 interlaminar space. Because the procedure requires a shallow approach to the epidural space, needle entry into the fascia is at least one level caudal to the proposed level. Once the epidural space is identified with the Touhy needle, the stimulating electrode is carefully advanced into position. Nearly all recent publications report the use of equipment provided by the Medtronic company for both percutaneous and laminotomy placed leads. The other manufacturer of SCS equipment is the Neuromed company, which produces a wide variety of stimulating electrodes.

The Medtronic Pisces Quad and the recently introduced Pisces Quad Plus leads (Fig. 40-1) are guided under fluoroscopic visualization to the appropriate level in a midline position or slightly to the affected side (Fig. 40-2). Trial testing with the ex-

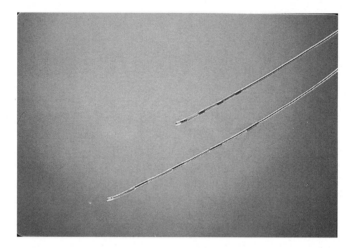

Fig. 40-1

Medtronic PISCES-Quad Plus Quadripolar Lead (*top*) has four 6-mm electrodes spaced 12 mm edge to edge. PISCES-Quad Lead (*bottom*) has four 3-mm electrodes spaced 6 mm apart. Each electrode is independently controlled. Leads are placed in epidural spaces through specially adapted 15-gauge Touhy needle that allows withdrawal and repositioning. *(Courtesy of Medtronic, Inc., Minneapolis.)*

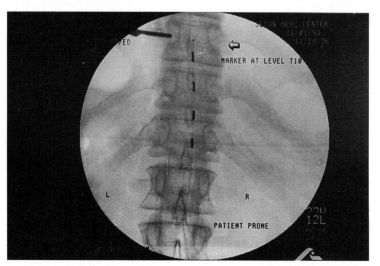

A

Fig. 40-2

A, Intraoperative fluoroscopic image of PISCES-Quad Plus lead placed to right of midline for treatment of right leg pain involving posterior thigh and calf.

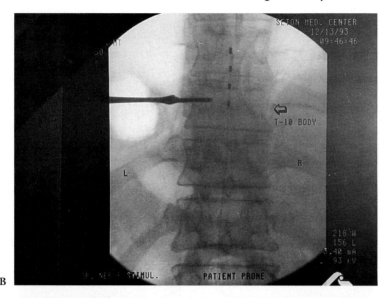

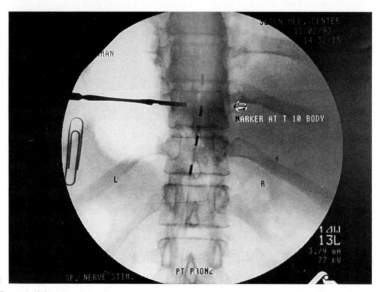

Fig. 40-2, cont'd

B, PISCES-Quad lead is centered at T9-T10 level and positioned to left of midline to stimulate left buttocks and hip. **C,** PISCES-Quad Plus is placed across midline in patient with bilateral leg pain. Activating multiple leads gives rise to broad stimulation patterns.

ternal screener (Fig. 40-3) allows the lead to be placed at the spinal cord level that produces paresthesias that overlap the patient's areas of pain. If adequate overlap is not obtained, SCS will not be successful. Only rarely is a percutaneous approach to the appropriate spinal level not achieved. The Medtronic Resume lead (Fig. 40-4) is then placed by laminotomy at the appropriate level. In our practice, the Resume lead had been used in patients who had previous success with a percutaneously placed lead but who have failed percutaneous revisions of a malpositioned lead and in patients for whom a percutaneous approach does not provide access to the epidural space.

After the lead is appropriately placed, it is anchored with nonabsorbable sutures, temporary wires connecting the lead to the generator are tunneled subcutaneously, and the wound is closed. The patient is discharged to home and trial testing proceeds for the next 5 days to 2 weeks. The patient is seen regularly in the office during the trial period so the wound can be checked and the stimulation parameters can be changed as needed. A positive response includes pain relief that the patient considers significant, an increase in activity level, a decreased need for pain medication, and frequently a much less disturbed sleep. For a small percentage of patients there will be good overlap of paresthesias with areas of

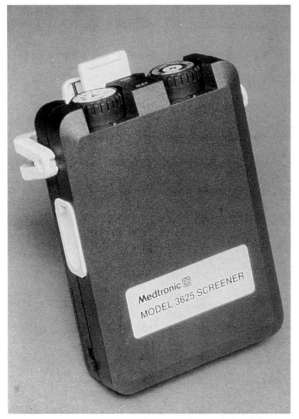

Fig. 40-3

Screener is connected to implanted lead by cable and subcutaneous connecting wires, both of which are discarded after trial period. Implanted electrode remains sterile during trial and is connected to permanent power source if trial is successful. Screener supplies power and electronic capabilities equal to permanently implanted power sources. *(Courtesy of Medtronic, Inc., Minneapolis.)*

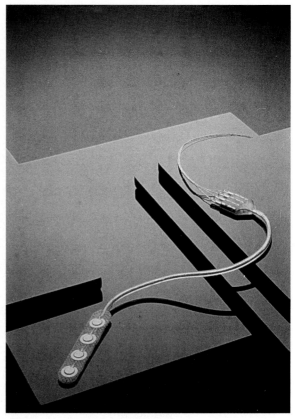

Fig. 40-4

RESUME lead contains four circular electrodes on 8 × 45 × 1.7 mm paddle. It is positioned in epidural space through small laminotomy incision. *(Courtesy of Medtronic, Inc., Minneapolis.)*

pain, but significant symptomatic relief will not be achieved. Such patients are deemed to have therapeutic failures, and the electrode is therefore removed. Occasionally, a patient will not obtain satisfactory stimulation and a revision of the electrode may be necessary. The use of the quadripolar leads during the testing phase is very helpful. Since reprogramming of the active electrodes usually provides at least partial coverage, the patient can determine whether the system relieves at least part of the pain. The electrode can be repositioned when the system is internalized.

The generator is also placed with the patient under local anesthesia with sedation. The pulse generator (Fig. 40-5) is placed in the upper quadrant of the abdomen or the upper buttocks, depending on the patient's preference. Most patients prefer the totally implantable system, but a radiofrequency-coupled system with an implanted receiver and external power supply is available if high power is required

(Fig. 40-6). Before the patient is discharged, settings of active electrodes, rate, voltage, and pulse width are optimized, and the patient is carefully taught how to operate the hand-held programmer and magnet that come with the unit and are used daily.

Many patients require minor adjustments in electrode settings over the first several weeks after implantation. These adjustments are made in the office by a nurse or some other trained member of the staff. Occasionally, patients report changes in stimulation patterns that cannot be reprogrammed to cover painful areas. In such cases, surgical revision of electrode position is required.

Future Applications

At our institution we have found SCS to be useful as the primary treatment in selected patients. For example, elderly patients with degenerative spinal stenosis and other concurrent medical problems have

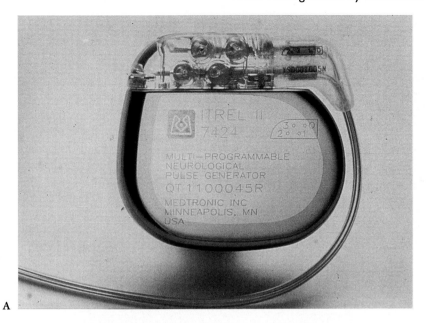

A

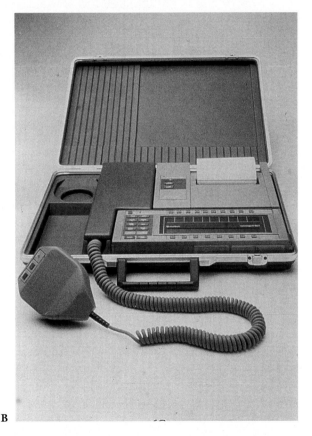

B

Fig. 40-5

A, Itrel II is an implanted power source with electronic parameters that are telemetry controlled. Unit is subcutaneously placed on torso. **B,** Amplitude, rate, pulse width, electrode selectability, and cycling on and off times are some of the features that can be controlled by noninvasive programming. Changes are made in the office by personnel trained in use of console programmer. Generator is connected to epidural electrode by subcutaneous cable. When battery is depleted, new unit is replaced surgically. *(Courtesy of Medtronic, Inc., Minneapolis.)*

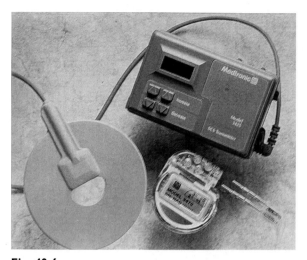

Fig. 40-6

X-TREL system consists of receiver (*bottom right*), which is placed subcutaneously; antenna (*bottom left*), which is positioned on skin over receiver; and external transmitter (*top*) with 9-volt battery as power source. *(Courtesy of Medtronic, Inc., Minneapolis.)*

returned to prior levels of activity after stimulator implant. Younger patients with multilevel degenerative disc disease and a poorly defined source of pain generation have also obtained relief with SCS for both upper and lower extremity pain.

In the future, SCS will be more reliable and predictable. Improvements in the design have already brought about the development of dual octapolar leads connected to a single power source. Placement on either side of the midline allows for bilateral as well as midline stimulation. This axial stimulation may allow for the treatment of back pain that is relatively resistant to stimulation with single multipolar electrodes. Pinpoint stimulation of the painful areas can be achieved, but the real challenge is the determination of the most appropriate electrode combinations out of the thousands that are available in such a system.[22] North et al.[36] have developed a computer-controlled system in which the patient determines the most appropriate settings. Barolat et al.[4] have pioneered the mapping of epidural stimulation, allowing for a more methodical placement of the stimulating electrode. Holsheimer et al.[14] have used computer modeling to determine which longitudinal fibers in the spinal cord are recruited by different contact combinations. Because SCS is based on pacemaker technology, one can envision future "smart" stimulators that can sense as well as pace, and thus provide pain relief on demand.

Summary

SCS is a technique that can greatly benefit a select group of patients. Neuropathic pain is notoriously difficult to treat, but some patients with this condition respond remarkably well to stimulation-produced analgesia. Although the technique is relatively simple to apply, good results are achieved only after extensive experience is obtained. Thus, appropriate candidates for treatment with SCS should be referred to multispecialty pain management centers, which can provide a team approach in providing care for these challenging patients.

References

1. Augustinsson LE, Sullivan L, Sullivan M: Physical, psychologic and social function in chronic pain patients after epidural spinal electrical stimulation, *Spine* 11:111, 1986.
2. Barolat G, Schwartzman R, Woo R: Epidural spinal cord stimulation in the management of reflex sympathetic dystrophy, *Stereotact Funct Neurosurg* 53:29, 1989.
3. Barolat G, Zeme S, Ketcik B: Multifactorial analysis of epidural spinal cord stimulation, *Stereotact Funct Neurosurg* 56:77, 1991.
4. Barolat G, et al.: Mapping of sensory responses to epidural stimulation of the intraspinal neural structures in man, *J Neurosurg* 78:233, 1993.
5. Broseta J, et al.: Spinal cord stimulation in peripheral arterial disease, *J Neurosurg* 64:71, 1986.
6. Broseta J, et al.: Chronic epidural dorsal column stimulation in the treatment of causalgia pain, *Appl Neurophysiol* 45:190, 1982.
7. Burton CV, et al.: Causes of failed surgery on the lumbar spine, *Clin Orthop* 157:191, 1981.
8. De la Porte C, Van de Kelft E: Spinal cord stimulation in failed back surgery syndrome, *Pain* 52:55, 1993.
9. Devulder J, et al.: Spinal cord stimulation in chronic pain: evaluation of results, complications, and technical considerations in sixty-nine patients, *Clin J Pain* 7:21, 1991.
10. Fiume D, et al.: Spinal cord stimulation (SCS) in peripheral ischemic pain, *Pace* 12:698, 1989.
11. Fox JL: Dorsal column stimulation for relief of intractable pain, problems encountered with neuropacemakers, *Surg Neurol* 2:59, 1974.
12. Franzetti I, et al.: Epidural spinal electrostimulatory system (ESES) in the management of diabetic foot and peripheral arteriopathies, *Pace* 12:705, 1989.
13. Freeman TB, Campbell JN, Long DM: Naloxone does not affect pain relief induced by electrical stimulation in man, *Pain* 17:189, 1983.
14. Holsheimer J, Struijk JJ, Rijkhoff NJM: Contact combinations in epidural spinal cord stimulation: a comparison by computer modeling, *Stereotact Funct Neurosurg* 56:220, 1991.

15. Hoppenstein R: Percutaneous implantation of chronic electrodes for control of intractable pain: preliminary report, *Surg Neurol* 4:171, 1973.

16. Jacobs JHM, et al.: Foot salvage and improvement of microvascular blood flow as a result of epidural spinal cord electrical stimulation, *J Vasc Surg* 12:354, 1990.

17. Kalin M-T, Winkelmüller W: Chronic pain after multiple lumbar discectomies—Significance of intermittent spinal cord stimulation, *Pain Suppl* 5:S241, 1990.

18. Koeze TH, Williams AC de C, Reiman S: Spinal cord stimulation and the relief of chronic pain, *J Neurol Neurosurg Psychiatry* 50:1424, 1987.

19. Krainick JU, Thoden U, Riechert T: Pain reduction in amputees by long-term spinal cord stimulation, long term follow-up over 5 years, *J Neurosurg* 52:346, 1980.

20. Kumar K, Wyant GM, Ekong CEU: Epidural spinal cord stimulation for relief of chronic pain, *Pain Clin* 1:91, 1986.

21. Kumar K, Nath R, Wyant G: Treatment of chronic pain by epidural spinal cord stimulation: a 10-year experience, *J Neurosurg* 75:402, 1991.

22. Law JD: Targeting a spinal stimulator to treat the "failed back surgery syndrome," *Appl Neurophysiol* 50:437, 1987.

23. Law JD, Kirkpatrick AF: Update: spinal cord stimulation, *Am J Pain Manage* 2:34, 1992.

24. Long DM: Electrical stimulation for relief of pain from chronic nerve injury, *J Neurosurg* 39:718, 1973.

25. Long DM, et al.: Electrical stimulation of the spinal cord and peripheral nerves for pain control: a 10-year experience, *Appl Neurophysiol* 44:207, 1981.

26. Mayer DJ, et al.: Analgesia from electrical stimulation in the brain stem of the rat, *Science* 174:1351, 1971.

27. Melzac R, Wall PD: Pain mechanisms: a new theory. *Science* 150:971, 1965.

28. Meglio M, et al.: Spinal cord stimulation in management of chronic pain, *J Neurosurg* 70:519, 1989.

29. Meyerson BA: *Electrostimulation procedures: effects, presumed rationale, and possible mechanisms.* In Bonica JJ, Lindblom U, Iggo A, editors: *Advances in pain research and therapy,* vol 5, New York, 1983, Raven Press.

30. Nashold BS Jr: *Electrical stimulation of the skin, peripheral nerves or dorsal columns for pain relief.* In Morley TB, editor: *Current controversies in neurosurgery,* Philadelphia, 1976, W.B. Saunders.

31. Nielson KA, et al.: Experience with dorsal column stimulation for relief of chronic intractable pain: 1968-1973, *Surg Neurol* 4:148, 1975.

32. North RB: *Spinal cord stimulation for intractable pain: indications and techniques.* In Long DM, editor: *Current therapy in neurological surgery,* Philadelphia, 1990, B.C. Decker.

33. North RB, Fischell TA, Long DM: Chronic stimulation via percutaneous inserted epidural electrodes, *Neurosurgery* 1:215, 1977.

34. North RB, et al.: Failed back surgery syndrome: 5-year follow-up after spinal cord stimulator implantation, *Neurosurgery* 28:692, 1991.

35. North RB, et al.: Spinal cord stimulation for chronic, intractable pain: superiority of "multi-channel" devices, *Pain* 44:119, 1991.

36. North RB, et al.: Patient-interactive, computer-controlled neurological stimulation system: clinical efficacy in spinal cord stimulator adjustment, *J Neurosurg* 76:967, 1992.

37. Pineda A: Dorsal column stimulation and its prospects, *Surg Neurol* 4:157, 1975.

38. Probst CH: Spinal cord stimulation in 112 patients with epi-/intradural fibrosis following operation for lumbar disc herniation, *Acta Neurochir* 107:147, 1990.

39. Racz GB, McCarron RF, Talboys P: Percutaneous dorsal column stimulator for chronic pain control, *Spine* 14:1, 1989.

40. Ray CD, editor: Electrical stimulation of the human nervous system for control of pain: Minneapolis Pain Seminar, *Surg Neurol* 4:61, 1973.

41. Ray CD, editor: Pain symposium: electrical stimulation of the human nervous system for the control of pain, *Surg Neurol* 4:61, 1975.

42. Reynolds DV: Surgery in the rat during electrical analgesia induced by focal brain stimulation, *Science* 164:444, 1969.

43. Robaina FJ, et al: Spinal cord stimulation for relief of chronic pain in vasospastic disorders of the upper limbs, *Neurosurgery* 24:63, 1989.

44. Sanchez-Ledesma MJ, et al.: Spinal cord stimulation in deafferentation pain, *Stereotact Funct Neurosurg* 53:40, 1989.

45. Scribonius L: De compositione medicamentorum liber. Translated in Kellaway P: The part played by electric fish in early history of bioelectricity and electrotherapy. *Bull Hist Med* 20:112, 1946.

46. Shatkin D, Mullett K, Hults G: Totally implantable spinal cord stimulation for chronic pain: design and efficacy, *Pace* 9:577, 1986.

47. Siegfried J: *Long-term results of electrical stimulation in the treatment of pain by means of implanted electrodes (epidural spinal cord and deep brain stimulation).* In Rizzi R, Visentin M, editors: *Pain therapy,* Amsterdam, 1983, Elsevier Biomedical Press.

48. Shealy CN, Mortimer JT, Reswick JB: Electrical inhibition of pain by stimulation of the dorsal columns: preliminary clinical report, *Anesth Analg* 46:489, 1967.

49. Simpson BA: Spinal cord stimulation in 60 cases of intractable pain, *J Neurol Neurosurg Psychiatry* 54:1296, 1991.

50. Spiegelmann R, Friedman W: Spinal cord stimulation: a contemporary series, *Neurosurgery* 28:65, 1991.

51. Sweet W, Wepsic J: Stimulation of the posterior column of the spinal cord for pain control: indications, technique and results, *Clin Neurosurg* 21:278, 1974.

52. Urban B, Nashold B: Percutaneous epidural stimulation of the spinal cord for relief of pain, *J Neurosurg* 48:323, 1978.

53. Zumpano BJ, Saunders RL: Percutaneous epidural dorsal column stimulation, *J Neurosurg* 45:459, 1976.

Chapter 41
Neurosurgical Approaches to Chronic Pain
Richard B. North

Failed Back Surgery Syndrome

> anatomic procedures
> augmentative procedures
> ablative procedures

Cancer Pain

> anatomic procedures
> augmentative procedures
> ablative procedures

Summary

Appendix: The Role of Spinal Cord Stimulation in Contemporary Pain Management

Pain is the most frequent complaint of patients presenting to the offices of physicians in general, and of spinal surgeons in particular. Some of the earliest neurosurgical procedures were developed for the relief of intractable pain, and over the past hundred years an extensive armamentarium has been developed. Pain of spinal origin is currently treated by a range of spinal, peripheral, and even intracranial procedures. As technology has advanced and the art and science of pain management have been refined, the results of neurosurgical procedures for pain have improved and morbidity has declined. Many surgeons and other physicians have a special interest in pain management and are trained in the full range of procedures described herein. This allows specific and appropriate treatments, some of which are directed at correcting the structural lesion responsible for the patient's pain and others at the pain *per se*. These issues are particularly important in a patient with pain of spinal origin.

Neurosurgical procedures for the relief of chronic, intractable pain may be divided into three categories: *anatomic procedures* to address a structural lesion causing pain; *augmentative procedures*, which treat the pain problem reversibly by electrical or chemical means; and *ablative procedures*, intended to block pain transmission by destroying parts of the nervous system. Table 41-1 gives examples of these procedures. Many are widely applicable, and adaptable to general neurosurgical practice, in the management of pain of spinal origin. Two common pain syndromes, failed back surgery syndrome (FBSS) and metastatic cancer involving the spine, will be used as illustrations (Table 41-2).

Certain general rules should be followed in patient selection. (1) There should be a documented, and ideally objective, basis for the patient's pain, such as computed tomographic or myelographically demonstrated root compression, arachnoiditis, or spinal metastatic disease. (2) Alternative treatment has been exhausted, is unacceptable or is medically contraindicated (e.g., physical or behavioral therapy, medical analgesic therapy). (3) Psychologic factors have been evaluated, and it has been established that there are no major psychiatric or personality disorders, overriding issues of secondary gain, serious drug habituation problems, or other abnormal illness behavior. (4) When feasible, temporary relief of

Table 41-1

Neurosurgical procedures for relief of pain of spinal origin

Anatomic	Augmentative	Ablative
Stabilization	Chemical	Open
Decompression	Infusion systems	Neurotomy
Reconstruction	Spinal epidural	Sympathectomy
	Spinal subarachnoid	Ganglionectomy
	Intraventricular	Rhizotomy
		Drezotomy
	Electrical stimulation	Cordotomy
	Transcutaneous	Myelotomy
	Implanted devices	Tractotomy
	Peripheral nerve	Closed
	Spinal cord	Percutaneous radiofrequency
	Intracerebral	Neurotomy (e.g. facet)
		Rhizotomy
		Cordotomy
		Cingulumotomy
		Percutaneous chemical
		Lytic subarachnoid block
		Stereotaxic hypophysectomy

pain should be demonstrated by a method analogous to the proposed treatment, before the permanent procedure. Neuroaugmentative procedures such as spinal cord stimulation and intraspinal narcotics may be tested with percutaneous temporary electrodes or catheters. Arguably, anatomic procedures such as spinal fusion may be tested indirectly by bracing. Ablative procedures may be tested by reversible, temporary local anesthetic blocks. These may have limited specificity and therefore limited positive predictive value; but if they are ineffective, they may be assumed to be accurate.

In general, anatomic (corrective) procedures are undertaken first, when there is reasonable certainty as to the structural basis for a patient's pain, and when the risk:benefit ratio and life expectancy of the patient warrant. Reversible neuroaugmentative procedures generally are considered before ablative procedures. The role of these procedures depends on specific clinical circumstance, as discussed below.

Failed Back Surgery Syndrome

Anatomic Procedures

When pain persists or recurs following lumbosacral spine surgery, reoperation may be appropriate. This assumes that a surgically correctable problem has developed since surgery (e.g., recurrent disc herniation), or that it was overlooked (e.g., retained disc fragment) or created iatrogenically (e.g., pars defect). Ideally, evaluation of such a case should include a review of all prior studies; when available, they often show that the indications for the original procedure were questionable.[9] The yield of surgery to correct a secondary problem, in this circumstance, will necessarily be reduced. Some cases of persistent pain relate to established nerve injury and will be refractory to secondary decompression or stabilization procedures.

We have reviewed our experience with reoperation on the lumbosacral spine, assessing outcome by disinterested third-party interview. Our overall experience with reoperation has been that the rate of "success" is approximately one third, and the morbidity significant.[12] We continue our efforts to refine diagnosis and patient selection for these procedures: for example, gadolinium-enhanced magnetic resonance imaging and three-dimensional computed tomography facilitate diagnosis of conditions such as epidural fibrosis and lateral recess and foraminal stenosis. It remains to be seen, however, whether this translates to improved results of reoperation.

Augmentative Procedures

Spinal cord stimulation was introduced 25 years ago as a reversible alternative to more invasive procedures such as spinal fusion or ablative surgery, for the relief of intractable pain. The use of spinal cord stimulation is discussed in detail in an article that appears as an appendix to this chapter. Therefore, only a few points are discussed here.

The earliest devices required a laminectomy for electrode placement. Subsequently, however, percutaneous methods were developed for placement of temporary electrodes. Trials with temporary electrodes enable the physician to demonstrate pain relief before implanting a permanent device and to map the epidural space for best electrode position. In addition, percutaneous techniques have been adapted to permanent electrode placement avoiding altogether the need for laminectomy. These devices have proven significantly more reliable, and clinical results have improved correspondingly. The rate of clinical failures (patient no longer using device as primary method of pain control) has been reduced significantly by contemporary devices.[11]

Table 41-2

Invasive procedures for intractable pain of spinal origin*

	Anatomic	Augmentative	Ablative
Failed back syndrome	Decompression, stabilization	Spinal cord stimulation	Radiofrequency facet denervation
Cancer pain	Debulking, decompression	Intrathecal narcotics	Rhizotomy, cordotomy, myelotomy

*Three broad categories of procedures are represented, for two common conditions.

In the failed back surgery syndrome, spinal cord stimulation has been reserved as a procedure of last resort for patients in whom surgical options have been exhausted. Typically, these patients are labeled with diagnoses such as "arachnoiditis" (with or without documented arachnoid fibrosis on diagnostic imaging studies) or "battered root syndrome." Using the same outcome measures as for reoperation, disinterested third-party interview, my colleagues and I have observed better results for spinal cord stimulation than reoperation for radicular symptoms of failed back surgery.[12,13] To the extent that patients undergoing spinal cord stimulation may have more impressive disease of longer duration, this comparison is all the more remarkable. Retrospective series, however, are awkward to compare; prospective, randomized study is required for more meaningful comparison.

The technical goal of achieving overlap of pain by stimulation paresthesias is more easily achieved for radicular pain than for axial pain. Furthermore, the former may be more neuropathic in origin, and the latter nociceptive—a distinction that may influence the response to stimulation. Targeting the low back in most patients requires careful psychophysical testing over a range of amplitudes, from first perception to discomfort or motor threshold, as described by Law.[6] Computerized systems have been developed to simplify this task, by interacting directly with the patient.[15] Routine treatment of axial pain by spinal cord stimulation, however, awaits further technical developments.[6]

Intraspinal opiate infusion has been employed in small numbers of patients with the failed back surgery syndrome and some encouraging results have been reported.[1] There have been no extended follow-up reports, however, and none have been assessed by disinterested third parties. Comparison with other therapies, therefore, is difficult. In patients with "arachnoiditis" who have demonstrated a tendency to react adversely, chronic subarachnoid infusion is problematic.[14] Before intraspinal opiate infusion is considered, the patient must first be an appropriate candidate for long-term opioid therapy in general. The patient should have appropriate trials of oral opioid therapy and fail either due to significant side effects or failure to achieve adequate analgesia. Only then should intraspinal delivery systems be considered.

Intracerebral stimulating electrode implantation is another reversible, nonablative technique that is occasionally useful in patients with the failed back surgery syndrome. Following extensive nerve-root injury, deafferentation may be so complete as to preclude the production of stimulation paresthesias in the painful area by spinal cord stimulation. In these patients, "deep brain stimulation" is a worthwhile alternative.

Ablative Procedures

Rhizotomy and Dorsal Root Ganglionectomy

Dorsal rhizotomy was reported in some early series as effective treatment for chronic, intractable lumbosacral radicular pain; but the series with the longest follow-up have reported a low yield.[8,17] An anatomic basis for persistent pain after rhizotomy was provided by the identification of ventral root afferents, with cell bodies in the dorsal root ganglia.[3] Extending rhizotomy to include dorsal root ganglionectomy so as to interrupt these ventral root afferents was expected to improve clinical results.

We have reviewed our experience with a series of patients with failed back surgery syndrome in whom dorsal root ganglionectomy was performed.[10] Patients were selected on the basis of their clinical presentation, suggesting a monoradicular pain syndrome; this was corroborated by diagnostic root blocks. A disinterested third party conducted follow-up interviews to assess outcome, a mean of 5.5 years following ganglionectomy. No patient was a long-term "success" (by definition requiring at least 50% sustained relief of pain, and patient satisfaction with the result). A minority of patients reported improvement in analgesic intake. Loss of sensory and motor function was reported frequently. Improvements in activities of daily living were recorded in a minority of patients.

Dorsal root ganglionectomy not only has a low yield, but also may reduce the yield of neuroaugmentative procedures. Destruction of primary afferents eliminates their presynaptic opiate receptors, which constitute half the receptors in the spinal cord. Furthermore, it destroys primary afferent fibers ascending in the dorsal columns of the spinal cord. This may compromise the results of spinal cord stimulation if, in fact, the mechanism of pain relief by stimulation involves the "dorsal columns."[2] In our ganglionectomy series, of seven patients who proceeded to trials of spinal cord stimulation, only one was ultimately successful. The usual yield is much higher in patients with monoradicular pain, who are a particularly favorable subgroup.

"Diagnostic" nerve blocks do not necessarily predict the results of an ablative or decompressive procedure. For example, nerve blocks performed distal to painful root or peripheral nerve lesions may give temporary relief.[5,21] Systemic effects of lidocaine (which can relieve, for example, post-ganglionectomy dysesthesias) may explain some, but not all, of these nonspecific results.[20]

Radiofrequency Facet Denervation

Radiofrequency lumbar facet denervations were developed more than 20 years ago as a treatment for intractable, mechanical low-back pain. In most reported patient series, high rates of success have been reported; but there has been limited long-term follow-up, objective outcome assessment, and analysis of prognostic factors. My colleagues and I have reviewed our experience in 82 patients with diagnostic lumbar facet blocks and percutaneous radiofrequency denervations, and have assessed long-term outcome by disinterested third-party interview. Of our patients who underwent diagnostic medial branch posterior primary ramus blocks, just over half reported at last 50% relief of pain and proceeded to permanent denervation. Of these patients, 45% reported at least 50% relief of pain 2 years after the procedure or at last follow-up (mean, 3 years). Only 13% of the patients who underwent only temporary blocks reported relief (i.e., spontaneous improvement or placebo effect) by at least 50% at same follow-up intervals. This represents a statistically significant difference, in favor of the patients undergoing denervation. We observed no complications from the procedure. This subject is covered in detail in Chapter 21.

Cancer Pain

Anatomic Procedures

A patient with cancer who has intractable pain due to spinal disease may, of course, require surgery to establish a tissue diagnosis or to treat instability or neurologic deficit. Absent these indications for surgery, if the pain is unresponsive to radiotherapy, chemotherapy and medical analgesics, the patient may be a candidate for palliative surgery. A wide range of anterior and posterior decompressive and stabilization procedures have been developed by spinal surgeons[19]; the details are beyond the scope of this chapter, but it is important to consider these procedures as the first step in pain management, if the patient's overall condition warrants. An anatomic, reconstructive procedure may have additional potential benefits, such as prevention of neurologic seque-

lae or deformity; this prospect of course influences the choice of therapy.

Augmentative Procedures

A metastatic lesion that causes a nociceptive pain problem commonly is responsive to intraspinal narcotic delivery even when systemic narcotics are ineffective.[18] If there is compromise of the normal cerebrospinal fluid circulation by metastatic spinal disease, this may preclude this type of neuroaugmentative procedure. When feasible, however, spinal epidural drug delivery offers one order of magnitude, and subarachnoid delivery two orders of magnitude, of dose advantage over systemic administration. The central side effects of systemic administration may be reduced or eliminated by this approach. Before any commitment is made to implantation of a permanent drug delivery system, patients may be tested individually by epidural or subarachnoid injection or infusion to establish that they respond to this form of treatment.

A wide range of drug delivery systems and catheters are used for intraspinal narcotic administration. An epidural catheter with a percutaneous extension is the simplest such system; it is appropriate if life expectancy is limited. The risk of catheter occlusion by fibrosis is lower, as is the cumulative risk of infection, in this circumstance. The cost of initial implantation is lower, but the maintenance costs of a percutaneous epidural system are higher than those of an implanted pump and subarachnoid catheter: ongoing nursing care is required, and higher doses of drug are needed. Despite the higher initial costs of the totally implanted system, it is more cost effective if life expectancy exceeds a few months. The simplest such device is passive, with a fixed infusion rate; it lacks versatility, but its initial cost is lower, and it has no life-limiting components requiring periodic replacement. Battery-powered, programmable devices allow noninvasive adjustment of infusion rate (and therefore of dosage) and complex infusion rate profiles (circadian variation, bolus administration). The longevity of these devices is limited by battery capacity, however, and their initial cost is high.

If intractable pain recurs due to progression of disease or the development of tolerance, spinal narcotics may be supplemented or replaced with other medications, such as local anesthetics. For cervical malignancies, which may be relatively refractory to spinal narcotics, a standard ventricular catheter with Ommaya reservoir or implanted infusion pump may be used to deliver medication centrally.[7,16]

Treatment with an implanted stimulator may be effective in a small number of cases of deafferentation or neurogenic pain, due to tumor invasion or the side effects of chemotherapy and/or radiotherapy. Radicular or segmental pain problems may be treated with spinal cord stimulation. For more widespread distributions of pain, implanted thalamic or periaqueductal gray electrodes may be effective. Like implanted drug delivery systems, these offer a reversible, nondestructive treatment option.

Ablative Procedures

When life expectancy is short, and when the expected or potential neurologic sequelae are acceptable, ablative procedures may be considered for the treatment of cancer pain. A straightforward example is sacral rhizolysis in an already incontinent patient. Percutaneous rhizotomy or neurotomy, using chemical, radiofrequency, or cryogenic techniques, is the simplest approach, but it is suited only to segmental or well-circumscribed pain problems. An anterolateral cordotomy addresses more extensive unilateral pain topographies, beginning several segments caudal and contralateral to the lesion. Open cordotomy is performed most often at upper thoracic levels; percutaneous cordotomy is most easily performed at C1-C2. Bilateral cordotomy may be appropriate for bilateral pain problems; but at C1-C2, when performed for lower cervical or high thoracic pain, it incurs a high risk of respiratory depression. When cordotomy is performed at high thoracic levels, although this complication is avoided, neurogenic bladder remains a risk. Midline (commissural) myelotomy is applicable to bilateral pain problems, and involves a single surgical procedure, but a more extensive, longitudinal, intradural exposure is required.[4]

Following an ablative procedure, delayed recurrence of pain may occur on the basis of deafferentation. This limits the role of these procedures in patients with longer life expectancies. Deafferentation pain, such as postcordotomy dysesthesias, may be more difficult to treat than the original, underlying pain problem.

As the use of high-dose systemic, intraspinal, and even intraventricular opiates has expanded, ablative procedures for cancer pain are performed less frequently. Neurosurgeons who have recently completed their training may not be familiar with many ablative procedures; of course, this limits their widespread application.

Summary

Neuroaugmentative and minimally ablative procedures are important additions to the armamentarium available for the management of chronic, intractable pain of spinal origin. These techniques may be employed earlier in the sequence of therapies, so they expand the population eligible for neurosurgical treatment. We should consider the overall treatment results and the overall "management morbidity" in a subject population, and not just in the surgical candidates. When we consider the potential benefits and the risks of alternative procedures, it is apparent that a greater emphasis on neuroaugmentative procedures will improve the results of treatment for chronic, intractable pain.

References

1. Auld AW, Maki-Jokela A, Murdoch DM: Intraspinal narcotic analgesia in the treatment of chronic pain, *Spine* 10:777-781, 1985.
2. Campbell JN, Davis KD, Meyer RA, North RB: The mechanism by which dorsal column stimulation affects pain: evidence for a new hypothesis, *Pain* 5:S228, 1990.
3. Coggeshall RE, Applebaum ML, Fazen M, et al.: Unmyelinated axons in human ventral roots, a possible explanation for the failure of dorsal rhizotomy to relieve pain, *Brain* 98:157, 1975.
4. Gybels JM, Sweet WH: *Neurosurgical treatment of pain*, Basel, 1989, Karger.
5. Kibler RW, Nathan PW: Relief of pain and paresthesiae by nerve block distal to a lesion, *J Neurol Neurosurg Psychiatry* 23:91, 1960.
6. Law JD: Targeting a spinal stimulator to treat the "failed back surgery syndrome," *Appl Neurophysiol* 50:437, 1987.
7. Labato RD, Madrid JL, Fatela LV, et al.: Intraventricular morphine for control of pain in terminal cancer patients, *J Neurosurg* 59:627, 1983.
8. Loeser JD: Dorsal rhizotomy for the relief of chronic pain, *J Neurosurg* 36:745, 1972.
9. Long DM, Filtzer DL, BenDebba M, Hendler NH: Clinical features of the failed-back syndrome, *J Neurosurg* 69:61, 1988.
10. North RB, Kidd DH, Campbell JN, Long DM: Dorsal root ganglionectomy for failed back surgery syndrome: a five year follow-up study, *J Neurosurg* 74:236, 1991.
11. North RB, Ewend MG, Lawton MT, Piantadosi S: Spinal cord stimulation for chronic, intractable pain: superiority of "multichannel" devices, *Pain* 44:119, 1991.
12. North RB, Campbell JN, James CS, et al.: Failed back surgery syndrome: five-year follow-up in 102 patients undergoing reoperation, *Neurosurgery* 28:685, 1991.

13. North RB, Ewend MG, Lawton MT, et al.: Failed back surgery syndrome: five-year follow-up after spinal cord stimulator implantation, *Neurosurgery* 28:692, 1991.

14. North RB, Cutchis P, Epstein JA, Long DM: Spinal cord compression complicating subarachnoid morphine administration: case report and laboratory experience, *Neurosurgery* 45:778, 1991.

15. North RB, Fowler KR, Nigrin DA, et al.: Automated "pain drawing" analysis by computer-controlled, patient-interactive neurological stimulation system, *Pain* 50:51, 1992.

16. Obbens EA, Hill CS, Leavens ME, et al.: Intraventricular morphine administration for control of chronic cancer pain, *Pain* 28:61, 1987.

17. Onofrio BM, Campa HK: Evaluation of rhizotomy: review of 12 years' experience, *J Neurosurg* 36:751, 1972.

18. Onofrio BM, Yaksh TL: Long-term pain relief produced by intrathecal morphine infusion in 53 patients, *J Neurosurg* 72:200, 1990.

19. Sundaresan N, Krol G, Digiacinto GV, Hughes JEO: *Metastatic tumors of the spine*. In Sundaresan N, Schmidek HH, Schiller AL, Rosenthal DI, editors: *Tumors of the spine: diagnosis and clinical management*, Philadelphia, 1990, W.B. Saunders Co., p 279.

20. Taub A: *Suppression of post-ganglionectomy dysesthesia by systemic lidocaine*, Presented to the American Pain Society, Washington, DC, 1986, as quoted in: Gybels JM, Sweet WH: *Neurosurgical treatment of persistent pain*, New York, 1989, Karger, p 123.

21. Xavier AV, McDanal J, Kissin I: Relief of sciatic radicular pain by sciatic nerve block, *Anesth Analg* 67:1177, 1988.

Appendix: The Role of Spinal Cord Stimulation in Contemporary Pain Management[*]

Spinal cord stimulation (SCS) was introduced 25 years ago as a reversible, nonablative technique for the management of intractable pain.[48] As initial, favorable experience with SCS was reported, it was adopted rather widely and uncritically. At that time, the indications for surgical intervention for the management of pain were not well understood. Our understanding of chronic pain and its management has since advanced considerably. Programs specializing in the field have proliferated, and behavioral and psychologic issues are emphasized in patient management, particularly selection for surgical procedures and implantation of devices.[9,30] The criteria for treatment of pain with a surgically implanted device have evolved empirically, as follows.

Implanted Devices For Intractable Pain

General Indications

1. There is an objective basis for the complaint of pain (e.g., myelographically documented lumbar arachnoid fibrosis).
2. Alternative therapy has been exhausted (e.g., medications, physical therapy/rehabilitation, spinal decompression or stabilization) or is unacceptable (e.g., microsurgical lysis of arachnoid adhesions, ablative procedures).
3. Psychiatric clearance has been obtained (in an attempt to rule out major psychiatric or personality disorder, issues of secondary gain, or a serious drug habituation problem).
4. For SCS, the topography of pain must be amenable to overlap by stimulation paresthesias (e.g., sciatica).[†] Routine placement of a temporary electrode to demonstrate relief addresses this issue.

The following have been reported as specific indications for spinal cord stimulation. They are listed in decreasing order of frequency of application and reported success rates.
1. Lumbar arachnoid fibrosis (arachnoiditis) or "failed back surgery syndrome" with radiculopathic pain, ideally predominating over axial low-back pain, in particular mechanical pain.[41]
2. Peripheral vascular disease, with ischemic pain.[2]
3. Peripheral nerve injury, neuralgia, or causalgia (including so-called reflex sympathetic dystrophy).
4. Phantom limb or stump pain.[17]
5. Spinal cord lesions, with well-circumscribed segmental pain.[45]

[*]Reprinted from North RB: *APS J* 2(2):91, 1993, with permission.
[†]References 5, 18, 19, 21, 36, 41, 44, 51, and 53.

Spinal Cord Stimulation Devices

Early SCS electrodes were relatively bulky devices, requiring a laminectomy for placement under direct vision into the dorsal epidural, endodural, or subarachnoid space.[4,36,52] Placement of such devices is problematic in several ways. First and foremost, it involves a surgical procedure simply to screen patients for permanent device implantation. Placing a laminectomy electrode in a "temporary" configuration, for subsequent removal or conversion to a permanent implant, represents a major commitment that may bias the patient and surgeon toward a permanent implant, even when the response is marginal. A laminectomy is itself painful; this may interfere with short-term assessment of relief by SCS, and in a patient with a preexisting chronic pain problem it carries some risk of precipitating a new problem. A laminectomy offers limited longitudinal access to the spinal canal for mapping potential electrode positions, and blindly manipulating a bulky electrode in the epidural space increases the risk of iatrogenic injury or hematoma.

In a typical patient with "failed back surgery syndrome" or "postlaminectomy syndrome," electrodes were initially implanted at upper thoracic levels to provide stimulation coverage of all segments below the array. This often resulted in uncomfortable local segmental effects; electrode placement more caudally afforded more specific coverage. Intraoperative test stimulation under local anesthesia was helpful in optimizing placement, but when a laminectomy was required, this was problematic, as the appropriate level was not known a priori in an individual patient. Finally, although a majority of patients report satisfactory pain relief, it is by no means universal, so screening with a temporary electrode, before implantation of a permanent device, is appropriate.

In order to address these problems, percutaneous techniques were developed for temporary electrode placement.[11,14,15] These techniques were adapted for permanent electrode implantation, obviating laminectomy in many patients.[38,55] Individual electrodes inserted independently tended to migrate, however, with respect to one another and with respect to the spinal cord, requiring surgical revision.[38] Modifications in lead design and anchoring techniques have ameliorated this. Arrays of electrodes have been developed for percutaneous placement; this precludes migration of one contact with respect to another.[23,41]

Contemporary arrays of spinal cord stimulating electrodes are supported by implantable, programmable pulse generators that allow noninvasive selection of stimulating anodes and cathodes. Formerly, this required surgical revision of electrode position or connector pin assignments. The topography of stimulation may thereby be adjusted after electrode implantation, under ordinary conditions of activity and posture, and ongoing readjustments are possible as the patient gains experience with the system. Contemporary programmable, multicontact systems rarely require surgical revision and are significantly more reliable than single-channel devices. Furthermore, they give sig-

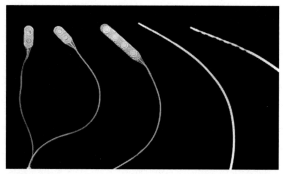

Fig. 41-A

Representative spinal cord stimulation arrays, bearing from one to four electrodes. In center is laminectomy array: the others may be inserted percutaneously, through Touhy needle.

nificantly better long-term clinical results.[41,45] Figure 41-A shows representative contemporary electrode designs of percutaneous as well as laminectomy type.

Clinical Assessment

It remains standard practice, and a condition for reimbursement by some third parties, that demonstration of pain relief with a temporarily implanted electrode precedes permanent implant. The criteria for proceeding with a permanent implant have varied: some authors have required as much as 70% reported pain relief [24,34] and others as little as 30%.[1] The percutaneous test phase has been as long as 2 months.[33] As few as 40% to 47%[49] of patients with temporary electrodes have gone on to receive permanent implants. At the other extreme, assessments of pain relief have been made during placement of the very first ("temporary") electrode, and the permanent device has been implanted in a single stage. It has been my practice to conduct a percutaneous trial over at least 3 days, with a disposable electrode, and to offer a permanent implant to a patient who reports at least 50% pain relief, while demonstrating improvement in activity and stable or improved use of analgesics.

Long-term results of SCS have been reported by a number of authors, using a number of different outcome measures. The early literature frequently described outcomes in poorly defined terms such as "excellent," "good," etc. Increasingly, the literature uses a broader range of outcome measures, defined more precisely, but they remain primarily patient self-reports. A wide variety of follow-up intervals, outcome measures, and interview techniques have been used (as summarized in Table 41-A); hence, comparisons or meta-analyses are difficult. The same is true, of course, of the literature on pain-relieving techniques in general.

One very important aspect of outcome assessment, which varies among clinical papers, is the source of follow-up information. We have always employed a disinterested third-party interview in reporting the results of spinal cord stimulation and other pain-relieving procedures.[29, 38-43] This methodology is reported increasingly,* but in a minority of studies in the literature on spinal cord stimulation. Disinterested third-party interview has been reported to reveal less optimistic results than hospital charts and surgeons' office records.[12,41]

Another important determinant of the rate of "success" is the number of patients considered—usually, the number receiving permanent implants, not the number of patients screened. In our experience, the rate of permanent implants has ranged from 78%[45] to 92%[41]; adjustment for this would be minor by comparison with other series, with rates as low as 40%[10] For other surgical procedures, success rates generally are reported in the literature in terms of the number of patients undergoing the definitive operation—not the number undergoing diagnostic procedures such as myelography or nerve blocks, whose morbidity is comparable to percutaneous temporary epidural electrode placement. Spinal cord stimulation has the advantage of a simple diagnostic test or trial that mimics the effects of the definitive procedure.

In addition to standard analog ratings of average pain intensity and pain relief, our patients also have given ratings of pain intensity as a function of time, using a six-point verbal rating scale.[35] In the great majority of patients with chronic pain, pain is a dynamic condition. Figure 41-B shows the average percentage of time spent at each intensity, reported by a series of patients receiving permanent implants, half of whom reported 50% or more relief of pain at long-term follow-up evaluation.[41] The percentage of time at the highest intensities has decreased severalfold, and the fraction of time with "no pain" or pain of low intensity has increased correspondingly.

We routinely consider other, secondary outcome measures, as summarized in Figure 41-C. Patients are asked to grade their impairment due to pain in performing various activities of daily living, they report their ongoing medication use, and they report neurologic symptoms (motor, sensory, and bladder/bowel function). Improvement is reported by a majority of patients in many activities of daily living. A majority of patients report reduction in or elimination of analgesic intake. A small number report increasing neurologic symptoms, but none have been attributed to implantation of the stimulator.

Certain favorable prognostic factors have been identified among the selected patients undergoing spinal cord stimulation, but beyond the routine selection criteria listed above, none have been observed uniformly or have achieved overriding significance. For example, women fared significantly better than men in two series,[41,46] but others have found no difference between the sexes.[16,19,34] Unilateral pain syndromes reportedly are more easily treated,[19,22,46] but this has not been observed uniformly.[41] Achieving stimulation overlap of the low back is recognized as technically difficult; most but not all[22] authors have not selected patients in whom low-back pain was the

*References 4, 12, 16, 19, 28, 37, 47, and 50.

Table 41-A

Summary of clinical literature on spinal cord stimulation

Author, Year	Number Screened	Number Implanted	Number Failed Backs	Follow-up Period, Mean	Follow-up Period, Range	Third-party Follow-up	"Excl/good" Results (≥ 50% Relief)	"Excl/good" FBSS Results
Blume, 1982		20	20		Up to 3 yr		70%	70%
Broseta, 1982		11		13 mo	3–20 mo		64%	
Burton, 1975	0	75	55	1 yr		Yes (mfr.)	59%	
Burton, 1977		198	186				43%	
Clark, 1975		13	6				54%	67%
De la Porte, 1983	94	36	36	36 mo	3–96 mo		60%	
de Vera, 1990	124	110	18				75%	
Demirel, 1984	48	33	11		2–5 yr		18%	
Devulder, 1990		45	23				78%	
Devulder, 1991		69	43		Up to 8 yr		55%	
Erickson, 1983	10	70			Up to 10 yr	Yes (60)	15–20%	
Hoppenstein, 1975		27	12				58%	64%
Hunt, 1975		13	5		9 mo–4 yr	Yes	15–31%	20–60%
Kälin, 1990			77				88%	88%
Koeze, 1987	0	26	5	28 mo			46–62%	
Krainick, 1989	126	91	5		Up to 5 yr		18%	
Kumar, 1986		60	54		6–60 mo		62%	
Kumar, 1991	121	94	56	40 mo	6 mo–10 yr	Yes	66%	
Law, 1983		81					36–80%	
Leclercq, 1981		20	20		1 –> 24 mo		50%	50%
LeRoy, 1981		49	49	30.7 mo	1–63 mo	No	60%	
Long, 1975		69	54		12–35 mo	Yes	18%	
Long, 1981		31	24		4–7 yr	Yes	73% @ 3y	
McCarron, 1987		22			3–24 mo		68%	
Meglio, 1989	109	64	19			No		23%
Meilman, 1989	20	12	20		Up to 3.5 yr		60%	60%
Mittal, 1987	31	26	21				46%	
Nielson, 1975	221	130	79		1 –> 35 mo	Yes	49%	46%
Pineda, 1975		76	56				43%	43%
Racz, 1989	0	26	18		12–42.7 mo	No	65%	
Ray, 1982		78	50	19.4 mo	3–64 mo		49%	
Richardson, 1979	36	22	12		1–3 yr		56%	
Richardson, 1991		136	136	45 mo		Yes (mfr.)	67%	67%
Robb, 1990	65	79	22		6 mo–5 yr		72%	69%
Sánchez-Ledesma, 1989	49	33	0	5.5 yr			57%	

(Continues)

Table 41-A

Summary of clinical literature on spinal cord stimulation (continued)

Author, Year	Number Screened	Number Implanted	Number Failed Backs	Follow-up Period, Mean	Follow-up Period, Range	Third-party Follow-up	"Excl/good" Results (≥ 50% Relief)	"Excl/good" FBSS Results
Shatin, 1986		116			0.9–13.3 mo	Yes (mfr.)	74% @ 6 mo-	
Shealy, 1975	0	80			7 mo–?	No	25%	15–45%
Shelden, 1975		27	3					67%
Siegfried, 1982	191	89	75	~ 4 y	1–8 yr		37%	
Simpson, 1991	24	56	7	29 mo	2 wk–9 yr		47%	
Spiegelmann, 1991	43	30	18	13 mo	3–33 mo	Yes	60%	
Sweet, 1974	100	98	33				21–42%	15–45%
Urban, 1978	20	7	9				86%	
Vogel, 1986	50	27	29		> 3 yr	No	18.6%	
Waisbrod, 1985		16	16	16 mo	6–30 mo	No	75%	
Winkelmüller, 1981	94	71	56			4 mo–7 yr		69%
Young, 1976		27	17		16–51 mo		66% ≥ 50%	
Young, 1978	14	51	25	38 mo	12–67 mo		65% ≥ 50%	

FBSS = failed back surgery syndrome. Third party follow-up: mfr.-device manufacturer. (From North et al.: Spinal cord stimulation for chronic, intractable pain: two decades' experience, *Neurosurgery* 32:384, 1993.)

chief complaint. With careful attention to the technical requirements of achieving low-back coverage, Law and Kirkpatrick have reported favorable results in this problematic subgroup of patients.[22]

In our experience with spinal cord stimulation over two decades, we have encountered no major morbidity (spinal cord injury, meningitis). Surgical wound infections, all superficial or extraspinal, have occurred in 5% of patients. All infections have cleared promptly after removal of hardware and a course of antibiotics; the device may then be reimplanted. Electrode migration or malposition requiring surgical revision occurred frequently with early SCS devices, particularly percutaneously inserted single electrodes. Contemporary percutaneously placed arrays and "multichannel" devices are much more forgiving of minor malposition, artifactual effects of implantation in the prone position, and even migration. The need for surgical revision of these devices is significantly less.[45]

Experimental Assessment

Spinal cord stimulation has a number of neurophysiologic effects: finite element modeling indicates that multiple pathways in the spinal cord are accessible for recruitment by longitudinally oriented, dorsal electrodes, and in vivo recordings confirm this.[8,13,20] It has been difficult to as-

certain which of these effects are necessary to achieving pain relief and which are epiphenomena. "Dorsal column" stimulation, the original name for SCS, reflects the proximity of the dorsal columns to midline electrodes; indeed, as shown by antidromic evoked activity recorded over peripheral nerves, primary afferents ascending in the dorsal columns are recruited by SCS.[54] Among the possible mechanisms of pain relief by SCS is frequency-related conduction block, occurring at branch points of primary afferents, with collaterals to dorsal horn.[6] The pain-relieving effects of SCS are in fact frequency dependent.[45]

The relief by SCS of ischemic lower-extremity pain is of particular interest, as it is accompanied by objectively demonstrable increases in lower-extremity circulation, reflected in measurements of tissue oxygenation.[3] These effects reportedly are blocked by sympathectomy or ventral rhizotomy and are not additive with the effects of hexamethonium or guanethidine, indicating that SCS inhibits sympathetic vasoconstriction.[25,26] The neurochemical mechanisms underlying the relief of pain by spinal cord stimulation have been the subject of a number of investigations, but it remains unclear which, if any, of the observed phenomena are necessary to achieving pain relief. In humans, SCS increases cerebrospinal fluid levels of substance P: its source may be inferred from microdialysis in the experimental animal, showing substance P release in re-

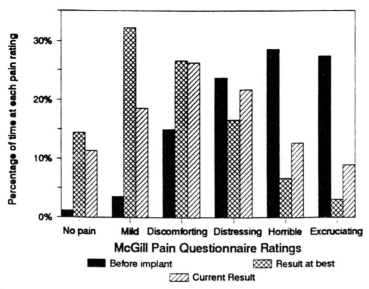

Fig. 41-B

Average ratings, by patients receiving permanent implants, of percentage of time spent at each level on standard six-point verbal pain rating scale. Fraction of time at highest intensities was reduced by more than half and fraction of time with "no pain" or pain on low intensity increased severalfold. *(From North et al.: Spinal cord stimulation for chronic, intractable pain: two decades' experience, Neurosurgery 32:384, 1993.)*

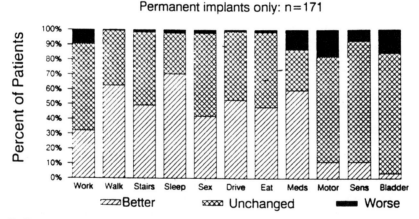

Fig. 41-C

Changes in patients' ratings of their abilities to perform various activities of daily living in terms of impairment due to pain, of ongoing medication use, and of reported neurologic symptoms. Percentage of patients reporting gains, losses, and no change is represented in stacked bar format. Most patients reported improvement in number of everyday acitivites and in medication use. *(From North et al.: Spinal cord stimulation for chronic, intractable pain: two decades' experience, Neurosurgery 32:384, 1993.)*

sponse to SCS or to peripheral noxious stimulation.[27] Serotonin release in the dorsal horn is also seen after SCS.[27]

Careful psychophysical studies of the effects of SCS on clinical and experimental pain and sensation[32] have shown decreases in cutaneous temperature discrimination, and in acute heat pain thresholds and pain ratings, within the area of stimulation-induced paresthesias. Studies of acute pain, of course, may not be relevant to the treatment of chronic pain. which in many cases follows neural injury or deafferentation. These studies are of interest, however, in characterizing both

therapeutic effects and side effects of SCS. Loss of normal protective sensations is undesirable in clinical application of SCS; fortunately, such effects are modest.

Stimulator Adjustment

Adjustment of contemporary programmable, multichannel implantable stimulation devices (technically, single-channel devices gated to multiple outputs) is a complex process that grows disproportionately as the number of

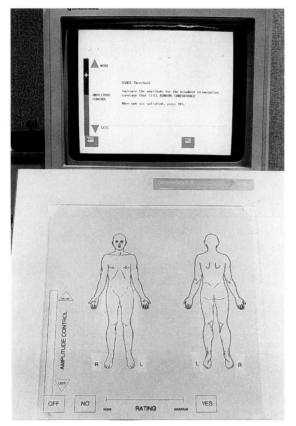

Fig. 41-D

Graphics tablet used by patients at our facility to enter pain drawings and corresponding outlines of stimulation paresthesias. Card on PC expansion bus is cabled to peripheral enclosure housing control circuitry for stimulators' radiofrequency transmitters. Patient controls, on top of peripheral enclosure, include three simple push buttons and two potentiometers. These controls have been designed to be larger and easier for patient to operate, as well as fewer in number than those of standard devices. *(From North et al.: Automated "pain drawing" analysis by computer-controlled, patient-interactive neurological stimulation system, Pain 50:51, 1992.)*

electrodes increases. Thorough testing over the full range of possible adjustments is extremely time consuming, if thresholds are to be measured precisely. Furthermore, there is a need to standardize methods of adjustment, and technical grading, of these devices to facilitate study and communication of results.

Like routine adjustment of stimulation amplitude and rate, this process may be managed by the patient, given appropriate supervision, means of control, and automated data collection and interpretation. For this purpose. we have developed a patient-interactive personal computer interface to standard, commercially available radiofrequency-coupled implants (Fig. 41-D). The patient controls have been designed for greater ease of operation than those of the standard external transmitter or programmer. A graphics tablet is used by the patient to enter "pain drawings" and corresponding outlines of the areas covered by stimulation paresthesias. These areas are compared and analyzed rapidly and automatically and ranked in order for everyday clinical use by the patient.[44]

Even contemporary "multichannel" devices are in fact single-channel stimulators gated to multiple electrodes. All experience with SCS to date has been with a simple, monotonic pulse train at fixed electrode combinations that may be changed only by manual control. Our computerized system, however, is capable of changing stimulation parameters (electrode combination, amplitude, and duration) in as little as 1 msec, effectively conferring true multichannel capabilities on these devices. This will permit a number of novel stimulation regimens—for example, alternating pulses between two electrode combinations whose effects are complementary. The system can vary the pulse parameters as well, as has been described in the literature on transcutaneous electrical nerve stimulation.[31] "Modulation" of the stimulus in the spatial and temporal domains may enhance the efficacy of SCS.

Automated, patient-interactive methods should facilitate routine use of implanted stimulation devices, and a standardized format with quantitative patient responses should facilitate communication between physicians as to technical goals and outcomes.

Discussion

The clinical results of SCS may be considered in the context of treatment alternatives: for the failed back surgery syndrome, the most common indication for SCS, the invasive treatment alternatives include reoperation for mechanical decompression or stabilization and ablative procedures (e.g., dorsal-root ganglionectomy). There has been no prospective comparison of these procedures, but we have reviewed our experiences.[40,42,43] retrospectively, using a standardized, disinterested third-party interview and questionnaire, differing only in technical details specific to treatment (e.g., stimulator settings for SCS patients). We have found that by comparison with other procedures, SCS has a substantially higher yield, in terms of patient ratings of pain relief, satisfaction with outcome, and ability to perform everyday activities.[43] Far fewer SCS patients report loss of functional capacity or neurologic function.[43] Any comparison of retrospective results is awkward, however, even among patients treated at the same center, for the same diagnosis; failed back surgery syndrome is a broad diagnostic category, and different selection criteria have been used for these procedures. Valid comparison requires a prospective, randomized study; we have begun such a protocol for reoperation and SCS.

Similar comparisons might be made between SCS and surgical procedures for other conditions enumerated above: e.g., dorsal-root entry-zone lesioning for postamputation pain syndromes or segmental pain following spinal cord injury; sympathectomy for "reflex sympathetic dystrophy"; or repeated reconstruction or amputation for painful end-stage peripheral vascular disease. The morbidity of SCS is so low that, assuming similar therapeutic efficacies, the ratio of potential benefit to risk favors SCS, indicating a therapeutic trial of SCS before such ablative procedures.

The cost effectiveness of SCS, considered apart from issues of pain relief per se, depends on (1) savings by comparison with alternative treatments and (2) return of patients to productive activities. The costs of SCS implantation reportedly are offset in part by reduction in medication use[1]; this is true not only of SCS, in the author's experience, but also of alternative procedures.[40,42,43] Significant increases in postoperative work capacity will recover SCS treatment costs quickly.[1] In the author's experience, a majority of patients under 65, in a series followed for a mean of over 7 years, have returned to work.[45] Rehabilitation-oriented programs, of course, likewise report high rates of return to work.[7]

A surgeon's perspective is, of course, procedure-oriented; procedures are applicable only to a select subset of patients. Physical therapy, rehabilitation, behavioral and psychologic techniques, as well as pharmacologic therapy, are applied routinely to these patients before and after surgery. Those who present for any procedure, including SCS, have "failed" these techniques by the cardinal criterion of pain relief, but they remain applicable as ancillary, complementary therapies, directed not only at relief of pain but at other aspects of the chronic pain problem. No procedure in isolation adequately addresses issues such as rehabilitation, major depression, or detoxification. Chronic pain and its management are multidimensional problems—the interplay of variable diagnoses, comorbidities, treatment combinations, and outcome measures is complex, and comparisons across different treatment modalities are overly simplistic and awkward. Overall, it may be that SCS offers the most favorable benefit:risk ratio of any procedure for conditions such as the failed back surgery syndrome, but noninvasive treatments are more widely applicable—even to patients who, for psychologic or other reasons, might be rejected for SCS.

Conclusions

Improvements in SCS devices, techniques, and patient selection over the past 20 years have enhanced the safety and efficacy of the procedure, suggesting an expanding role for SCS in the treatment of chronic, intractable pain. Percutaneous electrode placement has reduced morbidity, facilitated patient screening, and furthered the technical goal of matching stimulation paresthesias to the distribution of a patient's pain. Programmable implants have been developed to take full advantage of implanted electrode arrays. The morbidity of spinal cord stimulation is very low, and its benefit:risk ratio compares very favorably with alternative procedures. Careful patient selection and attention to alternative or ancillary noninvasive treatments are important to optimizing results.

References

1. Bel S, Bauer BL: Dorsal column stimulation (DCS): cost to benefit analysis, *Acta Neurochir* 52(Suppl):121, 1991.

2. Broseta J, Barbera J, DeVera J, et al.: Spinal cord stimulation in peripheral arterial disease, *J Neurosurg* 64:71, 1986.

3. Bunt TJ, Holloway GA, Lawrence P, et al.: Experience with epidural spinal stimulation in the treatment of end-stage peripheral vascular disease, *Semin Vasc Surg* 4:216, 1991.

4. Burton C: Dorsal column stimulation: optimization of application, *Surg Neurol* 4:171, 1975.

5. Burton CV: Session on spinal cord stimulation: safety and clinical efficacy, *Neurosurgery* 1:164, 1977.

6. Campbell JN, Davis KD, Meyer RA, North RB: The mechanism by which dorsal column stimulation affects pain: evidence for a new hypothesis, *Pain* 5:S228, 1990.

7. Cassisi JE, Sypert GW, Salamon A, Kapel L: Independent evaluation of a multidisciplinary rehabilitation program for chronic low back pain, *Neurosurgery* 25:877, 1989.

8. Coburn B, Sin W: A theoretical study of epidural electrical stimulation of the spinal cord. Part 1. Finite element analysis of stimulus fields, *Biomed Eng* 32:971, 1985.

9. Daniel M, Long C, Hutcherson M, Hunter S: Psychological factors and outcome of electrode implantation for chronic pain, *Neurosurgery* 17:773, 1985.

10. De la Porte C, Siegfried J: Lumbosacral spinal fibrosis (spinal arachnoiditis): its diagnosis and treatment by spinal cord stimulation, *Spine* 8:593, 1983.

11. Erickson DL: Percutaneous trial of stimulation for patient selection for implantable stimulating devices, *J Neurosurg* 43:440, 1975.

12. Erickson DL, Long DM: *Ten-year follow-up of dorsal column stimulation.* In Bonica JJ, editor: *Advances in pain research and therapy,* vol 5, New York, 1983, Raven Press, p 583.

13. Holsheimer J, Strujik JJ, Rijkhoff NJM: Contact combinations in epidural spinal cord stimulation: a comparison by computer modeling, *Stereotact Funct Neurosurg* 56:220, 1991.

14. Hoppenstein R: Electrical stimulation of the ventral and dorsal columns of the spinal cord for relief of chronic intractable pain, *Surg Neurol* 4:195, 1975.

15. Hosobuchi Y, Adams JE, Weinstein PR: Preliminary percutaneous dorsal column stimulation prior to permanent implantation, *J Neurosurg* 37:242, 1972.

16. Koeze TH, Williams AC, Reiman S: Spinal cord stimulation and the relief of chronic pain, *J Neurol Neurosurg Psychiatry* 50:1424, 1987.

17. Krainick JU, Thoden U, Riechert T: Pain reduction in amputees by long-term spinal cord stimulation: long-term follow-up study over 5 years, *J Neurosurg* 52:346, 1980.

18. Krainick TU, Thoden U: *Dorsal column stimulation.* In Wall PD, Melzack R, editors: *Textbook of pain,* New York, 1989, Churchill-Livingstone, p 701.

19. Kumar K, Nath R, Wyant GM: Treatment of chronic pain by epidural spinal cord stimulation: a 10-year experience, *J Neurosurg* 75:402, 1991.

20. Larson SJ, Sances A, Riegel DH, et al.: Neurophysiological effects of dorsal column stimulation in man and monkey, *J Neurosurg* 41:217, 1974.

21. Law JD: Targeting a spinal stimulator to treat the "failed back surgery syndrome," *Appl Neurophysiol* 50:437, 1987.

22. Law JD, Kirkpatrick AF: Pain management update: spinal cord stimulation, *Am J Pain Manage* 2:34, 1991.

23. Leclercq TA: Electrode migration in epidural stimulation: comparison between single electrode and four electrode programmable leads, *Pain* 20(Suppl 2):78, 1984.

24. Leibrock L, Meilman P, Cuka D, Green C: Spinal cord stimulation in the treatment of chronic low back and lower extremity pain syndromes, *Nebr Med J* 69:180, 1984.

25. Linderoth B, Fedorcsak I, Meyerson BA: Peripheral vasodilatation after spinal cord stimulation: animal studies of putative effector mechanisms, *Neurosurgery* 28:187, 1991.

26. Linderoth B, Gunasekera L, Meyerson BA: Effects of sympathectomy on skin and muscle microcirculation during dorsal column stimulation: animal studies, *Neurosurgery* 29:874, 1991.

27. Linderoth B, Gazelius B, Franck J, Brodin E: Dorsal column stimulation induces release of serotonin and substance P in the cat dorsal horn, *Neurosurgery* 31:289, 1992.

28. Long DM, Erickson DE: Stimulation of the posterior columns of the spinal cord for relief of intractable pain, *Surg Neurol* 4:134, 1975.

29. Long DM, Erickson D, Campbell J, North R: Electrical stimulation of the spinal cord and peripheral nerves for pain control, *Appl Neurophysiol* 44:207, 1981.

30. Long DM: A review of psychological considerations in the neurosurgical management of chronic pain: a neurosurgeon's perspective, *Neurosurg Q* 1:185, 1991.

31. Mannheimer C, Carlsson CA: The analgesic effect of transcutaneous electrical nerve stimulation (TNS) in patients with rheumatoid arthritis: a comparative study of different pulse patterns, *Pain* 6:329, 1979.

32. Marchand S, Bushnell MC, Molina-Negro P, et al.: The effects of dorsal column stimulation on measures of clinical and experimental pain in man, *Pain* 45:249, 1991.

33. Meglio M, Cioni B, Rossi GF: Spinal cord stimulation in management of chronic pain: a 9-year experience. *J Neurosurg* 70:519, 1989.

34. Meilman PW, Leibrock L, Leong FTL: Outcome of implanted spinal cord stimulation in the treatment of chronic pain: arachnoiditis versus single nerve root injury and mononeuropathy, *Clin J Pain* 5:189, 1989.

35. Melzack R: The McGill pain questionaire: major properties and scoring methods, *Pain* 1:277, 1975.

36. Nashold B, Somjen G, Friedman H: Paresthesias and EEG potentials evoked by stimulation of the dorsal funiculi in man, *Exp Neurol* 36:273, 1972.

37. Nielson KD, Adams JE, Hosobuchi Y: Experience with dorsal column stimulation for relief of chronic intractable pain, *Surg Neurol* 4:148, 1975.

38. North RB, Fischell TA, Long DM: Chronic stimulation via percutaneously inserted epidural electrodes, *Neurosurgery* 1:215, 1977.

39. North RB, Long DM: Spinal cord stimulation for intractable pain: eight-year followup, *Pain* 20(Suppl 2):79, 1984.

40. North RB, Kidd DH, Campbell JN, Long DM: Dorsal root ganglionectomy for failed back surgery syndrome: a five year followup study, *J Neurosurg* 74:236, 1991.

41. North RB, Ewend MG, Lawton MT, Piantadosi S: Spinal cord stimulation for chronic, intractable pain: superiority of "multichannel" devices, *Pain* 44:119, 1991.

42. North RB, Campbell JN, James CS, et al.: Failed back surgery syndrome: five-year followup in 102 patients undergoing reoperation, *Neurosurgery* 28:685, 1991.

43. North RB, Ewend MG, Lawton MT, et al.: Failed back surgery syndrome: five-year follow-up after spinal cord stimulator implantation, *Neurosurgery* 28:692, 1991.

44. North RB, Fowler KR, Nigrin DA, et al.: Automated "pain drawing" analysis by computer-controlled, patient-interactive neurological stimulation system, *Pain* 50:51, 1992.

45. North RB, Kidd DH, Zahurak M, et al.: Spinal cord stimulation for chronic, intractable pain: two decades' experience, *Neurosurgery* 32:384, 1993.

46. Richardson DE, Shatin D: *Results of spinal cord stimulation for pain control: long-term collaborative study.* Presented at American Pain Society, New Orleans, 1991.

47. Shatin D, Mullett K, Hults G: Totally implantable spinal cord stimulation for chronic pain: design and efficacy, *Pace* 9:577, 1986.

48. Shealy CN, Mortimer JT, Reswick JB: Electrical inhibition of pain by stimulation of the dorsal columns: preliminary clinical report, *Anesth Analg* 46:489, 1967.

49. Siegfried J, Lazorthes Y: Long-term follow-up of dorsal column stimulation for chronic pain syndrome after multiple lumbar operations, *Appl Neurophysiol* 45:201, 1982.

50. Spiegelmann R, Friedman WA: Spinal cord stimulation: a contemporary series, *Neurosurgery* 28:65, 1991.

51. Sweet WH, Wepsic JG: *Electrical stimulation for suppression of pain in man.* In Fields WS, editor: *Neural organization and its relevance to prosthetics,* New York, 1973, Intercontinental Medical Book, p 218.

52. Sweet W, Wepsic J: Stimulation of the posterior columns of the spinal cord for pain control, *Clin Neurosurg* 21:278, 1974.

53. Urban BJ, Nashold B: Percutaneous epidural stimulation of the spinal cord for relief of pain: long term results, *J Neurosurg* 48:323, 1978.

54. Yingling CD, Hosobuchi Y: Use of antidromic evoked potentials in placement of dorsal cord disc electrodes, *Appl Neurophysiol* 49:36, 1986.

55. Zumpano BJ, Saunders RL: Percutaneous epidural dorsal column stimulation, *J Neurosurg* 45:459, 1976.

Chapter 42
Use of the Morphine Pump for Pain Control
Robert J. Henderson

The purpose of this chapter is to introduce, define, and relate the use of intrathecal narcotics for the control of nonmalignant debilitating pain related to the spine. It is not meant to be an authoritative dissertation on the biochemistry or even physiology of how intrathecal narcotics work. This chapter will present a rationale for its use, complications encountered or known, and a review of how appropriately selected patients have responded to this form of therapy.

Technologic advances have provided clinicians with reliable, accurate, and programmable delivery systems for long-term infusion of spinally administered drugs (Figs. 42-1, 42-2, and 42-3). It is because of these advances and the impressive results of clinical studies for nonmalignant conditions that the use of intrathecal narcotics for nonmalignant pain disorders was approved by the FDA in February 1992. Because of these advances there has been a rapidly growing interest in long-term intraspinal infusional therapy for the control of chronic pain.

There are many publications that give the rationale for and the clinical uses of spinally administered narcotic (SAN) infusion therapy. However little is written about how to use, when to use, or how to address problems attendant to the use of SAN.

History and Rationale for Spinally Administered Narcotic

In 1973 Pert and Snyder discovered that opiate antagonism is discriminated by opiate receptor binding in the brain.[16] At about the same time Hughes and Terenius discovered opioid-like peptides endogenous to laboratory animals and humans.[8,18] In 1977, Atweh and Kuhar located opiate receptors not only in the brain but in the substantia gelatinosa of the spinal cord, by autoradiographic techniques.[2] This led to the discovery by Yaksh and Rudy in 1977 that direct injection of opiates into the spinal canal produce profound, naloxone-reversible analgesia in rats, and later in rats and monkeys.[20,21] This led to a report by Wang in 1979 of the successful intrathecal use of SAN in terminally ill cancer patients.[19] This spinal analgesia without attendant motor or autonomic blockade has been termed "selective spinal analgesia" by Michael Cousins.[6]

Patient Selection

What group of patients become candidates for SAN via an implantable programmable pump? I feel it is valid to consider all patients with multicentric pain that is not amenable to surgical correction; postoperative patients, for whom at least 2 years have passed since their last "corrective surgery" whose in-

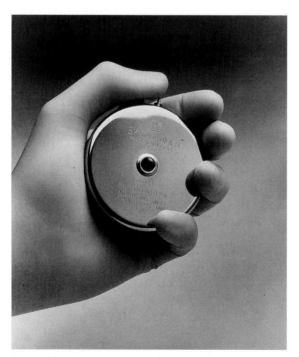

Fig. 42-1

Synchromed infusion pump from Medtronic, Inc., implanted under skin on patient's abdomen. Drug, placed in refillable reservoir inside pump, is delivered to its destination through small-diameter catheter inserted intrathecally and connected to pump. *(Courtesy of Medtronic, Inc., Minneapolis.)*

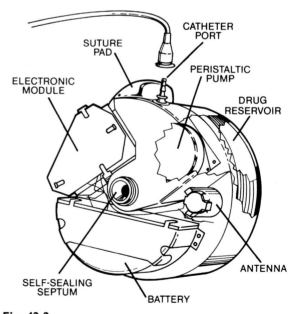

MEDTRONIC SYNCHROMED® INFUSION PUMP

Fig. 42-2

Major components of Synchromed pump. *(Courtesy of Medtronic, Inc., Minneapolis.)*

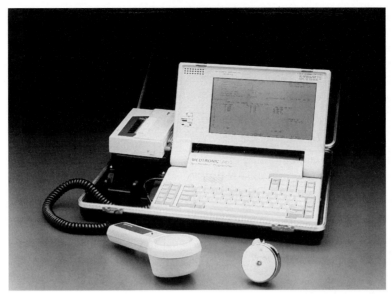

Fig. 42-3

Desktop computer programmer used to externally program and reprogram pump via radio signals with precise timing and accuracy. *(Courtesy of Medtronic, Inc., Minneapolis.)*

tractable, intolerable pain persists, and individuals who have documented multilevel discogenic pain (greater than three levels), thoracic disc disruption, intractable radiculopathy, arachnoiditis, neurofibromatosis, and phantom-limb syndrome.

SAN for nonmalignant pain remains controversial. There is concern regarding stabilization of drugs and whether their efficacy will decrease over time. There are reports in the literature of intraspinal infusional therapy in patients with nonmalignant pain, but long-term use in this population has not been adequately documented.*

In my experience a significant percentage (20% to 30%) of patients with long-term chronic pain who have been dependent on narcotics find an improved quality of life just by discontinuing their narcotic use and allowing their own endogenous endorphins to function again. This allows decreased pain in some patients, but more significantly, patients will find that they can tolerate their circumstances and be at a higher level of function emotionally, psychologically, and physically but without the undesirable side effects of exogenous narcotics. I prefer that candidates for the pump be narcotic-free prior to the time of implantation and prior to their test dose. Others such as Krames believe that patients should be "maxed out" on systemic exogenous narcotics demonstrating significant symptoms of chronic use (i.e., constipation, lethargy, somnolence, confusion, inani-

tion, etc.) and be considered candidates for neuroablative procedures prior to utilizing SAN.[12]

Prerequisites for Implantation

Prior to implantation of an intrathecal catheter with implantable pump the patient must be evaluated through a psychologically oriented pain program or its equivalent. There must be a complete and current review of all diagnostics. I have found that the vast preponderance of patients referred for consideration of pump implantation have correctable pathology and have responded to additional appropriate corrective surgery. The most common pathology is lateral recess stenosis, foraminal stenosis, pseudarthrosis, and discogenic pain in front of an intact posterior fusion mass.

The final prerequisite is that patients respond dramatically to an intrathecal test dose of morphine. The patient is admitted to the hospital for 23 hours and a 0.5-mg dose of preservative-free morphine is administered intrathecally through a translumbar approach. The pain response occurs over the first few hours and will continue in most cases for 12 to 48 hours. A positive response is not equivocal but "miraculous," meaning very clear cut. Initially I relied on responses to epidural morphine but found this to be less reliable, and it was more difficult to interpret the response.

The hospitalization is required so that adverse side effects or allergies to the morphine can be detected

*References 3, 5, 10, 12, 13, and 15.

and treated. These include apnea (it occurs during the 12- to 24-hour period postinjection), pruritus (treat symptomatically with diphenhydramine by mouth), and urinary retention. Naloxone (Narcan) will reverse all these side effects, but may have to be given repeatedly if needed.

Implant Procedure

Typically the implant procedure can be done under local anesthesia or regional blockade, although general anesthesia may be preferred for most patients.

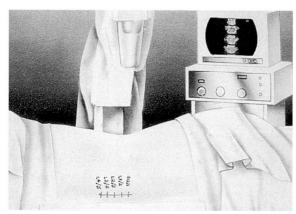

Fig. 42-4

Procedure begun by properly positioning patient in lateral recumbent position. Use digitalized C-arm fluoroscope to mark skin over identified levels, usually T12-L1 to L4-L5. Prepare and drape both back, flank, and abdomen to allow for simultaneous preparation of pocket site and catheter insertion site. Anteroposterior positioning of the C-arm fluoroscope is preferred (not shown). *(Courtesy of Medtronic, Inc., Minneapolis.)*

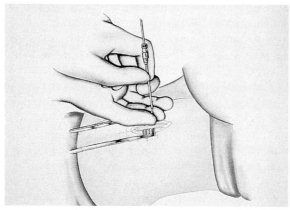

Fig. 42-5

Midline incision through skin and subcutaneous tissues down to aponeurosis is created. Touhy needle is inserted intrathecally, catheter is passed cephalad, and its position is checked with C-arm fluoroscope. Touhy needle is extracted over catheter and guidewire is withdrawn and cerebrospinal fluid is confirmed returning. *(Courtesy of Medtronic, Inc., Minneapolis.)*

The Synchromed pump is implanted subcutaneously in the right or left abdomen where there is sufficient skin and subcutaneous tissue to support the implanted system. The pump pocket site should be determined preoperatively. Consideration should be given to the amount of supportive tissue available, skin integrity, patient activity, clothing and belt lines, and other surgical therapies likely to be performed in the future.

It is important to remember once again that SAN is not the "panacea" for pain syndromes, but a valuable tool to be used judiciously to expand our network of effective treatments for pain. Nociceptive pain responds more completely to SAN than does neuropathic pain. Experimentation with adjuvant anesthetics (bupivacaine) with SAN has made some promising inroads into this most difficult conundrum (Figs. 42-4 to 42-11).

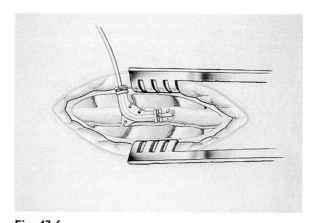

Fig. 42-6

Anchoring sleeve is secured to catheter and then to surrounding aponeurosis or ligament. *(Courtesy of Medtronic, Inc., Minneapolis.)*

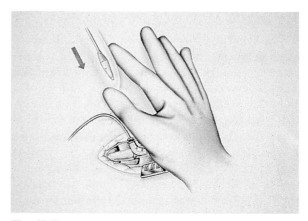

Fig. 42-7

Pocket has been created on abdomen and tunneling rod is passed from abdomen to posterior incision and used to draw connecting catheter to pocket site. *(Courtesy of Medtronic, Inc., Minneapolis.)*

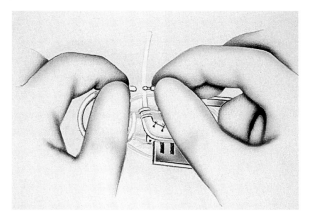

Fig. 42-8

At spinal incision site, both catheters are trimmed, leaving enough slack in connecting catheter for patient movement. Cathers are anastomosed over metal tube and secured. *(Courtesy of Medtronic, Inc., Minneapolis.)*

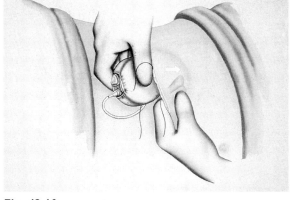

Fig. 42-10

Pump is inserted into prepared pocket, carefully placing any excess catheter under pump. *(Courtesy of Medtronic, Inc., Minneapolis.)*

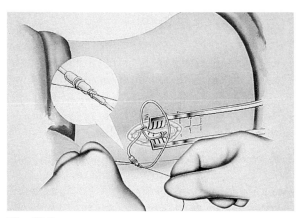

Fig. 42-9

Additional ligatures secure anastomosis within strain relief sleeve. *(Courtesy of Medtronic, Inc., Minneapolis.)*

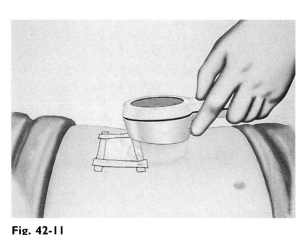

Fig. 42-11

Programming pump from desktop computer to infuse medication. *(Courtesy of Medtronic, Inc., Minneapolis.)*

Case Studies

Case 1

Intractable lower extremity pain developed in a 34-year-old white female with a history of multiple explorations, excisions, and resections in the lumbar spine for neurofibromatosis. She had some documented denervation in the lower extremities and partial loss of bladder control prior to the insertion of the intrathecal catheter for infusion of preservative-free morphine via the Synchromed programmable pump (Fig. 42-12). She has maintained a constant dosage of 22 to 23 mg per day at continuous rate for the past 18 months and is 32 months postinsertion of the pump. During the time since insertion she has required two revisions of her catheter—once

for migration into the epidural space and once for kinking. She was and continues to be extremely thin, but states she gained 20 lb in the 6 months following the insertion of the pump, which puts her at her stable weight of 92 pounds. Neither the patient nor her mother note any side effects from the morphine other than pain relief. The pump has allowed her to continue to care for her children and remain alert and cognitive, with a normal affect, all of which was not possible when she was taking exogenous systemic narcotics for her pain control.

Case 2

A 36-year-old white male had had multiple lumbar procedures, including a PLIF. Fusion status was excellent, as was decompression, but intractable back and leg pain persisted, which was thought to be due

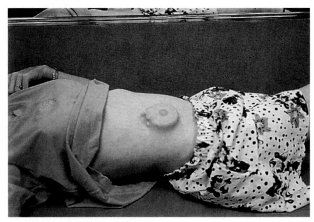

Fig. 42-12
Ninety-pound female with neurofibromatosis dramatically demonstrates pump position on abdominal wall.

in part to active epidural fibrosis. Prior to insertion of his pump he required multiple hospitalizations for conservative pain management. The pain was severely compromising his ability to perform or even to attend work. The intrathecal catheter and programmable pump was inserted 2 years ago. He is able to continue working and even to work overtime. Because his pain decreased, he was able to rehabilitate himself physically, and as a result lost a considerable amount of weight. He continues, 3 years postinsertion of the pump, on 4.4 mg per day of morphine at a continuous rate. His goals are to continue his self-administered rehabilitation program and eventually have the pump removed.

Case 3

A 68-year-old white male with a long history of multiple lumbar surgical procedures with intact fusions up to the second lumbar level has failed to respond to a dorsal column stimulator for intractable leg pain unilaterally. Intractable lumbar and bilateral leg pain subsequently developed. He responded to a test dose of morphine, and 2 years ago he had his intrathecal catheter and programmable pump implanted. For the first time in many years the patient had excellent pain relief that could have been improved with higher doses of morphine. But this was complicated by a significant sensitivity to the side effects of morphine—in his case, nausea and bladder retention. Pruritus resolved over a few days. His dose was gradually increased as tolerated. On two occasions his requirements for pain relief began increasing and were finally found to be secondary to extradural migration of his catheter. A trial of epidural morphine did not provide sufficient pain relief, and there were in-

creased side effects. The catheter was reinserted intrathecally both times. Two years post-insertion he maintains good pain relief and a marked increase in daily function. He pursues physical rehabilitation vigorously on a continuous daily dosage of 1.74 mg per day.

Case 4

A 41-year-old white male was diagnosed with multilevel discogenic pain involving the thoracic discs, with unremitting pain for 9 years. He had been unable to work for several years. Eighteen months after implantation of the pump he remains much more functional and has returned to employment as an independent businessman. His dose has been gradually increased over these 18 months to 8.5 mg per day at a continuous rate.

Complications

Because of the known and, more importantly, unknown complications associated with intrathecal SAN, insertion of the pump and catheter should be the last treatment alternative. Patients need to be acutely aware of the fact that we do not know the potential long-term ramifications of this procedure, but that the benefits usually outweigh the risks they are taking.

Death

Death is the most significant complication and has been the result of dosing errors when reprogramming dose instructions to the pump. There have been refilling errors when the drug was given through the contrast (direct access) port versus the reservoir port and miscalculations when altering concentrations of drug and miscalculations when administering bolus doses.

Infection

Infection is eventually unavoidable, particularly in an implant of this size with direct access into the central nervous system. Surprisingly, to date there have not been any reported serious infections extending into the spinal canal in patients with nonmalignant disease who are not immunocompromised. However, the more patients treated, the greater the likelihood of this occurring.

Mechanical problems

Coiling, kinking, fracture, leaking, and expulsion of the catheter from the intrathecal space are the practical problems that need to be considered most frequently when response to the pump is being compromised. Anteroposterior and lateral chest x-ray studies will demonstrate most of the catheter problems. Aspiration of cerebrospinal fluid through the direct access port confirms intrathecal placement of the catheter. When cerebrospinal fluid is not obtainable, infusion of dye through the direct access port with CT examination will confirm intrathecal placement of the catheter and its integrity in all but the rare case.

Pump Problems

Pump problems result from battery failure, rotor failure, exceeding pressure thresholds by overfilling cold infusate that expands when warmed to body temperature, or allowing too much air into the reservoir.

Clinical Observations

When intrathecal morphine is continuously infused, there is increased tolerance to the morphine dose that must be increased in order to maintain the same degree of pain relief. This is frequently noticed within the first few days, and will continue in stages for about 6 months. Accommodation to the adverse side effects such as nausea, pruritus, ileus, or urinary retention occurs within a few days of dosage increases. Oral diphenhydramine may diminish these effects. Naloxone will remedy urinary retention.

One of my patients reported the inability to sense heat either by touch or by taste. Therefore, he was repeatedly burning his mouth on hot coffee, his hands in hot water, etc. He did discern that he could smell the heat, and learned to visualize rising steam, etc., in an effort to protect himself. This loss of heat sense accompanied a very satisfactory relief of pain. The pain relief has persisted as has the loss of heat sensitivity.

Several male patients noted an exacerbation of sexual impotency, but none of them was disappointed in the trade-off for pain relief.

Overall, narcotics administered through an implantable programmable pump is a highly satisfactory salvage procedure. There is no discernible "drug" effect from the morphine, only analgesia—no drowsiness, no euphoria, no disorientation. All the patients exhibited and admitted to an improved quality of life. Use of exogenous narcotics was virtually nonexistent. Increased activity and function allowed many to return to work, increase their endurance for work, or be retrained for the work force. The number of required hospitalizations and visits to emergency rooms was markedly diminished in all cases, resulting in a significant long-term cost reduction in the care of these patients who were at the "end of the line."

Practice Considerations

When a physician decides to adopt intraspinal drug infusion in his/her practice, an allied health professional should be trained as an implant assistant. This individual is invaluable during all facets of the therapy, including preoperative patient education, surgical support, pump refilling, and long-term patient treatment.

Prior to implantation of the pump, the logistics of long-term patient treatment and pump refills must be determined. In many instances, pump refills are done as a routine office visit. Those involved must be trained in refilling the pump and adjusting dosage, and have access to a Synchromed programmer.

Inservicing of key hospital staff who must be informed include the operating room staff to ensure product availability and a smooth surgical procedure, pharmacy staff to provide the drug in preservative-free form, and floor nursing staff to provide patient care during the trial and operative procedure.

Summary

The practice of spinally administered narcotic infusion therapy is in a state of rapid development. New and better methods of patient selection, drug selection, and technique are being developed every day.

This subspecialty of pain control in spinal medicine is a very valuable tool. For decades the spine specialist has been faced with patients with intractable pain whom he/she could not help. Out of frustration, the surgeon has attempted to stretch the indications of his corrective operative procedures. This pump pain control technique offers a more humane and economical solution.

Because of the rapidly changing technology and economics of the medical care delivery system, there will be many socioeconomic issues that we face with regard to selection, overuse and abuse, authorization, and payment.

Pain control by this technique or others may be the best solution for many patients with spinal pain. Once pain is under control, patients can train and rehabilitate physically and psychologically. They can reestablish themselves in society and hopefully avoid major unsuccessful spine surgery.

References

1. Akahoshi MP, Furuike-McLaughlin T: Patient controlled analgesia via intrathecal catheter in outpatient oncology patients, *J Intravenous Nurs* 11:289, 1988.
2. Atweh SF, Kuhar MJ: Autoradiographic localization of opiate receptors in rat brain: 1. Spinal cord and lower medulla, *Brain Res* 124:53, 1977.
3. Auld AW, Maki-Jokela A: Intraspinal narcotic analgesia in the treatment of chronic pain, *Spine* 10:777-781, 1985.
4. Bedder MD: The anesthesiologist's role in neuroaugmentative pain control techniques: spinal cord stimulation and neuraxial narcotics, *Prog Anesthesiol* 4, 1990.
5. Coombs DW, Saunders RL, Gaylor MS: Relief of continuous chronic pain by intraspinal narcotics infusion via an implanted reservoir, *JAMA* 250:2336, 1983.
6. Cousins MJ, Mather LE, Glynn CJ, et al.: Selective spinal anesthesia, *Lancet* 1:1141, 1979.
7. Hassenbusch SJ, Pillay PK, et al.: Constant infusion of morphine for intractable cancer pain using an implanted pump, *J Neurosurg* 73:405, 1990.
8. Hughes J, Smith TW, Kosterlitz HW, et al.: Isolation of two related pentapeptides from brain with potent opiate activity, *Nature* 258:577, 1975.
9. Intraspinal drug delivery—surgical technique notebook, Minneapolis, 1991, Medtronic, Inc.
10. Jacobson L: Clinical note: relief of persistent postamputation stump and phantom limb pain with intrathecal fentanyl, *Pain* 37:317, 1989.
11. Krames ES: Intrathecal infusional therapies for intractable pain, Minneapolis, 1991, Medtronic, Inc.
12. Krames ES: Intrathecal infusional therapies for intractable pain: patient management guidelines, *J Pain Sympt Manage* 8:(1)36-46, 1993.
13. Krames ES, Gershow J, Glassberg A, et al.: Continuous infusion of spinally administered narcotics for the relief of pain due to malignant disorders, *Cancer* 56:696, 1985.
14. Onofrio BM: Long-term pain relief produced by intrathecal morphine infusion in 53 patients, *J Neurosurg* 72:200, 1990.
15. Penn RD, Paice JA: Chronic intrathecal morphine for intractable pain, *J Neurosurg* 67:182, 1987.
16. Pert CB, Snyder S: Opiate receptors demonstration in nervous tissue, *Science* 179:1011, 1973.
17. Portenoy RK: Chronic opioid therapy in nonmalignant pain, *Pain Sympt Manage* 5(1 Suppl): 546-562, 1990.
18. Terenius L, Wahlstrom A: Morphine like ligand in opiate receptors in human CSF, *Life Sci* 16:1759, 1975.
19. Wang JF, Nauss LA, Thomas JE: Pain relief by intrathecally applied morphine in man, *Anesthesiology* 50:149, 1979.
20. Yaksh TL: Analgetic actions of intrathecal opiates in cat and primates, *Brain Res* 153:205, 1978.
21. Yaksh TL, Rudy TA: Studies on the direct spinal action of narcotics in the production of analgesia in the rat, *J Pharmacol Exp Ther* 202:411, 1977.

Section 4
Sport-Specific Structural Injuries

Chapter 43
Baseball*
Robert G. Watkins

Biomechanics

Electromyographic Analysis of Hitters

Clinical Correlation

Dynamic Electromyographic Analysis of Torque Transfer in Pitchers

Treatment of Hitters with Lumbar Spine Injuries

*Portions of this chapter are taken from Watkins R, Dennis S, et al.: Dynamic EMG analysis of torque transfer in professional baseball pitchers. *Spine,* 14(4) 404-408, J.B. Lippincott Co., 1989.

Our evaluation of spinal problems in baseball players began with examining and interviewing every catcher in the National League. At that time, we found no catcher who admitted to having low-back pain (LBP). Examinations were normal, and histories were normal; in fact, the total lack of symptoms was different from what one would expect from ballplayers and the population in general.

The conclusions drawn from this initial evaluation were either (1) that catchers were closely screened early in their careers and eliminated from play if a back problem was noted, or (2) that squatting is a good position for the back. Certainly, the low incidence of lumbosacral pain and degenerative disease in populations in whom squatting is a common practice would lead one to believe that the squatting position of the catcher puts no undue stress on the lumbar spine.

Biomechanics

Physician visits for back pain are most commonly made by infielders. This is not unexpected. Infielders have a bending job. As in any lifting occupation, those with proper bending techniques usually have fewer problems than those with improper bending techniques. Infielders often take 100 ground balls in a rigorous practice day, repeatedly bending over. During a game, infielders stand, bent over in a ready position, inactive for certain periods of time. They are then suddenly required to perform extreme torsion and twisting motions of the lumbar spine, executing off-balance bending and lifting maneuvers. Fortunately, proper fielding mechanics are protective of the low back. While good coaching and good technique reduce the risk of low-back spasm, injury is often unavoidable. Many major-league baseball infielders have had lumbar spine problems for their entire careers.

Another interesting group of players are the hitters—that is, any team member who has to swing a bat. Hitters who take a lot of batting practice, swinging a heavy bat with great velocity, are certainly subject to lumbar spine injury. However, even the infrequent hitter (such as a pitcher), who may not have good hitting mechanics, is vulnerable to injury.

Lumbar spine problems in hitters begin with their eyes—the ability to see the ball is a critical factor in swing mechanics. Abnormal swing mechanics essentially involve a loss of body synchrony—that is, a loss of control between the hips and shoulders. Irregular, uncoordinated upper extremity and torso motion puts undue rotational strain on the lumbar spine. A lumbar spine injury in someone required to do this type of torsional activity further compounds the problem by producing stiffness, weakness, and asymmetry, which adds to the pain, preventing satisfactory healing. We refer to the biomechanics of hitting as an ocular-muscular reflex, a totally hybrid term referring to the triggering of bat mechanics and the muscles in a split-second response to what the hitter is able to see. If the hitter is not seeing the ball well, he may tend to open his hips too early. With the bat and upper torso lagging behind, sudden torsional movement occurs to catch up the shoulders and bat with the rest of the body. Poor visualization of the ball produces delays in hand and arm response.

To diagnose and treat lumbar spine problems in hitters, the physician should understand hitting mechanics. Proper swing mechanics require power in the legs and trunk; a rigid, solid cylinder of torque transfer; and fine muscle control of the arms and wrists.

Electromyographic Analysis of Hitters

For a scientific look at hitting, Ben Shaffer and colleagues performed electromyographic studies of trunk musculature in 18 professional baseball players from the Los Angeles Dodgers instructional training camp in Phoenix, AZ. Thirteen batters were right-handed, five were left-handed. Ages ranged from 19 to 44 years, averaging 22 years.

The Basmajian technique[4] was used to insert fine wire electrodes into the supraspinatus, triceps (lateral head), posterior deltoid, and middle serratus anterior (sixth rib) muscle of each subject's lead (forward) arm, as well as the lower gluteus maximus muscle of their trail (back) leg. Surface electrodes monitored right and left erector spinae, abdominal obliques, vastus medialis obliques (VMO), semimembranosus, and biceps femoris (long head) of the trail leg. A light-weight belt pack allowed for transmission of the electromyographic signals via FM telemetry to a recording console. Resting and maximum manual muscle test (MMT) recordings were made for each muscle.

Each subject was allowed to warm up until comfortable, and then hit six pitched fastballs (approximately 75 miles per hour).

Simultaneous high-speed motion picture photography using 16-mm film at 400 frames per second captured each swing. An electronic pulse marked the film and electromyogram, which allowed for film synchronization with the recorded electromyographic data.

The film was examined and divided into four discrete phases.

Phase I, windup, began as the lead heel left the ground, and ended as the lead toe reestablished contact with the ground.

Phase II, pre-swing, began as the lead forefoot struck the ground, and ended as the swing began.

Phase III, swing, was subdivided three times: into early, middle, and late, as determined by bat position. Early swing began as the bat moved forward, until it was perpendicular to the ground; middle swing continued until the bat was parallel with the ground; and late swing continued until contact was made with the ball.

Phase IV, follow-through, began with ball contact, and ended as the lead shoulder reached maximum abduction and external rotation.

The electromyographic data were then converted from analog to digital form by sampling 2500 times per second, and integrated by averaging groups of 200 samples per second.

Using a resting signal as baseline and a peak 1-second MMT at the 100% level, these records were then processed by computer to yield a relative activation figure. Activity patterns were assessed every 5 msec and expressed as a percentage of the activity recorded during the maximal MMT.

The mean percentage of MMT and standard deviations were obtained for each muscle throughout the swing. An Anova ($p < 0.5$) was performed to determine statistically significant differences between phases for each muscle, and between specific muscle groups. When the Anova revealed such differences, a post-hoc sequential Tukey multiple comparison test was done.

Results

Lower Extremities

Hamstring activity (biceps femoris and semimembranosus) was below 50% MMT in windup. During pre-swing, however, activity increased signficantly to 154% MMT and 157% MMT, respectively. Activity decreased significantly in early swing to 100% and 90% MMT, respectively, and continued declining throughout the remainder of the swing to its lowest level of 40% MMT in follow-through.

Lower gluteus maximus activity was lowest during windup (25% MMT) and increased significantly during pre-swing to 132% MMT. Activity remained high in early swing (125% MMT), decreased thereafter in middle swing (65% MMT), and decreased again in late swing (45% MMT). Activity decreased in follow-through to a low of 26% MMT.

Vastus medialis obliques activity increased significantly from windup (26% MMT) to pre-swing (63% MMT), and again from pre-swing to middle swing, where it peaked at 107% MMT. It diminished thereafter through late swing (97% MMT) and follow-through (78% MMT).

Trunk

During windup, activity in both erector spinae was low (24% MMT), but increased signficantly to > 90% MMT throughout the pre-swing, early swing, and middle swing. Activity then decreased in late swing (98% MMT lead, 85% MMT trail), to lower levels significantly during follow-through (58% MMT, 68% MMT). No significant difference was evident in activity between the lead and trail erector spinae during any phase.

As in the erector spinae, both abdominal obliques demonstrated relatively low levels of activity during windup (< 30% MMT). Activity jumped significantly to > 100% MMT in pre-swing and remained elevated throughout the remainder of the phase. No significant differences in activity were noted between lead and trail obliques.

Comparison of the abdominal obliques and erector spinae revealed a statistically significant difference in activity level only during the follow-through phase, when the abdominal obliques activity remained high (101% MMT, 134% MMT), relative to the decreasing erector spinae level (58%, 68% MMT).

Upper Extremities

Posterior deltoid activity increased signficantly from a low in the windup phase (17% MMT) to a high in pre-swing (101% MMT). Signal intensity subsequently decreased throughout the remainder of the swing, and this decrease was signficant between late swing (76% MMT) and follow-through (25% MMT).

The triceps demonstrated low activity in windup (25% MMT), which increased significantly in early (92% MMT) and middle (73% MMT) swing. Activity then declined significantly between middle swing and follow-through (23% MMT).

Supraspinatus activity remained relatively low (< 32% MMT) throughout the swing. The lowest activity occurred during windup (13% MMT), which revealed significantly less activity than either pre-, mid-, or late swing (32% MMT each).

Middle serratus activity remained low throughout swing (< 40% MMT), particularly during windup (18% MMT), which showed significantly less activity than either middle or late swing (39% MMT each).

Analysis

Windup

Activity levels during windup were relatively low except in the trail-leg hamstrings. During this period of single leg stance, hamstring activity maintained hip extension as weight shifted to the trail leg in preparation for the swing.

Pre-swing

The high level of activity in the hamstrings and lower gluteus maximus during pre-swing indicated their role in hip stabilization and initiation of power. Both lead and trail erector spinae and abdominal obliques were also quite active at this time for trunk stabilization and power transmission. As the body was lowered during pre- and early swing, posterior deltoid and triceps activity increased markedly, to maintain lead shoulder elevation.

Swing

During pre-swing and early swing, there was increased activity in the VMO, which prevented collapse of the increasingly flexed trail leg, and promoted push-off to facilitate force transfer. When weight was transferred to the lead leg, hamstring and gluteus maximus activity in the trail leg declined. Trunk activity in both erector spinae and obliques remained high throughout the swing, with erector spinae activity declining just prior to ball contact. This demonstrated the importance of the trunk in power transmission as the body uncoils.

Swing progression yielded decreasing, albeit relatively high, activity in the posterior deltoid and triceps, suggesting their likely positional role. Though they may contribute to power generation, their consistently decreasing levels throughout swing suggests they are not the main "drivers." The trunk muscles (erector spinae and obliques) played a very important role, not just in power transmission, but also in coordinating upper to lower extremity muscle function.

Follow-through

Activity levels in the lower and upper extremities were low during follow-through, except for the VMO, which maintained an extension force on the flexed trail knee. Back and abdominal oblique mus-

cle activity levels remained high, maintaining trunk rotation and stabilization.

Conclusions

A distinct pattern of muscle activity was observed during the batting swing. Lower extremity groups appear important in early pelvic stabilization and power generation. The hamstrings maintain hip stabilization in addition to contributing to the "thrust" provided to initiate rotation (uncoiling mechanism). Vastus medialis obliques activity increased throughout the swing, as the lower extremity pushed against the ground and through the bent knee to contribute the forward thrust of the pelvis and trunk.

The erector spinae and abdominal oblique muscles were extremely active in trunk stabilization and rotation for smooth power transfer. The lack of discernible activity differences between lead and trail spinae or obliques suggests their premier importance in torso stabilization and rotation rather than power generation per se. However, it is also possible that our use of surface electrodes for the obliques recorded information from both the internal and external oblique muscles, as these are relatively thin muscles next to one another. This may preclude the ability to discern a "coupling force" between the internal and external fibers, hence the lead and trail sides. Differences between the lead and trail erector spinae may have been similarly masked owing to their close proximity.

The posterior deltoid and triceps appeared to be more important to positioning than to power generation. The middle serratus anterior and supraspinatus did not significantly contribute to the swing.

The uncoiling of the woundup pelvis, trunk, and upper extremities on a stable base provides the power for the baseball batting swing. Of the muscles tested, there appears to be a sequence of activity from the lower extremities (most active group in pre-swing), through the trunk (highest in early swing), to the upper extremity muscle groups.

This sequence appears nearly identical to that observed in the golf swing, where initiation of the swing begins in the hip.[10] As in batting, electromyographic studies of the golf swing show the importance of the trunk in stabilization and power transfer.[15] The serratus anterior and supraspinatus are more active in the golf swing than during the batting swing; the posterior deltoid is less active.[9,16] This difference is most likely due to the higher position of the golf club, which requires scapular protraction and humeral abduction. The baseball bat is held in a more horizontally abducted position, thus there is relatively more activity in the posterior deltoid. The pectoralis major and latissimus dorsi may contribute to power in the golf swing by internally rotating and adducting the humerus. This position puts the arm in a stable position to transmit power to the ball. However, this study[16] did not monitor activity in these muscles. Future studies of additional upper-extremity muscle groups will be of great interest in furthering our understanding.

The following conclusions can be drawn from the electromyographic data obtained in our study of 18 professional baseball players.

1. Hamstring and lower gluteus maximus activity contributes signficantly to the stable base and the power of the thrust from which the torso "uncoils" during the swing.

2. Skilled batting relies on a coordinated transfer of muscle activity from the lower extremities to the trunk and finally to the upper extremities.

3. The increased muscle activity in the erector spinae and abdominal oblique throughout the swing suggests the importance of emphasizing abdominal and back exercises in a comprehensive exercise and conditioning program for baseball batters.

4. Unlike conclusions from previous studies the triceps and other muscles of the upper extremity appear most important in positioning the swing. Contribution of other upper extremity-muscles to power generation remains an area for future study.

5. This study provides a base line upon which further investigation of the baseball batting swing can be performed. Prevention and rehabilitation of batting injuries can be more specifically focused given an understanding of the biomechanics of the batting swing.

Clinical Correlation

For a more practical understanding of hitting, we turned to a hitting coach and skilled batter.[8,17]

Stance

The swing starts with the stance. The key to the proper baseball stance is balance. Every player's stance will be different; the ideal position is probably feet shoulder-width apart. The hitter may fashion a hole for the back foot, to push off with; he may change his position slightly from closed to open for an inside pitch. However, no matter what position the player assumes, no matter what he is doing before initiating the swing, controlling the hitting motion starts with a balanced stance. As the pitcher approaches the mound and begins his windup, the hitter coils up. This coiling maneuver brings the bat to the position required for the hitter to initiate the swing. Regardless of the initial batting position, most hitters bring the bat to a fairly standard position relative to the strike zone just before beginning the forward stride. The body is in position; the coiled hips and head are approximately level; the knees are slightly bent; there is some flexion of the lumbar spine; the shoulders are level; and the head is turned, chin against left shoulder, eyes gazing directly at the pitcher. Hand position will vary slightly, according to the player; 4 to 8 inches from the body, level to shoulder high, is usual. The bat position is approximately 45 degrees in the coiled stance, with the elbow level to the ground and out from the body. Hands held too far from the body may reduce the power of the swing. Holding the hands too low and too close to the body reduces bat speed and may reduce the contact zone.

In the coiled position just described, the hitter begins his swing with the forward arm motion of the pitcher. His eyes pick up the ball from the pitcher's hand and he begins to time his forward stride and swing. The key to hitting, obviously, is vision. If the hitter cannot see the ball, then he is guessing with the swing and will not be able to make contact. Not only is visual acuity critical, eye control and function are also important. The hitter must have clear binocular focus to see the ball and predict its location. The ball's speed prevents the hitter from following the ball all the way to the bat. The hitter should follow the ball as far as he can, and then make a prediction as to its line of projection. Without visualization, concentration, and focus, the hitter will fail to project the arrival point of the ball, resulting in inadequate ball contact. Balance and control are also determined by eye focus, as is any coordinated muscle activity. If the eyes are focused on one point, the body is better able to produce a coordinated, balanced motion than if the eyes are closed. Thus, successfully maintaining the stance requires balance, eye focus, and good body position. What happens before this coiling maneuver is not of great importance. However, body and head position in the coiled portion of the swing should place the bat in a reasonable position to begin the stride.

Stride

Ben Hines, Dodger batting coach, has presented five important aspects of the swing, starting with the stride:[8]

1. Back foot rotation in which the heel rotates out and the body pivots on the ball of the back foot.

2. Forward stride with the left foot.

3. Rapid hip and trunk rotation that repositions the navel from perpendicular to the pitch to parallel to the pitch.

4. Triangulation and extension of the arms.

5. Lateral wrist flexion.

Efficiency of motion is essential to the hitter[17]; he must avoid needless motion. Motion must be balanced and coordinated in the forward stride. The backward motion in the coiled position precedes the forward motion. The front leg initially rotates internally but the coil position will externally rotate the leg in the stride. The stride should be directly toward the pitcher. The weight shift during the hitting motion is very important as well. The weight stays on the heel of the back foot as the forward foot strides forward lightly on the ball of the forward foot. The left knee and leg, which are initially rotated internally, will then rotate externally, shifting the left knee into extension. The ability to lock the left knee and provide rigid resistance to body motion is important for keeping the rotational axis of the body centered. If the left knee flexes, the body weight will shift forward and the proper axis of rotation is lost. The foot will land evenly and it may be slightly open. Initially the knee is flexed slightly as the foot lands but will then lock in extension as the hips come through. The core of the swing action is the hitter's mid-section, where hitting power is generated.[17] Maintaining a center axis of motion and balance is critical in maintaining head position. Too much head motion will result in loss of coordination and visualization of the ball. A key to the stride and swing positions is locking the head to the center of axis of rotation. In the coiled position the bat is approximately at a 45-degree angle. As the bat comes through, there is a relative leveling of the bat, usually, of < 10 degrees of angulation. The pitch starts high because the pitcher is on the mound, throwing down. A difference of a certain number of degrees between the ball and the bat exists with the bat coming down as the ball comes down.

Rotation

The forward stride of the legs and the rotation of the hips is reasonably standard in speed and approach. The large muscles in these areas cannot be controlled quickly enough to allow the hitter to adjust to the faster speed of the pitch. One of the important parts of batting training techniques is the sudden, rapid hip twist in which the navel shifts from 90 degrees to the pitch to directly parallel to the pitch. This movement, in many ways, determines the bat speed and allows the hitter to be in a prime position to adjust to the speed and type of pitch. Therefore, stride length, hip rotation, and navel toward the pitcher is the same in virtually every pitch and must be a standardized, balanced, well-coordinated motion.

A question that is raised, however, is if these movements are well-coordinated, adjustments made accommodate different speed pitches in different pitch zones. An adjustable ratio of derotation of the body occurs as it leaves the coil position to the point of contact. With the power generated through the hip and belly rotation, fine control comes with the speed of the upper body uncoiling and the speed of elbow extension and wrist lateral flexion. Location of the pitch, of course, will vary tremendously and the fine adjustment takes place in these latter three aspects. Therefore, the upper body trails behind the derotation of the hips. Trailing behind does not imply that this is a helter-skelter, uncoordinated motion. Because the ratio of derotation of the upper body to the lower body must vary with the pitch, even more muscular trunk control is required to allow the proper rotation to take place. Therefore, the hitter must visualize the ball, in less than a second, to determine the ratio of derotation of the upper body and the position of the head, elbows, and hands for the point of contact with the ball. This requires excellant muscle control, balance, and coordination.

Retraining the muscles to fire and respond to changes in balance and coordination, and retraining the trunk muscles to maintain a tight, rigid but mobile control between the upper and lower body, is key to proper hitting. Lumbar pain that prevents proper rotation, by causing the muscles to work in an uncoordinated fashion, can have a devastating effect on the hitter's ability to deliver the bat to the ball. After hip rotation, with the upper body trailing slightly behind, under maximum muscle control, and at a specific ratio of derotation as determined by the pitch, the upper body rotates through to the point of ball contact. The head is level and goes down with the pitch; the eyes focus on the ball. The chin is against the left shoulder, and it will end up against the right shoulder after ball contact. Again, head motion equals poor efficiency.

At this point, with the bat coming through the strike zone, part of the key to proper mechanics shifts to the shoulders and upper arms. The arms should form a perfect triangle with the chest as the base, the two arms parallel as they extend out. Locking the left shoulder is of critical importance. Stabilization of the left shoulder allows extension of the left elbow and allows proper generation of bat speed.

The bottom hand pulls and anchors the bat, the top hand pushes and guides the bat. As the arms and elbows extend, the bat still trails behind with the wrists in the cocked position. Obviously, the mechanics of hitting, including the weight shift from the back foot to the forward foot, the position of the elbows, hands, wrists, and bat, must allow the hitter to delay his final committment of bat position as long as possible, while still allowing time to generate the necessary power and force. It is certainly possible to make contact with the ball with no trunk rotation and no power, but that is hardly going to produce sufficient results on the field.

The follow-through after ball contact is a natural part of the swing and is not of major consequence: weight will be shifted to the front foot, the left knee will be locked; good quadriceps function control of the front leg is imperative. The arms will be extended, the top hand will roll over at an appropriate time and should not be rushed too early.

Dynamic Electromyographic Analysis of Torque Transfer in Pitchers

Professional baseball pitching is one of the most demanding precision, high speed torsional activities in sports, and some of the most difficult lumbar spine problems are seen in baseball pitchers. Trunk stability is critical to a pitcher's throw, and any pain producing weakness and stiffness can lead to a potentially catastrophic injury. In an effort to better study the role of trunk musculature and lumbar injury in the professional baseball pitcher's performance, we attempted to evaluate electromyograms of trunk musculature in the Centinela Hospital Gait Laboratory.

With help from Harry Farfan, M.D., and professional pitchers, coaches, and trainers, we initially postulated that trunk fatigue produces increased lordosis of the lumbar spine and therefore places the shoulder and arm behind in the throwing motion. This leads to a high release point, with the ball rising in the strike zone and becoming easier to hit. Also, arm strain can result from using the arm muscles to try to catch up the arm to the trunk. Our goal was to provide a foundation for the analysis of pitching biomechanics, trunk conditioning, and rehabilitation that could be used to improve the efficiency of the athlete and decrease the incidence of injuries.

We first had to understand the normal patterns. Twenty nonprofessional athletes underwent electromyographic (EMG) analysis of trunk musculature while pitching. After considerable difficulty, problems with electrodes were worked out. This evaluation indicated a basic pattern of firing sequences needed for the pitching motion. The contrasting patterns indicated a sequence necessary for skilled performance.

Fifteen professional baseball pitchers from the Los Angeles Dodgers then volunteered for testing. They underwent EMG activity amplitude evaluation via surface electrode telemetry of their trunk musculature, including the abdominal obliques, rectuc abdominus, lumbar paraspinous, and gluteus maximus bilaterally. Proper electrode placement was established by a therapist and computerized telemetry evaluation.

The signals from the leads were transmitted using an FM-FM telemetry system that transmitted data from four muscles simultaneously. Correct electrode placement was confirmed via manual muscle testing as documented on an oscilloscope.

Each pitcher wore a battery-operated FM transmitter belt pack oriented to prevent restriction in bodily movement. Muscle activity patterns were synchronized with high-speed film (450 frames/sec) to obtain percent muscle activity values at each phase of the pitching motion.

The film was then synchronized for computer analysis using the following phase of pitching:

1. Trunk movement to hands apart
2. Hands apart to foot touch (leading leg)
3. Foot touch to maximum external rotation (dominant shoulder)
4. Maximum external rotation to ball release
5. Ball release to end follow-through

After warm-up and confirmation of the lead placement, each player was asked to do four runs consisting of 40 pitches, using proper throwing techniques at 60% to 70% of maximum velocity as measured by radar gun. Two separate series of runs were conducted, A and B, as delineated by the individual muscle groups tested.

Results

The key to evaluating even a homogeneous group of subjects is determining the consistency of trends and reproducible changes. In using only professional level pitchers, we found wide variance of delivery styles, physical characteristics, and techniques, which produced a wide range of absolute values, but consistent and predictable trends in muscle activity.

The nondominant rectus abdominus, lumbar paraspinous, and abdominal obliques all showed consistent and significant increases in activity over their dominant side partners at predictable phases.

RECTUS ABDOMINUS

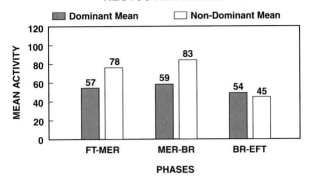

Fig. 43-1

Rectus abdominus activity during pitching phases from foot touch (FT) through end of follow-through (EFT). D = dominant side; ND = non-dominant side; MER = maximum external rotation; BR = ball release. *(From Watkins R, Dennis S, et al.: Dynamic EMG Analysis of Torque Transfer in Professional Baseball Pitchers. Spine, 14(4): 404-408, J.B. Lippincott Co., 1989.)*

LUMBAR PARASPINUS

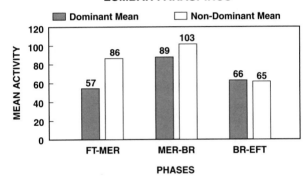

Fig. 43-2

Lumbar paraspinus activity during the pitching phases from foot touch (FT) through end of follow-through (EFT). D = dominant side; ND = non-dominant side. *(From Watkins R, Dennis S, et al.: Dynamic EMG Analysis of Torque Transfer in Professional Baseball Pitchers. Spine, 14(4): 404-408, J.B. Lippincott Co., 1989.)*

The glutei demonstrated bilateral increases consistent with the phases of pitching.

The nondominant rectus exhibited individual increases into the active phase of 5- to 20-fold with sustained increases throughout the active phase as high as 10-fold. The mean increase over the active phase through ball release for the nondominant rectus was 40% higher than that of the dominant side. In the actual cocking phase, foot touch to maximum external rotation, individual activity levels increased from 5 to 100, and 12 to 114, 2000% and 950% increases, respectively, from the prior phase on the nondominant side. At this same point, the dominant side was 35.5 and 11.5 (as compared with 100 and 114, respectively).

Four players demonstrated slightly dominant side predominance in cocking, two reversed or balanced in delivery, and all pitchers were in nondominant side control at the time of ball release and follow-through (Fig. 43-1).

The nondominant lumbar paraspinous demonstrated individual increases of 100% to 400% during the active phases, with an occasional subject showing dominant side increases as well. During the maximum cocking phase, through and including ball release, this nondominant muscle demonstrated a mean of 50% increase in activity over the dominant side. The dominant lumbar paraspinous was much more active than the rectus counterparts at an earlier phase. However, in every subject, during each of the active phases through ball release, the nondominant side demostrated increased activity. In the cocking phase, the mean increase was 51%, while in the delivery phase the mean was only 16% with generalized in-

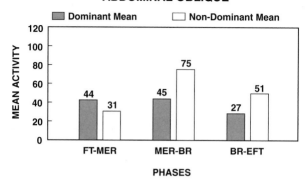

Fig. 43-3

Abdominal oblique activity during pitching phases from foot touch (FT) through end of follow-through (EFT). D = dominant side; ND = non-dominant side. *(From Watkins R, Dennis S, et al.: Dynamic EMG Analysis of Torque Transfer in Professional Baseball Pitchers. Spine, 14(4): 404-408, J.B. Lippincott Co., 1989.)*

GLUTEUS MAXIMUS

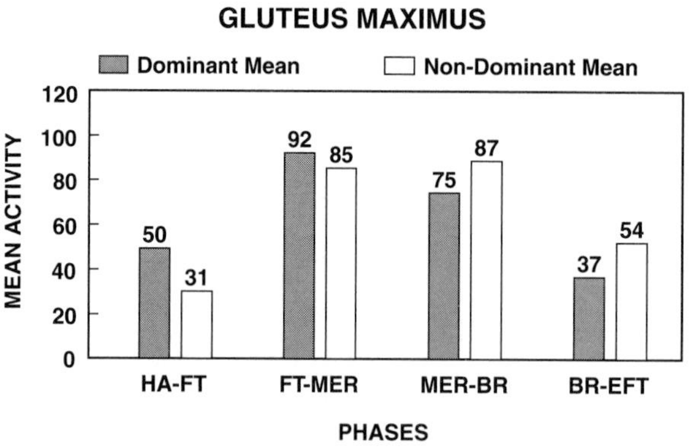

Fig. 43-4

Gluteus maximus activity during pitching phases from foot touch (FT) through end of follow-through (EFT). D = dominant side; ND = non-dominant side. *(From Watkins R, Dennis S, et al.: Dynamic EMG Analysis of Torque Transfer in Professional Baseball Pitchers. Spine, 14(4): 404-408, J.B. Lippincott Co., 1989.)*

creases overall on both sides and individual increases on the nondominant side from 6% to 250% (Fig. 43-2).

The abdominal obliques demonstrated consistent increases in the nondominant side as opposed to the dominant side during the active phases. Increases of 300% to 500% activity were seen in 9 of 16 pitches in the active phases, with increases in all pitchers on the nondominant side over the dominant side. Mean increases of 85% for all subjects and all runs were seen during the final three phases in the nondominant abdominal obliques, a greater increase than any other muscle or pair of muscles. A mean increase of 98% in the cocking phase alone is the largest mean increase of any pair of muscles, nondominant or dominant in any phase (Fig. 43-3).

The glutei fired bilaterally in an expected pattern, as seen by stance phases of the pitching motion. The dominant side bears all the weight initially as rotation begins, and as the stride begins during the cocking and acceleration phases, the nondominant side becomes equally active and must balance as the dominant side pushes through hip extension in the "controlled falling"[14] of delivery. The nondominant side remains flexed at the hip, the gluteus stabilizing the pelvis as the trunk derotates, and delivery and ball release follow (Fig. 43-4).

Analysis

It is common in spring training to see throwers, especially pitchers, having pain in the opposite side sacroiliac joint. This is due to torsional strain, probably in the lower facet joints, from the pitcher being unused to pitching over the winter break. There is a high incidence of back stiffness in throwers as they start to get their mechanical functioning back. Having referred discogenic or facet joint pain in the typical referred pain pattern—which is through the facet joint, across the posterior superior iliac spine, sacroiliac joint, and posterior ilium, and into the area of the greater trochanter—is a very common occurence. Development of secondary contractures, weakness, bursitis, tendinitis, and inflammations in the referred pain area can also occur. Often a pitcher will have greater trochanteric bursitis (sacroiliac joint pain), that produces its own secondary effects.

A key part of the rehabiitation of these players is not only to rehabilitate the back but also the secondary inflammatory effects that can produce the same biomechanical abnormalities in the pitching motion that lead to further injury. Indeed, the pain itself may prevent proper pitching and performance and lead to injury. True sciatica and muscle weakness in a leg produces a critically important dysfunction in a pitcher. It will produce severe abnormalities of his pitching motion, and put his arm, shoulder, and elbow in jeopardy. Sciatica, especially with associated pain with increasing intradiscal and interabdominal pressure, can produce severe dysfunction during the throwing motion.

The concept of trunk strengthening and control is not a new one. Over the years, however, most of the data have been collected in regard to the failed back, discogenic disease, and spondylolisthesis,[19] as opposed to athletic performance. The majority of the electromyographic data have been concentrated on posture, loading, and muscle effects on ligamentous and bony structures. Until recently, no reliable and/or accepted measurement of trunk strength has been available.

Our objective was developed with the concept of multiple applications. First was to document the firing sequence and activity levels of the trunk musculature in pitching at the professional level. Beginning with these baseline data, the application leads to using the trends and patterns in evaluating faulty biomechanics. We hoped for a successful rehabilitation tool, and, with continued refinement and growth of the database, to be able to evaluate new prospects and potential athletes.

A phase of coiling or rotational loading immediately before the cocking phase is one of the most important load components in the pitching motion. This phase loads the body so that the arm may both load and release with maximum power and efficiency. During this phase, the dominant gluteus maximus is the key, first working in neutral and slight extension for balance to allow maximum coiling as the stabi-

lizer of the pelvis and trunk, and immediately following as a powerful extensor to provide maximum power as transmitted through the leg. During these cocking and acceleration phases, which take less than 0.3 seconds,[5] the player goes through the phenomenon of "controlled falling".[14] This controlled falling sequence is a combination of deceleration and derotation of the trunk during maximum cocking and subsequent acceleration of the pitching arm to ball release and follow-through. These oppositional forces cause an imbalance and "fall" toward the dominant side, which must be resisted to maintain body position for both power and accuracy and to prevent injury within the trunk and arm.

It is during this transition that those nondominant-side trunk muscles become most important. The predominance of contralateral muscles to control rotation is a well-documented concept.[1,11] These paraspinal muscles act as stabilizers while the obliques act to initiate further flexion or rotation.[11] In other posture and loading studies of EMG back muscle activity using asymmetric loading on an increased angle at a fixed point, higher activity was found on the contralateral side of the lumbar region.[1]

In this situation of controlled falling, both rotational forces and gravity must be resisted. Asmussen,[2] and Asmussen and Klausen,[3] documented the counteraction of gravity to be maintained primarily by the back muscles only, but usually one set of muscles. In only 20% to 25% of the time do the abdominal muscles affect posture.[3] In applying this concept of trunk support and the rotational component involved in this activity, previous data completely support our findings. Donisch and Basmajian's work also documented this paradoxic activity of increased lumbar contralateral EMG function in axial rotation.[7] All of the previous studies using a form of external load have been of lifting resisted movements, or static postures,[1] In evaluating the trunk muscle function during active motion, the subject is measured in various postures and in transition, resisting his own acceleration and deceleration, and generating power through the trunk as in lifting. In all of the previous studies of rotation or transition, the contralateral rotations and trunk stabilizers have been most active in the work done.[1-3,7,11]

In analyzing the pitching data, we found the same patterns of muscle activity power exhibited as are seen in simple postural loading activities. We hypothesized, therefore, that we should be able to apply the concept of trunk strengthening for improved function and decreased injury in pitchers. Chaffin and Moulis[6] proposed that strengthening the deep back muscles relieves pressure on the intervertebral discs, and should therefore decrease injury during loading. Parnianpour and coworkers[13] recently documented the trunk movements, showing that fatigued muscles are slower and subsequently take longer to respond to change in loads. This demonstrated the phenomenon of compensation of secondary muscle groups causing loading in some injury-prone patients. Nordin and Kahanovitz have shown how men after disectomy have loss of 55% to 71% of isometric strength in flexion and extension, respectively.[12] Using these data and applying them to athletic injury as opposed to postoperative condition, it is crucial for a pitcher to have maximum strength to maintain his level of performance and avoid injury. The corollary to avoiding trunk injury is the concept that maintaining a strong trunk helps avoid arm, i.e., shoulder and elbow, stress by protecting it from the overuse and abnormal motion seen with poor trunk mechanics.

Returning to our initial objective, we have demonstrated a reproducible, consistent pattern despite delivery and physical variations. The applica-

tion of our objective in evaluating faulty biomechanics is represented in the differences as seen in Figs. 43-5 through 43-7. Player OH is an experienced player at the top of his craft and ability. Although his actual activity levels often are higher than the mean, they are highest in the nondominant oblique in all phases, and nondominant paraspinous and rectus in the torque phase of unloading before ball release. Compared with LG, a rising young player recently converted to a pitcher and currently developing his pitching biomechanics, one notes extremely irregular activity levels, off the scale and in no reproducible pattern consistent with the subject mean (Fig. 43-8).

One further comparison is SS, a professional outfielder who volunteered for the study. He participated as a pitcher, using the mound and attempting his best pitching biomechanics. His values are represented in Fig. 43-9, and one can easily note the vast differences in his values compared with both OH (Fig. 43-10) and the mean patterns. These values are of particular signficance in that this player is

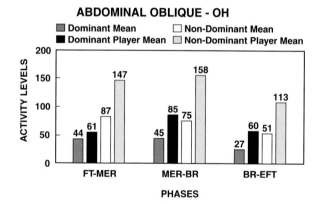

Fig. 43-5

Comparison of activity levels, mean versus individual player in individual muscles. O. H. is an experienced major league consistent pitcher. Each player means are dotted bar graphs. *(From Watkins R, Dennis S, et al.: Dynamic EMG Analysis of Torque Transfer in Professional Baseball Pitchers. Spine, 14(4): 404-408, J.B. Lippincott Co., 1989.)*

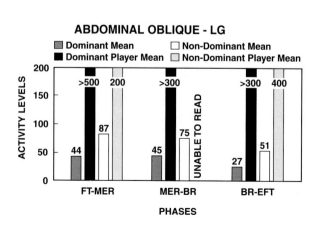

Fig. 43-6

Comparison of activity levels, mean versus individual player in individual muscles. LG - a minor league pitcher converted from infield position. *(From Watkins R, Dennis S, et al.: Dynamic EMG Analysis of Torque Transfer in Professional Baseball Pitchers. Spine, 14(4): 404-408, J.B. Lippincott Co., 1989.)*

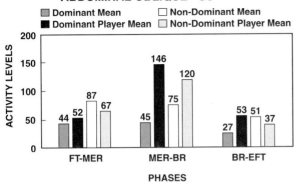

Fig. 43-7

Comparison of activity levels, mean versus individual player in individual muscles. SS - outfielder used as a comparison. *(From Watkins R, Dennis S, et al.: Dynamic EMG Analysis of Torque Transfer in Professional Baseball Pitchers. Spine, 14(4): 404-408, J.B. Lippincott Co., 1989.)*

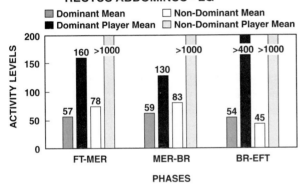

Fig. 43-8

Comparison of activity levels, mean versus individual player in individual muscles. L.G. is a new minor league pitcher converted from an infield position. *(From Watkins R, Dennis S, et al.: Dynamic EMG Analysis of Torque Transfer in Professional Baseball Pitchers. Spine 14(4): 404–408, J.B. Lippincott Co., 1989.)*

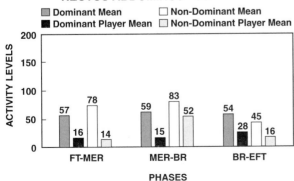

Fig. 43-9

Comparison of activity levels, mean versus individual player in individual muscles. S.S. is an outfielder used as comparison. *(From Watkins R, Dennis S, et al.: Dynamic EMG Analysis of Torque Transfer in Professional Baseball Pitchers. Spine, 14(4): 404-408, J.B. Lippincott Co., 1989.)*

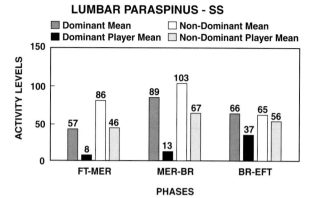

Fig 43-10

Comparison of activity levels, mean versus individual player in individual muscles. S.S. is an outfielder used as comparison. *(From Watkins R, Dennis S, et al.: Dynamic EMG Analysis of Torque Transfer in Professional Baseball Pitchers. Spine, 14(4): 404-408, J.B. Lippincott Co., 1989.)*

also a professional baseball player, yet has none of the fine-tuned activity biomechanics associated specifically with pitching. Therefore, what is the importance of demonstrating a mean firing sequence of trunk musculature? What is the importance of demonstrating the difference in firing sequence between a top level pitcher, a strong outfielder, and a rookie pitcher? All of these three athletes are strong with good musculature. The point is that trunk muscle coordination is as important as trunk muscle strength in being able to perform as a top level baseball pitcher. Coordinated strength is less fatiguing and more effective than uncoordinated strength. Therefore, a logical conclusion would be that a trunk-strengthening program that incorporates balancing and coordination while doing the strengthening can be more effective.

This last comparison leads to the possibility of using gait laboratory analysis as a predictive indicator for success as a pitcher as based on biomechanics and muscle activity. We accept the need for larger sampling of pitchers with particular emphasis on those who have continued success over time and fewest injuries. We would hope for this measurement to be an additional tool for evaluation of pitchers. The most important application of our objectives, however, is to use the complete data package—muscle activity levels, firing patterns, their trends and timing, and the high speed photographic techniques—to aid the athlete. By careful laboratory analysis, coupled with the evaluation of coaches and trainers, we can aid in the detection of biomechanical changes and, through rehabilitation or changes in technique, improve the efficiency of the athlete.

The use of this gait analysis for the injured ath-

lete in need of rehabilitation is an important concept. The significant association of the injured shoulder or elbow to the weak or injured lumbar spine needs to be further documented. Unfortunately, under laboratory conditions, we were unable to fatigue a pitcher in order to study the interaction of the arm and spine in this situation. It is an accepted concept in baseball that fatigue causes an early release point in the throwing motion, which in turn causes the ball to rise at the batter, making it easier to hit. This fatigue originates in a weak trunk, causing the arm to work harder, and predisposes it to injury. By using laboratory evaluation, we hope to aid in rehabilitation programs by emphasizing the role of trunk strength in shoulder rehabilitation.

Conclusions

The documentation of trunk activity in the dynamic state of baseball pitching clearly demonstrates a reproducible pattern of muscle function. This pattern impacts directly on the biomechanics of the throwing arm by controlling the stabilization and loading characteristics responsible for maximum power and control.

The implication of such a pattern is that athletes can be analyzed with the objective of maintaining and/or fine-tuning biomechanics, i.e., improvements or changes in technique can be based on objective data.

The rehabilitation of an injured athlete, whether it be shoulder, elbow, or back, can be better assessed with gait analysis. The use of objective physical data for goals and program documentation can add to a rehabilitation program. Also, with expanded data

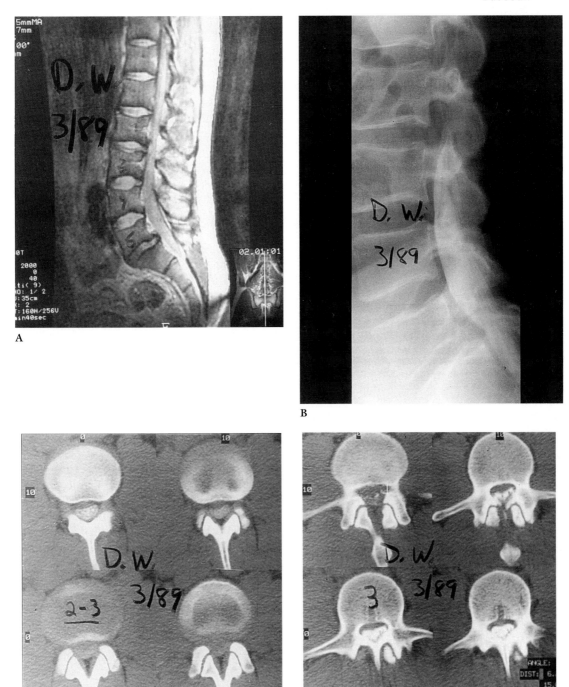

Fig. 43-11

This 32-year-old major-league infielder presented with severe back and radiating hip pain and hip weakness. He had no true sciatica. His pain was reproduced with a femoral nerve stretch. He had weakness in his hip area, but it was an ill-defined dermatomal pattern. **A,** The MRI demonstrated the extruded disc fragment at L2-L3. **B,C,D,** The myelogram and contrast CT scans demonstrate the large extruded fragment of the L2-L3 disc that was removed with a microscopic lumbar discectomy. The patient returned to full sports function.

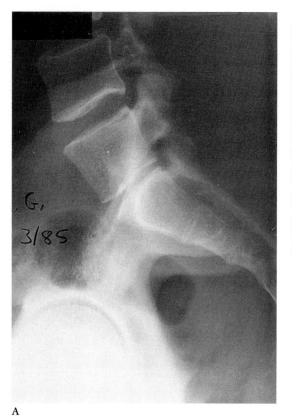

A

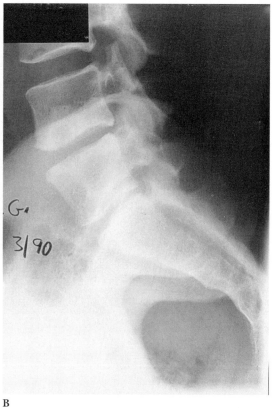

B

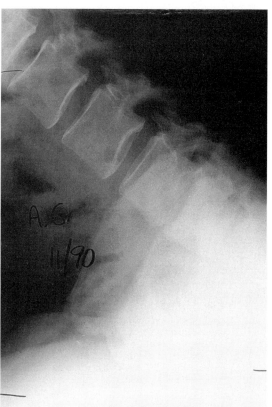

C

Fig. 43-12

A, This 28-year-old major-league infielder had an evaluation for mild mechanical back pain. **B,** Five years later (3/19/90), the patient was seen for a significant mechanical back pain. His diagnosis was degenerative disc disease. **C,** Eight months later, the patient had a marked increase in the narrowing of the disc space and an increase in spasms and symptoms.

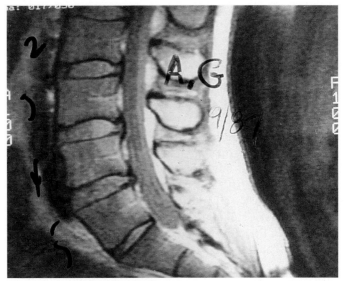

D

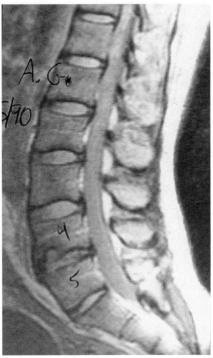

E

Fig. 43-12, cont'd

D, The MRI chronicles this change from 9/87, when the L4-L5
disc space did not look severely involved, to 5/90 **(E),** which
shows marked narrowing and a progressive Smorl's node. This
patient underwent a multiple disc-space aspiration for infection,
but no infection was identified. He had a percutaneous discectomy with more specimens sent for pathologic analysis. No infection was identified and the patient returned to play, painfree,
2 years after a proper trunk stabilization rehabilitation program.

and close association with productivity evaluation, determining predictive success outcome may not be an impossibility.

Treatment of Hitters with Lumbar Spine Injuries

Certainly, this encompasses the usual treatment methods of decreased inflammation, strengthening, stretching, and conditioning, with one added, very important component. Hitters personify the rehabilitation rule: take the instrument out of their hands to begin rehabilitation. Like a tennis player and other racquet sports players, a hitter, when he has a bat in his hands, is going to swing the bat basically the same way he has always swung the bat. If he has developed poor trunk mechanics over a period of time in response to an injury that is still painful, or as a compensation for contractures and weaknesses, he will not be able to change those mechanics as part of his rehabilitation as long as he is holding the bat. It is too inbred a learned response. Something that occurs in a split second and involves entire body muscle performance is very difficult to change. Thus, the following steps should be undertaken.

1. Take the bat out of his hands. You have got to take him away from home plate, out of baseball, onto the gym floor or the therapist's table, and begin a muscle retraining process that teaches muscles to fire and contract in response to trunk and upper extremity stimuli.

2. Start the trunk stabilization program. Progress to Level III stabilization training.

3. Teach muscles to maintain a tight muscle contraction throughout a full rotation.

4. Teach trunk musculature to relock the shoulders to the hips in a controlled, tight fashion.

5. Reestablish flexibility through contractures and provide full range of motion for the spine throughout the normal degrees of motion required to perform the activity.

6. Institute resistive PNF techniques where the hitter is rotating against resistance from the therapist or at the full range of motion; use isometric muscle control in a push-pull pattern for reestablishing muscle function; restore symmetry of muscle balance by strengthening the muscles on the opposite side.

7. Do rotational resistive exercises in the opposite direction.

8. Reevaluate the batting stance just as you reevaluate the approach for a golfer.

9. Assure the hitter is balanced and under control, that he has the ability to establish a tight, neutral spine position so that the spine is being held in an appropriate posture to produce a coordinated, balanced, strong swing.

10. Progress toward an aerobic conditioning program to achieve maximum aerobic shape.

After work on the floor— doing the stability exercises, the balancing and coordinating exercises, and the B&F techniques with a trainer — and after the therapist has established strong, tight, trunk control, good flexibility, balance, and has restored aerobic conditioning, then the therapist and the trainer work to institute initially the basics of bat mechanics while emphasizing the muscle strengthening and condition program.

At this point, the hitting coach can play a major role. The hitting coach and the trainer collaborate with the hitter to translate the new strength, flexibility, and coordination into the proper sports-specific activity. The hitting coach should be able to incorporate the new ideas and mechanisms established by the physical therapist to establish and improve a hitting technique that allows the hitter to swing and hit pain free. Slight changes suggested by the hitting coach, such as adjusting hand position on the bat, opening the stance, or emphasizing a different type of eye control for the hitter, can prove invaluable.

Changing the basic swing of a baseball player who has made it to the major leagues as a hitter is difficult. You can shorten up the swing, change the hand position, emphasize head control, discuss going to right field, change bat size, and other isolated techniques, and you are still left with the basic rehabilitation principles of establishing a strong, functional trunk that can transfer power from the legs to the end of a bat.

Rehabilitation of the infielder is much like rehabilitation of anyone with a lifting job. Proper infield techniques should be designed to protect the spine. The simple concept of squatting to gather a ground ball is good for backs. Bending over at the waist with the knees straight is bad lifting technique and lousy fielding technique. The ability to work in a bent-forward position is more proportional to quadriceps strength than back strength. Also, abdominal strengthening and extensor strengthening are important. The use of an abdominal binder in an infielder would not be inappropriate; if it does not restrict the range of motion it might add a bit of support in the off-balance, forward-bending position that is sometimes required.

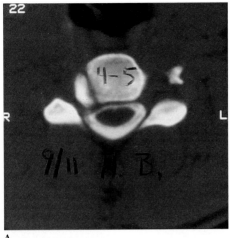

A

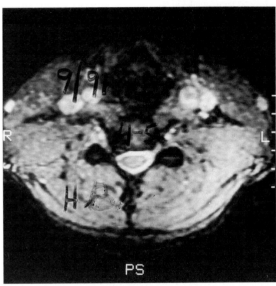

B

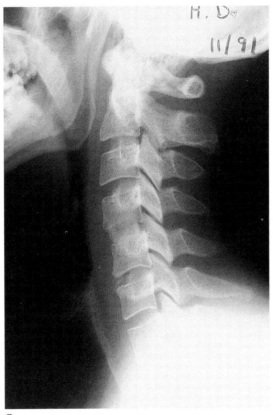

C

Fig. 43-13

A, This illustration shows the transverse section of the contrast CT scan in a 31-year-old professional baseball player with weak right shoulder abduction and clinical C5 root lesion. **B,** He underwent a successful anterior cervical fusion with solid healing. **C,** He had some problems with nerve-root irritation after returning to function, but has a solid fusion and full return of strength from the C5 nerve root.

Summary

In conclusion, not only must a baseball player have speed, strength, and flexibility in aerobic conditioning, but he must also have balance and coordination. The EMG studies of the baseball hitters, the EMG studies of the baseball pitchers, and every aspect of research done into the key activities in baseball indicate that it is not just strength, but is also the coordinated firing of muscles in exact patterns and sequences that equals the coordination necessary to perform the sport. The trunk stabilization program that we have advocated increases trunk strength and coordination. Balance and coordination must be included in any muscle strengthening techniques in order to achieve maximum performance of the player.

References

1. Andersson GBJ and others: Quantitative electromyographic studies of back muscle activity related to posture and loading, *Orthop Clin North Am* 8:85, 1977.
2. Asmussen E: The weight-carrying function of the human spine, *Acta Orthop Scand* 29:276, 1960.
3. Asmussen E, Klausen K: Form and function of the erect human spine, *Clin Orthop* 25:55, 1962.
4. Basmajian JV: *Muscles alive: their functions revealed by electromyography,* Baltimore, 1967, Williams & Wilkins.
5. Braatz JH: The mechanics of pitching, *J Orthop Sports Ther* 9(2):56, 1987.
6. Chaffin DB, Moulis EJ: An empirical investigation of low back strains and vertebral geometry, *J Biomech* 2:88, 1969.
7. Donisch EW, Basmajian JV: Electromyography of deep back muscles in man, *Am J Anat* 133:25, 1972.
8. Hines B: Los Angeles Dodgers batting coach, personal communication, 1992.
9. Jobe FW, Moynes DR, Antonelli DJ: Rotator cuff function during the golf swing, *Am J Sports Med* 14(5):388, 1986.
10. Jobe FW, Schwab DR: *30 exercises for better golf,* Inglewood, CA, 1986, Champion Press.
11. Morris JM and others: An electromyographic study of the intrinsus muscles of the back in man, *J Anat* 96(4):509, 1962.
12. Nordin M and others: *A comparative analysis of postoperative discectomy trunk strength and endurance.* Presented at the Federation of Spine Associations, Atlanta, GA, February 1988.
13. Parnianpour M and others: *The effect of fatigue on the motor output and patten of isodynamic trunk movement.* Presented at the Annual Meeting of the International Society for the Study of the Lumbar Spine, Florida, April 1988.
14. Perry J: Personal communication
15. Pink M: *The biomechanics of golf.* Presented at the 1990 PGA Teaching and Coaching Summit, Nashville, TN, November 1990.
16. Pink M, Jobe FW, Perry J: EMG analysis of the shoulder during the golf swing, *Am J Sports Med* 18(2):137, 1990.
17. Winfield D: New York Yankee baseball player, personal communication, 1991.

Chapter 44
Basketball

Joel M. Press
Mark S. Pfeil
Jeffrey L. Young

Spine Injuries in Basketball

Mechanisms of Injury

Specific Spine Injuries
    ligamentous strain and muscular
       strain/contusion
    spondylolysis/spondylolisthesis
    intervertebral disc injuries

Spine Stabilization

Spine Stabilization Exercise Programs

Criteria for Return to Play After
    Back Injury/Surgery

Since its inception at Smith College in Northhampton, Massachusetts, in 1894, basketball has gained tremendous popularity. A 1982 survey showed that approximately 25 million people participate in basketball yearly.[14] With increasing popularity, however, comes an increasing number of injuries. Basketball requires a combination of speed, strength, endurance, agility, balance, and coordination. Most injuries in basketball occur to the lower extremities.[1,7] However, there are a significant number of spinal injuries due to basketball. This chapter will outline the epidemiology of spine injuries in basketball, some possible mechanisms of injuries, sport-specific injuries and principles of rehabilitation, some specific examples of therapy used for two professional basketball players after spinal surgery, and return-to-play parameters after spine injuries or surgery.

Spine Injuries in Basketball

Low-back injuries secondary to basketball usually rank third behind ankle and knee injuries.[1,15] In one study of professional basketball players, back and hip injuries ranked second accounting for 11.5% of all injuries in basketball,[7] Zelisko and colleagues compared injuries in men and women professional basketball players and found the incidence of low-back injuries to be 13.0% and 8.2%, respectively.[15] Back injuries were the most common injury sustained by centers.[1,7] The roles of height and weight as contributory factors in low-back pain (LBP) in the general population remain controversial with some studies indicating contributory effects and others indicating no correlation.[5] The study by Apple and associates revealed that back injuries accounted for 15.2% of missed time playing.[1]

Mechanisms of Injury

Basketball is a sport with significant contact and numerous collisions. Falls and sudden twisting and torquing of the torso and extremities are quite common. As levels of competition increase, leaning, holding, and hand and boy checking become more frequent and accepted. The size of the athlete also increases significantly with higher levels of competition, with resultant exertion of larger forces on anatomic structures such as the spine. The repetitive pounding and twisting in basketball puts tremendous stress on the low back. The predominant activity in basketball is running, which is associated with lateral rotation, flexion, and extension of the lumbar spine. These motions can occur with rapid acceleration or deceleration as well as with sudden changes in direction of movement. Furthermore, there is often nonuniform loading of the intervertebral disc and posterior elements. This can occur when a player lands off balance after jumping to retrieve a rebound, or when body contact suddenly shifts the player's center of gravity (e.g., being fouled while attempting a jump shot or lay-up). The combinations of movements such as twisting, bending, and bending with rotation will result in increased stress and strain on a disc, especially with a superimposed load.[13] Similar stress can be placed on the posterior elements and spinal musculature.

Other contributing factors to back injuries in basketball could include poor conditioning, improper body mechanics, overuse, poor preworkout stretching, incomplete rehabilitation of injuries of the lower extremity, or unrecognized previous injury.[9,14] Another very significant, and often overlooked, cause of back injuries is insufficient hip, leg, and trunk strength, which becomes a greater factor as fatigue sets in and postural changes occur, placing additional stress on low-back structures.

Specific Spine Injuries

Ligamentous Strain and Muscular Strain/Contusion

The most common injury to the back in basketball is lumbosacral strain of ligamentous tissue or strain of paravertebral, pelvic, or flank musculature. Numerous ligaments support the structures of the low back, including the bones, intervertebral discs, vertebral bodies, and apophyseal joints. The history given for strains and sprains is that of sudden, rapid, rotational motion, often with flexion and/or extension, with pain ensuing at the time of the movement or shortly thereafter. A player may relate the onset of pain to pulling down a rebound while simultaneously landing off-balance on one foot, or rapidly changing the direction of pursuit when suddenly running into a pick set by another player. The clinical picture will depend on what ligamentous structure is damaged, how severe the injury is, and what, if any, associated muscular injury has occurred. Active motion will be limited and often painful. The pain if often located only in the back without radiation of symptoms to the buttock or leg.

In particular, strains of the apophyseal joints are quite common because of the significant amount of extension and hyperextension combined with the rotation of the spine that occurs in basketball. Two examples include a player shooting a jump shot, and a player "reaching back" for a rebound over his head

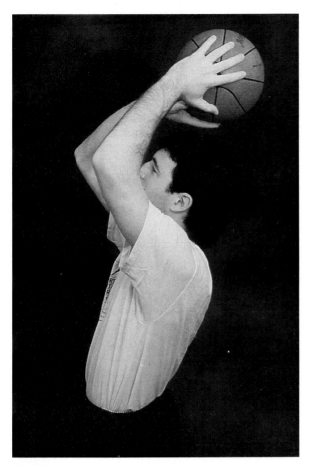

Fig. 44-1

A player shooting a jump shot with some increased extension in the lumbar spine.

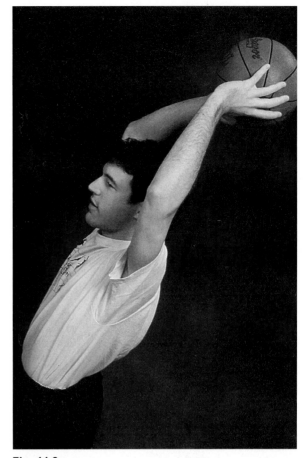

Fig. 44-2

A player reaching back for a rebound over his head with exaggerated lordosis of his lumbar spine.

(Figs. 44-1 and 44-2). Both activities demonstrate increased extension of the lumbar spine. Surrounding muscle spasm may be quite significant. Pain is more pronounced with passive extension and relieved with passive or gently active flexion.

Initial treatment for most back strains may be accelerated with the use of antiinflammatory modalities such as ice, electric stimulation, resting of the injured areas, supportive taping or strapping, and gently soft-tissue mobilization. Early gentle passive and active range of motion (ROM) may be encouraged to prevent soft-tissue contracture and maintain nutrition to the intervertebral discs with increasing flexibility and stretching as acute edema and inflammation resolve.

Lumbosacral contusions are also common and are the result of direct trauma from collisions or contact, which occur often in basketball. Treatment is similar

to ligamentous strains with the liberal use of ice, compression, antiinflammatory medications and modalities, rest, and rapid progression of ROM exercises.

Spondylolysis/Spondylolisthesis

Spondylolysis and spondylolisthesis are conditions seen in approximately 5% of the general population of the United States and are significant causes of LBP. [4] Athletics in general may predispose an individual to spondylolysis or injury to the pars interarticularis. These injuries are usually associated with repetitive stresses over a period of time, in particular hyperextension maneuvers, which occur frequently in basketball. Because of the torsion associated with hyperextension in basketball, athletes may develop unilateral spondylolysis. The player will typically complain of a dull aching pain in the lum-

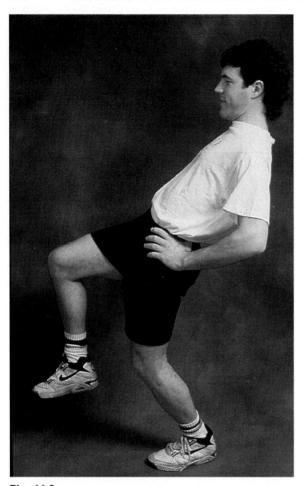

Fig. 44-3

A single leg hyperextension test causes pain with this maneuver in patients with spondylolysis or spondylolisthesis.

bosacral region that is worse with hyperextension activities, often relieved with flexion activities, and rarely causes leg symptoms. Examination will reveal a hyperlordotic position, hamstring tightness, and pain with extension of the hip and leg. The single leg hyperextension test may be positive (Fig. 44-3). Oblique radiographs may show the defect in the pars innerarticularis. Oftentimes a bone scan may be necessary for diagnosis if the radiographs are normal.

Treatment options are nicely outlined elsewhere and consist of a regimen of restricted activities, selective bracing, and an exercise program to strengthen abdominal muscles, decrease lumbar lordosis, and decrease hamstring inflexibility.[4, 8] Spine stabilization exercise as discussed elsewhere in this text is also necessary as part of the rehabilitation program before return to playing basketball.

Intervertebral Disc Injuries

Herniation of a lumbar disc and/or disc degeneration can be a problem in the basketball player. Repetitive torsional stresses can cause tearing of the anulus fibrosis and subsequent degenerative changes of the intervertebral disc, making them more susceptible to herniation. Flexion and rotational movements are often implicated in injury to the disc because of increased loading combined with shear stresses to the anulus. Disc herniation can often be treated with an aggressive nonsurgical rehabilitation program with excellent results[11]. However, for athletes competing at higher levels of basketball, disc herniations with significant leg pain and radiculopathy may warrant surgery for more rapid return to playing. When surgery becomes necessary, postoperative rehabilitation becomes crucial if the athlete is to return to playing basketball.

Spine Stabilization

Essential to the rehabilitation of all of the above injuries in basketball is stabilization of the spine musculature to protect the underlying injured or damaged areas. Both muscle strength and endurance of spinal musculature are essential for the back to withstand the multiple forces applied to it in basketball. Muscular strength, or maximal tension or force that can be generated by a muscle or group of muscles, is important statically (the ability to exert maximal force for an extended period of time), dynamically (the ability to repeatedly create forces to move or support a portion of the body weight for an extended period of time), and for explosive movements (the ability to exert a maximal, short burst of force).[6] Muscle endurance, or the ability of a group of muscles to work at less than maximal level for an extended period of time,[10] is important because of the continuous, aerobic nature of basketball.

Strength ratios for spinal extensor/flexor muscles very greatly.[2] The most commonly cited ratio is 1.3:1, indicating that the trunk extensors are 30% stronger than the flexors.[6] The generally accepted ratio for lateral flexion and rotation is 1:1.[6] The purpose of strengthening back musculature to approximate these ratios is to provide stability to the trunk and pelvis for the numerous rotational forces applied to the back during basketball. Specifics of spine rehabilitation programs are described elsewhere in this text. Similar stabilization programs are essential postop-

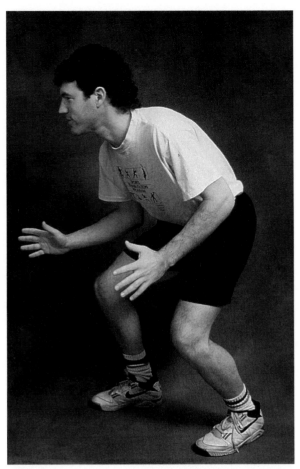

Fig. 44-4

The flex-forward posture of a player in a defensive position.

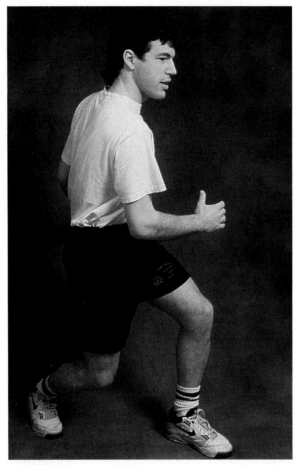

Fig. 44-5

A player in a defensive position starting to rotate at his spine to follow another player.

operatively to the athlete who has had spine surgery and wishes to return to playing basketball.

Some specific training issues need to be addressed in the spinal rehabilitation of basketball players. Because the sport entails many activities that may stress the spinal structures, such as sudden flexion or extension combined with rotation, specific playing techniques in spine-safe positions need to be stressed. Initially, evaluation of current playing technique needs to be addressed, including spine position when assuming a defensive position, identifying trouble spots of stance and movement, and determining spine-safe solutions to them. The new spine-safe movements of play are performed first in a controlled slow motion, then gradually increased to full speed as the new patterns become automatic.[3]

Two common problem areas in basketball are flexing forward in a defensive position and rotation of the back when turning side to side to cut toward the basket or follow another player defensively. (Figs. 44-4 and 44-5). Increased lumbar flexion can cause

increased stress on the anulus fibrosis and intervertebral disc. Repetitive flexion produces injuries over time that are progressively degenerative. Therefore, the less flexion a player places on this back, the more he protects his spine from recurrent stresses that produce these injuries.[3] Rotational injuries can cause posterior element dysfunctions as well as disc or nerve injury. The less a player rotates his back, the more he protects his spine from both acute injury and the recurrent stresses that produce spinal degeneration. Examples of more spine-safe positions are shown in Figs. 44-6 and 44-7.

Progression of any rehabilitation program for the spine in basketball players will require initial emphasis on performance patterns in slow motion to ensure that engrams are set with correct posture, positioning, and balance. Drills are then performed at increased speed and multiple repetitions to ensure that spine-safe activities can be maintained over time to avoid fatigue and regression to improper patterns and positions. Playing techniques need to be per-

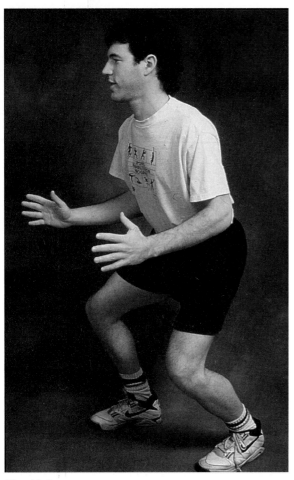

Fig. 44-6

A more spine-neutral position of a player in a defensive position with more of an upright posture and less flexion.

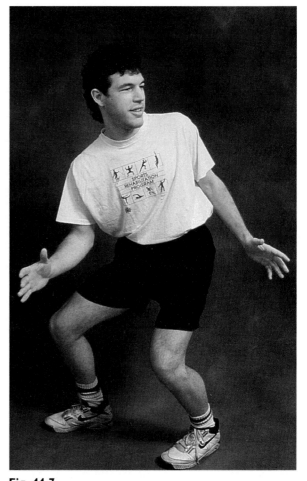

Fig. 44-7

A player moving in a defensive position and rotating at the ankles and knees to decrease some of the torque across the lumbar spine when changing directions and running.

fected so that they are automatic regardless of what stresses are applied suddenly to the player. Elements of surprise should be added after the motions are well engrained and proper strength and endurance have been obtained. An example may be doing sudden changes in direction drills while in a defensive posture.

Two examples of postoperative spine rehabilitation programs undertaken by two professional basketball players are outlined below.

Spine Stabilization Exercise Programs

Example 1: Player A is a 31-year-old NBA guard with the diagnosis of herniated lumbar disc at L4-L5. He underwent a lumbarlaminectomy at single

level in 1991. On day one postoperatively, the patient was walking short distances, increasing as tolerated. A progressive back stabilization program was initiated within the first few days postoperatively with emphasis on a neutral spine. He had been instructed preoperatively in the basics of spine stabilization and had undergone a rehabilitation program. Over the first 4 to 6 weeks, he progressed from a walk to a walk-run, ultimately reaching a 25-minute run at 7 miles per hour. No resistive extension of flexion activities were permitted until week 12. Back stabilization exercises were continued all along. After 12 weeks, trunk, shoulder, and hip stabilization exercises were added, always keeping the spine in neutral position. At 10 weeks postoperatively, the patient started with basketball activities after 30 to 40 minutes of exercise. These activities included dribbling, shooting, passing, and defensive foot work. There was very little rotation to the lumbar spine permitted. Aerobic and anaerobic conditioning were advanced. Progressive sport-specific activities were added that included flexion and extension of the lumber spine. Progressive resistance exercises were also increased. Advancement to 1:1, 2:2, 2:1, 3:2, 3:3, and 5:5 drills were initiated at 10 weeks postoperatively. The patient returned to competitive basketball at 13 weeks and played without symptoms for the rest of the year.

Example 2: Player B is a 26-year-old NBA guard who had an L5-S1 herniated disc with a large extruded fragment and S1 radiculopathy. He underwent a hemilaminotomy at L5-S1 level. He started walking regularly from postoperative day one. He was instructed to avoid sitting and driving for the first six weeks postoperatively and to avoid increased loading of the intervertebral disc. He was also instructed to do partial squats against the wall each day, and toe raises to maintain tone in the calf and quadriceps muscles. During the initial 4 weeks postoperatively, his walking increased to a brisk pace at 5 to 6 miles per day. At week six, he began progressive strengthening of the spine in the spine-neutral position. He also started a full stretching program, which was done daily, as well as soft-tissue mobilization techniques over the scar area. Selective modalities were used to prevent or alleviate any soreness from workouts. He also started working a Nautilus program. No over head weight lifting was permitted for the first two weeks of wight training. Aerobic exercise included the treadmill, exercise bike, and progressive walking on an incline from walk-jog to jog to jog-run to running at a 7.5 to 8 minute mile pace for 1.5 to 2 miles. All activities were done stressing the neutral spine position. Flexion and extension activities were started without resistance at 10 weeks. Flexion and extension activities with resistance were started at 12 weeks. From weeks 12 to 16 training consisted of intense aerobic and anaerobic programs, resistance training for the back musculature, and sport-specific basketball activities, including 1:1, 2:1, 2:2, 3:2, 3:3, and 5:5 drills. The patient returned to full activity at 16 weeks with excellent flexibility, strength, and endurance. He has continued playing professional basketball for the past 4 years, achieved All-Star status, and has had no recurrent low-back problems.

Criteria for Return to Play After Back Injury/Surgery

Return to playing basketball after spine injuries is predicated on a number of factors, including which structure was injured, the severity of the injury, what level of competition the athlete will be performing, what associated injuries have occurred, how complete the rehabilitation program has been, and what specific goals the patient has for further participation. Criteria for return to play in basketball should include resolution of pain symptoms, muscle spasms, and neurologic signs and symptoms, and normal strength and stability.[14] The patient should also have a maintenance program established to prevent further injury. Activities are typically upgraded incrementally starting with running, dribbling, and cutting with progression to jumping and shooting drills. Participation in practice sessions should start with only half-court maneuvers and proceed to full-court activities. Similarly, the player should move form limited playing time, gradually increasing to full activity.[14] Return to playing basketball after back surgery may take four to six months with proper rehabilitation. The two described cases show the potential for return to playing basketball, at its highest level, with well-defined surgery and aggressive focused rehabilitation. Return to playing basketball after a spinal fusion, in particular, is controversial.[12] The most significant concerns regard the possibility of accelerated disc degeneration of unfused segments adjacent to a successful fusion.

References

1. Apple DF, O'Toole J, Annis C: Professional basketball injuries, *Phys Sports Med* 10(1): 81, 1982.
2. Beimbaum DS, Morrissey MC: A review of the literature related to trunk muscle performance, *Spine* 13(6):655, 1958.
3. Cook T: The professional athlete, in *Spine: State Art Rev, Back School* 5(3):411, 1991.
4. Flemming JE: Spondylolysis and spondylolisthesis in the athlete, *Spine: State Art Rev* 4(2):339, 1990.
5. Frymoyer, JW, Gordon SL, editors: *New perspectives in low back pain*, American Academy of Orthopedic Surgeons Symposium, Chicago, 1988.
6. Glisan B, Hochschuler SH: General fitness in the treatment of prevention of athletic low back injuries, *Spine: State art rev* 4(2):287, 1990.
7. Henry JH, Lauear B, Neigut D: The injury rate in professional basketball, *Am J Sports Med* 10:16, 1982.
8. Micheli LJ, Hall JE, Miller ME: Use of modified Boston brace for back injuries in athletes, *Am J Sports Med* 8:351, 1980.
9. Moritz A, Grana WA: High school basketball injuries, *Phys Sports Med* 6:91, 1978.
10. Rasch PJ, Burke RK: *Kinesiology and applied anatomy: the science of human movement*, 1978.
11. Saal JA: Intervertebral disc herniation: advances in nonoperative treatment, *Phys Med Rehab: State Art Rev.* 4(2):175, 1990.
12. Shelokov, AP, Herring JA: Spinal deformities and participation in sports, *Spine: State Art Rev* 4(2):333, 1990.
13. Stith WJ: Exercise and the intervertebral disc, *Spine: State Art Rev* 4(2):259, 1990.
14. Yost JG Jr, Elfieldt HJ: *Basketball injuries*. In Nicholas JA, Herschman EB, editors: *The lower extremity and spine in sports*, St. Louis, 1986, Mosby.
15. Zelisko JA, Noble HB, Porter M: A comparison of men's and women's professional basketball injuries, *Am J Sports Med* 10:297, 1982.

Chapter 45
Bicycling
Michael J. Martin

The number of bicycles sold in the United States has increased tenfold since 1980,[5] and sales are expected to increase for some time. The reasons for the popularity of bicycling are many: the bike may be used as transportation or recreation by people of all ages; bicycling provides low-impact aerobic conditioning while strengthening the largest muscle groups in the body; and low-impact aerobic exercise is an ideal form of therapy, especially for patients with musculoskeletal problems that become symptomatic when engaged in high- or moderate-impact movement.

Back Pain and Bicycling

Back pain and bicycling may be related on two levels: (1) bicycling is regarded as a cause of back pain and pathology, and (2) bicycling assumes the role of rehabilitation for the patient with spinal pathology. No scientific data exist in the referenced medical literature pertaining to either subject. A few articles, nonscientific in their presentation and conclusions, exist in lay literature regarding back pain and its prevention in recreational bike riders.[3, 4, 11] Books devoted to the sport of racing and training mention back pain only briefly as a complication of improperly fitted componentry.[6, 10, 14] Back pain is commonly recognized in professional racing teams, usually attributed to ill-fitting equipment and inadequate training. This information exists primarily as "word of mouth" information in coaching and training circles.[5] Unfortunately, nothing is referenced in medical literature that addresses the incidence and prevalence of back pain in recreational or professional cyclists. In spite of being a frequently prescribed therapeutic modality by physicians and therapists, little data exist pertaining to the effect of bicycling on patients with lumbar pathology. The information available in the nonmedical literature deals primary with training, strengthening, stretching, and proper bike fit.

Pathology other than that found in the back can be responsible for similar symptomatology. Other conditions that are more common in cyclists that should be included in the differential diagnosis include ischial, trochanteric, and obturator bursitis; piriformis syndrome; pudendal nerve compression; prostatism; saddle sores; and inflammation of a pilonidal cyst.

Bicycle Design

A wide variety of bicycles are in use today. They include racing bikes, touring bikes, mountain bikes, "hybrid" bikes, tandems (bicycles built for two), motocross bikes, stationary bikes, recliners where the rider is positioned in a semirecumbent position, and other rare, custom or antique bikes. The majority can be classified into two groups based on the basic type of frame. First, racing and touring frames look like the bike frames we grew up with. Some technical variations exist between the two. Tandems are based on the traditional frame style of the racing and touring frames with modifications to increase strength and rigidity. The second type of frame is the mountain bike style, which is generally constructed to be smaller and better able to tolerate stresses and bumps than its on-road brethren. The division between the two types is not based solely on frame geometry but also on rider position in the saddle. Racing and touring frames, referred to as road frames here, have downward curved handle bars that necessitate a position of forward flexion of the lumbar spine and extension of the cervical spine (Fig. 45-1). Tandems usually are fitted with these types of handle bars as well. Mountain bikes have straight handle bars that require forward bend to a lesser degree than those above (Fig. 45-2). "Hybrids" and stationary "gym" bikes combine a road bike–type geometry frame with straight handle bars enabling a more upright posture for the rider, similar to the mountain bike posture. These positions represent both ends of the spectrum regarding body position in the saddle. Actually, the rider's position changes frequently during a ride, from extreme forward flex-

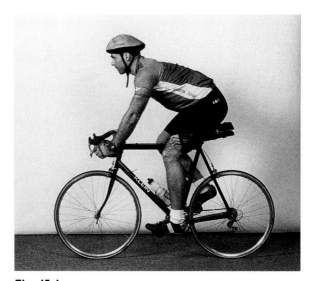

Fig. 45-1

Rider on road bike. Note the flexed lumbar spine and extended cervical spine. The thoracic and lumbar spines are flattened out. This "flat back" is a good position to prevent low-back discomfort and increase power output.

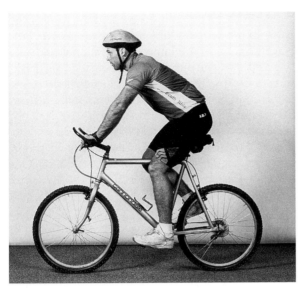

Fig. 45-2

Rider positioning on mountain bike. When compared with the position on the road bike, the rider is more upright. There is less flexion of the lumbar spine, while the back remains "flat."

ion to decrease wind resistance, to a more upright posture while climbing. Frequent position changes also decrease the incidence of muscle strain and overuse. Both road and mountain bikers will find themselves in these two positions, as well as all those in between, during the course of a ride.

Anatomy and Pathophysiology of Bicycling

The flexed position of the lumbar spine has several physiologic consequences. While the upright posture of human beings exposes the spine to stresses not seen elsewhere in nature, the spine is more adapted to a vertical posture than a horizontal one. As the rider's position becomes more aerodynamic, the spine becomes more horizontal. The paraspinal musculature, the musculature arising or inserting into the dorsolumbar fascia, and the abdominal wall musculature must provide the stability that the vertical position normally furnishes. For the paraspinal musculature, this is an eccentric muscle contracture, contrasting with its usual concentric type of contraction. The added stress of the position and the increased metabolic demand lead to muscle fatigue and pain. As the muscles fatigue, they become less able to maintain the more horizontal position. A return to the more vertical position may alleviate the pain and fatigue to some degree.

In addition to maintaining the spine in a more horizontal position, the back and its musculature must provide a stable "platform" from which the legs are able to supply prolonged power to the pedals. A pelvis that rotates laterally in the saddle quickly becomes uncomfortable where it contacts the saddle. It is also an inefficient way to pedal as the power is transmitted up to the lumbar spine instead of down to the pedals. As the muscles fatigue and weaken, the pelvis rotates laterally to an excessive degree and the ability of the legs to transmit force to the pedals is decreased. Without a stable platform, motion of the pelvis increases, as does the likelihood of soft-tissue injury. It is important to stabilize the pelvis to make the power output of the legs more efficient and to decrease the incidence of soft-tissue injury to the lumbar spine. As experience in patients with degenerative lumbar diseases has taught us, lumbosacral and pelvic stability are dependent on contributions from the abdominal wall musculature as well as from the paraspinal musculature, psoas/quadratutus lumborum complex, and pelvic girdle musculature. The rectus abdominus group and the obliques contribute significantly to pelvic stability.[2] Fatigue of the abdominal wall musculature also contributes to decreased pelvic stability.

As the lumbar spine moves into flexion, its normal lordosis is lost. Figs. 45-1 and 45-2 show the spine to be flat or even kyphotic. Normal flexion takes place to the greatest degree at the upper levels of the lumbar spine, with progressively smaller degrees caudally so that no flexion occurs at L5-S1. Flexion is achieved at each level by a combination of sagittal rotation and sagittal translation of each vertebral body on its inferior neighbor. As the spine becomes more horizontal, the end plates move toward the vertical, and sagittal translation is increased until an end point is reached; the inferior articular process contacts the superior articular facet of the level below. This forward translation is accompanied by sagittal rotation. Compression of the anterior aspects of the disc space and a distraction of the posterior disc elements occur. The facet joints are even further from the axis of rotation of the motion segment and move even more. The facet joint may slide 5 to 7 mm in the course of normal flexion.[7] This distraction of the facet joints results in an increase of the volume and cross-sectional area of the intervertebral foramina.

If the facet joints are flat and oriented at 90 degrees to the sagittal plane, an even distribution of forces is seen by the articular surfaces. If the joint surfaces are curved, the majority of the resistance to sagittal translation is provided by the medial aspect of the articular facets. As has been demonstrated, the degenerative changes of the facet joints begin in the medial third,[12] prolonged positioning in flexion may be expected to increase the rate and/or severity of these changes. The resistance to sagittal translation is primarily bony, as outlined above. The resistance to sagittal rotation is provided by a number of structures; the exact contribution of each one is somewhat controversial. Both mathematic models and serial sectioning studies in cadavers have been performed to assess the contributions of each structure.[1, 13] While the sectioning studies give an idea of the individual contribution of each ligament, the more probable conclusion is that the various structures act in unison. Mathematic analyses have estimated that the capsules of the facet joints provide 39% of the resistance to sagittal rotation, while the disc contributes 29%, the supraspinous and interspinous ligaments 19%, and the ligamentum flavum 13%.[1] These ligaments and the muscle/tendon units that cross the motion segment are placed in prolonged tension. While the stresses placed across these structures may be well below their fatigue limit, the repetitive submaximal stresses may result in fatigue failure of portions of each or selected structures. Any of these injured structures could then present clinically with posterior primary ramus-type pain that may take longer to resolve than the customary discomfort associated with muscle fatigue and prolonged positioning. Diagnosis may be made by a history of low-back or buttock pain that persists for hours or days after a ride. The pain is usually provoked by flexion or stretching of the injured area. There is usually tenderness over the interspace or facet joints. Treatment is directed at resting the area by avoiding the flexed position, applying ice, and taking non-steroidal antiinflammatory drugs (NSAIDs), as necessary, and strengthening the paraspinal musculature. Hyperextension exercises, in conjunction with a stabilization program, usually provide significant relief. The fit between the bike and rider should also be evaluated to ensure that improper positioning is not the source of the problem. The symptoms usually resolve within a few weeks with an aggressive strengthening program. Riding can usually be continued after a short period of rest.

The posterior aspect of the annulus is placed in tension as the spine is flexed. The tension is further increased by the increasingly posteriorly directed pressure exerted by the nucleus pulposus. The posterior anulus may be damaged by repetitive microtrauma, as outlined above. If the anulus is already incompetent or damaged, flexion of the spine may force nuclear material into the anular defect resulting in further incompetence and/or pain as the outer layers of the anulus become stretched. Prolonged flexion of the lumbar spine should probably be avoided in patients with symptomatic disc herniation and those less than six weeks postdiscectomy, as this position may force other loose nuclear material into the spinal canal. Patients with spinal stenosis, especially those with foraminal stenosis, may be expected to be free of their claudication symptoms as the area in the spinal canal and neuroforamina increases in the flexed position on the bicycle. Whether painful facet syndrome would be relieved or exacerbated by the flexed portion is unclear. While the flexed position would eliminate the weight-bearing function of the facets, this could be offset by their contribution to stabilizing sagittal translation. Asymptomatic spondylolysis and spondylolisthesis should remain so with proper rider/bike interface and conditioning.

The Proper Fit of Bike to Rider

An improperly fitted bike can lead to rapid muscle fatigue, overuse, and potential injury. Proper fitting of the rider to the bike can be complicated. Even when performed by a professional, considerable controversy exists as to the exact positioning of the components. For professional racers, a change of even a few millimeters may make the difference between a successful season and a debilitating injury.[6] The distance from pedal axle to the saddle, the distance of the saddle from the head tube, the elevation of the saddle above the handle bar stem, and angle of the saddle with the horizontal all affect the rider's position and therefore affect the incidence of back pain.

The first step in finding the proper bike fit is to select a bike with the correct frame size. A general rule of thumb is to multiply one's inseam, in inches or centimeters, by 0.65; this number is the frame size in inches or centimeters. If the rider is normally proportioned, the rest of the measurements of the bike should be appropriate. If the number falls between available sizes, it is best to pick a smaller frame. A smaller frame is lighter and stiffer than a larger frame and therefore more efficient to pedal. The bike with the smaller frame can be adjusted to the proper fit by altering saddle height, handle bar stem height, and length, as will be explained later.

A considerable amount of controversy surrounds calculating the correct saddle height,[6, 10] and it will not be addressed here. The inseam measurement multiplied by 0.883 should approximate the distance from the center of the bottom bracket (where the crank arms attach) to the top of the saddle. This is probably the most important measurement. A saddle position that is too high will result in lateral rocking of the pelvis and inefficient use of leg power. A position too low is also inefficient for the legs and can result in faster muscle fatigue or injury for the stabilizers of the pelvis.

The foot should be positioned on the pedal so the metatarsal heads are directly over the axle. If a noncleated shoe is worn, the toe clip cage should be adjusted to prevent the foot from moving too anteriorly. A cleated shoe or a clipless pedal system should be carefully adjusted, with the metatarsal heads over the pedal axle. The long axis of the foot should be parallel to the long axis of the bike. Excessive in-toeing or out-toeing may result in knee pain or injury.

Determination of the fore and aft positions of the saddle requires one or two assistants and a plumb line. With the rider in the saddle and the pedals at the 9 and 3 o'clock positions, one assistant holds the rider and bike while the second drops a plumb line from the tibial tubercle. The plumb line should fall somewhere between the axle of the pedal and 2 cm behind it. The exact position in this range is variable and depends on the type of riding to be done. Changes are made by moving the saddle forward or backward. A position that is too far forward results in increased flexion of the lumbar spine with a cramped look and feel in the saddle. A position that is excessively to the rear leads to increased hip flexion, anterior pelvic tilt, and the always unpleasant pudendal nerve paresthesias.

The length of the handle bar stem determines the distance the handle bars are from the rider. The stem length is not the portion that rises vertically from the head set but the piece that extends out at an acute angle to the head set. The length is variable, while height is less so. The measurement of handle bar position is much less scientific and depends to some degree on rider comfort. A rule of thumb is that while sitting on the bike with hands on the brake hoods, the handle bar should obscure the front axle. In addition to affecting the handling of the bike, a position too far in either direction will have consequences similar to those of a malpositioned saddle. Selecting the proper height of the stem is a balance of comfort and aerodynamics. Higher is more comfortable but causes increased drag; the converse is also true.

Most good bicycle shops have people skilled in fitting the bike to the rider. Several "fit kits," which provide a more scientific and reproducible fit, are also available on the market. Most books[6, 10, 14] on bicycle racing offer advice and insights into the controversies regarding fit. Approximately 97% of back pain in recreational cyclists can be linked to improper interface between the rider and bike and muscle fatigue/overuse.[11] Improper fit can be remedied with the assistance of a knowledgeable bike shop or with a commercially available "fit kit."

Conditioning and Training

Books devoted to racing and training as well as numerous periodicals deal with training concepts and strategies to prevent overuse injuries in the back.* Proper conditioning and training should decrease the incidence and severity of muscle fatigue and pain. In recreational riders, a program of lumbosacral stabilization exercises may help to provide a stable platform from which the legs can power the pedals. Improving the strength and endurance of all muscle groups that transverse the lumbosacral area to the pelvis and proximal femora is important. In the abdominal wall, the recti and obliques should be strengthened with isometric and isotonic exercises. Similarly, the quadratus lumborum/psoas groups should also be strengthened. Posteriorly, the paraspinals respond well to isometric and hyperextension exercises. Elite racers and endurance bikers generally are so strong about the hips and buttocks that generalized exercises aimed at stabilization do not adequately stress the less well-fit muscle groups in the abdominal wall. Each muscle group requires specific, isolated work so that its stronger neighbors do not protect them by virtue of increased strength and endurance. In short, a proportionally strengthened trunk, proper fit between the rider and bike, and an intelligent training schedule should eliminate most complaints of back pain.

It is essential that flexibility not be overlooked. Tight hamstrings and dorsolumbar fascia and musculature can all contribute to malposition in the saddle and muscle fatigue and pain. Stretching should be performed as part of the usual training regimen. Flexibility and stretching in the saddle are as important as stretches performed off the bike. A bike race or endurance ride may require the cyclist to spend 4 to 12 hours in the saddle. In ultraendurance events, like the Ride Across America, the riders may spend 20 hours in the saddle each day. Prolonged positioning of this duration can result in cramping, fatigue, and loss of muscle compliance, as well as joint stiffness. Stretching exercises for the back, shoulders, neck, arms, and legs are necessary to ensure comfortable and efficient cycling. Stretching restores the normal muscle fiber length, increases

* References 3, 4, 6, 10, 11, and 14.

blood supply to the stretched muscles, and helps maintain joint range of motion. It also provides a few seconds' rest. For rides shorter than 2 hours' duration, in-saddle stretching is usually not necessary. For rides longer than 2 hours, stretches may be performed every 20 to 30 minutes.[4] Cold weather has been demonstrated to contribute to decreased muscle and tendon compliance. If riding in cooler climates, proper insulation of the back will decrease the likelihood of overuse injury.

Summary

In short, bicycling is a safe, low-impact form of aerobic conditioning whether ridden for pleasure, transportation, exercise, or all three. The vast majority of all back symptomatology can be traced to improper bike fit, conditioning, or training regimen and, therefore, can be remedied relatively easily.

References

1. Adams MA, Hutton WC, Scott JRR: The resistance to flexion of the lumbar intervertebral joint, *Spine* 5:245, 1980.

2. Bogduk N, Twomey LT: *Clinical anatomy of the lumbar spine,* ed. 2, 1991, Churchill-Livingstone.

3. Bragman A: 10 common fitness questions answered, *Bicycling* 5:50, 1991.

4. Burke ER, Anderson B: Fast and loose, *Bicycling* 7:80, 1992.

5. Gorski M: Personal communication, Feb. 1994.

6. LeMond G, Gordis K: *Greg LeMond's complete book of bicycling,* 1987, Perigee.

7. Lewin T, Moffet B, Viidik A: The morphology of the lumbar synovial intervertebral joints, *Acta Morphol Neerlando-Scand* 4:299, 1962.

8. Macnab I, McCulloch J: *Backache,* ed. 2, 1990, Williams and Wilkins.

9. Pearcy M, Portek I, Shepard J: Three-dimentional x-ray analysis of normal movement in the lumbar spine, *Spine* 9:294, 1984.

10. Phinney D, Carpenter C, Nye P: *Training for cycling,* 1992,

11. Strickland B: Backs in the saddle, *Bicycling* 6:85, 1992.

12. Taylor JR, Twomey LT: Age changes in lumbar zygapophyseal joints, *Spine* 11:739, 1986.

13. Twomey LT, Taylor JR: Sagittal movements of the human lumbar vertebral column: a quantitative study of the role of the posterior vertebral elements, *Arch Phys Med Rehab* 64:322, 1983.

14. van der Plas R: *The bicycle touring manual,* 1993, Perigee.

15. White AA, Panjabi MM: *Clinical biomechanics of the spine,* ed 2, 1990, Lippincott.

Chapter 46
Dance
Richard D. Gibbs
Patricia H. Gibbs

Though dance in a variety of forms has been present since antiquity, medical study of the art is a new phenomenon. It was not until the early 1970's that data were collected on the epidemiology and treatment of dance injury. This may, in part, be owing to a reluctance of those involved in the art to interfere with the creative process through the application of science. Since that time, knowledge on the subject has accumulated, thanks to the work of a handful of investigators affiliated with major dance companies and ballet schools. Nevertheless, there is still much to be learned, particularly related to treatment and preventive strategies for dance injury.

A number of different dance forms exist, each with its own specific vulnerabilities and patterns of injury. Ballet, jazz, modern, and ethnic dance make up the majority of such dance forms. Ballet has been the most rigorously studied; thus, much of the information and analysis presented in this chapter deals with this form of dance.

The purpose of this chapter is to present information on spine injury in dancers. Discussion of epidemiology, pathogenesis, diagnosis, and treatment will focus on aspects specific to dance injury.

Epidemiology

There have been several major studies outlining patterns of dance injury. The first, published in 1978, surveyed professional ballet, modern, and jazz dancers on frequency of injury. Also polled were teachers, administrators, and physicians involved in the care of dancers.[16] The dancers themselves indicated that the spine was the most frequently inured body part. Conversely, the physicians, teachers, and administrators indicated that spine injury was only fourth in frequency, suggesting that dancers are aware of spine injuries but are not presenting the injury to teachers or physicians for attention.

Some evidence suggests that spinal injury is increasing in frequency in ballet dancers. In Thomasen's survey of ballet injuries between the years of 1958 and 1980, frequency of spine injury was 14.6%.[14] He also cites statistics from the Bolshoi Ballet, obtained by Volkov between 1965 and 1969, indicating a distribution of injury as follows: foot and ankle 71%, knee 12.2%, "all other" 16.5%. A survey of French ballet dancers from 1975 to 1980 revealed a 25% frequency of spine injury in males, and 20% in females, both ranking first as sites of injury.

The frequency of back injury reported in the French study is similar to our own observations at the San Francisco Ballet during the 1990 to 1991 season. Back injury comprised 24% of all injuries,

Table 46-1
Frequency of injury by body part, San Francisco Ballet, 11/90-5/91

Back	(total)	36	(19%)
	Lumbar spine	18	(9.5%)
	Cervical spine	10	(5%)
	Thoracic spine	8	(4%)
Foot		35	(18.5%)
Ankle		30	(16%)
Knee		19	(10%)
Hip		16	(8%)
Leg		7	(4%)
Other	(shoulder, leg, hand)	10	(5%)
	Total injuries	189	(100%)

making the spine the leading site of injury during that time (Table 46-1). Of interest, spine injury also appeared to be the most severe, with the greatest cost in terms of time lost from active participation in dance. The impression of greater disability due to spinal injury is supported by Micheli, who indicates that dancers in the Boston Ballet would frequently be eliminated from dance participation for months or even the entire season owing to back injury.[10]

A few epidemiologic studies of dancers categorize back injuries by diagnosis. Thomasen indicates that of 134 spine injuries, 36% were due to lumbar disc degeneration, 40% to herniated nucleus pulposus (HNP), 13% to spondylolysis/spondylolisthesis, 7% to cervical disc degeneration, 1% to cervical fracture, and 3% to "miscellaneous."[14] Washington found that of low-back injuries, 82% were a result of "musculoligamentous" injuries, 9% of HNP, 5% of "sciatica," and 4% of "Miscellaneous," including vertebral chip fracture.[16]

Risk Factors for Back Injury in Ballet

There are several biomechanical aspects inherent to ballet that predispose dancers to back injury. Most striking is the external rotation of the hips required of all ballet dancers. Referred to as "turn-out" by dancers, this bilateral 80 to 90 degree external rotation of the hips is the core of ballet technique. External rotation is maintained by the dancer through all training sessions and most dance sequences on the stage. The purpose of turn-out is both functional and artistically aesthetic. for example, the externally rotated leg can initiate movement with great ease in a 360-degree radius around the dancer. Additionally,

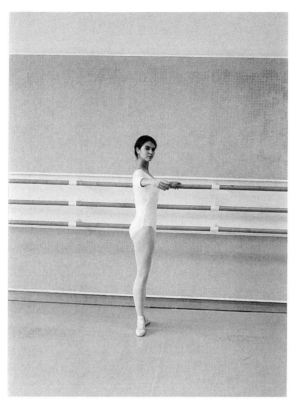

Fig. 46-1

Correct ballet placement. Hips are externally rotated and dancer is using firm abdominal musculature to maintain a neutral spine.

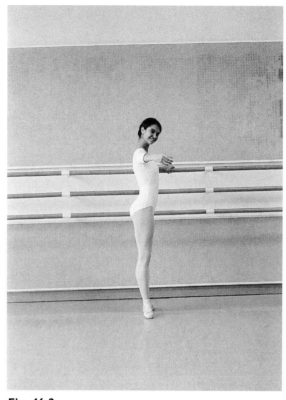

Fig. 46-2

Incorrect ballet placement. In an attempt to take stress off the hip capsule, the dancer has inadvertently tilted the pelvis anteriorly, which relaxes the iliofemoral ligament. The result is a hyperextension of the lumbar spine and nonengaged abdominal muscles.

turn-out allows the dancer to raise the leg higher (called "extension" by the dancer), because the externally rotated greater trochanter can clear the acetabular rim as the leg is lifted to the front and side. However, turn-out is also aesthetically necessary. An externally rotated leg presents a visually pleasing straight line rather than the bumpy contours of the knee and ankle that are seen when the leg is viewed in the anatomic position.

Foremost among the problems associated with turn-out is an incorrect compensatory hyperextension of the lumbar spine. The endeavor of turn-out is stressful enough to cause many students and dancers to incorrectly tilt the pelvis forward when the hips are externally rotated. In this way, the iliofemoral ligament is slightly relaxed and the dancer feels less strain in the hip capsule (Figs. 46-1 and 46-2). The result is a hyperextended lumbar spine with the associated effect of releasing the abdominal musculature to allow the low spine to extend. The dancer is left standing, moving, and lifting in a more weakened biomechanical alignment with excessive lumbar motion due to relaxed abdominal muscles.

The potential for lumbar injury can be imagined when considering the distribution of force as the dancer lands from a jump. In the hyperextended low back, the point of axial impact becomes the site of maximal posterior angulation in the lumbar spine. Each landing from a jump is associated with excessive axial loading rather than a distribution of force down a neutral spine and pelvis into the lower extremities, where quadriceps and hamstring muscles can share in the absorption of force. In the average ballet class, the dancer is required to perform at least 160 small jumps and 100 large jumps. Given that the advanced balled student takes two such classes a day, and that dancers usually work 6 days a week, this amounts to nearly 150,000 landings in each year of dancing. The cumulative stress on the low back, and resultant potential for injury in those dancers who hyperextend the lumbar spine, is plain to see.

A second biomechanical aspect of ballet that increases the risk of low-back injury is the arabesque position. This very common step is required of both men and women and involves standing on one leg while the other is extended posteriorly to a level of

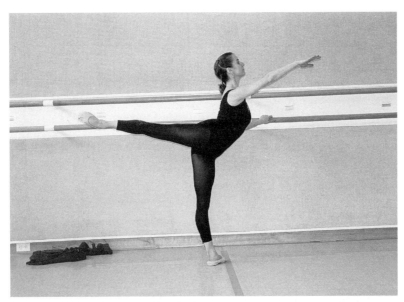

Fig. 46-3

The arabesque position.

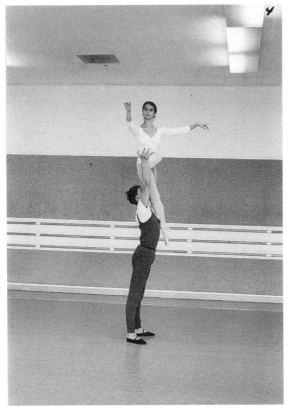

Fig. 46-4

A typical overhead lift. Note that the male has incorrectly allowed the lumbar spine to hyperextend.

at least 90 degrees while the back is maintained upright (Fig. 46-3). The position must be maintained for long periods of time in the slow work called adagio, and is also commonly used as a landing position in very forceful large jumps. Even in the most well-trained dancer who pays immaculate attention to good biomechanical alignment, there is a necessary forward tilting of the pelvis when the leg is raised to the required height. Again, the dancer is in a position of lumbar hyperextension with an undue load placed on the low spine.

Lifting is another element of the work that is risky for the low back. It is expected that male dancers be able to lift and then move gracefully with a female held overhead in various positions. In spite of adhering to techniques such as "lifting with the legs," and "getting your axis under the woman before the lift," the male dancer is clearly at risk for injury. Men are often observed setting the woman too far behind them while holding her overhead and then counterbalancing by hyperextending the lumbar spine (Fig. 46-4).

Lastly, the development of modern and jazz dance has made dancing somewhat more precarious in terms of injury. Even in classical ballet companies, the dancers are required to train and perform in these more modern styles. Although the movement in classical ballet is usually well-placed and symmetric, the Afro-Caribbean elements in jazz and modern dance require much off-balance work and forceful torquing of the upper body. The pelvis is often purposefully

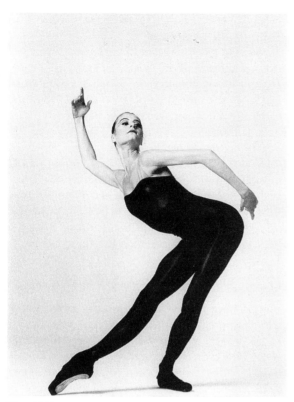

Fig. 46-5
Muriel Maffre of the San Francisco Ballet in a pose from the modern ballet repertory.

released to give a disjointed and modernistic look (Fig. 46-5).

No easy remedy exists for hyperextension of the lumbar spine in dance. By the time most dancers present with low-back injury, they have already trained for several years and find it difficult to change a body alignment they have worked with for so long. Thus, attempts to correct the forward pelvic tilt that results from the stress of turn-out is a difficult task. Also, steps that exacerbate lumbar hyperextension, such as arabesque, are a required and unchangeable part of the endeavor, as is the need for the dancer of today to do the disjointed and forceful work of jazz and modern dance.

These problems are compounded by the fact that dancers accept pain and disability as a normal part of their day. As a group, dancers are deeply devoted to their art form, and their determination to avoid missing work at all costs often keeps them from presenting with injury until the disability is severe. Studies on students and professionals show that up to 50% are working at any given time with injuries that restrict them.[4,12]

Specific Back Injuries in Dancers: Diagnosis and Treatment

Low-Back Strain

By far the most frequent back injury in multiple reports on dancers is acute low-back strain. This diagnosis implies low-back pain without neurologic signs or symptoms, occurring in the absence of specific radiologic findings. The diagnosis, of course, is inaccurate and includes injury to muscular, tendinous, and ligamentous structures in addition to facet injuries, degenerative disc disease, and probably mild cases of HNP and spondylolysis.

Despite the aforementioned difficulties in treating dancers, much can be done to prevent and treat the high incidence of this most common back injury. An emphasis can be placed on appropriate biomechanical alignment where possible. Good ballet teachers are eager to reduce injury and are usually willing to work with a physician in reinforcing to dancers the need to maintain a neutral spine and prevent lumbar hyperextension except where required by the assigned choreography. This alignment should be maintained not only when the dancer is standing, but throughout all movement and when lifting. Such factors as not forcing maximal turn-out of the hips too early in the training process and adequate stretching of the hip capsule are also important.

In our rehabilitation program at the San Francisco Ballet, the treatment of injury is three-tiered. First, the injury is assessed by the company physicians with the physical therapist present. It is important at this early stage to determine which dance movements may have caused the injury and what aspects of the individual dancer's technique may be exacerbating the injury. Because of the very specific requirements in the technique of classical ballet, our goal is to make the rehabilitation as ballet-specific as possible in addition to correcting any training errors in the dancer. In our program we have the advantage of having former professional dancers on the medical staff. Where this is not possible, assessing the injury with a ballet teacher present will help elicit any problems in the dancer's technique.

Second, the dancer is assigned to a physical therapist with a plan of treatment designed to be carried out using hip turn-out and a well-aligned, neutral lumbar spine. For example, one exercise to strengthen the abdominal musculature, including the obliques and hip extensors, uses the gym ball; the supine dancer externally rotates the hips and lifts the pelvis into proper alignment while balancing the turned-out feet on the ball. In addition to these therapeutic exercises, the physical therapist uses other techniques such as myofascial mobilization and proprioceptive neuromuscular facilitation.

The third tier of our rehabilitation program is an actual ballet class for the injured dancers that precedes their return to the normal company class. Here we maintain the exact format of a traditional ballet class, but the exercises (called "combinations" in ballet jargon) are tailored to the specific injury and to correcting any associated weakness in the dancer's technique. In the case of lumbar strain, the combinations that accentuate hyperlordosis of the lumbar spine, such as arabesque, are initially eliminated from the class. However, the ballet combinations that emphasize lower abdominal strength are done slowly and repeatedly. For example, the ballet steps that are called "tendu," "degage," "developpe," and "grand battement," when done to the front, are all variations of forward flexing the hip in a turned-out position while firmly maintaining the lower abdominal musculature. When done slowly and often, the dancer not only builds muscular strength but facilitates a disciplined recruitment of the appropriate musculature in the abdomen and leg.

At the same time, the standard ballet exercises that promote stretching of the lumbodorsal fascia and the hamstrings are done frequently. The combinations of grand port des bras with cambre (end-range flexion and extension at the waist while standing fully turned out at the hip) are repeated slowly while extra care is given to maintaining a neutral spine.

Because ballet is an art form, all the combinations in the rehabilitation ballet class are done to music. As in any proper ballet class, great emphasis is given to musicality, fluidity of movement, and exactness of movement.

In refractory cases of lumbar strain among San Francisco Ballet dancers, trigger-point and facet injections have been used with success. Micheli also suggests use of a spinal antilordotic device for rest and treatment of refractory low-back pain in dancers.[10]

Herniated Nucleus Pulposus

As in the general population, HNP is a less common cause of low-back pain in dancers than acute low-back strain. There are only scattered case reports describing medical care of dancers with this disorder. Micheli favors a conservative approach involving rest, use of an antilordotic brace, abstinence from lifting in male dancers, and physical therapy.[10] In the event that a concerted effort at conservative care is unsuccessful, surgery may be considered with the dancer's understanding that return to participation in dance is not guaranteed.

Thomasen cites 53 cases of HNP in dancers, six of whom underwent an unspecified surgical procedure, and all of whom were pain-free and able to dance again at an unstated postop interval.[14] On the other hand, Ende and Wickstrom describe the case of one dancer with HNP requiring surgery who has not returned to his profession.[7]

Two cases of lumbar HNP, documented by MRI scan, occurred during our 6-month study of the San Francisco Ballet. After 4 to 6 weeks of conservative treatment involving rest from ballet and intensive physical therapy, both individuals returned to full participation as principal dancers in the company.

Spondylolysis/Spondylolisthesis

Some evidence is present that lumbar spondylolysis occurs with greater frequency among ballet dancers than the general population, at a relative frequency of 4:1.[3] However, dance appears to have a relatively low risk for this disorder when compared with other athletic endeavors. For example, the incidence of spondylolysis in dancers is estimated at 11% to 20%,[10, 3] in swimmers at 23.7%, football linemen at 24%, and javelin throwers at 40% to 47.4%.[3] Nevertheless, one must maintain a high index of suspicion for this disorder among dancers.

The defect of the pars interarticularis is believed by most to represent a stress fracture due to the repetitive flexion, extension, and rotation required in dance.[15] Factors that may particularly predispose the female dancer to spondylolysis include amenorrhea and an associated decrease in bone density,[6] in addition to inadequate nutritional habits and eating disorders leading to poor bone health. Other factors associated with spondylolysis include family history of the disorder, ethnic background, and presence of spina bifida occulta.[13]

Diagnostic clues to the presence of spondylolysis in the dancer include complaints of pain occurring in spine extension, particularly positions such as arabesque (Fig. 46-3). If a dancer's low-back pain is unresponsive to an initial course of conservative care, a bone scan should be obtained. Plain films may be negative, but can help delineate the chronicity and location of the lesion and determine whether there is an associated spondylolisthesis.

Some controversy exists concerning appropriate treatment of acute and chronic spondylolysis in dancers. Micheli recommends treatment of acute pars defects through reduction and immobilization in a modified Boston brace until symptoms resolve.[10]

An attempt may be made at treatment of chronic spondylolysis/spondylolisthesis in a similar manner. Other authors have used strategies ranging from plaster immobilization[8] to simple abstinence from aggravating factors.[5] Most authors agree that chronic, refractory spondylolytic or spondylolisthetic defects must eventually be treated through spinal fusion.[8, 10, 14] There has been a report of three dancers who were able to return to full participation in dance 1 year following such a procedure.[10]

Scoliosis

The frequency of scoliosis in a group of professional female ballet dancers was found to be 24%.[15] This compares with a frequency of 3.9% in white female non-dancers. The prevalence of scoliosis in male dancers is unknown. Interestingly, the prevalence appears to be higher among ballerinas with a later onset of menarche or with higher scores on a scale of dieting behavior. This indicates, perhaps, that abnormal hormonal function paired with inadequate nutritional intake may predispose skeletal abnormalities such as scoliosis.

Scoliosis is not a contraindication to dance; however, appropriate treatment of progressive scoliosis may interfere with dance participation, and should not be delayed based on the desire to dance. Some authors are attempting intermittent bracing and/or electrospinal implantation for progressive scoliosis in dancers, with reported initial success.[9] Dancers with scoliosis not requiring surgery or bracing may be able to compensate impressively to allow little noticeable change in their technique.

Neck Strain

Little has been written about neck injury in dancers, and it appears to be of lesser significance than injuries to the lumbar spine. Dance, unlike collision sports, does not often involve cervical trauma. Most of the injuries to this area would be expected to arise from the rotational stress that occurs during "spotting" while performing rapid turns. (Dancers power multiple turns by whipping the head around to the front before each resolution of the torso.) However, head rotation depends primarily on motion between the first and second cervical vertebrae, while most cervical degenerative joint disease (DJD) occurs between the sixth and seventh cervical vertebrae.[11]

Of the 10 cervical spine injuries occurring in the San Francisco Ballet over 6 months, none required more than a few days off, and none involved cervical radiculopathy. All responded to various combinations of physical therapy, gentle manipulation, nonsteroidal antiinflammatory drugs, and cold or heat therapy.

Degenerative Joint Disease

A 1989 study of retired Scandinavian ballet dancers revealed an increased incidence of DJD in the hip, knee, and first metatarsal phalangeal (MTP) joints.[1] Unfortunately, the radiologic survey did not include the spine. Our impression based on spinal radiographs of professional dancers with back pain is that spinal DJD is probably increased relative to an age-matched population. Of five principal dancers aged late 20's to early 30's who obtained radiographs for low-back pain in one elite company, all had evidence of moderate to severe lumbar and/or thoracic DJD. A survey involving larger numbers, including asymptomatic individuals, would be helpful in determining actual prevalence of spinal osteoarthropathy in dancers.

Infections and Neoplasms

It is important to remember that the dance community includes a possibly larger proportion of individuals at risk for HIV infection than the general population, namely homosexual and bisexual males. While seemingly off the point in assessing acute athletic injury to the spine, it is critical to remain attuned to HIV risk factors when obtaining a history from these patients. Inquiry into the presence of night sweats, night pain, and frequent infections can point to the need for blood tests, purified protein derivative (PAD), and radiologic examination.

One professional ballet dancer known to our clinic had low-back pain initially attributed to musculotendinous injury. When the pain did not resolve after several weeks, spine films were obtained, showing a 6-cm soft-tissue shadow adjacent to the T12 vertebral body. Biopsy revealed this to be a T-cell lymphoma, while blood tests confirmed HIV infection. Following radiation and chemotherapy, the dancer has returned to full participation in ballet.

The Future of Dance Medicine

While the young discipline of dance medicine has developed a data base on the epidemiology of dance injury, it is evident that much remains to be learned about the appropriate and "dance specific" treatment of injury. Examples of questions that remain to be answered include (1) Is surgical treatment of common spinal problems such as HNP and spondylolisthesis truly possible in dancers who wish to continue their professional careers? (2) How does one promote the concept of the "neutral spine" in an activity that requires extremes of spinal flexion and extension? (3) Would modification of menstrual abnormalities in female dancers through the use of estrogen replacement therapy alter the incidence of spondylolysis or scoliosis? It might be hoped that defining answers to questions concerning an activity that stresses the spine to the limits of its capabilities would also shed light on issues with more general application to spinal medicine and patient care.

References

1. Andersson S and others: Degenerative joint disease in ballet dancers, *Clin Orthop Rel Res* 238:233, 1989.
2. Baillon JM: Articular and muscular lesions in dancers, *ACTA Orthop Belg* 49(1-2):112, 1983.
3. Bejjani FJ: Occupational biomechanics of athletes and dancers: a comparative approach, *Clin Pod Med Surg* 4(3):671, 1987.
4. Bowling A: Injuries to dancers: prevalence, treatment, and perceptions of causes, *BMJ* 298:731, 1989.
5. Ciullo JV, Jackson DW: Pars interarticularis stress reaction, spondylolysis, and spondylolisthesis in gymnasts, *Clin Sports Med* 4(1):95, 1985.
6. Drinkwater BL and others: Bone mineral content of amenorrheic and eumenorrheic athletes, *New Engl J Med* 311:277, 1984.
7. Ende LS, Wickstrom J: Ballet injuries, *Phys Sports Med* 10(7):101, 1982.
8. Howse J: Orthopaedists aid ballet, *Clin Orthop* 89:52, 1982.
9. Bergfeld, JA and others: Medical problems in ballet: a round table, *Phys Sports Med* 10(3):98, 1986.
10. Micheli LJ: Back injuries in dancers, *Clin Sports Med* 2(3):473, 1983.
11. Nixon JE: Injuries to the neck and upper extremities of dancers, *Clin Sports Med* 2(3):45, 1983.
12. Ryan AJ: *Epidemiology of dance injuries,* In Ryan AJ, Stephens RE, editors: *Dance medicine, a comprehensive guide,* Chicago, 1987, Pluribus Press.
13. Teitz CC: Sports medicine concerns in dance and gymnastics, *Clin Sports Med* 2(3):571, 1983.
14. Thomasen E: *Diseases and injuries of ballet dancers.* Arhus, 1982, Universitetsvorlagit I.
15. Warren MP and others: Scoliosis and fractures in young ballet dancers, *New Engl J Med* 314(21): 1348, 1986.
16. Washington EL: Musculoskeletal injuries in theatrical dancers: site, frequency, and severity, *Am J Sports Med* 6(2):75, 1978.

Chapter 47
Figure Skating
Joseph D. Fortin

Tenley Albright, M.D., who was the 1956 Olympic Gold Medalist in figure skating, provided a compelling description of the rigors of competitive figure skating when she described the attributes of a good skater as one who embodies "the balance of a tightrope walker, the endurance of a marathon runner, the aggressiveness of a football player, the agility of a wrestler, the nerves of a golfer, the flexibility of a gymnast, and the grace of a ballet dancer."[3]

Despite the large number of participants (the U.S. Figure Skating Association's membership is currently over 47,000) in a sport that imposes tremendous physical demands, there is a paucity of information regarding the rehabilitation of any figure skating impairment, most notably spinal injuries. The following factors further substantiate a need for systematic preventive/rehabilitative intervention for skaters: (1) Most competitive figure skaters begin training when they are physically immature.[6,8,27] (2) Competitive skaters train on the ice for 3 to 6 hours a day, 5 to 7 days a week.[6,15,27,34] (3) Trends toward off-ice training, involving such activities as weight training, dance, and aerobic activities, are increasing the hours a skater trains.[27,34] (4) The sport has become increasingly athletically demanding. In order to achieve top scores, single skaters must perform more double and triple jumps; pair skaters must execute more lifts and throws.[15] Prima facia, the successful quadruple toe-loop completed by Kurt Browning of Canada at the 1988 World Championships and the International Skating Union's recent decision to eliminate compulsory figures (allowing top athletes to concentrate exclusively on the freestyle events) will establish a greater precedence for athletic prowess in freestyle competition. (5) Perhaps no other sport places the same diversity of forces on such a narrow base of support.[25] (6) Only six studies have described the nature and incidence of competitive figure skating injuries.* Furthermore, the observation from three of these studies[5,6,40] were based on a relatively small number of athletes, and only two studies provided prospective data[21,39] (7) The significant rate of injury[5,38] and the severity of injury[5,6,20,39] (in terms of missed training days) to figure skaters suggests a need to evaluate predisposing factors and methods of rehabilitation.

Epidemiology

The differential effects that the type of skating, level of competition, and anthropometric variables have on patterns of figure skating injuries are yet unestablished. This is partly attributable to the con-

* References 5, 6, 20, 21, 39, and 40.

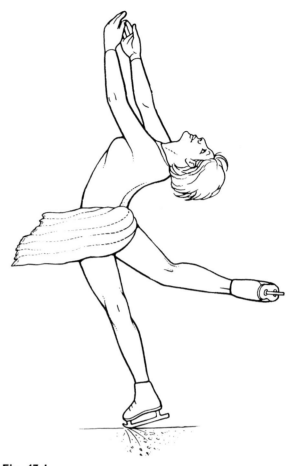

Fig. 47-1

Lay-back spin subjects the lumbar spine to combination of hyperextension and torsion forces. Ballistic nature of figure skating imparts complex array of stressors on lumbar spine of young participants.

flicting methods of data collection used in reports to date. Trends that indicate a relative susceptibility of pair skaters to injury[20,39] and the common types of injuries to skaters are beginning to coalesce.

The low-back region may account for one third of all figure skating injuries.[20] Consider the ballistic nature of competitive figure skating, including lifts, throws, jumps and spins which subjects its young participants to a barrage of axial skeletal stressors (Fig. 47-1). In the author's experience, low-back pain in skaters can result from facet syndrome, disc prolapse, sacroiliac joint dysfunction, occasionally symptomatic spondylitic defects, and rarely, compression fractures.[20]

Axial skeletal injuries to figure skaters undeniably warrant medical investigation when one also considers injuries to the pelvis and rib cage and the remainder of the spine.[5,6,20] Although the incidence of lower-extremity injuries is greatest,[5,6,20,39] the chronicity and recidivism associated with axial skeletal injuries may result in more missed training days.[6] Moreover, education on proper spinal mechanics may allow athletes to alleviate stressors applied to the appendicular skeleton while skating (see Fig. 47-8). Inadequate instruction on proper lifting technique may be responsible for injuries in pair skaters during lifting maneuvers.[38]

Biomechanics of the Lift

An overhead hand-to-hand press is a statuesque, core lift for pair skaters. The biomechanics of other lifts are not described herein but are all determined by the approach, the manner in which the male executes the lift, and the position of the female in the air.[34]

Sequential Motion of the Overhead Press

Fig. 47-2 provides the sequential motion sequence of the lift. The approach is face-to-face, with the skaters moving in opposite directions, the male forward and the female backward. This lift involves the male "pressing" his partner into an overhead position in front of him. To maximize leverage on the lift, they rotate their torsos close to each other and the male reaches "under' and across with his left hand. Their left hands join under her pelvis so he can control her center of mass during the lift. The opposite hands join overhead so that as the male rotates his female counterpart around his back and upward, she can assist in "pressing" herself to an upright position. Dismounting is simply a reversal of the lift as he lowers her with one hand "under" and one hand over in a counterclockwise rotation. He may also "throw" her from that position so that she completes one or two counterclockwise revolutions before landing on the back outside edge of the right skate. The landing is essentially the same as the axel landing described in a following section.

The anthropometric "matching" of pair teams becomes important when one considers the inordinate forces applied to the female's lumbar spine and pelvis as she is thrown by a male with a considerable difference in height and weight. Male partners ranked at a national level are on an average 4 to 5 years older than their female counterparts.[20,39]

Z-Axis Biomechanics of the Overhead Press

Coronal plane side-bending or Z-axis rotary motion is initially created in the lumbar spine of the male partner by the action of bending to one side and lifting with one upper extremity (see Fig. 47-2). This may cause excess lumbar torsion in the male athlete if the Z-axis moment is not partially counteracted by an opposing force applied by the contralateral "overhead" extremity. Torsional forces culminate as the male presses upward with the "underhand" and simultaneously rotates his partner's body toward the contralateral side of his body in an opposite side-bending direction of the trunk (with adduction of the overhead extremity). This "overhead extremity" must be intensely stabilized by sufficient scapulothoracic restraining force to oppose the side-bending moment, initially created by trunk bending. The co-contraction of the serratus anterior and middle trapezius muscles prevents X-axis or horizontal translatory motion of the scapula. Cocontraction of the latissimus dorsi and pectoralis minor muscles, as well as the remaining fibers of the trapezius muscles act to prevent Z-axis rotary motion of the scapula (i.e., cranial or caudad rotation). Latissimus dorsi activation also produces trunk rotation; opposing the left side-bending motion, which is created in the lumbar spine by the reaching under and lifting. The transversus abdominis muscle is another important trunk derotator (in the lift) vis-à-vis its attachments to the lumbodorsal fascia.[22] If the male is unable to control the rotational forces as he lifts the female up and around, torsional forces comparable to those on landing a jump are operable (see Fig. 47-2, *A, B, and C*).

In the female team member, the above muscle groups act bilaterally to allow her to assist in pressing herself to an upright posture. These kinematics can also prevent posterior displacement of her scapula on her thorax while she is maintaining her body in the overhead position. The scapulothoracic stabilizing forces converge on the spine at approximately the T4-T5 or T5-T6 motion segment, which may account for upper to midthoracic pain in pair skaters.[13,17]

X-Axis Biomechanics of the Overhead Press

Sagittal plane or X-axis rotary mechanics of the lift involve tensile forces applied by the weight of the female's body to the male's upper extremities. These forces, together with those from contributing body segments, generate anterior shear forces across the lumbosacral axis. These anterior forces are opposed by posterior restraining ones applied by concentric contractions of the hips and spine extensors. Attempts to assume an upright posture are also aided by extension at the knee and ankle. The largest moment arm in the sagittal plane is attained at the initiation of the lift, when the female's center of mass if farthest from the lifter's lumbosacral X-axis of rotation.[19] Completion of the lift to the overhead position does not involve large moments, but rather great coordination in maintaining those moments

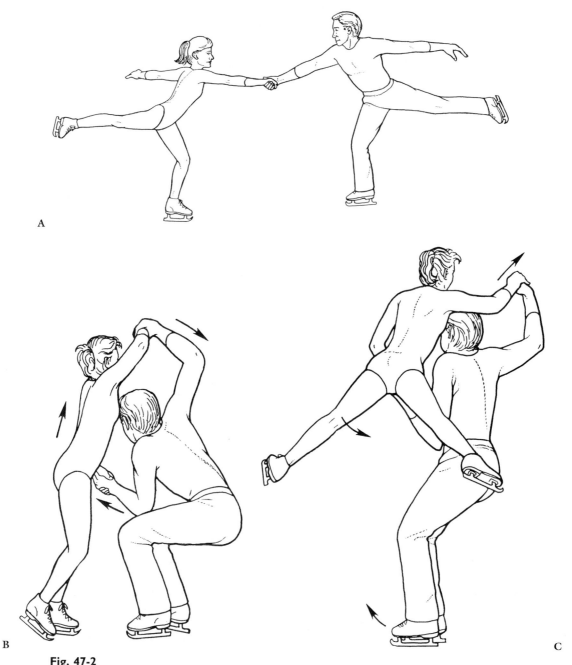

Fig. 47-2
Overhead hand-to-hand press lift. **A,** Approach. **B,** Initiation of lift. **C,** Lift.

near 0 (as the male keeps the female's center of mass aligned over his base of support).

Excess axial loading, from allowing the female's weight to remain too far from his base of support, may cause herniation of nuclear material through the end plates of the lumbar spine.[2,10,29,38]

Tight hip flexors can result in the male athlete completing the lift with the mechanically disadvantaged spine extensors rather than the more powerful gluteal muscles.[11,12,14,22,30] Since he cannot ex-

tend maximally through the hips, he is committed to completing the lift by hyperextending through the lumbosacral axis.[18,19] Hyperextension magnifies shear across the lower disc and forces the lumbosacral inferior articular processes to impact sharply on the subjacent laminae.[44] Tight pectoralis minor muscles, often found in conjunction with inflexible hip flexors, can also increase extension through the lumbar spine by preventing maximum flexion at the shoulder[28] (as he lifts his partner upward).

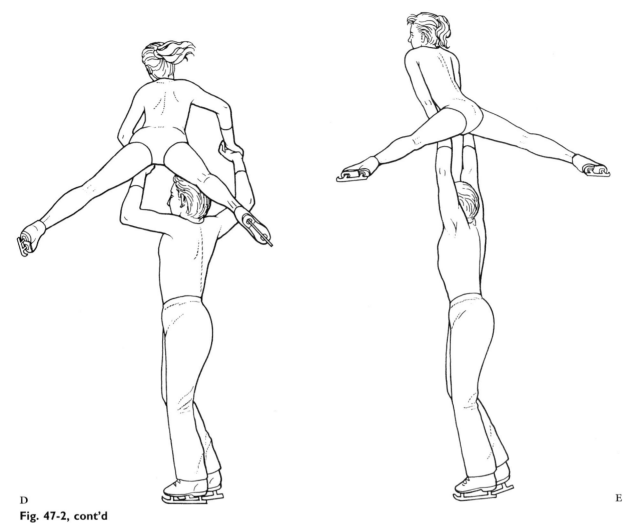

Fig. 47-2, cont'd

D, "Pressing" upward to overhead position. **E,** Final overhead position.

D

E

Biomechanics of the Jump

Multi-revolution jumps, with astonishing height and impeccable line, are the foundation of an elite freestyle figure skating program. Knowledge of jumping biomechanics is essential for understanding the complex muscle balancing and stabilization issues relevant to skaters.[37]

Sequential Analysis of the Axel Jump

A double axel jump (2.5 revolutions) is a requirement of any skater who desires to pass the Gold Test and compete at the senior National Championship level. The 1978 World Championship spectators witnessed for the first time in competition the completion of a triple axel (3.5 revolutions) by Vern Taylor of Canada. Midori Ito, of Japan, stunned the crowd at the 1989 World Championship as she became the first woman to complete a triple axel in competition—unveiling a new, unimaginable "gold standard" for women's freestyle competition.

Fig. 47-3 illustrates the sequential motion of the axel jump. The take-off for the axel jump originates from a left forward outside edge. An imaginary line of rotational direction from this edge is a counterclockwise circle. On the takeoff approach, the "free" right lower extremity and arms are flexed and circumducted upward and forward to accelerate the center of mass upward. Forceful right hip flexion, combined motions at the shoulders, and explosive extension at the left knee and hip are paramount to achieve optimal vertical velocity and jump height. Subsequently, the jump height determines the time in flight and secondarily the amount of revolution.

Angular momentum, necessary for spinning, must be conserved in flight so the skater "pulls in" the arms and right lower extremity (closer to the body's longitudinal axis of rotation). Accordingly, this maneu-

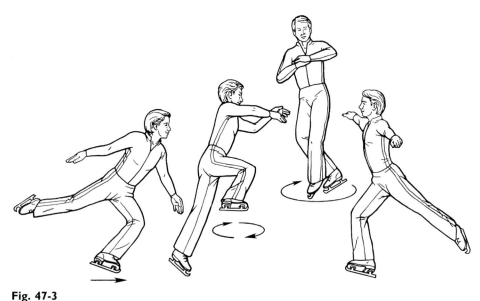

Fig. 47-3

Axel jump. (Reprinted with permission from the American Orthopaedic Society for Sports Medicine, 1990.)

ver serves to decrease the moment of inertia, thereby increasing the angular velocity required for spinning.

The jump is landed as the skater "checks out" by opening the upper extremities and left lower extremity while stepping down on a right back outside edge commensurate with the counterclockwise direction of rotation. Shoulder, knee, and hip strength relative to jump height have been previously elucidated.[37]

Jump Landing and Torsional Injury to the Lumbar Spine

The role of torsional forces in creating spine injury to skaters can be evidenced on examining the lumbar segmental motion of jump landing. Fig. 47-4 demonstrates the forces operating on the lumbar spine of the figure skater on landing a jump. Forces of axial loading on impact act to create shear forces in the planes of the lumbar discs. These forces, combined with the rotational momentum of the revolutions, apply torsional force concentrated at the neural arch. With trunk rotation, a lateral bending moment toward the side of the sharply apposed apophyseal joint is introduced in the disc (so-called coupled motion). Forced rotation of the sharply impacted facet beyond 2 to 3 degrees may simultaneously damage the facet, deform the neural arch, and disrupt the anulus, due to improper loading of the disc.[1,10,32,41,45] A priori, several cases familiar to the author are consequently illuminated—such as a 19-year-old male singles skater with a longstanding history of posterior element disease and a recent lumbar prolapsed disc, as well as a 23-year-old female pair skater with

a prior history of a traumatic spondylolisthesis due to skating. Other factors that magnify the risk of injury include poor dynamic stabilization mechanics in lifting, landing, or even takeoff (particularly in jumps such as the Lutz, in which the skater must turn against the inherent rotational momentum of the takeoff edge).

Sacroiliac Joint Dysfunction and Jump Landing

The mechanics of jump landing in figure skating may predispose some athletes to the development of sacroiliac (SI) joint dysfunction and possibly pain.[4,17,23,26,31,35,42,43] One can appreciate the extraordinary shear and torsional forces across this major weight-bearing joint from repetitively jumping and landing on one lower extremity, usually the right, and missed landings (which often result in the buttocks impacting directly on the ice).

Axial loading, transmitted on landing impact, from the bicondylar axis of the femur to the pelvis, can lead to innominate shear dysfunction.[23] The midstance position of landing on the right lower extremity places the sacrum in a right-facing torsion.[25] A preponderance of right-sided SI joint pain in clinical presentations is an almost inescapable conclusion, given the above combined kinetic factors.

The role of propulsion, spin, lift, and jump mechanics, as well as having more impact on one leg than the other in the development of low-back pain in skaters needs to be addressed in the rehabilitation and stabilization programs. For example, a skater

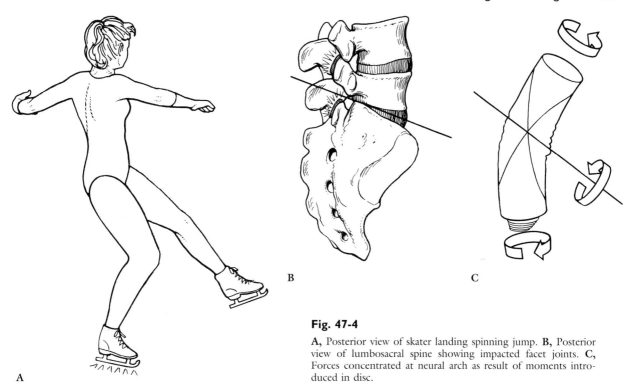

Fig. 47-4

A, Posterior view of skater landing spinning jump. **B,** Posterior view of lumbosacral spine showing impacted facet joints. **C,** Forces concentrated at neural arch as result of moments introduced in disc.

who develops a functional short leg and a secondary rotoscoliosis on the side on which jumps are consistently landed may be experiencing additional torsional forces. Therapeutic exercises and conditioning activities should be implemented to compensate for these and other functional biomechanical concerns.

Functional Restoration Program for Figure Skaters

Manual Medicine

In order initially to improve motion precisely where the restriction is, a patient with an adhesive capulitis of the shoulder may require passive range of motion with scapulothoracic stabilization prior to active mobilization. Similarly, a figure skater with an axial skeletal segmental motion aberrancy may need passive segmental motion prior to active mobilization.[24] This will often decrease pain and spasm, and expedite the athlete's aggressiveness in pursuing therapeutic exercise.[34] Athletes at the 1987 U.S. National Championships who presented with low-back pain responded immediately to manual medicine.[20] Following passive segmental mobilization (as indicated on presentation), active mobilization techniques (Fig. 47-5) should be initiated.

(The specifics of manual medicine as they apply to figure skaters are not the focus of this chapter.)

Muscle Balancing and Flexibility

Strength and flexibility imbalance about the hip and trunk in figure skaters with low-back pain may be a common finding.[20,40] This imbalance may arise from a combination of long hours of stroking in a flexed posture and repetitive unidirectional rotation, as well as landing on a dominant lower extremity.

Common Muscle and Flexibility Imbalances in Skaters

Muscle and flexibility imbalance often antagonizes the POOF (position of optimal function) in a static situation and unequivocally hinders optimal performance. Tight hip flexors and quadriceps with weak gluteal or quadriceps muscles will prevent maximal hip extension and decrease vertical velocity and height on jumps. It is common to find 15- to 20-degree hip flexion contractures in skaters.[18] Inflexible suboccipital muscles, long, weak longus colli/capitus muscles, and psoas or quadricep muscle contractures place the head forward with the pelvis in an anterior tilt. This muscle imbalance pattern also diminishes the male pairs skater's lift capacity by decreasing the range of posterior pelvic tilt. The resultant posture increases the moment of inertia and diminishes angular velocity attained on jumps and spins.

A common imbalance about the shoulder girdle includes tight pectoralis minor muscles, and weak

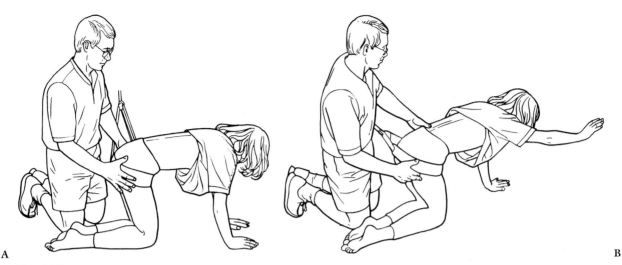

A   B

Fig. 47-5

"Cactus" Shumway, P.T., instructs athlete on active lumbar segmental mobilization. This 16-year-old singles skater has segmental motion aberrancy of lumbosacral spine involving flexion and right lateral bending. Lesion is commensurate with athlete's improper landing mechanics, which cause flexing and right lateral bending of trunk on impact of right lower extremity on ice. **A,** Quadruped position with hips stabilized (to prevent right lateral bending of lumbar spine). Pelvic belt, which is fixed to immobile object on athlete's left, resists any tendency for hips to shift right. **B,** Athlete raises right hand to introduce extension and left lateral bending in lumbar spine, which opposes her inherent segmental imbalance of flexion and right lateral bending. Therapist's hands ensure that proper motion occurs by providing kinesthetic cues to athlete.

rhomboid, lower trapezius, and serratus anterior muscles.[28] This inequity displaces the glenohumeral axis anteriorly by tilting the coracoid process forward, thus allowing the scapula to move posteriorly. The tilted position of the scapula is often the first indication of scapulothoracic imbalance or poor stabilization technique, particularly in pair skaters involved with lifting. The resultant moment arm created by shifting the weight of the shoulders forward in turn displaces the head forward and increases lumbar lordosis. Secondary amplification of scapulothoracic stabilizing forces across the upper and midthoracic spine may subsequently lead to thoracic facet joint dysfunction.[13,17] Each of these common imbalances should be considered during examination, and corrective exercises should be prescribed.

Case Studies in Muscle Balancing and Stabilization Activities for Skaters

Muscle balancing and flexibility assessment must be performed on each athlete concordant with their clinical presentation. The need for individual scrutiny, which cannot be obviated by a generic "protocol" therapeutic exercise program, is exemplified in the following cases.

Case 1 J.D. is a 16-year-old singles skater who has difficulty consistently landing jumps; her left lower extremity is "whipped" around, uncontrolled, and

she falls "in the circle" off the right back outside edge. J.D., therefore, repetitively, landed on her right hip and low back (Fig 47-6).

Muscle balancing and flexibility assessment revealed a weak right transverse abdominis, a short-weak left psoas major, and bilateral pronation. The right transversus abdominis[22] and left psoas major[28] were incapable of eccentrically checking left rotary trunk and hip motion, allowing the left lower extremity to whip around. Moreover, the tight left psoas muscle led to hyperextension through the lumbosacral axis and forced the upper torso to bend forward as the left lower extremity could not be extended further (as it attempted to complete its upward and counterclockwise rotation).

As shown in Fig. 47-7, the right transversus abdominis and external oblique were strengthened eccentrically with bent knee fall-outs while maintaining a POOF. The psoas muscle was stretched in the POOF and eccentrically strengthened.

Severe pronation also contributed to rotatory instability on landing. Pronation was corrected with rigid orthotics and POOF training. The POOF, by posteriorly displacing the center of gravity, placed a sufficient eccentric load on the anterior tibialis muscle to cantilever the longitudinal arch of the foot.

Through the above intervention, the skater was able to control the rotational momentum of the left lower extremity and improve her landing.

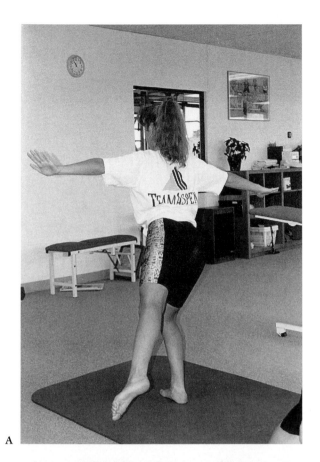

A

Fig. 47-6

A, Combination of weak right transversus abdominis muscle, inflexible, weak, left psoas muscle and pronation lead to an unstable landing position in this 16-year-old singles skater. The right external oblique did not eccentrically "check" left rotary trunk motion—allowing the left lower extremity to be "whipped-around" in an uncontrolled manner. **B,** Figure skating director and coach, Cindy Sullivan, works with an athlete to correct her landing mechanics. Note: The coach's left hand prevents the skater's left lower extremity, at the hip, from rotating further. The coach's right hand provides kinesthetic cues for the athlete to stabilize left lower extremity motion via eccentric action of the right abdominal muscles.

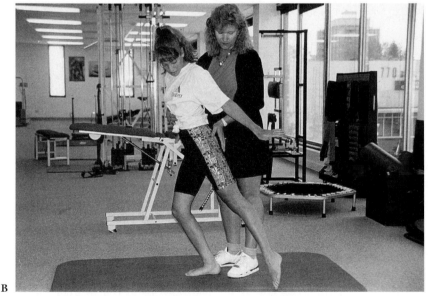

B

Case 2 J.W. is an 18-year-old singles skater with an SI joint dysfunction who has a tendency to "wrap" the landings (Fig. 47-8) or fall backward off the rear rocker of the skate. In either case, the result is to fail the landing, often with the buttocks impacting directly on the ice.

Manual muscle testing revealed a long, weak right gluteus medius muscle, which was responsible for the right lateral hip deviation and unstable pelvis on landing. The right gluteus medius was strengthened concentrically and eccentrically. Dynamic stabilization was then undertaken on the

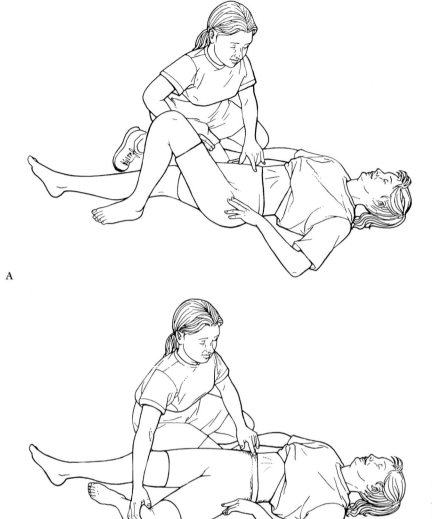

A

B

Fig. 47-7

A, Tammi Inglehart, P.T., instructs skater on bent-knee fall-out to strengthen the right transversus abdominis eccentrically. **B,** Skater must maintain posterior pelvic tilt and not allow pelvis to rotate toward left lower extremity as it "falls-out."

Heiden board by preferentially directing impact to the right lower extremity and eccentrically challenging the right gluteus medius (Fig. 47-9) to fortify landing control.

Dissociative Movement Therapy

Dissociative movement therapy (DMT) allows the figure skater the ability to diminish the loads on the axial skeleton and improve performance by using the extremities relatively autonomously in three dimensional space. Dissociative movement allows Ben Johnson or Carl Lewis to run the 100-m dash with a near straight line of linear progression. It also is responsible for the lyrical and "effortless" motions of the arms and legs of a premier ballerina, who gracefully spins and turns on stage while maintaining her "line" and "balance point."

Fig. 47-10 represents one application of DMT. The dowels (placed against the xiphisternum and pubic symphysis) force the athlete to adhere to the POOF while simulating theatrical arm motion she might make while in a spin or jump. If she does not keep her simulated spin or jump "centered," she is discouraged as she drops one or both dowels. The dowel method was popularized by David "Cactus" Shumway, P.T. Further discussion of DMT is beyond the scope of this writing.

Stabilization Exercises for Figure Skaters

Stabilization exercises provide a foundation for excelling in various figure skating maneuvers. Maintaining the POOF or finding the "balance point" (as skaters refer to it) is germane to preventing most of the errors that commonly occur, resulting in jump-

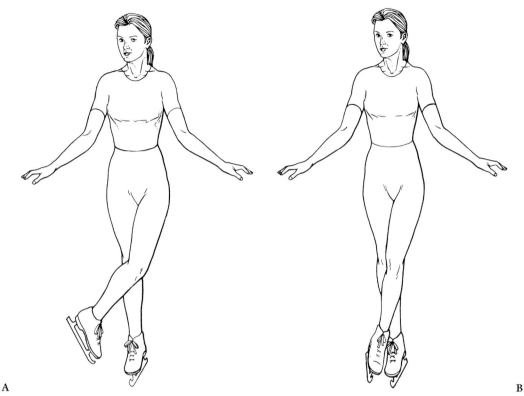

A   B

Fig. 47-8

A, Improper lower extremity position on landing: "wrapping it." Free lower extremity is excessively "wrapped" around landing one. *Note*: Right hip deviates right, which often results in falling to right (i.e., falling inside circle of clockwise rotation). Skater has clockwise direction of rotation and uses left leg for landing versus more common predominant counterclockwise rotation and right landing leg. **B,** Proper landing position of lower extremities. Pelvis is level and skater is on right back outside edge (congruent with counterclockwise direction of rotation in jumps).

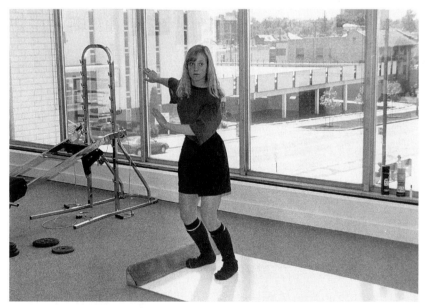

Fig. 47-9

Heiden board allows stabilization training in POOF concordant with stroking on ice. As athlete "skates" into stop (at end of board), she must also react to impact loading; not unlike landing a jump. This skater has a tendency to shift her right hip laterally on landing a jump on ice and was therefore instructed to use the right foot to the stop (to challenge the right gluteus medium muscle eccentrically). Right gluteus muscle weakness was implicated by her improper landing mechanics and manual muscle testing.

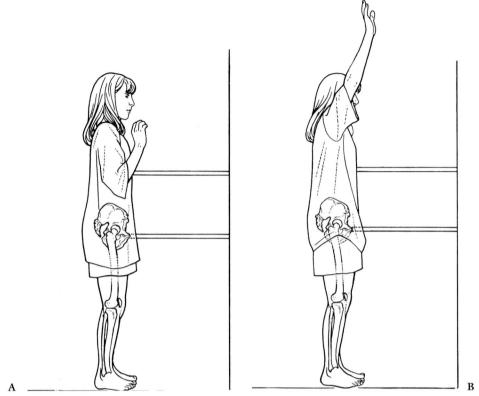

Fig. 47-10

Dissociative movement therapy with dowels. One dowel is placed against xiphisternum and wall and other against pubic symphysis and wall. Athlete is encouraged to maintain her POOF to prevent dowels from falling, while simulating theatrical arm motions. **A,** Beginning position. **B,** Final position with arms overhead.

A

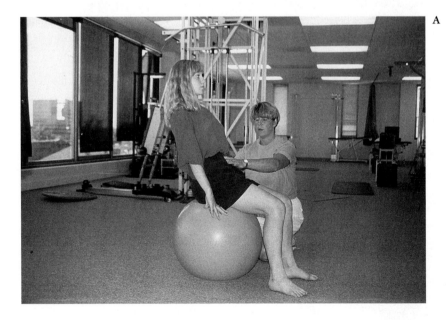

Fig. 47-11

Death spiral. Sequence of stabilization exercises to progressively approximate on-ice position of female. **A,** Upright POOF on a gymball.

execution mishaps.[36] Using the POOF to provide effective explosive hip and knee extension, and consequently to attain greater height and vertical velocity in jumps or lifts is one application for stabilization activities in figure skating. Controlling trunk flexion or side-bending during the takeoff, in mid-

flight, and on landing (to decrease the moment of inertia and prevent falling) is yet another of the innumerable applications for stabilization exercises.

Stabilization activities relevant to figure skating are legion, limited only by the confines of each therapist's creativity and ingenuity. The progression of

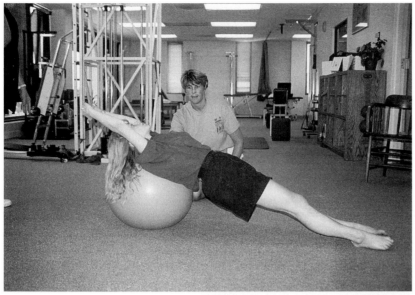

B

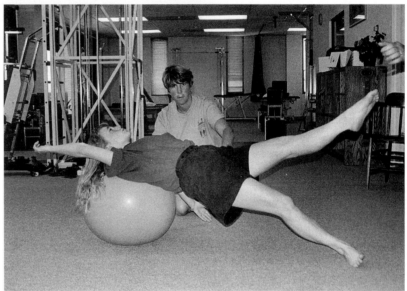

C

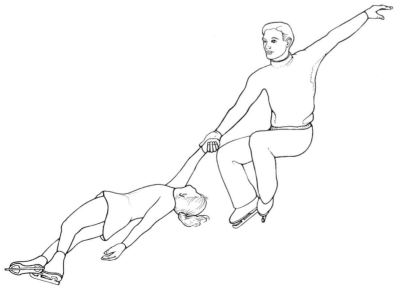

D

Fig. 47-11, cont'd

B, Bridging position. **C,** Unilateral support position congruent with on-ice position. **D,** Performing death spiral on ice. *Note*: Female's head is extended toward ice for artistic effect.

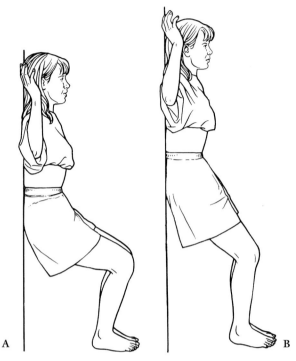

A   B

Fig. 47-12

Wall slides are excellent stabilization activity for skaters to develop hip and thigh strength. They can be performed with upper extremities against wall to provide pelvic and scapulothoracic stabilization simultaneously. **A,** Beginning. **B,** Completion.

exercises for the death spiral maneuver is exemplary. As Fig. 47-11 shows, this sequence involves progression from a POOF on a gymball, to a bridging position, and finally the on-ice unilateral support position requiring tremendous abdominal and trunk rotary strength.

Wall slides enhance the awareness of the POOF while simultaneously strengthening quadricep muscles and gluteal muscles for greater jump height and vertical velocity. Wall slides performed with the upper extremities against the wall directly counteract the aforementioned scapulothoracic imbalance often found in skaters (Fig. 47-12).

As shown in Fig. 47-13, cocontraction of the abdominal and erector spinae muscles, with Sports Cords activities, allows stabilization of the spine in the neutral position. This exercise prevents "breaking" at the waist or flexing the torso forward on landing jumps. Sports Cords or a Theraband can also be used to increase trunk and lower extremity rotatory strength to enhance jump control, height, and angular velocity (Fig. 47-14).

Once the athlete demonstrates the strength and coordination to maintain the POOF on wall slides and gymball activities, they are progressed to the Heiden board, plyometrics, Baps board, The Fitter,

and the Body Cycle. Ground reaction forces of the ice against the blade and boot limit the range of knee and hip extension attained on takeoff and jumps. The hip-knee-ankle mechanism necessitates a short and explosive take-off,[9] which is simulated by the action of the Heiden board and plyometrics.[7] These impact-loading exercises also enhance dynamic postural control for jump and flying-spin landings. The Baps board and The Fitter allow the athlete to work on proprioceptive capacity in a POOF to enhance control of the edges on takeoffs and landings. Dissociative training of the lower extremities (from pedaling with the pelvis level and the spine erect in a POOF) is combined with tremendous muscular endurance training on the Body Cycle (Fig. 47-15).

Weight Training for Figure Skaters

The relationship between knee, hip, and shoulder strength to jump height suggests a role for progressive weight training in figure skating.[37] Modified squats, reverse dumbbells, and cable crossovers form the foundation of the isotonic weight training program.[16] Antagonistic muscle action (such as biceps femoris and gastrocnemius) in "pre-stretching" prime movers (e.g., gluteus maximus and vastus medialis) must also be incorporated in the resistance equation.[9]

Return-to-Play Issues

The author uses the following algorithm to return the athlete to the ice, in conjunction with the aforementioned rehabilitation sequence. This algorithm, temporally, would be appropriate for an athlete with a facet joint syndrome or SI joint dysfunction uncomplicated by ligamentous injury or instability. The algorithm can be modified for returning figure skaters to the ice with other injuries.

One to two weeks after the implementation of the functional restoration program, concentrate on stroking, edges, and patchwork. At the end of the second week, begin various flexibility maneuvers such as the layback, but limit lumbar hyperextension and encourage a strict POOF. During week 3, concentrate on adding basic spins to footwork such as the back-, sit-, and camel-spins. During weeks 4 to 9, progressively, rather than impulsively, increase the difficulty of jumps and spins so that the build-up in torsional and axial loading is gradual. Torquing maneuvers should be discouraged until the athlete has demonstrated sufficient trunk and hip rotary strength.

For the jumps, the progression may be from a waltz, single, double, and triple revolutions to com-

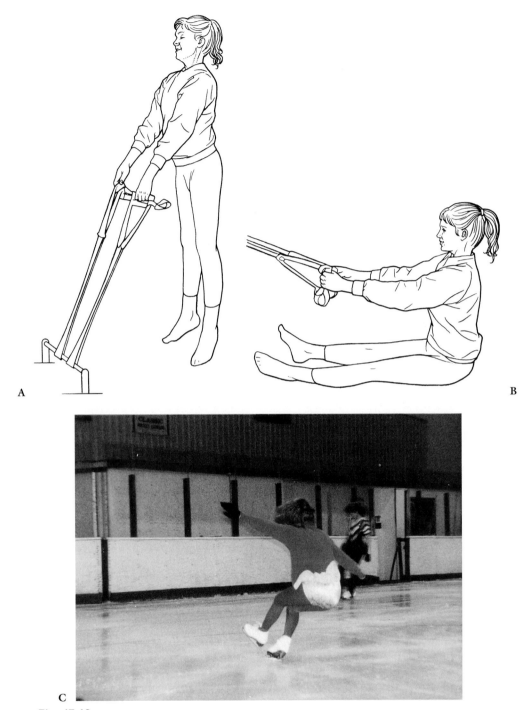

Fig. 47-13

Tremendous trunk stabilizing strength, provided by cocontraction of abdominal and erector spinae muscles, is necessary to control jump landings. Common cause of missed landings is tendency for torso to be thrust forward on impact with the ice. Concomitant concentric strengthening of abdominal muscles and eccentric strengthening of erector spinae muscles prevent this dilemma. **A,** Beginning position of Sports Cord abdominal strengthening. **B,** Completion. Note athlete is resisting tendency for torso to flex forward (as erector spinae muscles undergo a lengthening contraction) against resistance of cord. **C,** Lack of proper trunk stabilization leads to demise of this landing as athlete flexes her torso and loses her POOF. Note she falls in circle of counterclockwise rotation.

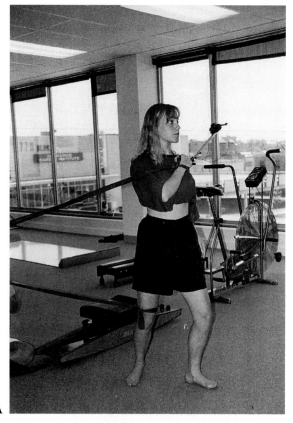
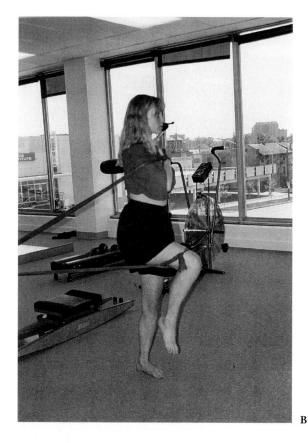

A   B

Fig. 47-14

Rotary strengthening of trunk and lower extremity to enhance jump control, height, and angular velocity. Athlete demonstrates take-off for an axel jump with Theraband for rotary stabilization. Once skater
masters the maintenance of the POOF (while simulating action of right lower extremity in takeoff), action of right upper extremity in takeoff is also incorporated in exercise (see Fig. 47-3). **A,** Beginning. **B,**
Completion.

bination jumps. Spins can be progressed from a combination that involves a transition on different feet
such as a sit-spin into a camel-spin, to a more difficult combination involving a transition on one foot,
such as a back-sit-spin into a back-camel-spin. Gradually, jumping and flying-spins can be added. Maneuvers such as the flying-sit-spin and death-drop,
which involve a great deal of axial loading with the
lumbar spine in a flexed posture, should be implemented toward the end of the return-to-play regimen.

Pair skaters, over 3 to 4 weeks into the program,
gradually progress from lifts that require little torsion (such as the tabletop) to those that require
greater torsion (such as the overhead hand-to-hand
press or a star lift). Finally, they work in the last several weeks of the protocol on throw jumps. For an
injured female skater, her male counterpart must be
cautioned to avoid inordinate height on throws to
diminish the impact loading. Again, they progress in
revolutions from singles to doubles.

The above protocol may be altered depending on
how a particular case plays out. This algorithm is
predicated on the athlete's condition, maturity, and
confidence. A skater with a torsion injury to the lumbar disc who continues to experience radicular pain
on landing jumps, may require a lumbar epidural
steroid injection before attempting further jumps. If
the injection is successful, one may wish to reexam-
ine the jump and landing mechanics of the athlete
in a harness. Further work on technique and rotary
strengthening of the hip and trunk muscles can then
be implemented, as indicated.

Injury Prevention

Prevention and training programs must match the
demands of a complex sport that requires speed,
agility, flexibility, and power.[34] The grueling efforts
of this routine come to fruition in the form of speed,
height, grace, and torquing momentum in such awe-

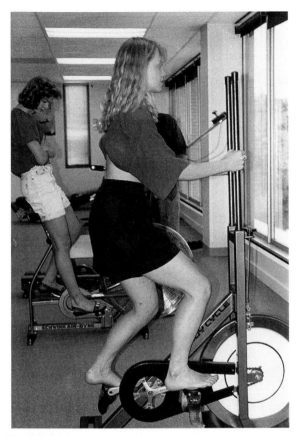

Fig. 47-15

Body Cycle. There is no seat, which necessitates extraordinary quadricep and gluteal muscle strength to maintain the POOF. Resultant strength is displayed on ice in such superbly theatrical maneuvers as multirevolution jumps and flying splits and spins.

inspiring, theatrical maneuvers as triple or quadruple jumps as well as flying-sit-spins or death-drops.

An example of a solid home program would be a 30-minute aerobic warm-up on a stationary cycle followed by 15 minutes of flexibility exercises and 20 minutes of gymball and Sports Cord activity. In addition to the daily home program, a cross-training program three to four times per week should be implemented. This may consist of ballet, circuit weight training, swimming, or cycling.

Activities on the ice are equally as important as exercise performed off the ice to prevent injury. Most elite skaters typically skate at least three sessions, 45 minutes to an hour, in one day. The first session should consist of warmup edges, patchwork, and footwork to build balance gradually and progressively move toward greater rotation. The athlete should slowly work toward the back-spin, as all jumps are based on counterclockwise or "back" rotation. Forward, clockwise rotation should not be eliminated, as this rotation may help to eliminate some of the rotary imbalance as a result of repetitive unidirectional torsion. Complex spins as the layback, camel, or combination spins can then be added. The athlete should be encouraged to maintain a position of optimal function so that all spins are well "centered."

The second session should involve more rapid motion, hard stroking, and build-up in the number of revolutions on jumps. More complex jumps and flying spins are finally added. The athlete may perform the short competition program during this session.

The final session of the day would involve the performance of the long program. The athlete should be leery of executing new or complex jumps or lifts at the beginning or end of training sessions, as this is when injuries often occur (Sullivan C, Sahlin N: personal communication, 1991). In addition, warmup stretching prior to practice is essential in preventing injury.

Summary

Understanding the specific mechanism of a figure skating injury is the key to successful treatment and prevention. The knowledge and benefits to be gained by the figure skating world through future, controlled, sport-science studies is unlimited. Investigating the mechanics of injury may delineate the exact relationship of injury to various maneuvers and predisposing factors. Equipment, such as boots, spotting harnesses, and protective headgear could be rigidly tested to elucidate a relationship to injury and injury prevention. The efficacy of various training methods, including the recently popularized cross-training methods, should be examined.

As sports science in figure skating is nascent, while the sport's popularity flourishes, there is a growing contribution to be made by the rinkside physician, through applying sound rehabilitation and stabilization principles in injury management and prevention.

References

1. Adams MA, Hutton WC: The relevance of torsion to the mechanical derangement of the spine, *Spine* 6:241, 1981.
2. Adams MA, Hutton WC: Gradual disc prolapse, *Spine* 10:524, 1985.
3. Albright TE: Editorial comment, *Am J Sports Med* 7:46, 1979.
4. Beal MC: The sacroiliac problem: review of anatomy, mechanics, and diagnosis, *J Am Osteopath Assoc* 81:667, 1982.

5. Brock RM, Striowski CC: Injuries in elite figure skaters, *Phys Sports Med* 14:111, 1986.

6. Brown PW, McKeag DB: Training, experience, and medical history of pairs skaters, *Phys Sports Med* 15:100, 1987.

7. Chu DA: Jumping into plyometrics, Champagne, IL; 1992, Leisure Press.

8. Davis MWW, Litman T: Figure skater's foot, *Minn Med* 9:647, 1979.

9. deBoer RW, et al.: Moments of force, power, and muscle coordination in speed-skating, *Int J Sport Med* 8:371, 1987.

10. Farfan HF, et al.: The effects of torsion on the lumbar intervertebral joints: the role of torsion in the production of disc degeneration. *J Bone Joint Surg* 52A:468, 1970.

11. Farfan HF: Muscular mechanism of the lumbar spine and the position of power and efficiency, *Orthop Clin North Am* 6:135, 1975.

12. Farfan HF: Biomechanical advantage of lordosis and hip extension for upright activities, *Spine* 3/4:336, 1978.

13. Farfan HF: The tired neck syndrome, Presented at Challenge of the Cervical Spine, First Annual International Conference, San Antonio, April, 1990.

14. Farfan HF, Gracovetsky S, Lamy C: Mechanism of the lumbar spine, *Spine* 6:243, 1981.

15. Ferstel J: Figure skating in search of the winning edge, *Sports Med* 7:129, 1979.

16. Fleck SJ, Kraemer WJ: *Designing resistance training programs*, Champagne, IL, 1987, Human Kinetics Books.

17. Fortin JD: Enigmatic causes of spine pain in athletes. In Watkins RG, editor: *The Spine and sports*, Chicago, Mosby Year-Book, (in press).

18. Fortin JD: Low back pain in weight lifters, *Arch Phys Med Rehab* 68:642, 1987.

19. Fortin JD: The biomechanical principles of preventing weight lifting injuries to the spine. In Watkins RG, editor: *The spine and sports*, Chicago, Mosby Year-Book, (in press).

20. Fortin JD, Roberts D: Competitive figure skating injuries, *Arch Phys Med Rehab* 68:642, 1987.

21. Garrick JG: Figure skating injuries, *Med Sci Sports Exerc* 14:141, 1982.

22. Gracovetsky S, Farfan HF, Lamy C: A mathematical model of the lumbar spine using an optimal system to control muscles and ligaments, *Orthop Clin North Am* 8:131, 1977.

23. Greenman PE: Innominate shear dysfunction in the sacroiliac syndrome, *Man Med* 2:114, 1986.

24. Greenman PE, editor: *Principles of manual medicine*, Baltimore, 1989, Williams & Wilkins, p 3.

25. Greenman PE: Clinical aspects of sacroiliac function in walking, *J Man Med* 5:125, 1990.

26. Grieve GP: The sacroiliac joint, *Physiotherapy* 62:385, 1976.

27. Hunter WN, Schumberth JM, McCrea JD: In-skate training brace for young beginning skaters, *J Am Podiatry Assoc* 71:643, 1981.

28. Janda V: *Muscles and cervicogenic pain syndromes*. In Grant R, editor: *Physical therapy of the cervical and thoracic spine*, New York, 1988, Churchill-Livingstone.

29. Jayson MIV, Herbert CM, Barks JS: Intervertebral disc: nuclear morphology and bursting pressures, *Ann Rheum Dis* 332:308, 1973.

30. Keagy RD, Brumlik J, Bergan JJ: Direct electromyography of the psoas major muscle in man, *J Bone Joint Surg* 48A:1377, 1966.

31. Kirkaldy-Willis WH, and Hill RJ: A more precise diagnosis for low back pain, *Spine* 4:102, 1979.

32. Lamy C, Kraus H, Farfan HF: The strength of the neural arch in the etiology of spondylolysis, *Orthop Clin North Am* 6:215, 1975.

33. MacDonald RS, Bell CMJ: An open controlled assessment of osteopathic manipulation in non-specific low-back pain, *Spine* 15(5):364, 1990.

34. McMaster WC, Liddle S, Walsh J: Conditioning program for competitive figure skating, *Am J Sports Med* 7:43, 1979.

35. Mierau DR, et al.: Sacroiliac joint dysfunction and low back pain in school-aged children, *J Manipulative Physiolther* 72:81, 1984.

36. Petkevich JM: Sports illustrated figure skating: championship techniques in New York, *Sports Illustrated.*, 1988.

37. Podolsky A, et al.: The relationship of strength and jump height in figure skaters, *Am J Sports Med* 18:400, 1990.

38. Rolander SD, Blair WE: Deformation and fracture of the lumbar vertebral end-plate, *Orthop Clin North Am* 6:75, 1975.

39. Smith AD, Ludington R: Injuries in elite pair skaters and ice dancer, *Am J Sports Med* 17:482, 1989.

40. Smith AD, Micheli LJ: Injuries in competitive figure skaters, *Phys Sports Med* 10:36, 1982.

41. Sullivan JD, Farfan HF: The crumpled neural arch, *Orthop Clin North Am* 6:199, 197.

42. Vleeming A, et al.: Relation between form and function in sacroiliac joint part II: Biomechanical aspects, *Spine* 15:113, 1990.

43. Walheim GG: Stabilization of the pelvis with the Hoffman frame, *Acta Orthop Scand* 55:319, 1984.

44. Yang KH, King AI: Mechanism of facet load transmission as a hypothesis for low back pain, *Spine* 9:557, 1984.

45. Yung-Hing K, Kirkaldy-Willis WH: The pathology of degenerative disease of the lumbar spine, *Orthop Clin North Am* 14(3): 491-504, July, 1983.

Chapter 48
Football
Robert M. Shugart

The game of football has become our nation's number one autumn sport. It is estimated that more than 1.5 million players will participate this year alone. It is a unique game that incorporates a variety of skills such as running, catching, blocking, and tackling. This diversity requires significant player contact and frequent high-velocity collisions. This can lead to severe and even life-threatening injuries. Current sources estimate approximately 1.2 million injuries per year in the United States. Prevention is of paramount importance not only to decrease injury rates, but also to help control costs in this era of cost containment. By understanding mechanics, specific injuries, conditioning, and rehabilitation, we can begin to prevent injuries and make football safer at all levels of play.

History

Obviously, the game of football as it is played today is much different from the original English game that dates back to approximately A.D. 1000. England was occupied by the Danes from A.D. 1016 to A.D. 1042. Some time after the Danish occupation, the story goes that workmen were digging in an old battlefield. They apparently unearthed the skull of a Dane and muttering about the unpleasant memories of the days of the Danish occupation, proceeded to kick the skull around the pasture. Boys, seeing this, sensed a new diversion and they continued the game. The skull, for obvious reasons, was eventually replaced with an inflated cow bladder, and thus the basic principle of football was born.

It was in the twelfth century that the game became officially known as "futballe." It remained strictly a kicking game until the year 1823. It was in that year that William Ellis picked up the ball and attempted to run with it. This eventually became incorporated to become the game now known as rugby.

True American football as it exists today has its roots based on a challenge between Harvard and McGill Universities in 1874. This game was played under "Boston game rules," which were a hybrid of soccer and rugby. This hybrid style became accepted as early American-style football, and its popularity increased. The forward pass was legalized in 1906 and refinements of the game have continued, culminating in the game we know today.

Injuries Seen Historically During Football

Twelfth century football had none but the most basic rules. At the time it was described as a "combination of soccer, vandalism, and mass modified homicide." Obviously, injuries were rampant and persisted through the centuries as the game continued to evolve and become more organized. However, little attention was given to these injuries in this initial period. Early American football was not exempt from its share of injuries.

An innovation in American football called the "flying wedge," instituted in the 1900s, led to an increasing number of severe injuries and deaths. Following a *Chicago Tribune* report of 18 deaths and 159 serious injuries during the 1905 season, President Roosevelt called for an end to the "brutality" in organized football, or elimination of the game altogether. Roosevelt's demands resulted in the formation of the National Collegiate Athletic Association (NCAA), the initiation of an organization to promote safety in football.

In 1869 when the first Princeton-versus-Rutgers game was played, no protective equipment was used. John W. Heisman is quoted as saying, "We had no helmets or pads of any kind; in fact, one who wore homemade pads was regarded as a sissy." Body padding and leather helmets were later added to the uniform for safety. And since that time, many revisions and changes have been made. It is a necessity for players to have properly fitted and functioning equipment. Today football players wear a complement of protection, including specially designed shoulder pads, helmets, and face masks, all of which are attempts to protect the players.[12] Guidelines for equipment are set by the National Operating Committee on Standards for Athletic Equipment (NOCSAE).

Mechanism of Injury

Football involves tackling and blocking as well as running and throwing the ball. The contact that occurs between players during these maneuvers can lead to a multitude of injuries. In the past decades, research has attempted to evaluate the cause of injuries in an effort to increase the safety of the sport. Early attempts were made to identify catastrophic football injuries. As previously mentioned, the NCAA was set up in 1905 at the request of President Roosevelt to make football a safer sport. Mueller and Schindler published a review of football fatalities from 1931 to 1986, and found that 90% of fatalities were a result of head or cervical spine injuries.[20] In order to better document the extent of head and neck injury, Torg established the National Football Head and Neck Registry in 1975.[34,35] Retrospective data were collected from 1971 and continue to be collected in a prospective fashion. Analysis of data has led to rule changes.

Torg found that a comparison of data from the periods 1959 to 1963 and 1971 to 1975 showed a significant increase in players rendered quadriplegic in the later 5-year period.[34,35] He attributed this change to the improved protective capabilities of the helmet mask unit, which encouraged the players to use the head as a primary point of contact in blocking and tackling. As a result of this information the National Federation of State High School (NFSHSA) and NCAA banned spearing or the use of the top of the helmet as the initial point of contact. Implementation of these rules at the high school and college level decreased permanent cervical quadriplegia from 34 in 1976 to 5 in 1984.[31]

Literature review gives significant information on how to minimize injuries. Tackling presents the greatest hazard for injuring the cervical spine and is the most dangerous activity in football.[17] It is this maneuver that is most likely to create unanticipated loads to the cervical spine. Defensive players have more permanent cervical cord injuries than offensive players, and the majority of the defensive players are injured while attempting to tackle.[19] In particular, defensive backs are at highest risk for cervical quadriplegia.[34] Therefore, by following appropriate rules and tackling techniques, avoiding head-first contact, and identifying activities that increase injury rates, appropriate changes can be made to increase football safety and decrease injury rates.

Cahill and Griffith have shown that at the college level, the greatest chance of injury per player minute occurred during the practice game.[4] Halpern et al. found that contact practice games generated the greatest risk of all practice activities at the high school level. Preseason practice is 5.4 times more likely to result in injury than in-season practice.[14] Blyth and Mueller[3] reported that when limited contact was used in practice, this significantly reduced the number of high school football injuries but did not appear to affect the win-loss record. He also showed that as the age of the coach increased, the injury rate of the team steadily decreased. Coaches who had a background of both high school and college football playing experience had teams with lower injury rates. The more assistant coaches on the football field, the lower the injury rate. Practice activity accounted for 51.1% of all injuries again at the high school level.[3] Zemper[37] noted that injuries occurred most often during the third quarter, as a result of inadequate warmup, and least often during the first quarter. Twenty percent of injuries occurred in noncontact categories, including sprinting, running, and lifting weights. He felt that many of these injuries probably could be avoided with the use of proper technique, conditioning, and stretching.

Review of Literature Related To Injuries

Review of the orthopedic literature as it pertains to spinal injuries identifies the cervical and lumbar region as being most susceptible to injury. Obviously, great emphasis has been placed on cervical spine injuries because of their catastrophic nature. Although the thoracic region may sustain injury, the frequency is noted to be quite low.

The cervical region is vulnerable in contact sports in general, and in football in particular. By its nature, football can lead to excessive loads to the cervical spine. Mechanisms of injury to the cervical spine in football can occur in flexion, extension, lateral stretch, axial loading, or a combination of these. Torg was able to demonstrate that the majority of cervical fractures and dislocations were due to axial loading.[31,32-34] Previously it was thought that flexion and extension were the most dangerous maneuvers. Albright et al. evaluated college freshman players and found that 32% had roentgenographic evidence of neck injuries.[2] X-ray studies were considered abnormal if there was a bony deformity of the posterior elements, fracture of the vertebral body, abnormality of the intervertebral disc, or instability. An age-matched control group who had never played football showed no such abnormalities.[2] In their review of head and neck injuries in college football, Albright et al. found that players with abnormal findings on screening examination (i.e., abnormal physical examination or x-ray films) were twice as likely to have a head or neck injury at some point in their college career as players with a normal screening examination.[1] The greater degree of abnormality on freshmen screening examination, the more severe the neck injury in college was likely to be. Linemen had the highest frequency of neck injuries. These investigators also found that once a head or neck injury occurred, the chance of being subject to a future injury was 42%. The overall incidence of collegiate head and neck injury in this study was 29%.[1]

It is not in the scope of this chapter to discuss in detail cervical fractures and dislocations and treatment. This will be discussed in depth in Chapter 104. However, they account for the majority of significant neurologic sequelae in the game of football.

Lumbar Spine

Low-back pain is a common presenting symptom among football players.[10] It has been reported to occur anywhere from 21% to approximately 27% of the time during a player's career. Wooden reported that 6% of high school players sustain lower-back injuries.[36] Over 20% of college football players will lose playing time because of a lumbar spine problem.[10,18,29] A survey of injuries in the National Football League showed a 12% incidence of spine injuries resulting in lost playing time.[24]

Low-back pain in football players can have many causes. Soft-tissue injury likely accounts for the majority of symptoms, and with treatment usually resolves over 4 to 6 weeks. Saal found that 70% of football-related lumbar spine problems involved the posterior elements, another 25% were injuries to the intervertebral disc.[25]

Lumbar spondylolysis occurs in approximately 6% of the adult population. It is reported to occur much more frequently in athletes participating in contact sports such as football.[10,15,18] The increased incidence is thought to be the result of repetitive forces being transmitted to the pars interarticularis.[10] Linemen who repeatedly hyperextend the spine in a three-point stance place additional stress on this area. The flexed position results in loss of lordosis and compression and narrowing of the disc spaces anteriorly, thus putting great stress on the pars interarticularis. The upward and forward drive and extension of the lumbar spine during contact puts shearing forces across the zygoapophyseal joints. This repetitive stress may cause a fracture through the pars interarticularis.[10] Other causes of injuries, such as weight training, may also be implicated in football players.[8,24] Ferguson et al. noted an incidence of 50% spondylolysis in interior linemen presenting with low-back pain.[10] Hoshina found that athletes with spondylolysis had greater body weight and back muscle strength, possibly allowing greater force to be exerted on the spine in hyperextension.[15] McCarroll et al. evaluated lumbar spondylolysis and spondylolisthesis in college football players.[18] They found an initial incidence of 13.1% and noted that a defect developed in 2.4% of players during their careers, for an overall incidence of 15.2%. However, none of the athletes with spondylolysis or spondy-

lolisthesis failed to complete their careers at the college level.[18]

Semon and Spengler also found no significant difference in time lost in practice or games between players with symptomatic spondylolysis and players who complained of low-back pain only.[29] In view of the data, players with spondylolysis should not necessarily be discouraged from the sport of football.

Although infrequently reported, lumbar disc disease can cause symptoms in football players. Day and Friedman found that down linemen were most commonly affected.[9] Radiculopathy is less obvious and the straight-leg-raise test is generally not striking. They recommended that surgical intervention be kept at a minimum after failure of consecutive therapy.[9] None of the individuals who had an open procedure were able to return to their former activity levels.

White (personal communication) has found that at professional and collegiate levels, players can return to play after laminotomy and discectomy for lumbar herniated nucleus pulposus, but this requires aggressive post-operative stabilization and strength training.

Preventing Injuries

Football is a physical contact sport and will therefore have associated injuries. However, this does not mean that significant improvement in injury reduction cannot be made. In the early years of football, fatal injuries led to changes in both rules and football gear. The football helmet has changed from simple leather protection to helmets that now must meet or exceed laboratory standards and guidelines (NOCSAE).[12] This has led to fewer neurotrauma fatalities.[9] Concerns that the helmet may be causing cervical cord injuries due to posterior edge impingement during forced hyperextension has been found to be unwarranted.[9,11,28] But one must understand that the helmet cannot be expected to protect the spinal cord or neck from injury. The helmet must not only meet acceptable standards, but it also must fit correctly if it is expected to function properly.

Shoulder pads are also very important and must fit properly to afford protection. Various types of shoulder pads are now manufactured, depending on position. Their primary function is to afford protection for the shoulder region. A common accessory is a cervical collar. Used appropriately, they appear to block cervical motion. However, their value has been questioned, and to date no studies on their efficiency have been done. In general, equipment must meet NOCSAE guidelines and fit well and be well maintained to afford maximum player protection.

It has been shown that appropriate rules changes and proper equipment can decrease injuries in football. The question is whether physical conditioning and training can also lead to fewer injuries in football, specifically spinal injuries. Cahill and Griffith found that total-body preseason conditioning significantly reduced the number and severity of knee injuries.[5] No studies are currently available on conditioning and its effect on spinal injuries in football, but one could logically assume that increased strength and flexibility as well as conditioning could potentially decrease these injuries and their recurrence.[13] Funk and Wells noted that the development of strong neck musculature could reasonably be expected to prevent many neck injuries, and exercises to develop neck strength should be a part of all preseason conditioning.[11] Cantu states that the neck can be strengthened and the risk of injury reduced.[6] While controversy exists as to whether the neck can be conditioned to withstand the maximum forces to which it is subject in contact sports, a neck exercise program as suggested by the National Football League (NFL) Management Council is universally agreed to minimize the risk of neck injury. Other authors have recommended low-back and neck strengthening, as well as stretching exercises for protective flexibility and range of motion in hopes of decreasing and preventing injuries.

Maroon et al. showed that with simple isotonic exercises, neck strength improved and neck circumference could be increased over 1 in. in 6 weeks in college football players.[16] The authors thought that proper conditioning of neck musculature may help reduce spinal cord injuries. It is therefore reasonable to assume that with physical conditioning and training one can afford protection to the cervical and lumbar spine by maintaining good flexibility, body mechanics, and increasing strength in the neck, shoulder unit, and lumbar region.

Rehabilitation and Stabilization Training

The first and foremost step in rehabilitation of cervical and lumbar injuries will be accurate diagnosis. History, physical examination, diagnostic tests, and imaging studies are paramount. Once an accurate diagnosis is made, appropriate short-term management can be initiated.

Following resolution of symptoms associated with the acute injury, it is important to place the player in a satisfactory rehabilitation program that will pre-pare him to return to football with satisfactory strength and flexibility that will help minimize further injury. At our institution we utilize a program termed "stabilization training." Whether it is applied to the cervical or lumbar region it is a program of education, strength, flexibility and movement patterns that attempts to decrease pain and protect the spine.[23] Muscle fusion involves the use of muscles to brace the spine and protect the motion segments from repetitive microtrauma and excessively high single-occurrence loads.[26,27] The goal of stabilization training is to obtain adequate strength and control of the spine to help minimize injury.[24,27]

Stabilization training is a tiered system that begins with simple non-weight-bearing supported positions and advances to complex functional activities. Initial training builds the foundation on which functional athlete-specific activities will be based. Basic stabilization training is quickly mastered by motivated athletes. Within a few short weeks they are advanced to functional athlete-specific activities. Here athletes can apply basic stabilization principles to the playing field.[27] This direct application of training principles to the football field is very important for athletes. They are much more willing to utilize stabilization techniques if they can see direct application to their sport.

The program of retraining athletes involves changing their current patterns of play to more safe spine patterns by evaluating current playing techniques.[26] A particular football activity can be broken down into segments, and trouble spots can be identified. A player can practice each segment using stabilization techniques and perform in a controlled environment, gradually increasing to full speed.[8] Once mastered, the player returns to the playing field. The new pattern becomes an engram so that the athlete will be able to continue to maintain a spine safe position while playing contact sports[27] (Figs. 48-1 and 48-2). Stabilization training techniques can be applied to either the cervical or lumbar region, the details of which will be covered in other chapters.[48]

These principles are applied not only to the playing field, but are also incorporated in a gym program with machines and free weights. The gym program serves three functions. It allows a player additional practice of stabilization techniques in a controlled gym environment. It also returns physical strength and endurance that was lost during the period of injury. Flexibility is also emphasized, and appropriate stretching techniques are used to maintain range of motion.

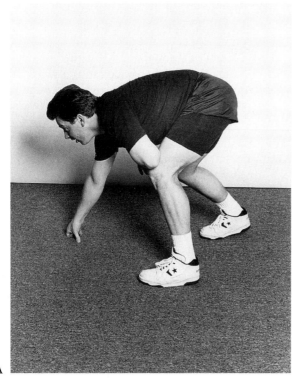

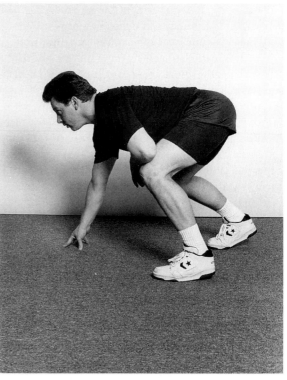

Fig. 48-1

A, Lineman in unsafe three-point stance, flexion promotes risk of spinal injury. **B,** Lineman in spine-safe three-point stance, which includes alignment of spine in position that reduces risk of injury.

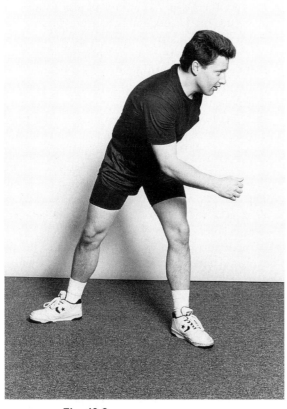

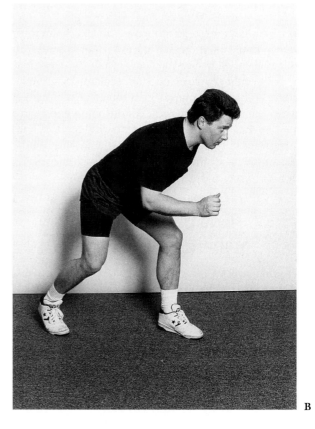

Fig. 48-2

A, Defensive back in unsafe spine position; turning upfield from back pedal with twisting back. **B,** Defensive back in safe spine position; turning upfield from back pedal with pivot and simultaneous hip and shoulder turn upfield.

By training the athlete in spine-safe patterns and increasing his strength and flexibility before returning to play, further injuries can be minimized.

Summary

The possibility of catastrophic injuries to the spine will always be present. To keep them to a minimum, players should be taught the proper blocking and tackling techniques, and rules prohibiting dangerous circumstances should be enforced. Continued improvement in player equipment should also result in fewer injuries. Finally, by encouraging proper conditioning, strengthening, and flexibility exercises, the number of football injuries can be reduced. Further research is still needed to evaluate other potential changes that might make football a safer sport.

References

1. Albright JP, McAuley E, Martin, RK, et al.: Head and neck injuries in college football: an eight-year analysis, *Am J Sports Med* 13:147, 1985.
2. Albright JP, Moses JM, Feldick HG: Nonfatal cervical spine injuries in interscholastic football, *JAMA* 236:1243, 1976.
3. Blyth CS, Mueller FO: Injury rates vary with coaching; *Physician Sportsmed* 3:45-50, 1974.
4. Cahill BR, Griffith EH: Exposure to injury in major college football, *Am J Sports Med* 17:183, 1979.
5. Cahill BR, Griffith EH: Effect of protection conditioning on incidence and severity of high school football knee injuries, *Am J Sports Med* 6:180, 1978.
6. Cantu RC: Head and spine injuries in the young athlete, *Clin Sports Med* 7:459, 1988.
7. Clarke KS, Powell JW: Football helmets and neurotrauma—an epidemiological overview of three seasons, *Med Sci Sports* 2:138, 1979.
8. Cook T: The professional athlete, *Occup Med State Art Rev* 7:87, 1992.
9. Day AL, Friedman WA: Observations on the treatment of lumbar disc disease in college football players, *Am J Sports Med* 15:72, 1987.
10. Ferguson RJ, McMaster JH, et al.: Low back pain in college football linemen, *J Sports Med* 2:63, 1974.
11. Funk FJ, Wells RE: Injuries of the cervical spine in football, *C.O.R.R.* 109:50, 1975.
12. Gieck J, McCue FC: Fitting of protective football equipment, *Am J Sports Med* 8:192, 1980.
13. Glisan B, Hochschuler SH: *General fitness in the treatment and prevention of athletic low back injuries. The Spine in sports,* Philadelphia, 1990, Hanley & Belfus, Inc.
14. Halpern B, Thompson N, et al.: High school football injuries: identifying the risk factors, *Am J Sports Med* 15:113, 1987.
15. Hoshina H: Spondylolysis in athletes, *Physician Sportsmed* 8(9):75, 1980.
16. Maroon JC, Kerin T, et al.: A system for preventing athletic neck injuries, *Physician Sportsmed* 77, 1977.
17. Maroon JC, Steele PB, Berlin R: Football head and neck injuries—an update, *Clin Neurosurg* 27:414, 1980.
18. McCarroll JR, Miller JM, Ritter MA: Lumbar spondylolysis and spondylolisthesis in college football players, *Am J Sports Med* 14:404, 1986.
19. Mueller FO, Blyth CS: Annual survey of catastrophic football injuries: 1977 to 1983, *Physician Sportsmed* 13(3):75, 1985.
20. Mueller FO, Schindler RD: Annual survey of football injury research 1931-1986, 1987; American Football Coaches Assoc, NCAA, and National Federation of State High School Assoc.
21. Nicholas JA, Rosenthal PP, Gleim GW: A historical perspective of injuries in professional football, *JAMA* 260:939, 1988.
22. Pritchett JW: High cost of high school football injuries, *Am J Sports Med* 8:197, 1980.
23. Robison R: The new back school prescription: stabilization training, part I. *Occup Med* 7:17, 1992.
24. Saal JA: Common American football injuries, *Sports Med* 12:132, 1991.
25. Saal JA: Rehabilitation of football players with lumbar spine injury (part 1), *Physician Sportsmed* 16(9):61, 1988.
26. Saal JA: Rehabilitation of football players with lumbar spine injury (part 2), *Physician Sportsmed* 16(10):117, 1988.
27. Saal JA: The new back school prescription: stabilization training, part II. *Occup Med* 7:33, 1992.
28. Schneider RC, Reifel E, Crisler HO, et al.: Serious and fatal football injuries involving the head and spinal cord, *JAMA* 177:362-367, 1961.
29. Semon RL, Spengler D: Significance of lumbar spondylolysis in college football players, *Spine* 6:172, 1981.
30. Sweeney T: Neck school: cervicothoracic stabilization training, *Occup Med* 7:43, 1992.
31. Torg JS, Vegso JJ, O'Neill MJ, et al.: The epidemiologic, pathologic, biomechanical, and cinematographic analysis of football-induced cervical spine trauma, *Am J Sports Med* 18:50, 1990.
32. Torg JS, Pavlov H, O'Neill MJ, et al.: The axial load teardrop fracture, a biomechanical, clinical and roentgenographic analysis, *Am J Sports Med* 19:355, 1991.
33. Torg JS, Sennett B, Vegso JJ, Pavlov H: Axial loading injuries to the middle cervical spine segment, *Am J Sports Med* 19:6, 1991.
34. Torg JS, Vegso JJ, Sennett B, Das M: The national football head and neck injury registry, *JAMA* 254:3439, 1985.
35. Torg JS, Truex R, Quedenfeld TC, et al.: The national football head and neck injury registry, JAMA 241:1477, 1979.
36. Wooden MJ: Preseason screening of the lumbar spine, *J Orthop Sport Phys Ther* 3:6, 1981.
37. Zemper ED: Injury rates in a national sample of college football teams: a 2-year, *Physician Sportsmed* 17:100, 1989.

Additional Readings

1. Barber FA: The lumbar spine in football, *Spine State Art Rev* 4:809, 1990.

2. Cantu RC: Catastrophic injuries in high school and collegiate athletes, *Surg Rounds Orthop* 62, 1988.

3. Cantu RC: Cervical spinal stenosis, challenging an established detection method, *Physician Sportsmed* 21 (9):57, 1993.

4. Duda M: Jets study: major injuries decrease, *Physician Sportsmed* 17(11):32, 1989.

5. Eismont FJ, Clifford J, et al.: Cervical sagittal spinal canal size in spine injury, *Spine* 8:663, 1984.

6. Feldick HG, Albright JP: Football survey reveals "missed" neck injuries, *Physician Sportsmed* 77, 1976.

7. Firooznia H, Jung HA, et al.: Sudden quadriplegia after a minor trauma. The role of pre-existing spinal stenosis, *Surg Neurol* 23:165, 1985.

8. Fourré M: On-site management of cervical spine injuries, *Physician Sportsmed* 19(4):53, 1991.

9. Goldberg B, Rosenthal PP: Injuries in youth football, *Physician Sportsmed* 12(8):122, 1984

10. Goldberg B, Rosenthal PP, et al.: Injuries in youth football, *Pediatrics* 81:255, 1988.

11. Grant TT, Puffer J: Cervical stenosis: a developmental anomaly with quadriparesis during football, *Am J Sports Med* 4:219, 1976.

12. Herzog RJ, Wiens JJ, et al.: Normal cervical spine morphometry and cervical spinal stenosis in asymptomatic professional football players, *Spine* 18(suppl):176, 1991.

13. Jackson DW, Lohr FT: Cervical spine injuries, *Clin Sports Med* 5:373, 1986.

14. Ladd AL, Scranton PE: Congenital cervical stenosis presenting as transient quadriplegia in athletes, *J Bone Joint Surg* 68A:1371, 1986.

15. Leidholt JD: Spinal injuries in athletes: be prepared, *Orthop Clin North Am* 4:691, 1993.

16. Matsuura P, Waters RL, Adkins RH, et al.: Comparison of computerized tomography parameters of the cervical spine in normal control subjects and spinal cord-injured patients, *J Bone Joint Surg* 71A:183, 1989.

17. Nuber GW, Schaffer MF: Clay shovelers' injuries, a report of two injuries sustained from football, *Am J Sports Med* 15:182, 1987.

18. Odor JM, Watkins RG, Dillin WH, et al.: Incidence of cervical spine stenosis in professional and rookie football players, *Am J Sports Med* 18:507, 1990.

19. Thompson N, Halpern G, Curl WW, et al.: High school football injuries: evaluation, *Am J Sports Med* 15:117, 1987.

20. Torg JS, Pavlov H, Genuario S, et al.: Neurapraxia of the cervical spinal cord with transient quadriplegia, *J Bone Joint Surg* 68A:1354, 1986.

21. Torg JS, Truex RC, Marshall J, et al.: Spinal injury at the level of the third and fourth cervical vertebrae from football, *J Bone Joint Surg* 59A:1015, 1977.

22. Torg JS, Pavlov H, et al.: Cervical spinal stenosis with cord neuropraxia and transient quadriplegia in athletes, *Surg Rounds Orthop* 9:19, 1987.

23. Watkins RG, Dillin WH, et al.: Cervical spine injuries in football players, *Spine State Art Rev* 4:391, 1990.

24. Watkins RG: Neck injuries in football players, *Clin Sports Med* 5:215, 1986.

Chapter 49
Golf

Kevin Finnesey

Back injuries are common in the game of golf, even though to some golf is not considered a physically demanding sport. It is a sport played by people of all ages and athletic abilities. A wide spectrum of injuries can occur.[1] Some players are in excellent physical condition, many are not. Even veteran touring professionals are subject to injury, although their injury patterns differ from those of novice, poorly conditioned players. This chapter will describe how back injuries occur during the golf swing as well as the prevention of such injuries. It stresses the importance that flexibility and strengthening have in the game of golf and includes various other "back savers" that the reader should find helpful.

Incidence and Etiology

Multiple injury patterns are common in the amateur as well as the professional golfer.[18] These include injuries to the back, shoulders, elbows (epicondylitis), wrists, and hands (hook of the hamate fractures),[6] as well as tibial stress fractures[5] and patellar osteochondral fractures.[10] Batt[1,2] conducted a survey of injuries in 461 amateur golfers, to which 193 responded. Of these, 57% reported a history of injuries, including wrist, back, muscle sprain, elbow, and knee problems. Overuse and poor technique were thought to be causes.

A number of specific back injuries are encountered in golfers. Most involve sprains and strains of joints and muscles in the low back. However, some unusual problems may occur that may be difficult to diagnose. Schultz and Leonard[17] described four patients with upper thoracic and shoulder pain associated with scapular winging. This was proven to be a stretch injury to the long thoracic nerve diagnosed by electromyography (EMG), and improved with exercise and range-of-motion exercises for the shoulder. Hsu[9] encountered six patients with back pain and chest pain in whom stress fractures developed in the ribs, which resulted from a pulled serratus anterior muscle during the golf swing. This was diagnosed with technetium-99 scintigraphy. Ekin and Sinaki[3] described the cases of three postmenopausal patients, all long-term golfers who sustained vertebral compression fractures during midswing.

Golf, unlike many sports, is an activity that is enjoyed well into late adult life and is often played more frequently as one gets older. Retired individuals have more time to enjoy the sport. These individuals may have preexisting degenerative skeletal conditions that can lead to overuse injuries due to the repetitive nature of the golf swing.[11] This emphasizes the importance of routine flexibility and strengthening exercises to avoid these injuries.

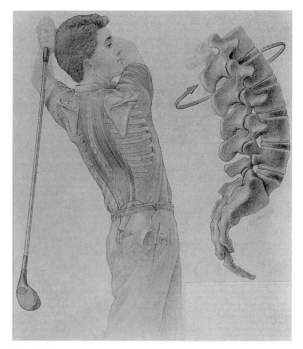

Fig. 49-1
Golf swing exerts considerable torsional forces on spine. *(From Stover C, Mallon W: Golf injuries: treating the play to treat the player, J Musculoskel Med 9:58, 1992.)*

The Warmup

As in other sports, warmup is important in preventing golf injuries to the spine.[4] Golfers who walk up to the first tee at 7 a.m. after a week of being sedentary, take out the driver, and take their hardest swing at the ball are likely to have an injury. More experienced players are well conditioned and have good muscle flexibility as well as strength. Safran et al.[15] examined the biomechanical role of warmup in preventing muscular injuries. Tears were produced in rabbit lower limb muscles that were preconditioned (stimulated before stretch) and nonstimulated controls. Elements examined included force and change of length required to tear the muscle, site of failure, and length tension deformation. He found that preconditioned muscles require more force to fail and stretched to a greater length before failure than controls. Length tension deformation curves showed that preconditioned muscles attained a lesser force at each length before failure, indicating an increase in elasticity. He concluded that preconditioned muscles can be stretched to greater length before failure and have a greater tendency to return to normal length after being stretched.

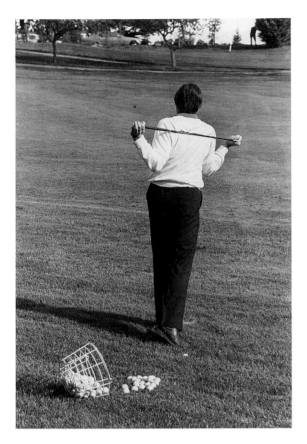

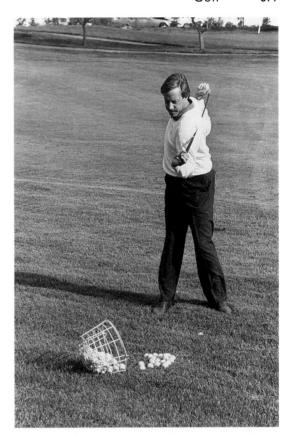

Fig. 49-2

To increase flexibility, hold club behind head across shoulders and rotate torso.

With respect to the spine, it can be inferred that with better flexibility and elasticity of the muscles, excessive stresses on the spine and trunk muscles are dissipated, thereby decreasing torsional loads on the intervertebral disc. The trunk muscles are the most common area injured during the golf swing. Pink et al.[14] demonstrated that these muscles are firing at a high and constant rate during most of the swing; this demonstrates the importance of conditioning these muscles.

As mentioned above, golf is a sport that produces excessive torsion or twisting of the back (Fig. 49-1). Considerable torque is required to produce an effective golf swing.

A proper warmup involves a few simple exercises before and after the golf game. Holding the club behind the head across the shoulders and slowly rotating the body to simulate a golf swing helps loosen up and stretch the shoulders, trunk, and hips (Fig. 49-2). Using a weighted club, or swinging two or three clubs at a time, also helps to loosen up. Hamstring and hip stretches can also be done (Figs.

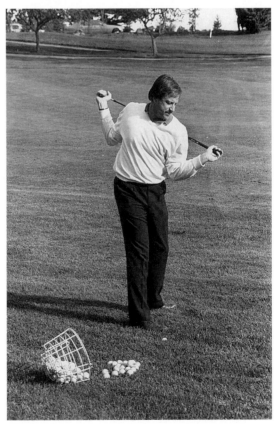

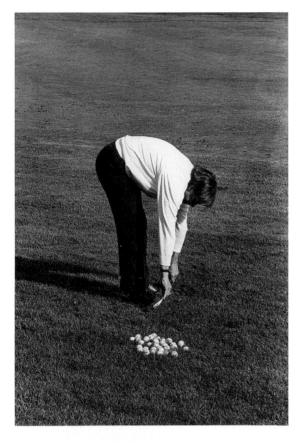

49-3 and 49-4). Any of the basic stabilization exercises given in Chapters 27 and 28 can be of great value.

Before starting the round of golf it is helpful to hit some practice shots (Fig. 49-5). Start with short, compact easy swings and work up to the longer shots gradually. Some players prefer to take one club, such as an 8-iron and hit shots with a half or three quarter swing. Again it defeats the purpose to pull out the driver immediately and hit the ball hard.

The Golf Swing

Learning the proper technique of the golf swing can also help to avoid injury. Swinging too hard and improperly can put unwanted stresses on the back. Touring professionals are able to generate tremendous club head speed through the hitting area (lower part of the arc of the swing) with little effort. This comes with years of practice and experience. The shoulders, torso, hips, knees, and ankles all should work in an effortless, interconnected, fluid-like motion. The goal is to limit the stresses in the low back and allow hip and shoulder turn to generate power.

Fig. 49-3
Hamstring stretch.

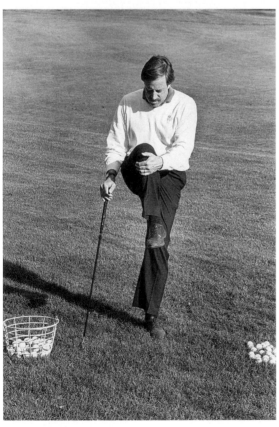

Fig. 49-4
Hip stretch.

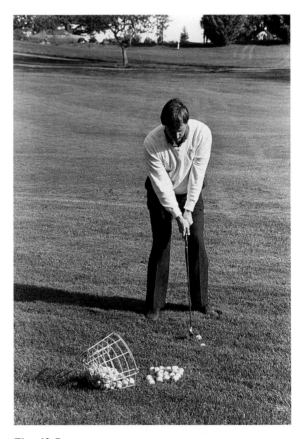

Fig. 49-5
Hit a few easy shots on range before play.

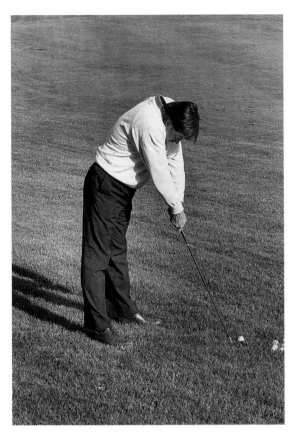

Fig. 49-6

Improper setup.

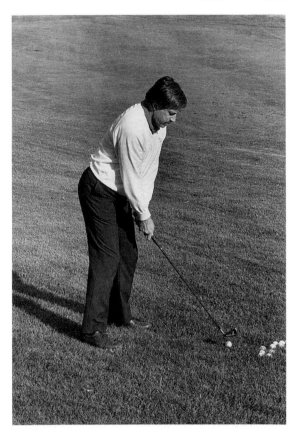

Fig. 49-7

Proper setup.

Inexperienced players tend to swing hard with the arms while keeping the legs and feet motionless and stiff, or to release the wrists too early, known as "swinging from the top." The novice will learn that a smooth, well-timed swing with the whole body working in unison can generate more power and accuracy than trying to swing hard with the arms only and "knock the cover off the ball."

The setup is an important prerequisite for a good swing. Proper stance and posture allow the swing to be generated effectively. This allows the golfer to be balanced and poised during the entire swing from take-away to follow-through.[7] The setup and swing should be routine and reproducible. When the pros seem to be fidgeting and waggling the hips just before swinging the club, they are concentrating on their setup.[7] These motions relieve tension and fine-tune the final address position.[13] If the feet are too wide, the knees tend to lock. This restricts the lower body during the swing. If the stance is too narrow, it is easy to lose one's balance during the swing. For a good setup, the feet should be approximately shoulder-width for mid-irons, slightly wider for long

irons and woods, slightly narrower for more lofted clubs. The spine should be straight, not hunched over, and tilted slightly forward so one's weight is distributed equally on the balls of the feet. The knees should be slightly bent and the shoulders relaxed (Figs. 49-6 and 49-7).

The take-away should be low, slow, and smooth.[13] Fast, jerky movements can cause sharp, sudden loading patterns on the muscles and discs. During the swing the trunk, or the area between the shoulder and the hips, responds to the shoulders and arms on one hand, and the hips and legs on the other. It follows what the shoulders and hips are doing.[19] At the top of the swing the back should be turned so it roughly faces the target. This requires considerable flexibility. On the follow-through one should be well balanced and facing the target (Fig. 49-8).

Videotaping one's swing can be very helpful.[12] Observing the swing from various angles with help from your golf professional, as well as slow-motion analysis can allow the golfer to visualize his or her mistakes graphically. Athletic trainers and physical therapists can also become involved in pointing out

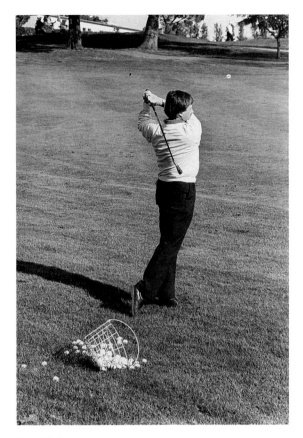

Fig. 49-8

Follow-through. This "classic swing" creates less hyperextension of lumbar spine in follow-through.

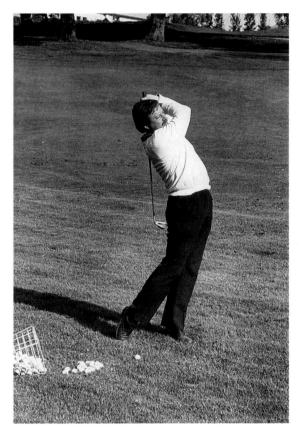

Fig. 49-9

Large turn and extended, arched lumbar spine produces "reverse C."

aggravating factors in the golf swing. They can also instruct the golfer in strength and flexibility exercise.[16] Sport-specific back schools are available at many spine centers, where back injuries are treated in addition to the patient being taught back awareness and body mechanics that can carry over into any sport or activity.

As indicated earlier in this chapter, considerable tensional forces are generated on the low back during the golf swing, and swinging too hard using improper techniques can produce injury. Stover and Mallon[18] illustrate two different types of golf swings. The first is known as the "modern swing." This consists of a large shoulder and hip turn on the back swing with an arched lumbar spine on the follow-through, commonly known as the "reverse C." This produces tremendous forces on the lumbar discs and other joints and takes them to the end range, where back injuries tend to occur. This is the swing pattern of many of the top touring pros today (Fig. 49-9).

Observing this physically demanding swing pattern, one can understand why *Golf Digest* reported

that 75% of all touring pros have experienced back injuries, even experienced players with extremely well-tuned and grooved golf swings. One can only imagine how this will affect the unconditioned amateur golfer.[8]

The second type of swing is known as the "classic swing." This swing involves less arching of the lower back on follow-through, with equal turn of the hips and shoulders. The lumbar spine is straighter on follow-through. The swing is also shorter. Reverting to this type of swing may be helpful for the recovering back-injured golfer (see Fig. 49-8). Instead of using hyperextension and torque of the lumbar spine to generate power, the golfer can emphasize hip turn and weight shifting of the lower body to generate power.

"Back Savers"

In addition to switching to the "classic swing," various other "back savers" are useful in maintaining a healthy back on the golf course. Bending at the knee

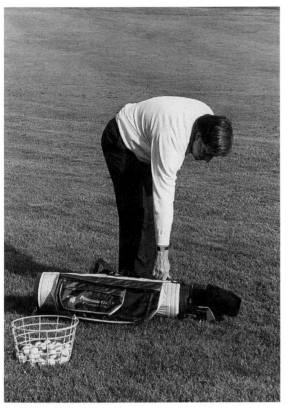

Fig. 49-10
Repeated bending to pick up bag.

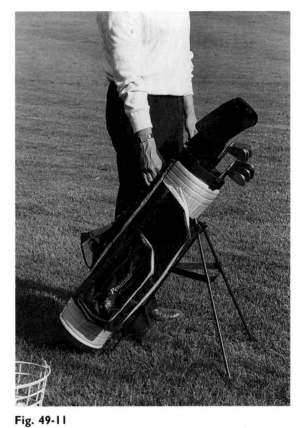

Fig. 49-11
Bag stand.

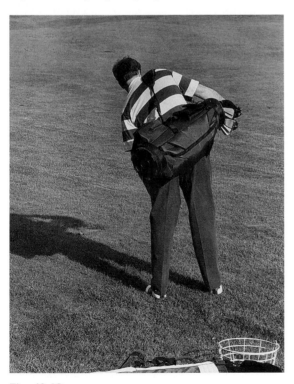

Fig. 49-12
Asymmetric posture carrying bag.

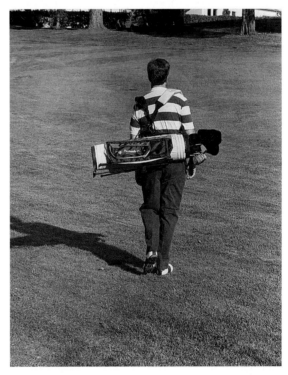

Fig. 49-13
"Izzo strap."

to tee up the ball or to pick the ball up out of the hole is suggested. Quadriceps strength is a prerequisite for this and all proper body mechanics in general (see Chapters 27 and 28). There are commercially available golf bag stands that reduce the amount of repeated bending to pick up the golf bag (Figs. 49-10 and 49- 11). There are also straps for the golf bag such as the "Izzo strap," in which two straps are used over the shoulders when carrying the bag instead of one, allowing one to walk with the back straighter when carrying the bag (Figs. 49-12 and 49-13).

Playing golf requires repetitive bending, lifting, walking, standing, and twisting. The proper body mechanics and postures for these activities are commonly taught in back schools. The strength, endurance, flexibility, and stabilization necessary to prevent injury can be learned through training (see Chapters 23, 25, 26, 27, and 28). Playing golf can reinforce such training and one's game can become more successful as a result.

Summary

Golf injuries are common but easily preventable with good warmup and attention to style. The basic principles of lumbar and cervical thoracic stabilization training are readily applicable to the game of golf.

Special thanks to Tom Toschi, Head Golf Professional, Peninsula Golf and Country Club, San Mateo, Calif.

References

1. Batt ME: Golfing injuries, an overview, *Sports Med* 16:64, 1993.
2. Batt ME: A survey of golf injuries in amateur golfers, *Br J Sports Med* 26:63, 1992.
3. Ekin JA, Sinaki M: Vertebral compression fractures sustained during golfing: a report of 3 cases, *Mayo Clinic Proc* 68:566, 1993.
4. Flock K, Gradinger R, Opitz G, Hipp E: Medical advice for golfers, *Fortschr Med* 107:7746, 1989.
5. Gregori AC: Tibial stress fractures in two professional golfers, *J Bone Joint Surg* 76B:157, 1994.
6. Gupta A, Risitano G, Crawford R, Burke F: Fractures of the hook of the hamate injury, *Injury* 20(suppl):284, 1989.
7. Hogan B: *Five lessons, the modern fundamentals of golf.* New York, 1957, Simon & Schuster.
8. Hochschuler S: *Back in shape: a back owner's manual.* Boston, 1991, Houghton Mifflin Co.
9. Hsu CY: Stress fracture of the ribs in amateur golfers diagnosed by Tc-99m MDP scintigraphy, *Kao Hsiung I Hsueh Ko Hsueh Tsa Chih* 9:381, 1993.
10. Isaacs CL, Schreiber FC: Patellar osteochondral fracture: the unforseen hazard of golf, *Am J Sports Med* 20(suppl):613, 1992.
11. Jobe FW, Schwab DM: Golf for the mature athlete, *Clin Sports Med* 10:264, 1991.
12. Leadbetter D: *The golf swing,* New York, 1990, Stephen Greene Press.
13. Norman G: *Shark attack! Greg Norman's guide to aggressive golf,* New York, 1988, Simon & Schuster.
14. Pink M, Perry J, Jobe FW: Electromyographic analysis of the trunk in golfers, *Am J Sports Med* 21:385, 1993.
15. Safran MR, et al.: The role of warmup in muscular injury prevention, *Am J Sports Med* 16:123, 1988.
16. Saunders HD: *Back injury prevention: role of strength and flexibility exercises.* In White AH, Anderson R: *Conservative care of low back pain,* Baltimore, 1991, Williams & Wilkins.
17. Schultz JS, Leonard JA Jr: Long thoracic neuropathy from athletic activity, *Arch Phys Med Rehab* 73:87, 1992.
18. Stover C, Mallon W: Golf injuries: treating the play to treat the player, *J Musculoskel Med* 9:58, 1992.
19. Toski B, Love O: *How to feel a real golf swing,* New York, 1988, Random House and Golf Digest/Tennis Inc.

Chapter 50
Ice Hockey
Paul J. Slosar, Jr.

Biomechanics of Skating
Basic Stabilization Training
Advanced Stabilization Training
Skating Drills
Passing/Shooting Drills
Collision Drills

The grace of ice hockey is best appreciated as players effortlessly glide over the frozen surface, snapping crisp passes from stick to stick. This tranquil environment is frequently shattered as opposition players intercede with locomotive force, reversing the forward progression of the puck. This interruption requires the offensive players to halt immediately, reverse direction, and pursue a defensive posture at full speed. It is now their turn to extract the puck forcefully from the opposing side. This relentless change of direction, coupled with frequent high-speed collisions, exerts a high toll on its participants.

Skating traces its roots to the Netherlands, with early reports dating back to the Middle Ages.[4] The first recorded hockey game was between two American colleges in 1894.[10] Professional hockey began in 1917 and its popularity has grown steadily since then. The American Hockey Association estimates that it has 300,000 youth players, and 12,000 teams.[10]

As player skill level increases with age, we find the most competitive athletes at the elite, college, semiprofessional, and professional levels. As players progress from pre–high school to professional ranks, the incidence rate of injuries increases dramatically, with the elite players averaging one injury per 7 hours of play.[11]

Hockey is a collision sport, and players must be prepared both to deliver and to withstand high-speed impacts, or checks. Typically players are involved in two types of checks. The high-speed open-ice check can be compared to a head-on collision between two cars. The other check involves one player being compressed between an opposition player and the boards, which are anchored in place. Players are more vulnerable in the boarding check as they have little room to escape a direct hit, and are often trapped in a compromising, nonphysiologic position at the time of impact. The boards themselves have a ridge, which is waist-high, where the fiberglass meets the baseboard. This ridge can also cause direct injury to exposed areas.

Contact accounts for the vast majority of ice hockey injuries. This contact may be from the puck, stick, ice, boards, goal post, or other players.[4,5] Overall, back injuries are a small percentage of injuries sustained in ice hockey. Several studies place the injuries to the trunk or back at 7% to 8%.[6,7] Although head and eye injuries have been reduced with improved helmets and face shields, catastrophic spinal injuries are still periodically reported.[12] Rule changes to reduce the incidence of cross-checking, boarding, and checking from behind have been instituted to reduce these injuries. It is the purpose of

this chapter to address the rehabilitation of acute back injuries in ice hockey in an effort to return the athlete to competition.

As hockey injuries result from impact, back injuries tend to be soft-tissue contusions, ligamentous sprains, and rarely bony fractures. Players wear protective girdle and shoulder pads, but the lower thoracic and upper lumbar spine can easily be exposed as players reach their arms away from their bodies. If the torso is turned or rotated as impact occurs, the abdominal and paraspinal musculature, as well as spinal ligamentous structure are pathologically stressed.

Most incidents of low-back pain in the athletes respond quickly to accepted forms of conservative treatment.[13] Most team trainers are familiar with the use of methods for the care of acute soft-tissue contusions.

The acute inflammatory phase can be controlled with analgesics, antiinflammatory medications, and the judicious use of muscle relaxants in addition to therapeutic cold methods. Rehabilitation now concentrates on restoring strength and flexibility, aerobic conditioning, and eventual return to full function. As mentioned previously, the basic requirement of these athletes is resumption of skating. After this is accomplished, the therapist must direct the training toward rotatory strength and balance. As the players pass and shoot the puck, they place a distinct torsional demand on the spine. Finally, strengthening will allow the hockey player to withstand and deliver body checks confidently as he anticipates returning to competition.

Biomechanics of Skating

The evaluation and rehabilitation of acute back injury in a competitive hockey player requires a basic understanding of the biomechanics of ice skating. Faster players have the advantage in hockey. Slower or unbalanced skaters are more vulnerable to injury and are less effective team players. Researchers have found that the fastest skaters tend to take longer and wider strides, and have a greater forward lean on the trunk and legs.[8] Slower skaters tend to skate straight-up, while the quicker, more balanced skaters lean forward at the waist with the back approaching a horizontal. As a skater fatigues, he/she tends to stand up.[3] This reflects fatigue of the quadriceps, hip extensors, and lumbar paraspinal muscle groups. The hockey player recovering from an acute back injury will fatigue these muscles more quickly; therefore, a rehabilitation program must concentrate on these areas.

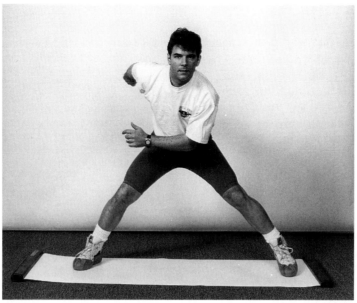

Fig. 50-1

Off-ice skating drill on a slideboard.

Basic Stabilization Training

Specific rehabilitation techniques for the hockey player with a nonoperative back injury must begin with a generalized program. We advocate the use of "Stabilization Training" as a multifaceted program that helps patients manage their low-back injury and prevent future recurrences.[9] The training program educates the athlete, while advancing flexibility, strength, coordination, and endurance training as the patient progresses. A therapist experienced in advanced stabilization techniques will be instrumental in returning the injured hockey player to competition. For a complete discussion of stabilization training, please see Robison[9] and Chapter 27 in this book.

Advanced Stabilization Training

After the hockey player has mastered the basics, advanced techniques specific to ice hockey should be employed. The first goal is resumption of skating. This is beneficial, for it allows resumption of aerobic conditioning and is the framework on which shooting and passing skills are rebuilt. The key muscles for trunk control are the abdominals and the spinal extensors.[1,2] Exhaustive detail to strengthening these groups is essential before skating drills begin. Hip flexors, quadriceps, hamstring, and gluteal muscles must also be strengthened, as these are critical for keeping the hockey player in a stable, crouched position with his back horizontal. Squat thrusts and weight lifting can be used as the patient advances. Rigorous abdominal strengthening is required to keep a neutral lumbopelvic tilt.

Skating Drills

Skating simulation is best accomplished with a slideboard (Fig. 50-1). This device allows the hockey player to begin off-ice skating posture drills under direct observation. The therapist can reinforce proper body mechanics while the athlete trains critical muscle groups and builds endurance.

In-line skating is a logical next step in training if the ice rink is unavailable. Again, the basics of stable zone body mechanics should be repetitively reinforced to make it instinctive for the athlete. In-line skating is an excellent off-season training adjunct, and is useful to the rehabilitating hockey player. The player should hold his hockey stick during in-line skating. This gives an accurate representation of his typical posture during games, and should be taken into account during this phase of rehabilitation. Videotaping the player's skating posture is valuable for providing direct visual feedback.

On-ice resistance drills will build skating strength and endurance. The player can skate forward, pushing against another player who provides resistance with his skates. Stop/start drills and skating around obstacles should follow.

Passing/Shooting Drills

All of the subsequent drills should be perfected while stationary before coupling them with skating. Passing and shooting require rotation of the spine. Attempt to minimize this torsional stress by absorbing the rotation at the hips, knees, and shoulders.

Maintaining rigid, tight control through the power portion of the swing is critical. Videotaping can also be useful at this juncture in rehabilitation.

Off-ice trunk rotation drills with a stick should be advanced, encouraging the player to rotate fully, as he would during a slap-shot. Stress the mechanics of a controlled swing and follow-through before concentrating on aim. Most players will fall into a swing pattern that has developed over many years and will not be able to alter it significantly.

Collision Drills

A player's return to competition will require him to tolerate body checks. As there is no way to specifically train for these events, the best way to minimize the trauma is to be conditioned. Elite hockey players possess the inherent strength and agility to avoid the contact when possible, and they stabilize themselves when a hit is unavoidable. The unseen or unanticipated collision is usually the most devastating. For that reason, reinforcing constant trunk control and muscle stabilization from the onset of training is critical. To prepare the player for these collisions, stand him on a narrow balance beam close to the floor. Toss a medicine ball at his trunk, not to catch, but to force him to withstand the impact while maintaining his balance. Add a blindfold, or have him close his eyes, during the drill, to create the element of surprise. Another creative way to simulate collisions is with a boxer's punching bag. Have the player attempt to remain neutral and stationary as the trainer swings the bag into him.

Using stabilization techniques during the off-season with healthy players may help prevent injuries while optimizing player potential.

References

1. Farfan H: Musculature mechanism of the lumbar spine in the position of power and efficiency, *Orthop Clin North Am* 6:135, 1975.
2. Gracovetsky S, Farfan H, Helleur C: The abdominal mechanism, *Spine* 10:317, 1985.
3. Greer N: *Biomechanics of skating.* In Casey MJ, editor: *Winter sports medicine,* Philadelphia, 1990, FA Davis Co. p 241.
4. Hornof Z, Napravnik C: Analysis of various accident rate factors in ice hockey, *Med Sci Sports* 5:283, 1973.
5. Hunter R: *Hockey.* In Reider B, editor: *Sports medicine, the school age athlete,* Philadelphia, 1991, WB Saunders Co., p 590.
6. Jorgensen U, Schmidt-Olsen S: The epidemiology of ice hockey injuries, *Br J Sports Med* 20:7, 1986.
7. Muller P, Biener K: Accidenti da hockey su ghiaccio, *Min Med* 66:1352, 1975.
8. Page P: *Biomechanics of forward skating in ice hockey,* master's thesis, 1975, Dalhousie University.
9. Robison R: *Stabilization techniques: the new back school prescription: stabilization training.* In White L, editor: *Back school,* 1991, Hanley & Belfus.
10. Sim FH, Simonet WT, Melton LJ, Lehn TA: Ice hockey injuries, *Am J Sports Med* 15:30, 1987.
11. Sutherland GW: Fire on ice, *Am J Sports Med* 4:264, 1976.
12. Tator CH, Edmonds VE: National survey of spinal injuries in hockey players, *Can Med Assoc J* 130:875, 1984.
13. Teitz CC, Cook DM: Rehabilitation of neck and low back injuries, *Clin Sports Med* 4:455, 1985.

Chapter 51
Spine Defense and the Martial Arts
Guido F. Schauer

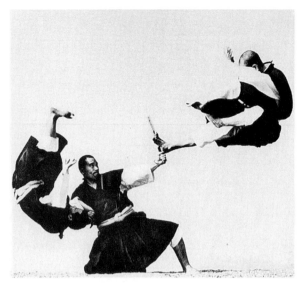

(From So D: Shorinji kempo: philosophy and techniques. Tokyo, 1970, Japan Publications, Inc., p 133.)

Introduction

This chapter explains the practice of martial arts as it relates to spine issues—and spine training as it relates to the martial arts. Martial arts practitioners must defend themselves, including their spines, against many hazards with potentially adverse effects, often under difficult conditions.[4,5,27] The challenge to the spine is not unlike that confronted by the other athletes,[6,23,24,29,32] patients with significant spine pathology,[22-24] and industrial workers.[18,21,32] Each requires skills in "spine defense" to contend with their conditions. This work will give the reader the "weapons" necessary to advise and treat those who face this challenge, especially in the context of martial arts practice.

For the most part, the practice of martial arts is based on principles that are healthful to the spine, and to the body as a whole,[13,31] and that help the individual to develop spinal skills. However, a number of hazards are often encountered, most of which arise out of inappropriate training or inadequate understanding.[4,5] The incorporation of spine training into the martial arts can help the practitioner avoid these hazards and may increase his/her martial arts skills as well.

The Martial Arts

The martial arts are practices that center on the ability to deal with physical, combative circumstances. Among other things, they may train the practitioner in confrontational and combative psychology, techniques, and tactics, both unarmed and armed with manually controlled and powered weaponry. Philosophically, martial arts practice cultivates harmony, especially personal harmony,* and helps the practitioner to come to terms with the sometimes harsh circumstances of life—and death.[7,28]

There are literally hundreds of styles of martial arts, most of which originated in East Asia hundreds and even thousands of years ago.[7,8] Each encompasses a set of foundational principles that dictate the style's training methods and technical skills. The various styles of martial arts incorporate many thousands of skills and variations, including those such as grabbing a pressure point, dodging a spear, reversing a joint lock, and throwing with a cane† (Figs. 51-1, *A* to *D*). Some styles have an eclectic origin and include a broader range of skills and techniques. A few are highly specialized, focusing on a particular situation of combat. Accordingly, a certain style may be more or less suited to a practitioner's preferences, physique, purposes, or other circumstances.

Spine Principles Relevant to Martial Arts Practice

Positioning for Load Tolerance

The spine's tolerance of loads varies with intraspinal positioning.‡ Within the spine's range of motion, one can clinically determine a position of optimal load tolerance (POLT), which is based on the particular spine's structure and physiologic state. This is the position in which loads stress the tissues most capable of handling them and that is least uncomfortable or symptomatic, especially with heavy loads. As the spine deviates from this position, its tolerance to loads decreases significantly. Another way of looking at this is in terms of a variable load tolerance range (VLTR). At low levels of loading, the spine can be moved through a greater range of motion without irritation or injury; whereas, with higher levels of loading, its tolerance is within a much narrower range. Thus, a vital component of success in training patients with difficult cases, who have narrower load tolerance ranges, and those who place high demands on their spines is the teaching of precise spine positioning control[15,22,23] (Fig. 51-2).

*References 7, 10, 13, 28, 31, and 33.
†References 2, 7, 8, 17, 28, 31, and 33.
‡References 1, 9, 11, 15, 18, 22 to 24, 30, 32, and 34.

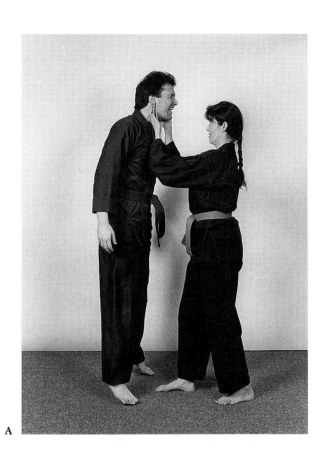

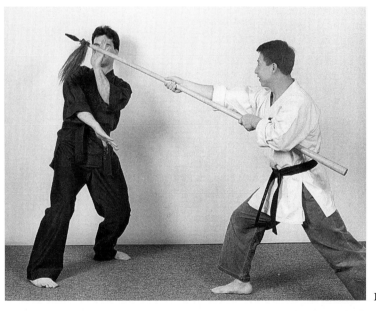

Fig. 51-1
Some of the many practices in the martial arts. **A,** Grabbing a pressure point. **B,** Dodging a spear.

When motion of the spine is imperative or desirable, the skillful individual may distribute movement over relevant spinal segments in relation to their capacity to tolerate loads with such positioning. Seg-mental positioning control is especially important for dancers, gymnasts, and patients with cervical spine pathology.[6,30] With such control, vulnerable segment motion can be decreased or eliminated.

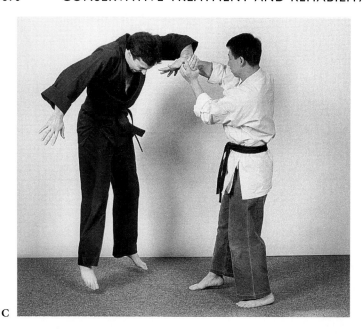

C

Fig. 51-1, cont'd
C, Reversing a joint kick.

Fig. 51-1, cont'd
D, Throwing with a cane.

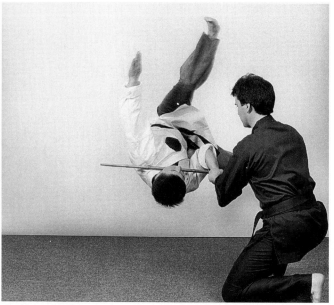

D

Bracing and Breathing Control

In order to provide direct support to the spine and minimize "give" into a compromised position, bracing is used.[22-24,32] Bracing is the active cocontraction of antagonistic muscles—in effect taking the "slack" out. This is especially important when unpredictable or quick changes in forces are anticipated, and may also be used to improve the accuracy or stability of positioning control.[19] The trunk can be further stabilized and spinal loading decreased through contraction of the diaphragm (against abdominal wall resistance), which pressurizes and "stiffens" the visceral cavity.[3,12,14,32,34] As it is strenuous, bracing should not be used when not needed.

Safe and effective bracing requires control over respiration as well. Sophisticated control over thoracic and diaphragmatic breathing is especially important in training patients with costovertebral and thoracic facet problems (Fig. 51-3).

Loading Preferences

Stresses the spine must endure increase with applied forces and their effective lever arms, or associated torques.[18,34] The spine is preferentially loaded axially,

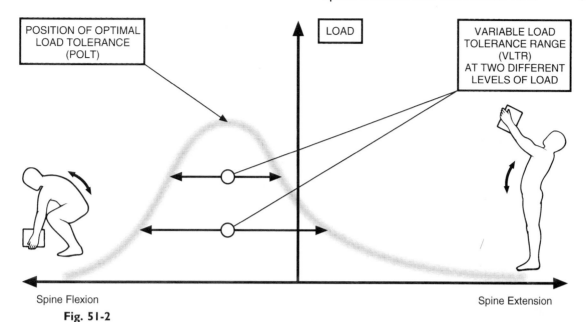

Fig. 51-2

Load tolerance with spine positioning. Simplified hypothetical "curve" for someone with flexion-bias POLT and sensitivity to spine extension.

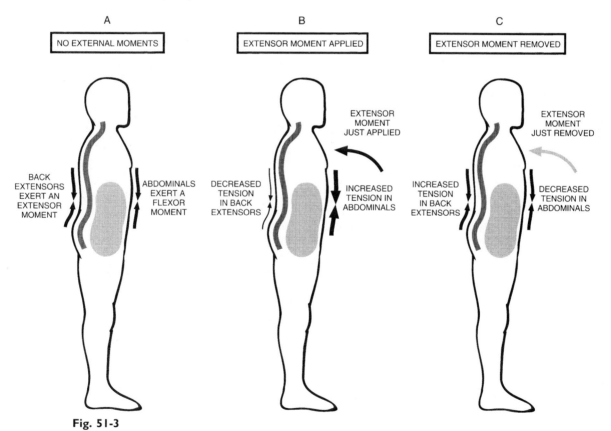

Fig. 51-3

Trunk bracing mechanism—sagittal plane only; visceral cavity pressure effects are not shown. An extensor moment is used for example. **A,** During bracing, antagonistic flexor and extensor moments counteract, or balance, one another. **B,** Suddenly applied extensor moment causes nearly immediate increase in tension in pretensed abdominals and corresponding decrease in tension in back extensors. The effect of bracing for suddenly applied moments is to minimize "give." **C,** Suddenly removed extensor moment causes nearly immediate increase in tension in pretensed back extensors and a corresponding decrease in tension in abdominals. The effect of bracing for suddenly removed moments is to minimize "lurching."

A   B

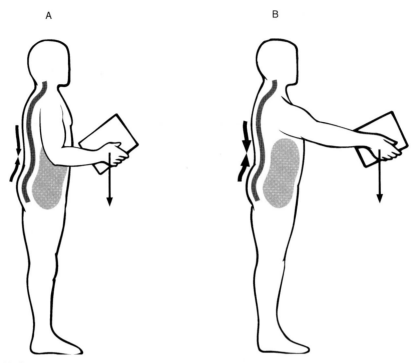

Fig. 51-4

Spine torque effects. Example is given for vertically oriented spine approximately aligned with gravity, for simplicity in considering forces and associated torques. Torque to spine increases as effective lever arm of force (in this case, a box) increases from *A* to *B:* As distance between line of action of applied force and spine increases, unilateral counterbalancing muscle tension and internal spinal stresses increase significantly. **A,** Less torque, muscle work, and stress to spine. **B,** More torque, muscle work, and stress to spine.

in alignment with these forces. Minimizing torques, whenever practicable, also decreases the amount of unilateral muscular activity required for the spine to maintain position. This is especially important for prolonged and static activities (Fig. 51-4).

In addition to their role in minimizing torques, the limbs can decrease loads to the spine through their action as springs or shock absorbers. However, their guarded use must be considered as much as proper use of the spine. All too often patients develop problems in other areas of their bodies, such as their knees, from deep knee bending[20] when lifting, because of the inappropriate fear that leaning itself will injure their spines,[18] when loss of good intraspinal positioning is the primary hazard.

Attending to Body Feedback

Though sensory feedback alone is inadequate to dictate proper spinal mechanics, it is an integral part of judging the correctness of technique.[15,22,30] Useful feedback about spinal irritation or other symptoms is important in determining the spine's POLT as well as its VLTR. The subtle awareness of the activity, or state of relaxation, of the paraspinal and other spine

and supportive muscles is also important, especially for improving sitting and cervical spine position holding tolerance.[18]

Preparing for Real Life

In order to control the spine properly in spite of the demands of many activities, preparation must occur in a number of areas.[22,23,30] Flexibility is important to allow peripheral joints to move through the relatively large ranges of motion in which they tolerate loads, as compared with spinal joints. Flexibility is also important for the proper distribution of inevitable spinal motion. Strength is required for the active control, or stabilization, of spinal movement.[32] Strength is also important for the limbs to act effectively within their full, safe ranges of motion. Endurance is important for lasting throughout activities, or the day.

However, mere physical capabilities are inadequate without the discipline, skills, reflexes, habit patterns, and problem-solving abilities needed to take advantage of them, consistently applying spinal strengths and avoiding vulnerabilities in real-life circumstances.[6,15,22-24,30,32]

Aspects of the Martial Arts that Are Healthful for the Spine

Background

The martial arts are among the oldest disciplines to train methodically in physical skills.[7,8,28,31] Hundreds of years of tested experience in movement and positioning, often under conditions of severe physical adversity, have led to certain advanced protective mechanisms for the spine, and the body as a whole. There is an obvious advantage to training in martial arts skills while not in combat; one can systematically develop fighting capability in a (more or less) controlled environment without many of the hazards of injury or death that combat situations often pose.

Many of the martial arts emphasize mind-body harmony.[*] This comes largely from their evolution through Zen and Taoism, which practice being "tuned-in" to and in natural agreement with one's reality.[†] Calming the mind and becoming focused on what is at hand is crucial to developing effective fighting abilities. Becoming "tuned-in" to one's body is a vital component for the care of the

---

[*]References 7, 10, 13, 17, 28, 31, and 33.
[†]References 7, 8, 10, 13, 28, 31, and 33.

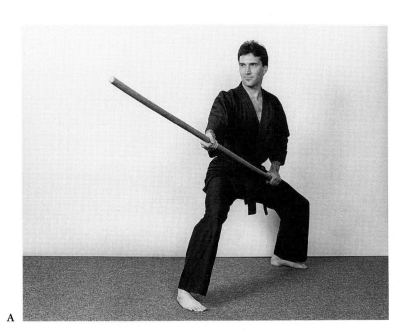

A

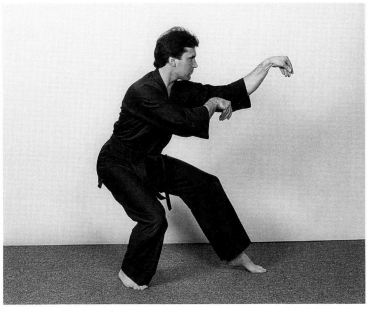

B

Fig. 51-5
Various stances common to many of the martial arts. **A,** Horse-riding stance. **B,** Cat stance.

spine.[15,22] As long as body information is properly interpreted, it is valuable to "listen to" for corrective action.

Many high-level practitioners developed an appreciation of the long-term and indirect implications of their practice.[13,31] Through this awareness, practitioners have traditionally integrated into their repertoire of skills many exercises primarily for health. Physical conditioning and the practice of martial skills for health as well as for combat is a natural extension of the philosophy of personal harmony. Promoting harmony in life is equivalent to minimizing harm in combat.

Martial Arts Practices that Employ Spinal Skills

Although each form of martial art emphasizes a particular set of skills and practices, there is considerable overlap in technical bases, especially concerning the use of the spine. The following describes some of the major skills and techniques that incorporate spinal skills.

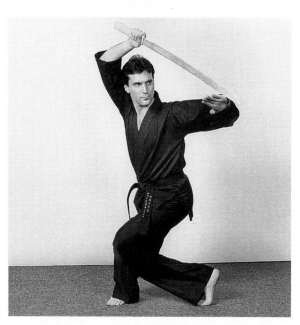

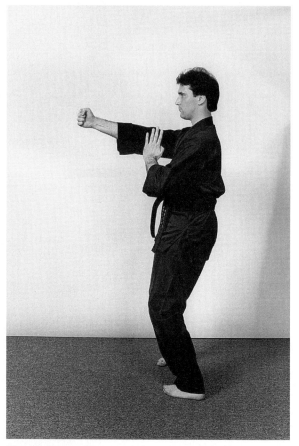

Fig. 51-5, cont'd
C, Crane stance. D, Crossed stance. E, Pigeon-toed stance.

Stance

The stance is the foundation of all martial arts techniques.* There are actually many different stances, each designed for various purposes. Common to each of them is a deliberate balance between efficiency, defensibility, spinal support, "preloading" of the legs, stability, and mobility (Fig. 51-5). Because they support offensive and defensive maneuvers alike, stances in the martial arts stress the powerful role of the legs and rarely compromise spine positioning.

Trunk Stability and Movement

Martial arts skills emphasize maintaining a stable "center," or trunk, whenever possible.[2,13,31,33] One can be more aware of one's surroundings and one's own state; one can also breathe more regularly and easily; accuracy and control in the execution of techniques are improved; and, "leading," or deceiving, opponents is easier. The limbs, acting as extensions of this center, "carry out" the bulk of the motion. This is consistent with the maintenance of good spine control.

Under certain circumstances, quick movements of the entire body are imperative. This is especially important for changing relative distance to the opponent, dodging an attack, jumping to launch an at-

*References 2, 13, 17, 28, 31, and 33.

tack, and recovering lost balance. Under such conditions, the legs drive, cushion, and adjust to minimize impact to the spine, which is often braced.

Bracing and Breathing

Many martial arts skills rely on the techniques of bracing and breathing.[13,17,31,33] Various methods include such applications as transmitting forces through the trunk, receiving a blow, falling, or lasting longer in combat. Forceful skills also use contraction of the diaphragm, or "pushing air down," to increase support. These skills can also minimize the impact of a blow to the trunk, because of effective "shielding" of internal organs and structures.

At a moment of intense exertion, practitioners often make a shouting (or other) sound.[17] Besides sometimes scaring the opponent, this technique is used to concentrate all of one's energy into one moment, and is used in offensive as well as defensive techniques. The glottis is generally not closed against forced expiration. This represents the most intense use of bracing with diaphragmatic breathing control applied to the support of the spine.

The relaxed and purposeful breathing of the martial artist is coordinated with these bracing techniques, emphasizing efficiency, preparedness for quick changes, and avoidance of or contending with side pains and "getting the wind knocked out." Some rather esoteric thoracic and diaphragmatic breathing skills are practiced as well, especially in conjunction with meditation.[13]

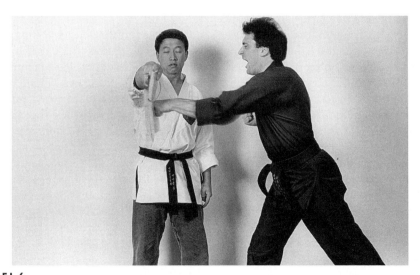

Fig. 51-6
In most attacks, and in the breaking of boards, the arm is supported by the trunk, which generally translates and rotates as a unit.

Transmitting Forces Through the Spine

In many offensive or countering skills, forces must be transmitted through the spine. The spine nearly always acts as a single-unit transmitter of power, as opposed to an actively twisting structure. For many upper-body techniques, such as head, elbow, or hand strikes, pushes, pulls, throws, and such attacks with weapons, the bulk of the power is generated in the legs and transmitted through the trunk to the arms.[19] The effectiveness of the attack depends on strong spine support, thus the spine's positioning is rarely compromised (Fig. 51-6).

Much of the overall positioning of the body is dictated by the training or fighting situation. As with stances, there is a balance between stability, defensibility, reach, power, etc. In order to improve efficiency and power, whenever possible, the spine is loaded as close to axially as circumstances and strategy allow; the trunk may be leaned in the direction of power. When loads cannot be axial, the forces of powerful strikes (thrusts) and throws are kept in planes approximately in line with the spine, minimizing rotational forces. Attacking from the center line is a common teaching.[2] Techniques that must employ rotational forces are generally quick, ballistic motions, inherently limited in support by the relative weakness of the extended arm, thus not having great impact on the spine. Therefore, the focus with any technique that transmits forces through the trunk is to minimize torques, and use the spine as efficiently and powerfully as possible, as a single unit in optimal positioning.

A "reverse use" of the trunk in transmitting power is found in spinning kicks. In performing these powerful attacks, momentum built up in the arms, in the usual ground-up direction, is transmitted back to the trunk and then to the spinning kicking leg to increase its rotational velocity and power. (Dancers and skaters similarly translate arm into body momentum in performing pirouettes.)[19,34]

The energy generated in motion is not always successfully expended against a striking bag or an opponent's body. Often techniques are practiced without a target; often an attack misses, is deflected, or must be retracted for safety. The energy of the attack must then be successfully controlled and absorbed by the attacker. Whenever practical, movements are cushioned, fluid, or have a circular follow-through. This allows the practitioner to absorb energy in the major muscles rather than in spinal structures, or to use the energy for the next attack.

Using the Trunk as a Massive Support

In kicking techniques, primary forces are not directly transmitted through the trunk. Rather, the trunk is used as a massive support, to "give weight" to the kick, increasing the kick's power. In these techniques the trunk is stabilized so that it may effectively act as a unit in support of the kick.

Contending with Imminent Forces

When an impending attack cannot be dodged, or if it is not advantageous to do so, the attack may be dealt with by jamming, blocking, cushioning, or deflecting it. If it is too late for that, one must prepare (if feasible) to absorb the blow as safely as possible. In each of these situations, some of the force of the attack must be taken in the spine. It is the role of the limbs to decrease forces, by lengthening time of contact or cushioning the attack.[19] Powerful attacks are also often yielded to by actively moving the entire body in the direction of force. The most threatening situation exists when the trunk is struck directly.[4,5,27] Many martial arts forms prepare for these occasions by training in special bracing, breathing, and positioning techniques. Some styles use exercises, called "iron body" training, to improve the ability to contend with landed attacks.[7]

Forces exerted on the body due to an inadequate attempt at a throw by an opponent are often defended against with bracing and counterattack. Powerful and successful throws are yielded to while countering.

Falling

Falls are a set of defensive techniques used, in effect, to "block" the floor from doing damage. There are four main classes of falling technique: break-falling, rolling, cushioning, and sliding.

Break-falling is used when one is thrown forcefully downward, or when there is little time to react. In break-falling techniques, the entire spine is forcefully braced in a position as close to optimal as possible. Usually cervical spine positioning deviates slightly from optimal positioning, to prevent the head or face from striking the floor. One never lands directly on the spine, but rather over large areas padded with muscle. The front fall is a good example of minimizing spinal "give" in spite of compelling forces. In this fall, only the forearms and the balls of the feet may strike the floor, in order to prevent weaker areas from making contact. The spine must

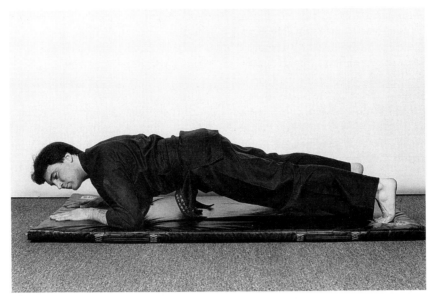

Fig. 51-7

Front break-fall. On contact with the floor, spine must be firmly braced and impact cushioned in muscles of arms.

be firmly braced, and the impact cushioned in the muscles of the arms (Fig. 51-7).

Rolling falls usually occur when one's body is projected mostly in a horizontal direction. During rolling, the spine cannot be positioned in a strict POLT. However, bending of the spine is distributed over its entirety, and the practitioner trains in not collapsing the normal curve.

Cushioning falls emphasize the use of the limbs as shock absorbers; they can only be used when there is ample time to preposition them. Sliding falls are also a milder form. They require no special spinal skills not already discussed.

Martial Arts Practices that May Be Hazardous to the Spine—and Their Solutions

It is ironic that martial arts practices should ever cause spine problems. One notable purpose of the martial arts is to prevent injury to the self, in spite of an opponent's ill intent. Practitioners who injure themselves are defeating their own purposes. Considering some of the injuries people sustain as a result of poor training, they might be better off not learning anything and taking their chances on the streets.

Training generally contains some inherent risks. One reason is that many skills closely simulate dangerous circumstances. Even with a methodical approach errors are not always avoidable. The demands placed on the spine may accidentally cause injury. However, most of the injuries sustained are the result of poor, inappropriate, or simply misguided training. These training problems should be recognized and taken into consideration in determining solutions to the errant practitioner's approach.

Ascertaining Potential Problems

In order properly to treat or train the martial arts practitioner who has spinal problems, it is important to obtain certain information about the nature of his/her abilities, pathology, and practice. One should consider the following: (1) What are the practitioner's particular sensitivities, pathology, and functional problems? Which activities exacerbate these? (2) What is the level of physical preparedness of the patient for the activities being pursued? Note any particular weakness, tightness, or difficulty. Ask the patient if any practices are particularly challenging. (3) What is the level of skill of the patient? Ask about the patient's teacher, training time, frequency and duration of sessions, and rank. Do not presume that high rank, such as a "black belt" or long training time, means that the patient has a high level of skill. For various reasons, some people remain locked into mediocrity, though they may have been training for many years. It is important to find out how effectively the patient applies martial arts spinal skills and how consistent he/she is—especially at intense levels of practice. The patient should be able to demonstrate good technique in each applicable category of problem areas discussed later in this chapter. (4) What were the patient's motivations before spine problems developed, and what are they now? Some patients incorrectly assume that they will no longer be able to do certain challenging activities, while others unrealistically cling to activities that their bodies may no longer tolerate. Methodical, safe practice is generally the best determinant of what will be possible. Help the patient to become comfortable with the uncertainty of not knowing the future. (5) What are the general personality traits of the martial arts practitioner? The approach the patient takes obviously makes a big difference.[23] The well-balanced, well-focused patient should easily be able to adjust to a better mode of training, once so instructed. (6) What are the goals and purposes of the patient's training? The demands placed on the spine are proportional to the demanding nature of skills as they are applied. The most hazardous circumstances exist when the practitioner must apply skills to real-life fighting. Some law-enforcement officers and those who must regularly walk into dangerous environments often have this concern. Competition can also be quite demanding[4,5]; in exhibitions, exceedingly challenging skills (hazardous, albeit impressive) are often attempted.[7,17] (7) What are the training circumstances of the patient—the approaches of the school, teacher, or other practitioners? Is it a controlled or uncontrolled environment? Would the teacher accommodate a spine-injured patient? What form of sparring practice is used? Do any training partners have an attitude problem? Are accidents likely to occur due to needless risks? Is the available equipment adequate for the challenges of training? For example, does the floor or matting have enough "give" for training in falling or jumping? (8) In what particular practices does the patient engage? In which martial arts style, specific classes of techniques (kicking, throwing, etc.), or other training is the patient involved? Some styles or training approaches are easier on the spine than others.

General Problematic Practice Methods

Nonincremental Training

Some people train without a gradual, step-by-step approach to the development of skills, or train in skills too advanced for their capabilities. When the practitioner is repeatedly overchallenged or not physically or mentally prepared for the difficulty of the tasks to be performed, there is likelihood of irritation or injury.

Overtraining

One common practice in many martial arts schools is to drill skills over and over. You get good at what you practice; if you practice doing a skill poorly, you will become good at doing it that way. Training beyond exhaustion, past the point of being able to correctly perform skills, is hazardous and develops poor judgment as well.

Training Without Focus

Training with a lack of intensity or "playing around" may also lead to injury. The practitioner may develop a poor sense of the real dangers of sparring or fighting, and reflexive spinal skills such as trunk bracing may not be drilled. Also, some more advanced exercises have a significantly smaller margin of error for safe performance. So while the skill itself may not seem so challenging, the potential for significant injury due to lack of focus may be greater.

Lack of Precautions

Martial arts skills that are inherently difficult to train in safely require certain precautions. Practitioners who do not make the effort to include these precautions predispose themselves, or others, to potential injury. Precautions important for the spine include the following: flooring with adequate "give" for jumping and falling, and with an appropriate amount of friction to prevent inadvertent falls; and proper matching of training partners, considering relative stature, skill, and control.

Ignoring Body Signals

An important skill is the ability to relegate some concerns or body signals in deference to the priorities of the circumstances of training or combat. The ability to continue in spite of often legitimate fears or pain can mean the difference between survival and death. When sustaining a broken arm in defense of one's life, one should fight aggressively, without succumbing to the pain, and guarding the arm, if possible. However, during practice it would be foolhardy to risk even greater injury when it is not necessary.

Hard training may at times be physically uncomfortable, though it is not injurious. It is important, however, to know the difference between the discomfort of muscular fatigue and stress on the cardiovascular system, and dysfunctional joint or nerve pains, which would be minimized or prevented.[4] Pain may be felt at times as a result of accidents or with a few legitimate practices in which the effects are not lasting.[16,26,28,33] However, the saying, "no pain, no gain," has no place in martial arts training. Perhaps "no strain, no gain" would be more appropriate.

Psychologic Considerations

Many people begin martial arts training because of a sense of insecurity, which may be based only partly in physical reality. In an attempt to prove to themselves and to others their apparent control and capabilities through martial skills, they often push themselves beyond their physical limitations, causing injury to themselves. Others are never satisfied and simply drive themselves too hard. People with this attitude tend to perform skills stiffly, with uncertainty, and with a higher rate of errors. Because they do not work in communion with themselves, they are also prone to ignore their bodies' warning signals.

Specific Areas with the Potential for Problems

Stretching

Many stretches inadequately elongate the intended muscles, and stressfully bend or twist the spine.

- Be wary of stretches in which it is impossible to avoid spine bending or twisting.

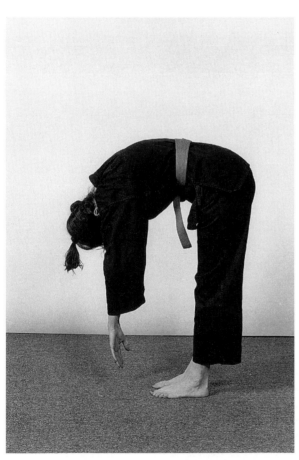
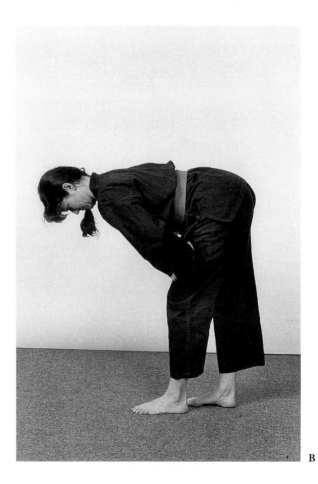

A   B

Fig. 51-8
Standing hamstrings stretch. **A,** Hazardous: Lumbar spine is flexed. In reaching for feet, stress is increased by weight of trunk and contraction of abdominals. **B,** Safer *and* more effective: Flexion occurs only at hip joint; trunk weight is supported; stretching one leg at a time increases stretch intensity without increasing back stress.

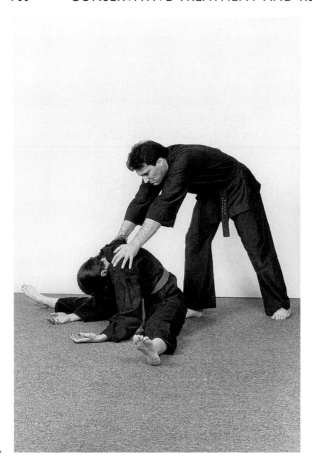

A

- Take notice of and minimize any avoidable spinal stresses.
- Take advantage of gravity, friction, and supports to aid stretching.
- Stretch hip and thigh muscles by moving the pelvis or supporting it.
- Stretch muscles that create motion in the sagittal plane and that are difficult to elongate one leg at a time.
- Do not reach the hand(s) for the foot (feet) if it involves any stressful or unnecessary spinal bending (Fig. 51-8).
- If you are inflexible, stretch more often with more controlled, isolated muscle stretches.
- With a partner, do only controlled stretches, which do not force spine bending or twisting (Fig. 51-9).
- In stretching the spine, do only stretches that are mild, supported, and not accentuated by gravity.

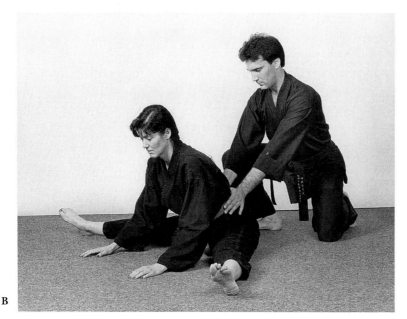

B

Fig. 51-9
Assisted sitting center splits stretch. **A,** Hazardous: Lumbar spine is forced into flexion by "helper." **B,** Safer *and* more effective: Force is applied at pelvis, allowing spine to remain in its POLT.

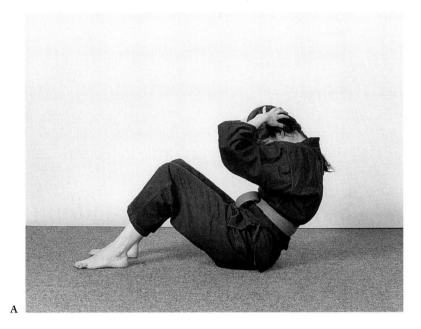

A

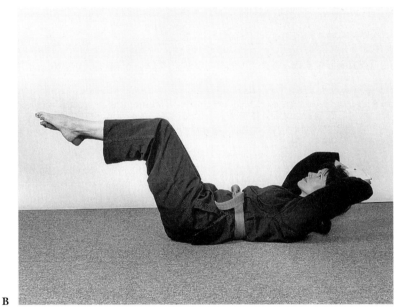

B

Fig. 51-10

Abdominal strengthening. **A,** Hazardous: full sit-ups can overstress spine. Spine is in heavy flexion; loading due to muscular contraction is compounded by gravity loading; ballistic (jerky) movement further increases spinal stresses. **B,** Safer *and* more effective: Aggressive but controlled partial sit-ups do not load spine out of its VLTR and better isolate abdominals.

Calisthenics

Some calisthenics that strengthen trunk and neck muscles compromise the structural capacities of the spine as well.

- Exercise muscles with the spine immobile, or moving in a small range near the POLT (Fig. 51-10).
- Increase intensity only when control has been gained.
- Avoid axial loading, if possible, especially if spinal motion is allowed.

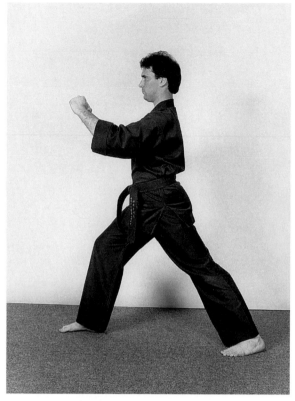
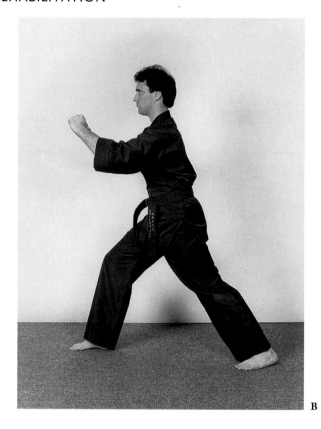

A   B

Fig. 51-11

Front stance with upright posture. **A,** Hazardous: Notable lumbar extension weakens support for upper body and can predispose posterior spinal elements to excessive stresses. **B,** Safer *and* stronger: Keeping spine in its POLT requires only subtle change in positioning.

Stances

Stances that maintain a fully upright trunk posture with the rear leg extended backward may extend and jeopardize the lumbar spine (Fig. 51-11).

- Improve the flexibility of the iliopsoas muscles.
- Shorten stance length or slightly bend the back leg to compensate for inextensibility of the hip joint.

Jumping and Moving Quickly

Quick, whole-body movements may cause shock to or inappropriate "give" in the spine.

- Use the legs to cushion and soften movements effectively.
- Brace adequately to counter forces that may move the spine.

Kicking

The positioning demands and momentum generated in many kicks can overwhelm the underprepared practitioner's ability to control the spine.

- Never kick higher than leg flexibility without spine involvement would allow.
- In the absence of complicating factors, mild spine bending may be acceptable.
- Be aware of increased vulnerability to injury at the height of a kick, on contact with a stable object, when missing a target, and when landing from a jumping kick.
- Especially with back and side leg position kicks, allow the trunk to lean with the pelvis.
- In kicks in which one's own hand is used as a target, do not reach for the foot unless spine positioning does not need to be compromised to accomplish the task (Fig. 51-12).
- In spinning kicks, commit any additional power-generating movements to the limbs.
- Emphasize regular stretching to meet the demands of high kicks.

Throwing

Throws that rely primarily on strength and leverage in challenging positions, if incorrectly performed, may dangerously compromise the spine.

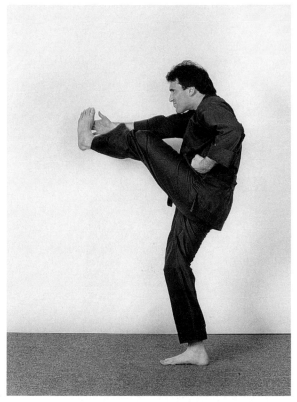

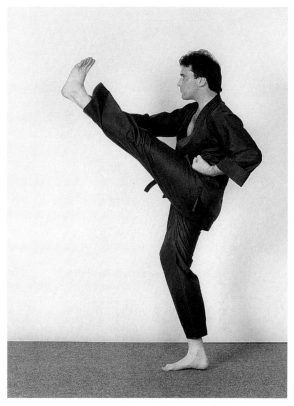

A   B

Fig. 51-12

Crescent kick, using the hand as a target. **A,** Hazardous: Lumbar spine may be forced into flexion and rotation by uncontrolled leg swing while reaching for the foot. **B,** Safer (and more deceptive): With spine in its POLT, hand need not reach foot, unless kicker is adequately flexible.

- Grab the opponent without compromising spine position.
- Adjust the legs, rather than spine, positioning in throwing smaller persons.
- Position for strength and control; do not "power through" an initially weak position (Fig. 51-13).
- If possible, take advantage of pressure point or joint attacks, momentum or balance upsetting.
- Minimize lifting by causing the opponent to spin or "jump" over.
- Minimize twisting through full use of the arms, legs, and trunk unit.
- Move with the falling opponent, if either person is still grabbing.

Falling

Many falls have small margins for error, due to sometimes exceedingly high impact forces or necessarily curved spine positioning on contact with the ground.

- Use floors with a firm top surface but plenty of "give" to allow for errors without fear of injury.
- Never do a fall that forces loss of body position control on contact with the floor.
- Avoid striking the floor with the unpadded, bony areas of the appendages or spine.
- The entire spine should be braced in its POLT, except to avoid head contact with the floor, especially in break-falls.
- In break-falls, all contact parts should strike the floor simultaneously.
- In break-falls, emphasize use of the limbs to absorb shock.
- Do not break-fall from a height at which technique and cervical spine muscle strength cannot prevent head rocking.
- Avoid overspinning and break-falling on the buttocks with the lumbar spine in flexion (Fig. 51-14).

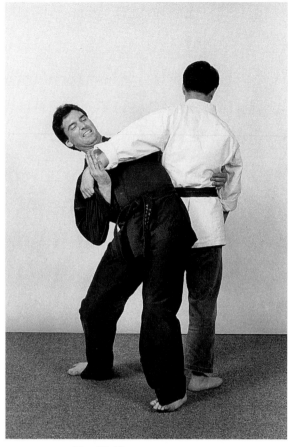
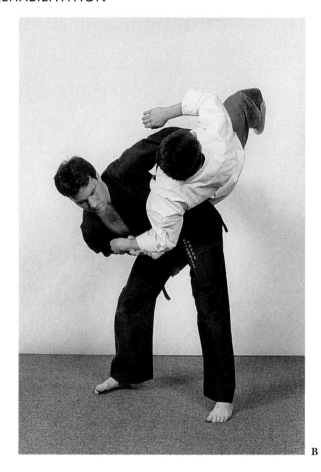

A   B

Fig. 51-13

Initiating a simple hip throw. **A,** Hazardous: Throw was attempted from weak starting position, with spine rotated, thrower straining to compensate for poor technique. **B,** Safer *and* more effective: This successful throw shows effective use of arms, legs, and trunk unit.

- Avoid rolling or falling on the neck or head.
- In rolling falls, emphasize even, mild bending of the spine.
- Roll only over the padded areas of the body.
- Do not compromise falling technique to expedite getting up.

Sparring

Some sparring situations may make it exceedingly difficult to maintain attention on spine control, and vulnerability to injury from accidents or uncontrolled opponent attacks can be high.

- Emphasize controlled attacks and clear-headedness.
- Never train in sparring at a speed or duration that can lead to poor technique.

- Emphasize sparring sessions that are focused on particular lessons of skill, as opposed to an all-out fray.
- Deliberately train in the ability to focus on spinal skills in any combative situation—however, slowly at first.

Special Problems of the Martial Arts Practitioner with Spine Pathology

Problems unique to the patient with spine pathology require further, more specific consideration for training. Some of the following problems may be "worked around" in the course of martial arts practice. However, it is highly advisable for the practitioner to learn the principles and subtle skills that proper spine training can address more directly. The

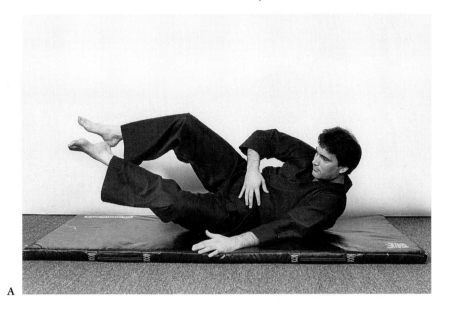

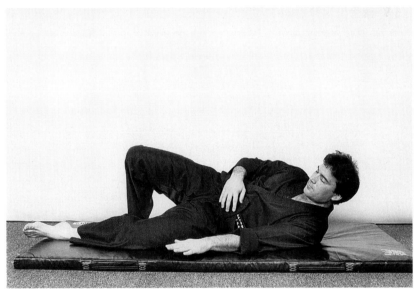

Fig. 51-14

Spinning break-fall. **A,** Hazardous: Avoid overspinning and break-falling on buttocks with lumbar spine in flexion. **B,** Safer: Correct landing position for spinning break-fall—spine is in its POLT, except for slight neck flexion; contact forces are distributed over padded areas of arm, leg, foot and trunk.

following are brief suggestions for some notable problems.

Nerve-Tension Sensitivity

Persons with significant nerve-tension sensitivity may have problems in safely performing many kicks and some stretches. In considering a patient's vulnera-

bilities, intraspinal position must be factored in along with limb positioning, as spine positioning sometimes significantly affects tension signs.[25,34] For example, some patients may have tension signs only with loss of lumbar lordosis.

- The angle at which symptoms are felt should indicate whether low kicks may be safely performed.

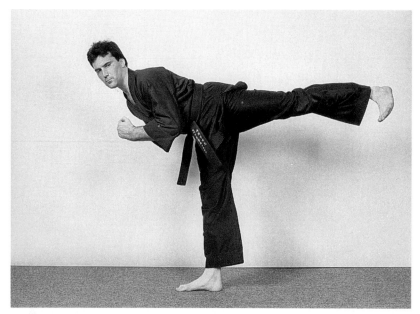

Fig. 51-15

In determining safety of performing kicks by nerve-tension-sensitive individuals, consider both kicking and standing leg angles relative to trunk.

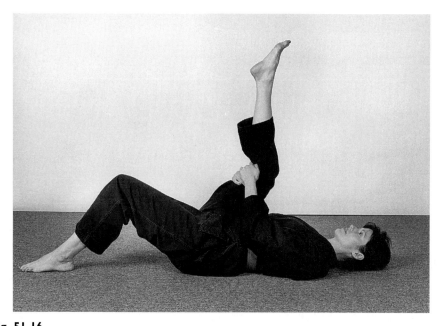

Fig. 51-16

To avoid nerve tension signs with hamstrings stretch try full hip flexion with incomplete knee extension (keeping spine in its POLT).

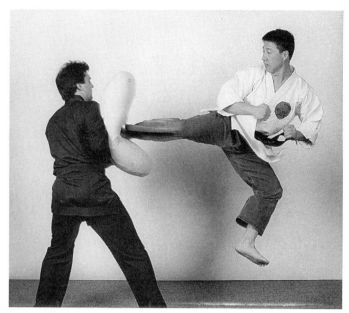

Fig. 51-17

Those with extension sensitivity must be able to avoid extension without error. This attack could be riskier to extension-sensitive kicker than to opponent.

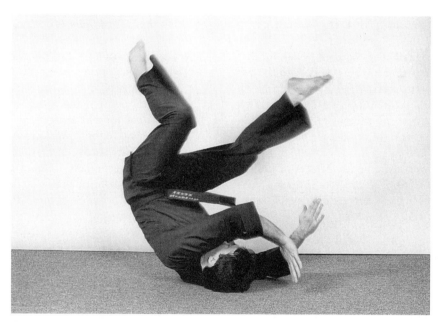

Fig. 51-18

Those with notable flexion sensitivity must avoid flexion without error. Rolling falls may not be practicable.

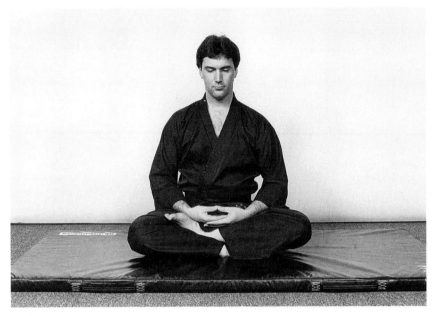

Fig. 51-19

Posture in seated meditation.

- In judging the safety of kicks, consider both kicking and standing leg angles relative to the trunk (Fig. 51-15).
- Since the hamstring muscles cross both the hip and knee joints, full flexion at the hip along with incomplete extension of the knee may be enough to cause an effective stretch without producing nerve tension problems (Fig. 51-16).
- Individuals with extreme hamstrings flexibility, or those with more severe tension signs, may not be able to achieve a stretch effectively without exacerbating symptoms.

Notable Spine-Position Sensitivity

People with significant sensitivity through part of their range of motion and those with significant range of motion limitations may find certain specific exercises and skills particularly difficult to perform without problems.

- Patients with sensitivity to spine extension or with a flexion-biased POLT (usually those with stenosis, spondylolisthesis, facet problems, etc.) are vulnerable in activities which tend to extend the hip and spine.[9,15,22,24]
- Those with extension sensitivity may be vulnerable in performing kicks during which the leg extends to the rear or side, in jumping skills, and with stance (Fig. 51-17).
- Patients with an extension-biased POLT or those with poor tolerance of spine flexion (many discogenic conditions)[15,22] should be cautious with many kicks, and may need to avoid rolling falls altogether (Fig. 51-18).
- Those with either a flexion- or extension-biased POLT, particularly those with a narrow VLTR, should be especially cautious with quick, strenuous, and ballistic actions.

Other Sensitivities

- Surface-pressure sensitivity in areas superficial to the spine, or in extremity muscles, may preclude many falling practices.
- Spasmodic, painful, or otherwise dysfunctional muscles secondary to nerve irritation or damage may require limiting the patient to milder forms of training.
- Patients with load sensitivity (not relieved by adjusting intraspinal positioning) should minimize ballistic movements and activities that are strenuous for the spine.

Relief Positioning

Positions of relief may be used to alleviate such problems as facet irritation, muscle spasms, or nerve impingement.[23,32] Practitioners with existing problems may have "picked up" various methods of "stretch" or "self-mobilization" in their encounters with medical practitioners or others with spine problems. Sometimes they themselves are unaware of how often, how forcefully, or even why they do these self-manipulations. Because of the greater vulnerability of the spine with extreme positioning, relief exercises should be reviewed for appropriateness or at least safety in manner of performance.

Appropriateness of Training

In considering the appropriateness of various activities, the vulnerability of the patient to problems must be weighed against his/her level of skill in avoiding them. The injured practitioner should not be dissuaded from training in the martial arts, unless avoiding problems become impossible. Realistically, the injured person may require an even greater level of martial arts and spinal skills in order to prevent further injury in the event of a real-life assault. Those who are strong and healthy are less in need of protective skills. For the injured, the appropriateness of training must be measured by weighing benefits against unavoidable risks.

Summary

This chapter stresses the importance and learnability of spinal skills soundly based on biomechanical principles *and* the awareness of subjective body feedback. It is naturally limited in depth because of the vastness of the considered subject. Other aspects of self-care and training may promote an increase in the tolerance and functionality of the spine; however, they cannot be oblivious to the vital protective mechanisms that are required in the martial arts, as well as any other physical activity. Martial arts skills implicitly rely on the safe and powerful use of a well-cared-for spine, and, therefore, must be in agreement with the principles of spine training. When charged with the care of the martial artist, the medical practitioner has a unique opportunity. It is the chance to teach the practitioner what is good for the spine as well as to help the martial artist to improve his/her skills in the martial arts (Fig. 51-19).

References

1. Adams MA, Hutton WC: The effect of posture on the lumbar spine, *J Bone Joint Surg* 67B:625, 1985.
2. Armstrong K, Fung J: *Wing chun kung fu,* Australia, 1980, K. Armstrong and J. Fung.
3. Bartelink DL: The role of abdominal pressure in relieving the pressure on the lumbar intervertebral discs, *J Bone Joint Surg* 39B:718, 1957.
4. Birrer RB, Birrer CD: Unreported injuries in the martial arts, *Br J Sports Med* 17:131, 1983.
5. Birrer RB, Halbrook SP: Martial arts injuries: the results of a five year national survey, *Am J Sports Med* 16:408, 1988.
6. Bryan N, Smith B: The ballet dancer. *Spine State Art Rev* 5:391, 1991.
7. Chow D, Spangler R: *Kung fu: history, philosophy, and technique,* ed 2, Hollywood, 1980, Unique Publications Co.
8. Corcoran J, Farkas E: *Martial arts: traditions, history, people,* New York, 1988, W.H. Smith Publishers, Inc.
9. Dunlop RB, Adams MA, Hutton WC: Disc space narrowing and the lumbar facet joints, *J Bone Joint Surg* 66B:706, 1984.
10. Fuller JR: Martial arts and psychological health, *Br J Med Psychol* 61:317, 1988.
11. Gordon SJ, et al.: Mechanism of disc rupture: a preliminary report, *Spine* 16:450, 1991.
12. Harman EA, et al.: Effects of a belt on intra-abdominal pressure during weight lifting, *Med Sci Sports Exerc* 21:186, 1989.
13. Jou TH: *The tao of tai-chi chuan: way to rejuvenation,* ed 2, Piscataway, NJ, 1983, Tai Chi Foundation.
14. Lander JE, Hundley JR, Simonton RL: The effectiveness of weight-belts during multiple repetitions of the squat exercise, *Med Sci Sports Exerc* 24:603, 1992.
15. Morgan D: Concepts in functional training and potential stabilization for the low back injured, *Top Acute Care Trauma Rehab* 2:8, 1988.
16. Olson GD, Seitz FC: An examination of aikido's fourth teaching: an anatomical study of the tissues of the forearm, *Percept Mot Skills* 71(3 pt 2):1059, 1990.
17. Oyama M: *This is karate,* ed 2, Tokyo, 1973, Japan Publications, Inc.
18. Pope MH et al., editors: *Occupational low back pain: assessment, treatment and prevention,* St. Louis, 1991, Mosby.
19. Rasch PJ, Burke RK: *Kinesiology and applied anatomy: the science of human movement,* ed 6, London, 1978, Henry Kimpton Publishers.
20. Reilly DT, Martens M: Experimental analysis of the quadriceps muscle force and patello-femoral joint reaction force for various activities, *Acta Orthop Scand* 43:126, 1972.
21. Riihimäki H, et al.: Radiographically detectable degenerative changes of the lumbar spine among concrete reinforcement workers and house painters, *Spine* 15:114, 1990.
22. Robison R: The new back school prescription: stabilization training, part 1, *Spine State Art Rev* 5:341, 1991.
23. Saal JA: Rehabilitation of sports-related lumbar spine injuries, *Phys Med Rehab State Art Rev* 1:613, 1987.
24. Saal JA: The new back school prescription: stabilization training, part 2, *Spine State Art Rev* 5:357, 1991.

25. Schnebel BE, Watkins RG, Dillin W: The role of spinal flexion and extension in changing nerve root compression in disc herniations, *Spine* 14:835, 1989.

26. Seitz FC, Olson GD, Stenzel TE: A martial arts exploration of elbow anatomy: ikkyo (aikido's first teaching), *Percept Mot Skills* 73(3 pt 2):1227, 1991.

27. Serina ER, Liew DK: Thoracic injury potential of basic competition taekwondo kicks, *J Biomech* 24:951, 1990.

28. So D: *Shorinji kempo: philosophy and techniques,* Tokyo, 1970, Japan Publications, Inc.

29. Swärd L, et al.: Back pain and radiologic changes in the thoraco-lumbar spine of athletes, *Spine* 15:124, 1990.

30. Sweeney T, et al.: Cervicothoracic muscular stabilization techniques, *Phys Med Rehab State Art Rev* 4:335, 1990.

31. Tam PFN: *Tai chi chuan: theory and practice,* Hong Kong, 1991, PBI Publications (Hong Kong) Ltd.

32. Twomey LT, Taylor JR, Oliver MJ: Sustained flexion loading, rapid extension loading of the lumbar spine, and the physical therapy of related injuries, *Physiother Pract* 4:129, 1988.

33. Westbrook A, Ratti O: *Aikido and the dynamic sphere.* Rutland, VT, 1970, Charles E. Tuttle Co., Inc.

34. White AA, Panjabi MM: *Clinical biomechanics of the spine,* ed 2, Philadelphia, 1990, J.B. Lippincott Co.

Chapter 52
Running
Arthur H. White

Contrary to popular belief running can be good for your health as well as your back. Studies have shown that runners have 40% more bone mineral content, weigh less, report better overall health, and have less disability then controls.[6]

Running does not seem to produce more short- or long-term injuries than other sports. One study found that only 2% of runners versus 2.4% of swimmers had severe pain in the hip or knee, and 16% of runners versus 20% of swimmers had mild to moderate pain.[7,14] A study of over 98 runners versus 365 nonrunners has demonstrated that runners have less physical disability than age-matched controls, require less medical care, and have less musculoskeletal disability. Therefore running may actually slow musculoskeletal aging.[1,7]

Running injuries have been recorded for several decades. Most of them have been overuse injuries such as stress fractures and muscles and ligament strains and sprains. Serious injuries rarely occur.

Running done properly is not bad for your back; it does not create arthritis of the knees or any other joints in an otherwise healthy individual. If there are already damaged joints then running on them can be detrimental. A nonrunner should have a musculoskeletal medical evaluation prior to starting running, and should use good, well-standardized training techniques.

In 1980 Jackson and Pagliano pointed out in a study of 1000 consecutive running injuries that only 1.1% were spine-related.[5] In 1970 Glick and Katch found that 9% of middle-aged joggers complained of back pain.[2]

Radiographic images of runners' spines do not demonstrate any greater degenerative abnormalities than the spines of the normal population. Guten has produced specific statistics on runners who had surgery for herniated discs with sciatica. Of the 10 runners studied, 8 returned to running and only 1 was unable to return to sports.[3]

Back injuries are not common to running. Well-trained runners have inherent protection because running done properly can develop and reinforce the lumbar protective mechanism. There have not been significant studies on improper running. Poorly trained runners or runners who have had no training at all and run sporadically may produce significant strains on their lumbar spine and precipitate injuries that would not occur if the runner trained properly.

Biomechanics of Injury

The impact forces from running can be as high as three times the individual's body weight.[15] These impact forces increase with stride length and when running down hill or on uneven terrain.

A 70-k runner taking 1175 steps per mile absorbs 220 tons of force.[10,15] If the runner is inadequately trained and utilizes his/her ankles, knees, and hips incorrectly, these forces can create significant microtrauma to the lumbar spine. If the runner is running in lordosis with excessive rotation his/her facet joints may become injured. It is well known that running creates hyperextension of the lumbar spine as the trailing leg leaves the ground. This hyperextension increases as the speed of running increases.

Each time the foot hits the ground there is a potential vibration and trauma transferred through the ankle, the knee, the hip, and into the spine. The force generated by heel strike is in excess of 2000 N.[8] If all links in the kinetic chain between the feet and the back are well trained and doing their job, the vibration or force will be dissipated equally and nontraumatically to each of the joints involved and the muscles that protect them.[10,11] If there is a weak link in the kinetic chain (a chronically sprained ankle, torn knee cartilage, or degenerated lumbar disc), that weak and unprotected joint may receive more than its share of the force and stress and is likely to undergo accelerated wear and tear. The result may be a permanent and significant injury that will prevent the individual from continuing athletic activities.

There is a significant decrease in disc height during running, despite the runner's experience.[13] The position of the pelvis seems to be a key factor in the distribution of stresses during running, as well as during stabilization training.[13]

It is not necessary to describe all the muscles that protect each joint and the potential joint-specific injuries that can occur. Lack of protection in the peripheral joints can generate ligament and muscle strain, and sprain in the early phases, acute arthritis in the subacute phases, and chronic arthritic changes in the end stages.

This stress can cause a disc to become symptomatic and require treatment. These repeated episodes of trauma exceed the reparative process and create enough local inflammation to become symptomatic.[4]

The specific pathologic process that occurs in any joint, including the facet joints of the lumbar spine, is well known. Repetitive microtrauma causes trabecular microfracture in the subchondral bone. There is subsequent internal remodeling of the architecture of bone that leads to stiffening of the sub-chondral area. This increases stress on the articular surfaces, which can lead to further cartilage break-down and subsequent joint degradation.[9,12]

As articular cartilage is damaged either by specific trauma from high-level athletic activities or from multiple microtrauma as described above, the fol-lowing changes occur. There is a loss of mu-copolysaccharide from the surface of the joint carti-lage, and the cartilage is weakened. With the loss of mucopolysaccharide, friction increases, lubrication decreases, and articular cartilage virtually begins to wear away. As the forces increase, osteophyte for-mation creates a greater surface area in the joint. If repair cannot keep up with the continued trauma, which is usually the case, the surface cartilage is vir-tually worn down to subchondral bone. The defects are filled in by the resultant repair scar, a reparative process that does not have the physiologic capabili-ties of protecting the joint. Further breakdown ul-timately results in a totally deformed and unsup-portive joint.[9]

Preventing Injury

All runners should be familiar with a few basic prin-ciples that can help them avoid injury and promote muscular skeletal health. These principles are dis-cussed below.

Most athletic injuries, especially those of runners are due to overuse. The greater number of miles that a runner runs per week, the higher the likelihood of injury. Many training periods per week promote a greater number of injuries. Therefore, to be totally safe, a runner should run only two or three times a week and for less than a total of 30 miles. Cross training provides excellent general conditioning and helps prevent injury.

Runners should be familiar with the "float" phase of running. This is the period when both feet are off the ground. The longer the float phase the greater the impact when the heel strikes the ground. This impact is responsible for most running injuries. Lengthening the stride, running down hill, or run-ning on uneven terrain increases the impact and is likely to lead to injury. Running uphill and shorten-ing the stride will decrease impact. Runners should take into consideration the above factors as well as surface, shoes, training schedule, warm-up, and weight training of the lower extremities as a part of the training program for running.

Most importantly with running or any other sport, training should be done slowly and painlessly. A base-line training level should be established based on previous experience, current strength, medical evaluation, and trial at moderate performance. If there is pain or stiffness following moderate perfor-mance, then a lower base line should be established. A base line should be the highest level of perfor-mance that can be attained without any residual symptoms. Too low a base line will slow the train-ing process excessively and psychologically work against the athlete.

Once the base line has been identified it is in-creased by 10% each week unless significant symp-toms develop. Occasionally, with high levels of per-formance, a 10% increase may cause minor symptoms for a day or two, but they should subside by the end of a week. If they do not, another week at the same level is in order.

Another basic well-accepted concept is cross train-ing. Exercising and traumatizing any one set of mus-cles or joints every day can lead to cumulative in-jury. Therefore, it is important to rest for at least 1 day after a very specific high-level activity. That is not to say that the athlete has to stop all training for a day or two. There are many other valuable activi-ties that the athlete can be doing. High-level ath-letes require flexibility, endurance, strength, and co-ordination. Rarely does a single sport or event tax all of these areas to the maximum. Sprinting, for ex-ample, develops maximum strength and coordina-tion but may not tax the maximum levels of flexi-bility and endurance. Cross training for the sprinter, therefore, could be more endurance running, flexi-bility training or weight training. Each athlete should work with his/her trainer and coaches to determine what the best cross-training activities would be for the sport in general and for the specific athlete's pos-itive and negative characteristics.

To prevent and treat spinal problems, the athlete should be doing specific training of the lumbar pro-tective mechanism at least 2 days a week. This is thoroughly covered in Chapter 22 on stabilization training. The coordinated utilization of muscles and movement patterns to protect the spine require high-level understanding and training. In general, however, there are certain muscles that need to have great strength and endurance to protect the spine during high-level athletics. These include all layers of the abdominal wall and gluteal, paraspinal, ham-string, and iliopsoas muscles. Flexibility of the ham-strings and hip joints is important for low-back pro-tection. The quadriceps muscles must be very strong so that the knees can be loaded in the flexed posi-tion repeatedly for long periods in order to allow hip flexion with a stable lumbar spine. In other words, the stress ordinarily placed on the lumbar spine in working and athletic activities needs to be transferred through the hips to the knees by a coordinated effort of strong abdominal, paraspinal, gluteal, and hamstring muscles. These muscles are used to find and hold the pelvis in a position that aligns the spine in a pain-free and stress-free range while running.

Rehabilitation

The rehabilitation of an injured runner first requires an extensive evaluation of the running style, mechanism of injury, physical examination, and aggravating and relieving factors (see Chapter 5). This is necessary to identify the pain generator and to provide a working diagnosis. Ankle and knee injuries in runners who run in excessive foot pronation or valgus can be prevented by commonly known corrective exercises and supports. By simply strengthening the weak side of a joint and stretching out the contracted side, one can overcome many of the chronic strains and sprains that occur. If there are already arthritic changes it may be too late to correct the mechanics of the joint adequately to return the runner to the high level that they expect. It is very difficult to train a runner to run with his/her knee or ankle in a position other than its normal one in contrast to the spine and pelvis, which can easily be altered and held in any available range.

With spinal problems it is difficult to identify the specific mechanism of injury. Observing the runner in action may help the clinician identify an excessive lordotic posture or unstabilized pelvic rotation and tilt. Recurring pain with sitting and bending may indicate a disc problem that can be better controlled by altering off-the-track activities rather than the actual running itself. A frankly herniated disc may be so severe that the vertical loading of running is impossible. In general, with improved spinal training most runners can modify the lumbar protective mechanism in order to stabilize themselves for improved running.

Runners are no more prone to herniating a disc than the average individual. The herniated disc virtually never occurs while running but is the result of improper body mechanics of bending, lifting, and sitting. If a herniated disc occurs, extreme levels of stabilization training may be necessary. Surgery, if necessary, accompanied by good spinal training, usually returns the athlete to normal running. These individuals frequently have good results with arthroscopic disc surgery.

The following intensive program of stabilization training applies to all nonneurologic sources of back pain.

Strength

Although the running muscles (calf, thigh, and hip) may be quite strong and have very good endurance in the long-distance runner, other muscles that contribute to the lumbar protective mechanism may not be as strong or have such great endurance. Specific work needs to be done on the abdominal, gluteal, and paraspinal muscles. Whereas a runner might have occasionally done a few sit-ups or crunches, he/she now may need to do several hundred a day. The paraspinal muscles are rarely specifically exercised in the running athlete. This requires some form of special equipment such as a Roman chair to do lumbar extension exercises or "back-ups." Most individuals can only do 20 or 30 repetitions of this exercise. Eventually the athlete with an injured lumbar spine should be able to do as many as 100 and perhaps 30 or 40 with a 20-lb weight held to the chest.

There are many easy ways to develop gluteal strength and musculature, such as climbing stairs two or three at a time. Eventually, the running itself becomes a spine-strengthening activity. Holding the pelvis in a new stabilized position while running reinforces the strength of the muscles of the lumbar protective mechanism.

Flexibility

Although the running athlete usually does a fair amount of stretching, an injured lumbar spine may continue to be stressed by tight hamstrings or tight hip joints, which transfer excessive forces to the lumbar spine. Extreme degrees of flexibility of the hamstring and hip joints can be protective to the low back. In the beginning, the runner may need to stretch as long as 30 minutes a day and then maintain this flexibility by performing at least a 5-minute warmup before and 5 minutes of slower running after every hard run.

Body Mechanics—Proprioception

The most difficult task for any athlete is to change his/her running style. He/she has developed success and style over years of repetition. Changing normal successful patterns is met with major resistance, both psychologically and physically. As the individual tries to change a style, performance will lag at first. With proper stabilization training, however, most athletes become more efficient and their success becomes greater when the new stabilization training becomes a natural process.

The analysis of a runner's stabilization is somewhat difficult. It requires a trained therapist, trainer, or physician either running with the patient, videotaping or standing next to a patient running on a treadmill. Obvious imbalance due to foot pronation and hip circumduction should be noted. Any irregularity in the alignment of the lower extremity joints as mentioned above will transfer undo forces to the lumbar spine. Some of these lower-extremity irregularities can be corrected by stretching, strengthening, or inserts. Ultimately, however, we have to teach the patient how to use his proprioception and muscles to hold the lumbar spine in a painless balanced range as other joints do the work.

Chapter 27 on stabilization gives the details of basic stabilization training. Once the basics are understood and working well in the training room, the runner must get out and practice stabilization while running. This may begin with fast walking and build through slow running to full running over months of practice.

Adjunctive Measures

When stabilization training is not working we need to add other tools to our armamentariam. One is injection procedures such as therapeutic blocks. Cortisone injections can be placed in the facet joint or in the epidural space to relieve inflammation and accelerate training. Corsets and braces can be used to stabilize a spinal condition temporarily while it is healing and while training to develop the strength and coordination to do without the external support. Manual therapy can assist in restoring normal range of motion of the spine to injured segments.

There are many pain control measures that can help training. These include acupuncture, ice, and massage. Many athletes are responsive to alternative approaches such as Rolfing, patterning, Feldenkreis, and Reike.

Although no one needs to give up running because of spinal problems, with good diagnostic studies and training techniques, an accurate diagnosis and successful rehabilitation program can be developed.

References

1. Eichner ER: Runner's macrocytosis: a clue to foot-strike hemolysis. Runner's anemia as a benefit versus runner's hemolysis as a detriment, *Am J Med* 78:321, 1985.
2. Glick J, Katch V: Musculoskeletal injuries in jogging, *Arch Phys Med Rehab* 51:123, 1970.
3. Guten G: Herniated lumbar disc associated with running: a review of 10 cases, *Am J Sports Med* 9:155, 1981.
4. Herring SA, Nilson KL: Introduction to overuse injuries, *Clin Sports Med* 6:225, 1987.
5. Jackson DW, Pagliano J: The ultimate study of running injuries, *Runner's World*, November:42, 1980.
6. Lane NE, Bloch DA, Jones HH, et al.: Long distance running, bone density and osteoarthritis, *JAMA* 255:1147, 1982.
7. Lane NE, Bloch DA, Wood PD, Fries JF: Aging, long-distance running and the development of musculoskeletal disability: a controlled study, *Am J Med* 82:772, 1987.
8. Lees A: A preliminary investigation in the shock absorptions of running shoes and shoe inserts, *Hum Movement Stud* 10:95, 1984.
9. Mankin H, et al.: Biochemical and metabolic abnormalities in articular cartilage from osteoarthritic human hips, *J Bone Joint Surg* 52A:424, 1970.
10. Mann RA: *Biomechanics of running.* In AAOS symposium on the foot and leg in running sport, September, 1980, St. Louis, 1982, Mosby.
11. Manter JT: Movements of the subtalar and transverse tarsal joints, *Anat Rec* 80:397, 1941.
12. Radin EL, Paul IL, Rose SM: Some mechanical factors in pathogenesis of osteoarthritis, *Lancet* 1:512, 1972.
13. Smith C: Physical management of muscular low back pain in the athlete, *Can Med Assoc* J 117:632, 1977.
14. Sohn R, Micheli LJ: The effect of running on the pathogenesis of osteoarthritis of the hips and knees, *Clin Orthop Relat Res* 198:106, 1985.
15. Ting AJ, King W, Yocum L, et al.: Stress fractures of the tarsal navicular in long distance runners, *Clin Sports Med* 7:89, 1988.

Chapter 53
Snow Skiing
Paul J. Slosar, Jr.

Snow skiing has grown in popularity over the past 20 years. Participants range from the very young to the elderly. Skiing demands aerobic conditioning, as well as strength and endurance. Skiers frequently encounter uneven terrain, and therefore a keen sense of balance is essential.

Competitive skiing has expanded from the traditional downhill slalom races to include free-style, ballet, moguls, and aerial events. While one would expect to see acute spinal injuries more frequently in freestyle aerialists, no well-documented prevalence studies have been published.[3] The two largest series place the prevalence rate of acute spinal injuries in the downhill skiing population at about 30%.[4,7] The severity of injury was highly variable, ranging from the simple (contusions and lumbar strains) to the catastrophic (injuries with neurologic loss). The most severe cases usually occurred as the result of a collision with stationary objects (rocks, trees, machinery, or other skiers). Margreiter et al. found a decreased rate of spinal injury in experienced skiers.[4] Each discipline of skiing places unique demands on the lumbar spine. Ballet, mogul, aerial, and slalom skiing, while unique sports, are not dissimilar. This discussion will therefore be generalized so that it may apply to the rehabilitation of an advanced snow skier. Specific adjustments for the individual skiing disciplines can be made with the input of ski-team trainers, therapists, and coaches.

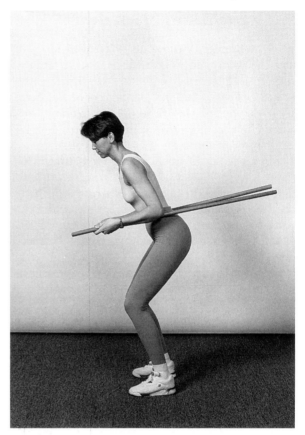

Fig. 53-1
Basic snow skiing position.

Mechanism of Injury

The basic mechanisms of injury to be considered are compression, rotation, and tension. While all three movements can occur while skiing, repetitive rotation or torsional spine movements are prevalent in Alpine skiing. It is this pathologic motion that is implicated in shear injuries to the annulus and disc.[2] It is of note that the first reported case of a herniated nucleus pulposus, as described by Mixter and Barr, was an injured skier.[6]

Biomechanics of Skiing

In an effort to understand better the injury patterns of competitive skiers, and formulate a sport-specific rehabilitation program, one must be familiar with the biomechanics of skiing. The skier is continuously adjusting to maintain balance. The center of gravity is somewhere below the pelvis, between the thighs. Expert skiers move their body parts efficiently to maintain proper balance. The arms are used as a balance–counterbalance system.[5] Stability is increased by lowering the center of gravity. This enables the skier to use an independent foot action for turning. The crouching, or tuck, position also reduces air friction.

The basic skiing position begins with the feet hip-width apart. The knees and ankles should be flexed for shock absorption and weight shifting. The hips are positioned above the boots. The trunk is bent slightly at the waist (Fig. 53-1). From this position, the skier can initiate turns and quickly react to terrain changes. This position forms a stable base in which weight is balanced to allow forward and backward weight shifts. A skier with a strong, agile base will ski efficiently, minimizing twisting upper body motions. It is these exaggerated trunk motions that tend to aggravate back pain.

Obviously, the freestyle ballet and mogul skiers will adopt markedly different body positions during their competitions. Nonetheless, they are still skiing down the hill, maintaining balance, and therefore are employing similar basic skills as the downhill racers.

Evaluating Back Injury

When evaluating the elite skier athlete with a back injury, the history will be most important. As with other competitive athletes, the injuries are usually either acute (sprains, contusions, anular tears or disc herniations) or chronic, repetitive overuse injuries. These chronic injuries may involve the anulus or disc, but may also be of more complex unclear etiology.

Most people do not sustain back injuries while skiing. Skiers who have a history of back pain may find that skiing will aggravate this symptom. If the skier's symptoms worsen by the day's end, then attention must be turned to evaluating the skier's strength, endurance, and body mechanics. This is especially common in recreational skiers who spend fewer than 10 days per year on the slopes. These skiers may also experience symptoms as they attempt to put on their skis and boots. This may be due to tight hamstrings and hip flexors, causing these skiers to overutilize their lumbar spines in flexion. Equipment advancements such as step-in boots and bindings may be helpful.

The paraspinal muscle spasm and pain that accompany the acute phase can be controlled with the judicious use of analgesics, antiinflammatory medications, muscle relaxants, and therapeutic methods, especially ice. As the acute phase of injury resolves, attention is turned to reconditioning and to reeducating the athlete.

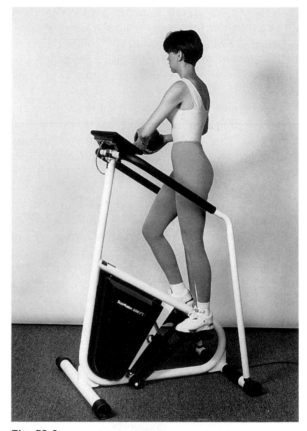

Fig. 53-2

Alternating from left to right trunk bias on stair climber.

Rehabilitation

The rehabilitation of competitive or recreational snow skiers will concentrate on specific muscle groups. Quadriceps strength is the cornerstone of the skier's program. Early focus on this muscle group along with the hip flexors, extensors, and external rotators will benefit the patient. If these muscle groups are weak, the skier may have difficulty controlling the position of his or her back. It is critical to keep these lower-extremity and pelvic girdle muscles well conditioned during the acute phases of a low-back injury. Flexibility of these lower-quadrant muscle groups is equally important. Improving the skier's strength at the cost of flexibility is to be avoided. All skiers, but especially the "weekend warriors," must be instructed on the importance of lower-extremity and back stretching before stepping into their boots and bindings.

The trunk muscles are crucial in force generation for turns as well as in stabilizing the skier over rough terrain.[5] The paraspinal, internal and external obliques, and rectus abdominous are the muscles that provide this power and stability. In essence, stabilization of the pelvis is the critical link for the skier. A stable pelvis provides the inherent resistance against which the legs may turn. High-level conditioning is extremely important for the weekend skier who insists on skiing at an advanced level. Critical attention to quadricep and hamstring strength, endurance, and flexibility is essential.

Stabilization training has the greatest potential to address the sports-specific demands of this high-level rehabilitation. The training stresses education, body mechanics, strength, flexibility, coordination, and endurance as program basics. A detailed description of stabilization training is found in Chapter 27. Proprioception and balance are critical elements of training for these athletes. Creative training techniques as discussed below will challenge the skier in sagittal, frontal, and transverse planes.

The competitive skier will modify the basic training specifically to address sport demands. As the neutral, or pain-free zone is defined, the athlete must begin to transfer this into his or her skiing. Early

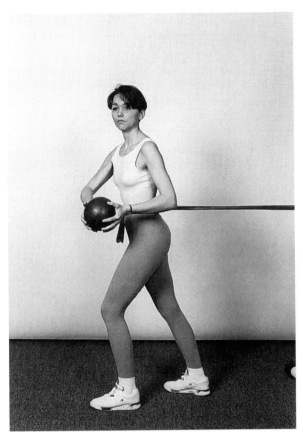

Fig. 53-3
Sports cord tied to patient and immovable object. Keeping pelvis straight and biasing shoulders, without lumbar rotation, reinforces formation of strong, stable base.

training on a slide board or lateral sled will give the skier a transition from the gym to the slopes. After the skier can maintain acceptable posture on the slide board for 15 to 20 minutes, the training should move outside the gym. Placing the athlete on a stair-climber machine and having him/her alternately sweeping his/her hands in an arc from left to right will improve balance, proprioception, and endurance (Fig. 53-2). Using a "sports cord" with the athlete's trunk and shoulders turned away from the pelvis reinforces the formation of a strong, stable base (Fig. 53-3).

Most competitive skiers participate in off-season skating-skiing drills using in-line skates. These skates are a tremendous training tool, and skiers of any level are encouraged to use them. The athlete may use ski poles and should begin on flat terrain. Direct feedback from the therapist or trainer will keep the athlete's spine in the proper neutral zone. Eventual progression to an inclined terrain will follow. Pylons are added to the course to simulate turning gates.

As the skier advances in the training, it will become necessary occasionally to use indoor sessions to cor-

rect technical problems seen during drills. Lapses usually occur as skiers tuck into a crouch without enough knee bend. Another difficult skill to master is reaching into the gate without excessive upper trunk rotation. Not only does this constitute poor stabilization form, but it also slows the skier down. Videotaping performance may also prove very useful.

Freestyle ballet and mogul skiers will consistently violate certain aspects of neutral spine mechanics during their routines. It may be more appropriate to view these competitors as gymnasts on skis. A trampoline can be used for coordination and balance drills. Most freestyle skiers will have some familiarity with off-season use of the trampoline.

The advanced weekend skier should be held to the same training ideals as the elite or professional athlete. Basic strength training of the quadricep, hamstring, abdominal, and paraspinal muscles must be accomplished. Most of these skiers should be able to hold a wall slide for 3 to 5 minutes and perform 100 to 200 abdominal crunches painlessly. Straight leg raising to 90 degrees should also be accomplished without pain.

Summary

As mentioned before, many skiers will experience back pain because they compromise their spines as they attempt to negotiate their equipment. By improving their flexibility and strength as well as utilizing proper equipment, most of this strain can be eliminated. Recreational skiing in a controlled fashion on groomed runs allows the skier to perform in a position of maximal comfort, essentially unloading the lumbar spine. Rehabilitating these patients to a safe and early return to the slopes is to be encouraged.

As the skier progresses through these drills, the rehabilitation training will transfer onto the ski slope. At this point, the athlete or coach will be more involved than the trainers or therapists. It is now the athlete's responsibility to prevent future injuries by maintaining a quality training program year-round.

References

1. Eriksson E: Ski injuries in Sweden: a one year survey, *Orthop Clin North Am* 7:3, 1976.
2. Farfan HF, Cossette JW, Robertson GH, et al.: The effects of torsion on the lumbar intervertebral joints: the role of torsion in the production of disc degeneration, *J Bone Joint Surg* 54A:469, 1970.
3. Frymoyer JW, Pope MH, Kristiansen T: Skiing and spinal trauma, *Clin Sports Med* 1:309, 1982.

4. Margreiter R, Raas E, Lugger LJ: The risk of injury in experienced alpine skiers, *Orthop Clin North Am* 7:51, 1976.

5. McMurtry JG: *Biomechanics of Alpine skiing.* In Maday MG editor: *Winter sports medicine,* Philadelphia, 1990, F.A. Davis Co., p 344.

6. Mixter WJ, Barr JS: Rupture of the intervertebral disc with involvement of the spinal canal, *N Engl J Med* 211:210, 1934.

7. Tapper EM: Ski injuries from 1939 through 1976: the Sun Valley experience, *Am J Sports Med* 6:114, 1978.

Chapter 54
Soccer
Lisa Steinkamp

Incidence of Injury

Soccer is the most popular sport in the world and is the fastest-growing team sport in the United States. Twenty-two million males and females of all ages currently participate in school, amateur, or professional soccer leagues.[6] Soccer's growing appeal can be attributed to its social and physical conditioning opportunities, as well as its relative inexpense and convenience.[11]

There are many factors involved in the computation of soccer injuries. An overall assessment of studies performed on soccer injuries reveals that injury rates increase with age and intensity of play, occurring more during games than practices; females have a higher incidence than males. Overuse injuries tend to occur during preseason and at the end of the season. Player position does not seem to matter, with the exception of the goalie position, where there is a higher incidence of injury.[6]

Depending on the study, anywhere from 64% to 88% of all soccer injuries reported involve the lower extremity. Head and upper-extremity injuries are proportionately greater in younger players. Although the incidence is low, most severe injuries appear to be induced through player contact and tackling, and tend to occur more in older players.[6] Back pain is infrequently reported, the highest incidence being presented in a study involving 14% of 496 players; however, any spine involvement should be approached seriously.[13]

Soccer is a challenging sport with respect to the spine due to its exploitation of trunk flexion, extension, and torsion, in addition to its capacity for running, cutting, jumping, landing, falling, and player contact.[2] Conditioning is important to avoid injuries. Soccer players need to maintain good cardiorespiratory status, flexibility, and strength, and should always warm up before play begins.

The vast majority of spine-related soccer injuries involve the lumbar spine.[14] The four predominant mechanisms of lumbar spine injuries are extension (Fig. 54-1), flexion (Fig. 54-2), torsion (Fig. 54-3), and compression (Fig. 54-4).[2] Excessive trunk extension can result in facet-joint injuries. Hyperflexion of the trunk adversely affects the intervertebral discs.[12] Torsional injuries to the spine implicate both the facets and the discs.[3] Repetitive impact such as occurs during jumping, heading, running, tackling, colliding, and falling can cause compressional injuries such as spondylosis, spondylolysis, and spondylolisthesis.[15] A biomechanical analysis of various soccer moves illustrates how these moves compromise

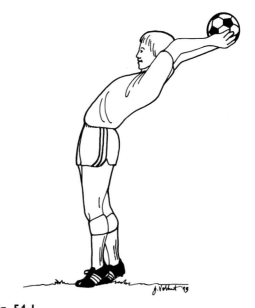

Fig. 54-1
Excessive trunk extension is required during many soccer moves, such as throw-ins.

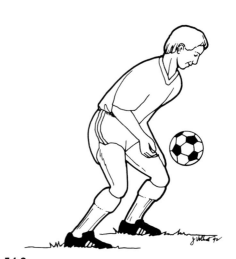

Fig. 54-2
Trunk hyperflexion is frequently utilized in soccer to trap and protect the ball.

the spine. Training tips are suggested to help protect the spine during these moves.

Kicking

The soccer kick can be initiated with the ball at a standstill, as in set plays, or while the ball is in motion, as in passes. Shooting also falls into this category. Ball contact can be made with the inside, outside, or full instep, or with the heel or medial aspect of the foot. The angle of approach and placements

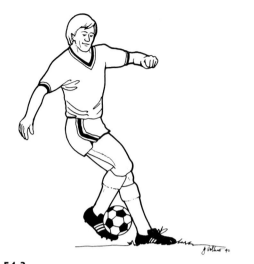

Fig. 54-3

Trunk torsion is inherent during such soccer moves as trapping, cutting, dribbling, and kicking.

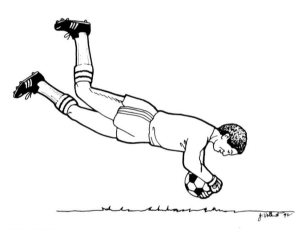

Fig. 54-4

Compressional injuries to spine can occur from running, jumping, falling, or player contact, especially while goalkeeping.

celeration during follow-through.[10] To allow for minimal trunk torque and maximum efficiency while ensuring neutral spine, the hip flexors must rotate with the pelvis throughout the kick. It is critical to have good overall flexibility in the spine musculature, as well as in the hamstring, quadricep, adductor, and gastrocnemius-soleus muscle groups. Flexible hip rotators during approach and foot plant, hip flexors during backswing, and hip extensors during follow-through are also important.

In terms of strength, emphasis should be placed on strong abdominals (including the obliques), gluteals, chest muscles (especially the pectorals), and spine musculature (especially the latissimus dorsi and paraspinals) for trunk stabilization, particularly during extreme motions of trunk flexion and extension. Strong quadriceps, hamstrings, adductors, abductors, and gluteals are important for both planting of the nonkicking leg, and acceleration and deceleration of the kicking leg. Soccer players need to be strong isometrically, concentrically, and eccentrically for stabilization, acceleration, and deceleration capabilities, respectively.

Dribbling

Fewer spine injuries are sustained during dribbling since it involves taking relatively shorter strides while contacting the ball with any available part of the foot.[1] However, to elude an opponent, feinting, which usually entails quick lateral movements, is necessary. These rapid changes in direction and speed can be stressful on the spine if it does not have time to react. To train for these situations, lateral motions with slight trunk flexion while maintaining neutral spine should be practiced. Strong gluteal, abdominal, chest, and upper-extremity muscle groups assist in stabilization; the spine musculature works statically. Strong quadriceps, hamstrings, gluteals, and hip adductors and abductors aid in holding a flexed knee position while performing lateral motions. Upper back and abdominal strength will help limit torquing at the waist.

Tackling

Tackling to take the ball away from an opponent demands sudden moves and can be accomplished with the foot, shoulder, or by sliding. Block tackles involve intercepting the ball with the tackling foot while most of the player's body weight is forward over the ball. Shoulder tackles entail lateral and rotational motions from the side or front as the player steals the ball.

of the planting foot, kicking foot, knee, and trunk, can vary depending on the direction, height, and distance desired for the ball. Power should originate from the lower-leg snap and not from the upper-leg swing.[5] Kicking incorporates ball approach, foot plant, body positioning with knee and trunk inclination, backswing, acceleration, ball contact, and follow-through. Most kicking injuries to the lumbar spine occur during long-distance kicks and are a result of excessive trunk extension during follow-through, especially when the kick is initiated from trunk flexion.[9] Other injuries to the spine can occur from pelvic torquing during any phase of the kick, impact during foot plant or ball contact, backswing into too much hip extension, or from ineffective de-

Slide tackling requires an oblique approach, sliding in front of the opponent while kicking the ball away. Spine injuries sustained during tackling moves are often due to improper contact with the opponent, but can also occur as a result of jarring during block tackles, excessive lateral or torquing motions during shoulder tackles, or as a consequence of poor falling techniques during slide tackles.[5] Quadriceps, hamstrings, gluteals, and spine muscles should be statically strong to maintain a flexed knee and trunk position during block tackles. Lateral motions should be practiced while maintaining neutral spine for shoulder tackling, and the player should have strong hip adductors and abductors as well as a strong upper body. Falling while stabilizing the spine should be practiced for slide tackling. Strong gluteals, abdominals, and spine muscles for spine stabilization are a necessity for all types of tackles. Flexibility is also important, especially in the hip flexors, extensors, abductors, adductors, and rotators during sliding and lateral motions.

Trapping

Trapping can be achieved with any part of the foot, thigh, or chest. The objective is to stop the ball, whether in the air or on the ground, and bring it under control. This usually involves relaxing and recoiling at contact the part of the body trapping the ball. Balance, quick reflexes, and ball control are essential. During foot and thigh traps, the body is centered over the ball. The most detrimental trap for the spine is the chest trap since the trunk is extended, then recoiled into flexion on ball contact to allow the ball to decelerate and drop in front of the player's feet.[1] For all traps, it is important to practice extremity isolation while maintaining neutral spine, during both acceleration and deceleration motions. Particularly for chest traps, it is necessary to have strong quadriceps, hamstrings, and gluteals for the starting position, and strong hip flexors and abdominals for the trunk motion from extension to flexion. Overall flexibility is vital to grant the range of motion required for trapping. Hip flexors need to be especially flexible during the starting position of a chest trap.

Heading

Heading is considered to be a type of trap but can also be employed to project the ball for purposes of passing, shooting, or clearing. Prior to ball contact, the trunk is extended, the chin is retracted, the cervical muscles are isometrically contracted, and the knees are flexed and widespread for balance. The ball is hit with a forward thrust of the trunk, head, and neck, making contact with the forehead. The head and neck should act as a single unit, with all power coming from the trunk.[5] Some players like to jump or dive while heading balls. To head a ball to the side, the body is rotated and the head is turned in the direction in which the ball is to travel. To head a ball backward, the knees are extended and the hips are driven forward at ball contact. Most injuries sustained during heading are either cervical in nature or are due to excessive trunk motion.[8] Cervical strength and stabilization are critical to prevent segmental movement during heading. Strong abdominal, gluteal, spine, chest, and anterior neck musculature are crucial to stabilize the spine. Flexible hip flexors are essential while the trunk is extended. Quadriceps, hamstrings, and gluteals should be strong to maintain the starting position. Since acceleration originates from the trunk, neck, and head, strength in the abdominals, hip flexors, and cervical muscles are important during the forward thrust.

Throw-ins

Throw-ins simulate heading in that there is an aggressive trunk drive from extension to flexion. The starting position is the same, with the trunk extended and the knees flexed and widely spread for balance. Throw-ins can be even more deleterious to the spine, since the lever arm is increased with the extension of both arms overhead, holding onto the ball. As the trunk is driven forward, the arms accelerate overhead, compounding the velocity imparted to the ball. The ball is released while it is overhead and both feet are on the ground. Follow-through is directed toward the target and requires deceleration of the trunk and arms after release of the ball.[1] Injuries can occur as a result of extreme trunk extension or flexion, trunk translation from extension to flexion, or from ineffective deceleration after ball release.[4] It is therefore important not only to be able to isolate the arms while stabilizing the spine, maintaining neutral spine from extension to flexion, but also to have strong abdominals concentrically and strong spine muscles eccentrically for the drive forward and follow-through, respectively. The strength and flexibility requirements discussed above for heading also apply to throw-ins.

Goalkeeping

Goalkeeping incorporates both catching and clearing skills. Catching can include any motion from flexing the trunk and kneeling for ground balls, to jumping and extending for overhead balls, to any motion in between. Catching also requires diving in random directions with full body extension, landing on the player's chest or side with elbows out front, rolling, and pulling the ball in to the chest. Clearing techniques involve ridding of the ball by kicking it, by punching it directly away or deflecting it overhead, or by throwing it underhand or overhand with elbow flexion or extension. All clearing techniques demand instant aim at any of a number of targets so agility is imperative. Since the objective is to protect the ball, the goalie is usually positioned in trunk flexion, bringing the ball to his/her chest, and recoiling the trunk to reduce the shock of the ball's impact. Injuries can occur in any of the above situations for many of the reasons we have already discussed. For example, during catching motions, excessive trunk flexion is requisite for ground balls, and the knees are extended to prevent the ball from rolling between them, so flexible hamstrings and spine muscles are critical. For high balls, excessive trunk extension is necessary, and for dive balls, landing is an additional hazard. Goalies should therefore work on absorbing the impact of the ball and ground with their bodies and on isolating their extremities while protecting the spine. With regard to clearing motions, deflecting the ball and overhead throws exploit trunk extension, while underhand throws abuse trunk flexion; strong abdominals are crucial during all. Kicking requires accelerated trunk movement from flexion to extension, so spine stabilization is essential. Fundamentally, goalies should attain appropriate flexibility and strength in their trunk and extremities to perform a wide variety of soccer moves effectively.

Rehabilitation Techniques and Progression of Return to Play

It has been shown that sport-specific prevention programs can help to reduce the risk of injury.[6] These programs should incorporate off-season conditioning maintenance, flexibility and strengthening exercises, warmup and cooldown periods, preparticipation and postinjury return-to-play medical evaluations, accurate injury diagnosis, and rehabilitation following the principles of specificity, recovery, and supervised progression.[7]

A basic clinical rehabilitative stabilization program for most spine injuries will take approximately 3 months. This will comprise the stages of pelvic tilt, bridging, partial situps, "dead bugs," and quadriped

exercises. Past this stage, exercises more specific to soccer begin to apply. For instance, with regard to throw-ins, the patient's progression should be from kneel-to-leanback exercises, to resisted diagonal kneeling, to throwing while sitting on a physioball, to medicine ball throwing from sitting to standing, followed by progression onto the field. Along with this advanced stabilization program, an upper-extremity weight program consisting of exercises such as chest row, chest press, leanback lat pulls, and wall-pulley stabilization exercises should be initiated.

For progression to dribbling and kicking, a similar program should be established advancing from kneel to leanback, to standing weightshift with resistance, to treadmill walking in neutral spine, to stationary dribbling, to manual resistance through kicking patterns with maintenance of neutral spine, and then onto the field with ball drills. Along with this stabilization program, there should be a lower extremity strengthening program consisting of modified hacksquats, modified leg press, Stairmaster, proprioceptive neuromuscular facilitation manuals, and wall-pulley stabilization exercises.

From the initiation of the stabilization program to the time the patient is allowed onto the field may take up to 3 months, depending on how long it takes for each phase to be accomplished successfully. Another month should be spent observing the player during practice, as he or she is slowly weaned into practice and then into a game situation.

Summary

The biomechanics of multiple soccer moves and of the vulnerable positions in which they place the spine are reviewed. The four most common mechanisms of lumbar spine injury are extension, flexion, torsion, and compression, which generally result in facet, disc, a combination of facet and disc, and spondylosis/spondylolysis/spondylolisthesis injuries, respectively. Strength, flexibility, and stabilization training are imperative to protect the spine against these injuries while playing soccer.

As soccer continues to gain popularity, it will become increasingly important for all involved, i.e., physician, physical therapist, athletic trainer, coach, parent, and player, to have a thorough understanding of its relevant biomechanics, potential mechanisms of injury, and treatment and prevention of these injuries. The more knowledge we have, and the younger we educate and train our soccer players, the more successful we may be at future injury prevention.

References

1. Bluth RG, editor: *Soccer: sports techniques,* Chicago, 1971, The Athletic Institute.

2. Farfan HF: *The biomechanics of lumbar injury in athletes.* Presented at Aggressive Rehabilitation of Back and Neck Pain in Athletes Conference sponsored by the Centinela Hospital Medical Center, Inglewood, CA, August 20-21, 1988.

3. Farfan HF: Effects of torsion on the intervertebral joints, *Can J Surg* 12:336, 1969.

4. Gracovetsky S: *Biomechanics of the lumbar spine.* Presented at Aggressive Non-surgical Rehabilitation of Lumbar Spine and Sports Injuries Conference sponsored by the San Francisco Spine Institute, San Francisco, March 23-25, 1989.

5. Ingels NB: *Coaching youth soccer,* Palo Alto, CA, 1975, Page-Ficklin Publishing Co.

6. Keller CS, Noyes FR, Buncher CR: The medical aspects of soccer injury, *Am J Sports Med* 15:230, 1987.

7. Kibler WB, Chandler TJ, Stracener ES: Muscoloskeletal adaptations and injuries due to overtraining, *Exerc Sport Sci Rev* 20:99, 1992.

8. Kurosawa H, Yamanoi T, Yamakoshi K: Radiographic findings of degeneration in cervical spines of middle-aged soccer players, *Skel Radiol* 20:437, 1991.

9. Olson JR, Hunter GR: Anatomic and biomechanical analyses of the soccer style free kick, *NSCA J* 7(6):4, 1985.

10. Pronk NP: The soccer push pass, *NSCA J* 13(2): 6, 77, 1991.

11. Ruege K: *Contemporary soccer,* Chicago, 1978, Contemporary Books, Inc.

12. Saal JA: Rehabilitation of sport related lumber spine injuries, *Phys Med Rehab State Art Rev* 1:613, 1987.

13. Schmidt et al: Injuries among young soccer players, *Am J Sports Med* 19:273, 1991.

14. Sward L, et al.: Back pain and radiologic changes in the thoracolumbar spine of athletes, *Spine* 15:124, 1990.

15. Weir MR, Smith DS: Stress reaction of the pars interarticularis leading to spondylolysis: a cause of adolescent low back pain, *J Adolesc Health Care* 10:573, 1989.

Chapter 55
Swimming

Andrew J. Cole
Richard E. Eagleston
Marilou Moschetti

Swimming remains the most prevalent sport in the United States.[14] It is an extremely popular form of exercise for recreation, competition, and rehabilitation. Current estimates reveal that over 28,000 people participate in U.S. Masters Swimming and over 2000 centers use aquatic techniques for rehabilitation.[78] Aquatic-related spine and associated musculoskeletal injuries are being seen in every-increasing numbers. Land-based exercise, swimming, or an inappropriate aquatic rehabilitation program can cause new spine injuries or exacerbate preexisting ones. Properly designed aquatic programs can be utilized to rehabilitate spinal injuries. Aquatic stabilization techniques and swimming programs may be used in conjunction with an aggressive, comprehensive land-based spine stabilization program or independently.[13,34]

Repetitive microtrauma from swimming is a primary cause of spine injury. It has been estimated that if the average competitive swimmer swims 5000 yards freestyle per day, 5 days each week, using 15 strokes per pool length, and breathes every other stroke, he/she will produce 600,000 arm movements, 300,000 cervical spine rotations, and 600,000 lumbar rotatory movements per year.[34] In addition, supplementary land-based flexibility and strength programs without attention to proper spine mechanics can either cause or contribute to spine injury and pain.[73] Mutoh et al.[61] retrospectively studied 66 elite Japanese aquatic athletes including competitive swimmers, divers, water polo players, and synchronized swimmers. The low back was the most common site of injury for all four groups, and 37.1% of the 19 competitive swimmers had chronic low-back pain. This finding is similar to Mutoh's 1983 study,[60] in which 33% of 51 Japanese swimmers had low-back pain. This is in contradistinction to Richardson's study in 1980,[70] in which shoulder pain was found to be the most common orthopedic problem in competitive swimming. Although all spinal structures are presumably at risk during swimming activities, the biomechanics of certain strokes predispose particular structures to increased risk.

Biomechanics of Spinal Injury

Of the four competitive strokes, freestyle and backstroke increase lumbar segmental axial rotation and thus torque forces most and therefore place the annulus fibrosus in particular jeopardy.[9,36,37,40] This risk factor would seem to decrease in importance with the improved stroke technique seen in elite swimmers. Although trained to roll their bodies as a unit (nonsegmentally),[23-26,77] minimizing torque

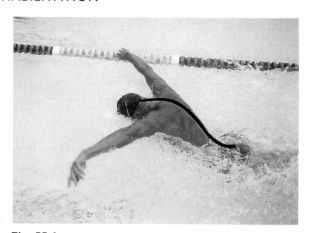

Fig. 55-1

Risk of lumbar facet pain increases with strokes that include an accentuated lumbar extension such as butterfly and breaststroke. *(From Moschetti M: AquaPhysics Made Simple, Aptos, CA, 1989, Aqua-Technics Consulting Group.)*

force across individual lumbar motion segments and also decreasing head drag forces, elite swimmers probably subject these segments to greater force per stroke. Thus, they paradoxically increase the chance of injury due to repetitive microtrauma.[9,17-20,29,54]

Lumbar Spine

The risk of lumbar facet pain increases with strokes that include an accentuated lumbar extension such as butterfly and breaststroke[77] (Fig. 55-1). In the performance of these two strokes, the elite athlete, in particular, is at risk due to an exaggerated undulation that increases sagittal motion—i.e., extension and flexion. This undulation compounds the risk of facet injury due to repetitive microtrauma. Even with the breaststroke, traditionally a controlled swimming style, advances in stroke technique have resulted in a significant increase in sagittal plane motion by emphasizing undulatory rather than linear, plane horizontal motion.[46] Although injury to the pars interarticularis may be seen more frequently in competitive divers,[72] many swimmers with a quiescent spondylolysis may become symptomatic due to the repetitive extensions that occur with breaststroke, butterfly, starts, and turns. Furthermore, the risk of developing a spondylolysis due to stress placed on the posterior column of the spine by these strokes remains unclear.

Thoracic Spine

Although injuries to the thoracic spine seem to occur less frequently and appear to be more easily rehabilitated, these structures are nonetheless at risk.

Most commonly seen is thoracic facet pain, especially with strokes that generate a great degree of increased segmental rotatory motion at particular thoracic motion segments, such as freestyle and backstroke. The extension required in butterfly and breaststroke may cause facet-joint dysfunction and pain. The pain, which may be caused by inflammation, results from repetitive facet compression, distraction, and shear forces.[24,25,28] We believe that during the pull phase, compressive forces are generated by the ipsilateral latissimus dorsi, scapular retractors, and long thoracic spinal extensor muscle groups. Ipsilateral thoracic spinal muscle groups produce an extension to counter the flexion of the latissimus dorsi. The contralateral thoracic spinal muscle groups stabilize the thoracic spine, preventing untoward lateral flexion toward the pull-phase side. Passive distractive forces affect the ipsilateral facet during the recovery phase due to activation of the ipsilateral scapular protractors, relaxation of the scapular retractors, inactivation of the latissimus dorsi, and relative relaxation of the thoracic spinal extensor muscle groups.[19,20,64,68,75]

Thoracic costovertebral joints may be injured due to significantly increased vital capacity and enhanced chest wall and rib motion. These joints may be further compromised by arm elevation and the consequent increased tension on the rib system. Additionally, faulty stroke mechanics resulting in increased rotation through the thoracic spine may also contribute to costovertebral joint pain.

Cervical Spine

The cervical spine is subjected to continuous repetitive microtrauma from the mechanics of breathing. Annular as well as facet injuries are most commonly seen with freestyle swimming due to the significant rotation required for side breathing.[19,20,28] Occasionally, a side-breathing technique is used during the butterfly, also placing the cervical segments at increased risk. Extension, which is seen with breaststroke and butterfly, increases the chance of cervical posterior element injury, resulting in cervical facet pain (Fig. 55-2). Cervical extension can also increase intradiscal pressure, compromising the intervertebral disc.[80] Although the backstroke requires little rotation for breathing, exceptional stabilization of the cervical segments in a relatively neutral position is needed to decrease drag forces. We therefore tend to see fewer intrinsic cervical segmental injuries from this stroke. However, muscular strain to the cervical dynamic stabilizing soft tissues such as the paraspinal muscle groups is common. Note should be made of the risk of catastrophic cervical spine injury due to

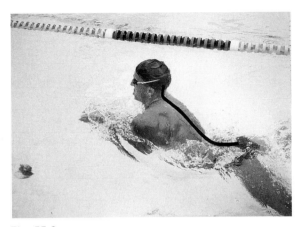

Fig. 55-2
Breaststroke requires repetitive end-range cervical extension for breathing, increasing risk of cervical posterior element injury, which can produce facet pain. *(From Moschetti M: AquaPhysics Made Simple, Aptos, CA, 1989, AquaTechnics Consulting Group.)*

impact loading.[3,41,47,49] The greatest potential for this type of injury occurs because of faulty start mechanics and less commonly with impact loading of the cervical spine during a missed turn—particularly during the backstroke, when the oncoming wall is not seen or overhead warning flags are not observed.[17,18,59]

Peripheral-Joint Mechanics and General Spinal Abnormalities

Peripheral-joint dysfunction can set off a cascade of motion changes throughout the spinal axis. In particular, the cervicothoracic and thoracolumbar transition zones are most commonly affected because they are the junction between the more mobile and less mobile sections of the spine.[28,66] Figure 55-3 presents that "motion cascade." For example, a shoulder injury such as rotator cuff tendinitis results in guarding and decreased range of motion of the shoulder.[24,27,28,75] The swimmer's arm cannot abduct and extend as it normally would[45] during recovery, resulting in decreased body roll, increased lumbar segmental motion, and an abnormally low head position from which to breathe.[23] Compensatory adaptive changes, which include cervical extension and rotation (Fig. 55-4) facilitated by increased range of motion from C3-C5, then occur.[28] The C5-T1 segments ultimately become hypomobile to compensate, and mid and low cervical pain results. Compensatory hypermobility from T2-T5 and hypomobility from T5-T7 and T10-L1 begin. Primary cervical, thoracic, and lumbar injuries and

Diagram 1. The Motion Cascade

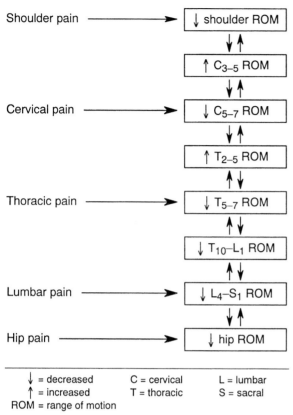

Shoulder pain ⟶ ↓ shoulder ROM

↑ C$_{3-5}$ ROM

Cervical pain ⟶ ↓ C$_{5-7}$ ROM

↑ T$_{2-5}$ ROM

Thoracic pain ⟶ ↓ T$_{5-7}$ ROM

↓ T$_{10}$–L$_1$ ROM

Lumbar pain ⟶ ↓ L$_4$–S$_1$ ROM

Hip pain ⟶ ↓ hip ROM

↓ = decreased	C = cervical	L = lumbar
↑ = increased	T = thoracic	S = sacral
ROM = range of motion		

Fig. 55-3

Peripheral-joint dysfunction sets off a "motion cascade" throughout the spinal axis; conversely, spine dysfunction can create peripheral-joint dysfunction. *(From Moschetti M: AquaPhysics Made Simple, Aptos, CA, 1989, AquaTechnics Consulting Group.)*

pain influence the spinal axis in a similar fashion. Hip, pelvis, and lumbar spine pain result in hypomobility of L4-S1 and ultimately at the T10-L1 transition zone. Adaptive changes then proceed up the axis and may even set the stage for a compensatory change in shoulder mechanics and ultimately cause a shoulder injury. Identification of the initial injury is important so that treatment can eliminate that problem as well as the secondary compensatory sites of dysfunction.[24]

Patients with Scheuermann's kyphosis were found to have increased pain during swimming, particularly during the butterfly stroke, as seen in a study by Wilson and Lindseth.[82] Of the four competitive strokes, the butterfly includes the greatest end-range extension of the diseased, less-mobile thoracic motion segments. Increased pectoral and associated chest and abdominal muscle contractions during the pull phase of a stroke like the butterfly may cause additional compressive forces that further damage anterior column structures.[7] However, because these muscles are also significantly active during the pull phase of the freestyle and breaststroke,[15,58,64,67,68] repetitive end-range extension microtrauma may be the primary biomechanical source of pain in the butterfly. Although patients with kyphosis can be managed conservatively with daily bracing, additional time out of the brace was suggested to allow continued swimming. So long as the butterfly stroke was avoided, no deleterious change was noted.[82] Additionally, be-

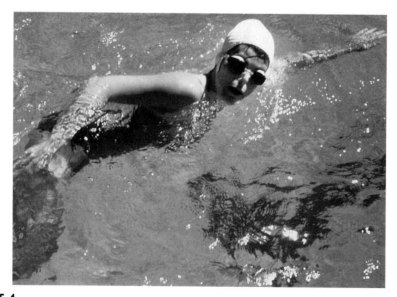

Fig. 55-4

Crane breathing during freestyle swimming. During crane breathing, suboccipital and cervical extension coupled with cervical rotation occurs in addition to cervical rotation. *(From Moschetti M: AquaPhysics Made Simple, Aptos, CA, 1989, AquaTechnics Consulting Group.)*

cause of the swimmer's horizontal position in the water and the buoyant effect of the water, the axial compressive forces on the spine[58] are significantly reduced. This positioning and buoyancy may therefore significantly mitigate the mechanical risk factors that may cause this condition to progress.

The prevalence of adolescent idiopathic scoliosis is approximately 2% to 3%.[79] In the athletic population, the average frequency of idiopathic scoliosis has been reported to be 2%,[53] and the incidence of functional scoliosis 33.5%.[51] The higher incidence of functional scoliosis in the athletic population may be due to larger unilateral torque forces developed in particular activities such as serving and throwing.[53] More recent work by Becker[5,6] has shown an incidence of 6.9% for idiopathic scoliosis and 16% for functional scoliosis in the screening of 336 swimmers at the Junior Olympic Swimming Championships, East, 1983. The 6.9% figure is roughly three times the reported incidence of structural idiopathic scoliosis, but the 16% figure is below the incidence reported by Krahl and Steinbruck.[51] However, 100% of the functional curves were toward the dominant-hand side, which according to Yeater et al. consistently produces greater pull-phase peak forces than the nondominant side.[83] Further studies summarized by Becker revealed histologic and morphologic changes in the paraspinal and gluteus muscles and secondary adaptation of supporting vertebral soft tissues and adaptive changes in muscles to meet specific repetitive functional demands.[8] However, if curve progression is truly facilitated by the unsymmetrical functional demands swimming places on the spine, then a therapeutic exercise program could theoretically be designed to counter them. Moreover, exercise alone is unable to inhibit the progression of a scoliotic curve,[6] and it remains to be shown whether it can accelerate curve progression. Additionally, the most recent advances in swimming technique, especially in the freestyle, emphasize symmetrical motion (e.g., alternate-side breathing) and minimize repetitive unilateral torsion and lateral flexion. Proper coaching should help to deemphasize further the potential effect of a stronger dominant side on the spine. We believe that swimming is not contraindicated for the adolescent with functional or idiopathic scoliosis. We recommend appropriate training by the patient's therapist and coach, both of whom should know swimming technique and mechanics. In fact, with proper technique, aquatic activity may help the scoliotic patient to maintain flexibility, strength, and endurance, while minimizing axial compressive forces and sheer forces on the spine.

Diagnosis and Treatment

The work-up and diagnosis of spine pain in swimmers is no different than that for any other athlete and has already been covered. The astute clinician has a thorough understanding of anatomy and stroke-specific functional biomechanics, which allows him/her to make a correct final diagnosis. In addition, the sports spine physician must be cognizant of the great physiologic and psychologic needs of elite competitive athletes. For example, highly competitive athletes require alternate training regimens during their rehabilitation programs to maintain peak flexibility, strength, and aerobic conditioning. Recreational swimmers may be more flexible in this regard. Therefore, the aggressiveness of a work-up and rehabilitation program should be geared to the level of an athlete's need. The need to make changes in land-based training and specific stroke mechanics as part of the rehabilitation process make close cooperation with the patient, therapist, and coaches imperative.[21,24-26,28,69,77]

Dynamic land-based stabilization training is a specific type of therapeutic exercise that can help patients gain dynamic control of segmental spine forces, eliminate repetitive injury to their motion segments (i.e., discs, facets, and related structures), encourage healing of injured motion segments, and possibly alter the degenerative process. The underlying premise is that motion segments and their supporting soft tissues react to minimize applied stresses and thereby reduce risk of injury. The goals of aquatic stabilization swimming programs incorporate these same elements but take into account the unique properties of the aqueous medium so that risk of spine injury is minimized. Aquatic stabilization swimming programs should minimize segmental trunk motion and shear forces; reinforce lumbar control; encourage hip, knee, and ankle propulsion; develop head and neck stability; and establish arm control and strength.[16,19,20,23,74]

Properties of Water

Buoyancy was first described by Archimedes (ca. 287-212 B.C.), who noted that the force exerted on an immersed object is equal to the weight of the liquid it displaces.[55,58] This unique property of water allows for depth-dependent graded elimination of gravitational and shear forces on the immersed patient. When patients are vertically immersed up to their necks, a reduction of gravitational forces of approximately 90% occurs.[32] A center of buoyancy can

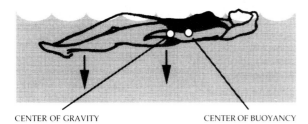

CENTER OF GRAVITY   CENTER OF BUOYANCY

Fig. 55-5

Center of buoyancy and center of gravity are located in two separate positions. *(From Moschetti M: AquaPhysics Made Simple, Aptos, CA, 1989, AquaTechnics Consulting Group.)*

be located in the region of the pleural cavity in supine patients. This center is distinct from the center of gravity, which is the point through which the force of gravity acts, and which is located at the level of the second sacral segment or anterior superior iliac spine (Fig. 55-5). In water, the more caudad the center of gravity, the greater the amount of spine extension is required to keep the patient afloat, that is, to place the center of buoyancy in an optimal position to balance downward forces at the center of gravity (Fig. 55-6). Conversely, a more cephalad center of gravity requires less spine extension to keep the patient afloat (Fig. 55-7). Buoyancy increases

Fig. 55-6

More caudad center of gravity requires greater spine extension to keep patient afloat. This extended spinal position creates potential pain problem for patients with facet pain or foraminal stenosis. *(From Moschetti M: AquaPhysics Made Simple, Aptos, CA, 1989, AquaTechnics Consulting Group.)*

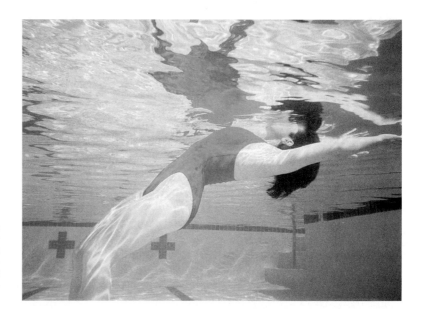

Fig. 55-7

More cephalad center of gravity requires less spinal extension to keep patient afloat but may increase intradiscal pressure and exacerbate discogenic symptoms. *(From Moschetti M: Aqua-Physics Made Simple, Aptos, CA, 1989, Aqua-Technics Consulting Group.)*

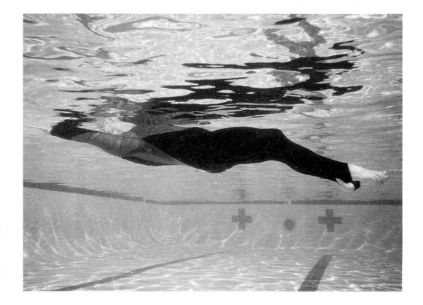

with decreasing depth and will have a greater effect on body parts that are positioned to produce longer lever arms. Therefore, the direction of motion of the body part, up, down, or horizontal, dictates whether buoyant force is used to assist, resist, or support it, respectively.[39,41,52]

The *specific gravity,* that is, relative density, of an object is defined as its weight relative to the weight of an equal volume of water. The specific gravity of water is 1.0. Humans float because their specific gravity is less than that of water. In humans, specific gravity increases with greater bone density and muscle mass and reduced body fat. Specific gravity decreases with less bone density and muscle mass and more body fat. Clearly, both buoyant forces and specific gravity play a critical role in patient positioning and energy consumption during aquatic therapeutic

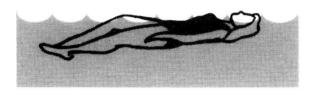

SPECIFIC GRAVITY IS LESS THAN 1.0 —
THUS THE HUMAN BODY WILL FLOAT

Fig. 55-8

Specific gravity of humans is less than that of water; thus human body floats in water. *(From Moschetti M: AquaPhysics Made Simple, Aptos, CA, 1989, AquaTechnics Consulting Group.)*

exercise programs[41,47,48] (Fig. 55-8). In fact, women can swim a given distance with approximately 30% less energy consumption that men because of their increased hydrodynamic lift and buoyancy. Their increased lift and buoyancy is due to their lower specific gravity and higher body fat.[57] The effect that gravity and buoyancy have on an immersed object is known as the metacentric principle. Gravity and buoyancy work in opposite directions: gravity downward and buoyancy upward. If these two forces are equal and opposite, no movement occurs. If, however, they are not equal, rotation of the object occurs until the forces once again balance. Therefore, careful assessment must be made of a patient's shape, relative density, and precise site of injury and pain to help avoid any undesirable movement through the injury site when positioning the patient for aquatic therapeutic exercise.[13]

Hydrostatic pressure is force per unit area and is measured in atmospheres. The greater the depth, the greater its effect on an immersed patient. It may enhance proprioceptive feedback and improve patients' kinesthetic awareness (Fig. 55-9). Hydrostatic pressure has many effects on the cardiovascular system, including increasing venous return and stroke volume. Hydrostatic pressure also has renal consequences such as changes in renal blood flow and ear, nose, and throat (ENT) effects including changes in sinus pressure. Appropriate cardiac, renal, and ENT precautions must be observed.*

*References 1, 4, 10, 11, 34, 35, 38, 44, 52, 56 to 58, 62, and 71.

Hydrostatic Pressure in Water

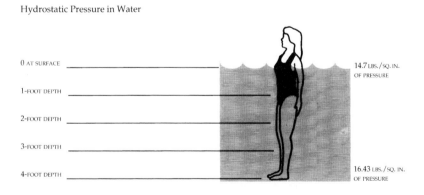

0 AT SURFACE

1-FOOT DEPTH

2-FOOT DEPTH

3-FOOT DEPTH

4-FOOT DEPTH

14.7 LBS./SQ. IN. OF PRESSURE

16.43 LBS./SQ. IN. OF PRESSURE

.433 POUNDS PER SQUARE INCH INCREASE IN HYDROSTATIC PRESSURE FOR EVERY ONE FOOT OF INCREASE IN DEPTH

AT 33 FEET DEEP, PRESSURE IS TWICE AS MUCH AS IT IS AT THE SURFACE

Fig. 55-9

Hydrostatic pressure progressively increases at greater depths and thus produces depth-dependent physiologic consequences in human body. *(From Moschetti M: AquaPhysics Made Simple, Aptos, CA, 1989, Aqua-Technics Consulting Group.)*

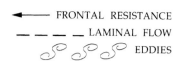

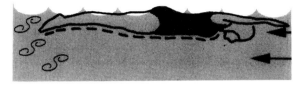

Fig. 55-10

Frontal resistance, laminar flow, and eddies created during prone swimming activities. *(From Moschetti M: AquaPhysics Made Simple, Aptos, CA, 1989, AquaTechnics Consulting Group.)*

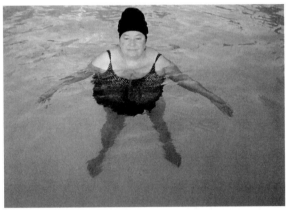

Fig. 55-11

Refraction causes visual distortion of submerged portion of body when viewed from above water. *(From Moschetti M: AquaPhysics Made Simple, Aptos, CA, 1989, AquaTechnics Consulting Group.)*

Viscosity is the frictional resistance of a fluid. Because water is more viscous than air, it offers a resistive force to movement that can assist in strengthening and conditioning patients as well as increasing their kinesthetic awareness. The faster the motion, the greater the resistance.[52,58] In fact, McArdle et al. point out that the energy cost of swimming a given distance is about four times greater than running the same distance.[57]

Turbulence is a force differential created by movement and is a result of frontal resistance, laminar flow, and drag (eddies, tail suction). Frontal resistance impedes forward progress of any body part. Ideally, a layer of water flows down the body while it is in motion. This laminar flow produces small low-pressure areas called "eddies," "tail sections," or "drag," which help dissipate frontal pressure caused when water is not able to "fill in" the streamlined parts of the body. Faster movement through water

results in greater drag and resistance, which increase the muscular work required for movement[52] (Fig. 55-10).

Refraction is a medium-dependent change in the speed of light causing visual distortion of submerged objects when viewed from above water. Refraction can make the acquisition of new skills, particularly those involving specific coordinated motions, more difficult. This effect is most profound in patients who have limited kinesthetic awareness[58] (Fig. 55-11).

Water temperature can affect cognitive function as well as cardiac, respiratory, and muscular effort through a variety of mechanisms, including various forms of heat transfer such as conduction, convection, and radiation. Oxygen consumption increases linearly with swimming speed, with the greatest consumption occurring in colder water due almost entirely to the energy cost of shivering to maintain core temperature. Therefore, the optimal temperature range for swimming is 28° C-30° C (82° F-86° F). Within this range, the metabolic heat generated during exercise is easily transferred to the water without causing an even greater energy cost due to cold-water stress.*

The advantages aquatic programs offer are directly related to the properties of water.[43] Graded elimination of gravitational forces through buoyancy allows the patient to train with decreased yet variable axial loads and shear forces. In essence, water increases the safety margin of patient postural error by decreasing the compressive and shear forces on the spine. The velocity of motion can be better controlled by water resistance, viscosity, buoyancy, and the training devices utilized. Buoyancy increases the available range of training positions. The psychologic outlook of athletes can be enhanced because rehabilitation occurs in their competitive environment. Many believe that a certain degree of pain attenuation takes place in the water because of the "sensory overload" generated by hydrostatic pressure, temperature, and turbulence.†

Aquatic Spine-Stabilization Techniques

The same principles of spine stabilization that have been discussed for land programs are applicable to

---

*References 2, 34, 41, 52, 56, 58, and 63.
†References 17, 18, 30, 31, 42, 48, 50, 52 to 58, 64 to 68, 72 to 74, and 76.

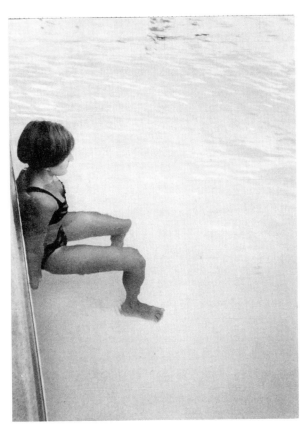

Figure 55-12

Wall sit develops isometric strength primarily in quadriceps and hamstring groups. Abdominal muscles are trained to hold appropriate dynamic posture. *(From Moschetti M: AquaPhysics Made Simple, Aptos, CA, 1989, AquaTechnics Consulting Group.)*

aquatic programs. Certain exercises that can be performed on land cannot be reproduced in water and vice versa. Aquatic programs can be designed for those unable to train on land or for those whose land training has plateaued. Aquatic stabilization was first described by Richard Eagleston in 1989.[33]

A set of six core aquatic stabilization exercises with three levels of difficulty has been designed to provide graded training of stabilization skills.[17-20,22,23,25,26] Table 55-1 and Figs. 55-12 to 55-25 illustrate a typical aquatic exercise progression for a patient with lumbar discogenic pain. Programs must be customized to meet the needs of each patient's unique spine pathology, related musculoskeletal dysfunctions, and comfort with the aquatic environment. Once mastered, a more advanced program is provided. Eventually, athletes can return to swimming programs that incorporate spine stabilization techniques.[17–20]

Rehabilitation Environment: Land versus Water

Accurate diagnosis of patients' spinal injuries and observation of their initial response to land-based stabilization helps determine further therapeutic exercise treatment options. A transition from dry to wet exercise conditions eliminates dry-land risks, establishes a supportive training environment, provides a new therapeutic activity, decreases the risk of pe-

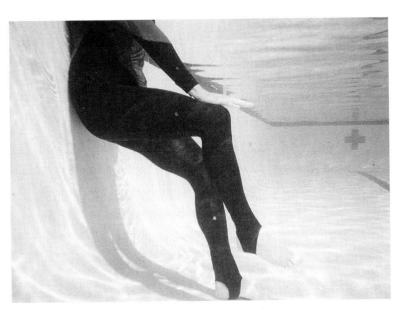

Fig. 55-13

Level 1 partial wall situps train muscles activated in wall sit and additionally challenge contralateral gluteals, ipsilateral hip flexors, and rotation abdominals, and paraspinals. *(From Moschetti M: AquaPhysics Made Simple, Aptos, CA, 1989, AquaTechnics Consulting Group.)*

Table 55-1

Aquatic stabilization exercises: progression for lumbar discogenic pain

Exercise	Level 1	Level 2	Level 3
Wall sit	Isometric 90-degree hip 90-degree knee 1-min hold	Isometric 90-degree hip 90-degree knee 3-min hold	Isometric 90-degree hip 90-degree knee 5-min hold
Partial wall situp	Isometric Hip flexion Unilateral Alternating 90-degree hip 90-degree knee 5-sec hold 60 sec/side	Isotonic Hip flexion Bilateral Simultaneous 45-degree hip 90-degree knee Repetitions: 2 min	Isotonic Hip flexion Bilateral Simultaneous 45-degree hip Knee: full extension Repetitions: 3 min
Modified superman	Face wall Hip extended to 20 degrees Knee: 45-degree static Unilateral 60 sec/side	Face wall Hip extended to 20 degrees Knee: full extension Unilateral 2 min/side	Face wall Hip extended to 20 degrees Knee: full extension Unilateral 3 min/side 3 lb/ankle cuffs
Water walk backward	Palms at side 3 min Slow speed*	Palms forward Abduct arms 45 degrees 5 min Moderate speed†	Palms forward Abduct arms 45 degrees Hand paddles 10 min Fast speed‡
Water walk forward	Palms at side 3 min Slow speed*	Palms forward Abduct arms 45 degrees 5 min Moderate speed2	Palms forward Abduct arms 45 degrees Hand paddles 10 min Fast speed‡
Quadruped	Therapist assist Prone Mask/snorkle Alternating Arms only 1 min Alternating Legs only 1 min	Therapist assist Prone Mask/snorkle Simultaneous or alternating Arm/leg 3 min	No assist Ski belt Prone Mask/snorkle Simultaneous or alternating Arm/leg 5 min

*Slow = 50% of potential maximum velocity.
†Moderate = 70% of potential maximum velocity
‡Fast = 85% of potential maximum velocity.

ripheral-joint injury, and allows a return to a prior activity. Moving from dry to wet environments should also be considered if patients have an intolerance to axial or gravitational loads or require increased support in the presence of a strength or pro-

prioceptive deficit. Remaining in a water-supported environment is appropriate if the dry environment exacerbates symptoms or the patient has an exclusive preference for the water. Transition from a wet to a dry environment should occur if patients are

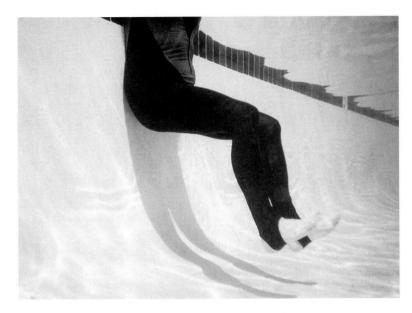

Fig. 55-14

Level 2 partial wall situps train bilaterally and isotonically hip flexors and hip extensors. Higher-level isometric conditioning continues for abdominal and paraspinal muscle groups. *(From Moschetti M: AquaPhysics Made Simple, Aptos, CA, 1989, AquaTechnics Consulting Group.)*

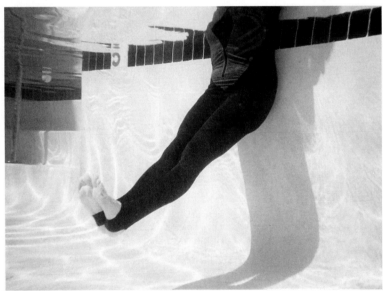

Fig. 55-15

Level 3 partial wall situps provide an incrementally greater challenge to all groups described in Fig. 55-14, level 2 exercise. *(From Moschetti M: AquaPhysics Made Simple, Aptos, CA, 1989, AquaTechnics Consulting Group.)*

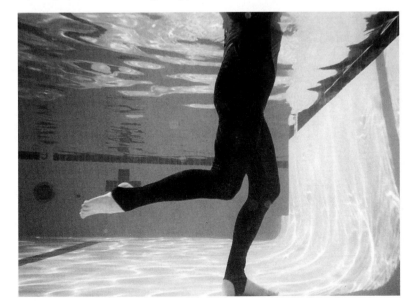

Fig. 55-16

Level 1 modified superman develops strength in ipsilateral hip flexors and extensors and contralateral gluteus medius, as well as isometric strength in abdominal and paraspinal stabilizers. *(From Moschetti M: AquaPhysics Made Simple, Aptos, CA, 1989, AquaTechnics Consulting Group.)*

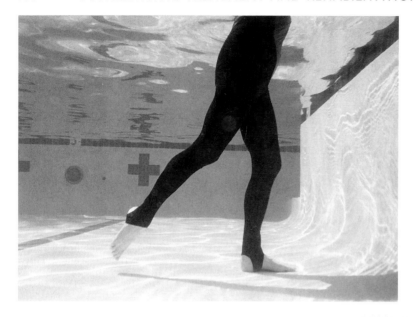

Fig. 55-17

Level 2 modified superman provides an incrementally greater challenge to all groups described in Fig. 55-16, level 1 exercise. *(From Moschetti M: AquaPhysics Made Simple, Aptos, CA, 1989, AquaTechnics Consulting Group.)*

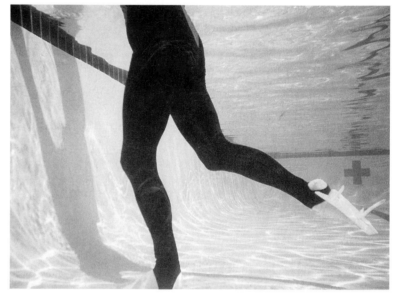

Fig. 55-18

Level 3 modified superman again incrementally enhances resistive exercise and training duration of activity for muscle groups previously described for this component of progression. *(From Moschetti M: AquaPhysics Made Simple, Aptos, CA, 1989, AquaTechnics Consulting Group.)*

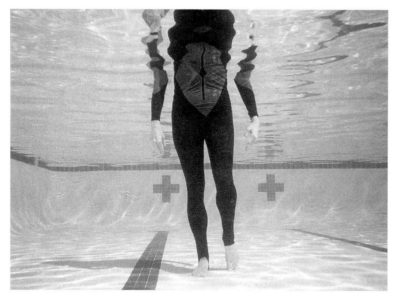

Fig. 55-19

Level 1 walking forward isometrically strengthens abdominal muscle groups and groups involved in maintaining proper posture. Isotonic strengthening occurs in muscles dynamically involved in gait. Walking backward provides similar strengthening pattern with greater emphasis on isometric paraspinal muscle conditioning. *(From Moschetti M: AquaPhysics Made Simple, Aptos, CA, 1989, AquaTechnics Consulting Group.)*

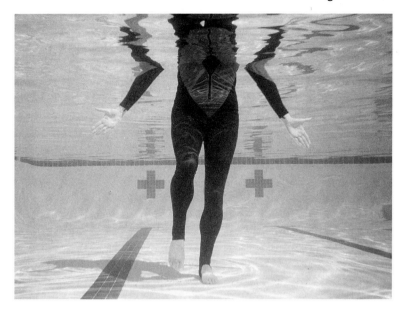

Fig. 55-20

Level 2 walking forward and backward provides incrementally greater challenge to all groups described in Fig. 55-19, level 1 exercise. *(From Moschetti M: AquaPhysics Made Simple, Aptos, CA, 1989, AquaTechnics Consulting Group.)*

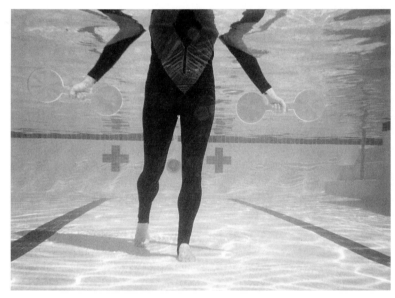

Fig. 55-21

Level 3 walking forward and backward incrementally enhances resistive exercise and training duration of activity for muscle groups previously described for this component of progression. *(From Moschetti M: AquaPhysics Made Simple, Aptos, CA, 1989, AquaTechnics Consulting Group.)*

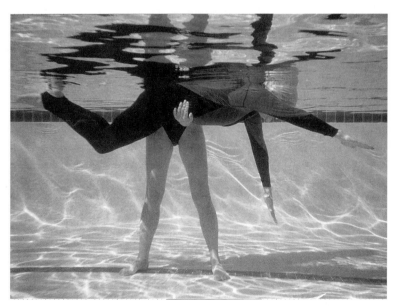

Fig. 55-22

Level 1 quadruped activities (arms only) challenge lumbar spine stabilizer groups isometrically and upper-extremity shoulder groups that produce flexion and extension isotonically. *(From Moschetti M: AquaPhysics Made Simple, Aptos, CA, 1989, AquaTechnics Consulting Group.)*

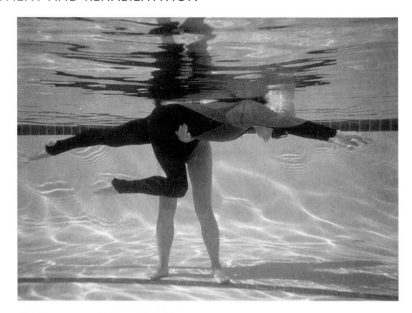

Fig. 55-23

Level 1 quadruped activities (legs only) challenge lumbar spine stabilizer groups isometrically and lower extremity hip flexors and extensors isotonically. *(From Moschetti M: AquaPhysics Made Simple, Aptos, CA, 1989, AquaTechnics Consulting Group.)*

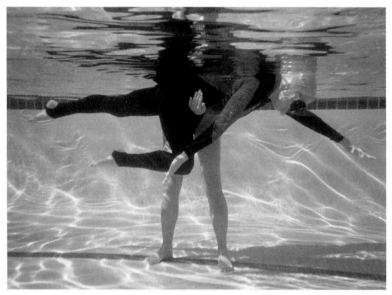

Fig. 55-24

Level 1 quadruped activities incrementally and isometrically challenge lumbar spine stabilizer groups and continue to train isotonically upper- and lower-extremity groups previously described in Figs. 55-22 and 55-23, level 1 exercise. *(From Moschetti M: AquaPhysics Made Simple, Aptos, CA, 1989, AquaTechnics Consulting Group.)*

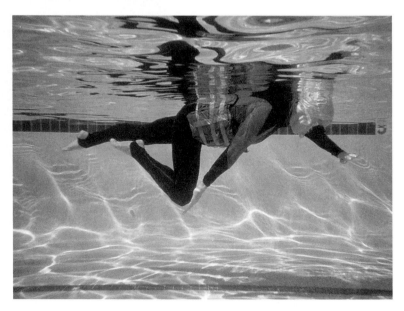

Fig. 55-25

Level 3 quadruped exercise again increases training intensity progression by requiring greater independence during performance of exercise. *(From Moschetti M: AquaPhysics Made Simple, Aptos, CA, 1989, AquaTechnics Consulting Group.)*

doing well in the water and need to return to land to most efficiently meet functional training needs in order to attain their ultimate competitive goals.[17-20] (See box below for specific contraindications for aquatic rehabilitation).[21,25,69]

Contraindications for Aquatic Rehabilitation

1. Fever
2. Cardiac failure
3. Urinary infections
4. Bowel and/or bladder incontinence
5. Open wounds
6. Infectious diseases
7. Contagious skin conditions
8. Excessive fear of water
9. Uncontrolled seizures
10. Colostomy bag or catheter used by patient
11. Cognitive/functional impairment that creates a hazard to the patient or others in pool
12. *Severely* weakened or deconditioned state that poses a safety hazard
13. *Extremely* poor endurance
14. *Severely* decreased range of motion that limits function and poses a safety hazard

Prone Swimming

Once patients' stabilization skills have progressed to the point at which a return to swimming is possible, a thorough analysis of stroke technique and its effect on spine motion is critical. The following overview will focus on lumbar spine injury and indicate the role that the cervical spine plays in the mechanics of lumbar aquatic motion.

In prone swimming, the head should be midline. Breathing should occur by turning the head, i.e., rotating the head along the axial plane. There should be no craning, that is, extending and rotating the cervical spine (see Fig. 55-4). Body roll also contributes to proper breathing mechanics and is essential in order to minimize dysfunctional cervical positioning and subsequent pain. The cervical spine should be kept in the neutral position along the sagittal plane since excessive extension causes the legs and torso to drop in the water while excessive flexion can cause a struggle for air.[17-20,23,25,26,28]

Upper-body arm position is evaluated by stroke phase (see box below). Freestyle is broken into three phases. The entry phase includes both hand entry and hand submersion ("ride"). The pull phase incorporates insweep, outsweep, and finish components. The recovery phase includes exit and arm swing.[77] There are several stroke defects that can cause poor lumbar mechanics. If the arm abducts beyond 180 degrees, lateral lumbar flexion is produced (Fig. 55-26). During the pull phase, decreased body rotation can cause lateral lumbar flexion and rotation, which stresses the lumbar spine. Inadequate triceps strength during the finish phase results in low arm recovery, which in turn generates secondary lateral flexion through the lumbar spine. During recovery, inadequate body roll causes the neck to crane, which results in a struggle for air and accompanying lateral flexion and rotation through the lumbar spine.[17-20,23-26,28]

Swimming Stroke Phases (Freestyle)

I. Entry phase
   A. Hand entry
   B. Hand submersion ("ride")

II. Pull phase
   A. Insweep
   B. Outsweep
   C. Finish

III. Recovery phase
   A. Exit
   B. Arm swing

Trunk motion is closely monitored for any primary or secondary lumbar flexion, both sagittal and coronal, or for axial rotation. If not corrected by simple changes in stroke mechanics, additional proprioceptive cues can be provided by taping the lumbar spine region. The tape pulls on the skin each time the lumbar spine moves in a segmental manner (i.e., when the patient generates excessive lumbar rotation or lateral lumbar flexion) (Fig. 55-27).

Flip turns are discouraged. Instead, stabilized turns are employed in which the patient initially comes to a vertical position before turning. This vertical position allows the patient the opportunity to stabilize the spine in preparation for changing direction. Eventually, a horizontal spin is incorporated into the turn and the vertical position is eliminated. Flip turns may then be resumed.[17-20,23,25,26,77]

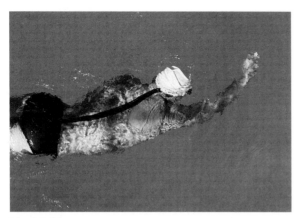

Fig. 55-26

Swimmer's arm abducts beyond 180 degrees during the entry phase of freestyle. This stroke defect creates lateral lumbar flexion and lumbar segmental rotation. *(From Moschetti M: AquaPhysics Made Simple, Aptos, CA, 1989, AquaTechnics Consulting Group.)*

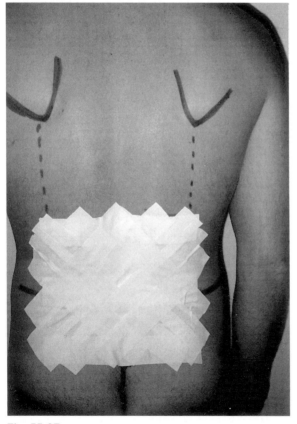

Fig. 55-27

Waterproof strapping tape can be applied to lumbar spine to reinforce lumbar proprioceptive awareness and help minimize lumbar rotation and lateral flexion. *(From Moschetti M: AquaPhysics Made Simple, Aptos, CA, 1989, AquaTechnics Consulting Group.)*

Supine Swimming

In the supine position, starting with a simple kicking program is best, with arms at the side since adequate stabilization can be easily maintained. Often, the use of fins is suggested to improve propulsion. While supine, extension of the cervical spine will induce lumbar extension. On the other hand, cervical flexion will cause the patient to "sit" in the water with lowered leg position and decreased propulsion. Extreme cervical extension or flexion are to be avoided in favor of a more neutral stabilized cervical posture[17-20,23-26,28,77] (Figs. 55-28 and 55-29).

Improving Stroke Technique

Problems with stroke technique can usually be solved with simple changes in stroke mechanics or by the addition of adaptive equipment. For example, a struggle for air can be resolved by the addition of a mask and snorkel. Trunk position can be improved by using the taping technique already mentioned. Poor propulsion can be remedied with an appropriate choice of fins. Hand paddles can provide better kinesthetic awareness of hand and arm position.[17-20,23,25]

Once basic stroke mechanics can be performed in a spine-safe manner, more complicated and challenging strokes and training regimens may be initiated. Patients might begin rigorous skulling programs for enhanced aerobic benefit. Or, aquatic running programs might be added.[12,81] The spine can be challenged with varied and graded axial loads by varying the depth in which patients train. A variety of other exercise options exist. The critical factor common to all aquatic therapeutic exercise programs is that they be performed with the lumbar spine in neutral position and well stabilized.[31,36,37,54,55]

Summary

Repetitive microtrauma from swimming and the land-based flexibility and strength programs that are performed without attention to proper spine mechanics can either cause or contribute to spine injury and pain. Because the spinal axis is essentially a force transmitter for peripheral-joint motion, both direct spinal injury as well as altered biomechanics at sites distant from the spine can change spinal mechanics and cause dysfunction and pain. A series of aquatic stabilization exercises have been designed that incorporate the intrinsic properties of water and

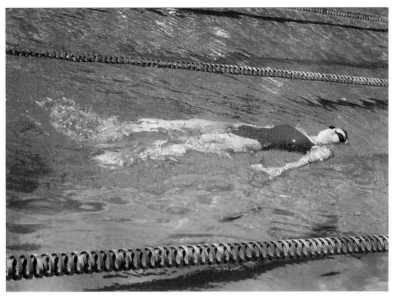

Fig. 55-28

While supine, cervical spine extension induces lumbar extension. *(From Moschetti M: AquaPhysics Made Simple, Aptos, CA, 1989, AquaTechnics Consulting Group.)*

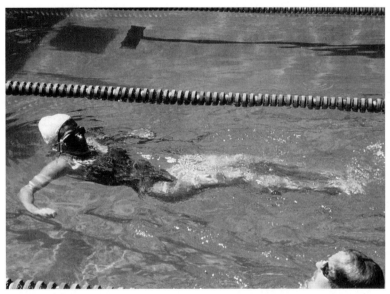

Fig. 55-29

While supine, cervical spine flexion induces lumbar flexion and "sits" in the water. *(From Moschetti M: AquaPhysics Made Simple, Aptos, CA, 1989, AquaTechnics Consulting Group.)*

enhance rehabilitative efforts. Once mastered, injured athletes can soon be advanced to spine-safe swimming. Close attention must be paid to proper swim stroke biomechanics and to the effect that abnormal mechanics may have on the spine. This attention ensures the most rapid rehabilitation of spinal disorders in the swimming athlete.

Acknowledgment

The authors would like to thank Sandra Pinkerton, Ph.D. (Director of Academic Activities at the Texas Back Institute Research Foundation, Plano, TX) and Anne Geddes (Scientific Publications Office, Baylor Research Institute, Dallas, TX) for reading and editing the manuscript.

References

1. Arborelius M Jr, et al.: Hemodynamic changes in man during immersion with head above water, *Aerospace Med* 43:592, 1972.

2. Astrand P, Rodahl K, editors: *Textbook of work physiology: physiological bases of exercise,* ed 3, New York, 1986, McGraw-Hill Book Co., p 654.

3. Bailes JE, et al.: Diving injuries of the cervical spine, *Surg Neurol* 34:155, 1990.

4. Becker B: *The physiologic consequences of aquatic exercise.* Presented at the American Academy of Physical Medicine and Rehabilitation Annual Meeting, San Francisco, November 16, 1992.

5. Becker TJ: Personal communication, 1991.

6. Becker TJ: *Scoliosis in swimmers.* In Ciullo JV, editor: *Clinics in sports medicine,* Philadelphia, 1986, WB Saunders Co., p 149.

7. Benson D, Wolf A, Shoji H: Can the Milwaukee brace patient participate in competitive athletics? *Am J Sports Med* 5:7, 1977.

8. Blount WP, Moe JH: *The Milwaukee brace,* Baltimore, 1978, Williams & Wilkins Co.

9. Bogduk N, Twomey LT: *Clinical anatomy of the lumbar spine,* ed 2, New York, 1991, Churchill-Livingstone.

10. Bove A: *Cardiovascular disorders and diving.* In Bove A, editor: *Diving medicine,* Philadelphia, 1990, WB Saunders Co., p 239.

11. Bove A, Davis J: *Pulmonary barotrauma.* In Bove A, editor: *Diving medicine,* Philadelphia, 1990, WB Saunders Co., pp 188-191.

12. Brennan D, Wilder R: *Deep water running: an instructors manual,* Houston, 1991, Houston International Running Center.

13. Campion M: *Introduction to hydrotherapy.* In Campion M, editor: *Adult hydrotherapy: a practical approach,* London, 1990, Heinemann Medical Books, p 3.

14. Canadian Olympic Association Report, 1982.

15. Clarys JP, Piette G: *A review of EMG in swimming: explanation of facts and/or feedback information.* In Hollander AP, Huijing PA, deGroot G, editors: *Biomechanics and medicine in swimming,* Champaign, IL, 1983, Human Kinetics Books, p 153.

16. Cole A, et al.: *Lumbar torque: a new proprioceptive approach,* Presented as a poster session at the Annual Meeting of the North American Spine Society, Keystone, CO, August 1-3, 1991,

17. Cole AJ: *Aquatic stabilization strategies.* Presented at the American Academy of Physical Medicine and Rehabilitation Annual Meeting, San Francisco, November 16, 1992.

18. Cole AJ: *The intrinsic properties of water.* Presented at the American Academy of Physical Medicine and Rehabilitation Annual Meeting, San Francisco, November 16, 1992.

19. Cole AJ: *Spinal pain in the elite competitive swimmer.* Presented at the Steadman Hawkins Foundation, Vail, CO, December 4-5, 1992.

20. Cole AJ: *Spine injuries in the competitive swimming athlete.* Presented at the American College of Sports Medicine Annual Meeting, Seattle, WA, June 4-5, 1993.

21. Cole AJ: When to call for help, *J Phys Ed Rec Dance,* January:55, 1993.

22. Cole AJ, et al.: The Portola Valley Scale: a classification system for aquatic exercise (manuscript in preparation).

23. Cole AJ, Eagleston RE, Moschetti ML: Getting backs in the swim, *Rehab Manage,* August/September: 62-70, 1992.

24. Cole AJ, Herring SA: *Role of the physiatrist in management of musculoskeletal pain.* In Tollison DC, editor: *The handbook of pain management,* Baltimore, 1994, Williams & Wilkins.

25. Cole AJ, Moschetti ML, Eagleston RE: *Lumbar spine aquatic rehabilitation: a sports medicine approach.* In Tollison DC, editor: *The handbook of pain management,* Baltimore, 1994, Williams & Wilkins.

26. Cole AJ, Moschetti ML, Eagleston RE: Aquatic rehabilitation for spine pain, *J Back Musculoskel Rehab.* Accepted for publication.

27. Cole AJ, Reid M: Clinical assessment of the shoulder, *J Back Musculoskel Rehab* 2(2):7, 1992.

28. Cole AJ, Stratton SA, Farrell JP: *Cervical spine athletic injuries: a pain in the neck.* In Press J, editor: *Physical medicine and rehabilitation clinics of North America,* Philadelphia, W.B. Saunders Co. 1994.

29. Cole AJ, Weinstein S: *Lumbar spine pain: a clinical approach,* Andover Medical Publishers (in press).

30. Costill D, Cahill P, Eddy D: Metabolic responses to submaximal exercise in three water temperatures, *J Appl Physiol* 22:628, 1967.

31. Councilman J: *The science of swimming,* Englewood Cliffs, NJ, 1968, Prentice-Hall, Inc., p 457.

32. Department of Health and Human Services: *Aqua dynamics: water exercises are the new way to stay in shape,* Washington, DC, 1986, Department of Health and Human Services.

33. Eagleston R: *Aquatic stabilization programs.* Presented at the Conference on Agressive Nonsurgical Rehabilitation of Lumbar Spine and Sports Injuries, San Francisco, San Francisco Spine Institute, March 23, 1989.

34. Eagleston R: Personal communication, Orthopedic and Sports Physical Therapy of Portola Valley, Inc., 1991.

35. Epstein M: Cardiovascular and renal effects of head-out water immersion in man, *Circ Res* 39:619, 1976.

36. Farfan H: Effects of torsion on the intervertebral joints, *Can J Surg* 12:336, 1969.

37. Farfan HF, et al.: The effects of torsion on the lumbar intervertebral joints: the role of torsion in the production of disc degeneration, *J Bone Joint Surg* 52A:468, 1970.

38. Farmer J, Jr: *Ear and sinus problems in diving.* In Bove A, editor: *Diving medicine,* Philadelphia, 1990, WB Saunders Co., p 200.

39. Genuario S, Negso J: The use of a swimming pool in the rehabilitation and reconditioning of athletic injuries, *Contemp Orthop* 20:381, 1990.

40. Goldstein JD, et al.: Spine injuries in gymnasts and swimmers: an epidemiologic investigation, *Am J Sports Med* 19:463, 1991.

41. Good R, Nickel V: Cervical spine injuries resulting from water sports, *Spine* 5:502, 1980.

42. Hansson T, Keller T, Manohar M: A study of the compressive properties of lumbar vertebral trabeculae: effects of tissue characteristics, *Spine* 12:56, 1987.

43. Haralson K: Therapeutic pool programs: clinical management, *Phys Ther* 5:10, 1985.

44. Holmer I: Physiology of swimming man, *Acta Physiol Scand Suppl* 407:1, 1974.

45. Kadaba MP, et al.: Intramuscular wire electromyography of the subscapularis, *J Orthop Res* 10:394, 1992.

46. Kenney S: Personal communication, Head Swim Coach, Stanford University Men's Swim Team, Palo Alto, CA, 1991.

47. Kewalramani L, Taylor R: Injuries to the cervical spine from diving accidents, *J Trauma* 15:130, 1975.

48. Kirby R, et al.: Oxygen consumption during exercise in a heated pool, *Arch Phys Med Rehabil* 65:21, 1984.

49. Kiwerski J: Cervical spine injuries caused by diving into water, *Paraplegia* 18:101, 1980.

50. Kolb M: Principles of underwater exercise, *Phys Ther Rev* 37:361, 1957.

51. Krahl H, Steinbruck K: *Sportsachaden and Sportverletzungen and der Wirbelsaule Arztebl:* Deutsch, 19, 1978.

52. Kreighbaum E, Barthels K: *Biomechanics: a qualitative approach for studying human movement,* ed 2, Minneapolis, 1985, Burgess Publishing Co., p 421.

53. Kuprian W: *Physical therapy for sports,* Philadelphia, 1982, WB Saunders Co., p 377.

54. Maglischo E: *Swimming faster,* Mountain View, CA, 1982, Mayfield Publishing Co., p 472.

55. Martin R: *Swimming: forces on aquatic animals and humans.* In Vaughan CL, editor: *Biomechanics of sport,* Boca Raton, FL, 1989, CRC Press, Inc., p 35.

56. Martin W, et al.: Cardiovascular adaptations to intensive swim training in sedentary middle-aged men and women, *Circulation* 75:323, 1987.

57. McArdle W, Katch F, Katch V: *Energy expenditure during walking, jogging, running, and swimming.* In McArdle W, Katch F, Katch V, editors: *Exercise physiology: energy, nutrition, and human performance,* Philadelphia, 1986, Lea & Febiger, p 158.

58. Miller F: *Fluids.* In *College physics,* ed 4, New York, 1977, Harcourt, Brace, Jovanovich, Inc., p 271.

59. Moschetti ML, Cole AJ: Risk management and facility issues in aquatic rehabilitation, *J Back Musculoskel Rehab.* Accepted for publication, 1994.

60. Mutoh Y: Mechanism and prevention of swimming injury, *Jpn J Sports Sci* 2:527, 1983.

61. Mutoh Y, Miwako T, Mitsumasa M: *Chronic injuries of elite competitive swimmers, divers, water polo players, and synchronized swimmers.* In Ungerecht VB, Wilke K, editors: *Swimming science,* Champaign, IL, 1988, Human Kinetics Books, p 333.

62. Neuman T: *Pulmonary disorders in diving.* In Bove A, editor: *Diving medicine,* Philadelphia, 1990, WB Saunders Co., p 233.

63. Nodel E, et al.: Energy exchanges of swimming man, *J Appl Physiol* 36:465, 1974.

64. Nuber G, et al.: Fine wire electromyography analysis of muscles of the shoulder during swimming, *Am J Sports Med* 14:7, 1986.

65. Panjabi M, et al.: Spinal ability and intersegmental muscle forces: a biomechanical model, *Spine* 14:194, 1989.

66. Paris S: The spine and swimming. *Spine State Art Rev* 4(2):351, 1990.

67. Piette G, Clarys JP: *Telemetric EMG of the front crawl movement.* In Terauds J, Bedingfield W, editors: *Swimming III,* Baltimore, 1979, University Park Press, p 153.

68. Pink M, et al.: The normal shoulder during freestyle swimming: an electromyographic and cinematographic analysis of twelve muscles, *Am J Sports Med* 19:569, 1991.

69. Reister VC, Cole AJ: Start active, stay active in the water, *J Phys Educ Rec Dance,* January:52, 1993.

70. Richardson A, Jobe F, Collins H: The shoulder in competitive swimming, *Am J Sports Med* 8:159, 1980.

71. Risch WD, et al.: The effect of graded immersion on heart volume, central venous pressure, pulmonary blood distribution and heart rate in man, *Pflugers Arch* 375:115, 1978.

72. Rossi F: Spondylolysis, spondylolisthesis and sports, *J Sports Med Phys Fitness* 18:317, 1978.

73. Saal J: *Rehabilitation of the injured athlete.* In DeLisa J, editor: *Rehabilitation medicine: principles and practice,* Philadelphia, 1988, JB Lippincott Co., p 840.

74. Saal J, Saal J: *Later stage management of lumbar spine problems.* In Herring S, editor: *Physical medicine and rehabilitation clinics of North America,* Philadelphia, 1991, WB Saunders Co., p 205.

75. Scovazzo M, et al.: The painful shoulder during freestyle swimming: an electromyographic cinematographic analysis of twelve muscles, *Am J Sports Med* 19:577, 1991.

76. Shirazi-Adl A, Ahmed A, Shrivastava S: Mechanical response of a lumbar motion segment in axial torque alone and combined with compression, *Spine* 11:914, 1989.

77. Sinnett E, Cole AJ: The biomechanics of the freestyle, backstroke, breaststroke, and butterfly swim strokes, *J Back Musculoskel Rehab* (in press).

78. United States Master's Swimming and YMCA of America: Personal Communication.

79. Weinstein SL: *Adolescent idiopathic scoliosis: prevalence and natural history.* In AAOS Instruct Course Lect, 37:115, 1989.

80. White A: *Clinical anatomy and biomechanics.* Presented at the meeting of the Cervical Spine and Upper Extremity in Sports and Industry, San Francisco, San Francisco Spine Institute, April 1, 1990.

81. Wilder R, Brennan D, Schotte D: Standard measure for exercise prescription for aqua running, *Am J Sports Med* 21:45, 1993.

82. Wilson F, Lindseth R: The adolescent swimmer's back, *Am J Sports Med* 10:174, 1982.

83. Yeater R, et al.: Tethered swimming forces in the crawl, breast, and back strokes and their relationship to competitive performance, *J Biomech* 14:527, 1981.

Chapter 56
Weight Lifting

Robert E. Windsor

Susan J. Dreyer

Jonathan P. Lester

Frank J. E. Falco

Athletic conditioning has evolved significantly over the past several decades. During the first half of this century the role of weight lifting in training for other sports was very limited. Weight lifting was thought to create athletes that were "muscle bound," slow, and possibly predisposed to injury.[54,57] During that era, only weight lifters lifted weights and were generally not considered to be athletes. Beginning in the late 1960s, weight lifting enjoyed increasing popularity as an auxiliary means of athletic conditioning. Today, weight lifting has assumed a dominant role in training athletes in almost all sports.[12]

The medical field was also slow to accept weight training as a valid means of conditioning. In 1945, DeLorme described a conditioning program that emphasized the use of progressive resistance exercises.[10] The DeLorme technique required an individual to begin with a fraction of his 10-repetition maximum (10 RM) and increase the weight lifted throughout the training session until he could no longer lift the weight. In 1951, Zineoff described the "Oxford technique" of conditioning, which was a modification of the DeLorme technique.[60] The Oxford technique required an individual to begin a training session with the 10 RM after appropriate warmup.

The terms *weight lifting* and *weight training* are commonly, but incorrectly, used interchangeably. *Weight lifting* refers to the competitive sport of Olympic weight lifting and power lifting. *Weight training* refers to a technique of using resistance exercises to promote overall fitness. Body building is a competitive sport emphasizing the development of a large symmetrical, well-proportioned physique.[12,17,47]

History of Weight Lifting

The earliest mention of resistance exercises is a drawing on the funerary chapel in Beni-Hassan, Egypt.[57] This drawing depicts three people in various stages of lifting a heavy bag overhead for exercise. In 1896 B.C. there is record of strength competitions taking place in what is now known as the British Isles. In the sixth century B.C., archeologic data indicate that Milo of Crotone hoisted a heifer calf on his shoulders daily and walked the length of the Olympic stadium until the calf was 4 years old. Milo is often credited with the development of progressive resistance exercises and was a six time Olympic champion.[54,57]

In the second century A.D., a celebrated physician named Galen developed a system of resistance training using implements such as the halters, or hand weights, to increase strength. His system also included heavy lifting, dumbbell exercises and person-to-person isometric contraction exercises. With the fall of the Roman empire and the beginning of the Dark Ages, weight training was lost for approximately 1000 years. Essentially all physical training during this time was focused on warfare.[57]

In 1531 Sir Thomas Elyot made reference to Galen's system of exercises. In 1544 Joachim Camerius wrote the *dialogue de gymnasius,* which encouraged boys to engage in strength competitions, lift weights, and climb ropes. The latter part of the sixteenth century and the seventeenth century saw a gradual rebirth of strength training philosophy, and by the eighteenth century, strong-man feats began springing up across London.[57]

Strength training did not become popular in Europe until the early nineteenth century. The Prussians had been defeated by Napolean in 1811 and were not allowed to arm themselves. A Prussian nationalist named Friedrich Ludwig Jahn began training Prussian soldiers using resistance exercises to emphasize strength development so that they would be better able to defend themselves. As this trend spread, "strong-man" competitions sprang up across Germany as well. One such "strong man," Fredrick Muller (known as the "Great Sandow") defeated the English strong-man team known as "Samson and the Cyclops" in 1889. This made him the most renowned strong man in England and caused England to become the center of strong men in Europe. In 1892 Florence Ziegfeld recruited the "Great Sandow" to the United States and in 1893 the "Great Sandow" performed at the Chicago World Fair. This ushered in the popularity of weight training in the United States.[57]

Modern-day amateur weight lifting had its birth in 1891, when the German Athletic Association was founded. It brought a large number of the local weight clubs under the guidance of a single governing body. Its first competition was in Cologne in 1893 and its first "World Championship" in Vienna in 1898. By 1900 it had over 300 clubs and 12,000 members.[57]

Beginning in 1896, three of the first four modern Olympics included a weight lifting competition. There was a rebirth of this sport in 1920, and it has continued until the present. The first U.S. National Powerlifting Championship was held in 1964, and in 1965 it was divided into a seniors and juniors competition. In 1969 the first National Collegiate Powerlifting Championship was held.[57]

Bodybuilding also became a growing sport around the turn of the century. Eugene Sandow sponsored physique contests for his students and

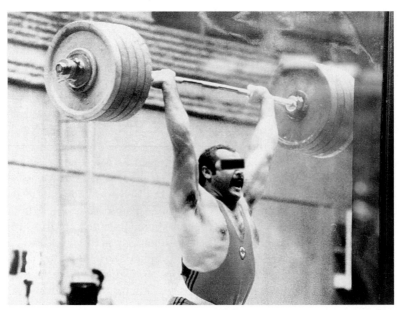

Fig. 56-1

Shoulder to overhead press in clean-jerk lift.

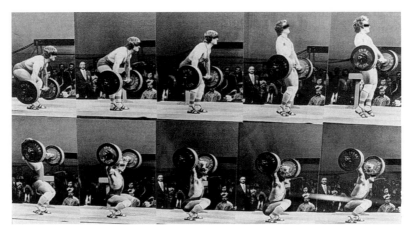

Fig. 56-2

Snatch lift. Athlete lifts bar directly overhead without stopping at shoulders, which is snatch portion of this Olympic lifting event. Next, athlete stands up maintaining bar overhead (not shown in this figure).

awarded them gold, silver, and bronze statuettes. The first physique contest held in the United States was in 1904. It was held in New York City and offered large cash prizes to the winners. The first Mr. America contest was held in 1939 and the first Mr. Universe contest in 1947.[57]

Description of Different Weight Lifting Styles

Bodybuilding is an artistic sport that emphasizes extreme muscularity, symmetry, and aesthetics. Body builders routinely engage in power lifting–type activities and emphasize a high repetition and moderate weight program. In addition, there is a greater emphasis on overall fitness and aerobic conditioning than in power lifting or Olympic lifting.[17,57]

Olympic weight lifting emphasizes speed, agility, and strength. It consists of the clean jerk and the snatch lifts. The clean jerk (Fig. 56-1) is a lift in which the weight bar is lifted from the floor to the shoulders and subsequently overhead. The snatch lift (Fig. 56-2) is a lift in which the weight bar is lifted from the floor directly overhead without stopping at the shoulders.[17,57]

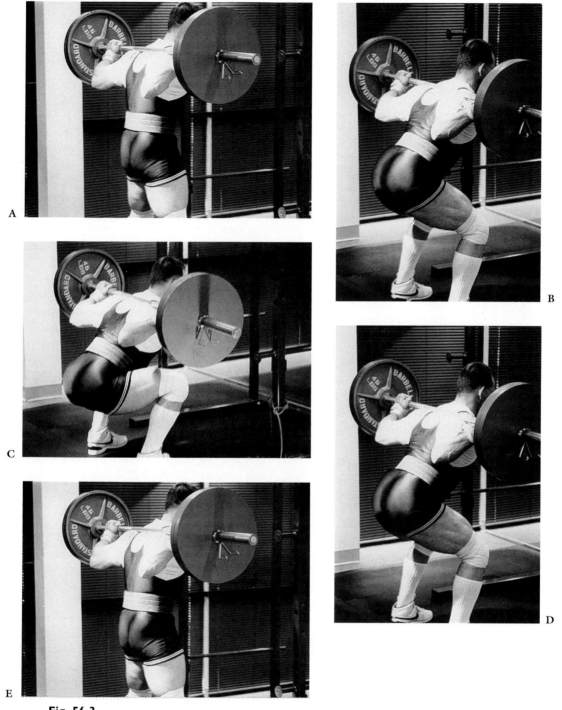

Fig. 56-3

Squat lift. **A,** Starting position. **B,** Half squat position. **C,** Full squat position. **D,** Rising from full squat position. **E,** Returning to starting position.

Power lifting emphasizes extreme power development with relatively little emphasis on speed or agility. Power lifting consists of the squat, bench press, and dead lift. The squat lift begins by holding the weight bar across the posterior-superior aspect of the shoulder girdles. The lifter then squats down to where the anterior thigh passes inferior to the horizontal plane of the patella in the squat position and then stands up. The bench press begins by a weight lifter lying supine on a bench and holding a weight bar in his hands with his shoulders flexed 90 degrees and the elbows completely extended. The bar is then slowly lowered to the chest and held there until it has become motionless prior to raising it to its starting position. The dead lift involves lifting a weight bar from the floor to waist level and then lowering it to the floor under control.[17,57]

Biomechanics of Power Lifting

The biomechanics of power lifting most closely resemble lifting biomechanics utilized in the workplace and during activities of daily living. Thus, a more detailed description of power lifting follows.

Proper power lifting technique is crucial to timely advancement in strength and prevention of injuries. There is a paucity of biomechanical data published on power lifting. While there are several accepted techniques for each lift, only the conventional methods will be described.

Squat

In the squat (Fig. 56-3), the lifter's heels should be slightly wider than shoulder width and the hips should be 30 to 45 degrees externally rotated. The hips should not externally or internally rotate substantially during the lift so that the knees flex in the same direction the feet are pointing. This helps maintain the lower extremities in physiologic position and thus decreases the torsional forces to the knees, hips, pelvis, and lumbar spine.[38]

The weight bar should be placed on the posterior-superior aspect of the shoulders and should not be allowed to roll significantly. The hands should be placed in a comfortable position with the thumb on the same side of the bar as the fingers (monkey grip) (Fig. 56-4). This seems to prevent injuries of the upper extremity if the bar rolls or if the lifter has to "dump" the weight for any reason.

Lumbar lordosis should be maintained throughout the lift to aid stability, facilitate erector spinae contraction, and possibly reduce the load on inert soft tissues.[16,31,55] The angle created by the coronal plane of the lifter's trunk and the horizontal plane of the floor (trunk-floor angle) should be as large as possible during the lift and at no time should it be less than 45 degrees.[8,45,46] The degree of forward lean of the trunk during the squat is directly proportional to the trunk extensor torque and indirectly proportional to the thigh extensor torque. Highly developed lifters attempt to minimize trunk lean and thus minimize trunk extensor torque while maximizing thigh extensor torque. McLaughlin mentions

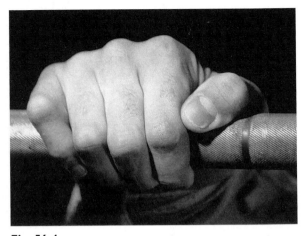

Fig. 56-4
Squat lift monkey grip. Notice that thumb is positioned on same side of bar as fingers.

a constant point during the lift at which the thigh-floor angle reaches 30.3 degrees, at which point the lifter is least able to generate vertical force. This point is known as a "sticking point."[46] The maximum amount of weight a lifter is able to lift through this point of the event is generally equal to his one-repetition-maximum (1RM).

Center of gravity should be kept 5 to 7 cm anterior to the heel-floor interface. If the center of gravity is maintained in the proper position then the ankles will not dorsiflex beyond 30 degrees, the knees will not flex beyond 120 degrees, and proper trunk mechanics can be maintained throughout the lift.[38]

Bench Press

In the bench press (Fig. 56-5) the lifter should keep his feet flat on the floor and his buttocks, shoulders, and head flat on the bench throughout the lift. Lumbar lordosis should be maintained and the scapulae should be kept in the fully retracted and "locked" position. This provides for maximum stability during the lift and may help prevent injuries to shoulder girdle and lumbar spine musculature.

The lifter begins the lift by supporting a weight bar in his hands with his shoulders flexed 90 degrees and his elbows completely extended. Hand position on the bar should be as wide as comfortable for maximum power production.[42] The lifter should have his thumbs in the opposed position ("club grip") (Fig. 56-6) to prevent the bar from rolling out of his hands and falling on his chest. The bar is then slowly and smoothly lowered to the chest and "paused" until it is no longer moving prior to lifting it back to its starting position. The path of the

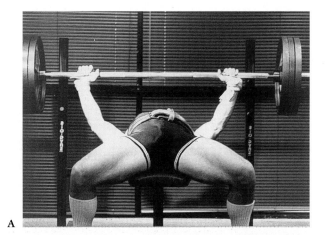

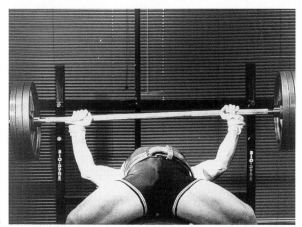

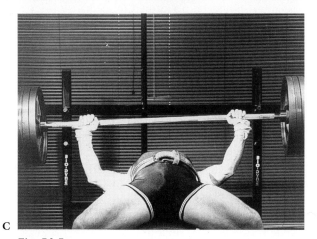

Fig. 56-5

Bench press. **A,** Starting position. **B,** Pause position. **C,** Press to starting position.

bar during descent should take a gentle arc with the concavity toward the head, and during ascent the path should be similar with the concavity toward the feet.[36] The bar should come to rest 2 to 5 cm superior to the sternoxiphoid junction. When the bar is on the chest, the shoulders should achieve a max-

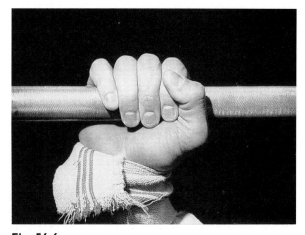

Fig. 56-6

Bench press club grip. Note that thumb is positioned on opposite side of bar as fingers.

imum abduction of 45 degrees. This degree of abduction initially increases as the bar is lifted from the chest and then decreases after the sticking point has been passed. The sticking point has been determined to be 12 cm or less from the surface of the chest.[42] Shoulder abduction at the termination of the lift is dependent on the lifter's hand position on the bar.

Dead Lift

At the beginning of the dead lift (Fig. 56-7), the lifter stands over the bar while it rests on the floor. The feet should be positioned slightly narrower than shoulder width in a neutral position, and the legs should be touching the bar during the quiet standing position. The lifter stoops and grasps the bar immediately outside of his legs with his dominant forearm pronated and his nondominant forearm supinated (reverse grip) (Fig. 56-8). Care should be taken during the stooping process to keep the bar as near the heel-floor interface as possible (i.e., minimize ankle dorsiflexion); the torso is in an erect posture similar to the squat; and the head is up (i.e., cervical spine slightly extended beyond neutral).[6] Prior to lifting the weight off the floor, the lifter should "pull the slack out" (i.e., fully extend the elbows and fully depress the shoulder girdles). This will help prevent injuries that may occur to soft tissues as a result of a sudden jerking force.

Once lift-off has occurred, there is a natural tendency to extend the knees faster than the hips, thus creating excessive forward lean. This tendency should be resisted. The lifter should attempt to shift his center of gravity posteriorly in an attempt to offset the anterior moment created by the loaded bar.

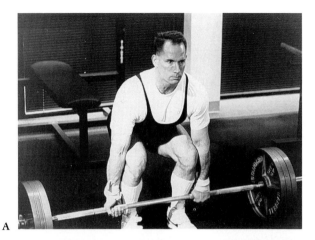

A

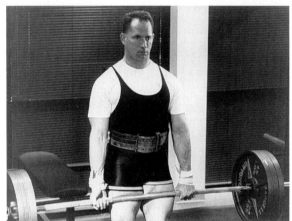

B

Fig. 56-7

Dead lift. **A,** Starting position. **B,** Finishing position.

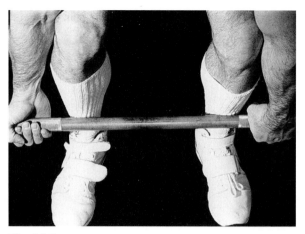

Fig. 56-8

Dead lift reverse grip. Note that dominant forearm (in this case the left forearm) is pronated and nondominant forearm supinated.

In addition, the lifter should strive to maintain the upright trunk posture and "head-up" position while concentrating on extending his hips and dragging the bar up the anterior aspect of his legs.[6]

Once the sticking point (infrapatellar region) has been passed, the ankles should begin to dorsiflex while the hips and knees continue to extend. The bar should continue to be dragged up the anterior aspect of the thighs until the lifter is in an erect posture. The bar should then be lowered in a controlled fashion using knee and hip flexion while keeping an upright trunk and head-up position.

Typical Training Methods of Power Lifting

Prophylactic Conditioning

The novice power lifter typically has several "weak links" in his musculoskeletal chain that are at risk for injury. These links should be identified and strengthened prior to launching into a rigorous power lift-

ing program. Typically, the novice should focus on overall flexibility, strengthening the rotator cuff and abdominal musculature, power lifting technique, and muscle balance.[12,17,29,34,54]

Overall flexibility may minimize mechanical stress placed on vulnerable tissues.[34,54] A good flexibility program should include the shoulder girdle musculature, calves, hamstrings, quadriceps, iliotibial band, hip adductors, hip flexors, gluteal musculature and abdominal obliques (Figs. 56-9 and 56-10). This program should be performed immediately prior to and at the termination of each workout. It should emphasize slow, sustained stretching and avoid bouncing, which may injure the musculotendinous unit.

Typical power lifting routines strive to increase shoulder girdle internal rotation and flexion strength, which may create a strength imbalance in the rotator cuff. To offset these changes, the rotator cuff should be trained twice weekly with emphasis on external rotation and abduction (Fig. 56-11). This will help maintain strength and balance in the rotator cuff and thus dynamic stability in the glenohumeral joint during lifting.

Specific prophylactic conditioning should also include the abdominal obliques (Fig. 56-12). The abdominal muscles may be trained daily without fear of overtraining. Strong abdominal oblique and transverse abdominal contraction during lifting has been demonstrated to help stabilize the lumbar spine as well as to create an extension moment at the lumbar spine.[23,40,44] This is via their attachment to the lumbodorsal fascia and the mechanical arrangement of this fascia.*

* References 9, 22, 27, 28, 30, 32, 43, 44, 55, and 56.

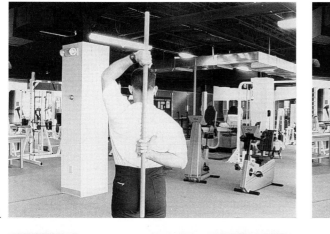

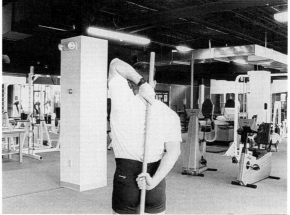

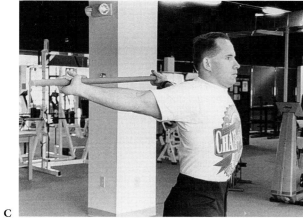

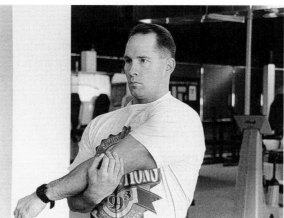

Fig. 56-9

Shoulder girdle stretching routine. **A, B, C,** Stretching anterior shoulder girdle. **D,** Stretching posterior shoulder girdle.

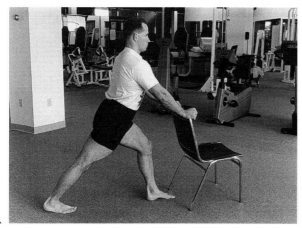

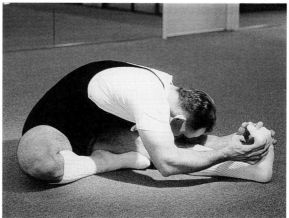

Fig. 56-10

Lower limb stretching routine. **A,** Calves. **B,** Hamstrings.

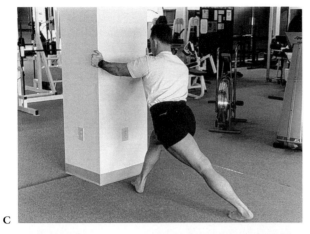

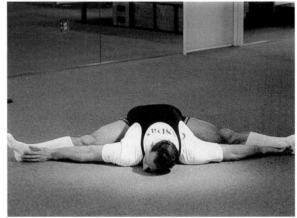

C

D

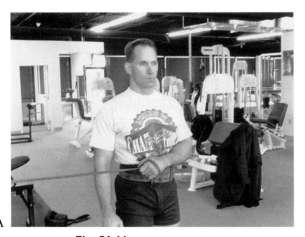

E

Fig. 56-10, cont'd
C, Iliotibial band. D, Hip adductors. E, Hip flexors.

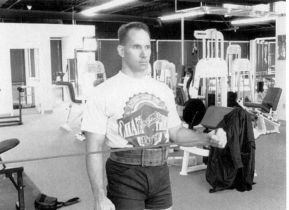

A

B

Fig. 56-11
Rotator cuff strengthening. A, B, Elastic band resistance for the novice lifter.

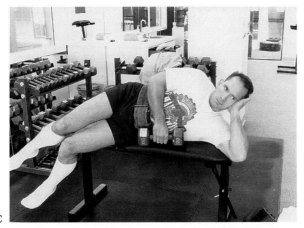

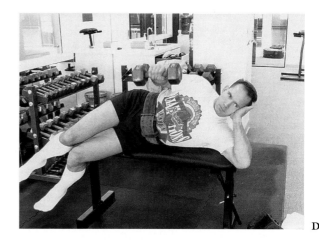

C   D

Fig. 56-11, cont'd

C, D, Weight resistance for the more experienced lifter.

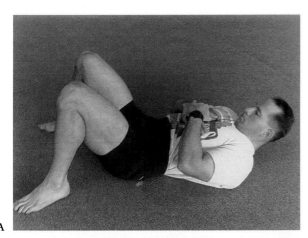

A

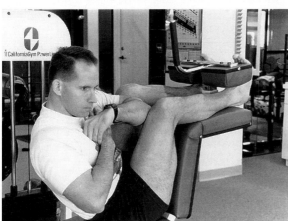

B

Fig. 56-12

Abdominal strengthening. **A,** Rectus isolation. **B,** Oblique isolation.

A beginning power lifting program is a general weight training program that emphasizes overall fitness and also power lifting technique. Heavy power lifts are not emphasized in this phase, since a novice power lifter is at increased risk for injury until he has had the opportunity to develop proper technique and sufficient remodeling of his bones, entheses, and musculotendinous junctions to withstand the load of heavy weights.*

As the lifter matures and his lifting techniques improve, he can gradually begin to increase the weight lifted and decrease the number of repetitions per set. During this phase he should gradually begin wearing a weight belt (Fig. 56-13). These belts appear to support the lumbar spine by augmenting the abdominal mechanism and creating an extension mo-

* References 1, 5, 18, 20, 21, 24, 25, 35.

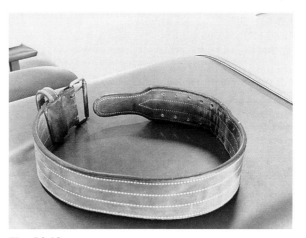

Fig. 56-13

Weight belt.

ment at the lumbar spine.[39] Once the lifter has demonstrated technical proficiency and adequate overall conditioning, then he may begin a serious power lifting program.

Cycle Training

A serious adult power lifter has typically been training for 1 to 2 years. He trains in cycles that last 8 to 10 weeks and coordinates these cycles with competitions. Generally, the bench press and squat are trained twice per week and the dead lift is trained once per week, although some lifters train squat only once per week and dead lift once every other week. The lifter will typically alternate "heavy" and "light" days, with the "heavy" days emphasizing heavier weights and fewer repetitions and the "light" days emphasizing lighter weights and more repetitions. The heavy days are designed to stress the muscle maximally to provide strength and a growth stimulus, while the light days are designed to allow the muscles to continue to heal and yet still receive a training stimulus. A lifter involved in cycle training seeks to achieve a one-repetition-maximum (within the cycle) once every 2 or 3 weeks. During weeks 2 and 3 prior to a major competition the lifter generally eliminates or significantly curtails the light day to allow for maximum healing of overtrained or injured muscles.[18,19,37] During the week prior to competition the lifter emphasizes rest and mental preparation for the upcoming competition.

Auxiliary Lifting Techniques

The elite power lifter has been training vigorously for many years and has reached a very highly developed state. He is able to employ auxiliary lifting techniques that should not be attempted by others. These include lifts based on the "overload principle," such as heavy "walk outs" and "half squats," "heavy negative bench press," and "heavy partial dead lifts." These auxiliary lifts are generally performed with 110% to 130% of the 1 RM and should be performed once per week to once per month during weeks 3 through 8 prior to a major competition. These lifts should not be performed more frequently than once per week and should not be performed in the 2 weeks prior to a major competition since muscles do not seem to be able to recuperate quickly enough. The intention of these lifts is to stimulate the bones, tendons, and contractile mechanism maximally to become stronger.

In between lifting cycles, the power lifter assumes a modified body-building routine. The emphasis is placed on overall fitness, including muscle balance, flexibility, and cardiovascular conditioning. Heavy joint-loading activities such as squats and dead lifts are still performed with significantly less weight and intensity. This is a healing phase.

Spine Injuries During Weight Lifting

Weight lifting–induced spine injuries are common and predictable in their scope; however, there is very little published about these injuries. As a result, much of the following information is drawn from my experience as a physician treating spine injuries and as a previously world-ranked power lifter. Power lifting will be used as a model since it comes closest to reflecting the methods used by the majority of strength athletes and industrial workers.

The incidence of spine injuries in weight lifting has not been well defined. In the adolescent population, all weight lifting–induced musculoskeletal injuries combined range from 7.1% to 39.4%, depending on the definition of injury.[4,36,47] No similar data are available for the adult population. I would estimate the incidence of weight-lifting-induced spine injury lasting greater than 1 week in noncompetitive males between the ages of 35 and 50 years old to range from 10% to 20%. However, I would estimate the incidence of these injuries in a similar population of competitive elite power lifters to be nearly 100%. The vast majority of these injuries occur in the lumbar spine.

The types of spine injuries suffered while lifting weights are predictable. These include myofascial strain, facet joint sprain, chronic facet joint dysfunction, disc injury with and without radiculopathy, spinous process fracture, vertebral body fracture, and possibly pars interarticularis fracture.[2,7,26,36,59] Myofascial strains and facet joint injuries make up the major portion of these injuries and are usually self-limited. The remainder of these injuries may cause prolonged pain, dysfunction and interference with training.

Spine injuries generally have one or more predisposing factors, including improper warmup, muscle strength or length imbalance, poor technique, overtraining, or skeletal imbalance such as leg length discrepancy or scoliosis. Other skeletal abnormalities that may predispose to injury include facet tropism, equinous deformity, subtalar hyperpronation, tarsal coalition, and pelvic asymmetry.

Myofascial Strain

True myofascial strain typically occurs in the superficial spinal erectors at the thoracolumbar or lumbosacral junction. This injury usually occurs during the dead lift or squat. The pain and dysfunction that occurs from this injury is usually self-limited and resolves spontaneously within 1 to 2 weeks with antiinflammatory modalities and modified activities. There may or may not be an associated ecchymosis.

Facet Joint Injury

A true facet joint sprain or chronic facet joint dysfunction with pain typically occurs in the midthoracic or thoracolumbar region. These injuries may also occur in the lumbar spine but are much more likely to be associated with a concomitant disc injury. A facet joint sprain is usually the result of a rotational movement during ascent in the squat or dead lift. Pain and dysfunction from this injury may last from several weeks to several months and occasionally may develop into a chronically painful condition. Facet joint dysfunction with pain may be the result of a facet joint sprain that has created a chronically dysfunctional joint or abnormal biomechanics resulting from scoliosis, leg length discrepancy, or facet tropism. When these injuries occur acutely, they usually involve only one side and only 1 or 2 levels.

Rehabilitation of facet joint injuries is dependent on their presentation. If an injury is acute and is associated with minimal pain and has not been preceded by other similar injuries then it generally will resolve spontaneously with 2 to 4 weeks with antiinflammatory modalities, modified rest, and progressive mobilization of the injured joint. The deep paraspinal and abdominal musculature should be adequately rehabilitated via standard stabilization-type exercises outlined in other areas of this book.[48-50] This exercise protocol should be followed by progressive conditioning of the superficial paraspinal muscles and lower extremities via sports-specific activities such as partial dead lifts, squats, and Roman chair hyperextensions. Additionally, predisposing factors and technique errors should be sought and corrected.

If the injury is chronic, recurrent, or severe it will probably take longer to improve and may not totally resolve. Rehabilitation efforts are similar to those mentioned above although they will generally need to be more intensive and may require the judicious use of facet joint cortisone injections if an inflammatory component to the injury is suspected. Occasionally, in severe chronic cases a diagnostic facet-joint nerve block followed by a facet joint nerve ablation may be required.[53]

Disc Injuries

Disc injuries usually occur in the lower lumbar spine and less commonly at the thoracolumbar junction. They are generally also the result of rotational movements during ascent in the dead lift or squat. These injuries can usually be managed by conservative means and rarely require surgery.[50,51]

Acute rehabilitation efforts focus on control of inflammation with cryotherapy and antiinflammatory medication. Heating modalities should be avoided for the first several days.[14,52] Pain should not be managed with narcotics unless the injury is severe. If narcotics are indicated, they should be used for a limited time only and in a scheduled manner. The patient should remain mobilized as much as possible and bed rest should be employed for no longer than 2 days, if at all.[11] Ideally, the patient should interrupt his workout schedule as little as possible except to "work around the injury" and reduce training intensity. During this phase of recovery, the patient should emphasize open-chain aerobic conditioning, abdominal crunches, and non-disc-loading upper-extremity and torso activities such as light pec-deck, standing cable tricep extensions, and preacher bench curls. McKenzie program activities should be used acutely to centralize radicular pain and help normalize segmental motion.[13,41]

Epidural cortisone injections (ESI) should be used if inflammatory radicular pain exists.[3] The authors do not use the "trial of three ESIs" concept. Performing ESIs under fluoroscopic guidance dramatically reduces the need for repeat injections. As a rule, if the first ESI does not work, then the third will not either.[15] Additionally, the "blind" (i.e., nonfluoroscopic) placement of an epidural needle during ESI has been demonstrated to be improper 25% of the time.[58]

Once radicular pain has resolved and segmental motion has improved, then standard stabilization activities should be employed. In the experienced weight-trained athlete this program can usually progress rapidly. Once the athlete is able to demonstrate adequate lumbar stability, gentle sports-specific disc-loading activities should be instituted. A weight belt should be worn at all times during this phase to augment the abdominal mechanism and lumbar extension moment.[39] Progression of activity should take place cautiously but as quickly as clinically acceptable. The athlete must be informed of typical warning signs and told of the importance of peripheralizing pain and neurologic signs. Home program activities should be performed on a daily basis and include McKenzie and stabilization activities.

Spinous Process Fractures

Spinous process fractures occur almost exclusively during the squat. These fractures generally involve C7 or T1.[33] They typically occur as the result of the weight bar suddenly rolling down the neck in an uncontrolled fashion during either ascent or descent. They may also occur at the top of the squat. This may occur if the lifter has rapidly ascended through the squat and the bar is allowed to bounce while resting on the back of the neck. This injury is usually heard and felt by the athlete. It is associated with the acute onset of localized pain and swelling and may be described by the athlete as a crunching or breaking sound and feeling. During either mechanism the injury may be prevented by not allowing the bar to roll or bounce and keeping the shoulder girdles adequately retracted and elevated to pad the spinous processes with contracted trapezius musculature. Usually there are no long-term consequences to this injury. It should be treated in the short term with antiinflammatory medication and copious ice. Squats should be avoided for approximately 2 weeks, during which time the lower extremities should be conditioned with activities that do not place stress on the neck, such as leg presses, hack squats, leg extensions, and leg curls. Approximately 2 weeks after the injury, the lifter should begin light squats again and advance over time as pain allows. During the next 4 to 6 weeks emphasis should be placed on the prophylactic measures mentioned above.

Vertebral Body Injuries

Weight-lifting-induced vertebral body injuries are rare. There are four cases mentioned in the literature of weight-lifting-induced lumbar apophyseal ring fractures in adolescents.[7] In adults, weight-lifting-induced vertebral body compression fractures are probably even more rare and are usually associated with other injuries. I have seen only two. Both cases involved elite lifters who were attempting maximum squat lifts and occurred when the lifters bounced at the bottom of the lift. Both lifters sustained a grade 1 L1 vertebral body compression fracture as well as other injuries. Associated injuries in both cases included patellar tendon ruptures and anterior cruciate injuries. One case included a dislocated ankle and bilateral open tibial fractures. These cases point out that care of other injuries may be the rate-limiting step in the overall recovery of the athlete who suffers from a weight-lifting-induced compression fracture. In addition, they demonstrate the importance of proper technique.

Care of a vertebral body compression fracture should include placing the athlete in a Thoracolumbosacral orthosis (TLSO) extension brace for approximately 3 months and significantly curtailing his activities for at least 2 to 4 weeks. The brace should be worn continuously for the first 3 to 4 weeks, at which time the athlete may be permitted to remove it only while bathing. During this period, pain control may require the judicious use of narcotics. At 2 to 3 weeks, narcotic medication should no longer be required and the athlete should increase his activities as pain permits while avoiding all axial and flexion loading forces.

Initially, all spine-loading activities should be avoided. If other injuries permit, open-chain aerobic conditioning is acceptable within the limits of pain. Approximately 6 weeks after the injury, the athlete is generally able to perform his activities of daily living in the brace without significant pain. At this point, it is acceptable to begin gentle conditioning activities of the upper and lower extremities that do not significantly load the spine and do not cause pain. In addition, at this point it is acceptable to begin gentle isometric abdominal conditioning activities within the brace. Conditioning activities should continue to be advanced within the limits of pain until the brace is removed at 3 to 4 months.

Once the brace has been removed, initial rehabilitation efforts should emphasize regaining segmental motion of the spine in general and the injured segments specifically. In addition, gentle stabilization activities should be initiated. Once the athlete has completed stabilization activities, it is acceptable to begin conditioning activities of the superficial paraspinal muscles. Approximately 6 months after the injury, the patient may begin very light squats and dead lift activities, advancing as tolerated.

Other Injuries

As of the writing of this chapter I have seen neither reports in the literature nor clinical cases of weight-lifting-induced fractures of the pars interarticularis. However, weight lifting does appear to be highly associated with its development, since its reported incidence in weight lifters is 36.2% compared to 5% to 10% for the normal population.[36]

I have treated six elite power lifters with a symptomatic spondylolisthesis. Of this group, four had defects at L5 with a grade 1 slip and the other two had defects at L4 with a slip. Two had a grade 1 slip and the other 2 had a grade 2 slip. No defects were acute at the time of presentation and no athletes gave a history of a traumatic event. All athletes had a degenerative disc at the level involved but no herniations were demonstrated by either CT scan or MRI. All had been complaining of low-back pain at the segment involved for greater than 2 years and all had activity-related unilateral or bilateral radicular pain. When they were not in a heavy portion of their training cycle they all had tolerable low-back pain only. However, when they began to train heavily, their back pain would increase and radicular pain would develop.

All six of these athletes were extremely competitive; therefore, relative rest was not an acceptable option to them. Flexion and stabilization activities were of no benefit in any of these cases. Four of the six athletes were able to achieve partial, temporary relief with McKenzie extension activities. The other two were able to get partial, temporary relief with manual mobilization of the involved segment. These athletes were followed for 9 to 21 months and all continued to compete despite the above-mentioned symptom complex.

Lumbar Stabilization in Power Lifting

Initially, the injured power lifter should be treated appropriately for the type, age, and severity of an injury as outlined above and in other areas of this book. When the active phase of injury rehabilitation begins it should include cardiovascular conditioning, appropriate stretching, extremity strengthening that does not present a substantial axial or rotational load to the lumbar spine, and the initial phases of lumbar stabilization outlined in other parts of this book. It is especially important to review proper lifting mechanics and breath control. By following these precautions, intraspinal pressures may be minimized and further injury may be avoided.

Conditioning should be advanced as rapidly as tolerated by the athlete. Signs that advancement may be taking place too rapidly include peripheralization of pain, return of dural tension sign, neurologic change in one or both lower extremities, or possibly worsening of dyskinetic segmental motion of the lumbar spine.

Once the lumbar stabilization program has reached the intermediate stages and the athlete is tolerating it without difficulty, sports-specific stabilization should begin. Initially, I recommend alternate-extremity bench press–type activities with the athlete standing, pushing on either Theraband tied to the wall at shoulder level or using a cable system with the pulley at shoulder level. The athlete should keep one foot forward and should keep the lumbar spine in a neutral posture. The athlete should be advanced in weight (or tension), repetitions, and time.

Once the athlete has been advanced at least twice in the standing bench press–type activities and is tolerating it without difficulty for at least three sessions, then Roman chair activities should be initiated. In this exercise, the athlete places his anterior pelvis prone on one pad and his posterior ankles under the other pads of the Roman chair and alternately eccentrically flexes and concentrically extends his lumbar spine against gravity. He should begin with at least two sets of 10 and advance in repetitions and sets as tolerated. After he has progressed to at least three to four sets of 20 repetitions without difficulty, weight should be applied to his posterior shoulder girdles or cervical spine.

Once the athlete is performing three to four sets of 20 repetitions with 20 to 30 lb without difficulty, it is time to progress to alternating one-arm lifts bent over supported rows. In this exercise the athlete bends at the waist with one foot forward. He places one hand on a flat utility bench and grasps a dumbbell that he can manage easily that is resting on the floor. While keeping the lumbar spine in a neutral posture, the dumbbell is lifted to the chest with a coupled scapular retraction and shoulder extension activity and then lowered back to the floor. Once again, this should be advanced until the athlete can perform 20 repetitions for three to four sets on each side at least three times per week.

Once this activity is well tolerated and the weight has been advanced at least twice, then it is time to begin partial dead lifts out of a rack. Initially, the bar should begin approximately 4 to 6 inches above the knees. Four to six sets of no more than 8 to 10 repetitions should be performed. Initially, this activity should occur with the bar only. Weight should be added and the bar should be progressively lowered toward the floor as tolerated. This activity must be advanced slowly and should be performed no more frequently than twice per week.

Once the dead-lift program has begun and is progressing without difficulty, then partial squats may begin. This program should also begin with the bar only. Initially, only quarter squats should be performed and only weight should be increased. Four to six sets of no more than 8 to 10 repetitions and no fewer than 4 to 6 repetitions should be performed. This program should occur no more frequently than twice per week. It is generally acceptable to progress to half squats once the squat program has progressed for six to eight training sessions without setback, the weight has been advanced at least five times, and both the therapist and athlete are comfortable with progressing to the next phase.

Once both the partial dead lifts and partial squats are being performed for at least four to six repetitions with at least 50% of the athlete's previous 1 RM with acceptable technique, minimal low-back pain and no lower-extremity pain, it is usually acceptable to progress to the full technique. Of course, with the progression from one phase to the next the weight should be reduced accordingly to evaluate how well the athlete will be able to handle it. Once it is determined that the athlete will do fine with the weight, then it is acceptable to progress with caution.

The most common reasons for an athlete's failing to progress through a program is attempting to advance too rapidly, failing to follow through with the core stabilization activities, and having unrealistic expectations about how rapid recovery will be. Once the athlete has recovered, the main identifiable reasons for relapse are not maintaining a flexibility program, proper warmup activities, proper lifting technique, and at least a basal stabilization program.

Summary

Weight training has permeated almost every aspect of athletics and has become an integral part of most sports-specific training. In addition, the weight-lifting sports of power lifting, body building, and Olympic lifting have become popular and well-defined sports.

Very little research exists on the kinetics and biomechanics of weight lifting. As a direct result, coaches and athletes are developing programs largely from empirical data. More research is needed on proper lifting technique, biomechanics, and injury epidemiology in order best to prevent injury and maximize performance gained through weight training.

References

1. Aggrawal N, et al.: A study of changes in the spine of weight lifters and other athletes, *British Journal of Sports Medicine* 13(2):58, 1979.
2. Alexander M: Biomechanical aspects of lumbar spine injuries in athletes: a review, *Can J Appl Sci* 10:1, 1985.
3. Benzon H: Epidural steroid injections for low back pain and lumbosacral radiculopathy, *Pain* 24:277, 1986.
4. Brady T, Cahill B, Bodnar L: Weight training-related injuries in the high school athlete, *Am J Sports Med* 10:1, 1982.
5. Brown A, McCartney N, Sale D: Positive adaptation to weight-lifting training in the elderly, *Am Physiol Soc* 69(5):1725, 1990.
6. Brown E, Abani K: Kinematics and kinetics of the dead lift in adolescent power lifters, *Med Sci Sports Exerc* 17:554, 1985.
7. Browne T, Yost R, McCarron R: Lumbar ring apophyseal fracture in an adolescent weight lifter, *Am J Sports Med* 18:533, 1990.
8. Capozzo A, et al.: Lumbar spine loading during half-squat exercises, *Med Sci Sports Exerc* 17:613, 1985.
9. Davis P: The use of intra-abdominal pressure in evaluating stresses on the lumbar spine, *Spine* 6:90, 1981.
10. DeLorme T: Restoration of muscle power by heavy resistance exercises, *J Bone Joint Surg* 27A:645, 1945.
11. Deyo R, Diehl A, Rosenthal M: How many days of bedrest for acute low back pain? A randomized clinical trial, *N Engl J Med* 315:1064, 1986.
12. DiNubile N: Strength training, *Clin Sports Med* 10:33, 1991.
13. Donelson R, Silva G, Murphy K: Centralization phenomenon, *Spine* 15:211, 1989.
14. Duncombe A, Hopp J: Modalities of physical therapy, vol 5, *Phys Med Rehab State Art Rev* 5:493, 1991.
15. El-Khoury G, et al.: Epidural steroid injection: a procedure ideally performed with fluoroscopic control, *Radiology* 168:554, 1988.
16. Farfan H: The biomechanical advantage of lordosis and hip extension for upright activity: man as compared with other anthropoids, *Spine* 3:336, 1978.
17. Fleck S, Kraemer W: Resistance training: basic principles (part 1 of 4), *Phys Sportsmed* 16:160, 1988.
18. Fleck S, Kraemer W: Resistance training: physiological responses and adaptations (part 2 of 4), *Phys Sportsmed* 16:108, 1988.
19. Fleck S, Kraemer W: Resistance training: physiological responses and adaptations (part 3 of 4), *Phys Sportsmed* 16:63, 1988.
20. Gleeson P, et al.: Effect of weight lifting on bone mineral density in premenopausal women, *J Bone Miner Res* 5:153, 1990.
21. Gracovetsky S, Farfan H, Lamy C: A mathematical model of the lumbar spine using an optimized system to control muscles and ligaments, *Orthop Clin North Am* 8:135, 1977.
22. Gracovetsky S, Farfan H, Helleur C: The abdominal mechanism, *Spine* 10:317, 1985.
23. Gracovetsky S, Farfan H, Lamy C: The mechanism of the lumbar spine, *Spine* 6:249, 1981.
24. Granhed H, Jonson R, Hansson T: Mineral content and strength of the lumbar vertebrae: a cadaver study, *Acta Orthop Scand* 60:105, 1989.
25. Granhed H, Johnson R, Hansson T: The loads on the lumbar spine during extreme weight lifting, *Spine* 12:146, 1987.

26. Granhed H, Morelli B: Low back pain among retired wrestlers and heavyweight lifters, *Am J Sports Med* 16:530, 1988.

27. Grew N: Intraabdominal pressure response to loads applied to the torso on normal subjects, *Spine* 5:149, 1980.

28. Grillner S, Nilsson J, Thorstensson A: Intra-abdominal pressure changes during natural movements in man, *Acta Physiol Scand* 103:275, 1978.

29. Grimby G: Progressive resistance exercises for injury rehabilitation, *Sports Med* 2:309, 1985.

30. Harman E, et al.: Intra-abdominal and intra-thoracic pressures during weight lifting and jumping, *Med Sci Sports Exerc* 20:195, 1987.

31. Hart D, Stobbe T, Jaraiedi M: Effect of lumbar posture on lifting, *Spine* 12:138, 1987.

32. Hemborg B, et al.: Intraabdominal pressure and trunk muscle activity during lifting-effect of abdominal muscle training in healthy subjects, *Scand Rehab Med* 15:183, 1983.

33. Herrick R: Clay-shoveler's fracture in power-lifting, *Am J Sports Med* 9:29, 1981.

34. Hershman E: The profile of prevention of musculoskeletal injury, *Clin Sports Med* 3:65, 1984.

35. Hutton W, Adams M: Can the lumbar spine be crushed in heavy lifting? *Spine* 7:586, 1982.

36. Johnson R: Low-back pain in sports, *Phys Sportsmed* 21:53, 1993.

37. Kraemer W, Fleck S: Resistance training: exercise prescription, *Phys Sportsmed* 16:69, 1988.

38. Landers J, Bates B, Devita P: Biomechanics of the squat exercise using a modified center of mass bar, *Med Sci Sports Exerc* 18:469, 1986.

39. Lander J, Simonton L, Giacobbe K: The effectiveness of weight-belts during the squat exercise, *Med Sci Sports Exerc* 22:117, 1990.

40. Macintosh J, Bogduk N, Gracovetsky S: The biomechanics of the thoracolumbar fascia, *Clin Biomech* 2:78, 1987.

41. Mackler L: Rehabilitation of the athlete with low back dysfunction, *Clin Sports Med* 8:4, 1989.

42. Madsen N, McLaughlin T: Kinematic factors influencing performance and injury risk in the bench press exercise, *Med Sci Sports Exerc* 16:376, 1984.

43. Mairiaux P, et al.: Relation between intra-abdominal pressure and lumbar moments when lifting weights in the erect posture, *Ergonomics* 27:883, 1984.

44. McGill S, Norman R: Potential of lumbodorsal fascia forces to generate back extension moments during squat lift, *J Biomed Eng* 10:312, 1988.

45. McLaughlin T: A kinematic model of performance of the parallel squat as performed by champion powerlifters, *Med Sci Sports Exerc* 9:128, 1977.

46. McLaughlin T, Lardner T, Dillman C: Kinetics of the parallel squat, *Res Q* 49:175, 1978.

47. Risser W: Musculoskeletal injuries caused by weight training, *Clin Pediatr* 29:305, 1990.

48. Robinson R: The new back school prescription: stabilization training, part 1, *Spine State Art Rev* 5:341, 1991.

49. Saal J: Rehabilitation of football players with lumbar spine injuries (part 2 of 2), *Phys Sportsmed* 16:117, 1988.

50. Saal J: The new back school prescription: stabilization training, part 2, *Spine State Art Rev* 5:357, 1991.

51. Saal J, Saal J: Nonoperative treatment of herniated lumbar intervertebral disc with radiculopathy, *Spine* 14:431, 1989.

52. Shelton G: *Principles of musculoskeletal rehabilitation.* In Mellion M, editor: *Sports injuries and athletic problems,* Philadelphia, 1988, Hanley & Belfus, Inc.

53. Silvers H: Lumbar percutaneous facet rhizotomy. *Spine* 15:36, 1990.

54. Stover C: Physical conditioning of the immature athlete, *Orthop Clin North Am* 13:525, 1982.

55. Styf J: Pressure in the erector spinae muscle during exercise, *Spine* 12:675, 1987.

56. Tesh K, Dunn J, Evans J: The abdominal muscles and vertebral stability, *Spine* 12:501, 1987.

57. Todd T: *Brief history of resistance exercises.* In Pearl B, Moran G, editors: *Getting stronger,* Bolinas, CA, 1986, Shelter Publications, Inc.

58. White A, Derby R, Wynne G: Epidural injections for the diagnosis and treatment of low-back pain, *Spine* 5:78, 1980.

59. Yoganandan N, et al.: Microtrauma in the lumbar spine: a cause of low back pain, *Neurosurgery* 23:162, 1988.

60. Zineoff A: Heavy-resistance exercises; the "Oxford technique," *Br J Phys Med* 14:129, 1951.

Chapter 57
Wrestling
Paul P. Vessa

Competitive wrestling embodies the ultimate test of physical endurance and mental fortitude. Participants are superbly fit because of grueling hours of practice and conscious weight control. Strength and endurance are maximized by adhering to a strict reduction in caloric intake while increasing metabolic demands through vigorous exercise. However, the physical demands of the sport have been associated with a high rate of significant injuries.[18] Various studies have documented these injuries among participants at all levels, including grammar school, high school, college, and olympic competition.* These injuries are varied and incorporate a broad spectrum of severity. Many authors have called attention to the incidence of both minor and major injuries to the spine.[5,12,16,23]

Moreover, the potential ramifications and long-term sequelae are greatest for these injuries. Although catastrophic injuries resulting in permanent neurologic deficits are uncommon, the potential for such an occurrence is daunting to any medical professional called to evaluate such a patient. Spinal injuries can be divided into those of the cervicothoracic spine and those of the lumbar spine.[23] Each presents a unique spectrum of injuries intrinsic to both the spinal anatomy and the wrestling holds and forces resulting in injury.

Wrestling has been cited by several investigators as the fifth most popular high school sport.[5,12,13,19] Its popularity has been consistent over the past two decades. Strauss and Lanese,[19] in their report to the *Journal of the American Medical Association*, thought that the consistent popularity resulted from the sport's ability to allow participants of all sizes to compete against individuals of equal weight. At the high school level alone it has been estimated to involve 300,000 to 400,000 athletes annually.[5,13,19] The sport involves essentially three different types of competitions. These include intercollegiate freestyle, international freestyle, and Greco-Roman. Intercollegiate freestyle wrestling dominates grammar school, high school, and collegiate competitions. This style of wrestling awards points for escaping while competing in the disadvantaged position (Fig. 57-1), and an additional point may be awarded to the wrestler who compiles excessive time while in control of his opponent (riding time) during the match. International freestyle is the style of wrestling seen in Olympic and World Cup competitions.[17] Differences are subtle between international and intercollegiate freestyle. Unlike intercollegiate freestyle, in international freestyle points are awarded neither

*References 4, 5, 7, 10, 12, 13, 16, 17, 19, and 23.

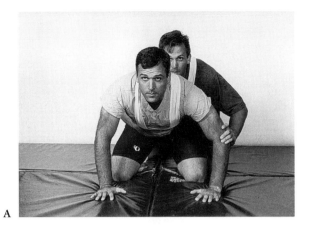

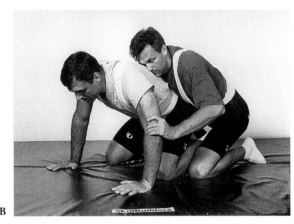

Fig. 57-1
Wrestlers demonstrating the disadvantaged or "down" position. **A,** From front. **B,** From side.

for dominating an opponent (excessive riding time) nor for escapes while competing in the disadvantaged position. The format for both styles is divided into three periods. During the first period both wrestlers are standing facing each other in the neutral position (Fig. 57-2). The next two periods are begun with each wrestler in the disadvantaged position. Greco-Roman wrestling, contrary to its name, began in France approximately 100 years ago and bears no relationship to the ancient Greek and Roman competitions; emphasis is placed on competing in the standing position with both wrestlers facing each other (neutral position), and any hold below the waist is prohibited from either forcing an opponent to the mat or holding an opponent in the disadvantaged position.[4,17] This variety of competition relies heavily on upper-body throws to bring an opponent to the mat, substantially increasing the potential for cervical spine injuries. Regardless, upper-body strength combined with mechanical leverage are essential techniques that are taught and practiced in all types of competitions. It is during the execution

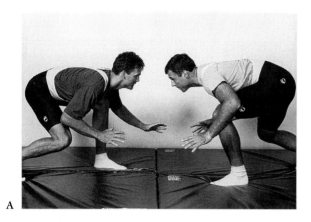

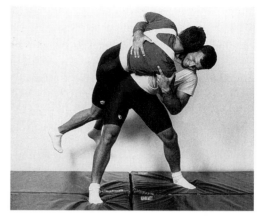

Fig. 57-3

Upper-body throws with resultant vulnerability of head, neck, and shoulders after opposing wrestler is swept off his feet.

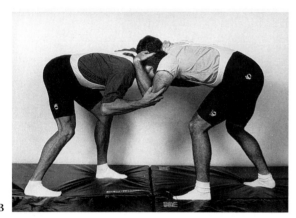

Fig. 57-2

Neutral position. **A,** Neutral or standing position. **B,** Neutral position with upper body engaged.

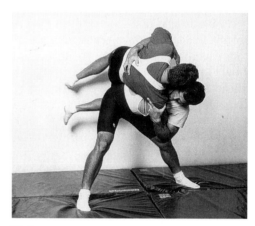

Fig. 57-4

Position of head and neck is most vulnerable.

of these techniques that potentially dangerous injuries can occur. Leveraging an opponent to the mat by controlling his head and neck is a commonly executed upper-body throw. The aggressor grabs his opponent around the neck and pulls him toward his chest while pivoting on his feet in order to sweep the opponent off his feet (Fig. 57-3). Considerable leverage is gained by pivoting and thrusting the pelvis against the lower abdomen while controlling the head and neck. While an opponent is off his feet, his head and neck are vulnerable on hitting the mat (Fig. 57-4). The potential exists for the weight of both wrestlers to come to bear on the neck and cranium. The result is excessive forces to the head and neck on contact with the mat. Head position at the point of contact will result in either pure axial loading if the contact occurs on the crown of the head and the vector of force is perpendicular to the mat, or various combinations of axial, lateral bending, and rotatory forces depending on the position of the head and the angle of the force vector to the mat.

This maneuver is referred to as "spearing the head and shoulders of a defenseless opponent" (see Fig. 57-4). Any maneuver that places an opponent in a physically compromised or potentially dangerous position is strictly forbidden. Referees are trained to recognize potentially dangerous positions and to intervene appropriately. Additionally, rules have been enacted that penalize any opponent who purposefully performs a dangerous maneuver such as "spearing" a defenseless opponent's head and shoulders to the mat.[23] This penalty results in an automatic loss of the match and the maximum points awarded to the opposing wrestler's team. These rules serve to prevent injuries; however, the rapidity with which maneuvers can occur may result in an accidental injury.

Lumbosacral injuries usually stem from hyperextension or hyperflexion forces. These result most often from attempts by the aggressor at controlling an opponent's lower extremities while competing in the standing (neutral) position (see Fig. 57-2). In intercollegiate and freestyle competitions, in which holds below the waist are permitted, forced hyperextension or hyperflexion injuries to the lumbosacral spine have been described. These will be discussed in more detail later under "Injuries to the Lumbar Spine."

Incidence of Occurrence

In a review of the injuries sustained by the University of Iowa wrestling team during the eight-season period from 1976 to 1984, Wroble and Albright[23] found an incidence of 176 injuries per 100 wrestlers per year. Furthermore, since the average squad encompasses 58 individual wrestlers, they determined that this represents two injuries per wrestler per year. Prior injury statistics by these authors were reported as 110 injuries per 100 wrestlers for the initial 6-year period. They thought that the sudden increase over the final two-year period could best be explained by improved record-keeping and more scrupulous attention to recording all injuries.[23] The actual number of significant injuries defined as greater than or equal to a 7-day loss of participation did not change. This study reported all injuries sustained by wrestlers, not just those to the spine. Table 57-1 represents a breakdown of injuries to the neck and back from the data of all injuries sustained by the University of Iowa wrestling team over an 8-year period. These figures are comparable to those previously reported in the literature. In 1978 Estwanik et al.[4] reported 9.6% neck injuries and 4% back injuries. In 1982 Snook[17,18] reported 5.5% neck injuries and 3.3% back injuries. Many studies combined injuries to the head, face, and neck, and therefore do not allow exact distinction between neck injuries and, for instance, facial lacerations and contusions. Requa and Garrick[13] reported an incidence of 34% for injuries

Table 57-1

Incidence of neck and back injuries, University of Iowa, 1976-1977 to 1983-1984

Total neck and back injuries	145
Total neck and back injuries per year	18
Total neck injuries	104 (12% of all wrestling injuries)
Total back injuries	41 (5% of all wrestling injuries)

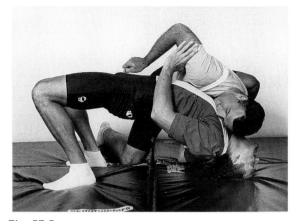

Fig. 57-5

"Bridging" move that results in large hyperextension forces to the cervical spine.

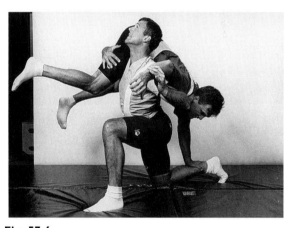

Fig. 57-6

Lifting move that results in large hyperextension forces to the lumbar spine.

to the spine and trunk, characterized as paraspinal strains of the cervical, thoracic, and lumbar regions. This represents 9.8 injuries per 100 participants and is the highest of all prior studies. The authors thought that maneuvers intrinsic to wrestling were principally the cause of this high rate. Moves requiring hyperextension of the spine (bridging, lifting, and pinning) (Figs. 57-5, 57-6, and 57-7), often against appreciable resistance, seemed to result in the highest number of paraspinal sprains and strains. Several studies have cited this mechanism of action and conclude that wrestling is second only to gymnastics in the occurrence of excessive hyperextension moments.[7,9] Additionally, repetitive hyperextension of the lumbosacral spine, especially against resistance, has been reported to result in a greater incidence of spondylolysis.[15] The orthopedic and radiologic literature is replete with studies concerning

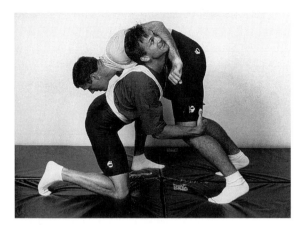

Fig. 57-7

Wrestlers demonstrating both lumbar hyperextension forces and cervical strain injury mechanisms.

the epidemiologic factors resulting in spondylolysis. Some studies have documented the statistically higher incidence of spondylolysis and radiologic abnormalities of the vertebral end plate that occurs in young athletes competing in sports theorized to result in repetitive hyperextension trauma to the spine. Rossi and Dragoni[15] and Hellstrom et al.[8] provided the most conclusive evidence in a radiologic and clinical study of the spine. In Hellstrom et al.'s study, competitive athletes were compared with nonathletes of similar age, body weight, and sex in a random and blinded fashion radiographically. Wrestlers and gymnasts were found to have the highest incidence of radiologic abnormalities exclusive of Schmorl's nodes. Specific findings included disc height reduction, abnormal configuration of the vertebral bodies (wedging, flattening, and increased anteroposterior diameter of the vertebral body), spondylolysis, and spondylolisthesis. This marked overrepresentation of radiographic abnormalities clearly indicates the impact that repetitive hyperextension stresses placed on the immature spine. Rossi and Dragoni[15] retrospectively reviewed 3132 records and x-ray films of competitive athletes suffering from low-back pain over a 26-year period. They found that competitive wrestlers had an incidence of spondylolysis five times that expected to occur in a nonathletic adult population. The long-term sequelae of these findings have not been adequately studied. Therefore, recommendations regarding the counseling of parents of children involved in elite-level wrestling and patients presenting with these radiologic abnormalities following injuries sustained while competing are not universally accepted. Clearly, patients with back pain and new-onset spondylolysis should be prevented from competing

and appropriately immobilized until the bilateral or unilateral pars interarticularis defects heal. However, should wrestlers with abnormal vertebral body configurations be prevented from competing? Arguments can be made that abnormalities discovered in asymptomatic individuals who for unrelated reasons underwent x-ray studies need not be pursued. Controversy arises when symptomatic wrestlers have documented vertebral-body abnormalities. It would seem medically prudent to exclude these patients from practice or future competition until an asymptomatic period can be documented; however, many believe that symptomatic patients who have several years of growth remaining as evidenced by their skeletal age and the appearance of ring apophyses should be forbidden to compete until skeletal maturity occurs.[6,21] Reports have circulated documenting acute injury to the vertebral ring apophysis in adolescents participating in sports that can result in heavy loads to the spine.[8,20,21] These reports specifically address wrestling, gymnastics, and water-ski jumping.[21] Some have construed these abnormalities as a variation of Scheuermann's disease occurring in the lumbar spine. Alexander[1] referred to this condition as a traumatic spondylodystrophy. He believed that unlike classic Scheuermann's disease, which typically presents from T7 to T10, this variant is often detected in and about the vicinity of L1. Marginal or minimal decrease in anterior vertebral height without undulation of the vertebral end plate are additional hallmarks of traumatic spondylodystrophy.[1,8,9,21] Unlike classic Scheuermann's disease less than three vertebrae are frequently involved, and involvement can occur at noncontiguous levels in the thoracolumbar spine.[9] Several studies have documented a traumatic etiology in this caudal variant of classic Scheuermann's disease. The occurrence has been reported to be minimal, representing only 3.3% of all Scheuermann's disease.[21] Dzioba and Gervin[3] reported on irreversible spinal deformity in Olympic gymnasts. It is recognized that lumbar Scheuermann's disease is more apt to result in low-back pain and therefore certainly would have an implication for the future. Sward et al.[21] investigated the occurrence of clinically significant back pain correlated with radiographic changes in wrestlers of the Swedish national teams. They discovered that reduced disc height, Schmorl's nodes, and change in configuration of vertebral bodies correlated with back pain in a statistically significant fashion. They hypothesized in two case reports of acute injury to the vertebral apophysis that an initial injury of the end plate results in loss of disc material through a defect in the cartilaginous layer between the anterior part of the ring apophysis and the vertebral body.[20] This loss of disc material then results in marked disc height reduction and potential segmental degeneration. Additional disc material herniation may therefore be prevented by restriction of activities until the ring apophysis fuses with the vertebral body. Schmorl's nodes, although frequently an incidental finding when discovered, are considered traumatically induced when they occur at the anterior margin of the vertebral body.[8,20] This is especially relevant when the nodes occur in the anterior part of the ring apophysis. Sward et al.'s[21] study reported this occurrence exclusively in athletes. The ethical considerations remain relevant today.

Granhed and Morelli[6] compared the incidence and prevalence of low-back pain among retired wrestlers to similarly aged men sampled at random. The lifetime incidence was reported to be 59% versus 31% in the control group. Interestingly, the wrestlers, although reporting a higher incidence of low-back pain had less back-related absenteeism at their jobs. Skeletal damage represented by obvious fractures and spondylolysis predictably resulted in clinically significant low-back pain in the future. Studies employing larger numbers of participants followed well into adult life in order to draw conclusions that are statistically significant need to be designed and undertaken to better predict which wrestlers must be kept from competing and which can safely return without fear of long-term sequelae.

Evaluation

A thorough understanding of spinal immobilization and transportation to the nearest medical facility for a series of comprehensive examinations and radiographic studies serves as the cornerstone of initial management. On presentation, a clinical history should be obtained if possible from the patient or from eyewitnesses. Specifically, the nature of the injury with regard to body position and the type of force exerted to result in injury should be ascertained.[23] For instance, an axial loading injury to the calvarium would tend to make an examining physician suspicious of a compression type of spinal injury, while twisting injuries to a flexed or extended spine typically result in posterior ligamentous strains of varying magnitude. Physical examination should incorporate an initial brief inspection searching for bruising or ecchymotic areas that may indicate the level of the injury. Careful but meticulous palpation of the entire spine should next be performed; areas of pain or palpable incongruities of the spinous

processes in unconscious patients should alert the examiner to potential areas of injury. A neurologic examination that attempts to localize the level of injury if a deficit exists should be performed. Rectal examination noting rectal tone and sacral sensation are important physical findings in partial cord injuries. Pathologic reflexes, including Babinski's sign and sustained ankle clonus portent a poor prognosis; however, if a neurologic injury is discovered, each examination should be concluded with a test of the bulbocavernosus reflex to determine the presence of spinal shock. Reflex contraction of the anal sphincter in response to stimulation of the glans or clitoris heralds the end of spinal shock and renders the neurologic examination an accurate reflection of the neurologic injury. All this information should be recorded in the patient's chart in order that repeat examinations can be compared to the original to detect trends for the better or the worse.[23]

All patients must receive a full cervical spine trauma series of x-ray films on initial presentation and x-rays of the thoracic or lumbosacral spine if the history and physical examination indicate a potential injury. X-ray films provide an easy and accurate assessment of the bony architecture of the injured spine.

Catastrophic injuries to the cervical spine and spinal cord have been reported in high school wrestling[14,24] and at the collegiate level.[22] Older wrestlers at the collegiate and Olympic levels sustain devastating subaxial cervical cord injuries with resultant fracture dislocation at or adjacent to the involved levels. Younger wrestlers, on the other hand can sustain complete cervical cord injuries without demonstrable damage to the bony architecture.[24] A diligent work-up must be performed on these patients in order to detect the level of injury. Myelographic examination has been supplanted by MRI scan to localize the level of injury; however, a complete block to myelographic contrast in a progressively worsening patient provides an excellent study to intervene operatively and decompress the cord.[24] It is for this reason that many centers may still proceed with a cervical myelogram as part of the work-up rather than depending solely on the findings of the MRI scan. Many feel that the myelogram, although certainly more invasive, provides a more dynamic study with regard to cord swelling and edema following catastrophic cervical spine injuries without concomitant bony injury. Furthermore, the studies can often complement each other, for instance, when an MRI scan defines additional pathology above the site of contract block on myelography.[2]

Injuries to the Lumbar Spine

Acute herniated nucleus pulposus in the lumbar spine rarely is reported as a result of a wrestling injury.[23] This may be largely due to the relatively young age of the participants and the structural characteristics of the vertebral body and disc complex. The nucleus pulposus in athletes 13 to 22 years of age are high in proteoglycan and well hydrated, providing an excellent construct to withstand compressive forces.[11] This hydraulic-like mechanism tends to be more resistant to compressive forces; while the firm attachment of Sharpey's fibers to the adjacent vertebral bodies and the laminated structure of the annulus are more resistant to tensile and shearing forces.[11] Therefore, injuries to the vertebral apophysis would be expected to occur before the disc complex is involved. Even in a mature spine the disc complex is far more resistant to pure compressive forces than the underlying superior vertebral end plate, which predictably deforms to result in compression fractures.[11]

Low-back injuries potentially can occur during any portion of the wrestling match. Although it would seem logical to conclude that as the match progressed fatigue would contribute to a higher occurrence in the later periods, studies have not shown this trend.[19] During the initial period of competition, the wrestlers face each other in a neutral position and spar to gain advantage. This is often referred to as the "takedown period" (see Fig. 57-3). In collegiate freestyle matches a successful takedown is performed by getting in deep on the opponent's legs then following through with your buttocks and legs. The classically executed single- or double-leg takedown necessitates a hyperextension moment on the lumbar spine as the wrestler attempts to keep his head square to his opponent while following through with his lower body. The counter or defensive move attempts to direct the head and shoulders away with one arm while exerting a downward force on the offensive wrestler's back to prevent proper follow-through. This downward force results from resting your chest and body weight on the offensive wrestler's back and extending your legs (see Fig. 57-7). The net effect of these opposing forces results in incredibly large shearing, tensile, compressive, and torsional stresses to the lumbosacral spine.[23] Additionally, while sparring, wrestlers are instructed to keep their feet apart, knees slightly bent, and most importantly, their head and shoulders square to their opponent. This position results in slight hyperextension of the spine and subsequent loading of the posterior elements (facet joints,

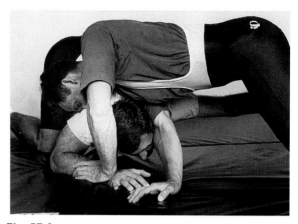

Fig. 57-8

Wrestlers demonstrating proposed etiology of cervical pinch injuries.

supraspinous and interspinous ligaments) as well as the powerful erector spinae musculature. These loaded structures are at risk for injury if a forceful twisting and flexion maneuver suddenly occurs. Repetitive trauma resulting in an overuse injury may occur, resulting in clinically significant injury after what may initially appear to be trivial trauma. Wroble and Albright[23] described this mechanism of action for low-back strains and sprains and cervical spine injuries. Cumulative spinal injuries can theoretically result in subclinical soft-tissue trauma or more likely clinically apparent soreness and immobility that resolves initially. Symptoms that persist beyond 2 to 3 weeks may represent more serious injury, requiring an accurate diagnosis and management. Jackson[9] reported that lumbosacral pain in athletes 18 years of age and younger lasting longer than 3 months nearly always resulted in the confirmation of a pars fracture, spondylolisthesis, growth-plate injuries, altered disc space anatomy, infection, or neoplasm. Persistent low-back pain (symptoms persisting longer than 3 months) in wrestlers 18 years of age and younger should raise a red flag in a practitioner's mind that a potentially serious injury has occurred.

Injuries to the Cervical Spine

Axial loads to the cervical spine occur frequently during takedowns, resulting in "pinch" injuries to the cervical roots or the brachial plexus[23] (Fig. 57-8). Forced extension or flexion combined with lateral deviation of the cervical spine can result in traumatic compression neuritis. The involved roots of the brachial plexus depend on the position of the cervical spine and the force directed to the area. Tearing and hemorrhage to facet joints or the less mobile interbody joints of Luschka in the cervical spine could result in fibrous scarring, further reducing the mobility of these structures and perhaps effectively increasing the chances of further injury.[23] Although undocumented, Wroble and Albright[23] did believe that there is a correlation between repetitive sprains and future injury.[19,22] Degenerative changes could then develop in these repetitively traumatized areas. Most injuries of this nature do not result in medical evaluation unless they fail to resolve over several weeks to months. Neurologic symptoms will consistently develop in a small group of patients with what may be considered trivial trauma, especially transient motor weakness. These individuals need lateral cervical spine x-ray studies and careful scrutiny of the neural canal diameter. Any patient whose Pavlov's ratio (the ratio between the vertebral body width and the width of the neural canal) is less than 0.8 should be advised that continued participation can potentially result in permanent neurologic injury. Although controversy has arisen regarding the accuracy of Pavlov's ratio, absolute canal diameters less than 10 mm in symptomatic patients should always exceed a practitioner's threshold for continued participation. Younger individuals should be excluded from any participation, and a discussion with the patient's parents regarding the serious consequences of noncompliance should be undertaken. This sheds some light on the circumstances a medical practitioner needs to appreciate when attempting to treat wrestlers. These athletes are usually highly motivated and conditioned to tolerate discomfort. Noncompliance is the rule rather than the exception when prescribing treatment regimens and rest. Wroble and Albright,[23] in a study of knee injuries in wrestlers in 1986, described this predictable noncompliance on the part of wrestlers to adhere to a prescribed rehabilitative regimen. They also described a relationship between noncompliance and subsequent recurrence of the injury. Albright[22,23] has described the "jamming" of the cervical spine resulting in stingers or burners in wrestlers and believes that following an initial injury these athletes are at greater risk for additional injury. Medical personnel are therefore forced to keep firm control over these patients. This is best accomplished by involving the coach in the wrestler's rehabilitation, since he is perhaps in the best position to enforce activity restrictions. Treatment plans should be outlined to the coach with particular emphasis on activity restriction and/or modification to ensure as strict compliance as possible to prescribed rehabilitation. Counseling of the coach and the individual wrestler with particular emphasis on the high incidence of reinjury and subsequent increased time lost from practice and competition when noncompliant is probably the most effective method to approach this delicate situation.

Treatment Overview

A treatment algorithm should be kept in mind when confronted with a wrestler with a spinal injury. Obviously the nature of the injury is the most important determinant of treatment options. However, most injuries will appear clinically similar initially unless serious neurologic compromise has occurred. Patients should undergo x-ray study initially more as a screening mechanism to detect individuals with structural disorders such as spondylolisthesis, endplate abnormalities, etc. All patients should be given a period of rest and observation with follow-up examination by a physician familiar with the initial examination. Persistent symptoms must be aggressively worked up with appropriate radiologic studies, including MRI or CT scan or tomography. Patients with negative radiologic studies and continued pain and immobility may then become candidates for trigger-point injections to relieve spasm. Costovertebral injections will often provide rapid and effective relief for thoracic paraspinal spasms occurring secondary to torsion injuries to the costovertebral joint. Fluoroscopically placed needles with instillation of contrast into the involved costovertebral joint followed by short-acting anesthetic and steroidal antiinflammatory agents should provide rapid pain relief. The relief of spasm and pain is often immediate, and gentle range-of-motion exercises can be instituted without aggravation of symptoms. Costovertebral pain is point-specific to palpation and generally is aggravated by deep inspiration.

Prevention of Spinal Injuries

Prevention of spinal injuries while wrestling should be the foundation on which most exercise programs are designed in both the practice and rehabilitative settings. Specific exercises that strengthen the muscles anterior to and posterior to the spine serve as the cornerstone for these programs.[23] Practice sessions should emphasize technique with regard to these exercises as well as the avoidance of potentially dangerous holds and throws. These exercises can easily be incorporated into the daily warmup routines that precede practice or competition. Each wrestler must undergo a comprehensive physical examination that pays particular attention to the mobility of the cervical and lumbosacral spine. Full painless range of motion is the minimal threshold for competition.

Athletes with prior spinal injuries will generally require more scrutiny and may require radiographic studies, depending on their particular circumstances.[23] It is always prudent to exclude a wrestler from competition temporarily if any question arises during the physical examination or if an incomplete history of a prior spinal injury is given. The inconvenience to the wrestler and the team is minimal and the information gained in the interim may be critical to the wrestler's future health.

Summary

Wrestling enjoys a significant popularity in this country, and injury statistics indicate that many physicians are likely to encounter an acutely or chronically injured athlete. Spinal injuries are frequent enough to demand an understanding of the types of injuries, their etiology, and their ramifications for the future for physicians treating and advising these patients. Lumbosacral injuries are dominated by paraspinal muscular strains that are usually self-limited in nature; however, persistent low-back pain may indicate a significant injury to the vertebral apophysis or end plate and pars interarticularis that will have a dramatic impact on the patient's future. Cervical injuries can occur along a severity spectrum from minor muscular strains to catastrophic cord injuries. Fortunately, the latter occur rarely. Neurologic symptoms should be aggressively evaluated to determine their etiology. Frequent recurrence of injuries or recurrence after trivial trauma should permanently exclude a wrestler from competition. Exercises to condition the muscles about the spine and proper instruction are necessary components to all wrestling programs. This should occur at all levels of competition in order to ensure safe competition while minimizing injuries to the spine.

References

1. Alexander CJ: Scheuermann's disease. A traumatic spondylodystrophy? *Skel Radiol* 1:67, 1977.
2. Aprill CN: *Myelography*. In Freimoyer, editor: *The adult spine: principles and practice*, New York, 1991, Raven Press, p 311.
3. Dzioba R, Gervin A: Irreversible spinal deformity in olympic gymnasts, *Orthop Trans* 8:64, 1984.
4. Estwanik JJ, Bergfeld J, Canty: Report of injuries sustained during the United States Olympic wrestling trials, *Am J Sports Med* 6:335, 1978.
5. Estwanik JJ, Bergfeld JA, Collins HR, Hall R: Injuries in interscholastic wrestling, *Phys Sportsmed* 8:121, 1980.
6. Granhed H, Morelli B: Low back pain among retired wrestlers and heavyweight lifters, *Am J Sports Med* 16:530, 1988.
7. Hartmann PM: Injuries in preadolescent wrestlers, *Phys Sportsmed* 5:79, 1978.
8. Hellstrom M, Jacobsson B, Sward L, Peterson L: Radiologic abnormalities of the thoraco-lumbar spine in athletes, *Acta Radiol* 31:127, 1990.
9. Jackson DW: Low back pain in young athletes: evaluation of stress reaction and discogenic problems, *Am J Sports Med* 7:364, 1979.
10. Kersey RD, Rowan L: Injury account during the 1980 NCAA wrestling championships, *Am J Sports Med* 11:147, 1983.
11. Kramer J: Intervertebral disk diseases, New York, 1990, *Georg Thieme Verlag*, p 14.
12. Lorish TR, Rizzo TD, Ilstrup DM, Scott SG: Injuries in adolescent and preadolescent boys at two large wrestling tournaments, *Am J Sports Med* 20:199, 1992.
13. Requa R, Garrick JG: Injuries in interscholastic wrestling, *Phys Sportsmed* 9:44, 1981.
14. Rontoyannis GP, Pahtas G, Dinis D, Pournaras N: Sudden death of a young wrestler during competition, *Int. J. Sport Med* 9:353, 1988.
15. Rossi F, Dragoni S: Lumbar spondylosis: occurrence in competitive athletes, *J Sports Med Phys Fit* 30:450, 1990.
16. Roy SP: Intercollegiate wrestling injuries, *Phys Sportsmed* 7:83, 1979.
17. Snook GA: Injuries in intercollegiate wrestling, *Am J Sports Med* 10:142, 1982.
18. Snook GA: A survey of wrestling injuries, *Am J Sports Med* 8:450, 1980.
19. Strauss RH, Lanese RR: Injuries among wrestlers in school and college tournaments, *JAMA* 248:2016, 1982.
20. Sward L, Hellstrom M, Jacobsson B, et al.: Acute injury of the vertebral ring apophysis and intervertebral disc in adolescent gymnasts, *Spine* 15:144, 1990.
21. Sward L, Hellstrom M, Jacobsson B, Peterson L: Back pain and radiologic changes in the thoraco-lumbar spine of athletes, *Spine* 15:124, 1990.
22. Torg JS, Booth RE, Albright JP, et al.: Symposium: athletic injuries to the cervical spine and brachial plexus, *Contemp Orthop* 9:65, 1984.
23. Wroble RR, Albright JP: Neck and low back injuries in wrestling, *Clin Sports Med* 5:295, 1986.
24. Wu WQ, Lewis RC: Injuries of the cervical spine in high school wrestling, *Surg Neurol* 23:143, 1985.

Index